AF668499

Cardiological Society of India

CARDIOLOGY

UPDATE 2025

DISCLAIMER

Authors contributing chapters to *"CSI Cardiology Update 2025"* are solely responsible for obtaining permission to reproduce any copyrighted material, including figures, tables, illustrations, or excerpts from other publications. All necessary permissions must be secured prior to submission.

Neither the Editor(s) nor the Publisher shall be held liable for any infringement of copyright or related rights arising from the content submitted by contributing authors. Responsibility for ensuring originality and proper permissions rests entirely with the authors.

Cardiological Society of India

CARDIOLOGY

UPDATE 2025

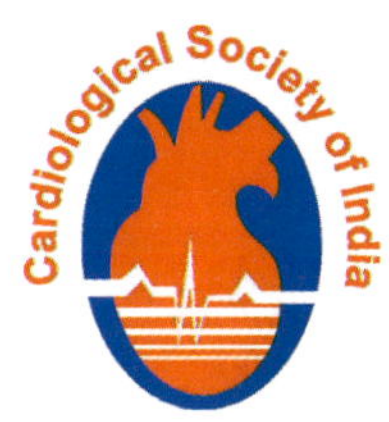

VOLUME 1

Editor-in-Chief

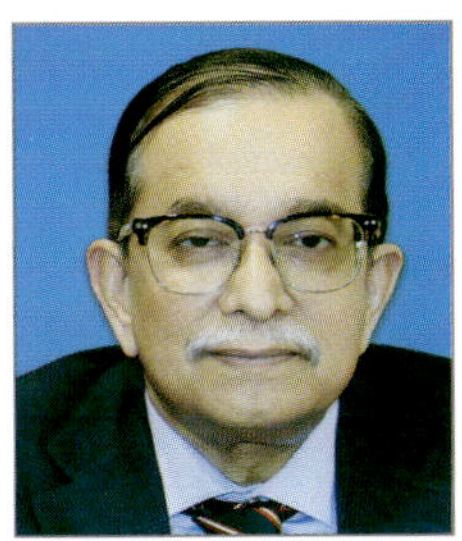

Dhiman Kahali
MD DM FESC FSCAI
Director – Interventional Cardiology
BM Birla Heart Research Centre
Kolkata, West Bengal, India
President Elect – Cardiological Society of India
Ex-Chairman – National Intervention Council, Cardiological Society of India (CSI)
Ex-Convener – STEMI Council, Cardiological Society of India (CSI)
Ex-Vice President – Cardiological Society of India (CSI) 2020–2024

Editorial Advisors

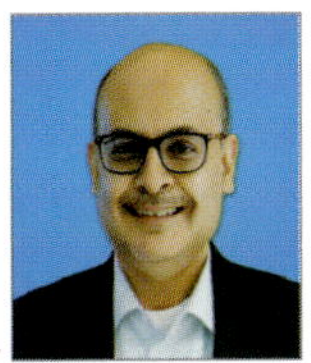

Debabrata Roy
MD DM(Cardiology) FACC FESC FSCAI FAHA
Senior Consultant Interventional Cardiologist
and Academic Coordinator
NH-RTIICS
Kolkata, West Bengal, India

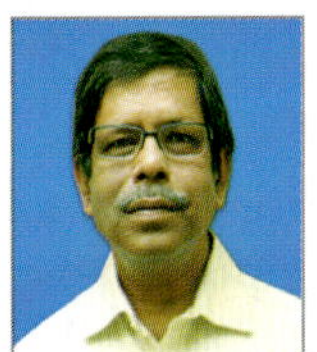

DP Sinha
MD DM FESC FSCAI FJCS
Director – Cardiac Services
Vivacity Hospital, Madhyamgram
Consultant Cardiologist, ILS Hospital
Dumdum, West Bengal, India

Associate Editors

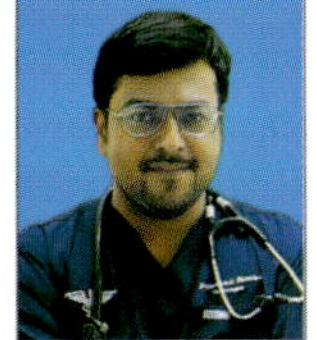

Navanil Biswas
MD(General Medicine) DrNB(Cardiology) MNAMS
FESC(Europe) FACC(USA) EECC Certified
Consultant Interventional Cardiologist
Apollo Multispeciality Hospitals
Kolkata, West Bengal, India

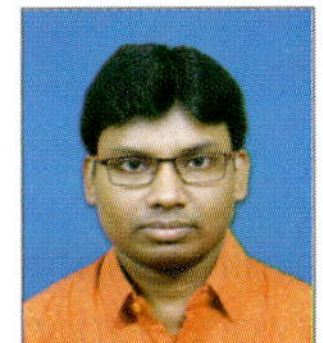

Debabrata Biswas
MBBS DNB(General Medicine)
DrNB(Cardiology)
Senior Registrar of Cathlab
NH-RTIICS
Kolkata, West Bengal, India

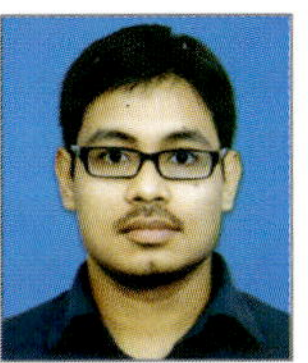

Kaushik Manna
MD(General Medicine) DM(Cardiology)
Consultant Cardiologist
Department of Cardiology
NH-RTIICS
Kolkata, West Bengal, India

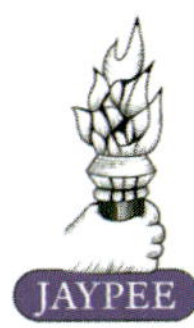

JAYPEE BROTHERS MEDICAL PUBLISHERS
The Health Sciences Publisher
New Delhi I London

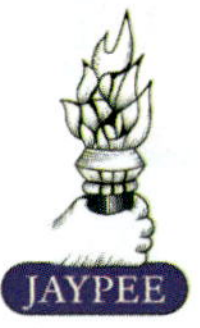

Jaypee Brothers Medical Publishers (P) Ltd

Headquarters
EMCA House, 23/23-B
Ansari Road, Daryaganj
New Delhi 110 002, India
Landline: +91-11-23272143, +91-11-23272703
+91-11-23282021, +91-11-23245672
e-mail: jaypee@jaypeebrothers.com

Corporate Office
4838/24, Ansari Road, Daryaganj
New Delhi 110 002, India
Phone: +91-11-43574357
Fax: +91-11-43574314
e-mail: jaypee@jaypeebrothers.com

Overseas Office
JP Medical Ltd.
83, Victoria Street, London
SW1H 0HW (UK)
Phone: +44-20 3170 8910
e-mail: info@jpmedpub.com

EU GPSR Authorised Representative
Logos Europe, 9 rue Nicolas Poussin
17000, La Rochelle, France
Phone: +33 (0) 6 67 93 73 78
e-mail: contact@logoseurope.eu

Website: www.jaypeebrothers.com
Website: www.jaypeedigital.com

Inquiries for bulk sales may be solicited at: jaypee@jaypeebrothers.com

***CSI Cardiology Update 2025 (Volume 1)* / Dhiman Kahali**

First Edition: **2026**

ISBN: 978-93-7202-345-9

Printed in India

Dedication

We dedicate this book to our parents and teachers for their inspiration, unwavering support, and guidance—for instilling in us the belief that with perseverance, we can overcome any challenge.

We are deeply grateful to our families—spouses and children—for their constant encouragement, patience, and for selflessly giving us the invaluable time needed to complete this demanding task.

We extend our heartfelt gratitude to our patients for their trust and for being an integral part of our journey.

Contributors

Editor-in-Chief

Dhiman Kahali MD DM FESC FSCAI
Director – Interventional Cardiology
BM Birla Heart Research Centre
Kolkata, West Bengal, India
President Elect – Cardiological Society of India
Ex-Chairman – National Intervention Council, Cardiological Society of India (CSI)
Ex-Convener – STEMI Council, Cardiological Society of India (CSI)
Ex-Vice President – Cardiological Society of India (CSI) 2020–2024

Editorial Advisors

Debabrata Roy MD DM(Cardiology) FACC FESC FSCAI FAHA
Senior Consultant Interventional Cardiologist and Academic Coordinator
NH-RTIICS
Kolkata, West Bengal, India

DP Sinha MD DM FESC FSCAI FJCS
Director – Cardiac Services
Vivacity Hospital, Madhyamgram
Consultant Cardiologist
ILS Hospital
Dumdum, West Bengal, India

Associate Editors

Navanil Biswas MD(General Medicine) DrNB(Cardiology) MNAMS FESC(Europe) FACC(USA) EECC Certified
Consultant Interventional Cardiologist
Apollo Multispeciality Hospitals
Kolkata, West Bengal, India

Debabrata Biswas MBBS DNB(General Medicine) DrNB(Cardiology)
Senior Registrar of Cathlab
NH-RTIICS
Kolkata, West Bengal, India

Kaushik Manna MD(General Medicine) DM(Cardiology)
Consultant Cardiologist
Department of Cardiology
NH-RTIICS
Kolkata, West Bengal, India

Contributing Authors

Abhijit Bharali MD
Assistant Professor
Department of Cardiology
Dr Ram Manohar Lohia Institute of Medical Sciences
Lucknow, Uttar Pradesh, India

Abhijit Chatterjee MD DM DipCard(Kolkata) DNB (Delhi)
Senior Consultant
Department of Cardiology
NH-RTIICS
Kolkata, West Bengal, India

Abhinandan Saha DNB
Postgraduate Resident
Apollo Multispecialty Hospital
Kolkata, West Bengal, India

Abhinit Gupta DM(Cardiology)
Associate Director
Department of Cardiac Sciences
Regency Hospital
Kanpur, Uttar Pradesh, India

Abhishek Dash DNB(Medicine) DrNB
Trainee
Department of Cardiology
Apollo Hospitals
Bhubaneswar, Odisha, India

Abhishek Garg MD DM
Resident
Department of Cardiology
Dayanand Medical College and Hospital
Unit-Hero DMC Heart Institute
Ludhiana, Punjab, India

Achukatla Kumar Pharm D
Senior Research Consultant
Department of Cardiology
Apollo Rajshree Hospitals
Indore, Madhya Pradesh, India

AD Arun Mohan MD
Cardiology Resident
Meenakshi Hospital
Thanjavur, Tamil Nadu, India

Adeeb Shakeel Sheikh MD(Medicine)
Senior Resident
Department of Cardiology, GMC
Kolhapur, Maharashtra, India

Aditi Rastogi DNB(General Medicine) DM(Cardiology)
Consultant Cardiologist and Assistant Professor
Department of Medicine
Rohilkhand Medical College and Hospital
Bareilly, Uttar Pradesh, India

Aditya Kapoor MD DM
Professor and Head
Department of Cardiology
Sanjay Gandhi Postgraduate Institute of Medical Sciences
Lucknow, Uttar Pradesh, India

Aditya Mulgaonkar MD
Fellow in Cardiac EP
Narayana Institute of Cardiac Sciences
Bengaluru, Karnataka, India

Adrita Banerjee MD(Medicine)
Consultant Physicians
Godrej Memorial Hospital
Mumbai, Maharashtra, India

Aftab Khan MD(Medicine) DM(Cardiology) DNB(Cardiology) FSCAI
Senior Consultant Interventional Cardiologist
InCharge – Electrophysiology Services
Apollo Multispeciality Hospitals
Kolkata, West Bengal, India

Ahitagni Banerjee MD MRCPCH(UK) DNB
Resident, Department of Cardiology
NH-RTIICS
Kolkata, West Bengal, India

Ajay Bahl FRCP DM
Professor
Postgraduate Institute of Medical Education and Research
Chandigarh, India

Ajay Kumar Pandey MD DM(Cardiology) FACC FESC FSCA
Consultant Interventional Cardiologist
Department of Cardiology
Galaxy Hospital
Varanasi, Uttar Pradesh, India

Ajay Kumar Sinha MD FESC FACC(Cardiology)
Director
Department of Preventive Cardiology
Jay Prabha Medanta Super Specialty Hospital
Patna, Bihar, India

Ajit Namdeorao Hange MD(Medicine)
Senior Resident
Department of Cardiology
GMC
Kolhapur, Maharashtra, India

Ajit S Mullasari MD DM
Chairman and Head
Department of Cardiology
Institute of Cardio Vascular Diseases
The Madras Medical Mission Hospital
Chennai, Tamil Nadu, India

A Kader Sahib MD DrNB MRCP(London)
Consultant Cardiologist
Apollo Specialty Hospitals
Trichy, Tamil Nadu, India

Akhilesh Dubey MD DM
Director
Department of Cardiology
Galaxy Superspeciality Hospital
Jabalpur, Madhya Pradesh, India

Akhilesh Kumar MD(Medicine) DrNB(Cardiology)
Associate Consultant
Department of Cardiology
Fortis Escort Heart Institute
New Delhi, India

AK Pancholia MD FACC FESC FCSI FISH FIMSA MAMS
Head
Department of Medicine, Clinical and Preventive Cardiology
Arihant Hospital
Indore, Madhya Pradesh, India

Akshay Ashok Bafna MD(Medicine) DM(Cardiology) FESC FCSI DGM(Geriatric Medicine)
Head
Department of Cardiology
GMC
Kolhapur, Maharashtra, India

Akshay Prashanth G MD DM
Assistant Professor
Department of Cardiology
Sri Ramachandra Institute of Higher Education and Research
Chennai, Tamil Nadu, India

AK Trivedi DM(Cardiology)
Director
Department of Cardiac Sciences
Regency Hospital
Kanpur, Uttar Pradesh, India

Amal Kumar Khan MD MNAMS DM
Former Professor
Department of Cardiology
WBMES
Visiting Consultant
Manipal Hospital, Salt Lake
Kolkata, West Bengal, India

Aman Asthana MD(Medicine)
Senior Resident
Department of Cardiology
North Eastern Indira Gandhi Regional Institute of Health and Medical Sciences
Shillong, Meghalaya, India

Amar Narayan Patnaik MD DM DNB
Senior Consultant Cardiologist
Star Hospitals
Formerly Professor of Cardiology
NIMS
Hyderabad, Telangana, India

Amartya Khan MD(Anesthesiology) DrNB
Critical Care Medicine Trainee
RN Tagore International Institute of Cardiac Sciences
Kolkata, West Bengal, India

Amitabha Chattopadhyay DCH DNB Fellowship in Pediatric Cardiology(Australia)
Chief Pediatric Cardiologist and Clinical Lead Eastern India
Department of Pediatric Cardiology
Narayana Superspeciality Hospital
Howrah, West Bengal, India

Amit Malviya MD DM
Additional Professor
Department of Cardiology
North Eastern Indira Gandhi Regional Institute of Health and Medical Sciences
Shillong, Meghalaya, India

Amit Sanghvi DM(Cardiology)
Consultant Interventional Cardiologist
Godrej Memorial Hospital, Criticare Asia Hospital
Mumbai, Maharashtra, India

Amit Vora MD DNB
Cardiologist
SR Mehta and KP Cardiac Institute
Mumbai, Maharashtra, India

Ampady Sreedhar MD(General Medicine) DM(Cardiology)
Consultant Interventional Cardiology
Department of Cardiology
St Gregorios Medical Mission Hospital
Parumala, Kerela, India

Amreen Dhindsa MD DNB(Cardiology)
Resident Internal Medicine
Wyne State university
Detroit Medical Center
Detroit, Michigan, USA

Anagh TS MD DM
Senior Resident
Department of Cardiology
Grant Government Medical College and Sir JJ Group of Hospitals
Mumbai, Maharashtra, India

Anees Thajudeen MD DM Fell Clin Electrophysiology(UCLA) CEPS
Head
Division of Heart Rhythm Disorders
Senior Consultant Cardiologist
KIMS Hospital
Thiruvananthapuram, Kerala, India

Col Anil Dhall Sena Medal MD(Medicine) DM(Cardiology) FACC FESC FAHA FRCP(Edinburgh) FSCAI FHRS FCSI
Professor and Head
Department of Cardiology
Janakpuri Super Speciality Hospital
New Delhi, India

Anil Mishra MBBS Dip in Cardiology(London) D Cardiac Medicine(London) MRCP(UK)
Director of Cardiology
BM Birla Heart Research Centre
Kolkata, West Bengal, India

Anil Yadav MD DM(Cardiology)
Associate Consultant Cardiologist
Department of Cardiac Sciences
Max Superspeciality Hospital
Saket, New Delhi, India

Animesh Mishra MD DM
Senior Professor and Head
Department of Cardiology
North Eastern Indira Gandhi Regional Institute of Health and Medical Sciences
Shillong, Meghalaya, India

Anirudh Mukherjee MD DM
Research Associate
Department of Cardiology
Advanced Cardiac Centre
Postgraduate Institute of Medical Education and Research
Chandigarh, India

Anish Chugh DM(Interventional Cardiology)
Interventional Cardiologist
Department of Cardiology
Chopda Medicare and Research Centre Private Limited/Magnum Heart Institute
Nashik, Maharashtra, India

Anish Kumar Khan DM(Cardiology) MD(Pulmonary Medicine) FCCP(USA) DAA(CMC Vellore) EDARM(HERMES)
Consultant Interventional Cardiologist and Pulmonologist
Visiting Consultant
Manipal Hospital, Salt Lake
Kolkata, West Bengal, India

Anita Saxena MD DM FACC
Vice Chancellor
Pt BD Sharma University of Health Sciences
Rohtak, Haryana, India

Ankit Kumar Sahu MD DM FACC FSCAI FICC
Additional Professor
Department of Cardiology
Sanjay Gandhi Postgraduate Institute of Medical Sciences
Lucknow, Uttar Pradesh, India

Ankur U MPharm MTech
Senior Safety Scientist, Project Coordinator
Safety Science Speciality in Pharmacology and Toxicology
Durham College
Oshawa, Canada

Lt Col Ankush Gupta MD DM(Cardiology)
Classified Specialist Medicine and Cardiologist
Department of Cardiology
Command Hospital Air Force
Bengaluru, Karnataka, India

Anuj Gupta MBBS
Junior Resident
All India Institute of Medical Sciences
Bhopal, Madhya Pradesh, India

Anupam Goel MD DM(Cardiology)
Director – Interventional Cardiology
Department of Cardiac Sciences
Max Superspeciality Hospital
Saket, New Delhi, India

Anupam Prakash MD(General Medicine) PGCC(Hospital Management) PDCDM FICP FAMS FACP FIACM FRCPE
Director, Professor and Head
Department of Medicine
Lady Hardinge Medical College and Associate Hospitals
New Delhi, India

A Purnanand MD DM
Consultant
Department of Cardiology
Purna Heart Institute
Vijayawada, Andhra Pradesh, India

Arif Nabi Bhat MD(Medicine) DM(Cardiology)
Consultant Interventional Cardiologist
Apollo Multispeciality Hospitals
Kolkata, West Bengal, India

Arijit Ghosh MD DM
Head
Department of Cardiology
Manipal Hospitals
Kolkata, West Bengal, India

Arijit Kumar Ghosh DM(Cardiology)
Professor and Head
Department of Cardiology
All India Institute of Medical Sciences
Nagpur, Maharashtra, India

Arindam Mitra MD(General Medicine) DM(Cardiology)
Senior Resident
Department of Cardiology
Medical College
Kolkata, West Bengal, India

Arindam Pande MD(Medicine) DM(Cardiology) FICC FESC FSCAI(USA) FACC(USA) FRCP(Glasgow)
Senior Consultant Cardiologist
Manipal EM Bypass Hospital
Kolkata, West Bengal, India

Arpita Katheria MD(Medicine) DM(Cardiology)
Assistant Professor
Department of Cardiology
Sanjay Gandhi Postgraduate Institute of Medical Sciences (SGPGIMS)
Lucknow, Uttar Pradesh, India

Arshad Nazir MD DM
Assistant Professor
Department of Cardiology
Sanjay Gandhi Postgraduate Institute of Medical Sciences
Lucknow, Uttar Pradesh, India

Arundhati MD(Pathology)
Associate Professor
Department of Pathology
Patna Medical College and Hospital
Patna, Bihar, India

Arun Gopalakrishnan MD DM
Additional Professor
Department of Cardiology
Sree Chitra Tirunal Institute for Medical Sciences and Technology
Thiruvananthapuram, Kerala, India

Lt Col Arun N DNB(Medicine) MNAMS DM
Senior Resident
Department of Cardiology
JMMC and RI
Thrissur, Kerala, India

Arup Dasbiswas MD DM(Cardiology) FCSI FICC FIAE FIAMS FICP FSCAI(USA) FACC(USA) FESC(Europe) FAPVS(Asia)
Emeritus Professor (Cardiology)
PKG Medical College and Hospital
Ex-Director
ICVS, IPGMER
Ex-Professor and Head
Department of Cardiology
IPGMER and SSKM Hospital
Kolkata, West Bengal, India

Arvind Kumar MD DM(Cardiology) FESC FICC FACC
Senior Consultant Interventional Cardiologist
Jeevak Heart Hospital
Patna, Bihar, India

Ashish Deshpande MD DM(Cardiology) FACC
Consultant Interventional Cardiologist
ORIION CitiCare Super Specialty Hospital
Ex-Professor and Head
MGM Medical College and Hospital
Aurangabad, Maharashtra, India

Ashish Jha MD
Professor (Jr)
Department of Cardiology
Dr Ram Manohar Lohia Institute of Medical Sciences
Lucknow, Uttar Pradesh, India

Ashish Kumar Jha MD DM(Cardiology)
Senior Consultant
Department of Cardiology
Heart Hospital
Patna, Bihar, India

Ashish Nabar MD DNB PhD
Cardiologist
SR Mehta and KP Cardiac Institute
Mumbai, Maharashtra, India

Ashok Kumar MD DM
Associate Professor
Department of Cardiology
Patna Medical College and Hospital
Patna, Bihar, India

Asharam Panda MD DM
Assistant Professor
Department of Cardiology
Dreams University and Institute of Health Sciences and Padmini Care Hospital
Cuttack, Odisha, India

Ashu Gupta MD
Medical Officer
State NCD Cell
Department of Health and Family Welfare
Government of Punjab
Punjab, India

Atul Mathur MD DM
Chairman Cardiology and Chief of Cathlab
Fortis Escorts Heart Institute
New Delhi, India

Atul Verma MD FHRS
Cardiologist and Cardiac Electrophysiologist
McGill University Health Centre
Montreal, Canada

Avani Jain MD
Medical Officer
DNS Hospital
Indore, Madhya Pradesh, India

Awadhesh K Sharma MD DM(Cardiology) FACC FSCAI
Professor
Department of Cardiology
LPSIC GSVM
Kanpur, Uttar Pradesh, India

Ayush Shukla MD DM FAPSIC FSCAI
Assistant Professor
Department of Cardiology
King George's Medical University
Lucknow, Uttar Pradesh, India

Bagirath R MD DNB(General Medicine) DM(Cardiology)
Senior Consultant Cardiologist
Director of Heart Transplant
Narayana Institute of Cardiac Sciences
Bengaluru, Karnataka, India

Col Balwinder Singh MD DM(Cardiology)
Classified Specialist Medicine and Cardiologist
Department of Cardiology
Military Hospital
Jaipur, Rajasthan, India

Behera Soumen Prasad MD(Medicine) DM(Cardiology) FSCAI
Assistant Professor
Department of Cardiology
Hi-Tech Medical College and Hospital
Rourkela, Odisha, India

Bhabatosh Biswas MS DNB MCh(Cardio Thoracic and Vascular Surgery)
Emeritus Professor
School of Health Sciences and Translational Research
Sister Nivedita University
Kolkata, West Bengal, India
Former Vice Chancellor – West Bengal University of Health Sciences

Bharat V Purohit DM FAPSIC FSCAI FACC FESC
Senior Consultant Cardiologist
Director – Cathlab
Yashoda Hospital
Hyderabad, Telangana, India

Bhavana M MD DrNB
Consultant Cardiology and Cathlab
Fortis Escorts Heart Institute
New Delhi, India

Bhavik S Shah MD DM(Cardiology) MRCP(UK)
Assistant Professor
Department of Cardiology
Seth GS Medical College and KEM Hospital
Mumbai, Maharashtra, India

Bhuban Majhi MD DM(Cardiology)
Professor
RG Kar Medical College
Kolkata, West Bengal, India

Bhuwan Chandra Tiwari MD
Professor and Head
Department of Cardiology
Dr Ram Manohar Lohia Institute of Medical Sciences
Lucknow, Uttar Pradesh, India

Bijay Narayan Jha MD(Medicine) Dip Cardiology FCSI FICP
Chief Health Director
Head
Department of Cardiology and Medicine
South Eastern Railway Central Hospital
Kolkata, West Bengal, India

Bijay Prakash Pandey MD DM(Cardiology)
Senior Interventional Cardiologist and Head
Chief of Cathlab
NH Superspeciality Hospital, Howrah
NH Multispeciality Hospital
Chunavati, West Bengal, India

Bijay Prakash Yadav DM(Cardiology)
Senior Consultant
Department of Cardiac Sciences
Regency Hospital
Kanpur, Uttar Pradesh, India

Biraja Prasad Beura MD DM
Assistant Professor
Department of Cardiology
MKCG Medical College and Hospital
Berhampur, Odisha, India

Bishav Mohan MD DM(Cardiology)
Professor and Head
Department of Cardiology
Dayanand Medical College and Hospital
Unit Hero DMC Heart Institute
Ludhiana, Punjab, India

Biswajit Majumder MD DM FACC FCSI FICP FICC
Professor and Head
Department of Cardiology
RG Kar Medical College and Hospital
Kolkata, West Bengal, India

Biswaranjan Mishra MD DM FCSI FIAE FICC
Senior Consultant Cardiologist
Max Diagnostic
Cuttack, Odisha, India

Bitan Mohanty MD DM
Senior Resident
Department of Cardiology
SCB Medical College
Cuttack, Odisha, India

B Kesavamoorthy MD DM
Head and Senior Interventional Cardiologist, Meenakshi Hospital
Thanjavur, Tamil Nadu, India

BKS Sastry MD DM FACC
Chairman
Renova Century Hospital
Hyderabad, Telangana, India

Blessvin Jino MD DM FNB
Consultant Interventional Cardiologist
Department of Cardiology
Meditrina Hospital
Kollam, Kerala, India

Calambur Narasimhan MD(General Medicine) DM(Cardiology)
Head of Electrophysiology
Senior Consultant Cardiology
Department of Electrophysiology
AIG Hospitals
Hyderabad, Telangana, India

CB Chandan MD
Assistant Professor
Department of Cardiology
Indira Gandhi Institute of Medical Science
Patna, Bihar, India

Chakrapani Vuppala MD
Associate Professor
Department of General Medicine
TRR Institute of Medical Sciences
Hyderabad, Telangana, India

Chandini Suvarna BDS Dip Clinical Research
Senior Research Fellow
Holy Family Hospital
New Delhi, India

Chandra Bhan Meena MD DM FACC FSCAI FESC MHRS MAPHRS
Senior Professor
Department of Cardiology
SMS Medical College
Jaipur, Rajasthan, India

Chandrakanta Mishra MD DM(Cardiology)
Professor
Department of Cardiology
SCB Medical College
Cuttack, Odisha, India

Charan Reddy KV MD DM
Consultant Interventional Cardiologist
Apollo Hospital
Navi Mumbai, Maharashtra, India

Chetan P Shah MD DM
Consultant Interventional Cardiologist and Head, Department of Cardiology
Criticare Asia Hospital
Mumbai, Maharashtra, India

Chhabi Satpathy MD DM FACC FSCAI FESC FCSI FICC FIAE
Professor and Head
Deaprtment of Cardiology
PMSSY Hospital
MKCG Medical College and Hospital
Berhampur, Odisha, India

Chitra Priyadarshini MD
Senior Resident
Department of Cardiology
Gauhati Medical College
Guwahati, Assam, India

C Narasimhan MD(General Medicine) DM(Cardiology)
Head of Electrophysilogy and Senior Consultant Cardiologist
AIG Hospital
Hydrabad, Telangana, India

C Venkata S Ram MD MACP FACC FASH
Director
Apollo Institute for Blood Pressure Management
Apollo Group of Hospitals
Hyderabad, Telangana, India
Professor of Internal Medicine
University of Texas Southwestern Medical Center
Dallas, TX, USA

DB Pahlajani DNB(Medicine) DNB(Cardiology) FSCAI
Head
Department of Cardiology
Breach Candy Hospital
Mumbai, Maharashtra, India

Debabrata Biswas MBBS DNB(General Medicine) DrNB(Cardiology)
Senior Registrar of Cathlab
NH-RTIICS
Kolkata, West Bengal, India

Debabrata Roy MD DM(Cardiology) FACC FESC FSCAI FAHA
Senior Consultant Interventional Cardiologist and Academic Coordinator
NH-RTIICS
Kolkata, West Bengal, India

Debasis Ghosh MD MRCP(London) FRCP(Edinburgh) FRCP(London) FACC(USA) FESC(Europe)
Senior Consultant
Department of Interventional Cardiology
Chief Federation Examiner for MRCP (UK)
Apollo Multispeciality Hospitals
Kolkata, West Bengal, India

Debasish Das MD
Postdoctoral Trainee
Department of Cardiology
NH-RTIICS
Kolkata, West Bengal, India

Debasree Gangopadhyay MD(Pediatrics) FNB(Pediatric Cardiology)
Consultant
Department of Pediatric Cardiology
NH-RTIICS
Kolkata, West Bengal, India

Debdatta Kar MD DM
Associate Consultant
BM Birla Heart Hospital
Kolkata, West Bengal, India

Debika Chatterjee MD
Cardiologist
NH RTIICS
Kolkata, West Bengal, India

Deepak Padmanabhan MD
Consultant Electrophysiologist
Narayana Institute of Cardiac Sciences
Bengaluru, Karnataka, India

Deepchand Raja MD DM DNB
Consultant Cardiologist and Clinical Lead – Cardiac Electrophysiology
Kauvery Hospital
Chennai, Tamil Nadu, India

Deepti Yadav MD DM
Consultant Interventional Cardiologist
Medanta – The Medicity
Gurugram, Haryana, India

Dharmendra Jain DM
Professor and Unit Head
Department of Cardiology
Institute of Medical Sciences
Banaras Hindu University
Varanasi, Uttar Pradesh, India

Dharmendra Kumar Singh DNB(Medicine) DM(Cardiology)
Senior Resident
Department of Cardiology
Bardhaman Medical College
Bardhaman, West Bengal, India

Dhiman Kahali MD DM FESC FSCAI
Director – Interventional Cardiology
BM Birla Heart Research Centre
Kolkata, West Bengal, India
President Elect – Cardiological Society of India
Ex-Chairman – National Intervention Council, Cardiological Society of India (CSI)
Ex-Convener – STEMI Council, Cardiological Society of India (CSI)
Ex-Vice President – Cardiological Society of India (CSI) 2020–2024

Dikshit Byomakesh MD(Medicine) DM(Cardiology) FNB(Interventional Cardiology)
Senior Consultant
Department of Cardiology
Apollo Hospitals
Bhubaneswar, Odisha, India

Dipak Ranjan Das MD DM
Professor
Department of Cardiology
SCB Medical College
Cuttack, Odisha, India

Dipankar Ghosh Dastidar DCH MD(Medicine) DM(Cardiology) FACC FESC FCSI FICP FSCAI
Associate Professor and Head
Department of Cardiology
Burdwan Medical College
Burdwan, West Bengal, India

D Nishtha BDS
Head and Consultant Clinical Research
Ubuntu Heart and Super Specialty Hospital
Bhopal, Madhya Pradesh, India

DP Sinha MD DM FESC FSCAI FJCS
Director – Cardiac Services
Vivacity Hospital, Madhyamgram
Consultant Cardiologist
ILS Hospital
Dumdum, West Bengal, India

D Seshagiri Rao MD DM
Former Head
Department of Cardiology
Nizam's Institute of Medical Sciences
Director
Department of Cardiology
Apollo Spectra Hospital
Hyderabad, Telangana, India

DS Gambhir MD DM FAMS FCSI FICC FCAPSC FSCAI FACC(USA)
Group Director
Department of Cardiology
Kailash Health Care Ltd
Director, Kailash Hospital and Heart Institute
Noida, Uttar Pradesh, India

Durlabh Debbarma MD(Medicine) DrNB(Cardiology)
Resident, Manipal EM Bypass Hospital
Kolkata, West Bengal, India

Farhin Iqbal MD
Associate Professor
Department of Cardiology
Gauhati Medical College
Guwahati, Assam, India

Ganesan Manohar MD DM(Cardiology)
Director
Department of Cardiology
MGM Malar Hospital
Former Professor
RGGGH and MMC
Chennai, Tamil Nadu, India

Ganesh Seth MD DM(Cardiology)
Associate Director
Department of Cardiology
Medanta Super Speciality Hospital
Lucknow, Uttar Pradesh, India

Gaurav Agarwal MD DM
Consultant, Department of Cardiology
Narayana Multispecialty Hospital
Kolkata, West Bengal, India

Gaurav Chaudhary DM FACC FSCAI
Professor of Cardiology
King George's Medical University
Lucknow, Uttar Pradesh, India

Gaurav Sharma MD(Medicine) DM(Cardiology)
Senior Resident
Department of Cardiology
GB Pant Institute of Postgraduate Medical Education and Research
New Delhi, India

Girish B Navasundi MD DNB
Senior Consultant Cardiologist
Apollo Hospital
Bengaluru, Karnataka, India

Girish MP MD DM
Professor, Department of Cardiology
GB Pant Institute of Postgraduate Medical Education and Research
New Delhi, India

G Justin Paul MD DNB(Medicine) DM DNB(Cardiology) FACC FESC FSCAI
Professor
Institute of Cardiology
Madras Medical College
Chennai, Tamil Nadu, India

G Kumar MD
Associate Professor
Department of Cardiology
Indira Gandhi Institute of Medical Science
Patna, Bihar, India

Gopala Krishna Koduru MD DM
Consultant Cardiologist
Aayush Hospitals
Vijayawada and Eluru
Andhra Pradesh, India

Guruprasad Datta Naik MD FACC FSCAI
Head
Department of Cardiology
Goa Medical College
Bambolim, Goa, India

Haresh Mehta MD(Medicine) DNB(Cardiology) FACC FESC FSCAI
Director – Interventional and Structural Cardiology
SL Raheja – Fortis Hospital
Mumbai, Maharashtra, India

Harikrishnan Sivadasanpillai DM FACC FRCP FAMS
Professor and Head
Department of Cardiology
Editor-in-Chief
Heart Failure Journal of India
Sree Chitra Tirunal Institute for Medical Sciences and Technology
Thiruvananthapuram, Kerala, India

Harilalith Kovvuri MD(General Medicine)
Senior Resident
Department of Cardiology
Sri Ramachandra Institute of Higher Education and Research
Chennai, Tamil Nadu, India

Harinder K Bali MD DM(Cardiology)
Chairman – Cardiac Sciences
Dean – Academics and Research
Livasa Hospitals
Chandigarh, India

Harishankar Pratap Singh Chandel MD DM
Director
Department of Cardiology
Aditya Superspeciality Hospital
Jabalpur, Madhya Pradesh, India

Harsh Chaudhary MD DrNB(Cardiology)
Interventional Cardiologist
Apollo CVHF Heart Institute, Ahmedabad
Apollo Hospital International
Gandhinagar, Gujarat, India

Harshit Khare MD DM(Cardiology)
Assistant Professor
Department of Cardiology
Sanjay Gandhi Postgraduate Institute of Medical Sciences
Lucknow, Uttar Pradesh, India

Hem Chandra Kalita MD(Medicine) DM(Cardiology)
Professor
Department of Cardiology
Assam Medical College and Hospital
Dibrugarh, Assam, India

Hetan C Shah MD DNB(Cardiology) FACC FSCAI(USA) FESC(Europe)
Professor
Department of Cardiology
Seth GS Medical College and KEM Hospital
Mumbai, Maharashtra, India

Himanshu Mahla MD DM
Associate professor
Department of Cardiology
SMS Medical College
Jaipur, Rajasthan, India

Himanshu Gupta MD DM
Associate Director
Department of Cardiology
Medanta Super Speciality Hospital
Lucknow, Uttar Pradesh, India

Hitinder Kaur MD
Director
Department of Health and Family Welfare
Government of Punjab
Punjab, India

HK Chopra MD DM FRCP FACC FISC FISCU FASE FCSI FIAE FIMSA
Senior Consultant Cardiologist
Medanta Moolchand Heart Institute
Chairman
CME Moolchand Medcity
New Delhi, India
Past President – National CSI

Hygriv B Rao MD DM FACC FESC
Senior Consultant Cardiologist and Director
Division of Electrophysiology and Pacing
KIMS Group of Hospitals
Hyderabad, Telangana, India

Jagdish Chander Mohan MD DM
Interventional Cardiologist
Department of Cardiology
Institute of Heart and Vascular Diseases
Jaipur Golden Hospital
Rohini, New Delhi, India

Jayanta Saha MD(General Medicine) DM(Cardiology)
Professor and Head
Department of Cardiology
Medical College
Kolkata, West Bengal, India

Jayanta Sharma MD FRCP(London, Glasgow, Edinburgh) FICP FIACM FIAMS FICCMD FCSI FGSI FACP
Senior Consultant
Apollo Multispecialty Hospital
Kolkata, West Bengal, India

Jebaraj MD MRCPCH(UK)
Senior Consultant and Clinical Lead – Pediatric Cardiology and Cardiac MRI
Kauvery Hospital
Chennai, Tamil Nadu, India

Jhala Darshan A MD DM
Interventional Cardiologist and Electrophysiologist
Lilavati Hospital and Research Centre
Mumbai, Maharashtra, India

Jhala Malav MD(General Medicine) DM(Cardiology) Postdoctoral Fellowship in Cardiac Electrophysiology
Interventional Cardiologist and Electrophysiologist
Lilavati Hospital and Research Centre
Mumbai, Maharashtra, India

Johann Christopher MD DNB FICI FACC
Consultant Cardiologist
Director – Cardiac Imaging
CARE Hospitals
Hyderabad, Telangana, India

Jonaki Pal MD
Resident
Department of Pediatric Cardiology
NH-RTIICS
Kolkata, West Bengal, India

JPS Sawhney DM FESC FACC FRCP
Chairperson
Department of Cardiology
Dharma Vira Heart Center
Sir Ganga Ram Hospital
New Delhi, India

JB Vincil Jito MD(Medicine)
Senior Resident
Department of Cardiology
Madras Medical College
Chennai, Tamil Nadu, India

Kajal Ganguly MD DM FACC
Consultant Interventional Cardiologist
Manipal Hospital
Kolkata, West Bengal, India

Kalyan Munde MD DM(Cardiology)
Professor and Head
Department of Cardiology
Grant Government Medical College and Sir JJ Group of Hospitals
Mumbai, Maharashtra, India

Karthikaa Saminathan MD DM DrNB(Cardiology)
Interventional Cardiologist
Department of Cardiology
Sri Muthukumaran Medical College Hospital and Research Institute
MGM Malar Hospital
Chennai, Tamil Nadu, India

Karthik Thangamuthu MD
Senior Resident
Department of Cardiology
Assam Medical College
Dibrugarh, Assam, India

Kashinath Ghosh Hazra MD DM DNB(Cardiology) MNAMS FNB(Interventional Cardiology)
Senior Consultant Interventional Cardiologist
NH-RTIICS
Kolkata, West Bengal, India

Kaushal Chhatrapati MD DM
Senior Interventional Cardiologist
Saifee Hospital
Mumbai, Maharashtra, India

Kaushik Manna MD(General Medicine) DM(Cardiology)
Consultant Cardiologist
Department of Cardiology
NH-RTIICS
Kolkata, West Bengal, India

Kaushik Mondal MD(Medicine) DM(Cardiology)
RMO, Department of Cardiology
Burdwan Medical College and Hospital
Burdwan, West Bengal, India

Kavish Chopda MD(Medicine) DM(Cardiology)
Resident
Department of Cardiology
Padmashree DY Patil Medical College
Mumbai, Maharashtra, India

Kayan Siodia DNB(Medicine) DNB(Cardiology) FSCAI
Cardiologist , PD Hinduja Hospital
Breach Candy Hospital
Raheja Hospital
Mumbai, Maharashtra, India

KK Talwar MD DM FAMS FACC FNA DSC(Hon. Causa)
Chairman
PSRI Heart Institute
PSRI Hospital
Sheikh Sarai, New Delhi, India

Koushik Chaki MBBS PGDCC
Associate Consultant
Department of Cardiology
Narayana Superspeciality Hospital
Howrah, West Bengal, India

K Roshan Rao MD DM FACC FESC FSACI
Senior Interventional Cardiologist and Head
Department of Cardiology
Apollo Rajshree Hospitals
Indore, Madhya Pradesh, India

Kumar Himanshu MD
Associate Professor
LPS Institute of Cardiology
Kanpur, Uttar Pradesh, India

Kumar Shubham MD
Associate Consultant
Division of Interventional Cardiology
Medanta Heart Institute
Medanta – The Medicity
Gurugram, Haryana, India

Lekha Adik Pathak MD(Medicine) DM(Cardiology) FRCP(Edinburgh)
Director and Head
Department of Cardiology
Nanavati Max Super Speciality Hospital
Mumbai, Maharashtra, India

Lipika Adhikari MD DM
Associate Professor
Department of Cardiology
RG Kar Medical College and Hospital
Kolkata, West Bengal, India

Madhupada Kiran Kumar DNB DrNB(Cardiology)
Associate Consultant
Department of Cardiology
Apollo Hospitals Jubilee Hills
Hyderabad, Telangana, India

Madhu Shukla MBBS Dip(Cardiology) PhD
Head of Noninvasive Cardiology
Department of Cardiology
Institute of Heart and Vascular Diseases
Jaipur Golden Hospital
Rohini, New Delhi, India

Mahadevan R MD DM
Senior Consultant
Department of Interventional Cardiology and Diabetology
Kauvery Hospital
Chennai, Tamil Nadu, India

Mahesh Babu MD DNB
Senior Consultant
Kauvery Hospital
Chennai, Tamil Nadu, India

Mahesh Nalin Kumar MD(Medicine) DNB(Cardiology) FRCP FACC FESC
Head and Senior Consultant Cardiology
Department of Cardiology
St Gregorios Medical Mission Hospital
Parumala, Kerela, India

Mahesh Rameshrao Deshpande MD DrNB FSCAI AFESC
Head
Department of Cardiology
Dr Hedgewar Rugnalay
RK Damani Medical College
Sambhajinagar, Maharashtra, India

Mahua Roy MD FNB
Senior Consultant Pediatric Cardiologist
NH-RTIICS
Kolkata, West Bengal, India

Mainak Mukhopadhyay MD MRCP DM FESC CCDS
Senior Interventional Cardiologist
Manipal Hospitals
Kolkata, West Bengal, India

Maitreyee Bhattacharyya MD DM
Assistant Professor
Department of Cardiology
Gauhati Medical College and Hospital
Guwahati, Assam, India

Mahima Saran MD DM(Cardiology)
Director
Department of Cardiology
Medanta Super Speciality Hospital
Lucknow, Uttar Pradesh, India

Manoj Bansal MD DM
Cardiologist
Care CHL Hospitals
Indore, Madhya Pradesh, India

Manoj Chopda MD DM(Cardiology)
Interventional Cardiologist and Founder
Chopda Medicare and Research Center Pvt Ltd
Nasik, Mahasrashtra, India

Manokar P MD DM FACC FRCP(Glasgow) FAHA FSCAI FESC FAPSIC FCSI FIMSA
Senior Interventional Cardiology
Clinical Lead – Heart Failure and Transplant Program
Kauvery Hospital
Chennai, Tamil Nadu, India

Manu Gupta MD
Senior Resident
Department of General Medicine
PCMS and RC
Bhopal, Madhya Pradesh, India

Manu Rajendran MD DM
Consultant Interventional Cardiologist
Department of Cardiology
Meditrina Hospital
Kollam, Kerala, India

Mayank Nausran MD
Senior Resident
Department of Cardiology
SMS Medical College
Jaipur, Rajasthan, India

Mayank Shami MD(Medicine) DM(Cardiology)
Senior Resident
Department of Cardiology
GB Pant Institute of Postgraduate Medical Education and Research
New Delhi, India

Md Amish Shikoh MD(Medicine)
Senior Resident
Department of Cardiology
North Eastern Indira Gandhi Regional Institute of Health and Medical Sciences
Shillong, Meghalaya, India

MD Asif Iqbal MD
Senior Resident
Department of Cardiology
ABVIMS and Dr RML Hospital
New Delhi, India

Meemansa Buch MD(General Medicine) DrNB(Cardiology)
Fellow in Interventional Cardiology
Manipal Hospitals
Bengaluru, Karnataka, India

Mitendra Singh Yadav MD DNB
Associate Director – Interventional Cardiology
Department of Cardiac Sciences
Max Superspeciality Hospital
Saket, New Delhi, India

M Mashhadi MD DM(Cardiology)
Interventional Cardiologist
Apollo CVHF Heart Institute
Apollo Hospital International Ltd
Ahmedabad, Gujarat, India

Mohamed Iesa M MD DM(Cardiology) DNB(Cardiology)
Senior Consultant Cardiologist
Iqraa International Hospital and Research Centre
Kozhikode, Kerala, India

Mohit D Gupta MD DM FAMS FACC(USA)
Director–Professor
Department of Cardiology
GB Pant Institute of Postgraduate Medical Education and Research
New Delhi, India

Mohsin Raj Mantoo MD DM
Assistant Professor
Department of Cardiology
All India Institute of Medical Sciences
New Delhi, India

Monika Bhandari MD DM FACC FESC FSCAI APSIC
Professor (Jr)
Department of Cardiology
King George's Medical University
Lucknow, Uttar Pradesh, India

Mrinal Kanti Das MD DM FICP FICC FCSI FACC FESC
Consultant Cardiologist
CK Birla Hospitals (BMB/CMRI)
Kolkata, West Bengal, India

MS Ravi MD DM(Cardiology)
Former Director
Department of Cardiology
Madras Medical College and Rajiv Ghandhi Government General Hospital
Chennai, Tamil Nadu, India

M Subroto MD DC DM FICC FIEIC FCPCI(Italy) FACC(USA) FSCAI(USA)
Professor and Head
Department of Cardiology
Director – Cathlab
Ubuntu Heart and Super Specialty Hospital
Bhopal, Madhya Pradesh, India

MU Rabbani DM FRCP(London, Edinburgh, Glasgow) FACC
Former Director and Head
Department of Cardiology
JN Medical College
Aligarh Muslim University
Aligarh, Uttar Pradesh, India

Muthiah Subramanian DM PDF CCDS CEPS-A MRCP(UK) FRCP(Edinburgh)
Cardiologist and Electrophysiologist
AIG Hospital
Hydrabad, Telangana, India

Nagendra Boopathy Senguttuvan MD(General Medicine) DM(Cardiology) FACC FSCAI Fellowship in Interventional Cardiology Fellowship in Structural Interventions
Professor
Department of Cardiology
Sri Ramachandra Institute of Higher Education and Research
Chennai, Tamil Nadu, India

Nakul Sinha MD DM FACC FSCAI FICC FCSI FAPSC
Chairman
Department of Cardiology
Max Healthcare, Lucknow (Erstwhile Sahara Hospital, Gomti Nagar)
Former Professor and Head
Cardiology, SGPGI
Lucknow, Uttar Pradesh, India

Navanil Biswas MD(General Medicine) DrNB(Cardiology) MNAMS FESC(Europe) FACC(USA) EECC Certified
Consultant Interventional Cardiologist
Apollo Multispeciality Hospitals
Kolkata, West Bengal, India

Brig Navreet Singh MD DM(Cardiology)
Consultant Medicine and Cardiologist
Military Hospital
Jalandhar Cantt
Jalandhar, Punjab, India

Nayanika Bose MS
Consultant Ophthalmologist and Microsurgeon
RG Kar Medical College and Hospital
Kolkata, West Bengal, India

Neha Chopra MD
Senior Resident
Department of Cardiology
Vardhman Mahavir Medical College and Safdarjung Hospital
New Delhi, India

Nikhil Agarwal DM
Senior Resident
Department of Cardiology
GB Pant Institute of Postgraduate Medical Education and Research
New Delhi, India

Nikhil Gadade MD(Medicine)
Senior Resident
Department of Cardiology
Government Medical College
Kolhapur, Maharashtra, India

Nikhil Gupta MBBS
Junior Resident
Department of Internal Medicine
Sir Ganga Ram Hospital
New Delhi, India

Nilay Tripathi DM(Cardiology)
Assistant Professor
Department of Cardiology
King George's Medical University
Lucknow, Uttar Pradesh, India

Nishad Chitnis MD MRCP DNB
Senior Consultant Cardiologist and Director
Division of Pacing and Electrophysiology
KIMS Group of Hospitals
Hyderabad, Telangana, India

Nishant Tripathy MD DM
Chairman
Department of Interventional Cardiology
HDNA Aarogyam Hospital
Patna, Bihar, India

Nitharsha Prakash M MD(General Medicine)
Senior Resident
Department of Cardiology
Sri Ramachandra Institute of Higher Education and Research
Chennai, Tamil Nadu, India

Col Nitin Bajaj MD DM(Cardiology)
Senior Adviser-Medicine and Cardiologist
Military Hosptial
Ahmedabad, Gujarat, India

Nitish Naik MD DM
Professor
Department of Cardiology
All India Institute of Medical Sciences
New Delhi, India

Nitish Prasad DNB(Medicine) DrNB(Cardiology)
Consultant Cardiologist
Apollo Hospitals
Bhubaneswar, Odisha, India

Padma Madhab Bisoi MD(General Medicine) DrNB
Resident
BM Birla Heart Hospital
Kolkata, West Bengal, India

Padmanabh Kamath MD DM(Cardiology)
Professor
Department of Cardiology, KMC
Mangaluru, Karnataka, India

Pankaj Sharma MSc PhD
Research Associate
Jawaharlal Nehru Centre for Advanced Scientific Research
Bengaluru, Karnataka, India

Pankaj Singh MD DNB(Cardiology)
Consultant
NH-RTIICS
Kolkata, West Bengal, India

PC Rath MD DM FICC FACC FESC FRCP(London, Edinburgh)
Director and Head
Department of Cardiology
Apollo Hospitals Jubilee Hills
Hyderabad, Telangana, India

PK Asokan MD DM FRCP FCSI FACC FESC FSCAI FICC
Senior Consultant Cardiologist
Director-Cardio Life Care
Fathima Heart Foundation
Kozhikode, Kerala, India

Pooja Sharma Gupta MD
Senior Resident
Department of Dermatology
PCMS and RC
Bhopal, Madhya Pradesh, India

Poyla Ghosh MBBS
Medical Officer
Department of Medicine
Command Hospital (Air Force)
Bengaluru, Karnataka, India

Prafulla Kerkar MD DM(Cardiology) FSCI FESC(Europe) FACC (USA)
Professor, Asian Heart Institute
Mumbai, Maharashtra, India

Prakas Chandra Mondal MD MRCP(UK, Ireland) MRRCPS(Glasgow) DM(Cardilogy) DNB(Cardiology) FACC(USA)
Director and Head
Department of Cardiology
Apolo Multispeciality Hospital
Kolkata, West Bengal, India

Pranabes Chakraborti MD(Medicine) DrNB(Cardiology)
Resident, Manipal EM Bypass Hospital
Kolkata, West Bengal, India

Pranab Jyoti Bhattacharyya MD DM
Professor
Department of Cardiology,
Gauhati Medical College and Hospital
Guwahati, Assam, India

Pranjal Raparia MD
Senior Resident
Department of Cardiology
Sanjay Gandhi Postgraduate Institute of Medical Sciences
Lucknow, Uttar Pradesh, India

Prasannakumar CK MD(Medicine) DM(Cardiology) FSCAI FACC
Professor and Head
Department of Cardiology
JMMC and RI
Thrissur, Kerala, India

Prasant Kr Sahoo MD DM FRCP(London and Glasgow) FACC FSCAI FESC FAPSIC FCSI FICC
Director
Department of Interventional Cardiology
Apollo Hospitals
Bhubaneswar, Odisha, India

Prashant Kumar Pandey 3rd Year Resident MD(Medicine)
Junior Resident
Department of General Medicine
Heritage Institute of Medical Sciences
Varanasi, Uttar Pradesh, India

Pratap Kumar MD
Senior Resident
Department of Cardiology
Institute of Medical Sciences
Banaras Hindu University
Varanasi, Uttar Pradesh, India

Prathap Kumar N MD DM FIC
Chief Interventional Cardiologist
Department of Cardiology
Meditrina Hospital
Kollam, Kerala, India
Course Director
Indo Japanese CTO Club (IJCTO)

Praveen Ashok Kumar MD DM(Cardiology)
Associate Consultant
Department of Cardiology
The Madras Medical Mission Hospital
Chennai, Tamil Nadu, India

Praveen Chandra MD DM
Chairman
Institute of Cardiac Science
Medanta – The Medicity
Gurugram, Haryana, India

Prayaag Kini MD(Medicine) DNB(Cardiology) Fellow(Interventional Cardiology) FSCAI
Additional Senior Consultant
Department of Cardiology
Sri Sathya Sai Institute of Higher Medical Sciences
Bengaluru, Karnataka, India

Preetam Thakur MD DM
Assistant Professor
Department of Cardiology
Indira Gandhi Medical College
Shimla, Himachal Pradesh, India

Prerna Garg MD DM MRCP
Senior Resident
All India Institute of Medical Sciences
New Delhi, India

Priyanka Agarwal MD DrNB PDF
Assistant Professor
Sri Jayadeva Institute of Cardiovascular Sciences and Research
Bengaluru, Karnataka, India

P Sabari Krishnan MD DM
Senior Interventional Cardiologist
Meenakshi Hospital
Thanjavur, Tamil Nadu, India

PS Banerjee MD DM(Cardiology) FACC
Chief Interventional Cardiologist
Manipal Hospital
Former Head
Department of Cardiology
Medical College
Kolkata, West Bengal, India
Past President
Cardiological Society of India

Puneet Rastogi MD DM
Professor and Head
Department of Cardiology
GR Medical College
Gwalior, Madhya Pradesh, India

P Vijay Shekar MD DM Fellowship in Electrophysiology
Consultant
Apollo Specialty Hospitals
Trichy, Tamil Nadu, India

R Archana MD(Medicine)
Senior Resident of Cardiology
Madras Medical College
Chennai, Tamil Nadu, India

Raghav R Nagpal MD
Consultant – Interventional and Structural Cardiology
SL Raheja – Fortis Hospital
Mumbai, Maharashtra, India

Raghu Cherukupalli MD
Clinical Director – Cardiology
Yashoda Hospital
Hyderabad, Telangana, India

Raghuram Palaparti MD DM
Consultant Cardiologist
Aayush Hospitals
Vijayawada and Eluru
Andhra Pradesh, India

Rahul Shewale DM(Interventional Cardiology)
Interventional Cardiologist
Department of Cardiology
Chopda Medicare and Research Centre Private Limited/Magnum Heart Institute
Nashik, Maharashtra, India

Raja Ramesh Nukavarapu MD DM FAPSIC FSCAI
Lead Interventional Cardiologist
Aster Ramesh Hospitals
Vijayawada, Andhra Pradesh, India

Rajarshi Halder MD(General Medicine)
Postdoctoral Trainee
Department of Cardiology
RG Kar Medical College
Kolkata, West Bengal, India

Rajat Kar MD DrNB(Cardiology)
Junior Interventional Cardiologist
NH Superspeciality Hospital, Howrah
NH Multispecialty Hospital, Chunavati
West Bengal, India

Rajeev Garg MD(Medicine) DNB(Cardiology) MNAMS FSCAI FESC FACC
Senior Interventional Cardiologist and Heart Failure Specialist
Aware Global Hospital
Hyderabad, Telangana, India

Rajeev Gupta MD DM(Cardiology)
Professor and Head
Department of Cardiology
Gandhi Medical College
Bhopal, Madhya Pradesh, India

Rajeev Gupta MD PhD
Chairman
Department of Preventive Cardiology and Medicine
Eternal Heart Care Centre and Research Institute
Jaipur, Rajasthan, India

Rajendra Kumar Jain MD DM FACC DIU(Paris)
Consultant Cardiologist and Head
Department of Cardiology
KIMS Hospitals
Secunderabad, Telangana, India

Rajesh Vijayvergiya MD DM FSCAI FACC FESC FISES
Professor
Department of Cardiology
Advanced Cardiac Centre
Postgraduate Institute of Medical Education and Research
Chandigarh, India

Rajiv Bajaj MD DM
Consultant
Vinay Vishal Healthcare
Roorkee, Uttarakhand, India

Rajiv Krishna MD DNB FACC
Consultant Intervention Cardiologist
Mediversal Multispeciality Hospital
Patna, Bihar, India

Rajneesh Kapoor MD DNB FACC
Chairman
Division of Interventional Cardiology
Medanta Heart Institute
Medanta – The Medicity
Gurugram, Haryana, India

Rakesh Yadav MD DM
Head
Department of Emergency Medicine
Professor
Department of Cardiology
All India Institute of Medical Sciences
New Delhi, India

R Alagesan MD(General Medicine) DM(Cardiology)
Retired Professor and Head
Department of Cardiology
Madras Medical College
Chennai, Tamil Nadu, India

Ramesh Thakur MD
Former Professor
Department of Cardiology
LPS Institute of cardiology
Kanpur, Uttar Pradesh, India

Ramya Pechetty MD DM
Interventional Cardiologist
Apollo Spectra Hospital
Hyderabad, Telangana, India

Ranabrata Sen MD(Medicine) DrNB(Cardiology)
Consultant Cardiologist
Department of Cardiology
NH-RTIICS, Kolkata
Subham Hospital, Cooch Behar
West Bengal, India

Ranjit K Nath MD DM FACC FESC FCSI FSCAI
Director, Professor and Head
Department of Cardiology
ABVIMS and Dr RML Hospital
New Delhi, India

Rathindra Nath Karmakar MD DM
Consultant
Department of Cardiology
Narayana Multispecialty Hospital
Kolkata, West Bengal, India

Ratul Ghosh MD DM
Senior Resident
Department of Cardiology
RG Kar Medical College and Hospital
Kolkata, West Bengal, India

Ravi Vishnu Prasad MD(Medicine) DM(Cardiology)
Associate Professor
Department of Cardiology
Indira Gandhi Institute of Medical Science
Patna, Bihar, India

Reeta Varyani MD(Medicine) DNB(Cardiology) Fellow(Interventional Cardiology) FSCAI
Senior Consultant and In-Charge
Department of Cardiology
Sri Sathya Sai Institute of Higher Medical Sciences
Bengaluru, Karnataka, India

Rishika Mehta MD(Pediatrics) DrNB(Pediatric Cardiology)
Pediatric Cardiologist
Department of Pediatric Cardiology
Narayana Superspeciality Hospital
Howrah, West Bengal, India

R Krishna Kumar MD DM FAHA
Professor and Head
Department of Pediatric Cardiology
Amrita Institute of Medical Sciences and Research Centre
Cochin, Kerala, India

Rohan Patel DNB(Medicine)
Senior Resident
Department of Cardiology
Dharma Vira Heart Centre
Sir Ganga Ram Hospital
New Delhi, India

Ronak Sheth MD FNB(Pediatric Cardiology)
Consultant Pediatric Cardiologist
Fortis Hospitals
Mumbai, Maharashtra, India

Ronak V Ruparelia DNB(Medicine) DNB(Cardiology)
Hon. Cardiologist
Bankers Super Speciality Hospital
Vadodara, Gujarat, India

Roopali Khanna MD DM
Professor
Department of Cardiology
Sanjay Gandhi Postgraduate
Institute of Medical Sciences
Lucknow, Uttar Pradesh, India

R Praveen Babu MD(General Medicine) DNB(Cardiology)
Associate Professor
Department of Cardiology
Vinayaka Missions Medical College
Karaikal, Puducherry, India

RR Mantri DM(Cardiology)
Co-Chairperson
Department of Cardiology
Dharma Vira Heart Centre
Sir Ganga Ram Hospital
New Delhi, India

Ruchit Shah DNB(Medicine) DNB(Cardiology) Fellowship Interventional Cardiology S Korea Training in TAVR Mitraclip LA(USA)
Honorary Assistant Professor
Department of Cardiology
Grant Government Medical College
and Sir JJ group of hospitals
Consultant Cardiologist
Saifee, Jaslok, Breach Candy Hospital
Mumbai, Maharashtra, India

Ruman Kugashiya MD DNB
Fellow Cardiology
Batra Hospital and Medical
Research Centre
New Delhi, India

Sabarish S MD DM
Associate Consultant Cardiologist
Institute of Cardio Vascular Diseases
Madras Medical Mission
Chennai, Tamil Nadu, India

Sachin Narendra Patil MD(Medicine) DNB(Cardiology)
Consultant Cardiologist
Sachin Multispeciality Hospital
Kolhapur, Maharashtra, India

Sadhanandham Shanmugasundaram MD(General Medicine) DNB(Cardiology)
Professor, Department of Cardiology
Sri Ramachandra Institute of Higher
Education and Research
Chennai, Tamil Nadu, India

Sajeet Kumar Verma DM
Assistant Professor
King George's Medical University
Lucknow Uttar Pradesh, India

Saket Ramraika MD(Medicine)
3rd Year Resident (DM)
Department of Cardiology
King George's Medical University
Lucknow, Uttar Pradesh, India

Sameer Dani MD DM(Cardiology)
Director
Department of Cardiology Services
Apollo CVHF Heart Institute,
Ahmedabad
Apollo Hospital International
Gandhinagar
Gujarat, India

Sameer Gupta FACC
Director
Cardiac Cath Lab
Metro Group of Hospitals
Noida, Uttar Pradesh, India

Samhita Purandare DNB(Medicine) DNB(Cardiology)
Assistant Professor
Padmashree DY Patil Medical College
Mumbai, Maharashtra, India

Samriddhi Yasha MD
Resident, Department of Cardiology
RG Kar Medical College and Hospital
Kolkata, West Bengal, India

Sandeepan Saha MD
Assistant Professor
Department of Cardiology
Dr Ram Manohar Lohia Institute of
Medical Sciences
Lucknow, Uttar Pradesh, India

Sandipta Ray MD DM
Senior Interventional Cardiologist
Manipal Broadway Hospital
Kolkata, West Bengal, India

Sangeeta Dhir MDS(Periodontology) Fellow ICOI(USA) Fellow(Diabetes India)
Consultant
Dentistry and Clinical Research
Max Superspeciality Hospital
Saket, New Delhi, India
Chairperson
Diabetes India Oral Health Group

Sanjana R Badami MD DM
Junior Consultant
Department of Cardiology
KIMS Hospitals
Secunderabad, Telangana, India

Sanjay Tyagi MD(Medicine) DM(Cardiology) FAMS FICP FCSI FICA FRCP(Edinburgh) FSCAI FESC FACC(USA)
Dr BC Roy National Awardee
Senior Consultant
Academic Advisor (Head) and
Clinical Director
Department of Cardiology
Apollo Hospitals, Northern Region
New Delhi, India
President
Cardiological Society of India

Sanjeev Asotra MD DM
Professor, Department of Cardiology
Indira Gandhi Medical College
Shimla, Himachal Pradesh, India

Sanjeev Kumar MD
Professor
Department of Cardiovascular
Radiology and Endovascular
Interventions
All India Institute of Medical Sciences
New Delhi, India

Sanjiv Sharma MD DM(Cardiology)
Senior Consultant Cardiology
Batra Hospital and Medical Research
Centre
New Delhi, India

S Anne Princy MD DM
Assistant Professor
Department of Cardiology
Tamil Nadu Government Multi Super Speciality Hospital
Chennai, Tamil Nadu, India

Sarita Rao MD DM FACC FSACI
Senior Interventional Cardiologist and Director – Cathlab
Department of Cardiology
Apollo Rajshree Hospitals
Indore, Madhya Pradesh, India

Satish K Parashar MD FACC FCSI FIAE
Director
Department of Non-invasive Cardiology, Heart Institute
Lajpat Nagar, New Delhi, India

Sathish S Reddy MD DM
Professor and Head, Department of Cardiac Electrophysiology
Sri Jayadeva Institute of Cardiovascular Sciences and Research
Bengaluru, Karnataka, India

Satya Narayan Routray MD DM FACC FESC FSCAI
Former Head, Department of Cardiology, SCB Medical College
Cuttack, Odisha, India

Satya Prasad Mahapatra MD DM(Cardiology)
Senior Resident
Department of Cardiology
Sanjay Gandhi Postgraduate Institute of Medical Sciences
Lucknow, Uttar Pradesh, India

Satyavan Sharma MD DM FACC FAMS FESC FSCAI
Honorary Consultant Cardiologist
Bombay Hospital and Medical Research Centre
Mumbai, Maharashtra, India

Satyavir Yadav MD DM
Associate Professor
Department of Cardiology
All India Institute of Medical Sciences
New Delhi, India

Satyendra Tewari MD DM FACC FSCAI FESC FAPSC FCSI FICC
Professor
Department of Cardiology
Sanjay Gandhi Postgraduate Institute of Medical Sciences
Lucknow, Uttar Pradesh, India

Saumitra Ray MD FRCP FESC FACC FSCAI FCSI FICP
Consultant Cardiologist
Manipal Hospitals
Kolkata, West Bengal, India

Saumya Sagar MD
Assistant Professor
Department of Medicine
Lady Hardinge Medical College and Associate Hospitals
New Delhi, India

Sayar Ahmad Pandit MD DM
Assistant Professor
Department of Cardiology
LPSIC GSVM
Kanpur, Uttar Pradesh, India

S Bhushan MD DNB
Assistant Professor
Department of Cardiology
All India Institute of Medical Sciences
Bhopal, Madhya Pradesh, India

Shabbir Ali Shaik MD DM FNB FESC
Consultant Interventional Cardiologist
AIG Hospitals
Hyderabad, Telangana, India

Shaheen Ahmad MD DM(Cardiology)
Director
Department of Cardiology
Jay Prabha Medanta Super Specialty Hospital
Patna, Bihar, India

Shamshad Alam MD DM(Cardiology)
Associate Director
Department of Cardiology
Medanta Heart Institute
Jay Prabha Medanta Super Specialty Hospital
Patna, Bihar, India

Shanmugasundaram Somasundaram MD DM(Cardiology)
Former Professor of Cardiology
Stanley and Madras Medical Colleges
Chennai, Tamil Nadu, India

Shantanu Deshpande MD(Medicine) DM(Cardiology) DNB(Cardiology)
Head
Department of Cardiology
Padmashree DY Patil Medical College
Mumbai, Maharashtra, India

Sharad Chandra DM FACC FESC FSCAI FAPSIC FCSI
Professor
Department of Cardiology
King George's Medical University
Lucknow, Uttar Pradesh, India

Sharath K Kumar MD DM
Cardiologist
Department of Electrophysiology
AIG Hospitals
Hyderabad, Telangana, India

Shibba Takkar Chhabra MD DM
Professor
Department of Cardiology
Dayanand Medical College and Hospital
Unit-Hero DMC Heart Institute
Ludhiana, Punjab, India

Shilanjan Roy MD(Medicine) MRCP(UK) DM(Cardiology) FSCAI FAPSIC
Senior Consultant
Department of Interventional Cardiology
Charnock Hospital
Former Assistant Professor
Department of Cardiology
KPC Medical College and Hospital
Kolkata, West Bengal, India

Shishir Soni MD DM FACC
Assistant Professor
Department of Cardiology
NSCB Medical College
Jabalpur, Madhya Pradesh, India

Shishu Shankar Mishra MD FAIMS MCAM DoCM FCCP FIAE FICC FCSI
Professor and Director
SOA University, Bhubaneswar
Professor and Director
Dreams University and Institute of Health Sciences and Padmini Care Hospital
Director
Med-n-Heart Clinic
Cuttack, Odisha, India

Shitij Chaudhary MD
Senior Resident
Department of Cardiology
All India Institute of Medical Sciences
New Delhi, India

Shreya Gupta MD DM
Medical Officer
Department of Cardiology
ABVIMS and Dr RML Hospital
New Delhi, India

Shyam Prasad Sahoo MD
Trainee
Department of Radiodiagnosis
JSS Medical College and Hospital
Mysuru, Karnataka, India

Shyam S Kothari MD DM
Professor
Department of Cardiology
UN Mehta Institute of Cardiology
Ahmedabad, Gujarat, India

Siddarth Varshney MD DM
Consultant Interventional Cardiologist
Medanta – The Medicity
Gurugram, Haryana, India

Siddhartha Mani MD DM(Cardiology)
Consultant Cardiologist
Department of Cardiology
NH-RTIICS
Kolkata, West Bengal, India

Sivasubramanian Ramakrishnan MD DM
Professor
Department of Cardiology
All India Institute of Medical Sciences
New Delhi, India

SK Dwivedi MD DM FACC FESC FSCAI
Director
Department of Interventional Cardiology
Medanta Super Speciality Hospital
Lucknow, Uttar Pradesh, India

Snehal Kulkarni MD DrNB(Cardiology) FACC
Director
Department of Pediatric Cardiac Sciences
Fortis Hospital
Mumbai, Maharashtra, India

Somil Verma MD DM
Consultant Cardiologist
Medanta Super Speciality Hospital
Lucknow, Uttar Pradesh, India

Somnath Maji MD
Resident
Department of Cardiology
RG Kar Medical College and Hospital
Kolkata, West Bengal, India

Somya Mahlawat MD DM(Cardiology)
Assistant Professor
Department of Cardiology
King George's Medical University
Lucknow, Uttar Pradesh, India

Sonali Sharma MSc[Biochemistry(Med)] PhD[Biochemistry(Med)]
Professor
Department of Biochemistry
RUHS College of Medical Sciences
Rajasthan University of Health Sciences
Jaipur, Rajasthan, India

Sridhar Kasturi MD DM FACC FESC FSCAI FICC
Head
Department of Cardiology and Cardiothoracic Surgery
KIMS – Sunshine Hospitals, Begumpet
Secunderabad, Telangana, India

Srina Ray MBBS
Junior Fellow – ICU
Epsom and St Hilier Hospital
Sutton, United Kingdom

SR Sharath Shanmugam MD(General Medicine) DM(Cardiology)
Postgraduate
Sri Ramachandra Medical College
Chennai, Tamil Nadu, India

Subhashis Dey MD(Medicine) DRNB(Cardiology)
Assosciate Consultant
Department of Cardiology
Narayana Multispeciality Hospital
Barasat, West Bengal, India

Subhasis Roy Chowdhury MD DM FSCAI
Director-Cath Lab, Manipal Hospitals
Kolkata, West Bengal, India

Subir Sen MD DM(Cardiology)
Senior Interventional Cardiologist
Manipal Broadway Hospital
Kolkata, West Bengal, India

Subrahmanya Murti V MD DM
Senior Specialist
Department of Cardiology
Aster CMI Hospital
Bengaluru, Karnataka, India

Sucheta Barman MD(Pediatrics) DrNB(Pediatric Cardiology)
Senior Resident
Department of Pediatric Cardiology
IPGMER
Kolkata, West Bengal, India

Sudarshan K Vijay MD DM
Professor
Department of Cardiology
Dr Ram Manohar Lohia Institute of Medical Sciences
Lucknow, Uttar Pradesh, India

Suman Bhandari MD DM FACC FESC FSCAI FIMSA
Director
Department of Cardiology
Fortis Escort Heart Institute
New Delhi, India

Sumang Mohan MD
Senior Resident
Department of Cardiology
Sanjay Gandhi Postgraduate Institute of Medical Sciences
Lucknow, Uttar Pradesh, India

Sumanta Chatterjee MD
Consultant Cardiologist
Manipal Hospitals
Kolkata, West Bengal, India

Sumanyu Suresh MD
Senior Resident
Department of Cardiology
Sree Chitra institute for Medical Sciences and Technology
Thiruvananthapuram, Kerala, India

Sumit Kumar MD DM
Assistant Professor
All India Institute of Medical Sciences
New Delhi, India

Sunandan Sikdar MD DM FACC
Consultant
Department of Cardiology
Narayana Multispecialty Hospital
Kolkata, West Bengal, India

Sundar Chidambaram MD DNB DM FNB FESC FSCAI
Consultant Interventional Cardiologist and Endovascular Specialist
Kauvery Hospital
Chennai, Tamil Nadu, India

Sunil Lhila MD DM
Consultant Interventional Cardiologist
Department of Cardiology
NH-RTIICS
Kolkata, West Bengal, India

Sura Kishore Mishra MD DM(Cardiology)
Professor and Head
Department of Cardiology
SCB Medical College
Cuttack, Odisha, India

Sushil Kumar MD DM(Cardiology)
Consultant
Department of Cardiology
Jay Prabha Medanta Super Specialty Hospital
Patna, Bihar, India

Suvadeep Biswas MD
Resident
Department of Cardiology
RG Kar Medical College and Hospital
Kolkata, West Bengal, India

Tanmay Mukhopadhyay MD DM(Cardiology)
Associate Professor
Department of Cardiology
Burdwan Medical College and Hospital
Burdwan, West Bengal, India

TR Muralidharan MD(Medicine) DM(Cardiology) FACC FESC
Director, Institute of Cardiac Sciences
SRM Global Hospital
Kattankulathur, Tamil Nadu, India

Tapan Ghose MD(Medicine) DNB(Cardiology) DNB FNB MNAMS FIMSA FCSI FASCAI FACC
Senior Director and Head
Department of Cardiology
Head – Clinical Research and Academics
Fortis Flt Lt Rajan Dhall Hospital
New Delhi, India

Tapas K Kundu PhD FNASc FASc FNA
Professor
Transcription and Disease Laboratory
Molecular Biology and Genetics Unit
Jawaharlal Nehru Centre for Advanced Scientific Research
Bengaluru, Karnataka, India

Thomas Alexander MD DM
Head
Department of Cardiology
Kovai Medical Center and Hospital
Coimbatore, Tamil Nadu, India

Trinath Kumar Mishra MD DM FCSI FACC
Professor
Department of Cardiology
MKCG Medical College and Hospital
Berhampur, Odisha, India

Ujjwala Tulluri MD DrNB(Cardiology)
Resident
Asian Heart Insititute
Mumbai, Maharashtra, India

Umesh Tripathi MD DM(Cardiology)
Assistant Professor
Department of Cardiology
King George's Medical University
Lucknow, Uttar Pradesh, India

Umeshwar Pandey MD DM
Professor
Department of Cardiology
LPS Institute of Cardiology
Kanpur, Uttar Pradesh, India

Upadhyay Aditya Chandradhar MD DM
Assistant Professor
Department of Cardiology
Dr Ram Manohar Lohia Institute of Medical Sciences
Lucknow, Uttar Pradesh, India

Vadivelu Ramalingam MD DM
Consultant Interventional Cardiologist
McGill University Health Centre
Montreal, Canada
Velammal Medical College Hospital and Research Institute
Madurai, Tamil Nadu, India

Vaidehi Agarwal MD DNB
Fellow Cardiology
Batra Hospital and Medical Research Centre
New Delhi, India

Varsha Rakshitha Prakash MD(Medicine) DM(Cardiology) PDF(Cardiac Electrophysiology)
Cardiologist and Cardiac Electrophysiologist
Department of Cardiology
MS Ramaiah Memorial Hospital
Bengaluru, Karnataka, India

Varshini Neethi Mohan
Department of Humanities and Social Sciences, IIT Madras
Chennai, Tamil Nadu, India

Venkata RS Subrahmanya Sarma MD DM
Consultant Cardiologist
Aayush Hospitals
Vijayawada and Eluru
Andhra Pradesh, India

Vibhav Sharma MD DM
Consultant
Department of Cardiology
Amrita Institute of Medical Science and Research
Faridabad, Haryana, India

Vibhav Sharma MD DM
Consultant
Department of Cardiac Sciences
Max Superspeciality Hospital
Saket, New Delhi, India

Vidya PL DM(Cardiology)
Junior Consultant
Department of Cardiology
Sri Sathya Sai Institute of Higher Medical Sciences
Prasanthigram, Andhra Pradesh, India

Vidyut Jain MD FACC FSCAI FRCP FESC
Consultant Cardiologist
Choithram Hospital
Indore, Madhya Pradesh, India

Vijay Bang MD DM FCSI FESC FSCAI FACC
Senior Interventional Cardiologist
Lilavati Hospital and Research Center
Honorable Professor and Head
Grant Medical College and
Sir JJ Group of Hospitals (Former)
Mumbai, Maharashtra, India

Vikash Kumar Maurya MD
Senior Resident
Department of Cardiology
Institute of Medical Sciences
Banaras Hindu University
Varanasi, Uttar Pradesh, India

Vikas Singh DM FACC FSCAI FAPSIC FCSI FICP
Consultant Intervention Cardiologist
Mediversal Multispeciality Hospital
Patna, Bihar, India

Vilas Magarkar MD DM FSCC-FSCAI(USA) FESC(Europe) FCSI(India)
Head, Department of Cardiology
Seth Nandlal Dhoot Hospital
Aurangabad, Maharashtra, India

Vinay Bhardwaj MD DM
Assistant Professor
Department of Cardiology
Indira Gandhi Medical College
Shimla, Himachal Pradesh, India

Vinay Kumar Sajja MD
Associate Consultant Cardiologist
Yashoda Hospital Hitech City
Hyderabad, Telangana, India

Vineeta Ojha MD DM
Assistant Professor
Department of Cardiovascular Radiology and Endovascular Interventions
All India Institute of Medical Sciences
New Delhi, India

Vipin Kumar MD DM(Cardiology) FACC FSCAI
Senior Consultant Interventional Cardiologist
Ruban Memorial Hospital
Patna, Bihar, India

Vishal Batra MD DM(Cardiology)
Professor
Department of Cardiology
GB Pant Institute of Postgraduate Medical Education and Research
New Delhi, India

Viveka Kumar MD DM FACC FSCAI FCSI
Director
Department of Cardiology
Max Hospital
Saket, New Delhi, India

Vivek Chaturvedi MD DM FACC
Senior Consultant and Professor
Department of Cardiology
Amrita Institute of Medical Science and Research
Faridabad, Haryana, India

VK Bahl MD DM(Cardiology)
Head
Department of Cardiovascular Sciences and Research
Metro Group of Hospitals
Noida, Uttar Pradesh, India

V Murugesan MD(General Medicine) DM(Cardiology)
Consultant Cardiologist
Rohini Hospitals
Thanjavur, Tamil Nadu, India

VS Prakash MD(Medicine) DM(Cardiology) PDF(Cardiac Electrophysiology) FACC FESC FSCAI FISE
Interventional Cardiologist
Cardiac Electrophysiologist and Head
Department of Cardiology
Chief – Arrhythmia Services
MS Ramaiah Memorial Hospital
Bengaluru, Karnataka, India

Preface

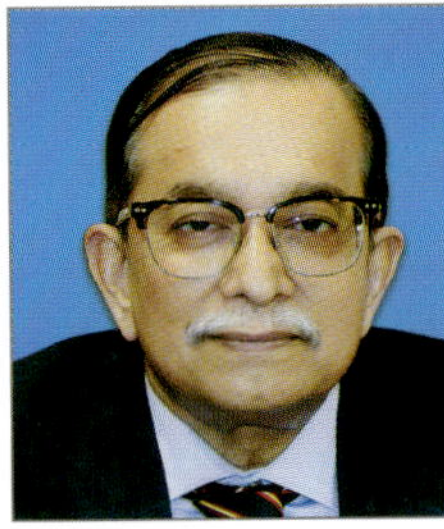

Dhiman Kahali MD DM FESC FSCAI
Director – Interventional Cardiology
BM Birla Heart Research Centre
Kolkata, West Bengal, India
President Elect – Cardiological Society of India
Ex-Chairman – National Intervention Council, Cardiological Society of India (CSI)
Ex-Convener – STEMI Council, Cardiological Society of India (CSI)
Ex-Vice President – Cardiological Society of India (CSI) 2020–2024

A very warm greeting from the Cardiological Society of India (CSI). It gives me immense pleasure to present the *"CSI Cardiology Update 2025"*, a thoughtfully curated compilation that reflects the dedication, expertise, and collective spirit of the CSI fraternity.

This annual publication stands as a valuable reference for clinicians, researchers, and students of cardiovascular medicine. The CSI Cardiology Update continues its tradition of offering evidence-based insights and practical perspectives on emerging developments in cardiology.

Each edition builds upon the legacy of its predecessors, striving to capture the dynamic evolution of cardiovascular science and practice.

The 2025 edition encompasses a wide array of topics ranging from preventive cardiology, clinical trials, and diagnostic innovations to cutting-edge interventional procedures and heart failure management. Each chapter, contributed by leading experts from across the country, is designed to serve as a trusted guide for practicing cardiologists and trainees alike.

Our mission through this publication remains clear—to provide cardiologists with a comprehensive resource that enhances their clinical practice and encourages continual learning. The carefully structured chapters aim to deliver clarity, conciseness, and clinical relevance, ensuring that the content remains both practical and academically sound.

I extend my sincere gratitude to all the contributors for their time, knowledge, and commitment for maintaining the highest standards of academic excellence. My special thanks go to the editorial team for their meticulous efforts in conceptualizing, reviewing, and refining each section to perfection. Their hard work and collaboration have made this publication possible.

I would also like to acknowledge the unwavering support of the CSI leadership, the scientific committee, and our publishing partners for their professional excellence in producing this volume.

A special note of heartfelt appreciation goes to *Dr Debabrata Roy, Dr Kaushik Manna, and Dr Debabrata Biswas* for their unwavering support and dedicated efforts in ensuring the timely completion and successful delivery of the *"CSI Cardiology Update 2025"*. Their commitment and guidance have been instrumental in bringing this publication within the permitted time schedule.

It is my hope that *"CSI Cardiology Update 2025"* will serve as an enduring source of insight and inspiration for cardiologists, fellows, and students alike. May it guide you to deliver even better care, deepen your understanding, and empower your practice toward a healthier and stronger cardiovascular future.

Contents

VOLUME 1

SECTION 1: PREVENTIVE CARDIOLOGY

1. **Improving Community-level Cardiac-health Awareness through School-based Education Program in India** 3
   Debabrata Biswas, Debabrata Roy

2. **Air Pollution and Cardiovascular Disease in India: Current Perspective** 8
   Debabrata Biswas, Kaushik Manna, DP Sinha

3. **Can We Cancel Out the Excess Cardiovascular Risk Caused by Chronic Kidney Disease?** 12
   Farhin Iqbal, Chitra Priyadarshini

4. **Smoking Cessation: Never too Early, Never too Late!** 17
   Saumitra Ray, Sumanta Chatterjee, Srina Ray

SECTION 2: HYPERTENSION

5. **Implications of Systolic Blood Pressure Time in Target Range** 25
   AK Trivedi, Abhinit Gupta, Bijay Prakash Yadav

6. **Artificial Intelligence: An Emerging Tool for the Diagnosis and Management of Hypertension** 29
   C Venkata S Ram

7. **Clinical Management of Primary Aldosteronism** 37
   Dharmendra Jain, Vikash Kumar Maurya, Pratap Kumar

8. **Implications of Myocardial Interstitial Fibrosis in Hypertensive Heart Disease** 43
   Debasis Ghosh, Navanil Biswas

9. **Renovascular Hypertension: Kidney Intrinsic Mechanism as Novel Target** 47
   Manu Gupta, Anuj Gupta, Pooja Sharma Gupta, Rajeev Gupta

10. **The Complexity of Resistant and Refractory Hypertension** 56
    Somya Mahlawat, Umesh Tripathi, Sharad Chandra

SECTION 3: CARDIOMETABOLIC

11. **Slowing Cardiovascular Aging by Promoting Cardiometabolic Health** 69
Bhabatosh Biswas, Pankaj Sharma, Tapas K Kundu

12. **Obesity and Cardiovascular Diseases** 76
Amit Malviya, Md Amish Shikoh, Aman Asthana, Animesh Mishra

13. **Myocardial Abnormalities Across the AHA-ACC Heart Failure Spectrum in Diabetic Patients** 83
Umeshwar Pandey, Kumar Himanshu

SECTION 4: DYSLIPIDEMIA MANAGEMENT

14. **Implications of Lipid-lowering Therapy for Premature Coronary Artery Disease** 89
AK Pancholia

15. **The Challenges in Reducing Non-high-density Lipoprotein Cholesterol** 95
Arvind Kumar, Vipin Kumar

16. **Particle Number and Characteristics of Lipoprotein(a), Low-density Lipoprotein, and ApoB: Perspectives on Contributions to Atherosclerotic Cardiovascular Disease** 101
JPS Sawhney, Rohan Patel

17. **Childhood LDL Cholesterol, Non-HDL Cholesterol and Adult Atherosclerotic Cardiovascular Events** 105
Rajeev Gupta, Sonali Sharma

SECTION 5: HEART FAILURE

18. **Worsening Heart Failure: Definition and Management** 117
Dhiman Kahali, Debdatta Kar, Padma Madhab Bisoi

19. **Pulmonary Hypertension in Heart Failure: The Good, the Bad, and the Ugly** 126
A Purnanand

20. **Progression from Pre-heart Failure, Heart Stress to Subclinical Heart Failure** 132
Arpita Katheria, Ankit Kumar Sahu, Aditya Kapoor

21. **Immunology of Heart Failure: Deconstructing Inflammatory Risk** 138
Amal Kumar Khan, Anish Kumar Khan, Amartya Khan

22. **Iron Deficiency States and Effective Iron Repletion Strategies in Chronic Heart Failure** 146
Ankit Kumar Sahu, Arshad Nazir, Pranjal Raparia

23. **Risk Scores in the Management of Heart Failure** 157
Ashish Jha, Abhijit Bharali

24. **Issues in Reversing Advanced Heart Failure** 164
Awadhesh K Sharma, Sayar Ahmad Pandit

25. **Early Initiation of GDMT in HFrEF: Accelerating Outcomes with Timely Evidence-based Titration** 169
Dikshit Byomakesh, Behera Soumen Prasad

26. **Mixed Cardiogenic-vasodilatory Shock** 174
Biswajit Majumder, Somnath Maji, Suvadeep Biswas, Ratul Ghosh

27. **Chronic Right-sided Heart Failure and Tricuspid Regurgitation: "No Longer a Forgotten Entity"** 180
Chandrakanta Mishra

28. **Neuromodulation Interventions in the Management of Heart Failure** 192
Manoj Bansal

29. **Congestion and Diuretic Resistance in Worsening Heart Failure** 198
HK Chopra

30. **Role of Imaging in Heart Failure Risk Stratification** 205
Haresh Mehta, Raghav R Nagpal, Kayan Siodia

31. **Can Left Ventricular Wall Strain Predict Heart Failure?** 212
Jagdish Chander Mohan, Madhu Shukla

32. **Medical Therapy of Cardiogenic Shock: Contemporary Use of Inotropes and Vasopressors** 220
Kashinath Ghosh Hazra, Ahitagni Banerjee

33. **Continuum of Preshock to Classic Cardiogenic Shock** 230
MU Rabbani

34. **Triaging of Patients of Acute Decompensated Heart Failure** 236
Pranab Jyoti Bhattacharyya, Maitreyee Bhattacharyya

35. **Gut Hypothesis of Heart Failure: Role of Gut Microbiota–Derived Metabolites** 241
Puneet Rastogi

36. **Diuretic Potentiation Strategies in Acute Heart Failure** 246
SK Dwivedi, Somil Verma

37. **Approaches in Heart Failure with Mildly Reduced and Preserved Ejection Fraction** 254
Vidyut Jain, Avani Jain

38. **Characteristics and Outcomes of Patients with Valvular Cardiogenic Shock** 259
Sumanyu Suresh, Harikrishnan Sivadasanpillai

39. **Hemodynamic Assessment by Right Heart Catheterization in Management of Heart Failure** 267
Bijay Prakash Pandey, Rajat Kar

SECTION 6: CARDIOMYOPATHY

40. **Sudden Cardiac Death in Hypertrophic Cardiomyopathy** 275
R Alagesan, C Narasimhan, Muthiah Subramanian

41. **Polygenic Inheritance in Hypertrophic Cardiomyopathy** 289
Ajay Bahl

42. **Dual (Ischemic and Nonischemic) Cardiomyopathy: A Wolf in Sheep's Clothing** 292
Chandra Bhan Meena, Himanshu Mahla, Mayank Nausran

43. **Vasovagal Syncope: What Treatment Can We Offer in 2025?** 300
Nishad Chitnis, Hygriv B Rao

44. **Role of Clonal Hematopoiesis in the Pathogenesis of Dilated Cardiomyopathy** 306
Ganesan Manohar, Karthikaa Saminathan

45. **Dilated Cardiomyopathy in Systemic Immune-mediated Diseases** 313
Ganesh Seth, Mahima Saran, Himanshu Gupta

46. **Arrhythmia-induced Cardiomyopathy** 318
Arindam Mitra, Aditi Rastogi, Jayanta Saha

47. **Alcoholic Cardiomyopathy** 326
Shishu Shankar Mishra, Biswaranjan Mishra, Asharam Panda

SECTION 7: CONGENITAL HEART DISEASE

48. **Expanding Future of Sinus Venosus Atrial Septal Defect Closure** 335
Rishika Mehta, Amitabha Chattopadhyay

49. **Clinical Risk Assessment and Prediction in Congenital Heart Disease Across the Lifespan** 342
Anita Saxena

50. **Early Intervention for Tetralogy of Fallot, but at What Cost?** 348
Mahua Roy, Sucheta Barman

51. **Novel Imaging Techniques for Congenital Heart Disease** 353
D Seshagiri Rao, Ramya Pechetty

52. **Evaluation and Management of Chronic Heart Failure in Children and Adolescents with Congenital Heart Disease** 373
Jonaki Pal, Debasree Gangopadhyay

53. **Advancing New Solutions for Adult Congenital Heart Diseases-related Heart Failure** 381
Prafulla Kerkar, Ujjwala Tulluri

54. **Care for Congenital Heart Disease in India: The Evolving Landscape** 386
R Krishna Kumar

55. **Echocardiography for Childhood Left Ventricular Noncompaction** 393
Sura Kishore Mishra, Bitan Mohanty

56. **Adults with Congenital Heart Disease: What Every Cardiologist Should Know About Their Care?** 398
Arun Gopalakrishnan, Shyam S Kothari

57. **Quest for a Lifelong Pulmonary Valve in Repaired Tetralogy of Fallot** 408
Ronak Sheth, Snehal Kulkarni

SECTION 8: VALVULAR HEART DISEASE

58. **Multiparametric Approach to Asymptomatic Aortic Stenosis** 419
Ajay Kumar Pandey, Nikhil Gupta, Prashant Kumar Pandey

59. **Secondary Mitral Regurgitation: Phenotypes, Proportionality, and Evolving Management** 424
Arijit Ghosh, Arup Dasbiswas, Subhasis Roy Chowdhury, Mainak Mukhopadhyay

60. **Mitral Annular Disjunction in Mitral Valve Prolapse** 433
Biswaranjan Mishra

61. **An Update on High-gradient Moderate Aortic Stenosis** 439
Debika Chatterjee

62. **Comprehensive Risk Phenotyping in Aortic Stenosis** 443
Dipankar Ghosh Dastidar

63. **When to Treat Young and Low-risk Patients with Aortic Stenosis** 451
Gopala Krishna Koduru, Raghuram Palaparti, Venkata RS Subrahmanya Sarma

64. **Acute Rheumatic Fever and Rheumatic Heart Disease: A Continuum (Recent Advances)** 456
Mohit D Gupta, Girish MP, Gaurav Sharma, Mayank Shami

65. **Comprehensive Approach to Aortic Valve Pathophysiology by Fibro-Calcific Imaging** 473
Johann Christopher, Raja Ramesh Nukavarapu

66. **Reimagining Valvular Heart Disease Management: Insights from the 2025 ESC/EACTS Guidelines** 481
Mrinal Kanti Das

67. **Rheumatic Heart Disease in India: An Imperative Tale to Tell** 486
Sanjeev Asotra, Vinay Bhardwaj, Preetam Thakur

SECTION 9: CARDIO-OBSTETRICS

68. **Cardiac Interventions during Pregnancy** 499
S Anne Princy, R Archana, G Justin Paul

69. **Antepartum Cardiovascular Risk Assessment and Management of High-risk Cardiac Delivery** 505
Monika Bhandari, Saket Ramraika

70. **Understanding and Managing Heart Failure during Pregnancy—What is New in Peripartum Cardiomyopathy?** 515
Roopali Khanna, Sumang Mohan, Harshit Khare

71. **Hypertensive Disorder of Pregnancy and Long-term Cardiovascular Outcome** 520
S Anne Princy, G Justin Paul

72. **Understanding and Managing Anticoagulant during Pregnancy in Women with Heart Valves** 528
Abhishek Garg, Shibba Takkar Chhabra

SECTION 10: CORONARY ARTERY DISEASE

73. **Sarcopenia and Coronary Microvascular Dysfunction** 537
Nakul Sinha

74. **Spontaneous Coronary Artery Dissection** 540
Prakas Chandra Mondal

75. **Platelet Biology and Function: Plaque Erosion versus Rupture** 545
Ranjit K Nath, MD Asif Iqbal, Shreya Gupta

76. **Coronary Artery Aneurysm: A Therapeutic Dilemma** 549
Ramesh Thakur, Kumar Himanshu

77. **Atherosclerosis, Aortic Dissection, and Peripheral Artery Disease: New Therapeutic Targets** 554
Akhilesh Kumar, Suman Bhandari

SECTION 11: CARDIAC ARRHYTHMIA

78. VT Ablation as Stand Alone Procedure without ICD in Stable Scar VT in Mild or Moderate LV Dysfunction 565
Anees Thajudeen

79. Atrial Fibrillation and Long-term CV Outcome 570
Bhuban Majhi, Rajarshi Halder

80. Effect of Left Atrial Dyssynchrony on Long-term Clinical Outcomes during Cardiac Resynchronization Therapy 575
Anil Mishra

81. Divergence from Guideline Directed Management of Cardiac Implantable Electronic Device Infections 584
Ashish Nabar, Amit Vora

82. Leadless Pacing: Past, Present, and Future 591
Aftab Khan, Navanil Biswas, Arif Nabi Bhat

83. Atrial Fibrillation in Heart Failure: Role of Catheter Ablation 598
Sharath K Kumar, Calambur Narasimhan

84. Ventricular Tachycardia Ablation in the Emergency Setting 612
Aditya Mulgaonkar, Deepak Padmanabhan

85. Prevention of Sudden Cardiac Death beyond Automated External Defibrillators and Implantable Cardioverter Defibrillators 620
Girish B Navasundi

86. Pulsed Field Ablation—in Present Perspective 625
Vadivelu Ramalingam, Atul Verma, KK Talwar

87. Para-Hisian Ventricular Arrhythmias 634
Sathish S Reddy, Priyanka Agarwal

SECTION 12: IMAGING

88. Risk Stratification with Coronary Computed Tomography Angiography-derived Fractional Flow Reserve and Fractional Flow Reserve Gradient 641
Lekha Adik Pathak, Ronak V Ruparelia

89. Role of Multimodality Imaging in Multivalvular Heart Disease 646
Rajendra Kumar Jain, Sanjana R Badami

90. **Role of Left Atrial Indices in Management of Chronic Severe Asymptomatic Aortic Regurgitation** 657
Satish K Parashar

91. **Application of Emerging Hybrid Intracoronary Imaging Technologies in Clinical Practice and Research** 664
Harilalith Kovvuri, Nagendra Boopathy Senguttuvan

92. **Current Concepts and Clinical Implications of Coronary Artery Calcification** 670
Satyavan Sharma

93. **Cardiac CT: Emerging Role in Microvascular Dysfunction** 677
VS Prakash, Varsha Rakshitha Prakash

94. **Role of Cardiac Imaging for Optimizing Medical Therapy** 684
Vilas Magarkar

Index *i1–i13*

VOLUME 2

SECTION 13: ST-ELEVATION MYOCARDIAL INFARCTION (STEMI)

95. **P2Y12 Inhibitor Pretreatment in STEMI** 693
Amar Narayan Patnaik

96. **ST-elevation Myocardial Infarction Revascularization in India: Lessons Learned from Punjab (Mission AMRIT)** 696
Ashu Gupta, Hitinder Kaur, Bishav Mohan

97. **Cardiac Magnetic Resonance Evaluation of Left Ventricular Remodeling after Myocardial Infarction** 703
Vineeta Ojha, Sanjeev Kumar

98. **Recurrent Thrombosis after Myocardial Infarction** 711
Sundar Chidambaram, Manokar P, Mahesh Babu, Mahadevan R, Deepchand Raja, Jebaraj

99. **STEMI Revascularization in India: Lessons Learnt from Tamil Nadu—5 Years Experience** 715
S Anne Princy, JB Vincil Jito, G Justin Paul

100. **Thrombolysis in STEMI in the Primary PCI Era: Current Relevance in India** 723
Padmanabh Kamath

101. **STEMI Revascularization in India—Lessons Learnt from Goa** 729
Guruprasad Datta Naik

102. **Role of Novel Risk Factors in ST-segment Elevation Myocardial Infarction Among Young Women** **735**
M Mashhadi, Sameer Dani, Harsh Chaudhary

103. **Transition from ST-segment Elevation Myocardial Infarction to Occlusion Myocardial Infarction** **739**
Rajiv Bajaj

104. **ST-elevation Myocardial Infarction Revascularization in India: Role of Thrombolysis in Ambulance** **746**
Mohsin Raj Mantoo, Chandini Suvarna, Sivasubramanian Ramakrishnan

105. **Addressing Delays in Reperfusion Therapy—Developing Chest Pain Clinics: A New Initiative from STEMI India** **749**
Thomas Alexander, Varshini Neethi Mohan, Ajit S Mullasari

106. **Advanced Cardiac Patches in the Treatment of Myocardial Infarction** **752**
Nitharsha Prakash M, R Praveen Babu, V Murugesan

SECTION 14: CORONARY INTERVENTION

107. **Thrombus Aspiration in Primary Angioplasty** **761**
BKS Sastry

108. **Evaluation of Microvascular Dysfunction during Diagnostic Coronary Angiography** **765**
B Kesavamoorthy, P Sabari Krishnan, AD Arun Mohan

109. **Prevention of Progression of Obesity and Cardiometabolic Disease: Intervention in School-aged Children** **773**
Bhuwan Chandra Tiwari, Sandeepan Saha

110. **Diagnosis and Management of Coronary Artery Perforation** **779**
Chetan P Shah, Charan Reddy KV

111. **Coronary Physiology by Different Approaches for Guiding Percutaneous Coronary Intervention** **782**
DB Pahlajani, Kayan Siodia

112. **Interventional Treatment for Left Main Bifurcation In-stent Stenosis** **792**
DS Gambhir

113. **Management of Drug-eluting Stent ISR** **798**
Gaurav Chaudhary, Sajeet Kumar Verma, Ayush Shukla

114. **Bailout Strategies in Chronic Total Occlusion Percutaneous Coronary Intervention** **809**
Prathap Kumar N, Manu Rajendran, Blessvin Jino

115. Metal-less Percutaneous Coronary Intervention: Current Evidence, Techniques, and Future Directions 817
Madhupada Kiran Kumar, PC Rath

116. Percutaneous Coronary Intervention in High-risk Renal Disorders: Strategies for Renal Protection 825
PK Asokan

117. Effect of Anatomical and Viability-guided Completeness of Revascularization on Clinical Outcomes in Ischemic Cardiomyopathy 834
Rajesh Vijayvergiya, Anirudh Mukherjee

118. Dual Antiplatelet Therapy in CKD: Duration and Bleeding Risk in Post-percutaneous Coronary Intervention Patients 845
Satyendra Tewari, Satya Prasad Mahapatra

119. Technological Progress in Treating Calcified Coronaries 850
Sridhar Kasturi

120. Expanding the Indications of Multivessel Angioplasty: Review of Emerging Evidence and Clinical Implications 862
Vijay Bang, Kaushal Chhatrapati, Ashish Deshpande

SECTION 15: STRUCTURAL INTERVENTION

121. Transcatheter Aortic Valve Replacement in Heart Failure 873
Ajit S Mullasari, Praveen Ashok Kumar

122. Antithrombotic Selection Post-left Atrial Appendage Occlusion 881
Bhavana M, Atul Mathur

123. Predictors of Outcome of Reinterventions after TAVR 886
Bharat V Purohit, Vinay Kumar Sajja

124. Implications of Left Bundle Branch Block in Aortic Stenosis beyond Pacemaker Implantation 891
Raghu Cherukupalli, Chakrapani Vuppala

125. Imaging of Transcatheter Valve Failure: An Update 901
Manoj Chopda, Kavish Chopda, Anish Chugh, Rahul Shewale

126. Transcatheter Treatment of Pure Aortic Regurgitation: Current Evidence, Challenges, and Future Directions 910
Prasant Kr Sahoo, Nitish Prasad, Abhishek Dash, Shyam Prasad Sahoo

127. Changing Context and Goals for Transcatheter Mitral Therapy 923
Deepti Yadav, Siddarth Varshney, Praveen Chandra

128. **Unveiling Right Ventricle Remodeling Following Tricuspid Valve Intervention** 928
Rajneesh Kapoor, Kumar Shubham

129. **Resolving the Unmet Need for Treatment of Tricuspid Regurgitation** 932
Sadhanandham Shanmugasundaram, Akshay Prashanth G

130. **Bleeding after Transcatheter Structural Valve Interventions** 939
Shabbir Ali Shaik

SECTION 16: HOT TOPICS

Part 1: Heart Failure

131. **Mitral Regurgitation in Heart Failure** 955
A Kader Sahib, P Vijay Shekar

132. **Aging in Heart Failure** 963
Ashish Kumar Jha

133. **Consequences of Discontinuing Long-term Drug Treatment in Patients with HFrEF** 966
Rohan Patel, RR Mantri

134. **Tackling Metabolic Defects in Heart Failure with Preserved Ejection Fraction** 970
Vikas Singh, Rajiv Krishna

135. **Timing of Physical Activity and Cardiovascular Health: Walk the Talk!** 973
Prayaag Kini, Reeta Varyani

136. **Impact of the EAT-Lancet Diet in Preventing Heart Failure** 977
Subhashis Dey

137. **Controversies and Conundrums in Cardiac Cachexia** 980
Sunandan Sikdar, Rathindra Nath Karmakar, Gaurav Agarwal

138. **Therapeutic Inertia in Treating Heart Failure with Reduced Ejection Fraction** 984
Vipin Kumar, Arvind Kumar

139. **ARNI-induced Hypotension in HFrEF: A Feared Side Effect or a Marker of Modifiable Risk?** 989
Arindam Pande, Durlabh Debbarma, Pranabes Chakraborti

140. **Why have We Not been Able to Demonstrate Reduced Mortality in Patients with HFmrEF and HFpEF?** 993
Ravi Vishnu Prasad, G Kumar, CB Chandan

141. **HFrEF and HFpEF: How they Differ in Advanced Heart Failure—A Global Perspective** 999
Ranabrata Sen, Subhashis Dey, Kaushik Manna

142. **Decongestion in Acute Heart Failure—Beyond the Diuretic-centred Paradigm** **1002**
MS Ravi, TR Muralidharan, SR Sharath Shanmugam

143. **Hepatic Biomarker Abnormalities in the Cardiac Intensive Care Unit Proposed Criteria for Cardiohepatic Syndrome** **1005**
K Roshan Rao, Sarita Rao, Achukatla Kumar

144. **Bridging Atrial and Ventricular Failure Through Biomarkers** **1012**
Mahesh Rameshrao Deshpande

145. **Therapeutic Options in Ambulatory Advanced Heart Failure** **1017**
Hetan C Shah, Bhavik S Shah

146. **Hypoalbuminemia and Heart Failure: State-of-the-Art 2025** **1022**
Mainak Mukhopadhyay, Sandipta Ray, Subhasis Roy Chowdhury, Arijit Ghosh, Kajal Ganguly

147. **Implications of Atrial Fibrillation for GDMT in Heart Failure** **1026**
Ayush Shukla, Nilay Tripathi

148. **Why has it been Challenging to Modify Kidney Disease Progression in Patient with Heart Failure?** **1032**
Pankaj Singh, Debasish Das

Part 2: Hypertension

149. **Supranormal Left Ventricular Ejection Fraction, Concentric Remodeling, and Long-term Survival** **1035**
Viveka Kumar, Anil Yadav, Mitendra Singh Yadav, Sangeeta Dhir, Anupam Goel

150. **Brain Pathways in Blood Pressure Regulation** **1039**
Akhilesh Dubey, Shishir Soni, Harishankar Pratap Singh Chandel

151. **Low-renin Hypertension: Current Understanding and Future Directions** **1044**
Shilanjan Roy

152. **Sodium, Interstitium, Lymphatics, and Hypertension—A Tale of Hydraulics** **1047**
Tapan Ghose

153. **Arterial Stiffness as a Predisposing Factor for Chronic Kidney Disease** **1051**
Shantanu Deshpande, Samhita Purandare

Part 3: Coronary Artery Disease

154. **Association between Coronary Artery Spasm and Atherosclerotic Disease** **1055**
Subhasis Roy Chowdhury, Arijit Ghosh, Mainak Mukhopadhyay

155. **Prognostic Significance of Peri-infarct Ischemia** 1058
Brig Navreet Singh, Lt Col Ankush Gupta, Col Nitin Bajaj, Col Balwinder Singh

156. **Hemorrhagic Myocardial Infarction: Pathophysiology, Diagnosis, and Clinical Implications** 1061
Col Anil Dhall

157. **Stent Failure after Percutaneous Coronary Intervention in Diabetes Mellitus** 1066
Lipika Adhikari, Samriddhi Yasha

158. **Red Blood Cells as a New Target for Atherosclerotic Cardiovascular Disease** 1072
Sachin Narendra Patil

159. **Residual Chest Pain after Percutaneous Coronary Intervention** 1076
Ranabrata Sen, Siddhartha Mani

Part 4: Dyslipidemia Management

160. **Enhancing High-density Lipoprotein Function to Prevent Atherothrombosis** 1080
Debabrata Biswas

161. **Cholesterol Screening and Management in Young Adults** 1085
Shamshad Alam, Ajay Kumar Sinha, Shaheen Ahmad, Sushil Kumar

Part 5: Ischemic Heart Disease

162. **Role of Vitamin D in Heart Disease** 1089
Bijay Narayan Jha, Dharmendra Kumar Singh

163. **Testosterone and Cardiovascular Health** 1095
Jayanta Sharma, Abhinandan Saha

164. **Primary Prevention for Intermediate Risk** 1100
Ashok Kumar, Nishant Tripathy, Arundhati

165. **Exposomes in the Ischemic Heart Disease—beyond Traditional Risk Factors** 1103
Prasannakumar CK, Lt Col Arun N

166. **Interaction between Dietary Calcium and Vascular Calcification** 1111
Mohamed Iesa M

167. **Stabilizing Stable Coronary Artery Disease without Beta-blockers** 1115
Nikhil Agarwal, Girish MP, Mohit D Gupta, Vishal Batra

Part 6: Structural Intervention

168. **Closing Patent Foramen Ovales to Prevent Stroke: A False Sense of Security** 1121
Ruchit Shah, Anagh TS, Kalyan Munde

Part 7: Heart and Brain

169. **Left Atrial Stiffness in Cryptogenic Stroke** 1125
Vibhav Sharma, Vivek Chaturvedi

Part 8: Cardiac Arrhythmia

170. **Which Patients with Nonischemic Cardiomyopathy should Receive a Defibrillator?** 1130
Vaidehi Agarwal, Ruman Kugashiya, Sanjiv Sharma

171. **Predicting Risk of Sudden Cardiac Death in Hypertrophic Cardiomyopathy: Role of Radiomics** 1134
Akshay Ashok Bafna, Adeeb Shakeel Sheikh, Ajit Namdeorao Hange, Nikhil Gadade

172. **Anticoagulation for Atrial Fibrillation in Patients with Intermediate Stroke Risk: Is the Gray Zone Becoming Less Gray?** 1141
Vibhav Sharma, Satyavir Yadav

173. **Should We Stop Prescribing Digoxin?** 1146
Navanil Biswas, Nayanika Bose

Part 9: Amyloidosis

174. **Linking Amyloid Burden to Prognosis** 1150
Kayan Siodia

175. **Predicting the Future for Amyloid Light Chain Amyloidosis in Patients with Cardiac Involvement** 1153
Jhala Malav, Jhala Darshan A

SECTION 17: TOP 10 PAPERS

176. **The Year in Cardiovascular Medicine (2025): The Top 10 Papers in Diabetes and Metabolic Disorders** 1161
Neha Chopra, Shitij Chaudhary, Nitish Naik

177. **Top Papers of 2025 on Antithrombotic** 1168
PS Banerjee, Tanmay Mukhopadhyay, Kaushik Mondal

178. **Top 10 Lipid Trials of 2024–2025** 1177
Prerna Garg, Sumit Kumar, Rakesh Yadav

179. **Top 10 Papers of 2024 on Intervention** 1182
Subrahmanya Murti V, Sameer Gupta, VK Bahl

SECTION 18: VIEWPOINT

Part 1: Obesity Paradox is a Fact

180. An Unexpected Relationship Between Body Weight and Health Outcomes (Proponent) 1195
Mahesh Nalin Kumar, Ampady Sreedhar

181. Myth or Reality (Opponent) 1198
M Subroto, D Nishtha, Ankur U, Rajeev Gupta, S Bhushan

Part 2: Time Matters When Considering Treatment for Patients with Mitral Regurgitation

182. Time Matters When Considering Treatment for Patients with Mitral Regurgitation (Proponent) 1205
Rajeev Garg

183. Time Matters When Considering Treatment for Patients with Mitral Regurgitation (Opponent) 1208
Dipak Ranjan Das

184. CHA_2DS_2-VASc of 1: Not Same for Every Patient with AFib 1211
Chhabi Satpathy, Trinath Kumar Mishra, Biraja Prasad Beura

185. How to Resolve the Prosthesis–Patient Mismatch Debate? 1215
Harinder K Bali, Amreen Dhindsa

186. Artificial Intelligence will Replace Clinical Cardiology: Against the Motion 1221
Abhijit Chatterjee

SECTION 19: MISCELLANEOUS

187. Takayasu Arteritis: What is New? 1225
Sanjay Tyagi

188. Treatment of Obstructive Sleep Apnea and its Impact on Cardiovascular Disease 1234
Arijit Kumar Ghosh, Vidya PL, Poyla Ghosh

189. Participation in Sports by Athletes with Cardiovascular Disease 1245
Ashish Deshpande

190. Donor Selection for Heart Transplantation in 2025 1252
Bagirath R, Meemansa Buch, Sabarish S

191. **Antithrombotic Therapies in Patients with Peripheral Artery Disease** **1258**
Hem Chandra Kalita, Karthik Thangamuthu

192. **Cardiology Training in India: Past, Present, and Future** **1263**
Kajal Ganguly, Sandipta Ray, Mainak Mukhopadhyay, Subir Sen

193. **Recent Insights into Native Valve Infective Endocarditis** **1266**
Satya Narayan Routray, Dipak Ranjan Das

194. **Pulmonary Hypertension—No Longer an Orphan Disease** **1271**
Shanmugasundaram Somasundaram

195. **Unraveling the Unsolved Mysteries of the Athletic Heart** **1284**
Sudarshan K Vijay, Upadhyay Aditya Chandradhar

196. **Cardiac Sarcoidosis and Management** **1291**
Sunil Lhila, Debasish Das, Koushik Chaki

197. **Marantic Endocarditis** **1299**
Saumya Sagar, Anupam Prakash

198. **Epilepsy and the Heart—Can "Brain Arrhythmia" Lead to Cardiac Arrhythmia?** **1305**
Adrita Banerjee, Amit Sanghvi

Index ***i1–i15***

SECTION

1

Preventive Cardiology

Section Outline

1. **Improving Community-level Cardiac-health Awareness through School-based Education Program in India**
   Debabrata Biswas, Debabrata Roy
2. **Air Pollution and Cardiovascular Disease in India: Current Perspective**
   Debabrata Biswas, Kaushik Manna, DP Sinha
3. **Can We Cancel Out the Excess Cardiovascular Risk Caused by Chronic Kidney Disease?**
   Farhin Iqbal, Chitra Priyadarshini
4. **Smoking Cessation: Never too Early, Never too Late!**
   Saumitra Ray, Sumanta Chatterjee, Srina Ray

CHAPTER 1

Improving Community-level Cardiac-health Awareness through School-based Education Program in India

Debabrata Biswas, Debabrata Roy

ABSTRACT

Cardiovascular diseases (CVDs) have emerged as the leading cause of mortality in India, due to rapid urbanization, lifestyle changes, and socioeconomic disparities. This paper explores the importance of community engagement in CVD prevention and presents a school-based intervention led by the Cardiological Society of India (CSI) in West Bengal. The program integrated teacher training, student-led campaigns, and culturally rooted activities such as dramas, debates, and art to promote cardiac health awareness. Students acted as peer educators, extending preventive messages to families and communities. The initiative demonstrated significant improvements in knowledge and dietary choices, emphasizing schools as powerful platforms for community-based health education. By combining scientific content with cultural participation, this model offers a sustainable, scalable framework for strengthening cardiovascular health awareness and prevention across diverse Indian communities.

Keywords: Cardiovascular diseases, community engagement, school-based intervention, health education, preventive cardiology.

INTRODUCTION

As in many low- and middle-income countries, cardiovascular diseases (CVDs) have become the leading cause of death in India, overtaking many communicable diseases. With rapid urbanization, lifestyle shifts, aging, and changes in diet and physical activity, India is undergoing a strong epidemiologic transition toward noncommunicable diseases (NCDs), particularly CVDs.[1] In 2016, noncommunicable diseases (NCDs) were responsible for 63% of all deaths in India, with CVD contributing 27% of this burden. Among individuals aged 40–69 years, CVDs alone accounted for 45% of total deaths.[2] Early recognition of risk factors, community awareness, and preventive strategies are essential to curb this rising burden. Community involvement is vital for estimating the burden of CVDs, identifying locally relevant risk factors, formulating preventive strategies that are culturally appropriate, as well as widely acceptable, and ultimately implementing them effectively.

RECENT EPIDEMIOLOGIC TRANSITIONS IN CARDIOVASCULAR DISEASES IN INDIA

India is in the midst of a profound epidemiologic transition, wherein CVDs have supplanted infectious diseases as the dominant cause of morbidity and mortality. This shift, shaped by rapid urbanization, evolving lifestyles, and widening socioeconomic disparities, reflects a broader transformation in the country's health landscape.

■ Escalating Burden of Cardiovascular Disease

Cardiovascular disease now contributes to more than one-quarter of all deaths in India, with ischemic heart disease and stroke as the principal drivers. The years of life lost to CVD rose dramatically from approximately 23.2 million in 1990 to 37 million in 2010, with significant toll of premature mortality.[1,3]

■ Transformation of the Urban–Rural Gradient

Historically, CVD risk factors—such as obesity, hypercholesterolemia, sedentary lifestyles, and dietary excesses—were more pronounced in urban and affluent populations, while rural communities were relatively spared. However, recent nationally representative surveys demonstrate a striking convergence, with risk factors such as overweight, hypertension, and diabetes rising more rapidly among disadvantaged groups, including rural residents, those with lower education, and the less wealthy.[4] Data from NFHS-5 (2019–2021), compared with NFHS-4 (2015–2016), show sharper absolute and relative increases in overweight, diabetes, and hypertension in rural populations.[4] Longitudinal evidence from South India further corroborates this, with incidence rates of hypertension and type 2 diabetes in rural areas now comparable to, or exceeding, those in urban cohorts.[5] This epidemiologic "catch-up" phenomenon necessitates intensified public health interventions in rural communities, which often face additional barriers of limited infrastructure, low awareness, and constrained access to healthcare.

Shifting Socioeconomic Gradient

Traditionally, higher socioeconomic status (SES)—wealthier and better-educated groups—were strongly associated with obesity, hypertension, and diabetes in India.[6] In recent years, however, this gradient has reversed, with the steepest rise in CVD risk factors occurring among lower SES groups.[4] Affluent populations have benefited from increasing health literacy, preventive healthcare access, and improvements in control of blood pressure, diabetes, cholesterol, and tobacco use.[7] In contrast, lower SES groups—both in urban slums and rural areas—continue to face escalating risks, compounded by poor health literacy, limited medical access, unhealthy diets, occupational exposures, and entrenched tobacco use.[8] Evidence from the India State-Level Disease Burden Initiative (2017) reveals significantly higher CVD mortality among individuals with lower education and income levels,[9] while the ICMR–INDIAB study highlights the growing concentration of hypertension and diabetes in disadvantaged populations, where treatment and control rates remain the lowest.[10] This inversion of the socioeconomic gradient underscores the urgency of equity-focused policies that expand affordable primary care, enhance risk factor screening, and implement community-based prevention programs.

Younger Age of Onset

Perhaps most concerning is the earlier age of CVD onset in India compared to high-income countries. The INTERHEART study reported a mean age of first myocardial infarction of just 53 years among South Asians, nearly a decade earlier than the 58–63 years observed in other regions.[11] Similarly, the CREATE registry documented that nearly half of Indian patients with acute coronary syndrome were younger than 55 years.[12]

This early onset is driven by the so-called "Asian Indian phenotype," marked by central obesity, insulin resistance, type 2 diabetes, and dyslipidemia.[13] Lifestyle determinants—physical inactivity, tobacco use, and unhealthy diets—alongside genetic predispositions, including elevated lipoprotein(a), further accelerate risk accumulation.[14]

The socioeconomic consequences are profound, as CVD disproportionately strikes individuals in their most productive years, amplifying the economic burden on families and society. This reality highlights the imperative for earlier screening, aggressive management of cardiometabolic risks, and the integration of preventive strategies from young adulthood.

GAPS IN AWARENESS, KNOWLEDGE, ATTITUDES, AND PRACTICES

Myths and misconceptions related to CVD are widespread in India, as is the knowledge regarding healthcare access, economic cost, healthcare workforce constraints, and health insurance/social protection. Therefore, community engagement in healthcare delivery is imperative to address these issues.

Knowledge, Attitudes, Practices (KAP) Surveys

A survey in the CARRS cohort (Delhi and Chennai) found that while individuals knew about common cardiovascular risk factors, knowledge of symptoms and monitoring was inconsistent. Attitudes toward nonphysician health workers and digital/text interventions were positive, but preventive practices were limited.[15] In periurban Karnataka, college students had poor awareness of CVD risk factors, with mean knowledge scores of 21/50, highlighting significant misconceptions.[16]

A study conducted among adolescent school students in Kolkata, West Bengal, highlights a significant "knowledge-behaviour gap" regarding CVD prevention. Only 18% perceived themselves at risk, under 30% exercised regularly, and over half showed unhealthy eating patterns. Strikingly, students with good CVD-related knowledge were less likely to maintain healthy eating habits, showing that awareness alone doesn't drive behavior. Targeted interventions are needed to bridge this gap.[17]

Factors-associated with Poor Awareness and Control

Barriers included financial constraints, limited manpower, and cultural challenges.[18]

GOVERNMENT INITIATIVES IN AWARENESS AND PREVENTION OF CARDIOVASCULAR DISEASE IN INDIA

The Government of India has recognized the rising burden of CVDs and other NCDs and has launched a range of programs to strengthen awareness, early detection, and preventive care.

- *NPCDCS (National Programme for Prevention and Control of Cancer, Diabetes, Cardiovascular Diseases and Stroke)*: Launched in 2010, NPCDCS is the flagship initiative for NCDs, focusing on health promotion, opportunistic and population-based screening, early diagnosis, treatment, and referral services through primary health centers and district hospitals.[19] It also emphasizes lifestyle modification, training of health workers, and establishment of NCD clinics. By 2022, more than 66 million individuals had been screened for hypertension and diabetes under NPCDCS.[20]
- *National Action Plan on NCDs*: Developed in alignment with WHO's global NCD targets, this plan sets measurable goals such as a *30% reduction in tobacco use, 25% reduction in hypertension prevalence*, and *25% reduction in premature mortality* from NCDs by 2025.[21] It emphasizes population-wide behavior change, health education, and promotion of healthy lifestyle practices.
- *Community-based Assessment Checklist (CBAC)*: As part of NPCDCS, the CBAC tool is used by frontline workers (ASHAs and ANMs) to screen individuals above 30 years for risk factors like tobacco use, obesity, high blood pressure, and family history of NCDs. This facilitates early identification of high-risk individuals and their linkage to higher facilities.[22]
- *Ayushman Bharat—Health and Wellness Centers (HWCs)*: Over 1.5 lakh subcenters and PHCs are being transformed into HWCs to provide comprehensive primary healthcare. These centers offer population-based screening for hypertension and diabetes, counseling services for lifestyle modification, and referral to higher-level facilities.[23] The program also aims to create a continuum of care, making preventive services more accessible to rural and underserved populations.
- *Regulatory and policy measures*: India has enacted strong regulatory steps such as the Cigarettes and Other Tobacco Products Act (COTPA), pictorial health warnings on tobacco packs, bans on advertising, and restrictions on smoking in public places.[24] Dietary risk reduction measures include FSSAI-led trans-fat elimination and salt reduction campaigns, alongside awareness drives like Fit India Movement and Eat Right India.[25]

COMMUNITY AS THE TARGET FOR HEALTHCARE INTERVENTION STRATEGIES

Community involvement is crucial in accurately estimating the burden of CVDs in India, where diverse socioeconomic, cultural, and geographical factors shape health outcomes.

While government initiatives focus on the state or district level, they tend to overlook substantial small-area and household-level clustering in CVD risk factors, thereby limiting their effectiveness. A study using data from the National Family Health Survey (2019–2021) found that for hypertension, diabetes, and obesity, *small areas* (villages or urban blocks) accounted for far more geographical variability than districts did—e.g., over 50% of variation in hypertension was attributable to small areas versus ~14% to districts.[26] Community involvement programs can help overcome the shortfall of national CVD control strategies by addressing *small-area and household-level clustering of risk factors*. Local initiatives—driven by community health workers, self-help groups, and peer networks—can map neighborhood-specific risks, provide targeted education, and deliver household-centered interventions. Community-based approaches improve screening, awareness at the microlevel, and help formulate prevention and management strategies tailored to local cultural practices and socioeconomic realities.

Thus, community involvement helps in:

- *Accurate estimation of CVD burden*: Engaging communities enables the collection of locally relevant data on prevalence of risk factors such as hypertension, diabetes, tobacco use, unhealthy diets, and physical inactivity, which often remain underreported in national statistics.
- *Awareness and behavior change*: Active participation also fosters awareness and recognition of modifiable risk factors, empowering individuals to adopt healthier behaviors.
- *Culturally appropriate prevention strategies*: Community-driven insights help in designing preventive strategies that are culturally appropriate, accessible, and sustainable, ensuring better compliance and long-term impact.
- *Involvement of local stakeholders*: By involving local stakeholders—schools, self-help groups, panchayats, and nongovernmental organizations—preventive interventions can be effectively implemented and monitored, bridging the gap between policy formulation and real-world practice.

Ultimately, community participation not only strengthens epidemiological surveillance but also builds ownership and accountability in the fight against CVD in India.[27]

CHALLENGES TO COMMUNITY-LEVEL AWARENESS

- *Low health literacy*: Many individuals fail to recognize cardiovascular risk factors or grasp the "silent" progression of hypertension and diabetes until serious complications emerge.
- *Socioeconomic and cultural constraints*: Out-of-pocket costs for screening, diagnostic services, and travel, along with the opportunity cost of missing work, act as deterrents. In addition, entrenched norms surrounding diet, gender roles, and reliance on traditional medicine limit the uptake of preventive measures.

- *Geographic disparities*: Remote and rural areas often lack adequate infrastructure, consistent medical personnel, and diagnostic capacity, leading to uneven access to care.
- *Implementation gaps*: Government programs, though well-intentioned, are frequently underfunded, understaffed, and weakly supervised, restricting their effectiveness at scale.
- *Data and monitoring deficiencies*: Limited availability of subdistrict incidence data and insufficient longitudinal tracking of awareness or behavioral trends hinder the development of precise, evidence-based strategies.[27]

SCHOOL AS A COMMUNITY HUB FOR HEALTH INTERVENTIONS

Schools are crucial in preventing NCDs as they reach children at a formative stage when lifelong habits are developed. By integrating health education into curricula and fostering supportive environments with nutritious meals, physical activity, and antitobacco policies, schools promote healthy behaviors reinforced by teachers and peers. The Teach BP program, implemented in a majority Black and low-income Virginia school, demonstrated this potential—students showed a 62.7% improvement in recognizing hypertension and a 92.1% increase in understanding its impact on the body. Beyond academics, schools act as community hubs, engaging families and local organizations, and their accessibility and scalability create a ripple effect that extends behavior change into communities, making them ideal for sustainable, community-based health interventions.[28]

CARDIOLOGICAL SOCIETY OF INDIA INITIATIVE TO COMMUNITY-LEVEL AWARENESS GENERATION

With the above context in mind, the Cardiological Society of India (CSI), an organization dedicated to the well-being of humanity, launched a pilot program on CVD awareness in selected schools and communities in West Bengal. The dual goals of the initiative were to improve the actual state of CVD and to enhance the level of awareness among the population at large about the centrality of the issue.

The project comprised a multitude of activities, including central and regional workshops, health check-ups, health fair, student-led health campaigns, reading festival, etc.

The plan of intervention in this project was:

- Addressing the knowledge gap on CVD and lifestyle measures needed to mitigate it by providing available literatures—preparation of an easy-to-understand manual for training the teachers.
- Providing practice materials like coloring books and videos to students and encouraging them to draw pictures and write short essays on CVD prevention.
- Helping the teachers to organize the students to take up the leadership in the movement and creating community awareness through organizing campaign in the localities with placards and posters, organizing dramas and debates, and organizing meetings with the community members including parents.

Key Characteristics of the Program

- *Strong student leadership*:
    - Students were the central drivers of the project, taking ownership and leading initiatives.
    - Their leadership ensured the movement reached beyond school boundaries into homes and communities.
    - Empowered children to act as *peer educators* and *community ambassadors* for prevention of CVD.
- *Cultural and interactive engagement*:
    - Used *dramas, debates, and role-play* to make the issue relatable and memorable.
    - Involved *parents and community representatives* through structured meetings and dialogues.
    - Reinforced awareness by embedding health education into cultural expressions familiar to the community.
- *Family and community involvement*:
    - Extended impact beyond individual learning to household decision-making.
    - Parents and local leaders became partners in promoting cardiovascular health.
    - Encouraged a *collective sense of responsibility* across multiple social layers.
- *Holistic and sustainable approach*:
    - Combined *scientific education, participatory learning, and cultural reinforcement*.
    - Ensured knowledge was not only understood but also acted upon.
    - Designed for long-term sustainability by integrating schools, families, and communities in a single framework.

Major Achievements of the Program

Students not only understood the subject, the teachers taught, but also showed interest in applying it in the real world.

CONCLUSION

India is in the midst of a significant epidemiologic transition, with CVD risk factors extending beyond urban or affluent segments to involve rural and lower SES populations. Awareness at the community level is therefore imperative—not just for detection, but for prevention. Government initiatives like NPCDCS, Ayushman Bharat, and the national NCD action plans lay an important foundation.

NGO, academic, and local community efforts complement them. For going forward, it is critical to reach rural, less educated, less wealthy populations with culturally sensitive, accessible messages and services. The project conducted by the CSI demonstrates that community-driven, school-based initiatives can significantly enhance awareness and transform behaviors related to health and environmental risks. Strong student leadership, reinforced through cultural activities and community engagement, fostered both individual and collective responsibility for healthier practices as evidenced by over 90% improvement in hygiene behaviors and widespread reduction in junk food consumption. More of such culturally rooted, community-led approaches are needed in addressing public health challenges at the microlevel (household/community), especially in the face of the changing epidemiology of CV risk factors.

REFERENCES

1. Prabhakaran D, Jeemon P, Roy A. Cardiovascular Diseases in India: Current Epidemiology and Future Directions. Circulation. 2016;133(16):1605-20.
2. World Health Organization. (2016). Cardiovascular diseases. WHO India. [online] Available from https://www.who.int/india/health-topics/cardiovascular-diseases [Last accessed October, 2025].
3. Loitongbam L, Surin WR. The Rising Burden of Cardiovascular Disease and Thrombosis in India: An Epidemiological Review. Cureus. 2024;16(11):e73786.
4. Wetzel S, Geldsetzer P, Mani SS, et al. Changing socioeconomic and geographic gradients in cardiovascular disease risk factors among Indians aged 15-49 years - evidence from nationally representative household surveys. Lancet Reg Health Southeast Asia. 2023;12:100188.
5. Vasan SK, Antonisamy B, Gowri M, et al. Prevalence, incidence and predictors of cardiovascular risk factors: longitudinal data from rural and urban South India and comparison with global data. BMJ Open Diabetes Res Care. 2020;8(1):e001782.
6. Samuel P, Antonisamy B, Raghupathy P, et al. Socio-economic status and cardiovascular risk factors in rural and urban areas of Vellore, Tamilnadu, South India. Int J Epidemiol. 2012;41(5):1315-27.
7. Gupta R, Gupta VP. Hypertension epidemiology in India: lessons from Jaipur Heart Watch. Curr Sci. 2009;97(3):349-55.
8. Marmot M, Allen J, Bell R, et al. WHO European review of social determinants of health and the health divide. Lancet. 2012;380(9846):1011-29.
9. India State-Level Disease Burden Initiative CVD Collaborators. The changing patterns of cardiovascular diseases and their risk factors in the states of India: The Global Burden of Disease Study 1990–2016. Lancet Glob Health. 2018;6(12):e1339-51.
10. Anjana RM, Deepa M, Pradeepa R, et al. Prevalence of diabetes and prediabetes in 15 states of India: results from the ICMR–INDIAB population-based cross-sectional study. Lancet Diabetes Endocrinol. 2017;5(8):585-96.
11. Yusuf S, Hawken S, Ounpuu S, et al. Effect of potentially modifiable risk factors associated with myocardial infarction in 52 countries (the INTERHEART study): case-control study. Lancet. 2004;364(9438):937-52.
12. Xavier D, Pais P, Devereaux PJ, et al. Treatment and outcomes of acute coronary syndromes in India (CREATE): a prospective analysis of registry data. Lancet. 2008;371(9622):1435-42.
13. Misra A, Khurana L. The metabolic syndrome in South Asians: epidemiology, determinants, and prevention. Metab Syndr Relat Disord. 2009;7(6):497-514.
14. Enas EA, Chacko V, Pazhoor SG, et al. Dyslipidemia in South Asian patients. Curr Atheroscler Rep. 2007;9(5):367-74.
15. Singh K, Kondal D, Mohan D, et al. Community-level knowledge, attitudes, and practices regarding cardiovascular diseases in India. Indian Heart J. 2024;76(6):376-84.
16. Kotian SP, Kulkarni P, Ganesh KS, et al. Knowledge about cardio-vascular disease and its risk factors among college-going youth near Bengaluru, India. Int J Noncommunicable Dis. 2021;6(1):29-33.
17. Kumar S, Ray S, Roy D, et al. Exercise and eating habits among urban adolescents: a cross-sectional study in Kolkata, India. BMC Public Health. 2017;17(1):468.
18. George A, Badagabettu S, Berra K, et al. Prevention of Cardiovascular Disease in India: Barriers and Opportunities for Nursing. J Clin Prev Cardiol. 2018;7(2):72-7.
19. Government of India. Operational Guidelines: National Programme for Prevention and Control of Cancer, Diabetes, Cardiovascular Diseases and Stroke (NPCDCS). Ministry of Health and Family Welfare; 2013.
20. Press Information Bureau. Progress under NPCDCS: Over 66 million screened for diabetes and hypertension. Government of India; 2022.
21. Ministry of Health and Family Welfare. National Action Plan and Monitoring Framework for Prevention and Control of NCDs in India. Government of India; 2013.
22. Gupta R, Joshi P, Mohan V, et al. Epidemiology and causation of coronary heart disease and stroke in India. Heart. 2008;94(1):16-26.
23. Ministry of Health and Family Welfare. Ayushman Bharat for Comprehensive Primary Health Care through Health and Wellness Centres. Government of India; 2018.
24. Reddy KS, Arora M, Shrivastava S, et al. Implementation of tobacco control law in India: gaps and opportunities. Indian J Public Health. 2012;56(4):267-73.
25. Food Safety and Standards Authority of India (FSSAI). Eat Right India Movement. Government of India; 2019.
26. Ko S, Oh H, Subramanian SV, et al. Small Area Geographic Estimates of Cardiovascular Disease Risk Factors in India. JAMA Netw Open. 2023;6(10):e2337171.
27. Ndejjo R, Hassen HY, Wanyenze RK, et al. Community-Based Interventions for Cardiovascular Disease Prevention in Low-and Middle-Income Countries: A Systematic Review. Public Health Rev. 2021;42:1604018.
28. Hundley J, Olson K, Rocha C, et al. Partnering With Schools for Community-Based Health Interventions: How Educating Children Improves Hypertension Awareness. Ochsner J. 2025;25(1):34-43.

CHAPTER

2

Air Pollution and Cardiovascular Disease in India: Current Perspective

Debabrata Biswas, Kaushik Manna, DP Sinha

ABSTRACT

Air pollution is a critical public health challenge in India, with fine particulate matter (PM2.5) emerging as a major driver of cardiovascular disease (CVD) morbidity and mortality. Despite notable declines in household air pollution, ambient PM2.5 levels continue to rise, disproportionately affecting marginalized populations. The cardiovascular impact of PM2.5 is mediated through multiple mechanisms, including oxidative injury, systemic inflammation, autonomic imbalance, metabolic dysfunction, and heightened thrombogenicity. Government initiatives such as the National Clean Air Programme and Pradhan Mantri Ujjwala Yojana have shown promise but face enforcement and equity barriers. Sustainable progress demands stricter regulation, clean energy expansion, and community participation to reduce India's escalating cardiovascular burden from air pollution.

Keywords: Air pollution, cardiovascular disease, PM2.5, public health policy, India.

INTRODUCTION

Air pollution is one of the most pressing global public health challenges of the 21st century. The World Health Organization (WHO) estimates that over 7 million premature deaths annually are attributable to ambient plus household air pollution (HAP).[1] Cardiovascular diseases (CVDs) are the principal contributor to air pollution-related mortality. Worldwide, the average life expectancy is shortened by approximately 1.8 years due to the combined effect of ambient as well as HAP.[2] Fine particulate matter (PM2.5), the most important mediator of air pollution-related health hazards, exerts systemic effects beyond the lungs, increasing the risk of ischemic heart disease, stroke, arrhythmias, heart failure, and hypertension.[3] Ecological and economic transitions over the past century have led to a disproportionate burden of PM2.5 exposure in countries like India.

AIR POLLUTION BURDEN IN INDIA

The Global Burden of Disease (GBD) study has identified ambient air pollution (AAP) as the second leading risk factor for mortality in India in 2019.[4] Air pollution levels in India have demonstrated a marked upward trajectory, with the annual population-weighted mean concentration of PM2.5 increasing from 27 μg/m^3 in 1998 to 44 μg/m^3 in 2022—substantially exceeding the World Health Organization's recommended limits. Seasonal exacerbations during winter months are particularly evident in the rural northern states, secondary to crop residue burning. Multiple drivers, including accelerated industrialization, rapid urbanization, agricultural practices, climate variability, and demographic expansion, have intensified both the complexity and magnitude of pollution sources.[5]

In 2019, air pollution was responsible for an estimated 1.67 million deaths, accounting for 17.8% (95% UI 15.8–19.5) of total mortality in India. Between 1990 and 2019, mortality attributable to HAP declined by 64.2% (52.2–74.2), whereas deaths linked to ambient PM2.5 and ambient ozone pollution rose sharply by 115.3% (28.3–344.4) and 139.2% (96.5–195.8), respectively. The economic burden of air pollution in 2019 was considerable, with estimated losses of US$28.8 billion (21.4–37.4) from premature mortality and US$8.0 billion (5.9–10.3) from morbidity-related productivity reductions, collectively representing 1.36% of India's gross domestic product (GDP).[6]

CHANGING ECOLOGY OF AIR POLLUTION IN INDIA

Addressing air pollution in India requires going beyond pollutant monitoring to incorporate socioeconomic and geographic determinants. Marginalized groups—such as Scheduled Castes, Other Backward Classes, and low-income rural households—bear a disproportionate burden due to reliance on biomass fuels and proximity to industrial or agricultural emission sources. A one standard deviation increase in the prevalence of Scheduled Caste and Other Backward Class households was linked with rises in PM2.5 levels of 0.127 μg/m^3 (95% CI 0.062–0.192) and 0.199 μg/m^3 (95% CI 0.116–0.283), respectively. Marked urban-rural and source-specific variations highlight the need for an environmental justice framework tailored to India's socioenvironmental realities.[7]

Namdeo et al. analyzed aerosol trends in India from 2001–2019 using satellite-derived Aerosol Optical Depth (AOD) and ground-level PM2.5 data, reporting significant increases—particularly over the Indo-Gangetic Plain, with sharp winter and postmonsoon peaks driven largely by biomass burning. The second decade showed steeper AOD rises and wider urban–rural gaps. While AOD and PM2.5 correlated well in regions such as Kanpur, variability in others like Delhi emphasized the importance of expanding ground-level monitoring.[8]

AIR POLLUTION COMPOSITION AND ITS HEALTH IMPACT

Air pollution is a complex mixture of gaseous pollutants such as ozone, oxides of nitrogen (NOx), ammonia (NH3), sulfur dioxide (SO_2), nonmethane volatile organic compounds (NMVOCs), and particulate pollutants (elemental and organic carbon, hydrocarbon, transition metal, microbes, lipopolysaccharide, etc.).[9] The health impact of PM2.5 is determined by its aerodynamic classification: <10 mm [thoracic particles (PM10), <2.5 mm [fine particles (PM2.5)], <0.1 mm (ultrafine particles), and between 2.5 and 10 mm [coarse (PM2.5–10)].

Among all air pollutants, PM2.5 has been identified as a substantial public health concern.[10] Sources of PM2.5 in India are mainly industrial and residential (>60%), including vehicular emissions, coal-based power plants, industrial processes, biomass burning, and construction dust.[11] Evidences suggest that short-term rises in PM2.5 are consistently associated with a 0.4–1.0% increase in daily all-cause and cardiovascular mortality per 10 μg/m^3 elevation. Whereas, long-term exposure leads to an approximate 10% increase in all-cause mortality per 10 μg/m^3 elevation of PM2.5.[12]

PM2.5 AND ATHEROSCLEROSIS: PATHOGENETIC MECHANISMS[13]

- *Oxidative stress*: PM2.5 induces oxidative stress by generating reactive oxygen and nitrogen species through mechanisms such as NADPH oxidase activation, eNOS uncoupling, and mitochondrial dysfunction. This oxidative burden leads to LDL oxidation, foam cell apoptosis, vascular smooth muscle cell proliferation, and extracellular matrix deposition, thereby driving plaque growth, intimal hyperplasia, and vascular remodeling.
- *Inflammation*: PM2.5 activates leukocytes, endothelium, and the NLRP3 inflammasome, driving cytokine release, macrophage polarization, ECM degradation, and plaque destabilization, while also stimulating leukopoiesis and systemic arterial inflammation.
- *Autonomic and neuroendocrine dysfunction*: PM2.5 induces autonomic and neuroendocrine dysfunction by reducing heart rate variability, activating sympathetic and neurohormonal vasoconstrictive pathways, impairing parasympathetic balance, and disrupting central neural control through inflammation and blood–brain barrier injury.
- *Metabolic alterations*: PM2.5 drives metabolic dysfunction by inducing dyslipidemia, impairing HDL function, and promoting LDL/ox-LDL-mediated vascular inflammation and endothelial injury, thereby accelerating atherosclerosis.
- *Enhanced thrombogenicity*: PM2.5 enhances thrombogenicity by promoting platelet activation, impairing fibrinolysis, and driving IL-6/TNF-α mediated coagulation, thereby increasing the risk of atherothrombotic events.

CHALLENGES IN ADDRESSING AIR POLLUTION

Tackling air pollution in India is a multifaceted challenge that demands sustained, coordinated efforts from multiple stakeholders. Key barriers include:

- *Weak enforcement*: Environmental regulations are poorly enforced, allowing widespread noncompliance among industries, transport sectors, and other polluting sources. Moreover, India's air quality standards remain less stringent than WHO guidelines, limiting their effectiveness.
- *Rapid urbanization*: Accelerated urban growth has intensified energy demand, vehicular emissions, and industrial activity in densely populated cities, making air quality management increasingly difficult.
- *Socioeconomic constraints*: Widespread poverty, limited access to clean energy, and inadequate rural infrastructure perpetuate both HAP and AAP, further worsening the crisis.[5]

GOVERNMENT INITIATIVES TO CURB AIR POLLUTION

Air pollution remains a critical environmental and public health challenge in India, requiring coordinated efforts from the government, industry, civil society, and individuals. To address this, the Government of India has undertaken several policies and programs:

- *The National Clean Air Programme (NCAP), 2019*:[14] The program sought to reduce PM concentrations by 20–30% by 2024, based on source apportionment studies conducted across 102 cities nationwide.
- *Promotion of clean energy*: Complementing NCAP, the government has introduced policies such as the adoption of *BS-VI fuel standards*, phasing out of coal-based power plants, and a strong push toward *renewable energy expansion*, targeting 500 GW of renewable capacity by 2030, with 190 GW already achieved as of 2024.[15]
- The *Pradhan Mantri Ujjwala Yojana (PMUY)*[16] has distributed clean cooking gas (LPG) connections to millions of households, reducing reliance on biomass fuels. This program aimed at addressing HAP, which remains a major contributor to health hazards in rural and periurban areas.
- On the urban front, measures like *odd-even vehicular policies* in Delhi and the promotion of *green transport initiatives* such as electric vehicles and hydrogen fuel adoption reflect attempts to curb vehicular emissions.
- The launch of the *Air Quality Index (2015)* further enhances transparency by providing easily understandable data on air quality and raising public awareness about health risks.[17]

Despite these commendable efforts, challenges persist in terms of implementation, enforcement, and sustained monitoring. Weak regulatory compliance, infrastructure gaps, rapid urbanization, and socioeconomic disparities hinder progress. Technological innovations like air purifiers, HEPA filters, and cleaner fuels offer short-term relief, but long-term success will depend on stricter enforcement, infrastructure upgrades, and widespread behavioral changes. Ultimately, achieving cleaner air in India requires a multisectoral approach that combines policy action, technological innovation, and active citizen participation.

INITIATIVE BY THE CARDIOLOGICAL SOCIETY OF INDIA

The *Cardiological Society of India (CSI)* launched a pilot program in schools and communities of West Bengal to raise awareness on air pollution and its health impact. The initiative had dual objectives—improving pollution awareness and promoting active community participation. Key interventions included developing simple manuals for teachers, providing creative learning tools such as coloring books, videos, and apps for students, and encouraging activities like drawing, essay writing, and use of air quality apps.

The program followed a three-tiered plan: Teacher training workshops with CSI experts, student-centered interactive sessions, and student-led campaigns that extended the message into households and local communities. Strong student leadership was a hallmark of the project, reinforced by cultural activities—dramas, debates, poster campaigns, and community meetings—which helped translate school-based learning into broader community action.

CONCLUSION

Air pollution has emerged as a major contributor to cardiovascular morbidity and mortality in India, largely mediated by PM2.5. Despite policy measures such as NCAP, PMUY, and clean energy initiatives, weak enforcement and socioeconomic disparities hinder progress. The changing ecology of air pollution, shaped by rapid urbanization, industrial growth, and socioeconomic inequities across urban and rural populations, further complicates mitigation efforts. Sustainable improvement will require stricter regulation, technological innovation, and equitable access to clean energy. Community-based initiatives, such as those led by the CSI, highlight the importance of awareness and citizen participation. A coordinated, multisectoral approach is essential to mitigate air pollution and reduce its cardiovascular burden.

REFERENCES

1. World Health Organization. (2021). Air pollution. [online] Available from https://www.who.int/health-topics/air-pollution [Last accessed October, 2025].
2. State of Global Air. How does air pollution affect life expectancy around the world? [online] Available from https://www.stateofglobalair.org/resources/report/how-does-air-pollution-affect-life-expectancy-around-world [Last accessed October, 2025].
3. Burnett R, Chen H, Szyszkowicz M, et al. Global estimates of mortality associated with long-term exposure to outdoor fine particulate matter. Proc Natl Acad Sci U S A. 2018;115(38):9592-7.
4. Fuller R, Landrigan PJ, Balakrishnan K, et al. Pollution and health: a progress update. Lancet Planet Health. 2022;6:e535-e47.
5. Kurmi OP, Adhikari TB, Tyagi SK, et al. Addressing air pollution in India: Innovative strategies for sustainable solutions. Indian J Med Res. 2024;160(1):1-5.
6. India State-Level Disease Burden Initiative Air Pollution Collaborators. Health and economic impact of air pollution in the states of India: the Global Burden of Disease Study 2019. Lancet Planet Health. 2021;5(1):e25-e38.
7. deSouza PN, Chaudhary E, Dey S, et al. An environmental justice analysis of air pollution in India. Sci Rep. 2023;13:16690.
8. Namdeo P, Chakraborty T, Chakraborty A. Two decades of aerosol trends over India: Seasonal characteristics and urban-rural dynamics. Environ Res Lett. 2024;19(12).
9. Rajagopalan S, Al-Kindi SG, Brook RD. Air Pollution and Cardiovascular Disease: JACC State-of-the-Art Review. J Am Coll Cardiol. 2018;72(17):2054-70.
10. McDuffie E, Martin R, Yin H, et al. Global Burden of Disease from Major Air Pollution Sources (GBD MAPS): A Global Approach. Res Rep Health Eff Inst. 2021;2021(210):1-45.

11. Guo H, Kota SH, Sahu SK, et al. Source apportionment of PM2.5 in North India using source-oriented air quality models. Environ Pollut. 2017;231(Pt 1):426-36.
12. Brook RD, Rajagopalan S, Pope CA 3rd, et al.; American Heart Association Council on Epidemiology and Prevention, Council on the Kidney in Cardiovascular Disease, and Council on Nutrition, Physical Activity and Metabolism. Particulate matter air pollution and cardiovascular disease: An update to the scientific statement from the American Heart Association. Circulation. 2010;121(21):2331-78.
13. Montone RA, Rinaldi R, Bonanni A, et al. Impact of air pollution on ischemic heart disease: Evidence, mechanisms, clinical perspectives. Atherosclerosis. 2023;366:22-31.
14. Council on Energy, Environment and Water (CEEW) and Urban Emissions. How robust are urban India's clean air plans? An assessment of 102 cities. [online] Available from https://www.ceew.in/publications/how-robust-are-clean-air-plans-in-urban-india-102-cities-assessment [Last accessed October, 2025].
15. Energy Transition Commission. Roadmap to India's 2030 decarbonization target. [online] Available from https://www.teriin.org/sites/default/files/files/Roadmap-to-India-2030-Decarbonization-Target.pdf/ [Last accessed October, 2025].
16. Ranjan, R., & Singh, S. Household cooking fuel patterns in rural India: pre-and post-Pradhan Mantri Ujjwala Yojana. IJHD. 2020;14(3):518-526.
17. Central Pollution Control Board, Ministry of Environment, Forest and Climate Change, Government of India. National Air Quality Index (AQI). [online] Available from https://cpcb.nic.in/National-Air-Quality-Index/ [Last accessed October, 2025].

CHAPTER

3

Can We Cancel Out the Excess Cardiovascular Risk Caused by Chronic Kidney Disease?

Farhin Iqbal, Chitra Priyadarshini

ABSTRACT

Chronic kidney disease (CKD) confers a disproportionately high burden of cardiovascular morbidity and mortality, often exceeding the risk associated with progression to end-stage renal disease (ESRD). Epidemiological data consistently demonstrate that patients with CKD have a two- to four-fold higher risk of major adverse cardiovascular events (MACE) compared to the general population, even after accounting for traditional risk factors such as diabetes and hypertension. This excess risk is driven not only by conventional mechanisms—atherosclerosis, hypertension, and metabolic dysregulation—but also by CKD-specific factors including uremic toxins, mineral-bone disorder, chronic inflammation, anemia, and oxidative stress. Evidence suggests that while aggressive risk factor modification, renin–angiotensin–aldosterone system inhibition, statin therapy, novel agents such as sodium-glucose cotransporter-2 inhibitors (SGLT-2i), glucagon-like peptide-1 receptor agonists (GLP-1RA), and mineral metabolism management reduce cardiovascular events, residual risk persists. This chapter evaluates the pathophysiological mechanisms underlying excess CV risk, clinical implications, and therapeutic strategies for reducing cardiovascular risk in CKD, while critically examining whether it can truly be "canceled out".

Keywords: Chronic kidney disease (CKD), cardiovascular risk, nontraditional risk factors, multifactorial intervention.

INTRODUCTION

Chronic kidney disease (CKD) affects nearly 10–15% of the global adult population and is strongly linked to cardiovascular disease (CVD). Many patients with CKD die from CVD before reaching end-stage kidney failure.[1-3] While CKD is traditionally studied for its role in progression to end-stage renal disease (ESRD) requiring dialysis or transplantation, mounting evidence highlights a more pressing reality: The risk of death from CVD far exceeds the risk of kidney failure for most patients with CKD. Cardiovascular mortality in advanced CKD is 10–30 times higher than in the general population.[4] Early stages of CKD are linked to increased heart failure, arrhythmias, and sudden cardiac death. Traditional cardiovascular risk factors only partly explain the high rates seen in CKD patients. Other contributors such as inflammation, vascular calcification, and metabolic changes are unique to kidney dysfunction.[5,6]

Randomized controlled trials have shown that managing risk factors such as diabetes,[7-9] hypertension,[10-12] and hyperlipidemia[11-13] can slow the progression of kidney function decline and lower the rates of cardiovascular events and mortality in individuals with CKD. Nevertheless, it remains unclear to what extent modern multifactorial interventions can attenuate or completely offset the excess cardiovascular risk associated with CKD.

PATHOPHYSIOLOGY OF EXCESS CARDIOVASCULAR RISK

The pathophysiology of excess cardiovascular risk in CKD is complex. Traditional risk factors such as hypertension, diabetes, dyslipidemia, obesity, and smoking are highly prevalent in CKD populations. However, CKD introduces nontraditional risk factors that significantly contribute to cardiovascular risk. These include chronic inflammation, oxidative stress, endothelial dysfunction, vascular calcification, anemia, and mineral-bone disorder.[5,6] Patients with advanced CKD often develop volume overload that continuously affects the cardiovascular system, causing left ventricular hypertrophy and heart failure. High sympathetic activity in both dialysis-dependent and nondialysis patients is common, contributing to left ventricular hypertrophy, heart failure, and other cardiovascular complications.[14] Due to mineral bone disease in CKD patients (CKD-MBD), there is increased FGF23 (fibroblast growth factor) and PTH (parathormone), both of which have been proven to cause increased LV mass and calcification of coronary arteries causing CV complications.[15] Anemia is another important reason of increased CV mortality in CKD patients as a result of multiple factors such as decreased erythropoietin production, chronic inflammation, uremia, and iron deficiency.[16]

THERAPEUTIC STRATEGIES TO REDUCE CARDIOVASCULAR DISEASE RISK

Management of cardiovascular (CV) risk in CKD requires a multifaceted and individualized approach that integrates pharmacological therapy with lifestyle interventions. Optimal care involves simultaneous targeting of both traditional risk factors and nontraditional CKD-specific factors including anemia and mineral-bone disorder.

Lifestyle interventions, although often underemphasized, remain fundamental. Dietary sodium restriction, smoking cessation, physical activity, and weight management improve BP control and reduce overall CV risk.[17-22] A heart-healthy diet—adapted for CKD—has shown measurable benefit. The Mediterranean diet, rich in plant-based foods and unsaturated fats, supports cardiovascular health—as demonstrated by Lambert et al.[17]

Blood pressure control remains central to risk reduction, with strong evidence supporting the role of renin-angiotensin-aldosterone system (RAAS) inhibition. Angiotensin-converting enzyme inhibitors (ACEi) and angiotensin receptor blockers (ARB) are first-line therapies and reduce both renal progression and CV outcomes.[23-27] In resistant hypertension, mineralocorticoid receptor antagonists (MRAs) may be beneficial, though their use is often constrained by hyperkalemia.

Lipid-lowering therapy is also a cornerstone. The SHARP trial demonstrated that a combination of simvastatin and ezetimibe reduced major cardiovascular events by 17% compared to placebo, with the effect most pronounced in those with atherosclerotic disease.[28] Current practices therefore favor statin therapy in CKD patients not on dialysis. Evidence in dialysis-dependent CKD is less persuasive. Although statins reduce LDL cholesterol, this has not consistently translated into reduced cardiovascular events. Randomized trials reported that benefits seen in earlier stages of CKD were attenuated in patients on dialysis.[29,30]

Glycemic management is crucial in diabetic CKD, but recent evidence has shifted the paradigm. *SGLT-2 inhibitors* have shown remarkable benefits independent of glycemic control. In the DAPA-CKD trial,[31] dapagliflozin reduced kidney failure and CV death irrespective of diabetes status, and the EMPA-KIDNEY trial[32] confirmed empagliflozin's ability to reduce kidney disease progression and CV mortality across a broad CKD population. *GLP-1 receptor agonists* have demonstrated cardiovascular protection, particularly in patients with diabetes. In the LEADER trial, liraglutide significantly reduced major adverse cardiovascular events (MACE) in high-risk patients with type 2 diabetes, including those with CKD.[33] Ashraf et al. further highlighted these benefits in diabetic CKD populations.[34] Similarly, the REWIND trial showed that dulaglutide lowered cardiovascular event rates in patients with type 2 diabetes and multiple risk factors, including kidney disease.[35] Although evidence in nondiabetic CKD remains limited, Rhee et al. suggested that GLP-1 receptor agonists may slow eGFR decline.[36]

Finerenone, a novel nonsteroidal MRA, has further expanded the therapeutic landscape. The FIDELIO-DKD [37] and FIGARO-DKD [38] trials demonstrated that finerenone reduced kidney disease progression and CV events in diabetic CKD, with a lower incidence of hyperkalemia than traditional MRAs. These data support its growing role in clinical practice for high-risk CKD patients.

Anemia and mineral-bone disorder (MBD) are major drivers of cardiovascular morbidity in CKD, contributing to vascular calcification, remodeling, and myocardial strain. Anemia arises from reduced erythropoietin, iron deficiency, and inflammation. While erythropoiesis-stimulating agents (ESAs) improve hemoglobin and quality of life, studies have observed that targeting higher hemoglobin increased cardiovascular events.[39-41] Careful dosing and iron supplementation are therefore essential to balance efficacy and safety.

Mineral-bone disorder, characterized by dysregulated phosphate, calcium, and vitamin D metabolism, accelerates vascular calcification and cardiovascular risk.[15] Evidence indicates that phosphate binders improve phosphate control and reduce vascular burden, while vitamin D supplementation may mitigate calcification and offer additional cardiovascular benefits.

CAN EXCESS CARDIOVASCULAR RISK CAUSED BY CHRONIC KIDNEY DISEASE BE NEUTRALIZED: INSIGHTS FROM RECENT STUDIES

Studies have consistently demonstrated the value of addressing individual factors in CKD: Effective management of modifiable risk factors—including diabetes, hypertension, and hyperlipidemia can significantly attenuate the progression of kidney function decline in patients with CKD. Beyond renoprotection, such interventions have also been associated with substantial reductions in the incidence of major cardiovascular events and overall mortality[7-13]. The SPRINT trial[42] showed that intensive SBP lowering (<120 mm Hg) reduced cardiovascular events and mortality in CKD patients without accelerating renal decline, while lipid-lowering studies confirmed that reducing LDL-C reduced major vascular events in patients with advanced CKD.[28]

Recent studies have explored whether multifactorial interventions can offset the excess cardiovascular risk associated with CKD. The UK Biobank study highlighted that adherence to the "Life's Essential 8" score—an updated American Heart Association metric incorporating diet, physical activity, smoking, BMI, lipids, glucose, blood pressure, and sleep duration—was associated with significant reductions in cardiovascular events and mortality in CKD and non-CKD populations alike.[43]

Geng and colleagues conducted a large prospective cohort study involving >20,000 Chinese adults with CKD but without prior cardiovascular disease, with a follow-up duration of 12.2–12.8 years, to evaluate whether optimal control of traditional cardiovascular risk factors could attenuate adverse outcomes.[44] The investigators specifically focused on strict control of systolic blood pressure (SBP <130 mm Hg), low-density lipoprotein cholesterol (LDL-C <100 mg/dL), and fasting blood glucose (FBG <110 mg/dL). Patients with all three factors optimally controlled had no excess cardiovascular risk compared with non-CKD controls. Hazard ratios (HRs) for myocardial infarction, stroke, and all-cause mortality were 0.80, 0.93, and 1.10, respectively, for patients with all 3 risk factors controlled. Furthermore, every additional controlled risk factor conferred incremental benefits: Each factor reduced CKD progression risk by 12% and CVD event risk in a dose-dependent manner. Importantly, the study demonstrated significant reductions in myocardial infarction (HR 0.43), stroke (HR 0.39), and all-cause mortality (HR 0.61) among those with three controlled risk factors compared with CKD patients with none.

More recently, Ling et al. provided compelling real-world evidence from the Chinese cohort, encompassing over 6,000 CVD patients with CKD and nearly 9,300 matched non-CKD controls, followed for a median of 5.6 years.[45] Their findings showed that patients with CKD who achieved blood pressure and glycemic targets while receiving renin–angiotensin system inhibitors had no excess all-cause or cardiovascular mortality compared with non-CKD individuals. This was particularly evident in CKD stage 3a and 3b, where hazard ratios approached unity for both short- and long-term outcomes.

A notable inference from these studies is the contribution of nontraditional, CKD-specific risk factors, including oxidative stress, inflammation, uremic toxins, anemia, and disturbances of mineral-bone metabolism. While these mechanisms have traditionally been regarded as major determinants of the heightened cardiovascular risk in CKD, emerging evidence indicates that their adverse effects may, to a considerable extent, be mediated through interactions with conventional risk factors. Consequently, stringent control of systolic blood pressure, LDL-C, and fasting blood glucose may indirectly attenuate the influence of these nontraditional pathways. This interaction could account for the observed attenuation of excess cardiovascular risk in the study cohort relative to controls when recommended therapeutic targets were achieved.

CONCLUSION

Cardiovascular disease remains the leading cause of mortality among patients with chronic kidney disease, with the heightened risk arising from both conventional and CKD-specific mechanisms. While the complete elimination of this excess cardiovascular risk remains debatable, evidence from studies by Geng et al. and Ling et al. strongly suggests that stringent control of traditional risk factors can substantially neutralize the additional cardiovascular risk associated with CKD. This suggests that comprehensive management of these parameters not only reduces the incidence of myocardial infarction, stroke, and mortality but also slows CKD progression in a dose-dependent manner.

Nevertheless, questions remain about the long-term sustainability of these benefits, their applicability across diverse populations, and the contribution of nontraditional mechanisms that may independently influence outcomes. Future research in broader and more diverse cohorts may provide insights into how traditional and nontraditional factors interact. Clinically, the priority should be aggressive and sustained optimization of SBP, LDL-C, and FBG as a central strategy for improving outcomes in CKD patients. By achieving these targets, clinicians may indeed be able to cancel out the excess cardiovascular risk imposed by CKD and align patient outcomes more closely with those of the general population.

REFERENCES

1. Weiner DE, Tighiouart H, Amin M, et al. Chronic kidney disease as a risk factor for cardiovascular disease and all-cause mortality. J Am Soc Nephrol. 2004;15(5):1307-15.
2. Chen J, Budoff MJ, Reilly MP, et al. Coronary artery calcification and risk of cardiovascular disease and death among patients with chronic kidney disease. JAMA Cardiol. 2017;2(6):635-43.
3. Muntner P, He J, Astor BC, et al. Traditional and nontraditional risk factors predict coronary heart disease in chronic kidney disease. J Am Soc Nephrol. 2005;16(2):529-38.
4. Koppara NK, Medooru KK, Yadagiri LA, et al. Oxidative stress, inflammation, and endothelial dysfunction in diabetic and nondiabetic chronic kidney disease predialysis patients. Indian J Nephrol. 2023;33(6):420-6.
5. Almquist T, Jacobson SH, Mobarrez F, et al. Lipid-lowering treatment and inflammatory mediators in diabetes and chronic kidney disease. Eur J Clin Invest. 2014;44(3):276-84.
6. Peter WLS, Guo H, Kabadi S, et al. Prevalence, treatment patterns, and healthcare resource utilization in non-dialysis-dependent chronic kidney disease patients with and without anemia in the United States. BMC Nephrol. 2018;19(1):67.
7. Wheeler DC, Stefánsson BV, Jongs N, et al. Effects of dapagliflozin on major adverse kidney and cardiovascular events in patients

with diabetic and non-diabetic chronic kidney disease: a prespecified analysis from the DAPA-CKD trial. Lancet Diabetes Endocrinol. 2021;9(1):22-31.

8. Tuttle KR, Lakshmanan MC, Rayner B, et al. Dulaglutide versus insulin glargine in patients with type 2 diabetes and moderate-to-severe chronic kidney disease (AWARD-7): a multicentre, open-label, randomised trial. Lancet Diabetes Endocrinol. 2018;6(8):605-17.
9. Cherney DZI, Dekkers CCJ, Barbour SJ, et al. Effects of the SGLT2 inhibitor dapagliflozin on proteinuria in non-diabetic patients with chronic kidney disease (DIAMOND): a randomised, double-blind, crossover trial. Lancet Diabetes Endocrinol. 2020;8(7):582-93.
10. Qiao Y, Shin JI, Chen TK, et al. Association between renin-angiotensin system blockade discontinuation and all-cause mortality among persons with low estimated glomerular filtration rate. JAMA Intern Med. 2020;180(5):718-26.
11. Agarwal R, Sinha AD, Cramer AE, et al. Chlorthalidone for hypertension in advanced chronic kidney disease. N Engl J Med. 2021;385(26):2507-19.
12. Charytan DM, Sabatine MS, Pedersen TR, et al. Efficacy and safety of evolocumab in chronic kidney disease in the FOURIER trial. J Am Coll Cardiol. 2019;73(23):2961-70.
13. Baigent C, Landray MJ, Reith C, et al. The effects of lowering LDL cholesterol with simvastatin plus ezetimibe in patients with chronic kidney disease (Study of Heart and Renal Protection): a randomised placebo-controlled trial. Lancet. 2011;377(9784):2181-92.
14. Hausberg M, Lang D, Levers A, et al. Sympathetic nerve activity in renal transplant patients before and after withdrawal of cyclosporine. J Hypertens. 2006;24(5):957-64.
15. Levin A, Bakris GL, Molitch M, et al. Prevalence of abnormal serum vitamin D, PTH, calcium, and phosphorus in patients with chronic kidney disease: results of the Study to Evaluate Early Kidney Disease. Kidney Int. 2007;71(1):31-8.
16. van der Velde M, Matsushita K, Coresh J, et al. Lower estimated glomerular filtration rate and higher albuminuria are associated with all-cause and cardiovascular mortality: a collaborative meta-analysis of high-risk population cohorts. Kidney Int. 2011;79(12):1341-52.
17. Lambert K, Cullen V, Jones B, et al. Novel insights and practical strategies for health professionals to improve the uptake of plant-based diets in people with chronic kidney disease. Kidney Res Clin Pract. 2025;44(2):153-62.
18. Ricardo AC, Anderson CA, Yang W, et al. Healthy lifestyle and risk of kidney disease progression, atherosclerotic events, and death in CKD: findings from the Chronic Renal Insufficiency Cohort (CRIC) Study. Am J Kidney Dis. 2015;65(3):412-24.
19. Bahnson J, Knowler WC, Bertoni AG, et al. Effect of a long-term behavioural weight loss intervention on nephropathy in overweight or obese adults with type 2 diabetes: a secondary analysis of the Look AHEAD randomised clinical trial. Lancet Diabetes Endocrinol. 2014;2(10):801-9.
20. Howden EJ, Leano R, Petchey W, et al. Effects of exercise and lifestyle intervention on cardiovascular function in CKD. Clin J Am Soc Nephrol. 2013;8(9):1494-501.
21. Michishita R, Matsuda T, Kawakami S, et al. Accumulation of healthy lifestyle behaviors prevents the incidence of chronic kidney disease in middle-aged and older males. Environ Health Prev Med. 2016;21(3):129-37.
22. Van Huffel L, Tomson C, Ruige J, et al. Dietary restriction and exercise for diabetic patients with chronic kidney disease: a systematic review. PLoS One. 2014;9(11):e113667.
23. Burnier M, Lin S, Ruilope LM, et al. Effect of angiotensin receptor blockers on blood pressure and renal function in patients with concomitant hypertension and chronic kidney disease: a systematic review and meta-analysis. Blood Press. 2019;28(6):358-74.
24. Kim-Mitsuyama S, Ogawa H, Matsui K, et al. An angiotensin II receptor blocker-calcium channel blocker combination prevents cardiovascular events in elderly high-risk hypertensive patients with chronic kidney disease better than high-dose angiotensin II receptor blockade alone. Kidney Int. 2013;83(1):167-76.
25. Tomlinson LA, Abel G, Chaudhry A, et al. ACE inhibitor and angiotensin receptor-II antagonist prescribing and hospital admissions with acute kidney injury: a longitudinal ecological study. PLoS One. 2013;8(11):e78465.
26. Huang RS, Cheng YM, Zeng XX, et al. Renoprotective effect of the combination of renin-angiotensin system inhibitor and calcium channel blocker in patients with hypertension and chronic kidney disease. Chin Med J (Engl). 2016;129(5):562-9.
27. Cheung AK, Chang TI, Cushman WC, et al. Executive summary of the KDIGO 2021 clinical practice guideline for the management of blood pressure in chronic kidney disease. Kidney Int. 2021;99(3):559-69.
28. SHARP Collaborative Group. Study of Heart and Renal Protection (SHARP): randomized trial to assess the effects of lowering low-density lipoprotein cholesterol among 9,438 patients with chronic kidney disease. Am Heart J. 2010;160(5):785-94.
29. Stanifer JW, Charytan DM, White JA, et al. Benefit of ezetimibe added to simvastatin in reduced kidney function. J Am Soc Nephrol. 2017;28(10):3034-43.
30. Fitchett D, Inzucchi SE, Cannon CP, et al. Empagliflozin reduced mortality and hospitalization for heart failure across the spectrum of cardiovascular risk in the EMPA-REG OUTCOME trial. Circulation. 2019;139(11):1384-95.
31. Heerspink HJL, Stefánsson BV, Correa-Rotter R, et al; DAPA-CKD Trial Committees and Investigators. Dapagliflozin in patients with chronic kidney disease. N Engl J Med. 2020;383(15):1436-46.
32. EMPA-KIDNEY Collaborative Group. Effects of empagliflozin on progression of chronic kidney disease: a prespecified secondary analysis from the EMPA-KIDNEY trial. Lancet Diabetes Endocrinol. 2024;12(1):39-50.
33. Marso SP, Daniels GH, Brown-Frandsen K, et al; LEADER Trial Investigators. Liraglutide and cardiovascular outcomes in type 2 diabetes. N Engl J Med. 2016;375(4):311-22.
34. Ashraf T, Bai S, Kumar A, et al. Safety and efficacy of semaglutide in type 2 diabetes mellitus and chronic kidney disease: a meta-analytic review. Ann Med Surg. 2025;87(4):2278-85.
35. Sattar N, Lee MM, Kristensen SL, et al. Cardiovascular, mortality, and kidney outcomes with GLP-1 receptor agonists in patients with type 2 diabetes: a systematic review and meta-analysis of randomised trials. Lancet Diabetes Endocrinol. 2021;9(10):653-62.
36. Rhee JJ, Han J, Montez-Rath ME, et al. . Comparative effectiveness of SGLT2 inhibitors versus GLP-1 receptor agonists in patients with type 2 diabetes and mild/moderate chronic kidney disease. Diabetes Obes Metab. 2024;26(4):1273-81.
37. Bakris GL, Agarwal R, Anker SD, et al; FIDELIO-DKD Investigators. Effect of finerenone on chronic kidney disease outcomes in type 2 diabetes. N Engl J Med. 2020;383(23):2219-29.
38. Pitt B, Filippatos G, Agarwal R, et al; FIGARO-DKD Investigators. Cardiovascular events with finerenone in kidney disease and type 2 diabetes. N Engl J Med. 2021;385(24):2252-63.
39. Singh AK, Szczech L, Tang KL, et al. Correction of anemia with epoetin alfa in chronic kidney disease. N Engl J Med. 2006;355(20):2085-98.

40. Gong W, Huang J, Zhu T, et al. Functional iron deficiency anemia and mortality in chronic kidney disease: the NHANES III follow-up study. Ren Fail. 2023;45(2):e223-31.
41. Locatelli F, Hannedouche T, Fishbane S, et al. Cardiovascular safety and all-cause mortality of methoxy polyethylene glycol-epoetin beta and other erythropoiesis-stimulating agents in anemia of CKD. Clin J Am Soc Nephrol. 2019;14(12):1701-10.
42. SPRINT Research Group, Wright JT Jr, Williamson JD, et al. et al. A randomized trial of intensive versus standard blood-pressure control. N Engl J Med. 2015;373(22):2103-16.
43. Tang R, Wang X, Li X, et al. Adherence to Life's Essential 8 and incident chronic kidney disease: a prospective study of 147,988 UK Biobank participants. Am J Clin Nutr. 2023;118(4):804-11.
44. Geng T, Xu W, Gao H, et al. Relationship between control of cardiovascular risk factors and chronic kidney disease progression, cardiovascular disease events, and mortality in Chinese adults. J Am Coll Cardiol. 2024;84(14):1313-24.
45. Ling Y, Ruan X, Jing L, et al. Association of guideline-directed management of chronic kidney disease with mortality among patients with cardiovascular disease: insights from a multi-center cohort in China. Atherosclerosis. 2025;403:119133.

CHAPTER 4

Smoking Cessation: Never too Early, Never too Late!

Saumitra Ray, Sumanta Chatterjee, Srina Ray

ABSTRACT

Tobacco smoking is one of the most serious health hazards with detrimental effects on almost all organs. Cardiovascular system is one of the most badly affected systems, and tobacco is one of the most important preventable factors for myocardial infarction. Stroke and peripheral vascular disease are also many fold more prevalent in smokers compared to nonsmokers. The silver lining is that once smoking is quitted, most of these adverse effects recede, some partially and some completely, with variable time frames. Various effective ways are now available for successful smoking cessation. So, it is never too early and also never too late to stop smoking.

Keywords: Smoking, cardiovascular disease, cessation.

INTRODUCTION

Over the decades, the area of debate and concern keep encircling around the most important health concern that is "smoking". The global platform is almost continuously trying every day and night to refrain the youth from consumption of tobacco and the subsequent effect. Smoking is a leading risk factor, and important modifiable risk factor for cardiovascular diseases.[1,2] Smoking causes >8 million deaths worldwide each year[3] and among adults aged 30–44 years who died from IHD, 38% of deaths were attributed to smoking.[4] The rising critical scenario is alarming as smokers tend to get attacked by multiple ailments involving almost all organs.

It has been noted that the sudden emergence and popularity of smoking came up in the era of World War I and II when cigarettes were distributed among the soldiers during stressful situations and the first advertisement in 1933 made it evident as a potent euphoriant among the younger generation.

However, even after statutory warning with bold color on the packets of cigarettes, youth get attracted to the ecstasy of the smoke and continue to be in the aura.

HARMFUL SUBSTANCES IN TOBACCO

The main components of the smoke of cigarettes are classified into two phases, the particulate phase and the gaseous phase. The particulate phase contains nicotine, benzopyrene, cadmium, arsenic, and lead. The gaseous phase contains carbon monoxide, nitrosoamines, vinyl chloride, acrolein, and acetaldehyde. Free radicals and peroxynitrite anion from the vapor phase of cigarette smoke activate ECs by inducing endothelial selectins, ICAM-1, VCAM-1, and platelets. There is high concentration of free radical generation in tobacco smoke, which causes harm to molecular level in human body. Cigarette smoke-induced cGAS is mainly activated by cytosolic-free mtDNA released through minority MOMP.

SMOKING-RELATED AILMENTS

One of the burning issues in the global platform is the tobacco smoking and its consequences. It poses a major health concern having a direct causal relationship for a number of ailments such as cardiovascular diseases, lung cancer, reproductive disorders, and osteoporosis among others. Major concern lies in cardiovascular and pulmonary diseases, with rising incidence of sudden cardiac death, acute myocardial infarction, unstable angina, stroke, and peripheral artery diseases. The pulmonary diseases range from lung cancer, emphysema, certain interstitial lung diseases, bronchiolitis, pulmonary Langerhans cell histiocytosis, and increased susceptibility to pneumonia. Even reproductive health gets jeopardized with erectile dysfunction, reduced fertility rate in women, high incidence of lower birth weight, premature birth, and ectopic pregnancy. Some other concerns are cataract, rheumatoid arthritis, and early menopause. Also, oropharyngeal and esophagogastric carcinomas are more frequent in smokers.

SMOKING AND CARDIOVASCULAR DISEASES

Cigarette smoking accounts for about 20% of cardiovascular deaths in the United States. It has wide range of risk burdens from risking the patient to coronary aneurysm to increasing the chance of atherosclerosis. The population attributable risk for myocardial infarction is 35.5% for current smokers, which is a close second in terms of importance to ApoB/Apo A1 ratio. The ischemic events increase as nicotine has the intrinsic tendency to increase the heart rate, blood pressure, and myocardial workload and directly causes endothelial dysfunction by impairment of nitric oxide release. Ultimately, the vasodilatation is hampered. Cigarette smoke activates endothelial cells promoting the adhesion of monocytes/lymphocytes and platelets to inflammatory endothelium. Smoking by pregnant ladies also increases the chance of congenital heart disease in the babies including coarctation of aorta and tetralogy of Fallot.

The major adverse effects of smoking on cardiovascular system:

- Increased blood pressure and heart rate
- Arrhythmia
- Hypercoagulable state
- Hypoxemic state
- Higher low density lipoprotein level

The thrombotic and polycythemic status in smokers produces high CRP and fibrinogen level. Insulin resistance and chronic inflammation contribute to coronary events more in smokers. It also increases the risk of nephrosclerosis and malignant hypertension.

Smoking also interferes with revascularization therapy for acute myocardial infarction. After thrombolysis, the reocclusion rate is four-fold higher in smokers who continue smoking than in those who quit. The risk of reocclusion of a coronary artery after angioplasty or of occlusion of a bypass graft is increased in smokers.

Aune et al. analyzed 12 cohort studies for sudden cardiac death (1,055 episodes in 138,273 participants), among current, former, and never smokers. A 300% increase in the relative risk of sudden cardiac death among current smokers and a 38% increase in risk in former smokers were noted compared to never smokers.[5]

Smoking is associated with higher risk of peripheral arterial disease compared to coronary arterial disease and stroke, and the risk is last to go after smoking cessation.

SMOKING CESSATION: NEVER TOO EARLY, NEVER TOO LATE!

It has been shown that once a smoker quits smoking, many of the adverse parameters tend to normalize very soon, some within days, and some within a year. So, even a life-long smoker should be encouraged to quit smoking, as it is never too late.

In the ELSA-Brasil study,[6] 14,103 participants without clinical CVD were enrolled of whom 1,844 were current smokers, 4,121 were former smokers, and 8,138 never smoked. Among former smokers, hsCRP and carotid intima-media thickness levels and odds of ankle-brachial index ≤1.0 and CAC >0 were lower with increasing time since quitting. Among current smokers, number of cigarettes per day (intensity) was positively associated with hsCRP and CAC >0 after adjusting for duration of smoking.

At the same time, to get back a presmoking state of health may take decades, and so the cessation of smoking should be embarked upon as soon as the opportunity comes. The best outcome, of course, is obtained if a person never starts to smoke.

Light ex-smokers having a CVD risk similar to that of never-smokers relatively soon after smoking cessation. For heavy ex-smokers, >25 years might be required for the residual CVD risk to align with that of never-smokers.

The reduction in all-cause mortality has been observed across all ages and is higher in those who discontinue smoking early.

Table 1 of timeline of benefit of smoking cessation emphasizes this point.

TABLE 1: Timeline of health benefits following smoking cessation.

Timing	Health benefits
Within 20 minutes of last cigarette	Blood pressure, pulse rate, and temperature come down to normal level
Within 8 hours	Carbon monoxide in blood decreases and oxygen increases
Within 24 hours	Risk of heart attack decreases
Within 48 hours	Food tastes and smells better
Within 2 weeks	Coughing, congestion, and shortness of breath decrease
Within 1 year	Risk of heart disease decreases by 50%
Within 10–15 years	Risk of dying prematurely approaches to that of normal person

A PRACTICAL APPROACH TO CESSATION OF SMOKING

American College of Cardiology recently published a consensus document on tobacco cessation management.[7]

The five steps to approach the issue are to ask the patient about tobacco use, to assess the dependence level, to advise to stop smoking, to offer and explain the help support and treatments available, and lastly to keep a close follow-up.

The clinician must ask the patient whether he is a current smoker (regular or sporadic), ex-smoker or never smoker. In the first category, an assessment should be done regarding the smoke year, how soon after waking up in the morning the person takes his first puff and whether he tried to quit smoking before. They should be informed about the health risks of tobacco and the benefits of quitting at any stage. Behavioral therapy, group therapy, pharmacotherapy, etc., should be discussed in detail, usually by an expert counselor. Those who agree to be treated should be given the most appropriate therapy under close supervision and after successful treatment, they should be followed up to prevent any possible relapse. Those who deny treatment in the first place should be encouraged to have further sessions in future.

The former smokers should be assessed for chance of relapse and should be monitored. The life-long nonsmokers should be assessed for any passive smoking and informed and counseled against that.

The need for the idealism came for the rising concern of the health situation. It has been reported that the overall scenario is alarming with the CV risk of 20% in smokers. Smoking cessation is a psychosocial and planned decision of an individual. The 5A's of smoking cessation as mentioned above are: (1) Ask about tobacco use, (2) advise to quit, (3) assess readiness to quit, (4) assist in connecting to tobacco treatment, and (5) arrange follow-up to review progress toward quitting. As smoking cessation may reduce cardiovascular risk [8,9] guideline strongly recommends cessation of smoking for primary and secondary prevention of CVD[7,10]

The most important effect of nicotine replacement therapies, with cultural, social, and counseling approach was the significant fall in smoking rate in the global population from 32.7% in 2000 to 22.3% in 2020. [4] One of the earliest antismoking campaigns got a tag line of "SMOKING KILLS", which became extremely popular. The need for psychosocial support along with pharmacotherapy will ultimately help individuals to reach their goal.

NONPHARMACOLOGIC SUPPORT

Stressing on group counseling can give the moral support before the quit day, and development of coping skills and suggestions for relapse prevention are integral parts of the goal. Different nongovernment organizations organize and sponsor educational platforms to promote smoking cessation activities. Pamphlets, statutory warnings, discussion during brand, and promotional activities are crucial step to promote smoking cessation.

PHARMACOLOGICAL SUPPORT

Some drugs such as nicotine replacement, bupropion, and varenicline are already in use to aid smoking cessation. Off-label drugs which are coming in the market are clonidine, nortriptyline, and topiramate.

Nicotine replacement therapies—5 types used mainly lozenges, polacrilex gum, transdermal system, nasal spray, and nicotine inhalers. Others getting highlighted are toothpicks and e-cigarettes.

Nicotine Replacement Therapy

This is used to reduce the intensity of withdrawal symptoms, usually given on the scheduled day of quitting. Transdermal system provides a steady concentration throughout the day and is very common in use nowadays. Some other formulations with episodic dosing are also in use. Common practice is a patch plus regimen, as whenever a smoker quits smoking the constant urge needs to be suppressed by the steady level of nicotine. Nicotine polacrilex gum contains 2–4 mg bound to resin containing a buffering agent which improves delivery. Generally, blood level peaks after 30 minutes and the higher dose is reserved for heavy smokers.

Dose recommendation—each gummies every 2–3 hours for 1–6 weeks.

Adverse effects—temporomandibular joint disease, trauma to dental appliances, sore jaw, oral irritation, ulcers and excess salivation, hiccups from swallowed nicotine, nausea, vomiting, abdominal pain, constipation, diarrhea, palpitation, and headache. In patients with dental appliances, usually it is avoided.

Transdermal nicotine patch—generally achieve nicotine level about 40–50%, at least 4 weeks therapy to be given, the patches to be worn at night.

Nicotine inhaler—particle, not delivered to lung, usual dosing 6–16 cartridges/day for 6–12 weeks followed by gradual reduction over next 6–12 weeks. The adverse effect is bronchospasm in individuals with reactive airways disease.

Bupropion

This is an antidepressant, which potentiates dopaminergic and noradrenergic signaling. It is more effective with nicotine replacement therapy (NRT). Dose—150 mg daily for 3 days then, 150 mg twice daily for 7–12 weeks. Therapy given for >1 year resulted in sustainable quits.

Adverse effects include dry mouth, insomnia, agitation, headache, high blood pressure, and reduction of seizure threshold.

Varenicline

It is the partial agonist at alpha 4 beta 2 nicotine receptor. By occupying the nicotine receptor, it prevents nicotine from acting and thus can reduce rewarding and reinforcement effects associated with it. It prevents relapse and is to be taken orally 0.5 mg once daily for 3 days, then twice daily for 4 days, then 1 mg twice daily for 3 months. An additional 3 months can be given.

Adverse events which are notified include nausea, insomnia, visual disturbance, syncope and skin reactions, and worsening cardiovascular symptoms.

There have been recorded cases that *bupropion* and *varenicline* are associated with suicidal events.

SMOKING CESSATION AND EFFECTS ON DIFFERENT DISEASE STATES

Heart Failure

Smoking is a well-known risk factor for heart failure (HF), as well as a contributor to the disease process that primarily lead to HF. Smoking along with different contributory factors showed direct causal relationship to left ventricular hypertrophy and cardiac dysfunction.[9] In addition, recent studies have found that current smokers have at least double the risk of developing HF compared with never smokers.[11-13] The risk becomes almost four-fold higher among smokers who smoke 25 or more cigarettes per day.[10]

Coronary Artery Diseases

Smoking increases the hypercoagulability of blood and increases the chances of coronary events. It has also effects on generating free radicals and hastening the process of CVD.

Literature says it takes almost 25 years stoppage of cigarettes to return to normal risk category of CVD comparing to smokers. Smokers generally have upregulation of cytokine receptor like factor 1, which causes oxidative stress and inflammation. Smoking causes narrowing of coronary vessels and frequent rupture of plaques.

Aortic Aneurysm

The degeneration of intima media, the important layer that integrates and stabilizes the aortic wall, plays an important role in the pathogenesis of aortic diseases. The media consists of a lamellar unit structured by smooth muscle cells, elastin, and collagen, and thus loss of any of these components would result in a damaged media in which a tear or dilation happens, hence disrupt the aortic wall and eventually cause aortic dissection or aneurysm.[14] An extensive body of literature reported that excess cigarette smoke stimulates macrophages' production of matrix metalloproteinase, thereby degenerating the elastin and collagen and leading to incidence of aortic diseases.[15-17] Furthermore, some basic research reported aortic dissection preceded the formation of atherosclerosis,[18] which indicates certain components of the pathogenesis of aortic dissection could be independent from atherosclerosis. Thus, we understand the mechanism of aortic aneurysm and subsequent dissection which can be prevented to a greater extent by cessation of smoking.

E-CIGARETTES

Electronic nicotine delivery systems are called e-cigarettes. They ate also known as vaping pens or vaping devices.

Its rising popularity among youth and an alternative to conventional smoking is a concern. This is generally a battery-operated heating device containing a cartridge which heats the liquid nicotine and generates the flavored steam. Different strengths are available with 24 mg being the highest strength and zero strength with almost no nicotine is also available.

The main components again are cadmium, nickel hydrocarbons, tolueneacetaldehyde, and acetone. Some find it an alternative solution to smoking, but it has almost similar side effect profile like smoking. It is contraindicated in pregnancy, and its use should be restricted as much as possible.

The entry to the market was in 2004 when China first introduced an alternative to conventional smoking with the aim of relieving the heavy smokers. E-cigarettes are only a support system for the motivated individuals who are determined enough to quit smoking but definitely not an alternative.

CONCLUSION

Even within few minutes of stoppage of cigarettes, the body responds in a positive way.

The blood pressure and pulse rate decrease, and after some weeks, the hypercoagulability improves with risk of coronary events decreasing in a steady way. Smoking cessation is of utmost importance at present to refrain society from further damage. The youth needs to understand the direct effect of smoking on cardiovascular death and its prevention. At present, there are currently 1 billion smokers over the world, and it emphasizes the massive movement we need to promote smoking cessation.

REFERENCES

1. Virani SS, Alonso A, Aparicio HJ, et al; American Heart Association Council on Epidemiology and Prevention Statistics Committee and Stroke Statistics Subcommittee. Heart disease and stroke statistics-2021 update: a report from the American Heart Association. Circulation. 2021;143(8):e254-743.
2. Teo KK, Ounpuu S, Hawken S, et al; INTERHEART Study Investigators. Tobacco use and risk of myocardial infarction in 52 countries in the INTERHEART study: a case-control study. Lancet. 2006;368(9536):647-58.

3. Murray CJ, Aravkin AY, Zheng P, et al; GBD 2019 Risk Factors Collaborators. Global burden of 87 risk factors in 204 countries and territories, 1990-2019: a systematic analysis for the Global Burden of Disease Study 2019. Lancet. 2020;396(10258): 1223-49.
4. Organization WH. WHO global report on trends in prevalence of tobacco use 2000-2025. World Health Organization; 2020.
5. Aune D, Schlesinger S, Norat T, et al. Tobacco smoking and the risk of sudden cardiac death: a systematic review and meta-analysis of prospective studies. Eur J Epidemiol. 2018;33(6):509-21.
6. Kianoush S, Yakoob MY, Al-Rifai M, et al. Associations of Cigarette Smoking With Subclinical Inflammation and Atherosclerosis: ELSA-Brasil (The Brazilian Longitudinal Study of Adult Health). J Am Heart Assoc. 2017;6(6):e005088.
7. Arnett DK, Blumenthal RS, Albert MA, et al. 2019 ACC/AHA guideline on the primary prevention of cardiovascular disease: a report of the American College of Cardiology/American Heart Association Task Force on Clinical Practice Guidelines. Circulation. 2019;140(11):e596-646.
8. Jha P. The 21st century benefits of smoking cessation in Europe. Eur J Epidemiol. 2013;28(8):617-9.
9. Jha P, Ramasundarahettige C, Landsman V, et al. 21st-century hazards of smoking and benefits of cessation in the United States. N Engl J Med. 2013;368(4):341-50.
10. Visseren FLJ, Mach F, Smulders YM, et al; ESC National Cardiac Societies; ESC Scientific Document Group. 2021 ESC Guidelines on cardiovascular disease prevention in clinical practice. Eur Heart J. 2021;42(34):3227-337.
11. Kamimura, Cain LR, Mentz RJ, et al. Cigarette smoking and incident heart failure: insights from the Jackson Heart Study. Circulation. 2018;137:2572-82.
12. Banks, Joshy G, Korda RJ, et al. Tobacco smoking and risk of 36 cardiovascular disease subtypes: fatal and non-fatal outcomes in a large prospective Australian study. BMC Med. 2019;17:128.
13. Ahmed AA, Patel K, Nyaku MA, et al. Risk of heart failure and death after prolonged smoking cessation: role of amount and duration of prior smoking. Circ Heart Fail. 2015;8:694-701.
14. Nakashima Y, Kawada S, Ueda T, et al. Pathophysiology of Aortic Dissection and Abdominal Aortic Aneurysm. In: Cardio-Aortic and Aortic Surgery, Keio University International Symposia for Life Sciences and Medicine. Springer, Tokyo; 2001.
15. Norman PE, Curci JA. Understanding the effects of tobacco smoke on the pathogenesis of aortic aneurysm. Arterioscler Thromb Vasc Biol. 2013;33:1473-7.
16. Sugamura K, Keaney JF, Jr. Nicotine: linking smoking to abdominal aneurysms. Nat Med. 2012;18:856-8.
17. Perlstein TS, Lee RT. Smoking, metalloproteinases, and vascular disease. Arterioscler Thromb Vasc Biol. 2006;26:250-6.
18. Saraff K, Babamusta F, Cassis LA, et al. Aortic dissection precedes formation of aneurysms and atherosclerosis in angiotensin II-infused, apolipoprotein E-deficient mice. Arterioscler Thromb Vasc Biol. 2003;23:1621-6.

SECTION

2

Hypertension

Section Outline

5. **Implications of Systolic Blood Pressure Time in Target Range**
   AK Trivedi, Abhinit Gupta, Bijay Prakash Yadav
6. **Artificial Intelligence: An Emerging Tool for the Diagnosis and Management of Hypertension**
   C Venkata S Ram
7. **Clinical Management of Primary Aldosteronism**
   Dharmendra Jain, Vikash Kumar Maurya, Pratap Kumar
8. **Implications of Myocardial Interstitial Fibrosis in Hypertensive Heart Disease**
   Debasis Ghosh, Navanil Biswas
9. **Renovascular Hypertension: Kidney Intrinsic Mechanism as Novel Target**
   Manu Gupta, Anuj Gupta, Pooja Sharma Gupta, Rajeev Gupta
10. **The Complexity of Resistant and Refractory Hypertension**
    Somya Mahlawat, Umesh Tripathi, Sharad Chandra

CHAPTER

5

Implications of Systolic Blood Pressure Time in Target Range

AK Trivedi, Abhinit Gupta, Bijay Prakash Yadav

ABSTRACT

Hypertension is a major modifiable risk factor for cardiovascular disease worldwide, traditionally managed through isolated blood pressure (BP) measurements. Emerging evidence highlights the superiority of time in target range (TTR)—the proportion of time BP remains within an optimal range—as a dynamic and comprehensive metric for assessing BP control and predicting cardiovascular outcomes. Studies demonstrate that higher TTR correlates with reduced risks of major cardiovascular events, heart failure, renal complications, dementia, and mortality across diverse populations. Advances in digital technology and artificial intelligence (AI) now enable automated, longitudinal TTR monitoring, facilitating personalized hypertension management beyond sporadic clinical measurements. Despite promising benefits, key challenges remain including defining optimal TTR thresholds tailored to specific populations, preserving BP stability, validating digital tools, and integrating these approaches into real-world clinical practice cost-effectively. Addressing these research gaps is critical to improving hypertension care and reducing global cardiovascular disease burden. Adoption of TTR-guided management, combined with AI-supported digital health solutions, promises a more precise, equitable, and impactful approach to BP control and cardiovascular risk reduction.

Keywords: Hypertension, blood pressure control, time in target range, cardiovascular disease, major adverse cardiovascular events (MACE), public health.

INTRODUCTION

Hypertension remains a leading modifiable risk factor for cardiovascular disease (CVD), contributing significantly to global morbidity and mortality.[1] Elevated blood pressure (BP) is directly associated with increased risk of ischemic heart disease, stroke, and premature death.[2] Traditional approaches to hypertension management have primarily focused on achieving target BP levels based on sporadic office measurements; however, novel metrics, such as *Time in Target Range* (TTR)—the proportion of time a patient's BP remains within an optimal range—have emerged as important predictors of clinical outcomes.[3] Moreover, this emerging evidence suggests that a more comprehensive approach, considering BP dynamics over time, may offer improved cardiovascular protection.

THE LIMITATIONS OF TRADITIONAL BP MEASUREMENT

Conventional BP management strategies often rely on isolated BP readings obtained in a clinical setting. These measurements may not accurately reflect an individual's BP profile due to factors such as white-coat hypertension, masked hypertension, or variability related to daily activities.[4,5] Furthermore, relying solely on achieving target BP levels at a single point in time may overlook the significance of BP fluctuations and the cumulative impact of uncontrolled hypertension. Ambulatory blood pressure monitoring (ABPM) involves noninvasive, automated 24-hour monitoring and provides a more comprehensive evaluation of BP. It has an advantage to detect patterns such as sustained, white-coat, and masked hypertension, while also recording nocturnal BP and dipping status, which are strong predictors of cardiovascular risk. Compared to office readings, ABPM correlates better with target organ damage, cardiovascular outcomes, and helps in tailoring treatment more effectively.[4]

THE CONCEPT OF TIME-IN-TARGET RANGE

Beyond average BP values, to address the limitations of traditional BP measurement, the concept of "TTR" has emerged as an important parameter for assessing BP control.[6] TTR represents the percentage of time that a patient's BP remains within a predefined target range. It provides dynamic monitoring versus static average values and a more comprehensive assessment of BP control by considering both the magnitude and duration of BP elevations or reductions.[3]

CLINICAL EVIDENCE SUPPORTING TTR

Recent studies have demonstrated the clinical benefits of achieving high BP-TTR in various patient populations. In individuals with hypertension and high cardiovascular risk, higher TTR has been associated with reduced risk of major adverse cardiovascular events, renal health, and mortality, while a low TTR indicates unstable or poorly managed BP. This dynamic measurement complements ABPM and can be a valuable tool in guiding treatment and enhancing long-term outcomes.[7,8]

The JACC Asia Study: SBP-TTR and Cardiovascular Outcomes

A recent study published in *JACC: Asia* by *Han et al.* investigated the association between systolic blood pressure TTR (SBP-TTR) and cardiovascular outcomes in a community-based population. The study included 9,552 participants from the Kailuan community in China. The researchers found that for every standard deviation (SD) increase in SBP-TTR, there was a significant reduction in the risk of CVD, premature CVD, and premature death. When an SBP target of 110–130 mm Hg was modeled, a 1-SD increase in SBP-TTR was associated with even greater reductions in these adverse outcomes. These findings suggest that TTR can serve as a useful indicator of effective BP control and may have important implications for clinical practice **(Fig. 1)**.[3]

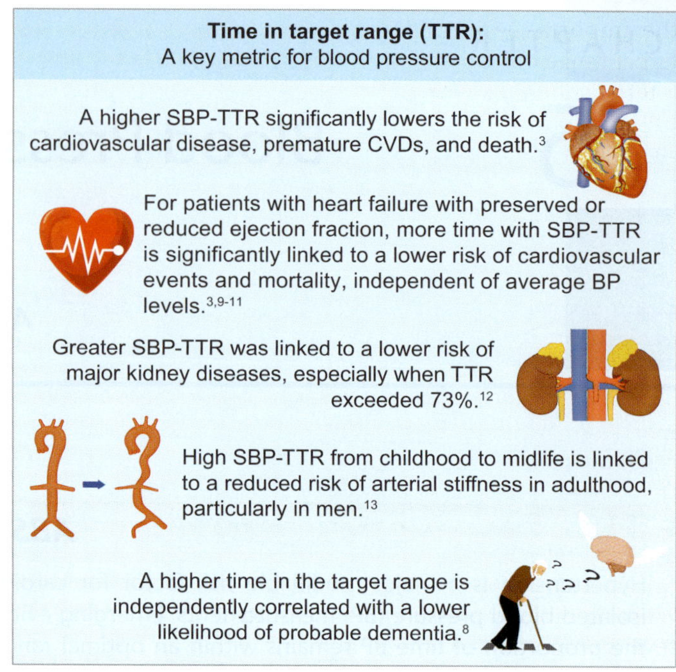

FIG. 1: Time in target range (TTR) and health outcomes.

Time in Target SBP Range and Its Prognostic Significance in Heart Failure

Huang et al. determined the association between BP control and clinical outcomes among patients with heart failure with preserved ejection fraction. They reported that in patients with heart failure with preserved ejection fraction, spending more time within the SBP target range was significantly linked to a lower risk of cardiovascular events and mortality, independent of average BP levels, with the strongest benefit seen in younger patients.[8] Similarly, in patients with heart failure, achieving a greater TTR has been linked to improved outcomes **(Fig. 1)**.[3,9,10]

Fu et al. performed a posthoc analysis of the *STICH* (Surgical Treatment for Ischemic Heart Failure) *trial*, which included 2,136 patients with ischemic cardiomyopathy. Using a systolic BP target range of 110–130 mm Hg, TTR was calculated by linear interpolation. Their findings indicated that a higher TTR was strongly associated with reduced all-cause mortality, suggesting that TTR may serve as a useful surrogate marker of long-term systolic BP control in patients with ischemic cardiomyopathy **(Fig. 1)**.[11]

In a secondary analysis of the *SPRINT* trial, researchers examined SBP targets of <120 mm Hg (intensive control) versus <140 mm Hg (standard control) among hypertensive individuals with elevated cardiovascular risk. Results demonstrated that maintaining a greater time within the SBP target range (TTR) was independently correlated with a lower likelihood of probable dementia. These findings suggest that TTR could represent a valuable and clinically feasible marker of long-term BP management and dementia risk assessment in older adults with hypertension **(Fig. 1)**.[8]

In a retrospective cohort analysis of participants from the *SPRINT* and *ACCORD-BP* trials, SBP TTR was linked to adverse cardiovascular and kidney outcomes in adults with hypertension. After adjusting for demographics, risk factors, and study characteristics, greater TTR was associated with a lower risk of major kidney events. The relationship between TTR and kidney risk was nonlinear: The risk declined between TTR levels of 0 and 42%, remained stable up to 73%, and then decreased further when TTR exceeded 73% **(Fig. 1)**.[12]

Wang et al., investigated the independent association between long-term SBP-TTR from childhood to midlife and arterial stiffness in adulthood. They used brachial-ankle pulse wave velocity (baPWV) as a measure of arterial stiffness, where higher baPWV values indicate greater vessel stiffness. Their findings revealed that individuals with higher SBP-TTR over this extended period had a significantly reduced risk of arterial stiffness in midlife. This protective relationship remained significant even after accounting for average SBP levels and SBP variability. The study highlights the importance of maintaining SBP within the optimal target range consistently from early life to reduce the risk of arterial stiffening later in life, independently of mean BP or BP fluctuations. Notably, this association was particularly significant in men **(Fig. 1)**.[13]

Blood Pressure Variability, TTR, and Risk Prediction

Blood pressure variability (BPV) remains an independent risk factor for adverse outcomes. However, combined assessment—high BPV plus low TTR—identifies patients at the highest risk for major cardiovascular events and mortality. Maintaining both high TTR and low variability provides maximal protection.[14]

Practical Considerations for Implementing TTR

While TTR offers a promising approach to BP management, several practical considerations need to be addressed before widespread implementation.

- *BP measurement techniques*: Accurate and reliable BP measurements are essential for calculating TTR. The use of calibrated wearable BP measurement devices may facilitate seamless integration of TTR into clinical practice.[15]
- *Measurement practicality*: Determining how often BP should be measured for accurate TTR evaluation is essential. Home BP monitoring (HBPM) offers greater reproducibility and practicality for tracking TTR over time compared to ABPM. However, ABPM provides additional insights into nighttime BP variations and 24-hour patterns. The optimal frequency of BP measurements needed to enhance SBP-TTR accuracy, while avoiding unnecessary burden on patients, remains uncertain.[15]
- *Frequency and duration of assessment periods*: Recommended frequent, longitudinal measurement for representative TTR calculation, often over months or longer. The optimal duration of SBP-TTR assessment periods needs to be established. Ensuring frequent, accurate measurements, patient engagement, and correct thresholds remains a practical hurdle.[16]
- *Diastolic BP targets*: In addition to SBP, optimal diastolic BP targets should also be considered. Extremely low diastolic BP has been associated with increased adverse cardiovascular events.[17,18] The 2018 European Society of Cardiology (ESC)/European Society of Hypertension guidelines recommend a diastolic BP target of between 70 and 80 mm Hg for patients with all risk levels.[19]
- *Mean BP and pulse pressure*: Mean BP and pulse pressure have also been associated with poor cardiovascular outcomes.[20,21] Further research is needed to determine how these parameters can be incorporated into TTR-based BP management strategies.
- *Age and comorbidities*: Uniform targets (<130/80 mm Hg) are now recommended regardless of age, sex, or chronic conditions (e.g., chronic kidney disease and diabetes).[22] Further research is needed to determine how sex and ethnicity may affect TTR and how these factors should be considered in clinical practice.

TTR VERSUS OTHER METRICS OF BP CONTROL: CLINICAL IMPLICATIONS

Compared to average BP or single-point metrics, TTR provides superior prognostic value for adverse outcomes. It allows clinicians to assess both medication efficacy and overall BP stability. TTR's ability to integrate variability makes it a preferred tool for future management strategies.[23]

FUTURE DIRECTIONS AND RESEARCH NEEDS

- *Digital technology and AI integration*: Digital monitoring, individualized TTR targets, and AI-supported management are shaping hypertension care. AI can automate TTR assessment using longitudinal BP data, detect poor treatment compliance, and identify patients needing more intensive BP control. These tools reduce reliance on single, potentially unreliable measurements taken during acute illness or with poor technique.[24]
- *Research gaps*: Further research is needed to refine TTR-based BP management strategies and address the practical considerations outlined above. Studies should focus on:
  - Optimal TTR thresholds by population subgroup, how to preserve BP stability, and real-world integration strategies require further study.[3]
  - Evaluating the impact of TTR-based interventions on cardiovascular outcomes
  - Developing and validating digital tools for TTR assessment and management
  - Assessing the cost-effectiveness of TTR-based BP management strategies
  - Advance integration of digital precision health and task-sharing models in HTN care. Use digital tech and AI for personalized, continuous BP monitoring, and automated TTR assessment.
  - Identify and define optimal TTR thresholds tailored to diverse populations and address global disparities in hypertension awareness, diagnosis, treatment, and control.
  - Research how to maintain long-term BP stability in different settings.
  - Evaluate the impact of TTR-based interventions on cardiovascular outcomes through prospective studies.
  - Conduct implementation research to optimize healthcare workforce training and system reforms for hypertension management.

- *Policy impact and public health*: Promote guidelines development, inclusive of local context, patient engagement, and multidisciplinary approaches. Population-level TTR monitoring may enhance public health interventions and reduce the burden of CVD.[25]

By embracing a more dynamic and comprehensive approach to BP management, we can improve cardiovascular outcomes and reduce the global burden of hypertension.

CONCLUSION

Time in target range represents a new approach to BP management, shifting from isolated readings to a more dynamic assessment of control. Studies suggest that higher BP TTR is linked to better cardiovascular outcomes. Despite practical challenges, integrating TTR into clinical practice could enhance hypertension care and reduce CVD burden. Since effective BP control is crucial for preventing heart disease and early mortality, TTR now serves as a meaningful risk metric in current guidelines. Regular monitoring, maximizing TTR, and minimizing variability should guide clinical and policy decisions.[22]

ACKNOWLEDGMENT

We sincerely thank Dr Poonam Kushwaha, Associate Professor, RMCH and RC, Kanpur, for her invaluable role in editing and contributing to the writing of this chapter.

REFERENCES

1. Zhou B, Perel P, Mensah GA, et al. Global epidemiology, health burden and effective interventions for elevated blood pressure and hypertension. Nat Rev Cardiol. 2021;18(11):785-802.
2. Mohammad R, Bansod DW. Hypertension in India: a gender-based study of prevalence and associated risk factors. BMC Public Health. 2024;24(1):2681.
3. Han X, Liu S, Zhou X, et al. Systolic Blood Pressure Time in Target Range and Cardiovascular Disease and Premature Death. JACC Asia. 2024;4(12):987-96.
4. Muntner P, Shimbo D, Carey RM, et al. Measurement of Blood Pressure in Humans: A Scientific Statement From the American Heart Association. Hypertension. 2019;73(5):e35-e66.
5. Pickering TG, Hall JE, Appel LJ, et al. Recommendations for blood pressure measurement in humans and experimental animals: part 1: blood pressure measurement in humans: a statement for professionals from the Subcommittee of Professional and Public Education of the American Heart Association Council on High Blood Pressure Research. Circulation. 2005;111(5):697-716.
6. Fatani N, Dixon DL, Van Tassell BW, et al. Systolic Blood Pressure Time in Target Range and Cardiovascular Outcomes in Patients With Hypertension. J Am Coll Cardiol. 2021;77(10):1290-9.
7. Wang H, Song J, Liu Z, et al. Time in Target Range for Blood Pressure and Adverse Health Outcomes: A Systematic Review. Hypertens Dallas Tex 1979. 2025;82(3):419-31.
8. Huang X, Deng S, Xie W, et al. Time in target range of systolic blood pressure and cognitive outcomes in patients with hypertension. J Am Geriatr Soc. 2024;72(2):423-32.
9. Chen X, Orom H, Hay JL, et al. Differences in Rural and Urban Health Information Access and Use. J Rural Health Off J Am Rural Health Assoc Natl Rural Health Care Assoc. 2019;35(3):405-17.
10. Tian X, Zhang Y, Chen S, et al. Systolic blood pressure time in target range within 24 hours and incident heart failure: insights from the real-world setting. Hypertens Res. 2025;48(1):223-32.
11. Fu G, Zhou Z, Jian B, et al. Systolic blood pressure time in target range and long-term outcomes in patients with ischemic cardiomyopathy. Am Heart J. 2023;258:177-85.
12. Buckley LF, Baker WL, Van Tassell BW, et al. Systolic Blood Pressure Time in Target Range and Major Adverse Kidney and Cardiovascular Events. Hypertens Dallas Tex. 1979. 2023;80(2):305-13.
13. Wang Y, Qi H, Jia H, et al. Long-Term Time in Target Range for Systolic Blood Pressure Since Childhood and Midlife Arterial Stiffness. JACC Asia. 2025;5(1):101-12.
14. Feng Z, Li Y, Wang C, et al. Combined effect of time in target range and variability of systolic blood pressure on cardiovascular outcomes and mortality in patients with hypertension: A prospective cohort study. J Clin Hypertens. 2024;26(6):714-23.
15. Jones DW, Ferdinand KC, Taler SJ, et al. 2025 AHA/ACC/AANP/AAPA/ABC/ACCP/ACPM/AGS/AMA/ASPC/NMA/PCNA/SGIM Guideline for the Prevention, Detection, Evaluation and Management of High Blood Pressure in Adults: A Report of the American College of Cardiology/American Heart Association Joint Committee on Clinical Practice Guidelines. Circulation. 2025;CIR.0000000000001356.
16. Schlaich MP. Time in Target Range: the Future of Assessing Adequacy of Blood Pressure Control? Hypertension. 2023;80(2):314-5.
17. Bangalore S, Messerli FH, Wun CC, et al. J-curve revisited: an analysis of blood pressure and cardiovascular events in the Treating to New Targets (TNT) Trial†. Eur Heart J. 2010;31(23):2897-908.
18. Gaffney B, Jacobsen AP, Pallippattu AW, et al. The Diastolic Blood Pressure J-Curve in Hypertension Management: Links and Risk for Cardiovascular Disease. Integr Blood Press Control. 2021;14:179-87.
19. Li J, Somers VK, Gao X, et al. Evaluation of Optimal Diastolic Blood Pressure Range Among Adults With Treated Systolic Blood Pressure Less Than 130 mm Hg. JAMA Netw Open. 2021;4(2):e2037554.
20. Abbott TEF, Pearse RM, Archbold RA, et al. Association between preoperative pulse pressure and perioperative myocardial injury: an international observational cohort study of patients undergoing non-cardiac surgery. Br J Anaesth. 2017;119(1):78-86.
21. Zeng J, Zheng G, Li Y, et al. Preoperative Pulse Pressure and Adverse Postoperative Outcomes: A Meta-Analysis. J Cardiothorac Vasc Anesth. 2020;34(3):624-31.
22. Ohya Y, Sakima A. JSH2025 guidelines new viewpoints. Hypertens Res. 2025;1-3.
23. Li W, Gnanenthiran SR, Schutte AE, et al. Blood pressure time at target and its prognostic value for cardiovascular outcomes: a scoping review. Hypertens Res. 2024;47(9):2337-50.
24. Priyadarsini GS, Taha S, Lashari UG, et al. Digital health monitoring: examining the effectiveness of wearable devices in managing hypertension. a bibliometric analysis. South East Eur J Public Health. 2025;5311-57.
25. Ndejjo R, Hassen HY, Wanyenze RK, et al. Community-Based Interventions for Cardiovascular Disease Prevention in Low-and Middle-Income Countries: A Systematic Review. Public Health Rev. 2021;42:1604018.

Artificial Intelligence: An Emerging Tool for the Diagnosis and Management of Hypertension

C Venkata S Ram

ABSTRACT

Hypertension remains a major global health concern, affecting over one-third of adults worldwide. While progress in understanding the pathophysiology of hypertension has slowed down in recent years, artificial intelligence (AI) has created opportunities to improve hypertension care via precision medicine. AI algorithms have the ability to integrate and analyze vast multimodal datasets, including electronic health records, electrocardiograms, and wearable device outputs, to predict hypertension risk, enable early diagnosis, and personalize treatment strategies. AI can also facilitate individualized treatment recommendations based on environmental and patient-specific factors, including comorbidities and genetic traits, and shows promise in enhancing medication adherence and lifestyle modification through autonomous coaching systems. These innovations could promote anticipatory, patient-centered care and reduce long-term cardiovascular risks and healthcare costs at the community level. This chapter outlines the current status of AI in hypertension management and expounds on evolving challenges and potential solutions.

Keywords: Algorithms, artificial intelligence, blood pressure, cardiovascular disease, deep learning, hypertension, machine learning.

INTRODUCTION

Hypertension remains one of the most significant modifiable risk factors for cardiovascular disease and premature mortality worldwide. Notably, low- and middle-income countries, including India, have experienced a steady increase in the prevalence of hypertension since 1990.[1,2] Despite its high burden, hypertension continues to be underdiagnosed and inadequately managed: Only about 50% of individuals with hypertension are aware of their condition, fewer than half of those diagnosed receive treatment, and merely one in five achieve optimal blood pressure (BP) control.[3]

Traditional approaches to hypertension management have certain disadvantages. These include missed diagnoses due to asymptomatic presentation, limited access to routine screening and monitoring, poor adherence to treatment regimens, and a lack of personalized therapeutic strategies.[4-6] Innovative solutions and emerging technologies, particularly artificial intelligence (AI), have the potential to address these inherent limitations **(Fig. 1)**.[2]

FUNDAMENTALS OF ARTIFICIAL INTELLIGENCE IN MEDICINE

Artificial intelligence has rapidly become a transformative force in modern medicine. Various AI models, each offering unique capabilities and applications, have been developed and implemented across healthcare domains. The most commonly employed models include:

- *Machine learning (ML):* ML involves the use of algorithms trained on clinical data to identify patterns, make predictions, and support automated decision-making. Common ML algorithms include decision trees, random forests, support vector machines, and neural networks.[2]
- *Deep learning (DL):* A specialized subset of ML, DL utilizes multilayered neural networks to process complex, high-dimensional data such as medical images and unstructured clinical text. DL models have demonstrated superior performance in tasks such as image interpretation and natural language processing.[2,7]

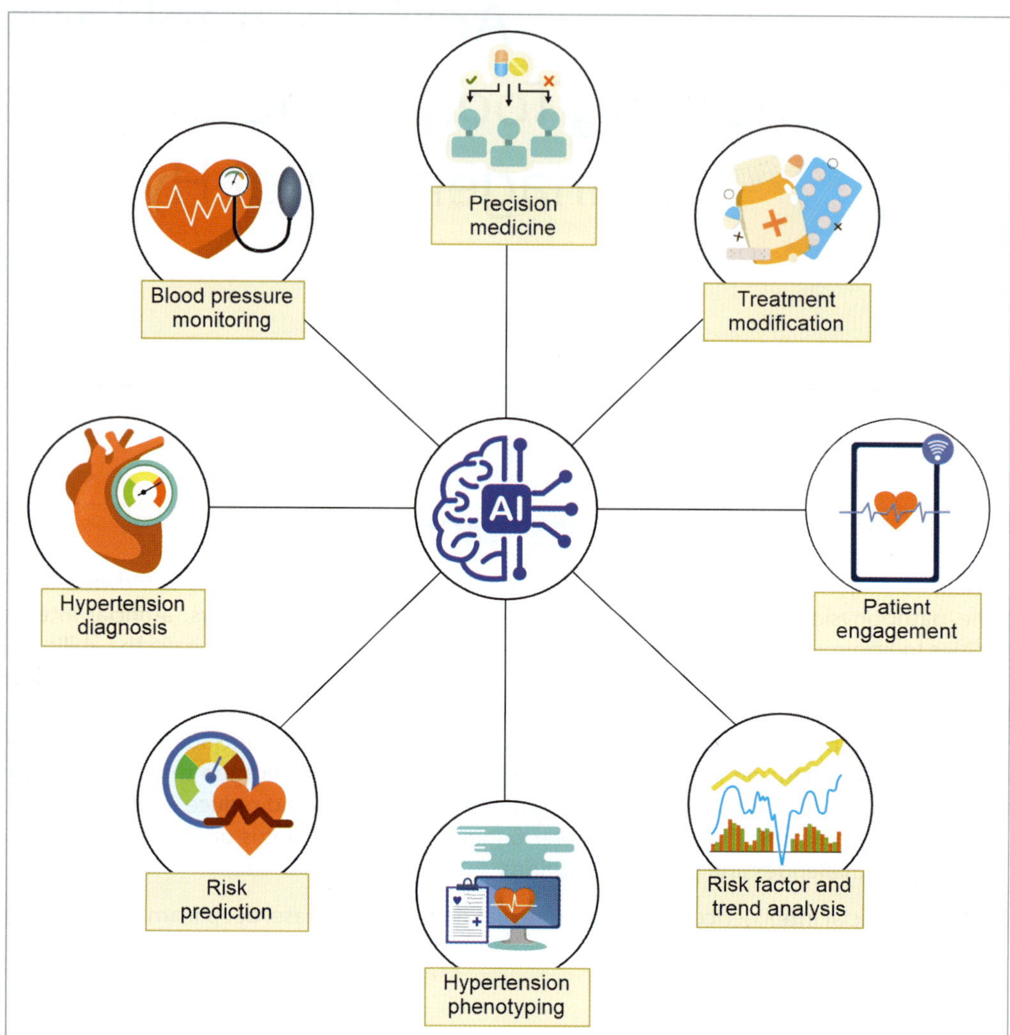

FIG. 1: Multifaceted applications of AI in hypertension management.

- *Generative AI and large language models (LLMs):* Recent advancements in generative AI, including LLMs, have introduced new capabilities such as natural language understanding, clinical note generation, and AI-assisted decision-making.[8]

In the context of hypertension, ML- and DL-based AI algorithms can be applied to a wide range of clinical tasks. Supervised learning algorithms, including regression models, classification trees, and neural networks, are trained on labeled datasets and can be used to predict hypertension risk, facilitate diagnosis, and enable patient stratification.[9] In contrast, unsupervised learning algorithms study unlabeled data to identify previously unrecognized patterns, allowing for the discovery of novel patient phenotypes and subgroups and improving our understanding of the heterogeneity within hypertensive populations.[9,10] Reinforcement learning, which determines optimal actions through feedback and reward mechanisms, can be employed to tailor personalized treatment regimens, including the dynamic adjustment of antihypertensive therapies.[2] Together, these AI methodologies have enabled not only predictive modeling and diagnostic support but also novel approaches to BP monitoring **(Table 1)**.[11]

BLOOD PRESSURE MEASUREMENT AND MONITORING

Blood pressure is traditionally measured in clinical or home settings using an inflatable cuff. However, this traditional approach fails to capture short-term BP variability, causing clinically significant fluctuations related to daily activities, stress, or circadian rhythms to be overlooked. Furthermore, phenomena such as the "white coat effect", where patient anxiety can result in elevated readings, may lead to misdiagnosis or inappropriate treatment modifications.[12,13]

Artificial intelligence is completely transforming BP monitoring through wearable devices. AI algorithms can

TABLE 1: Comparison of traditional versus AI-enhanced hypertension management.

Aspect	Traditional methods	AI-enhanced methods
Blood pressure monitoring	Manual measurement at home or in the clinic	Continuous and automated measurement with wearable devices
Risk prediction	Risk scores (e.g., Framingham score)	Machine learning-based, including multifactorial risk assessment
Treatment	Guideline-based management	Personalized, dynamic, and adaptive
Patient engagement	In-person, pamphlets	Digital, interactive, tailored, and easily accessed on demand

improve the accuracy of BP measurement with automatic oscillometric BP monitors. AI-based noninvasive, automated, cuff-less BP monitors have now arrived for the clinic, offering advantages such as ease of use and improved adherence to repeated BP measurements. By using continuous, noninvasive sensing technologies—such as photoplethysmography (PPG), mechanoelectrical sensors, and piezoelectric systems—wearables such as smartwatches can collect real-time physiological data, including pulse waveforms, heart rate, and blood flow dynamics.[14-17] The ML algorithms embedded within these systems can analyze the collected signals to estimate BP values, identify trends, and generate actionable health insights.[18] Using a DL approach, Chu et al.[19] developed an AI system capable of estimating arterial BP from PPG signals. In a related study, Li et al.[20] designed a wearable device featuring a flexible piezoelectric sensor array, a dynamic pressure adjustment unit, and a sophisticated signal processing module driven by advanced ML algorithms. This device analyzed pulse waveforms and could forecast BP up to a week in advance with an error margin under 10 mm Hg. Another recent study demonstrated that ChatGPT 4.0 can effectively interpret ambulatory BP monitoring data, achieving accuracy rates of 87% for hypertension detection, 89% for identifying nocturnal hypertension, and 81% for recognizing nocturnal dipping behavior.[21] Interestingly, data obtained via ultrasound, CT, and thermal imaging have also been analyzed via AI to estimate BP. Luo et al.[22] used an ML model to predict systolic and diastolic BP based on hemoglobin signals obtained through transdermal optical imaging with a smartphone camera, achieving 94.8% and 95.8% accuracy, respectively.

Beyond such hardware, AI also forms the basis of mobile health (mHealth) platforms that integrate data from wearable devices, electronic health records (EHRs), and patient-reported outcomes. Through these systems, users can self-monitor their BP, receive automated alerts for hypertensive episodes, and access personalized health recommendations.[16] For instance, some AI models can notify the patient (and, when integrated with clinical systems, alert healthcare providers) when a potentially dangerous BP spike is detected, thus facilitating timely intervention and reducing the risk of acute adverse cardiovascular events.[23] In the future, continued advancements in sensor design, signal processing algorithms, and clinical validation will be crucial for incorporating these tools into routine hypertension management in clinical practice.

RISK PREDICTION AND DETECTION OF HYPERTENSION

Artificial intelligence-based technologies are often superior to traditional statistical approaches in handling large amounts of complex, multidimensional data. Thus, they are emerging as vital tools for individual-level risk assessment and population-level surveillance.[24]

Contemporary ML models for hypertension risk stratification incorporate diverse data sources, including demographic information, clinical measurements, genetic profiles, behavioral patterns, and environmental exposures, frequently showing enhanced predictive performance compared to conventional models. For instance, one study utilizing health check-up data and the Light Gradient Boosting Machine (LightGBM) algorithm demonstrated that variables such as age, triglyceride levels, and alkaline phosphatase levels are key predictors of hypertension, achieving high predictive accuracy.[25,26] In a related study, Liao et al.[27] designed a predictive model for hypertension and hyperlipidemia utilizing data from electronic medical records (EMRs). Similarly, Sau et al.[28] trained the AIRE-HTN algorithm using over 1.1 million electrocardiogram (ECG) recordings from approximately 190,000 individuals. This algorithm could forecast the onset of hypertension as well as associated cardiovascular and kidney-related risks based solely on ECG data, enabling earlier medical interventions and mitigating future health complications. Notably, some modern AI systems that combine genetic data with imaging and clinical information have also been found to estimate 10-year cardiovascular risk more accurately than traditional risk scoring methods.[29] Such ML models have demonstrated success in predicting the onset of hypertension within 1 year in normotensive populations, enabling proactive interventions for high-risk individuals.[30] Additionally, interactive web-based risk prediction tools, powered by ML and interpretability features such as Shapley Additive Explanations (SHAP), support shared decision-making by making risk assessments understandable and actionable for both clinicians and patients.[25]

At the population level, AI enables comprehensive epidemiological modeling and forecasting. By analyzing large-scale datasets—such as EHRs, national health surveys, registries, and biobank data—ML can automate risk screening, monitor disease prevalence, and project future hypertension trends.[31] For instance, Zhao et al.[32] showed that various ML algorithms can successfully predict the risk of incident hypertension in sample populations, even in the absence of detailed clinical and genetic variables. Such insights could support strategic public health planning, enabling more efficient resource allocation and targeted interventions.[26,33,34]

Finally, the predictive powers of AI can also be used to uncover novel genetic markers and environmental risk factors associated with hypertension. By integrating multi-omics data with environmental and lifestyle variables, DL models can uncover previously unrecognized biomarkers and causal pathways.[18] Notably, Hrytsenko et al. developed nonlinear ML prediction models to detect the risk of hypertension using demographic and clinical variables and polygenic risk scores (PRSs).[35] These capabilities provide deeper insights into hypertension pathophysiology and pave the way for precision prevention strategies.[18]

PHENOTYPING OF HYPERTENSION

Artificial intelligence is enabling the improved diagnosis and phenotyping of hypertension by leveraging large-scale health data and advanced pattern recognition techniques to deliver faster, more accurate, and individualized assessments. Using EHR-derived clinical data, ML models such as neural networks and decision trees have demonstrated diagnostic accuracies of up to 95% for early hypertension detection.[36,37] These models excel at identifying subtle patterns and trends across large, heterogeneous datasets, often revealing associations that may be missed through conventional clinical wisdom. Therefore, AI can support more objective and timely diagnoses, particularly in primary care and high-volume clinical settings.[36,37]

Imaging and Detection of Target Organ Damage

Deep learning models are capable of interpreting a variety of inputs from imaginal modalities—such as retinal scans, ECG, and vascular imaging—to detect hypertensive target organ damage. This includes the early identification of complications such as left ventricular hypertrophy, retinal microvascular changes, and vascular remodeling.[23] A recent systematic review demonstrated that AI-based retinal image analysis can enable the early detection and grading of hypertensive retinopathy, offering higher accuracy, consistency, and potential for earlier clinical intervention than manual evaluation.[38]

Differentiating Primary and Secondary Hypertension

Accurately distinguishing between primary (essential) and secondary hypertension remains challenging for clinicians. Drawing on high-dimensional datasets—including laboratory results, imaging studies, genetic profiles, and longitudinal patient histories—AI models can identify patterns indicative of secondary hypertension in hypertensive individuals.[2,39] In 2021, researchers developed a two-stage DL framework that uses natural language processing (NLP) to analyze clinician notes and integrates structured laboratory data to diagnose common causes of secondary hypertension, such as primary aldosteronism, thyroid disease, nephritis/nephrotic syndrome, and aortic stenosis.[40] Meanwhile, an XGBoost-based model tested on retrospective EMR data also exhibited excellent discrimination capacity in predicting secondary hypertension caused by renovascular hypertension, primary aldosteronism, thyroid dysfunction, and aortic stenosis.[41] By automating the rapid and accurate differential diagnosis of secondary hypertension, such models could facilitate clinical decision-making and targeted BP management.

ARTIFICIAL INTELLIGENCE-DRIVEN PRECISION MEDICINE AND THERAPEUTIC OPTIMIZATION

Precision hypertension treatment can be achieved by customizing therapeutic strategies based on the individual genetic, clinical, and lifestyle characteristics of each patient. Unlike traditional, standardized treatment, precision medicine acknowledges the complex interactions between genetic predispositions, environmental exposures, and behavioral factors, which influence both hypertension onset and patient-specific therapeutic responses. AI can realize this vision and support individualized care decisions by processing vast, multimodal datasets.[42,43]

Personalized Antihypertensive Therapy

Artificial intelligence technologies, particularly ML models, enable the personalization of antihypertensive treatment by optimizing drug selection, dosage, and predicting treatment efficacy.[44] These models recommend tailored therapeutic regimens based on patient-specific inputs such as medical history, genetic profiles, comorbidities, and prior treatment outcomes to maximize clinical benefits while minimizing the risk of adverse effects and drug interactions.[18,43] The PRECISION model, developed using data from the SPRINT and ACCORD BP trials, assesses 59 variables including kidney function and comorbidities to personalize treatment targets and identify individuals who could benefit most from intensive BP lowering.[45] Meanwhile, a LASSO-based ML model forecasts individual BP responses to different antihypertensive medications, enabling rational drug selection.[46]

Beyond initial therapy recommendations, AI systems can also adapt treatment plans dynamically in response to evolving clinical trajectories. Some AI models can detect early deviations from expected treatment responses and suggest timely adjustments.[18,43] In fact, ML models have been deployed to forecast patient trajectories and proactively adjust treatment plans before clinical deterioration.[18] A reinforcement learning model trained on over 11 years of EHR data was found to accurately predict the need for transitioning from mono- to dual or triple therapy in hypertensive individuals with type 2 diabetes, supporting the shift toward anticipatory care.[47]

Integration with Omics Technologies

A major advancement in hypertension care is the integration of AI with omics technologies such as genomics, proteomics, and metabolomics. AI algorithms can identify genetic variants or molecular signatures associated with drug responses, side effects, and resistance, thus enabling refined risk stratification and the selection of targeted therapies.[2,18,43] When applied to multi-omics datasets, ML can reveal disease mechanisms and potential therapeutic targets, enabling the development of integrated systems biology frameworks.[48] Such AI-based systems biology approaches can uncover previously unknown molecular networks and causal genotype–phenotype–environment interactions, enabling biomarker-driven interventions.[49] By combining multi-omics data, AI can identify rare monogenic forms of hypertension and deepen our understanding of polygenic hypertension, in which numerous genetic loci interact with environmental and behavioral factors.[12,24] Studies are combining PRS with clinical and microbiome parameters to improve hypertension risk prediction on an individual level beyond genetics alone.[50] Such integrated approaches could facilitate a more precise and biologically informed, lucid classification of hypertension. By aligning therapy with the unique characteristics of each patient and adapting care over time, AI-driven precision medicine could support the proactive and personalized management of hypertension across the disease continuum.[24]

PATIENT ENGAGEMENT, ADHERENCE, AND BEHAVIORAL MODIFICATION

In addition to direct use by clinicians, AI can also help patients by improving engagement and facilitating behavioral modifications. Today, AI-powered chatbots and virtual assistants can deliver real-time, personalized support and education for hypertension patients, providing instant responses to common questions, customized information on hypertension management, and timely reminders for medication intake and BP monitoring.[12,24] By leveraging NLP and ML, such platforms could understand user intent, adapt to individual communication styles, and respond empathetically, thereby improving patient satisfaction, trust, and engagement.[24,51] Thus, healthcare providers and patients can become copartners in disease prevention and treatment.

Integration with mHealth and Lifestyle Interventions

Integrating AI technologies with mHealth and telehealth platforms is a valuable way to offer personalized lifestyle guidance. By analyzing real-time data from wearable devices, EHRs, and self-reported behaviors, AI systems can generate tailored recommendations on dietary habits, physical activity, sleep quality, and stress management based on patient-specific risk profiles. In a cohort of hypertensive adults managed over 24 weeks, a fully autonomous AI-driven lifestyle coaching platform that delivered such personalized guidance led to average reductions of approximately 8.1 and 5.1 mm Hg in systolic and diastolic BP, respectively.[52] Such platforms could allow patients to exert control of their own health status, eliminating the need for continuous clinician involvement.

Improvement of Medication Adherence and Empowerment

Artificial intelligence technologies can also enhance medication adherence and promote patient self-efficacy.[53,54] Automated reminders, educational messaging, and interactive interfaces help patients consistently follow their prescribed medication regimens and recommended lifestyle changes. AI-powered platforms can provide users with feedback on their progress, including BP control trends, reinforcing motivation, and encouraging sustained behavioral changes.[53] One digital intervention combining tailored text messaging and interactive voice messaging for hypertension patients achieved high user engagement over a 12-week period, with participants reporting improved awareness and motivation to take their medications.[55] A recent meta-analysis of 74 randomized controlled trials (covering >92,000 patients) found that mHealth interventions significantly improved medication adherence in hypertension, contributing to better BP control.[56] These studies show that through intelligent automation and data-driven personalization, AI can empower patients to take a proactive role in managing their condition, ultimately improving health outcomes.

CHALLENGES AND LIMITATIONS

Despite the immense potential of AI, its clinical integration is hindered by some critical challenges.[57] The first technical barrier is related to the limited availability of large, well-annotated, and representative datasets for training AI models, which can compromise model accuracy.[45] Additionally, AI models remain prone to overfitting (perform well on training data but poorly on new data) and underfitting (are too simple to capture key patterns).[29] Importantly, most complex algorithms have a "black box" nature and suffer from a lack of transparency because users cannot see their internal workings or how they arrive at their predictions or decisions, which undermines trust among clinicians and patients. Operational integration into clinical workflows also poses a major challenge, since several AI tools cannot be incorporated easily into EMR systems due to interoperability issues and the lack of universal data standards.[57]

From an ethical perspective, the use of AI in medicine raises concerns about patient privacy, informed consent, and data security. Legal uncertainties also persist, particularly around liability and accountability when AI systems influence medical decisions. Equity is another critical concern, since AI tools may perform poorly in marginalized populations if they are not trained on diverse datasets and thereby perpetuate health disparities and gaps in care. Finally, regulatory guidelines for AI in healthcare are still evolving, and tools such as AI-powered BP monitors still need to be standardized and validated in real-world settings.[57] Finally, questions arise regarding who is the custodian of medical records—AI technology, healthcare providers, or patients?

FUTURE DIRECTIONS AND RESEARCH PRIORITIES

As AI continues to evolve, its role in hypertension management will expand.[58] To fully harness the potential of AI in hypertension management, multidisciplinary collaboration, transparent algorithm design, equitable access, and strong regulatory structures will be essential. One key priority is the development of explainable AI tools, such as SHAP, which will help clarify how AI models generate their outputs.[12] For the long-term success of AI systems, we need a roadmap for responsible and equitable deployment, ensuring data quality, reproducibility, algorithmic transparency, and ethical oversight. Therefore, it is essential to train models and validate them in diverse populations. Additionally, we must focus on the integration of multimodal data, including clinical records, genetic information, imaging data, and wearable sensor outputs, as this could enable better risk prediction, the identification of new hypertension subtypes, and deeper insights into disease mechanisms. Institutions can collaborate to train models without sharing raw data, preserving patient confidentiality and data ownership. Further, prospective clinical trials and real-world validation studies must be conducted to determine how AI tools perform in diverse, real-life settings and identify barriers to clinical integration. Collaborative intelligence, where AI supports healthcare practitioners instead of replacing them, could help in enhancing diagnostic accuracy, streamlining workflows, and improving patient education. Active collaboration among clinicians, patients, technologists, and policymakers is needed to drive these efforts **(Fig. 2)**.[59,60]

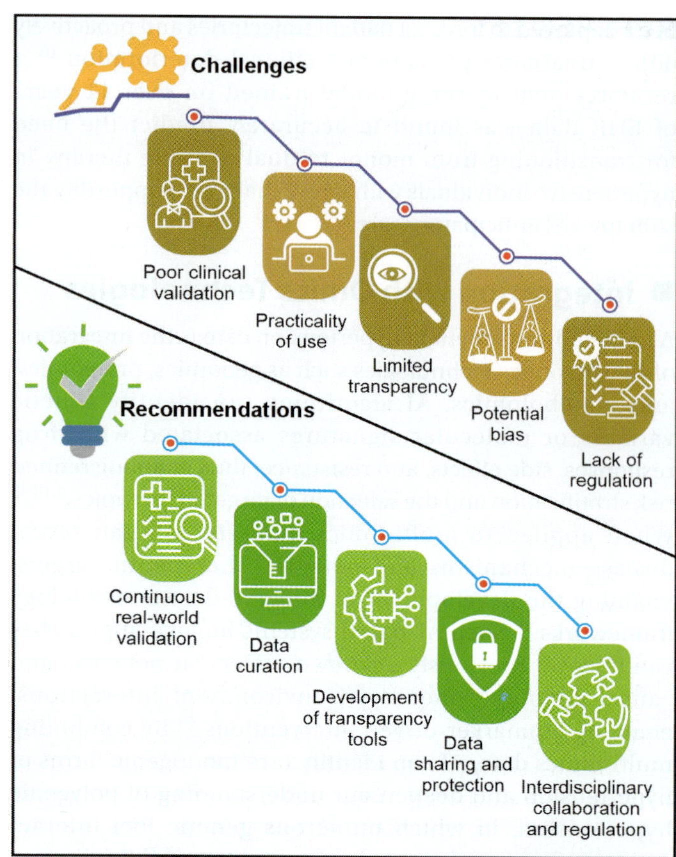

FIG. 2: Challenges and best practices for the application of AI in hypertension management.

CONCLUSION

Artificial intelligence is revolutionizing hypertension management through personalized, data-driven strategies that surpass traditional treatment approaches. Through advanced ML and DL algorithms and large-scale data integration, AI can facilitate hypertension risk prediction, early diagnosis, continuous monitoring, and individualized therapy, improving BP control and patient outcomes. Clinicians can leverage AI-powered decision-making tools that enhance diagnostic precision and optimize treatment plans based on patient-specific factors. As digital health technologies advance, AI can bridge care gaps at both the individual and population levels, supporting precision medicine and improving hypertension outcomes for millions globally. Continued collaboration among healthcare providers, data scientists, patients, and regulatory bodies will be essential to align AI tools with evolving clinical needs. Yes, AI is rapidly reshaping our lives. However, it cannot completely replace human traits—compassion and empathy—which are the two legs of medical care. AI may also inspire the medical practitioners to live and work for a deeper purpose and fulfillment. Interestingly, AI technologies actually enhance empathetic awareness and moral foundations of health care; however, such qualities are best translated directly by the medical community.

ACKNOWLEDGMENT

The author thanks Ms Zeba Sohel Khatri for her immense assistance in proofreading the manuscript, editing, and in the references verification process.

REFERENCES

1. Mills KT, Stefanescu A, He J. The global epidemiology of hypertension. Nat Rev Nephrol. 2020;16(4):223-37.
2. Chaikijurajai T, Laffin LJ, Tang WHW. Artificial Intelligence and Hypertension: Recent Advances and Future Outlook. Am J Hypertens. 2020;33(11):967-74.
3. Kario K, Okura A, Hoshide S, et al. The WHO Global report 2023 on hypertension warning the emerging hypertension burden in globe and its treatment strategy. Hypertens Res. 2024;47(5):1099-102.
4. Kario K. Management of Hypertension in the Digital Era: Small Wearable Monitoring Devices for Remote Blood Pressure Monitoring. Hypertension. 2020;76(3):640-50.
5. Zhou X, Zhang X, Gu N, et al. Barriers and Facilitators of Medication Adherence in Hypertension Patients: A Meta-Integration of Qualitative Research. J Patient Exp. 2024;11:23743735241241176.
6. Parati G, Lombardi C, Pengo M, et al. Current challenges for hypertension management: From better hypertension diagnosis to improved patients' adherence and blood pressure control. Int J Cardiol. 2021;331:262-9.
7. Mohsen F, Ali H, El Jahh N, et al. Artificial intelligence-based methods for fusion of electronic health records and imaging data. Sci Rep. 2022;12:17981.
8. Yu P, Xu H, Hu X, et al. Leveraging Generative AI and Large Language Models: A Comprehensive Roadmap for Healthcare Integration. Healthcare (Basel). 2023;11(20):2776.
9. Layton AT. AI, Machine Learning, and ChatGPT in Hypertension. Hypertension. 2024;81(4):709-16.
10. Cai A, Zhu Y, Clarkson SA, et al. The Use of Machine Learning for the Care of Hypertension and Heart Failure. JACC Asia. 2021;1(2):162-72.
11. Karnik A, Yang E. Artificial Intelligence to Improve Blood Pressure Control: A State-of-the-Art Review. Am J Hypertens. 2025;38(8):519-26.
12. Armoundas AA, Ahmad FS, Attia ZI, et al. Controversy in Hypertension: Pro-Side of the Argument Using Artificial Intelligence for Hypertension Diagnosis and Management. Hypertension. 2025;82(6):929-44.
13. Mizuno H, Choi E, Kario K, et al. Diagnostic Accuracy of Office Blood Pressure Measurement and Home Blood Pressure Monitoring for Hypertension Screening Among Adults: Results From the IDH Study. J Am Heart Assoc. 2023;12(24):e030150.
14. Manga S, Muthavarapu N, Redij R, et al. Estimation of Physiologic Pressures: Invasive and Non-Invasive Techniques, AI Models, and Future Perspectives. Sensors (Basel). 2023;23(12):5744.
15. Tan P, Xi Y, Chao S, et al. An Artificial Intelligence-Enhanced Blood Pressure Monitor Wristband Based on Piezoelectric Nanogenerator. Biosensors (Basel). 2022;12(4):234.
16. Sinou N, Sinou N, Koutroulakis S, et al. The Role of Wearable Devices in Blood Pressure Monitoring and Hypertension Management: A Systematic Review. Cureus. 2024;16(12):e75050.
17. Tsoi K, Yiu K, Lee H, et al. Applications of artificial intelligence for hypertension management. J Clin Hypertens (Greenwich). 2021;23(3):568-74.
18. Visco V, Izzo C, Mancusi C, et al. Artificial Intelligence in Hypertension Management: An Ace up Your Sleeve. J Cardiovasc Dev Dis. 2023;10(2):74.
19. Chu Y, Tang K, Hsu YC, et al. Non-invasive arterial blood pressure measurement and SpO2 estimation using PPG signal: a deep learning framework. BMC Med Inform Decis Mak. 2023;23:131.
20. Li J, Jia H, Zhou J, et al. Thin, soft, wearable system for continuous wireless monitoring of artery blood pressure. Nat Commun. 2023;14:5009.
21. Alam SF, Thongprayoon C, Miao J, et al. Advancing personalized medicine in digital health: The role of artificial intelligence in enhancing clinical interpretation of 24-h ambulatory blood pressure monitoring. Digit Health. 2025;11:20552076251326014.
22. Luo H, Yang D, Barszczyk A, et al. Smartphone-based blood pressure measurement using transdermal optical imaging technology. Circ Cardiovasc Imaging. 2019;12(8):e008857.
23. Alam SF, Gonzalez Suarez ML. Transforming Healthcare: The AI Revolution in the Comprehensive Care of Hypertension. Clin Pract. 2024;14(4):1357-74.
24. Dzau VJ, Hodgkinson CP. Precision Hypertension. Hypertension. 2024;81(4):702-8.
25. Du J, Chang X, Ye C, et al. Developing a hypertension visualization risk prediction system utilizing machine learning and health check-up data. Sci Rep. 2023;13:18953.
26. Islam SMS, Talukder A, Awal MA, et al. Machine Learning Approaches for Predicting Hypertension and Its Associated Factors Using Population-Level Data From Three South Asian Countries. Front Cardiovasc Med. 2022;9:839379.
27. Liao B, Jia X, Zhang T, et al. DHDIP: An interpretable model for hypertension and hyperlipidemia prediction based on EMR data. Comput Methods Programs Biomed. 2022;226:107088.
28. Sau A, Barker J, Pastika L, et al. Artificial Intelligence-Enhanced Electrocardiography for Prediction of Incident Hypertension. JAMA Cardiol. 2025;10(3):214-23.
29. Cho JS, Park JH. Application of artificial intelligence in hypertension. Clin Hypertens. 2024;30(1):11.
30. Kanegae H, Suzuki K, Fukatani K, et al. Highly precise risk prediction model for new-onset hypertension using artificial intelligence techniques. J Clin Hypertens (Greenwich). 2020;22(3):445-50.
31. Chen S, Yu J, Chamouni S, et al. Integrating machine learning and artificial intelligence in life-course epidemiology: pathways to innovative public health solutions. BMC Med. 2024;22:354.
32. Zhao H, Zhang X, Xu Y, et al. Predicting the Risk of Hypertension Based on Several Easy-to-Collect Risk Factors: A Machine Learning Method. Front Public Health. 2021;9:619429.
33. Naik A, Nalepa J, Wijata AM, et al. Artificial intelligence and digital twins for the personalised prediction of hypertension risk. Comput Biol Med. 2025;196(Pt A):110718.
34. Khamissi FZ, Sun L, Johnson P, et al. Machine Learning and Artificial Intelligence for Research on Hypertension. Am J Hypertens. 2025;38(11):867-71.
35. Hrytsenko Y, Shea B, Elgart M, et al. Machine learning models for predicting blood pressure phenotypes by combining multiple polygenic risk scores. Sci Rep. 2024;14:12436.
36. Gudigar A, Kadri NA, Raghavendra U, et al. Automatic identification of hypertension and assessment of its secondary effects using artificial intelligence: A systematic review (2013-2023). Comput Biol Med. 2024;172:108207.
37. Datta S, Morassi Sasso A, Kiwit N, et al. Predicting hypertension onset from longitudinal electronic health records with deep learning. JAMIA Open. 2022;5(4):ooac097.
38. Kankrale R, Kokare M. Artificial intelligence in retinal image analysis for hypertensive retinopathy diagnosis: a comprehensive review and perspective. Vis Comput Ind Biomed Art. 2025;8:11.
39. Adeleke O, Adebayo S, Aworinde H, et al. Machine learning evaluation of a hypertension screening program in a university workforce over five years. Sci Rep. 2024;14:30255.
40. Wu L, Huang L, Li M, et al. Differential diagnosis of secondary hypertension based on deep learning. Artif Intell Med. 2023;141:102554.

41. Diao X, Huo Y, Yan Z, et al. An Application of Machine Learning to Etiological Diagnosis of Secondary Hypertension: Retrospective Study Using Electronic Medical Records. JMIR Med Inform. 2021;9(1):e19739.
42. Sethi Y, Patel N, Kaka N, et al. Precision Medicine and the future of Cardiovascular Diseases: A Clinically Oriented Comprehensive Review. J Clin Med. 2023;12(5):1799.
43. Layton A. A Heart-to-heart with ChatGPT: AI Applications in Hypertension. Am J Hypertens. 2025 ;38(9):621-7.
44. Khude H, Shende P. AI-driven clinical decision support systems: Revolutionizing medication selection and personalized drug therapy. Adv Integrative Med. 2025;12(4):100529.
45. Shimbo D, Shah RU, Abdalla M, et al. Transforming Hypertension Diagnosis and Management in The Era of Artificial Intelligence: A 2023 National Heart, Lung, and Blood Institute (NHLBI) Workshop Report. Hypertension. 2025;82(1):36-45.
46. Yi J, Wang L, Song J, et al. Development of a machine learning-based model for predicting individual responses to antihypertensive treatments. Nutr Metab Cardiovasc Dis. 2024;34(7):1660-9.
47. Oh SH, Lee SJ, Park J. Precision Medicine for Hypertension Patients with Type 2 Diabetes via Reinforcement Learning. J Pers Med. 2022;12(1):87.
48. Lin M, Guo J, Gu Z, et al. Machine learning and multi-omics integration: advancing cardiovascular translational research and clinical practice. J Transl Med. 2025;23(1):388.
49. Wu Y, Xie L. AI-driven multi-omics integration for multi-scale predictive modeling of genotype-environment-phenotype relationships. Comput Struct Biotechnol J. 2025;27:265-77. [Erratum in: Comput Struct Biotechnol J. 2025;27:1089.]
50. Aryal S, Manandhar I, Mei X, et al. Combating hypertension beyond genome-wide association studies: Microbiome and artificial intelligence as opportunities for precision medicine. Camb Prism Precis Med. 2023;1:e26.
51. Hare AJ, Chokshi N, Adusumalli S. Novel Digital Technologies for Blood Pressure Monitoring and Hypertension Management. Curr Cardiovasc Risk Rep. 2021;15:11.
52. Leitner J, Chiang PH, Agnihotri P, et al. The Effect of an AI-Based, Autonomous, Digital Health Intervention Using Precise Lifestyle Guidance on Blood Pressure in Adults With Hypertension: Single-Arm Nonrandomized Trial. JMIR Cardio. 2024;8:e51916.
53. Funes Hernandez M, Babakhanian M, Chen TP, et al. Design and Implementation of an Electronic Health Record-Integrated Hypertension Management Application. J Am Heart Assoc. 2024;13(2):e030884.
54. Korb-Savoldelli V, Tran Y, Perrin G, et al. Psychometric Properties of a Machine Learning–Based Patient-Reported Outcome Measure on Medication Adherence: Single-Center, Cross-Sectional, Observational Study. J Med Internet Res. 2023;25:e42384.
55. Kassavou A, Mirzaei V, Brimicombe J, et al. A Highly Tailored Text and Voice Messaging Intervention to Improve Medication Adherence in Patients With Either or Both Hypertension and Type 2 Diabetes in a UK Primary Care Setting: Feasibility Randomized Controlled Trial of Clinical Effectiveness. J Med Internet Res. 2020;22(5):e16629.
56. Yap HJ, Lim JJJ, Tan SD, et al. Effectiveness of digital health interventions on adherence and control of hypertension: a systematic review and meta-analysis. J Hypertens. 2024;42(9):1490-504.
57. Padmanabhan S, Tran TQB, Dominiczak AF. Artificial Intelligence in Hypertension: Seeing Through a Glass Darkly. Circ Res. 2021;128(7):1100-18.
58. Amaratunga D, Cabrera J, Sargsyan D, et al. Uses and opportunities for machine learning in hypertension research. Int J Cardiol Hypertension. 2020;5:100027.
59. El-Geneedy M, El-Din Moustafa H, Khater H, et al. A comprehensive explainable AI approach for enhancing transparency and interpretability in stroke prediction. Sci Rep. 2025;15(1):26048.
60. Mueller FB. AI (Artificial Intelligence) and Hypertension Research. Curr Hypertens Rep. 2020;22(9):70.

CHAPTER 7

Clinical Management of Primary Aldosteronism

Dharmendra Jain, Vikash Kumar Maurya, Pratap Kumar

ABSTRACT

Primary aldosteronism (PA) is the most prevalent cause of secondary hypertension and is associated with increased cardiovascular and renal morbidity. Early detection and appropriate clinical management can lead to significant outcomes, including hypertension resolution and reduced organ damage. Recent guidelines and trials have refined diagnostic algorithms, expanded indications for adrenal venous sampling (AVS), and optimized surgical and pharmacologic therapies. This chapter offers a comprehensive update on the clinical approach to PA, including screening protocols, biochemical confirmation, subtype differentiation, and tailored treatment strategies, integrating evidence from recent studies and expert consensus.

Keywords: Primary aldosteronism, secondary hypertension, adrenal vein sampling, spironolactone, adrenalectomy.

INTRODUCTION

Primary aldosteronism (PA), once considered a rare endocrine disorder, is now recognized as the most common form of secondary hypertension, with a prevalence ranging from 5 to 10% in the general hypertensive population and up to 20% among those with resistant hypertension,[1,2] It is characterized by autonomous aldosterone secretion, leading to sodium retention, potassium wasting, and suppression of plasma renin activity. If left undiagnosed or untreated, PA is associated with significantly increased risks of cardiovascular events, atrial fibrillation, stroke, chronic kidney disease, and all-cause mortality—risks that are disproportionate to the degree of hypertension alone.[3]

Advances in diagnostic strategies over the past decade, particularly the refinement of the aldosterone-to-renin ratio (ARR) as a screening tool, have made early detection more accessible and accurate. The current paradigm emphasizes the importance of subtype differentiation—between unilateral aldosterone-producing adenoma (APA) and bilateral adrenal hyperplasia (BAH)—which critically determines therapeutic pathways, including the decision between surgical adrenalectomy and medical therapy.[4] Adrenal vein sampling (AVS) remains the gold standard for subtyping, although recent innovations such as steroid profiling and molecular imaging may soon transform diagnostic workflows.[5]

Guidelines from international societies continue to evolve, incorporating emerging genetic insights, updated criteria for confirmatory testing, and individualized approaches to long-term follow-up. The clinical relevance of diagnosing and treating PA has been strengthened by growing evidence demonstrating improved cardiovascular and renal outcomes following appropriate management.[6] This chapter provides an updated, comprehensive overview of the clinical evaluation, diagnosis, and management of PA, with emphasis on practical implementation and current best practices in endocrinology and hypertension care.

CLINICAL EVALUATION AND SCREENING

Effective screening for PA is crucial, as timely diagnosis enables curative or disease-modifying interventions. Clinical evaluation begins with identifying at-risk individuals. Current guidelines suggest that all individuals with hypertension be screened for PA by measuring aldosterone and renin and determining the aldosterone to renin ratio, and that subsequent clinical care be guided by the results.[7] The recommended diagnostic workup remains overly complex, potentially delaying or denying curative treatment for many patients. The guidelines advocate for confirmatory testing and AVS in most cases to distinguish between unilateral and bilateral PA. This process, while thorough, is resource-intensive, requires specialized expertise, and is not universally accessible, particularly in rural or underserved regions. In resource-limited settings, screening should be prioritized in patients with resistant hypertension, hypertension with spontaneous or diuretic-induced hypokalemia, hypertension with adrenal incidentalomas, or early-onset hypertension, particularly if accompanied by a family history of early-onset hypertension or stroke **(Table 1)**. Additionally, patients with atrial fibrillation and no other identifiable cause should be evaluated, as PA may be a hidden contributor.[8]

The preferred initial screening test is the *plasma ARR*, a sensitive and cost-effective method for detecting autonomous aldosterone secretion. Elevated ARR values, particularly when paired with a high plasma aldosterone concentration (>10 ng/dL) and suppressed renin, are suggestive of PA. However, false positives can occur, especially under conditions such as low sodium intake or interfering medications.[9] Therefore, clinicians are advised to manage antihypertensive medications carefully—preferably switching to agents with minimal impact on ARR, such as verapamil or hydralazine—at least two weeks prior to testing.[10]

Recent studies have improved our understanding of factors influencing ARR interpretation. For instance, older adults and patients with chronic kidney disease may have altered baseline renin levels, which can skew results.[11] Additionally, time of day, posture, and dietary sodium can impact the accuracy of the ARR. A standard approach involves obtaining the blood sample in the morning after patients have been ambulant for at least 2 hours and seated for 5–15 minutes.

In populations with high prevalence of hypertension and limited access to AVS, repeated ARR testing and confirmatory protocols (e.g., saline suppression) may be relied upon for diagnosis. Proper screening thus serves as the foundation for targeted subtype classification and eventual treatment strategy.

CONFIRMATORY TESTING

Following an elevated ARR, confirmatory testing is essential to establish the diagnosis of PA and exclude false positives. These tests aim to assess whether aldosterone secretion is truly autonomous and not suppressed by physiological cues such as sodium loading or ACE inhibition **(Table 2)**. Among the commonly used tests, the saline infusion test (SIT) is often preferred due to its balance of accuracy and practicality. A postinfusion plasma aldosterone concentration >10 ng/dL suggests PA. The captopril challenge test (CCT) is simpler and suitable in outpatient settings. The fludrocortisone suppression test (FST) remains the most sensitive but is labor-intensive and less widely available.[12] Recent studies have highlighted that confirmatory tests may be omitted in select high-risk patients, such as those with spontaneous hypokalemia, PAC > 20 ng/dL, and suppressed renin, particularly when AVS is planned.[13] Standardizing test protocols improves diagnostic yield and minimizes variability.[14]

Subtype Differentiation

Once the diagnosis of PA is confirmed, the next critical step is to determine whether the condition is due to unilateral aldosterone excess—most commonly an APA—or BAH. Subtype differentiation is essential, because it guides treatment decisions: Unilateral disease is potentially curable with adrenalectomy, while bilateral disease is best

TABLE 1: Indications for screening for primary aldosteronism (PA) in high-risk groups to facilitate early diagnosis and appropriate management.

Clinical scenario	Rationale for screening
Resistant hypertension	High prevalence of PA among patients requiring ≥3 antihypertensives
Hypertension with hypokalemia	Suggests mineralocorticoid excess, particularly when spontaneous or diuretic-induced
Adrenal incidentalomas	May represent aldosterone-producing adenomas even in normotensive individuals
First-degree relatives of patients with PA	Genetic forms of PA (e.g., familial hyperaldosteronism) are increasingly recognized
Early-onset hypertension (especially <40 years)	Suggests secondary hypertension; PA is a key reversible cause

TABLE 2: Confirmatory tests for primary aldosteronism.

Test	Mechanism	Key feature
Saline infusion test (SIT)	Sodium loading to suppress aldosterone	Preferred in most centers
Captopril challenge test (CCT)	Angiotensin-converting enzyme (ACE) inhibition to reduce aldosterone	Safe, outpatient-friendly
Fludrocortisone suppression test (FST)	Mimics physiologic aldosterone suppression	Most sensitive, used in complex cases

Note: These tests aim to verify autonomous aldosterone secretion after initial screening, with choice influenced by local expertise, patient tolerance, and resource availability.

managed with mineralocorticoid receptor antagonists (MRAs).[15]

Imaging (CT/MRI)

Adrenal computed tomography (CT) is often the first step to detect adrenal masses. However, its accuracy is limited, especially in patients over 35 years of age. Nonfunctioning adrenal nodules are common in this group and may be misinterpreted as the source of aldosterone excess.[16] Additionally, small APAs may be missed on imaging. Thus, reliance solely on imaging can lead to misdiagnosis and inappropriate therapy.

Adrenal Vein Sampling

Adrenal vein sampling remains the gold standard for differentiating unilateral from bilateral disease. It involves catheterizing both adrenal veins and measuring aldosterone and cortisol levels. A lateralization index (ratio of aldosterone/cortisol from one side vs. the other) >4 typically indicates unilateral aldosterone production.[17]

Although AVS is technically challenging and not universally available, it is crucial for accurate subtyping. Current guidelines recommend AVS for nearly all patients considering surgery, especially when imaging is inconclusive or bilateral nodules are present.[18]

To improve success rates, AVS is often performed under ACTH stimulation, which reduces pulsatile hormone secretion and facilitates interpretation. Novel steroid profiling methods using liquid chromatography-mass spectrometry (LC-MS) are emerging as potential noninvasive alternatives, but these remain investigational.[19]

Emerging Tools

Recent studies have explored 11C-metomidate PET-CT imaging as a functional method to localize aldosterone-producing tissue. This modality may complement AVS in specific cases but requires further validation.[20]

In select young patients (<35 years) with spontaneous hypokalemia, marked aldosterone excess, and a unilateral lesion on CT, AVS may be skipped due to high pretest probability of unilateral disease.[12]

TREATMENT

The primary goal in the treatment of PA is to normalize aldosterone levels, control blood pressure, correct hypokalemia, and mitigate cardiovascular and renal complications. Treatment depends on the underlying subtype—*unilateral disease* (typically an APA) or *BAH*—as determined by AVS **(Flowchart 1)**.

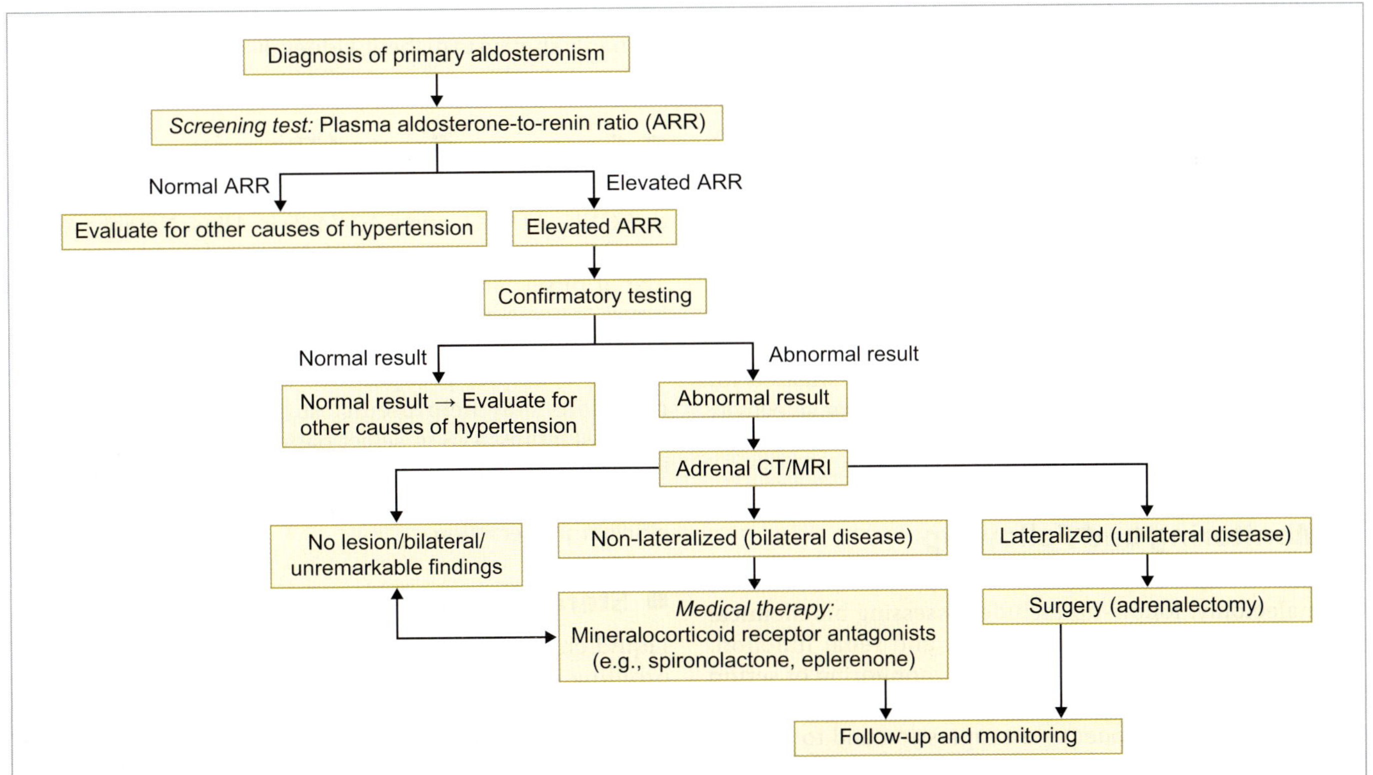

FLOWCHART 1: Diagnostic and management algorithm for primary aldosteronism (PA).

Note: Screening with the aldosterone-to-renin ratio (ARR) is followed by confirmatory testing by saline infusion test (SIT), captopril challenge test (CCT), fludrocortisone suppression test (FST), adrenal computed tomography (CT) or magnetic resonance imaging (MRI), and treatment with adrenalectomy for unilateral disease or mineralocorticoid receptor antagonists (MRAs, e.g., spironolactone and eplerenone) for bilateral or indeterminate disease.

Surgical Management

Laparoscopic adrenalectomy is the treatment of choice for patients with unilateral PA. When performed in appropriately selected patients, it offers significant clinical and biochemical success. Complete normalization of blood pressure occurs in about 30–40% of patients, while others show substantial improvement with reduced antihypertensive drug burden.[21]

Recent studies suggest that surgical intervention not only improves hypertension but also reverses target organ damage, including left ventricular hypertrophy and microalbuminuria.[22] Predictors of good surgical outcomes include younger age, shorter duration of hypertension, absence of diabetes, and fewer antihypertensive medications preoperatively.

Importantly, surgical outcomes should be evaluated using the PASO (Primary Aldosteronism Surgical Outcome) criteria, which define complete and partial clinical and biochemical success postadrenalectomy.[23]

Medical Management

Patients with BAH or those unsuitable for surgery are managed with MRAs, typically spironolactone or eplerenone.

- Spironolactone is highly effective but may cause dose-dependent side effects such as gynecomastia, menstrual irregularities, and sexual dysfunction due to its antiandrogenic properties.
- Eplerenone is more selective for the mineralocorticoid receptor and has fewer hormonal side effects but is costlier and may require higher dosing.

  Mineralocorticoid receptor antagonists reduce blood pressure and correct hypokalemia, but recent evidence emphasizes their role in reducing cardiovascular risk, including atrial fibrillation and left ventricular mass, even in the absence of overt hypokalemia.[24] Some patients may require combination therapy with other antihypertensives.

Newer agents such as esaxerenone and finerenone, which are nonsteroidal MRAs, are being investigated for use in PA. These drugs may offer greater receptor selectivity and reduced side effect profiles, although their use in PA specifically is still under clinical investigation.[25]

Monitoring and Follow-up

All patients require lifelong monitoring post-treatment. After adrenalectomy, follow-up includes assessing biochemical cure, blood pressure normalization, and renal function. In medically treated patients, regular monitoring of serum potassium, creatinine, blood pressure, and aldosterone levels is essential to ensure adequate suppression and to prevent hyperkalemia or renal impairment.

Patients should also undergo periodic cardiovascular assessment [e.g., echocardiography (ECG)] and evaluation for recurrence in case of adrenal nodular regrowth or medication noncompliance.

Individualized, subtype-directed therapy remains the cornerstone of optimal management. With proper diagnosis and treatment, patients with PA can experience significantly improved quality of life and long-term outcomes.

NEWER THERAPEUTIC INSIGHTS

While adrenalectomy and MRAs remain the mainstay of treatment in PA, several emerging therapies and precision medicine approaches are shaping the future of PA management.

Nonsteroidal Mineralocorticoid Receptor Antagonists

Traditional steroidal MRAs such as spironolactone and eplerenone, while effective, are often limited by side effects and dosing concerns. Newer nonsteroidal MRAs such as esaxerenone and finerenone have demonstrated superior selectivity and reduced off-target hormonal effects.

Esaxerenone has shown efficacy in lowering blood pressure and suppressing aldosterone-driven activity in hypertensive patients with confirmed or suspected PA. In a phase III Japanese trial, esaxerenone was not only effective but also well tolerated, offering an alternative for those who cannot tolerate spironolactone.[26] Finerenone, although primarily studied in diabetic kidney disease, is being explored for its role in aldosterone-mediated organ damage in PA.[27]

Genotype-directed Therapy

Recent advances in genomics have identified mutations such as *KCNJ5*, *ATP1A1*, and *CACNA1D* in APAs. Notably, *KCNJ5* mutations are associated with larger adenomas, younger age of onset, and better postsurgical outcomes.[28] In the future, genetic profiling could guide both the diagnosis and individualized treatment of PA.

For example, preoperative identification of *KCNJ5* mutations may help predict surgical responsiveness or justify skipping AVS in select patients.[29] Ongoing trials are investigating whether targeted pharmacologic inhibition of these mutated pathways can suppress autonomous aldosterone secretion.

Steroid Metabolite Profiling

Liquid chromatography–mass spectrometry-based steroid profiling of plasma or urine can potentially differentiate between unilateral and bilateral forms of PA. Profiling specific aldosterone precursors and metabolites like 18-oxocortisol and 18-hydroxycortisol shows promise as a noninvasive adjunct or alternative to AVS.[30] While not yet standardized, this could reduce the need for invasive testing in the future.

Molecular Imaging

11C-metomidate PET-CT is an emerging imaging technique targeting CYP11B2, the enzyme responsible for aldosterone synthesis. It enables functional localization of aldosterone-producing tissue and may complement or even replace AVS in certain patients.[31] However, high cost and limited availability currently restrict its widespread use.

LONG-TERM MONITORING AND OUTCOMES

Long-term monitoring in patients with PA is essential to ensure sustained therapeutic efficacy, prevent recurrence, and mitigate cardiovascular and renal complications. Monitoring strategies differ slightly based on whether the patient underwent surgical adrenalectomy or is managed medically with MRAs.

Post-adrenalectomy Monitoring

Patients who undergo unilateral adrenalectomy should be evaluated for biochemical and clinical cure using the PASO criteria, including normalization of blood pressure and plasma aldosterone levels without medication. Blood pressure, serum potassium, and estimated glomerular filtration rate (eGFR) should be assessed every 3–6 months during the first year and annually thereafter.[32] Periodic assessment for contralateral adrenal compensation or recurrence is recommended, especially if hypertension returns.[33]

Renal function may transiently decline postoperatively due to correction of glomerular hyperfiltration, but this typically stabilizes. Patients with persistent hypertension despite biochemical cure may benefit from ongoing antihypertensive therapy and cardiovascular risk management.[34]

Medical Therapy Follow-up

Patients treated with MRAs require lifelong follow-up to monitor blood pressure, serum potassium, renal function, and signs of under- or overtreatment. Dose adjustments are frequently necessary, especially in the elderly or those with chronic kidney disease. Patients should be monitored every 3–4 months during the first year and then semiannually.[7]

Repeat ARR or plasma aldosterone measurements may help assess treatment adequacy, particularly if symptoms or hypertension persist. Cardiovascular evaluations, including echocardiography and electrocardiography, are advised at regular intervals to track reverse remodeling and rhythm abnormalities.[6]

Appropriate and consistent follow-up reduces long-term risks of stroke, myocardial infarction, atrial fibrillation, and end-stage renal disease, which are otherwise elevated in untreated PA patients.

CONCLUSION

Primary aldosteronism has outgrown its historical label as a "rare zebra" and galloped into the mainstream of secondary hypertension. With a prevalence rivaling type 2 diabetes in specific subgroups and an outsized impact on cardiovascular and renal outcomes, PA demands vigilance, precision, and timely intervention.

The modern clinician now has an expanding toolkit: Sensitive screening with the ARR, nuanced confirmatory tests, gold-standard AVS, and increasingly precise imaging and molecular diagnostics. Treatment, too, has evolved—from a binary choice between surgery and spironolactone to a spectrum that includes genotype-guided strategies, selective MRAs, and even targeted imaging.

However, the core principle remains unchanged: Diagnosing PA early and treating it appropriately alters lives—lowering blood pressure, reversing cardiac hypertrophy, preserving renal function, and preventing strokes. In a field where misdiagnosis can lead to decades of unnecessary pill-burden and end-organ damage, PA stands as both a challenge and an opportunity for curative care. As we enter an era of endocrine precision medicine, managing PA is no longer about controlling numbers—it is about unmasking a silent saboteur, restoring hormonal harmony, and ultimately giving patients their cardiovascular future back. A small gland, perhaps—but with mighty consequences.

REFERENCES

1. Wrenn SM, Vaidya A, Lubitz CC. Primary aldosteronism. Gland Surg. 2020;9(1):14.
2. Reincke M, Bancos I, Mulatero P, et al. Diagnosis and treatment of primary aldosteronism. Lancet Diabetes Endocrinol. 2021;9(12): 876-92.
3. Georgios M. (2018). Hypertension, Atrial Fibrillation and Aldosteronism-A study of interplay, predictors and outcome. [online] Available from https://gupea.ub.gu.se/handle/2077/54954?show=full [Last accessed October, 2025].
4. Wu VC, Chueh SC, Chang HW, et al. Bilateral aldosterone-producing adenomas: differentiation from bilateral adrenal hyperplasia. QJM. 2008;101(1):13-22.
5. Buffolo F, Monticone S, Williams TA, et al. Subtype diagnosis of primary aldosteronism: is adrenal vein sampling always necessary?. Int J Mol Sci. 2017;18(4):848.
6. Byrd JB, Turcu AF, Auchus RJ. Primary aldosteronism: practical approach to diagnosis and management. Circulation. 2018;138(8): 823-35.
7. Adler GK, Stowasser M, Correa RR, et al. Primary aldosteronism: an endocrine society clinical practice guideline. J Clin Endocrinol Metabol. 2025;110(9):2453-95.
8. Pan CT, Tsai CH, Chen ZW, et al. Atrial fibrillation in primary aldosteronism. Hormone Metabol Res. 2020;52(06): 357-65.

9. Funder JW, Carey RM, Mantero F, et al. The management of primary aldosteronism: case detection, diagnosis, and treatment: an endocrine society clinical practice guideline. J Clin Endocrinol Metabol. 2016;101(5):1889-916.
10. Rossi GP, Rossi FB, Guarnieri C, et al. Clinical management of primary aldosteronism: an update. Hypertension. 2024;81(9):1845-56.
11. Hamada K, Taniguchi Y, Shimamura Y, et al. Serum level of soluble (pro) renin receptor is modulated in chronic kidney disease. Clin Experiment Nephrol. 2013;17(6):848-56.
12. Wolley MJ, Stowasser M. New advances in the diagnostic workup of primary aldosteronism. J Endocr Soc. 2017;1(3):149-61.
13. Bressan A. (2023). Cardiovascular risk assessment and diagnostic work-up in rare diseases: focus on hyperaldosteronism and primary antibody deficiency. [online] Available from https://tesidottorato.depositolegale.it/handle/20.500.14242/182190 [Last accessed October, 2025].
14. Kaplan NM. Analysis of screening and confirmatory tests in the diagnosis of primary aldosteronism. J Hypertens. 2006;24(9):1899.
15. Pintus G, Seccia TM, Amar L, et al. Subtype identification of surgically curable primary aldosteronism during treatment with mineralocorticoid receptor blockade. Hypertension. 2024; 81(6):1391-9.
16. Siemińska L, Siemińska K, Marek B, et al. Adrenal tumours and subclinical adrenal hyperfunction. Endokrynologia Polska. 2024;75(6):630-42.
17. Parasiliti-Caprino M, Bioletto F, Ceccato F, et al. The accuracy of simple and adjusted aldosterone indices for assessing selectivity and lateralization of adrenal vein sampling in the diagnosis of primary aldosteronism subtypes. Front Endocrinol. 2022;13:801529.
18. Quencer KB. Adrenal vein sampling: technique and protocol, a systematic review. CVIR Endovasc. 2021;4(1):38.
19. Papathomas TG, Sun N, Chortis V, et al. Novel methods in adrenal research: a metabolomics approach. Histochem Cell Biol. 2019;151(3):201-16.
20. Chen Cardenas SM, Santhanam P. 11C-metomidate PET in the diagnosis of adrenal masses and primary aldosteronism: a review of the literature. Endocrine. 2020;70(3):479-87.
21. Flammia RS, Anceschi U, Tufano A, et al. Minimally invasive partial vs. total adrenalectomy for the treatment of unilateral primary aldosteronism: a systematic review and meta-analysis. J Clin Med. 2022;11(5):1263.
22. Cohen DL, Wachtel H, Vaidya A, et al. Primary aldosteronism in chronic kidney disease: blood pressure control and kidney and cardiovascular outcomes after surgical versus medical management. Hypertension. 2023;80(10):2187-95.
23. Miller BS, Turcu AF, Nanba AT, et al. Refining the definitions of biochemical and clinical cure for primary aldosteronism using the primary aldosteronism surgical outcome (PASO) classification system. World J Surg. 2018;42(2):453-63.
24. Cohen JB, Bancos I, Brown JM, et al. Primary aldosteronism and the role of mineralocorticoid receptor antagonists for the heart and kidneys. Ann Rev Med. 2023;74(1):217-30.
25. Satoh F, Ito S, Itoh H, et al. Efficacy and safety of esaxerenone (CS-3150), a newly available nonsteroidal mineralocorticoid receptor blocker, in hypertensive patients with primary aldosteronism. Hypertens Res. 2021;44(4):464-72.
26. Ito S, Itoh H, Rakugi H, et al. Double-blind randomized phase 3 study comparing esaxerenone (CS-3150) and eplerenone in patients with essential hypertension (ESAX-HTN Study). Hypertension. 2020;75(1):51-8.
27. Uslar T, Sanfuentes B, Muñoz I, et al. Real-world outcomes of finerenone in primary aldosteronism. Eur J Endocrinol. 2025;192(5):K50-3.
28. Fernandes-Rosa FL, Williams TA, Riester A, et al. Genetic spectrum and clinical correlates of somatic mutations in aldosterone-producing adenoma. Hypertension. 2014;64(2):354-61.
29. Chan CK, Yang WS, Lin YH, et al. KCNJ5 somatic mutations are associated with better Long-Term outcomes in patients with unilateral primary aldosteronism. J Clin Endocrinol Metabol. 2025;110(9):e2918-e2928.
30. Szatko A, Toboła A, Falhammar H, et al. Advances in the biochemical diagnostics of primary aldosteronism: from immunoassays to steroidomics and proteomics. Front Endocrinol. 2025;16:1548344.
31. Wu X. The Role of Cell Adhesion Molecular 1 (CADMI) and 11C-Metomidate Pet CT in Molecular Pathogenesis and Diagnosis of Primary Aldostonism (Doctoral dissertation, Queen Mary University of London.). [online] Available from https://qmro.qmul.ac.uk/xmlui/handle/123456789/77234 [Last accessed October, 2025].
32. Meyer A, Brabant G, Behrend M. Long-term follow-up after adrenalectomy for primary aldosteronism. World J Surg. 2005; 29(2):155-9.
33. Sywak M, Pasieka JL. Long-term follow-up and cost benefit of adrenalectomy in patients with primary hyperaldosteronism. Br J Surg. 2002;89(12):1587-93.
34. Carter Y, Roy M, Sippel RS, et al. Persistent hypertension after adrenalectomy for an aldosterone-producing adenoma: weight as a critical prognostic factor for aldosterone's lasting effect on the cardiac and vascular systems. J Surg Res. 2012;177(2): 241-7.

CHAPTER 8

Implications of Myocardial Interstitial Fibrosis in Hypertensive Heart Disease

Debasis Ghosh, Navanil Biswas

ABSTRACT

Hypertensive heart disease (HHD) represents one of the most common manifestations of chronic hypertension and is one of the major contributors to cardiovascular morbidity and mortality worldwide. While left ventricular hypertrophy has traditionally been regarded as its defining feature, emerging evidence indicates that diffuse myocardial interstitial fibrosis (MIF) is the pivotal lesion driving functional impairment and adverse clinical outcomes. Fibrosis causes stiffening of the myocardium, disrupts contractility, impairs conduction, and compromises coronary microvascular reserve, thereby contributing to diastolic dysfunction, systolic failure, arrhythmias, as well as ischemia. Its development is mediated by an intricate interplay of mechanical overload, activation of the renin–angiotensin–aldosterone system, pro-fibrotic cytokines, immune responses, and genetic and metabolic factors.[1]

Diagnosis of myocardial fibrosis has now advanced beyond invasive biopsy toward noninvasive strategies such as cardiac magnetic resonance (CMR) with T1 mapping and extracellular volume (ECV) fraction estimation, echocardiographic strain imaging, and circulating biomarkers of collagen turnover. While optimal blood pressure control remains fundamental to prevention, pharmacological blockade of the renin–angiotensin–aldosterone system and mineralocorticoid receptor antagonism have recently shown the ability to regress fibrosis. Novel therapies, including sodium–glucose cotransporter-2 inhibitors, pirfenidone, and antifibrotic agents targeting collagen cross-linking, are under active investigation. Recognition of myocardial fibrosis as the central determinant of clinical progression in HHD emphasizes the need to integrate early detection and targeted antifibrotic therapy into clinical practice.

Keywords: Hypertension, myocardial interstitial fibrosis, hypertensive heart disease.

INTRODUCTION

Hypertension affects *>1.3 billion individuals* worldwide and is the *leading global cause of cardiovascular morbidity and mortality*. Hypertensive heart disease (HHD) is the structural and functional cardiac response to chronic pressure overload, traditionally characterized by concentric left ventricular hypertrophy (LVH). However, the adverse clinical outcomes observed in patients with HHD are not fully explained by hypertrophy alone. Many athletes exhibit physiological LVH without developing heart failure or arrhythmias, highlighting that hypertrophy per se is not pathogenic.[2]

Over the last two decades, *myocardial interstitial fibrosis (MIF)* has emerged as the central pathological substrate linking hypertension to adverse outcomes. Excessive deposition of fibrillar collagen within the myocardial extracellular matrix alters ventricular compliance, reduces contractile efficiency, disrupts electrical conduction, and impairs coronary microvascular function. Fibrosis is now recognized as the main driver of heart failure with preserved ejection fraction (HFpEF), as well as progression to reduced ejection fraction (HFrEF), atrial fibrillation, ventricular arrhythmias, and sudden cardiac death in hypertensive patients.

With advances in noninvasive imaging and biomarkers, myocardial fibrosis can be detected earlier, quantified more accurately, and monitored longitudinally. This has enabled better risk stratification and facilitated therapeutic strategies that go beyond blood pressure control to specifically target the fibrotic process. *In this chapter, we review the histopathological basis, mechanisms, clinical consequences, diagnostic approaches, and therapeutic implications of myocardial fibrosis in HHD, highlighting its central role in determining outcomes.*

HISTOPATHOLOGICAL BASIS OF MYOCARDIAL FIBROSIS IN HYPERTENSIVE HEART DISEASE

The myocardium is composed of cardiomyocytes embedded within an *extracellular matrix (ECM)* that provides structural integrity, mechanical support, and coordinated electrical propagation. The ECM is primarily formed by fibrillar collagens, with *type I* providing tensile strength and *type III* imparting elasticity. In health, collagen turnover is tightly regulated by a balance between synthesis by fibroblasts and degradation by matrix metalloproteinases.[3]

Hypertension disrupts this equilibrium, leading to excessive collagen deposition and architectural disarray. Fibrosis in HHD manifests in three distinct but overlapping patterns: (1) *Reactive interstitial fibrosis*, characterized by diffuse expansion of the interstitium without preceding cell loss; (2) *perivascular fibrosis*, involving concentric collagen accumulation around intramural vessels; and (3) *replacement fibrosis*, where necrotic or apoptotic myocytes are substituted by dense scar tissue. Among these, diffuse interstitial fibrosis is considered the most characteristic lesion of HHD.

Fibroblasts, which account for two-thirds of myocardial cell numbers despite forming only a minority of myocardial volume, play a central role. Under hypertensive stress, resident fibroblasts undergo phenotypic transformation into myofibroblasts, acquiring contractile properties and enhanced secretory capacity. Myofibroblasts secrete large amounts of type I and III collagen, express α-smooth muscle actin, and exhibit prolonged survival, thereby sustaining the fibrotic process. Cross-linking of collagen fibers, mediated by lysyl oxidase, further stiffens the ventricular wall and makes fibrosis resistant to degradation, amplifying its pathophysiological impact.

MECHANISMS OF FIBROSIS IN HYPERTENSIVE HEART DISEASE

Myocardial fibrosis in HHD arises from a complex interplay of hemodynamic load, neurohormonal activation, inflammatory signaling, and genetic or metabolic predispositions.[4]

- *Mechanical factors:* Chronic pressure overload increases wall stress, which activates mechanosensitive signaling in cardiac fibroblasts. Integrins and stretch-sensitive receptors stimulate fibroblast proliferation, enhance collagen gene expression, and suppress collagenase activity. The degree of wall stress correlates with regional variation in collagen deposition, with endomyocardial biopsies demonstrating transmural gradients of fibrosis in hypertensive patients.
- *Neurohormonal pathways:* The renin-angiotensin-aldosterone system (RAAS) is the dominant neurohormonal driver of fibrosis. Angiotensin II directly stimulates fibroblast proliferation, myofibroblast differentiation, and collagen synthesis, while simultaneously reducing collagen degradation. It also promotes oxidative stress and cytokine release. Aldosterone acts via mineralocorticoid receptors to induce perivascular and interstitial collagen deposition, independent of blood pressure effect. Experimental models of hyperaldosteronism reproduce the fibrotic phenotype, which can be attenuated by mineralocorticoid receptor antagonists. Endothelin-1 acts synergistically with RAAS to promote fibroblast contractility and matrix remodeling.
- *Cytokines and growth factors:* Transforming growth factor-β (TGF-β) serves as the master regulator of fibrogenesis. It activates Smad signaling, induces connective tissue growth factor (CTGF), and sustains the persistence of myofibroblasts. CTGF acts downstream to amplify collagen synthesis and fibrosis progression.
- *Inflammation and immune activation:* Hypertension induces low-grade sterile inflammation within the myocardium. Activated peripheral blood mononuclear cells infiltrate cardiac tissue, releasing cytokines such as interleukin-6 and tumor necrosis factor-α that stimulate fibroblast activity. Oxidative and nitrosative stress further perpetuate fibroblast activation and collagen deposition.
- *Genetic and environmental modifiers:* Individual susceptibility to fibrosis varies, influenced by genetic polymorphisms in the angiotensin-converting enzyme (*ACE*) gene and angiotensin II receptor subtypes. Environmental and metabolic comorbidities—including salt sensitivity, obesity, diabetes, and chronic kidney disease—accelerate fibrotic remodeling. Sex differences are also recognized; premenopausal women appear relatively protected, possibly due to estrogen's antifibrotic effects.

Taken together, these mechanisms explain why myocardial fibrosis is both ubiquitous in hypertensive patients and heterogeneous in extent, distribution, and clinical impact **(Flowchart 1)**.

CLINICAL CONSEQUENCES OF MYOCARDIAL FIBROSIS

Myocardial interstitial fibrosis is increasingly recognized as the pivotal determinant of adverse outcomes in HHD, mediating the transition from asymptomatic structural remodeling to overt clinical syndromes. By altering the mechanical, electrical, and vascular properties of the myocardium, fibrosis contributes to a broad spectrum of pathological consequences.[5]

One of the earliest and most important effects is the development of *diastolic dysfunction*, which arises from the accumulation of stiff type I collagen fibers within the ECM. This reduces ventricular compliance, impairs relaxation, and elevates filling pressures, ultimately leading to *HFpEF*—a syndrome highly prevalent in elderly hypertensive patients. As fibrosis advances, particularly in the form of replacement

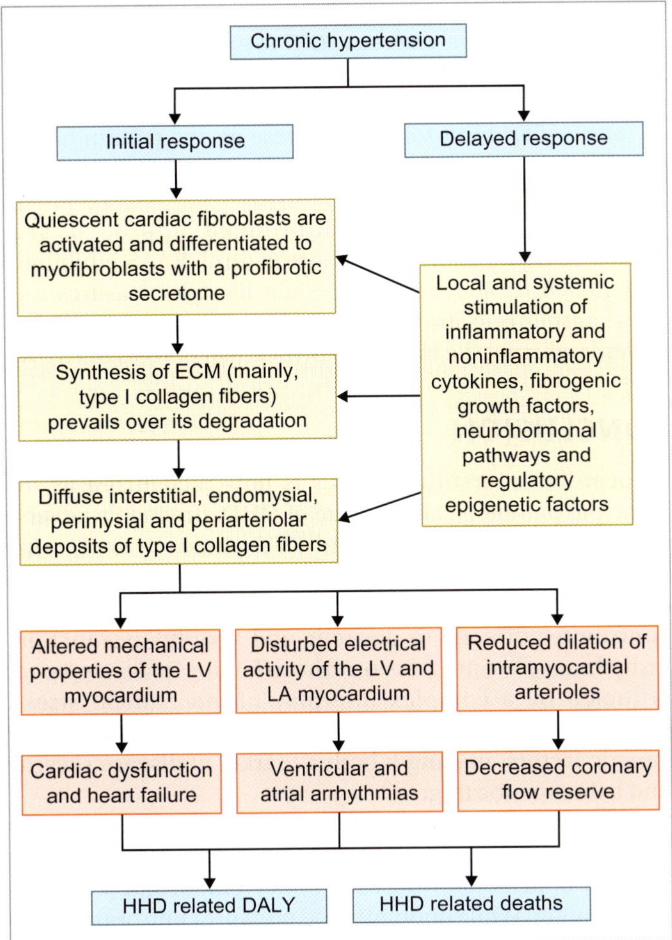

FLOWCHART 1: Pathogenesis of myocardial fibrosis in hypertensive heart disease.

scarring, *systolic dysfunction* may develop. The disruption of normal myocyte alignment and force transmission reduces contractile efficiency, contributing to progressive ventricular dilation and the evolution toward *HFrEF*.

In addition to impairing mechanical function, fibrosis profoundly disrupts the electrical properties of the myocardium. Patchy interstitial and replacement fibrosis slow conduction velocity, increase heterogeneity, and promote re-entry circuits. These changes create a vulnerable substrate for *atrial fibrillation* and malignant *ventricular arrhythmias*, both of which are common in hypertensive populations. Furthermore, *perivascular fibrosis* thickens the adventitia of intramural coronary arteries, reduces lumen diameter, and diminishes coronary flow reserve. The resulting microvascular dysfunction contributes to angina-like symptoms and ischemia even in the absence of epicardial coronary stenosis.

Collectively, these structural and functional derangements underscore fibrosis as the central mediator of progression in HHD and the strongest predictor of clinical outcomes.

DIAGNOSIS AND ASSESSMENT OF FIBROSIS

The definitive method for diagnosing MIF is histological quantification of collagen volume fraction in endomyocardial biopsy samples. Collagen fibers, stained with picrosirius red and viewed under polarized light, can be directly measured to provide a precise estimate of fibrotic burden. However, biopsy is invasive, limited by sampling error, and impractical for routine use, prompting a shift toward noninvasive approaches.[6]

- *Echocardiography* remains the most accessible tool for evaluating functional consequences of fibrosis. While traditional measures such as wall thickness and chamber dimensions are nonspecific, strain and strain-rate imaging can detect subclinical myocardial dysfunction related to interstitial collagen deposition, often preceding overt changes in ejection fraction.
- *Cardiac magnetic resonance (CMR)* has emerged as the gold-standard noninvasive imaging modality for tissue characterization. Late gadolinium enhancement (LGE) provides excellent sensitivity for focal replacement fibrosis but underestimates diffuse disease. In contrast, T1 mapping and calculation of ECV fraction allow accurate quantification of diffuse interstitial fibrosis, with values strongly correlating with biopsy findings. ECV has also been shown to predict adverse outcomes in patients with hypertension and heart failure.
- *Circulating biomarkers* offer a complementary and easily repeatable means of assessing fibrotic activity. Peptides reflecting collagen synthesis, such as the carboxy-terminal propeptide of procollagen type I (PIP) and the amino-terminal propeptide of procollagen type III (PIIINP), as well as degradation markers such as collagen type I telopeptide (CITP), have been validated as surrogates of ECM turnover. Tissue inhibitor of metalloproteinases-1 (TIMP-1) reflects impaired collagen breakdown, and elevated levels of these biomarkers correlate with both histological fibrosis and clinical outcomes. Emerging candidates, including galectin-3 and soluble ST2, may provide incremental prognostic value.

Thus, an integrated diagnostic approach that combines advanced imaging modalities with serum biomarkers provides a comprehensive assessment of fibrotic burden. This enables early detection, risk stratification, monitoring of disease progression, and evaluation of therapeutic efficacy in HHD.

THERAPEUTIC STRATEGIES

The primary goal in HHD is optimal blood pressure control, which reduces afterload, limits LVH, and slows progression of myocardial remodeling. However, numerous studies have demonstrated that blood pressure lowering alone is insufficient to prevent or reverse myocardial fibrosis. This recognition has shifted therapeutic focus toward targeting the cellular and molecular mechanisms driving fibrogenesis.

- *Renin-angiotensin-aldosterone system inhibition* forms the cornerstone of antifibrotic therapy. ACE inhibitors and angiotensin receptor blockers (ARBs) reduce fibroblast activation, suppress collagen synthesis, and improve ECM turnover beyond their hemodynamic effects. Clinical studies have shown significant reductions in biopsy-measured collagen volume fraction and improvements in diastolic function with these agents. Mineralocorticoid receptor antagonists (MRAs), such as *spironolactone and eplerenone,* directly counteract aldosterone-mediated collagen deposition and perivascular fibrosis. Their antifibrotic effects translate into reduced heart failure hospitalizations and improved survival, as demonstrated in large outcome trials.[7]
- *Non-RAAS antihypertensive agents* may exert indirect benefits. Beta-blockers, by reducing sympathetic activation, and calcium channel blockers, through vasodilatory effects, attenuate hypertensive remodeling, although their specific antifibrotic efficacy remains less robust compared to RAAS blockade.
- *Lifestyle modification* provides important adjunctive benefit. Sodium restriction lowers intravascular volume and reduces myocardial collagen turnover, while weight loss, regular aerobic exercise, and optimal management of diabetes and chronic kidney disease mitigate the metabolic and inflammatory drivers of fibrosis.
- *Emerging therapies* are now targeting fibrosis directly at the molecular level. Antifibrotic agents such as pirfenidone, already approved for pulmonary fibrosis, have demonstrated early promise in attenuating myocardial fibrosis and improving diastolic function in pilot studies. *Sodium-glucose cotransporter-2 (SGLT-2) inhibitors,*[8] beyond their established cardiovascular benefits, reduce myocardial fibrosis in experimental models and are being investigated as modulators of ECM remodeling in hypertensive heart failure. Other novel approaches include *inhibitors of lysyl oxidase (LOX)* to prevent collagen cross-linking and stiffening, *monoclonal antibodies against pro-fibrotic cytokines*, and *therapies targeting fibroblast-to-myofibroblast transition.* These agents remain largely investigational but represent the future direction of antifibrotic management.[9]

Taken together, a multipronged approach that combines rigorous blood pressure control, RAAS inhibition, mineralocorticoid receptor blockade, lifestyle measures, and novel antifibrotic strategies offers the most promising path toward reducing the burden of myocardial fibrosis in HHD.

CONCLUSION

Myocardial interstitial fibrosis is now recognized as the principal pathological substrate of HHD, driving its adverse clinical consequences beyond LVH alone. By increasing myocardial stiffness, impairing contractile efficiency, and disrupting electrical and microvascular integrity, fibrosis contributes directly to diastolic and systolic dysfunction, arrhythmias, and progression to heart failure. Its development is fueled by a complex interplay of mechanical stress, neurohormonal activation, inflammation, and metabolic and genetic factors, making it both a marker of disease severity and a therapeutic target.[10]

Advances in noninvasive imaging and biomarker assessment have greatly improved the ability to detect and quantify fibrosis, allowing earlier intervention and better risk stratification. While optimal blood pressure control and RAAS inhibition remain the foundation of therapy, these alone are insufficient to halt or reverse fibrotic remodeling. Future strategies will need to integrate novel antifibrotic agents, metabolic modulators, and lifestyle interventions alongside established therapies. A paradigm shift from focusing solely on blood pressure reduction toward targeting fibrosis itself offers the best opportunity to improve outcomes and reduce the long-term burden of HHD.

REFERENCES

1. Weber KT. Fibrosis in hypertensive heart disease: focus on cardiac fibroblasts. J Hypertens. 2004;22:47-50.
2. González A, López B, Ravassa S, San José G, Latasa I, Butler J, et al. Myocardial interstitial fibrosis in hypertensive heart disease: from mechanisms to clinical management. Hypertension. 2024;81:218-28.
3. Díez J. Mechanisms of cardiac fibrosis in hypertension. J Clin Hypertens. 2007;9:546-50.
4. Williams B, Mancia G, Spiering W, Agabiti Rosei E, Azizi M, Burnier M, et al. 2018 ESC/ESH Guidelines for the management of arterial hypertension. Eur Heart J. 2018;39:3021-104.
5. McDonagh TA, Metra M, Adamo M, Gardner RS, Baumbach A, Böhm M, et al. 2021 ESC Guidelines for the diagnosis and treatment of acute and chronic heart failure. Eur Heart J. 2021;42:3599-726.
6. Puntmann VO, Carr-White G, Jabbour A, Yu CY, Gebker R, Kelle S, et al. T1 mapping and extracellular volume in cardiovascular disease: novel imaging biomarkers. J Am Coll Cardiol. 2017;69:177-92.
7. Pitt B, Zannad F, Remme WJ, Cody R, Castaigne A, Perez A, et al. The effect of spironolactone on morbidity and mortality in patients with severe heart failure. N Engl J Med. 1999;341:709-17.
8. McMurray JJV, Solomon SD, Inzucchi SE, Kober L, Kosiborod MN, Martinez FA, et al. Dapagliflozin in patients with heart failure and reduced ejection fraction. N Engl J Med. 2019;381:1995-2008.
9. Ishida J, et al. Pirfenidone in heart failure with preserved ejection fraction: a randomized phase 2 trial. Hypertension. 2021;77:1119-28.
10. Lewis GA, Schelbert EB, Williams SG, Cunnington C, Ahmed F, McDonagh TA, et al. Biological and therapeutic insights into myocardial fibrosis in heart failure. Nat Rev Cardiol. 2021;18:127-44.

CHAPTER

9

Renovascular Hypertension: Kidney Intrinsic Mechanism as Novel Target

Manu Gupta, Anuj Gupta, Pooja Sharma Gupta, Rajeev Gupta

ABSTRACT

Renovascular disease (RVD) accompanied by blood pressure elevation is a cause of secondary hypertension. Renal artery stenosis (RAS) is recognized as a major cause of renovascular hypertension (RVH) and RVD. RVH might present as a progressive disease associated with diffuse atherosclerosis, leading to loss of renal function. Potential therapeutic targets in RVH include oxidative stress, microvascular disease, inflammation, mitochondrial injury, and cellular senescence.

Keywords: Renal artery stenosis (RAS), renovascular hypertension (RVH), renovascular disease (RVD), renin–angiotensin–aldosterone system (RAAS), reactive oxygen species (ROS), nitric oxide (NO), nicotinamide-adenine dinucleotide phosphate (NADPH), monocyte chemoattractant protein (MCP-1), nuclear factor-kappa B (NF-κB), tumor necrosis factor-alpha (TNF-α), glomerular filtration rate (GFR), mesenchymal stem cells (MSCs), tissue inhibitor matrix metalloproteinase (TIMP-1), plasminogen activator inhibitor (PAI-1), granulocyte-colony stimulating factor (G-CSF), angiotensin-converting enzyme inhibitors (ACEi), angiotensin-II receptor blockers (ARBs), angiotensin-1 (AT1), antiapoptotic B-cell lymphoma-2 (BCL2) and Bcl-xl, endothelial progenitor cells (EPCs), blood oxygen level-dependent (BOLD), sodium-glucose cotransporter-2 (SGLT-2)-inhibitors.

INTRODUCTION

Constriction of renal artery triggers renin release and elevated arterial pressure with a key role of the renal system in blood pressure (BP) regulation[1] leading to renovascular hypertension (RVH).

Even in unilateral renovascular disease (RVD), damage devlops both in the poststenotic kidney and in the non-stenotic contralateral kidney, due to reduced renal perfusion and activation of inflammatory mechanisms, prothrombotic mechanisms, and metabolic perturbations.[2] Atherosclerotic RVD can be bilateral[3] in about half of these patients.

The common precipitating causes for hemodynamically significant RVD are atherosclerotic lesions and are usually in the proximal third of the vessel, followed by fibromuscular diseases.[4] Currently, RVD is considered to contribute to ~5% of cases of hypertension and over 10% of patients initiating renal replacement therapy with no other identifiable primary cause.[5,6] RVD can be discovered as an incidental finding in elderly patients.[7] Cardiovascular risk is magnified in these patients,[8] but may alternatively present as an insidious, progressive disease that threatens kidney viability. Its presence magnifies cardiovascular risk by several folds, which in turn is often the cause of mortality in these patients.

Interactions of the renin–angiotensin–aldosterone system (RAAS) with vasodilator nitric oxide (NO) and vasoconstrictor prostaglandins seem to cause the development of RVH and renal injury.[9] In atherosclerotic RVD, associated atherogenic factors and dysregulated metabolic elements complicate these mechanisms and amplify intrarenal damage[10-12] and microvascular rarefaction.[13-15]

Renin–angiotensin–aldosterone system activation is a hallmark of RVD but may be transient. Its regulatory role in the sustenance of RVH may be subsequently abetted by elevated PGF2α-isoprostanes, potent vasoconstrictors, and oxidative stress biomarkers.[16] Within the poststenotic kidney, chronic RAAS activation also drives inflammation, microvascular loss, and fibrosis.[17] Indeed, blockade of the angiotensin-II angiotensin-1 (AT1) receptor stabilizes poststenotic kidney function.[17] Although the poststenotic kidney exhibits a remarkable capacity for decreasing its metabolic activity and sustaining perfusion,[18] severe stenoses overwhelm this capacity, aggravating renal scarring and microvascular remodeling, which may render renal damage irreversible. The magnitudes of RVH and renal injury may be exacerbated by coexisting atherosclerosis or essential hypertension, and neither is necessarily directly related to stenosis severity.[19]

MECHANISMS INTRINSIC IN KIDNEY

Oxidative Stress

Reactive oxygen species (ROS) regulate renal pathophysiology as important second messengers in renal physiology, but when in excess they overwhelm the antioxidant defenses and increase oxidative stress. An ischemic insult induces oxidative stress, which favors the quenching of NO leading to microvascular endothelial dysfunction,[2,16] as ROS abundance activates redox-dependent inflammatory and growth factors, unleashing progressive remodeling of the renal microvascular architecture that includes intimal thickening and luminal narrowing.[20,21]

Resolution of RVD decreases oxidative stress, improves antioxidant defenses, increases the bioavailability of NO, and improves vascular function and hypertension control,[22] supporting a multistep pathophysiological cascade. As such, targeting ROS[23-25] as a sole or coadjuvant intervention reads as a logical strategy in RVD.

Inflammation

Renal inflammation plays an important role in the pathogenesis of RVD and bears negative consequences for the kidney and other organs, leading to interstitial lymphocyte and macrophage infiltration.[26] Expression of proinflammatory cytokines such as monocyte chemoattractant protein (MCP-1), nuclear factor-kappa B (NF-κB), and raised tumor necrosis factor-alpha (TNF-α),[27-29] are associated with B-T cell and macrophage infiltration.[30,31] Renal biopsies from patients with severe RVD reveal macrophage infiltration and fibrosis.[32]

Furthermore, renal vein samples from stenotic swine[33] and human[34] kidneys show increased levels of inflammatory cytokines that portend acute kidney injury and impaired renal function and correlate with neutrophil gelatinase-associated lipocalin levels, reflecting kidney and systemic inflammation and ischemia.[35] Systemic C-reactive protein and peripheral leukocyte levels are also elevated[36] and associated with a higher prevalence of coronary artery disease and mortality.[37] In pigs with atherosclerotic RVD, restoration of renal arterial patency failed to attenuate renal inflammation or improve renal function,[38] and proinflammatory cytokines release inversely correlates with renal functional recovery,[33] underscoring the dominant role of inflammation in RVD. Similarly, in patients with RVD, restoration of arterial flow does not reverse tissue inflammatory and injury markers or improve renal function.[39]

Congruently, intrarenal infusion of mesenchymal stem cells (MSCs), which possess important anti-inflammatory properties, preserves stenotic kidney structure and function.[30,40,41]

Fibrogenic Pathways

Progressive glomerulosclerosis, interstitial fibrosis, and tubular atrophy are commonly seen in chronically ischemic kidneys and correlate with progression to renal insufficiency.[42] Profibrotic factors such as transforming growth factor-beta (TGF-β), tissue inhibitor matrix metalloproteinase (TIMP-1), and plasminogen activator inhibitor-1 (PAI-1) are all upregulated in stenotic kidneys.[38,43] Positive crosstalk between TGF-β and MCP-1 signaling in mesangial cells promotes ROS production and progressive renal disease, and its abrogation reduces fibrosis and atrophy in experimental RVD.[44] TGF-β upregulation in poststenotic kidneys is particularly evident when remodeling is completed.[32] Expression of its downstream mediator SMAD2/3 increases persistently in the stenotic kidney and instigates interstitial fibrosis,[28] while TIMP-1 inhibits extracellular matrix degradation and promotes collagen deposition,[43] and PAI-1 modulates angiotensin-II-mediated hypertensive injury.[43] Therefore, targeting these profibrotic cascades may blunt fibrosis and renal dysfunction in RVD. Therapeutic interventions that proved to be efficacious in ameliorating stenotic kidney fibrosis in experimental RVD include cell-based therapies,[30,31,45,46] mitoprotective drugs,[29,47] granulocyte-colony stimulating factor (G-CSF),[48] MCP-1 inhibitors,[27] angiotensin-converting enzyme inhibitors (ACEi)/angiotensin-II receptor blockers (ARBs), and triple therapy,[17] among others.

Atherosclerosis

The atherogenic process has a strong influence on the development of renal injury before the build-up of obstructive lesions, as atherosclerotic RVD associates with a greater incidence of progressive extrarenal vascular disease and renal dysfunction than nonatherosclerotic RVD.[42,49] Increased circulating lipids and their oxidation products deposit in the kidneys and promote glomerular, tubulointerstitial, and podocyte damage, resulting in proteinuria and loss of kidney function.[50] Systemic atherosclerosis also impacts vascular wall and microvascular remodeling, as coexisting atherosclerosis in swine RVD promotes oxidative stress, inflammation, and fibrosis.[2]

Atherosclerosis also impacts therapeutic outcomes. Revascularization of a nonatherosclerotic stenotic swine renal artery improves renal blood flow and restores function,[51] but its protective effects are dramatically blunted when atherosclerosis is superimposed.[38] Specifically, microvascular rarefaction and fibrosis persist after renal angioplasty, which may underlie the often inconsistent outcomes of revascularization in atherosclerotic RVD.[52,53] Importantly, these data imply that the obstruction per se is not the sole insult and that early injurious mechanisms in the atherosclerotic process are likely perpetuated independent of ischemia, warranting a refinement of therapeutic strategies. Indeed, intrarenal cell-based or proangiogenic therapies may improve renal recovery and hypertension without resolution of the vascular obstruction.[45,54,55]

Renin–angiotensin–aldosterone System Activation

The experiments of Goldblatt showing reduced renal perfusion in canine two-kidneys-one-clip-1 set the stage for the application of this approach in other translational animal platforms such as rats and pigs.[16,56] These observations were supported by showing that RAAS blockade can delay the development of hypertension, and AT1 receptor knockout two-kidneys-one-clip mice fail to develop hypertension.[57] In the two-kidneys-one-clip model, the contralateral kidney is exposed to elevated systemic perfusion pressures, which favor natriuresis, prevents renin release, and suppresses the rise in systemic pressures, sustaining reduced perfusion and increasing renin release from the stenotic kidney.

The effects of the RAAS in RVD include vasoconstriction and increased vascular resistance, sodium retention, and aldosterone release.[58,59] Furthermore, angiotensin-II contributes to renal vascular remodeling, inflammation, and fibrosis, as well as target organ injury (e.g., left ventricular hypertrophy). Thus, RAAS modulators (e.g., ACEi and ARBs) can achieve a multilevel renoprotection by regulating several aspects of renal injury.

Microvascular Disease

A healthy renal microvasculature is critical for the function and nutrition of the kidney. Studies showed that dysfunction and remodeling of the renal microvessels, mainly in the cortex, precede overt obstructive lesions in the renal arteries[10,60] supporting microvascular injury as a central pathophysiological trait of RVD. In turn, obstructive lesions aggravate microvascular disease by accelerating small vessel remodeling and loss not only in the cortex but also in the medulla.[61] Swine RVD leads to a decreased density of cortical[38] and medullary[62] microvessels in the stenotic kidney, which, depending on their size, affects interlobular, afferent, efferent, glomerular, or peritubular vasculature.[54]

Although microvessels may sustain renal function early in RVD,[63] concurrent progression of oxidative stress, inflammation, and fibrosis can compromise their function, morphology, and repair.[64,65] The small vessels are leaky vessels with abnormal morphology and increased tortuosity,[29,30] underscoring progressive microvascular disease as an important determinant of renal hemodynamics, filtration, and possibly tubular function,[2,24,66] whereas their replenishment prevents and reverses microvascular damage and restores stenotic kidney function[61,67] and can be improved by coadjuvant-targeted proangiogenic interventions.[67,68]

Endothelial Dysfunction

A healthy endothelial barrier is pivotal for the homeostasis of vascular tone, permeability, and fluid balance,[65] serving as both targets and sources of vasoactive compounds such as NO, prostacyclin, angiotensin-II, or endothelin-1. A central mechanism of endothelial dysfunction is the ROS-mediated quenching of NO. This leads to sustained vasoconstriction, a hallmark of endothelial dysfunction that can reduce renal perfusion, impair oxygen and nutrient delivery, and increase vascular permeability, with consequent disruptions of fluid balance between intra- and extravascular spaces.

Furthermore, a healthy endothelium has anti-inflammatory properties, whereas endothelial dysfunction promotes its interaction with circulating inflammatory cells and the generation of chemokines.[69] A dysfunctional endothelium may also facilitate thrombogenic activity via the upregulation of adhesion molecules and disruption of procoagulant and fibrinolytic activity.[70]

Senescence

In response to insults, cells undergo proliferation arrest and complex molecular changes and might develop a pathogenic senescence-associated secretory phenotype that disseminates inflammation and disrupts tissue repair.[71] While short-term cellular senescence may be renoprotective, sustained senescence ultimately contributes to both acute and chronic renal ischemic injury. In mice with unilateral RVD selective clearance of p16$^+$ senescent (primarily epithelial) cells alleviated renal damage,[72] yet broad-range clearance of both p16$^+$ and p21$^+$ cells was even more efficient. Cellular senescence was also observed in the human poststenotic kidney, suggesting that this process is conserved.[73] In swine RVD, cellular senescence was accompanied by mitochondrial injury[74] and impaired self-healing.[75] However, neither mitochondrial protection nor cell-based therapy[76] fully mitigated cellular senescence, supporting the development of specific senolytic strategies to repair senescent kidneys.

Apoptosis

Programmed cell death occurs primarily in the thick ascending limb and may serve as a protective mechanism to induce tubular remodeling and atrophy.[77] Decreased renal perfusion responds by activating the heme oxygenase-1 system, which exerts antiapoptotic action via mechanisms involving decreased caspases-3 and -9 activities, and increased expression of the antiapoptotic B-cell lymphoma-2 (BCL2) and Bcl-xl.[78] However, this defense mechanism is attenuated in the milieu of concurrent atherosclerosis, likely secondary to activation of NF-κB and decreased intracellular protein degradation.[43]

Tubular cell apoptosis is partly induced by angiotensin-II through AT1 and AT2 receptors and TGF-β, which promotes transcription of the proapoptotic genes *FAS* cell surface death-receptor, *FAS* ligand, and *BCL2*-associated-X apoptosis regulator.[79] Renal mitochondrial damage can also instigate apoptosis through mitochondrial permeability transition pore (mPTP) opening and activation of caspase-3 and -9.[80]

Apoptosis is partially reversible until fibrosis begins[81] and contributes to inflammation and vascular loss, leading to global renal atrophy and perpetual parenchymal damage.[82] Endothelial progenitor cells (EPCs) recruited to the stenotic kidney to participate in renal repair[31,34] also undergo apoptosis,[83] suggesting that its activation impairs renal repair.

Strategies that preserve the poststenotic kidney were associated with attenuation of apoptosis, including intrarenal administration of EPCs[31] or MSCs,[30] intravenous infusion of mitoprotective drugs[29,47] or G-CSF,[48] oral simvastatin supplementation,[83] or intraperitoneal injection of ACEi. In mice with ischemia–reperfusion injury, the antiapoptotic insulin-like growth factor-1 and ZVAD-FMK (a caspase inactivator) prevented the early onset of renal apoptosis, inflammation, and tissue injury.[82]

Mitochondrial Injury

Renal tubular cells are rich in mitochondria, and mitochondrial injury and dysfunction bear harmful consequences on multiple cell functions. Activation of AT2 receptors in the inner mitochondrial membrane stimulates production of mitochondrial ROS and apoptosis of renal tubular cells.[79] Ischemia and oxidative stress trigger mPTP opening favoring release of cytochrome-c into the cytosol[84,85] and thereby apoptosis. In patients with RVD, urinary levels of mitochondrial injury markers correlate with changes in renal function after renal arterial revascularization, implicating mitochondria in renal injury.[86] Renal revascularization acutely raises urinary mitochondrial DNA, likely reflecting reperfusion-elicited renal mitochondrial injury that in turn inhibits renal recovery.[87]

Pertinently, drugs protecting cardiolipin, an inner membrane phospholipid that prevents formation of the mPTP and improves the efficiency of the electron transport chain, attenuated microvascular rarefaction and improved renal function in swine RVD.[29,47] These drugs exerted beneficial effects on the myocardium,[88,89] underscoring the potential of mitoprotection to ameliorate target organ damage. In patients with RVD, adjunctive mitoprotection during renal revascularization attenuated postprocedural hypoxia, increased renal blood flow, and improved GFR,[90] positioning mitoprotection as a novel therapeutic option.

Hypoxia

The kidney is highly perfused with oxygenated blood and can autoregulate blood flow until reductions in arterial diameter reach 75%. Therefore, whole-organ ischemia is rare.[91]

Blood oxygen level-dependent (BOLD)-MRI, which evaluates intrarenal deoxyhemoglobin levels,[92-94] has been employed to assess renal oxygenation. Besides basal oxygenation, functional hypoxia is based on a response to furosemide, with a blunted increase in poststenotic kidney oxygenation indicating attenuated basal oxygen consumption related to tubular transport.[62] Under normal conditions, the renal medulla functions at levels close to hypoxia and in RVD may be protected by adaptive maintenance of tissue perfusion relative to cortical blood flow.[95] Even under relatively severe conditions, the kidney tissue can persist in a "hibernating" state, characterized by apoptosis and tubular atrophy, which is potentially reversible if renal blood flow is restored.[28,96] However, BOLD-MRI demonstrated increased swine cortical and medullary hypoxia during gradual renal arterial occlusion[97] and chronic RVD,[47,98] associated with renal dysfunction.[62] Similarly, in patients with RVD, despite preserved cortical oxygenation, hypoxia develops in deep medullary regions,[93] although tissue oxygenation is relatively well-preserved,[18] partly due to renal ability to reduce solute filtration and reabsorption, and thereby oxygen consumption.[99,100] Nevertheless, in severe RVD, decreased cortical oxygenation[97,101] suggests potentially irreversible tubular injury.[93]

THERAPEUTIC INTERVENTIONS

Revascularization Strategies

Catheter-based interventions (e.g., angioplasty, with and without stenting) are nowadays the intervention of choice since they are minimally invasive and involve faster recovery than surgery; however, surgical revascularization (e.g., bypass) is limited to patients in whom a percutaneous approach may be infeasible. Such interventions constituted primary treatments for RVD a few decades ago, driven by the rationale that the resolution of the obstruction should offset hypertension and deterioration of renal function, an assumption fueled by promising preliminary reports.[102-105] However, two major prospective randomized clinical trials, the Angioplasty and Stenting for Renal Artery Lesions (ASTRAL, 806 patients[53]) and the Cardiovascular Outcomes in Renal Atherosclerotic Lesions (CORAL, 947 patients[106]), clearly demonstrated that renal angioplasty and stenting did not confer a significant benefit for the prevention of clinical events when added to comprehensive medical therapy. Although a significant proportion of patients included had only modest stenoses,[107] the data revealed added substantial risks by the intervention with limited evidence of clinical benefit in terms of hypertension or recovery of renal function.

These conclusions, however, do not absolve the vascular obstruction from the pathophysiology of RVD. Clearly, RVD results from a long process that can affect the kidneys beyond the obstruction and during the build-up of the plaques. Hence, the pathophysiological processes distal to the stenosis are unlikely to be fully addressed by revascularization. An integrated understanding of the disease process supports the notion that the rate of progression and severity of the renal parenchymal damage tamper the success of interventional strategies and reinforces a need for a more refined and likely tailored approach. For example, studies show that early diagnosis and adequate revascularization could impact BP control, recovery, prevention, or preservation of renal function and improve patient survival.[108] Also, ancillary studies in the ASTRAL population suggest that specific subpopulations of patients might benefit from angioplasty, depending on their basal renal function or cardiovascular status.[109,110] In particular, recurrent congestive heart failure and pulmonary edema are considered indications for stenting in RVD.[111]

In a recent study,[112] we found in patients with RVD significant remodeling of the renal microvascular architecture, with signs of defective angiogenesis and microvascular repair, underscoring intrarenal microvascular disease as an important pathophysiological component of RVD. Furthermore, these findings extend and affirm preclinical data on the capacity of therapeutic strategies (e.g., angiogenic and mitoprotection)[38,62,67,68,98] targeting the renal parenchyma as a standalone and/or as a coadjuvant to stenting to be considered as a potential clinical approach.

Traditional Drugs

Atherosclerotic RVD may be managed effectively with medical therapy and remain undetected in many hypertensive patients when BP and renal function are well controlled.[113] Antihypertensive drugs, statins, aspirin, and withdrawal of tobacco use are associated with a significant reduction in cardiovascular risk[114] and have been integrated in large randomized clinical trials such as the CORAL and ASTRAL.[53,106] Results from these trials suggest that the benefits of optimized medical therapy over periods of 2–5 years are equivalent to those obtained upon addition of renal artery revascularization.[115]

Many patients with RVD have preexisting hypertension,[116] which can be well-controlled with moderate antihypertensive therapy,[113] including ACEi and ARBs. In swine RVD, an ARB exerts greater protective effects on the renal microvasculature compared to triple therapy.[17] In RVD rats, despite reduction in filtration, renal structural integrity was preserved and recovered after removal of the clip or discontinuation of ACEi.[117] Overall, these drugs are well-tolerated in patients with RVD[106,118] and provide important mortality benefits.[119]

However, although many patients can be managed without revascularization,[120] RVD treated with medical therapy alone often progresses.[121,122] The CORAL[106] and ASTRAL[53] trials reported 16 and 22% progression rates, respectively, in both therapy arms (medical therapy with or without renal revascularization), underscoring the importance of close monitoring of RVD patients treated with medical therapy.

Blood pressure control should be accompanied by appropriate lipid management, antiplatelet therapy, glycemic control, and lifestyle changes, including diet, exercise, and smoking cessation.[123] Statins decrease the development and progression of RVD, possibly independent of lipid lowering.[124] In swine RVD, chronic simvastatin supplementation attenuated poststenotic kidney microvascular remodeling[13] and renal EPC apoptosis, underscoring their capacity to preserve renal repair mechanisms.[83]

Newer Therapeutic Approaches

Sodium-glucose Cotransporter-2 Inhibitors

Landmark clinical trials have revealed the benefits of sodium-glucose cotransporter-2 (SGLT-2)-inhibitors in patients with chronic kidney disease.[125] Given their ability to lower arterial stiffness, and improve endothelial function, renal inflammation, and hypoxia[126] renoprotective efficacy in RVD would be a reasonable assumption, of SGLT-2 inhibitors. Possibly, their combination with other therapeutic interventions such as ACEi[127] or glucagon-like peptide-1 receptor agonists[126] could be useful, but additional studies are needed to determine the role of SGLT-2 inhibitors in patients with RVD.

Cell-based Therapies

Cell-based therapies can ameliorate kidney damage in experimental RVD. MSC-derived extracellular vesicles also improved renal structure and function in experimental RVD,[46,128] but studies are needed to determine their efficacy in humans.

CONCLUSION

Exciting developments may selectively restore homeostasis and improve patient management. Emerging techniques and technologies are available and have the potential in RVH. For example, single-cell sequencing,[72] cytometry by time-of-flight, or site-specific urinary EVs[129] might help pinpoint the renal cellular site of damage and Clustered Regularly-Interspaced Short Palindromic Repeats to edit dysregulated genes, while mitochondrial transplantation[130] may replenish exhausted energy sources. Artificial intelligence techniques may differentiate the poststenotic kidney from other forms of kidney damage and identify those likely to benefit from specific interventions.

Studies are also needed to compare novel strategies side by side to select the most effective, which might be guided by the dominant pathophysiology in individual patients (e.g., microvascular loss vs. inflammation).

In patients with RVD, potent medications are available to control BP with renal artery revascularization. Ongoing research will continue guiding efforts for mechanistic-based treatments for RVD as the complex set of intrinsic mechanisms that interact and often synergize in RVD makes renal pathophysiology challenging.

REFERENCES

1. Goldblatt H, Lynch J, Hanzal RF, et al. Studies on experimental hypertension: I. The production of persistent elevation of systolic blood pressure by means of renal ischemia. J Exp Med. 1934;59:347-79.
2. Chade AR, Rodriguez-Porcel M, Grande JP, et al. Distinct renal injury in early atherosclerosis and renovascular disease. Circulation. 2002;106:1165-71.
3. Stanley JC, Whitehouse WM Jr. Occlusive and aneurysmal disease of the renal arterial circulation. Dis Mon. 1984;30:1-62.
4. Textor SC, Misra S, Oderich GS. Percutaneous revascularization for ischemic nephropathy: the past, present, and future. Kidney Int. 2013;83:28-40.
5. Fatica RA, Port FK, Young EW. Incidence trends and mortality in end-stage renal disease attributed to renovascular disease in the United States. Am J Kidney Dis. 2001;37:1184-90.
6. Greco BA, Breyer JA. The natural history of renal artery stenosis: who should be evaluated for suspected ischemic nephropathy? Semin Nephrol. 1996;16:2-11.
7. de Mast Q, Beutler JJ. The prevalence of atherosclerotic renal artery stenosis in risk groups: a systematic literature review. J Hypertens. 2009;27:1333-40.
8. Conlon PJ, Little MA, Pieper K, et al. Severity of renal vascular disease predicts mortality in patients undergoing coronary angiography. Kidney Int. 2001;60:1490-7.
9. Welch WJ, Patel K, Modlinger P, et al. Roles of vasoconstrictor prostaglandins, COX-1 and -2, and AT1, AT2, and TP receptors in a rat model of early 2K,1C hypertension. Am J Physiol Heart Circ Physiol. 2007;293:H2644-9.
10. Chade AR, Bentley MD, Zhu X, et al. Antioxidant intervention prevents renal neovascularization in hypercholesterolemic pigs. J Am Soc Nephrol. 2004;15:1816-25.
11. Chade AR, Best PJ, Rodriguez-Porcel M, et al. Endothelin-1 receptor blockade prevents renal injury in experimental hypercholesterolemia. Kidney Int. 2003;64:962-9.
12. Wilson SH, Chade AR, Feldstein A, et al. Lipid-lowering-independent effects of simvastatin on the kidney in experimental hypercholesterolaemia. Nephrol Dial Transplant. 2003;18:703-9.
13. Chade AR, Zhu X, Mushin OP, et al. Simvastatin promotes angiogenesis and prevents microvascular remodeling in chronic renal ischemia. FASEB J. 2006;20:1706-8.
14. Chade AR, Zhu XY, Grande JP, et al. Simvastatin abates development of renal fibrosis in experimental renovascular disease. J Hypertens. 2008;26:1651-60.
15. Zhu XY, Chade AR, Rodriguez-Porcel M, et al. Cortical microvascular remodeling in the stenotic kidney: role of increased oxidative stress. Arterioscler Thromb Vasc Biol. 2004;24:1854-9.
16. Lerman LO, Nath KA, Rodriguez-Porcel M, et al. Increased oxidative stress in experimental renovascular hypertension. Hypertension. 2001;37:541-6.
17. Zhang X, Eirin A, Li ZL, et al. Angiotensin receptor blockade has protective effects on the poststenotic porcine kidney. Kidney Int. 2013;84:767-75.
18. Gloviczki ML, Glockner JF, Lerman LO, et al. Preserved oxygenation despite reduced blood flow in poststenotic kidneys in human atherosclerotic renal artery stenosis. Hypertension. 2010;55:961-6.
19. Lerman LO, Taler SJ, Textor SC, et al. Computed tomography-derived intrarenal blood flow in renovascular and essential hypertension. Kidney Int. 1996;49:846-54.
20. Simeoni M, Borrelli S, Garofalo C, et al. Atherosclerotic-nephropathy: an updated narrative review. J Nephrol. 2021;34:125-36.
21. Dobrek L. An outline of renal artery stenosis pathophysiology—a narrative review. Life (Basel). 2021;11:208.
22. Parildar M, Parildar Z, Oran I, et al. Nitric oxide and oxidative stress in atherosclerotic renovascular hypertension: effect of endovascular treatment. J Vasc Interv Radiol. 2003;14:887-92.
23. Chade AR, Krier JD, Rodriguez-Porcel M, et al. Comparison of acute and chronic antioxidant interventions in experimental renovascular disease. Am J Physiol Renal Physiol. 2004;286:F1079-86.
24. Chade AR, Rodriguez-Porcel M, Herrmann J, et al. Beneficial effects of antioxidant vitamins on the stenotic kidney. Hypertension. 2003;42:605-12.
25. Chade AR, Rodriguez-Porcel M, Herrmann J, et al. Antioxidant intervention blunts renal injury in experimental renovascular disease. J Am Soc Nephrol. 2004;15:958-66.
26. Truong LD, Farhood A, Tasby J, et al. Experimental chronic renal ischemia: morphologic and immunologic studies. Kidney Int. 1992;41:1676-89.
27. Zhu XY, Chade AR, Krier JD, et al. The chemokine monocyte chemoattractant protein-1 contributes to renal dysfunction in swine renovascular hypertension. J Hypertens. 2009;27:2063-73.
28. Cheng J, Zhou W, Warner GM, et al. Temporal analysis of signaling pathways activated in a murine model of two-kidney, one-clip hypertension. Am J Physiol Renal Physiol. 2009;297:F1055-68.
29. Eirin A, Li Z, Zhang X, et al. A mitochondrial permeability transition pore inhibitor improves renal outcomes after revascularization in experimental atherosclerotic renal artery stenosis. Hypertension. 2012;60:1242-9.
30. Eirin A, Zhu XY, Krier JD, et al. Adipose tissue-derived mesenchymal stem cells improve revascularization outcomes to restore renal function in swine atherosclerotic renal artery stenosis. Stem Cells. 2012;30:1030-41.
31. Eirin A, Zhu XY, Li Z, et al. Endothelial outgrowth cells shift macrophage phenotype and improve kidney viability in swine renal artery stenosis. Arterioscler Thromb Vasc Biol. 2013;33:1006-13.
32. Gloviczki ML, Keddis MT, Garovic VD, et al. TGF expression and macrophage accumulation in atherosclerotic renal artery stenosis. Clin J Am Soc Nephrol. 2013;8:546-53.
33. Eirin A, Ebrahimi B, Zhang X, et al. Changes in glomerular filtration rate after renal revascularization correlate with microvascular hemodynamics and inflammation in swine renal artery stenosis. Circ Cardiovasc Interv. 2012;5:720-8.
34. Eirin A, Gloviczki ML, Tang H, et al. Inflammatory and injury signals released from the post-stenotic human kidney. Eur Heart J. 2013;34:540-8a.
35. Eirin A, Gloviczki ML, Tang H, et al. Chronic renovascular hypertension is associated with elevated levels of neutrophil gelatinase-associated lipocalin. Nephrol Dial Transplant. 2012;27:4153-61.
36. Saeed A, Herlitz H, Nowakowska-Fortuna E, et al. Oxidative stress and endothelin-1 in atherosclerotic renal artery stenosis and effects of renal angioplasty. Kidney Blood Press Res. 2011;34:396-403.
37. Safak E, Wilke C, Derer W, et al. Long-term follow-up of patients with atherosclerotic renal artery disease. J Am Soc Hypertens. 2013;7:24-31.
38. Eirin A, Zhu XY, Urbieta-Caceres VH, et al. Persistent kidney dysfunction in swine renal artery stenosis correlates with outer cortical microvascular remodeling. Am J Physiol Renal Physiol. 2011;300:F1394-401.
39. Saad A, Herrmann SMS, Crane J, et al. Stent revascularization restores cortical blood flow and reverses tissue hypoxia in atherosclerotic renal artery stenosis but fails to reverse

inflammatory pathways or glomerular filtration rate. Circ Cardiovasc Interv. 2013;6:428-35.
40. Eirin A, Zhang X, Zhu XY, et al. Renal vein cytokine release as an index of renal parenchymal inflammation in chronic experimental renal artery stenosis. Nephrol Dial Transplant. 2014;29:274-82.
41. Saad A, Dietz AB, Herrmann SMS, et al. Autologous mesenchymal stem cells increase cortical perfusion in renovascular disease. J Am Soc Nephrol. 2017;28:2777-85.
42. Keddis MT, Garovic VD, Bailey KR, et al. Ischaemic nephropathy secondary to atherosclerotic renal artery stenosis: clinical and histopathological correlates. Nephrol Dial Transplant. 2010;25:3615-22.
43. Chade AR, Rodriguez-Porcel M, Grande JP, et al. Mechanisms of renal structural alterations in combined hypercholesterolemia and renal artery stenosis. Arterioscler Thromb Vasc Biol. 2003;23:1295-301.
44. Warner GM, Cheng J, Knudsen BE, et al. Genetic deficiency of SMAD3 protects the kidneys from atrophy and interstitial fibrosis in 2K1C hypertension. Am J Physiol Renal Physiol. 2012;302:F1455-64.
45. Chade AR, Zhu X, Lavi R, et al. Endothelial progenitor cells restore renal function in chronic experimental renovascular disease. Circulation. 2009;119:547-57.
46. Eirin A, Zhu XY, Puranik AS, et al. Mesenchymal stem cell-derived extracellular vesicles attenuate kidney inflammation. Kidney Int. 2017;92:114-24.
47. Eirin A, Ebrahimi B, Zhang X, et al. Mitochondrial protection restores renal function in swine atherosclerotic renovascular disease. Cardiovasc Res. 2014;103:461-72.
48. Nogueira BV, Palomino Z, Porto ML, et al. Granulocyte colony stimulating factor prevents kidney infarction and attenuates renovascular hypertension. Cell Physiol Biochem. 2012;29:143-52.
49. Chrysochou C, Kalra PA. Epidemiology and natural history of atherosclerotic renovascular disease. Prog Cardiovasc Dis. 2009;52:184-95.
50. Roumeliotis S, Georgianos PI, Roumeliotis A, et al. Oxidized LDL modifies the association between proteinuria and deterioration of kidney function in proteinuria diabetic kidney disease. Life (Basel). 2021;11:504.
51. Favreau F, Zhu XY, Krier JD, et al. Revascularization of swine renal artery stenosis improves renal function but not the changes in vascular structure. Kidney Int. 2010;78:1110-8.
52. Bax L, Woittiez AJJ, Kouwenberg HJ, et al. Stent placement in patients with atherosclerotic renal artery stenosis and impaired renal function: a randomized trial. Ann Intern Med. 2009;150: 840-8, W150-1.
53. ASTRAL Investigators; Wheatley K, Ives N, et al. Revascularization versus medical therapy for renal-artery stenosis. N Engl J Med. 2009;361:1953-62.
54. Chade AR, Tullos NA, Harvey TW, et al. Renal therapeutic angiogenesis using a bioengineered polymer-stabilized vascular endothelial growth factor construct. J Am Soc Nephrol. 2016;27:1741-52.
55. Chade AR, Zhu XY, Krier JD, et al. Endothelial progenitor cells homing and renal repair in experimental renovascular disease. Stem Cells. 2010;28:1039-47.
56. Lerman LO, Schwartz RS, Grande JP, et al. Noninvasive evaluation of a novel swine model of renal artery stenosis. J Am Soc Nephrol. 1999;10:1455-65.
57. Cervenka L, Horacek V, Vaneckova I, et al. Essential role of AT1A receptor in the development of 2K1C hypertension. Hypertension. 2002;40:735-41.
58. Palm F, Onozato M, Welch WJ, et al. Blood pressure, blood flow, and oxygenation in the clipped kidney of chronic 2-kidney, 1-clip rats: effects of tempol and angiotensin blockade. Hypertension. 2010;55:298-304.
59. Lerman LO, Textor SC, Grande JP. Mechanisms of tissue injury in renal artery stenosis: ischemia and beyond. Prog Cardiovasc Dis. 2009;52:196-203.
60. Chade AR, Krier JD, Galili O, et al. Role of renal cortical neovascularization in experimental hypercholesterolemia. Hypertension. 2007;50:729-36.
61. Chade AR, Kelsen S. Reversal of renal dysfunction by targeted administration of VEGF into the stenotic kidney: a novel potential therapeutic approach. Am J Physiol Renal Physiol. 2012;302:F1342-50.
62. Ebrahimi B, Li Z, Eirin A, et al. Addition of endothelial progenitor cells to renal revascularization restores medullary tubular oxygen consumption in swine renal artery stenosis. Am J Physiol Renal Physiol. 2012;302:F1478-85.
63. Levy BI. Microvascular plasticity and experimental heart failure. Hypertension. 2006;47:827-9.
64. Eirin A, Lerman LO. Darkness at the end of the tunnel: poststenotic kidney injury. Physiology (Bethesda). 2013;28:245-53.
65. Chade AR. Renal vascular structure and rarefaction. Compr Physiol. 2013;3:817-31.
66. Rodriguez-Porcel M, Krier JD, Lerman A, et al. Combination of hypercholesterolemia and hypertension augments renal function abnormalities. Hypertension. 2001;37:774-80.
67. Chade AR, Kelsen S. Renal microvascular disease determines the responses to revascularization in experimental renovascular disease. Circ Cardiovasc Interv. 2010;3:376-83.
68. Guise E, Engel JE, Williams ML, et al. Biopolymer-delivered vascular endothelial growth factor improves renal outcomes following revascularization. Am J Physiol Renal Physiol. 2019;316:F1016-25.
69. Ter Maaten JM, Damman K, Verhaar MC, et al. Connecting heart failure with preserved ejection fraction and renal dysfunction: the role of endothelial dysfunction and inflammation. Eur J Heart Fail. 2016;18:588-98.
70. Yau JW, Teoh H, Verma S. Endothelial cell control of thrombosis. BMC Cardiovasc Disord. 2015;15:130.
71. Zhang L, Pitcher LE, Yousefzadeh MJ, et al. Cellular senescence: a key therapeutic target in aging and diseases. J Clin Invest. 2022;132:e158450.
72. Kim SR, Puranik AS, Jiang K, et al. Progressive cellular senescence mediates renal dysfunction in ischemic nephropathy. J Am Soc Nephrol. 2021;32:1987-2004.
73. Kim SR, Zou X, Tang H, et al. Increased cellular senescence in the murine and human stenotic kidney: effect of mesenchymal stem cells. J Cell Physiol. 2021;236:1332-44.
74. Kim SR, Eirin A, Zhang X, et al. Mitochondrial protection partly mitigates kidney cellular senescence in swine atherosclerotic renal artery stenosis. Cell Physiol Biochem. 2019;52:617-32.
75. Chen XJ, Kim SR, Jiang K, et al. Renovascular disease induces senescence in renal scattered tubular-like cells and impairs their reparative potency. Hypertension. 2021;77:507-18.
76. Kim SR, Jiang K, Chen X, et al. Selective kidney targeting increases the efficacy of mesenchymal stromal/stem cells for alleviation of murine stenotic-kidney senescence and damage. J Tissue Eng Regen Med. 2022;16:550-8.
77. Gobe GC, Axelsen RA, Searle JW. Cellular events in experimental unilateral ischemic renal atrophy and in regeneration after contralateral nephrectomy. Lab Invest. 1990;63:770-9.
78. Botros FT, Olszanecki R, Prieto-Carrasquero MC, et al. Induction of heme oxygenase-1 in renovascular hypertension is associated with inhibition of apoptosis. Cell Mol Biol (Noisy-le-grand). 2007;53:51-60.

79. Bhaskaran M, Reddy K, Radhakrishanan N, et al. Angiotensin II induces apoptosis in renal proximal tubular cells. Am J Physiol Renal Physiol. 2003;284:F955-65.
80. Niimi K, Yasui T, Hirose M, et al. Mitochondrial permeability transition pore opening induces the initial process of renal calcium crystallization. Free Radic Biol Med. 2012;52:1207-17.
81. Meyrier A, Hill GS, Simon P. Ischemic renal diseases: new insights into old entities. Kidney Int. 1998;54:2-13.
82. Daemen MA, van 't Veer C, Denecker G, et al. Inhibition of apoptosis induced by ischemia-reperfusion prevents inflammation. J Clin Invest. 1999;104:541-9.
83. Lavi R, Zhu XY, Chade AR, et al. Simvastatin decreases endothelial progenitor cell apoptosis in the kidney of hypertensive hypercholesterolemic pigs. Arterioscler Thromb Vasc Biol. 2010;30:976-83.
84. Szeto HH. First-in-class cardiolipin-protective compound as a therapeutic agent to restore mitochondrial bioenergetics. Br J Pharmacol. 2014;171:2029-50.
85. Baines CP. The molecular composition of the mitochondrial permeability transition pore. J Mol Cell Cardiol. 2009;46:850-7.
86. Eirin A, Saad A, Tang H, et al. Urinary mitochondrial DNA copy number identifies chronic renal injury in hypertensive patients. Hypertension. 2016;68:401-10.
87. Eirin A, Herrmann SM, Saad A, et al. Urinary mitochondrial DNA copy number identifies renal mitochondrial injury in renovascular hypertensive patients undergoing renal revascularization: a pilot study. Acta Physiol (Oxf). 2019;226:e13267.
88. Eirin A, Ebrahimi B, Kwon SH, et al. Restoration of mitochondrial cardiolipin attenuates cardiac damage in swine renovascular hypertension. J Am Heart Assoc. 2016;5:e003118.
89. Eirin A, Williams BJ, Ebrahimi B, et al. Mitochondrial targeted peptides attenuate residual myocardial damage after reversal of experimental renovascular hypertension. J Hypertens. 2014;32:154-65.
90. Saad A, Herrmann SMS, Eirin A, et al. Phase 2a clinical trial of mitochondrial protection (Elamipretide) during stent revascularization in patients with atherosclerotic renal artery stenosis. Circ Cardiovasc Interv. 2017;10:e005487.
91. Evans RG, Gardiner BS, Smith DW, et al. Intrarenal oxygenation: unique challenges and the biophysical basis of homeostasis. Am J Physiol Renal Physiol. 2008;295:F1259-70.
92. Ebrahimi B, Gloviczki M, Woollard JR, et al. Compartmental analysis of renal BOLD MRI data: introduction and validation. Invest Radiol. 2012;47:175-82.
93. Textor SC, Glockner JF, Lerman LO, et al. The use of magnetic resonance to evaluate tissue oxygenation in renal artery stenosis. J Am Soc Nephrol. 2008;19:780-8.
94. Warner L, Glockner JF, Woollard J, et al. Determinations of renal cortical and medullary oxygenation using blood oxygen level-dependent magnetic resonance imaging and selective diuretics. Invest Radiol. 2011;46:41-7.
95. Lerman LO, Bentley MD, Fiksen-Olsen MJ, et al. Pressure dependency of canine intrarenal blood flow within the range of autoregulation. Am J Physiol. 1995;268:F404-9.
96. Abdi A, Johns EJ. Importance of the renin-angiotensin system in the generation of kidney failure in renovascular hypertension. J Hypertens. 1996;14:1131-7.
97. Juillard L, Lerman LO, Kruger DG, et al. Blood oxygen level-dependent measurement of acute intrarenal ischemia. Kidney Int. 2004;65:944-50.
98. Ebrahimi B, Eirin A, Li Z, et al. Mesenchymal stem cells improve medullary inflammation and fibrosis after revascularization of swine atherosclerotic renal artery stenosis. PLoS One. 2013;8:e67474.
99. Heyman SN, Khamaisi M, Rosen S, et al. Renal parenchymal hypoxia, hypoxia response and the progression of chronic kidney disease. Am J Nephrol. 2008;28:998-1006.
100. Textor SC, Lerman LO. Paradigm shifts in atherosclerotic renovascular disease: where are we now? J Am Soc Nephrol. 2015;26:2074-80.
101. Warner L, Gomez SI, Bolterman R, et al. Regional decreases in renal oxygenation during graded acute renal arterial stenosis: a case for renal ischemia. Am J Physiol Regul Integr Comp Physiol. 2009;296:R67-71.
102. Dorros G, Prince C, Mathiak L. Stenting of a renal artery stenosis achieves better relief of the obstructive lesion than balloon angioplasty. Cathet Cardiovasc Diagn. 1993;29:191-8.
103. Dorros G, Jaff MR, Mathiak L, et al. Stent revascularization for atherosclerotic renal artery stenosis. 1-year clinical follow-up. Tex Heart Inst J. 1998;25:40-3.
104. Dorros G, Jaff M, Mathiak L, et al. Four-year follow-up of Palmaz-Schatz stent revascularization as treatment for atherosclerotic renal artery stenosis. Circulation. 1998;98:642-7.
105. Dorros G, Jaff M, Jain A, et al. Follow-up of primary Palmaz-Schatz stent placement for atherosclerotic renal artery stenosis. Am J Cardiol. 1995;75:1051-5.
106. Cooper CJ, Murphy TP, Cutlip DE, et al. Stenting and medical therapy for atherosclerotic renal-artery stenosis. N Engl J Med. 2014;370:13-22.
107. Green D, Vassallo D, Handley K, et al. Cardiac structure and function after revascularization versus medical therapy for renal artery stenosis: the ASTRAL heart echocardiographic sub-study. BMC Nephrol. 2019;20:220.
108. Dorros G, Jaff M, Mathiak L, et al. Multicenter Palmaz stent renal artery stenosis revascularization registry report: four-year follow-up of 1,058 successful patients. Catheter Cardiovasc Interv. 2002;55:182-8.
109. Chrysochou C, Green D, Ritchie J, et al. Kidney volume to GFR ratio predicts functional improvement after revascularization in atheromatous renal artery stenosis. PLoS One. 2017;12:e0177178.
110. Green D, Ritchie JP, Chrysochou C, et al. Revascularization of atherosclerotic renal artery stenosis for chronic heart failure versus acute pulmonary oedema. Nephrology (Carlton). 2018;23: 411-7.
111. Bhalla V, Textor SC, Beckman JA, et al. Revascularization for renovascular disease: a scientific statement from the American Heart Association. Hypertension. 2022;79: e128-43.
112. Klomjit N, Zhu XY, Eirin A, et al. Microvascular remodeling and altered angiogenic signaling in human kidneys distal to occlusive atherosclerotic renal artery stenosis. Nephrol Dial Transplant. 2022;37:1844-56.
113. Rihal CS, Textor SC, Breen JF, et al. Incidental renal artery stenosis among a prospective cohort of hypertensive patients undergoing coronary angiography. Mayo Clin Proc. 2002;77:309-16.
114. Mann JF, Gerstein HC, Pogue J, et al. Renal insufficiency as a predictor of cardiovascular outcomes and the impact of ramipril: the HOPE randomized trial. Ann Intern Med. 2001;134:629-36.
115. Textor SC, Herrmann SM. Evidence and renovascular disease: trials and mistrials? Am J Kidney Dis. 2017;70:160-3.
116. Hajjar I, Kotchen TA. Trends in prevalence, awareness, treatment, and control of hypertension in the United States, 1988–2000. JAMA. 2003;290:199-206.
117. Gröne HJ, Warnecke E, Olbricht CJ. Characteristics of renal tubular atrophy in experimental renovascular hypertension: a model of kidney hibernation. Nephron. 1996;72:243-52.
118. Chrysochou C, Foley RN, Young JF, et al. Dispelling the myth: the use of renin-angiotensin blockade in atheromatous renovascular disease. Nephrol Dial Transplant. 2012;27:1403-9.

119. Hackam DG, Duong-Hua ML, Mamdani M, et al. Angiotensin inhibition in renovascular disease: a population-based cohort study. Am Heart J. 2008;156:549-55.
120. Chabova V, Schirger A, Stanson AW, et al. Outcomes of atherosclerotic renal artery stenosis managed without revascularization. Mayo Clin Proc. 2000;75:437-44.
121. Dean RH, Kieffer RW, Smith BM, et al. Renovascular hypertension: anatomic and renal function changes during drug therapy. Arch Surg. 1981;116:1408-15.
122. Caps MT, Zierler RE, Polissar NL, et al. Risk of atrophy in kidneys with atherosclerotic renal artery stenosis. Kidney Int. 1998;53:735-42.
123. Herrmann SMS, Saad A, Textor SC. Management of atherosclerotic renovascular disease after Cardiovascular Outcomes in Renal Atherosclerotic Lesions (CORAL). Nephrol Dial Transplant. 2015;30:366-75.
124. Cheung CM, Patel A, Shaheen N, et al. The effects of statins on the progression of atherosclerotic renovascular disease. Nephron Clin Pract. 2007;107:c35-42.
125. Heerspink HJL, Berger S, Gansevoort RT, et al. Will SGLT2 inhibitors be effective and safe in patients with severe CKD, dialysis, or kidney transplantation. Clin J Am Soc Nephrol. 2023;18:1500-2.
126. Yau K, Dharia A, Alrowiyti I, et al. Prescribing SGLT2 inhibitors in patients with CKD: expanding indications and practical considerations. Kidney Int Rep. 2022;7:1463-76.
127. Lytvyn Y, Kimura K, Peter N, et al. Renal and vascular effects of combined SGLT2 and angiotensin-converting enzyme inhibition. Circulation. 2022;146:450-62.
128. Eirin A, Zhu XY, Jonnada S, et al. Mesenchymal stem cell-derived extracellular vesicles improve the renal microvasculature in metabolic renovascular disease in swine. Cell Transplant. 2018;27:1080-95.
129. Santelli A, Sun IO, Eirin A, et al. Senescent kidney cells in hypertensive patients release urinary extracellular vesicles. J Am Heart Assoc. 2019;8:e012584.
130. Rossi A, Asthana A, Riganti C, et al. Mitochondria transplantation mitigates damage in an in vitro model of renal tubular injury and in an ex vivo model of DCD renal transplantation. Ann Surg. 2023;278:e1313-26.

CHAPTER 10

The Complexity of Resistant and Refractory Hypertension

Somya Mahlawat, Umesh Tripathi, Sharad Chandra

ABSTRACT

Resistant hypertension (RH) is defined as uncontrolled blood pressure despite optimal triple-drug therapy, while refractory hypertension (RfH) persists despite five or more agents. RH arises from complex neurohormonal, renal, and vascular mechanisms and is linked to high cardiovascular risk. Effective management integrates lifestyle modification, optimized pharmacotherapy, and emerging options such as aldosterone synthase inhibitors, renal denervation, and baroreflex activation therapy.

Keywords: Resistant hypertension, refractory hypertension, apparent treatment-resistant hypertension, pseudo-resistance, aldosterone synthase inhibitors, renal denervation, baroreflex activation therapy.

INTRODUCTION

Resistant hypertension (RH) refers to blood pressure that remains above the target level despite treatment with at least three different classes of antihypertensive drugs. These typically include a long-acting calcium channel blocker, a renin–angiotensin system inhibitor (such as an ACE inhibitor or an ARB), and a diuretic, all prescribed at optimal or maximally tolerated doses. The term also encompasses patients whose blood pressure is adequately controlled, but only through the use of four or more antihypertensive medications—a condition described as controlled resistant hypertension.[1-3]

The term *apparent treatment-resistant hypertension* (aTRH) is applied when patients seem to meet the criteria for resistant hypertension (RH) based on office blood pressure values and prescribed therapy, but potential secondary contributors to pseudo-resistance have not been ruled out. Factors commonly responsible for pseudo-resistance include:[4]

- Inaccurate blood pressure measurement, resulting in spuriously elevated values.
- The white-coat effect, where office readings are high but home or ambulatory measurements are normal.
- Therapeutic inertia, reflecting inadequate intensification or optimization of treatment.
- Poor adherence to prescribed medication, which continues to be a major obstacle to effective blood pressure control.

At the more severe end of the spectrum is *refractory hypertension* (RfH), which is characterized by persistent uncontrolled blood pressure despite treatment with at least five antihypertensive drugs, including both a thiazide-like diuretic (such as chlorthalidone) and a mineralocorticoid receptor antagonist (such as spironolactone), prescribed at maximally tolerated or optimal doses.[5]

These definitions have been summarized in **Table 1**.[1,2,5]

A meta-analysis conducted by Jacques and colleagues, which included 91 studies and >3.2 million participants, estimated the worldwide prevalence of RH at 10.3%.[6] The 2025 American Heart Association (AHA) and American College of Cardiology (ACC) guidelines report that RH affects roughly 8.5–20% of adults with hypertension in the United States. The condition is closely linked with risk factors such as older age, obesity, chronic kidney disease (CKD), and diabetes mellitus. It is also observed more frequently in Black individuals, largely attributable to disparities in healthcare access and socioeconomic determinants.[7,8]

Patients with RH face substantially increased cardiovascular and renal risk. Compared with those whose blood pressure is well controlled, RH is associated with at least a 50% higher likelihood of myocardial infarction, stroke, progression to end-stage kidney disease, and cardiovascular death. According to the 2024 European Society of Cardiology (ESC) guidelines, the prevalence of RH in clinical practice is approximately 10–20%, with affected patients exhibiting a two- to six-fold higher risk of major adverse cardiovascular and renal events.[9-11]

TABLE 1: Key terms and summarized definitions.

Term	Definition
Resistant hypertension (RH)	BP above goal despite ≥3 antihypertensive agents of different classes with at least one of them being a diuretic at maximum or maximally tolerated doses
Controlled resistant hypertension	BP at goal on ≥4 antihypertensive medications at maximal or maximally tolerated doses
Apparent treatment-resistant hypertension	Term used when adherence, medication dose, or out-of-office BP is not documented; and pseudo resistance not excluded in a patient on ≥3 antihypertensive agents.
Refractory hypertension (RfH)	BP uncontrolled despite ≥5 antihypertensive agents of different classes (including a thiazide-like diuretic such as chlorthalidone and spironolactone) at maximal or near-maximal doses
Pseudo-resistance	Falsely elevated BP due to factors such as poor measurement technique, white-coat effect, undertreatment, clinical inertia, or medication nonadherence
White-coat resistant hypertension	Office BP uncontrolled but out-of- office BP controlled in a patient on ≥3 antihypertensive drugs

PATHOGENESIS OF RESISTANT HYPERTENSION

Resistant hypertension develops through a complex interplay of neurohormonal overactivity, vascular dysfunction, renal abnormalities, and immune-inflammatory pathways. External factors such as diet, excess body weight, and associated comorbidities interact with an individual's genetic background to influence vulnerability to the condition. Recognizing these interdependent mechanisms is crucial for designing preventive strategies, optimizing treatment approaches, and ultimately improving patient outcomes.[12,13] The major pathophysiological contributors are outlined in **Figure 1**.

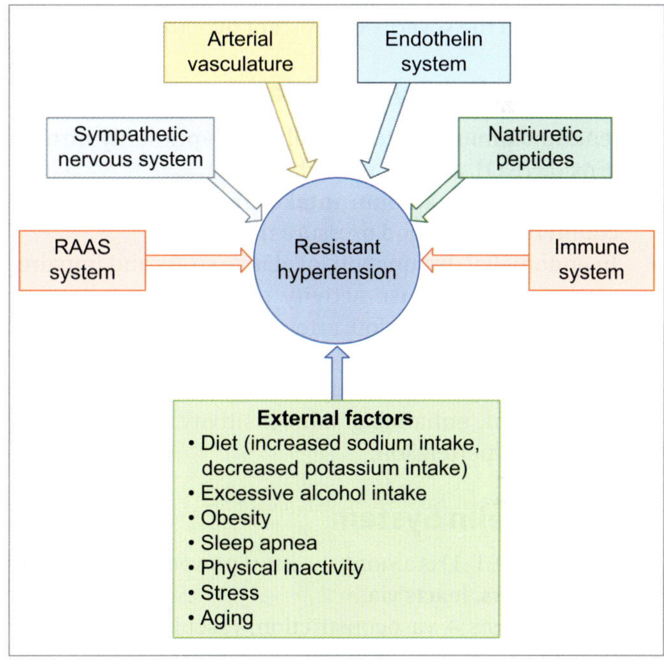

FIG. 1: Pathogenesis of resistant hypertension.

CONTRIBUTING FACTORS

Resistant hypertension is influenced by a combination of modifiable and non-modifiable determinants.[14] Key contributors include:

- Excess dietary sodium and insufficient potassium intake
- Obesity, physical inactivity, and heavy alcohol consumption
- Diabetes mellitus and the metabolic syndrome
- Chronic kidney disease (CKD)
- Obstructive sleep apnea (OSA)
- Advancing age and psychosocial stress

These elements frequently act in combination. For instance, diabetes accelerates renal impairment, while OSA augments sympathetic activation and aldosterone secretion—together sustaining elevated blood pressure.[15,16]

PATHOPHYSIOLOGICAL MECHANISMS

Renin–angiotensin–aldosterone System

The Renin-angiotensin-aldosterone System (RAAS) plays a pivotal role in blood pressure control through regulation of fluid balance, sodium and potassium handling, and vascular tone.

- A decline in blood pressure stimulates renin release from the kidney, initiating the conversion of angiotensinogen to angiotensin I.
- Angiotensin-converting enzyme (ACE) then generates angiotensin II, a potent vasoconstrictor.
- *Angiotensin II actions include:*
  - Promoting sodium and water reabsorption
  - Stimulating aldosterone release
  - Causing vasoconstriction
  - Activating thirst and antidiuretic hormone (ADH) secretion
  - Blunting baroreceptor sensitivity

In resistant hypertension, RAAS hyperactivity drives volume expansion and vascular resistance. This effect is often amplified by arterial stiffness, endothelial dysfunction, sympathetic nervous system (SNS) hyperactivity, and salt sensitivity.[13]

Sympathetic Nervous System

While the SNS normally mediates short-term blood pressure responses, sustained activation contributes to chronic hypertension.

- Induces vasoconstriction, increasing peripheral resistance
- Elevates heart rate and cardiac output
- Enhances renal sodium reabsorption
- Impairs baroreceptor regulation

Excessive SNS drive is particularly evident in obesity and correlates with the severity of resistant hypertension.[12,17]

Endothelial Dysfunction

The endothelium regulates vascular tone primarily through nitric oxide (NO), a major vasodilator.[18]

- Normally, high sodium intake triggers NO release to counterbalance blood pressure rise.
- In endothelial dysfunction, oxidative stress and impaired nitric oxide synthase activity reduce NO availability, causing vasoconstriction, arterial stiffening, and elevated resistance.
- Low potassium intake further aggravates endothelial impairment, enhancing salt sensitivity and the risk of resistant hypertension.

Endothelin System

Endothelin-1 (ET-1) is among the most powerful endogenous vasoconstrictors. It acts via:

- *ETA receptors* → vasoconstriction, vascular hypertrophy, fibrosis
- *ETB receptors* → vasodilation and ET-1 clearance

In resistant hypertension, increased ET-1 activity—especially via ETA receptors—leads to sodium retention, aldosterone release, vascular remodeling, and target-organ injury. Elevated ET-1 levels are commonly observed in obesity, diabetes, and CKD.[19,20]

Natriuretic Peptides

Atrial natriuretic peptide (ANP) and brain natriuretic peptide (BNP) exert protective effects against hypertension by:

- Promoting sodium and water excretion
- Causing vasodilation
- Increasing glomerular filtration rate (GFR)
- Reducing circulating volume

In resistant hypertension, these beneficial mechanisms are often blunted due to peptide breakdown or receptor insensitivity, limiting their antihypertensive effects.[12,14]

Immune and Inflammatory Mechanisms

Chronic low-grade inflammation also contributes to resistant hypertension.

- T cells and macrophages infiltrate vascular and renal tissues, promoting oxidative stress, fibrosis, and endothelial dysfunction.
- Inflammatory mediators further enhance RAAS and SNS activity, while diminishing NO bioavailability.

These immune-mediated pathways are particularly relevant in salt-sensitive and autoimmune-related forms of resistant hypertension.[12-14]

INTERCONNECTED PATHWAYS

The mechanisms underlying resistant hypertension do not function independently but are tightly interlinked.[21]

- Activation of the RAAS enhances sympathetic activity and amplifies inflammatory cascades.
- Persistent sympathetic stimulation increases renin release and contributes to endothelial injury.
- Inflammatory processes intensify oxidative stress, further diminishing nitric oxide availability.
- Vascular stiffening and endothelial dysfunction impair renal sodium handling, thereby heightening salt sensitivity.

DIAGNOSTIC CHALLENGES

Evaluating resistant hypertension (RH)[22] requires careful differentiation between *true* RH and conditions that only mimic resistance. Secondary hypertension, which accounts for roughly 5–10% of cases, must be systematically excluded.[9,23,24] Primary aldosteronism represents the most frequent endocrine cause yet often remains underdiagnosed, whereas atherosclerotic renal artery stenosis is the predominant renovascular contributor. In patients with suggestive clinical features, diagnostic imaging—starting with renal Doppler ultrasonography and followed, when appropriate, by CT or MR angiography—should be pursued.[25] A comprehensive list of secondary causes is outlined in **Table 2**.

Equally important is recognizing *apparent* RH, which may arise from technical errors or patient-related factors. Inaccurate blood pressure measurement, inappropriate cuff size, the white-coat effect, and poor adherence to therapy are frequent culprits. Standardized office protocols and confirmation with home or ambulatory monitoring are crucial to avoid overdiagnosis. In elderly patients and those with advanced CKD, arterial calcification can also falsely elevate readings.

Medication nonadherence is one of the most common contributors, affecting nearly one-third of patients.[26] Objective assessments—such as witnessed dosing or drug level assays—are more dependable than questionnaires

TABLE 2: Causes of secondary hypertension and diagnostic workup.[15,18,23,25]

Cause	Diagnostic tests
Chronic kidney disease (CKD)	eGFR urine albumin
Primary hyperaldosteronism	• 24-hour urine aldosterone ≥12 ng/day • Suppressed plasma renin activity ARR
Renovascular hypertension	• Doppler ultrasound • CT angiogram • MR angiography (MRA)
Coarctation of aorta	Physical examination (e.g., radio-femoral delay, BP differential)
Pheochromocytoma	Plasma free metanephrines
Cushing syndrome	• 24-hour urine free cortisol • Dexamethasone suppression test
Congenital adrenal hyperplasia (CAH)	17-hydroxyprogesterone
Acromegaly	• IGF-1 levels • Glucose suppression test
Thyroid dysfunction	Thyroid function test
Hyperparathyroidism	Calcium and PTH levels
Obstructive sleep apnea (OSA)	Polysomnography

or pill counts, and given that adherence can vary over time, repeated evaluation is often necessary. Screening for comorbidities, particularly obstructive sleep apnea, is also essential, as it frequently coexists with RH.[8,9]

Implementing a systematic, stepwise diagnostic strategy helps distinguish true RH from pseudo-resistance, prevents misclassification, and directs patients toward the most appropriate treatment pathway.

MANAGEMENT STRATEGIES

Resistant hypertension remains a therapeutic challenge, with many patients failing to achieve adequate blood pressure control despite optimized triple-drug therapy. Successful management requires a comprehensive approach that integrates lifestyle modification, elimination of contributing substances, stepwise pharmacological escalation, and structured follow-up. Substances known to interfere with blood pressure control include over-the-counter supplements, recreational drugs, and prescription medications such as oral contraceptives, immunosuppressants, and antidepressants. In carefully selected patients with uncontrolled blood pressure despite medical optimization, device-based therapies such as renal denervation may be considered.[27] A summary of management pathways is provided in **Flowchart 1**.

LIFESTYLE INTERVENTIONS

Lifestyle optimization is regarded as the cornerstone of RH management, endorsed by both the American (ACC/AHA) and European (ESC/ESH) hypertension guidelines. Evidence from recent network meta-analyses shows that non-pharmacological interventions alone can reduce office systolic BP by approximately 7 mm Hg—an effect comparable to adding another antihypertensive medication.[28]

DIETARY STRATEGIES

Dietary Approaches to Stop Hypertension and Mediterranean Diets

Both emphasize fruits, vegetables, legumes, whole grains, low-fat dairy, fish, and lean proteins, while limiting red meat, refined sugars, and processed foods. These dietary approaches consistently reduce systolic BP by 5–10 mm Hg and lower long-term cardiovascular risk.[28,29]

Sodium Restriction

- *ACC/AHA 2025:* <2,300 mg/day (ideal target: 1,500 mg/day).[30]
- *ESC 2024:* <2 g/day (~5 g salt), with tolerable limits up to 4 g/day.[31]

Potassium Supplementation

Enhancing potassium intake through diet (fruits, vegetables, and salt substitutes) can counteract sodium effects and reduce BP. This approach should be applied cautiously in advanced CKD to avoid hyperkalemia.

PHYSICAL ACTIVITY AND WEIGHT MANAGEMENT

Exercise Prescription

- *ACC/AHA 2025:* 75–150 min/week of aerobic or resistance activity.[30]

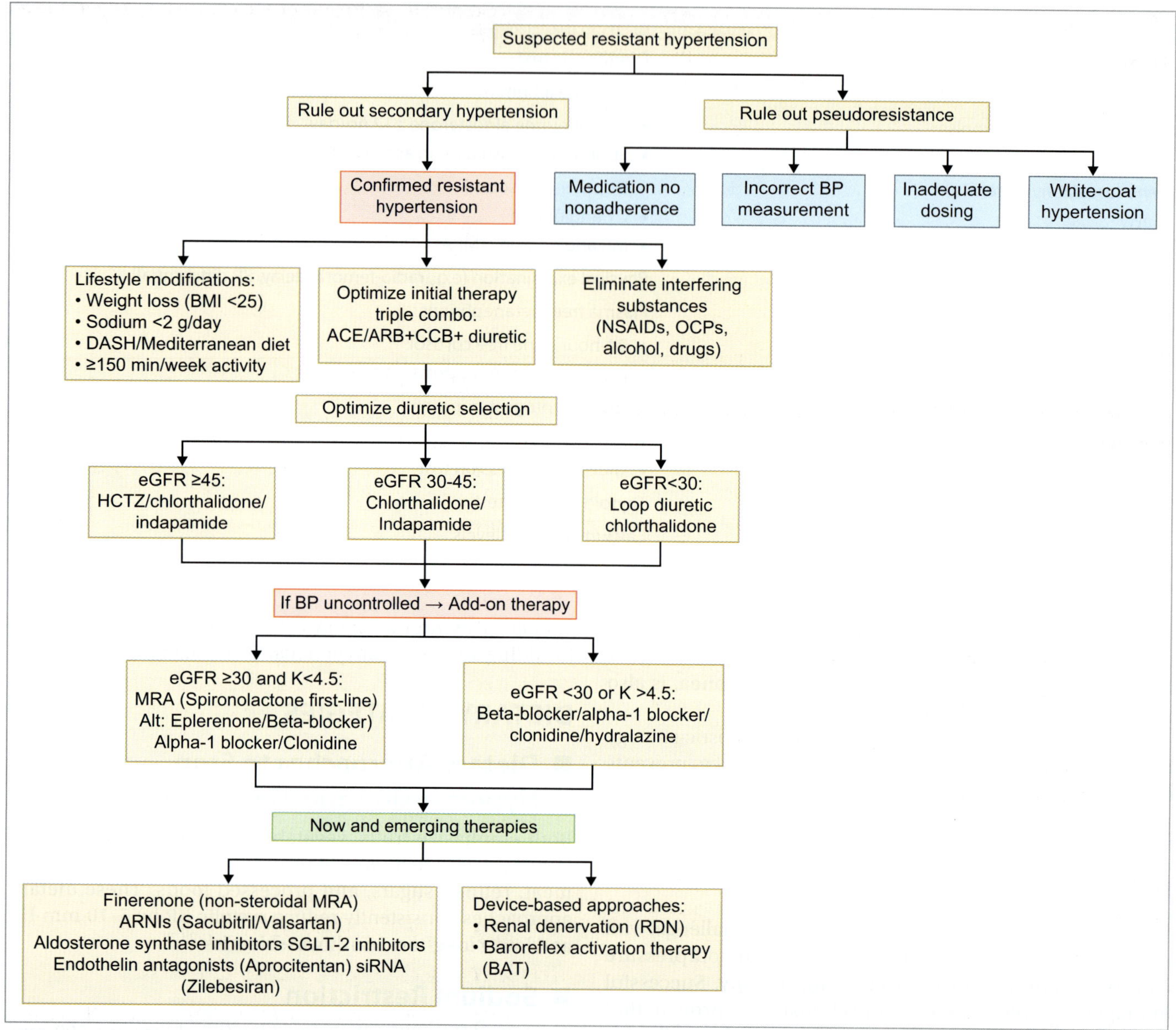

FLOWCHART 1: Management of resistant hypertension.

- *ESC 2024:* ≥150 min/week of moderate activity or 75 min/week of vigorous exercise. Aerobic training reduces systolic BP by up to 7–8 mm Hg, resistance training by approximately4–5 mm Hg.[31] Clinical trials (TRIUMPH, EnRicH) confirm that structured exercise lowers ambulatory BP and improves cardiometabolic and psychological outcomes.[32,33]

Weight Reduction

- *ACC/AHA:* ≥5% weight loss in overweight/obese patients.[30]
- *ESC:* Maintain BMI 20–25 kg/m² and waist circumference <94 cm (men) or <80 cm (women).[31] The GATEWAY trial demonstrated that bariatric surgery in RH patients significantly improved BP control, partly through mechanisms beyond weight loss, such as reduced sympathetic activity and better volume regulation.[34]

Alcohol, Smoking, and Stress

- *Alcohol:* ACC/AHA advises moderation (≤2 drinks/day for men, ≤1 for women); ESC favors abstinence for maximal cardiovascular benefit.[30,31]
- *Smoking:* Complete cessation is strongly recommended (Class I), reducing overall cardiovascular risk despite modest direct BP effects.[30,31]
- *Stress management:* Yoga, meditation, and relaxation therapies are increasingly recognized as effective adjunctive measures.[30,31]

Sleep and Obstructive Sleep Apnea

Obstructive sleep apnea (OSA) is highly prevalent among RH patients. Continuous positive airway pressure (CPAP) improves BP control, especially in severe OSA or those with abnormal nocturnal dipping. ESC guidelines also recommend screening OSA patients for secondary causes such as primary aldosteronism, given the bidirectional link between sleep disorders and hypertension.[31]

PHARMACOLOGICAL STRATEGIES

Optimal drug therapy for RH requires rationalization of initial treatment and a structured, stepwise addition of further agents. Both ACC/AHA and ESC/ESH guidelines emphasize ensuring that triple therapy is maximized before escalation.[30,31]

Optimization of Baseline Therapy

- *Triple-drug backbone:* A renin–angiotensin system blocker (ACEi/ARB), a dihydropyridine calcium channel blocker, and a diuretic—ideally as a single-pill combination to improve adherence.
- *Diuretic choice tailored to kidney function:*
  - *eGFR ≥45 mL/min/1.73 m^2:* Hydrochlorothiazide (dose escalation may be useful).
  - *eGFR 30–45:* Prefer chlorthalidone or indapamide for stronger and longer effects.
  - *eGFR <30:* Indapamide ineffective; chlorthalidone may work at higher doses; loop diuretics (furosemide, torsemide, and bumetanide) are first-line.

The CLICK trial confirmed that chlorthalidone lowered systolic BP by approximately 10 mm Hg in stage 4 CKD (mean eGFR 23), supporting its use even in advanced renal dysfunction.[35]

Fourth-line: Mineralocorticoid Receptor Antagonists

- *Spironolactone* is the gold standard, proven in PATHWAY-2 to reduce BP more effectively than placebo, bisoprolol, or doxazosin.[36] The ReHOT trial reinforced its superiority over clonidine.[37]
- *Limitations:* Risk of hyperkalemia and renal impairment; hormonal side effects (gynecomastia, impotence, menstrual irregularities).
- *Eplerenone:* More selective, fewer hormonal side effects but weaker, shorter-acting, and costlier.
- *Novel non-steroidal mineralocorticoid receptor antagonists:*
  - *Finerenone:* Demonstrated cardiovascular and renal protection in *FIDELIO-DKD* and *FIGARO-DKD,* though its BP-lowering effect was modest.[38,39]
  - *Esaxerenone:* Effective BP reduction with lower hyperkalemia risk; approved in Japan.
  - *Ocedurenone:* In late-phase trials, showing promising efficacy and safety.

Beyond Mineralocorticoid Receptor Antagonists: Individualized Add-on Therapy

When BP remains uncontrolled despite optimized triple therapy, intensified diuretic regimens, and mineralocorticoid receptor antagonists (MRAs), treatment should be individualized.

- *β-blockers:* Appropriate when indicated (post-MI, HFrEF, and tachyarrhythmias). Cardio-selective agents (bisoprolol, nebivolol, and metoprolol succinate) are preferred. Although less effective than spironolactone in PATHWAY-2, they remain essential in select populations.[36]
- *α-blockers:* Extended-release doxazosin can be useful, particularly in patients with coexisting BPH. However, *ALLHAT* raised concerns about increased heart failure risk, and side effects such as orthostatic hypotension limit widespread use.[40]
- *Centrally acting agents:* Drugs such as clonidine or moxonidine are options when others fail. *ReHOT* showed clonidine was inferior to spironolactone but still effective. Adverse effects—sedation, dry mouth, rebound hypertension—restrict use, though transdermal delivery may improve tolerability.[37]
- *Direct vasodilators:* Hydralazine and minoxidil are last-resort agents for refractory cases. Their use is limited by side effects (fluid retention, reflex tachycardia, and sympathetic activation), necessitating co-administration with diuretics and β-blockers.[27]

NEW AND EMERGING PHARMACOLOGICAL THERAPIES

A considerable proportion of patients with RH remain uncontrolled despite optimized standard therapy, prompting interest in novel pharmacological agents that target both established and emerging blood pressure pathways.

Angiotensin Receptor–Neprilysin Inhibitors

Sacubitril/valsartan [angiotensin receptor–neprilysin inhibitor (ARNI)] simultaneously enhances natriuretic peptide signaling and suppresses the RAAS. Beyond its established role in heart failure, post-hoc analyses of the *PARAGON-HF* trial and smaller hypertension-specific studies have shown clinically meaningful BP reductions even in patients already receiving multiple agents. By improving natriuresis, vasodilation, and vascular compliance, ARNIs may serve as a promising adjunct in RH, although large-scale dedicated trials are still limited.[41]

Aldosterone Synthase Inhibitors

These agents reduce aldosterone production without altering cortisol, offering a potential alternative to MRAs.

- *Baxdrostat (BrigHtn trial):* Achieved a placebo-adjusted systolic BP reduction of approximately 11 mm Hg at the 2 mg dose, with good tolerability and no effect on cortisol.[42]
- *Lorundrostat (Target-HTN trial):* Demonstrated dose-dependent reductions in BP and serum aldosterone, independent of baseline renin status. While efficacy was encouraging, interindividual variability in response suggests the need for personalized approaches.[43]

Together, these findings suggest aldosterone synthase inhibitors could become valuable options for patients intolerant of spironolactone or eplerenone.

Sodium-glucose Cotransporter-2 Inhibitors

Initially developed for type 2 diabetes, agents such as empagliflozin, dapagliflozin, and canagliflozin[44] have demonstrated cardiovascular and renal benefits that extend beyond glycemic control. Their antihypertensive effect is modest (average systolic BP reduction of 4–5 mm Hg), as observed in EMPA-REG OUTCOME and CREDENCE. Mechanisms include osmotic diuresis, reduced arterial stiffness, and improved endothelial function. Given their established role in heart failure and CKD, sodium-glucose cotransporter-2 (SGLT-2) inhibitors are now being evaluated specifically in RH populations.[45,46]

Endothelin Receptor Antagonists

Blocking endothelin-1, a potent vasoconstrictor, is a compelling therapeutic strategy.

- Earlier endothelin receptor antagonists (ERAs) (e.g., bosentan, ambrisentan) were limited by hepatotoxicity or fluid retention, and darusentan failed in resistant hypertension trials.
- *Aprocitentan,* a dual ETA/ETB antagonist, has shown the most promise.[47] In the *PRECISION trial,* it reduced systolic BP by approximately 3.8 mm Hg over placebo at 4 weeks, with sustained effects over 48 weeks and rebound hypertension upon withdrawal. Ambulatory monitoring confirmed efficacy. Peripheral edema (9–18%) was the most frequent side effect, but overall tolerability was acceptable, supporting its potential role in long-term RH management.[48]

Central and Novel Neurohormonal Targets

- *Firibastat,* an aminopeptidase A inhibitor that blocks angiotensin III within the brain, was tested in the *FRESH trial* but did not demonstrate superiority over placebo after 12 weeks. Its clinical relevance remains uncertain.[49]
- Additional experimental strategies include:
  - *Dopamine β-hydroxylase inhibitors* (e.g., etamicastat), designed to suppress sympathetic activity.
  - *Xanthine oxidase inhibitors* (e.g., allopurinol), aimed at reducing vascular stiffness. These remain early in development with limited clinical data.[50,51]

Ribonucleic Acid-based and Gene Therapies

- *Zilebesiran,* an siRNA molecule targeting hepatic angiotensinogen synthesis, represents a novel long-acting approach. Phase II studies demonstrated durable reductions in systolic BP (~22 mm Hg after 8 weeks) lasting several months after a single dose. The *KARDIA-1* and *KARDIA-2* trials confirmed sustained efficacy both as monotherapy and in combination regimens, while *KARDIA-3* is currently evaluating its utility in high-risk patients with uncontrolled hypertension.[52-54]
- *Vaccination strategies* directed against angiotensin I or II are under early investigation, aiming to provide long-term suppression of hypertensive pathways and reduce lifelong dependence on daily oral therapy.[55]

DEVICE-BASED THERAPIES IN RESISTANT HYPERTENSION

Although pharmacological advances have improved blood pressure (BP) management, a proportion of patients with RH continue to remain uncontrolled. For this group, device-based strategies have been developed to complement medical therapy by directly targeting neurohumoral mechanisms underlying hypertension. The two modalities most extensively investigated are *renal denervation (RDN)* and *baroreflex activation therapy (BAT).*

Renal Denervation

Renal denervation (RDN) is a minimally invasive, catheter-based procedure designed to disrupt sympathetic nerve fibers surrounding the renal arteries. Since sympathetic overactivity contributes to renin release, sodium retention, vasoconstriction, and elevated vascular tone, interrupting these pathways can help restore BP control.[56]

Mechanism of Action

- *Efferent fibers:* Promote renin secretion, sodium reabsorption, and vasoconstriction.
- *Afferent fibers:* Stimulate central sympathetic activity, increasing systemic vascular resistance. Renal denervation attenuates both components, thereby lowering RAAS activation, enhancing natriuresis, and reducing overall sympathetic drive.

Evidence from Clinical Trials

Initial enthusiasm was tempered by the *SYMPLICITY HTN-3 trial*, which showed no benefit over sham therapy. However, subsequent studies with improved devices and trial designs have confirmed consistent efficacy:

- *SPYRAL HTN-OFF MED/ON MED:* Radiofrequency RDN reduced office systolic BP by approximately 10 mm Hg, with parallel improvements in ambulatory BP in both untreated and treated hypertensive patients.[58,59]
- *RADIANCE-HTN SOLO/TRIO:* Ultrasound-based RDN lowered daytime ambulatory systolic BP by -6.3 mm Hg compared with placebo.[57,60,61]
- *GLOBAL SYMPLICITY registry:* Demonstrated durable reductions of -18/11 mm Hg in office BP sustained at 36 months.[62]

While BP reductions are modest, they are comparable to adding an additional antihypertensive agent. RDN is most appropriate for carefully selected patients with confirmed RH, particularly those intolerant to polypharmacy, poorly adherent to complex regimens, or with refractory disease.

BAROREFLEX ACTIVATION THERAPY

Baroreflex activation therapy (BAT) is an implantable system that modulates autonomic tone centrally by electrically stimulating baroreceptors in the carotid sinus. Unlike RDN, which acts at the renal level, BAT restores autonomic balance by suppressing sympathetic outflow and enhancing parasympathetic activity.[63]

Mechanism of Action

Baroreceptors in the carotid sinus and aortic arch normally sense arterial wall stretch and modulate autonomic activity. In chronic hypertension, their responsiveness is blunted, allowing persistent sympathetic activation. BAT devices (e.g., *Barostim neo*) deliver chronic electrical stimulation to the carotid sinus, mimicking natural baroreceptor activation. This results in:

- Reduced sympathetic tone and increased vagal drive
- Vasodilation and improved renal sodium excretion
- Lower systemic vascular resistance and heart rate
- Sustained reductions in BP

Evidence from Clinical Studies

- *DEBuT-HT trial:* Provided proof of concept, showing reductions of approximately 30/20 mm Hg in office BP among RH patients.[64]
- *Rheos pivotal trial:* Demonstrated significant BP lowering but raised safety concerns due to early device-related complications (nerve injury, surgical risks, and respiratory issues).[65]
- *Barostim neo trials:* Device refinements, including unilateral carotid stimulation with a smaller system, have improved safety and maintained BP-lowering efficacy.[66]
- *Meta-analyses and registry data:* Report consistent, durable office systolic BP reductions of 20–30 mm Hg over several years.

Baroreflex activation therapy appears particularly useful in advanced CKD, where RDN may be less effective. However, due to limited large-scale outcomes data, current guidelines recommend reserving BAT for highly selected patients managed in specialized centers.[67]

Refractory Hypertension

Refractory hypertension represents the most severe and uncommon form of blood pressure dysregulation. It is defined as uncontrolled hypertension despite treatment with at least five antihypertensive agents of different classes, including a long-acting thiazide-like diuretic (such as chlorthalidone) and a mineralocorticoid receptor antagonist (spironolactone or eplerenone). Unlike resistant hypertension—which is relatively frequent—RfH is rare, affecting fewer than 5% of patients seen in specialized referral centers.[5]

Patients with RfH often display a distinctive clinical profile. They are more likely to be younger, female, and share traditional risk factors seen in resistant hypertension—such as chronic kidney disease, diabetes, obesity, and Black ethnicity—but typically present with more advanced target-organ injury, including left ventricular hypertrophy and heart failure with preserved ejection fraction.

Pathophysiologically, RfH appears to diverge from resistant hypertension. Since diuretic therapy is already maximized, persistent hypertension is less attributable to fluid overload and more strongly linked to neurogenic mechanisms. Studies suggest that exaggerated sympathetic activation underpins this phenotype, supported by findings of elevated resting heart rates, greater arterial stiffness, and increased urinary norepinephrine levels compared with controlled hypertensive patients.[5]

Management remains particularly challenging, as most available pharmacological classes have already been exhausted. Traditional sympatholytic agents such as clonidine may offer some benefit but are limited by tolerability issues. This therapeutic gap has intensified interest in *device-based approaches*—notably renal denervation (RDN) and baroreflex activation therapy (BAT)—which directly modulate sympathetic activity. These strategies, currently being evaluated in resistant hypertension, may prove especially valuable in the refractory subgroup, where sympathetic overdrive appears to be the defining feature.

CONCLUSION

Refractory hypertension remains a rare but formidable clinical entity, demanding innovative treatment strategies that move beyond conventional pharmacology. By targeting the central role of sympathetic activation, emerging device-based therapies may hold the key to improving outcomes in this challenging population.

REFERENCES

1. Carey RM, Calhoun DA, Bakris GL, W et al. Resistant hypertension: detection, evaluation, and management: a scientific statement from the American Heart Association. Hypertension. 2018;72(5):e53-90.
2. Romano S, Rigon G, Albrigi M, et al. Hypertension, uncontrolled hypertension and resistant hypertension: prevalence, comorbidities and prescribed medications in 228,406 adults resident in urban areas: a population-based observational study. Intern Emerg Med. 2023;18(8):1951-9.
3. Acelajado MC, Calhoun DA. Aldosteronism and resistant hypertension. Int J Hypertens. 2011;2011:837817.
4. Calhoun DA, Jones D, Textor S, et al. Resistant hypertension: diagnosis, evaluation, and treatment: a scientific statement from the American Heart Association Professional Education Committee of the Council for High Blood Pressure Research. Hypertension. 2008;51(6):1403-19.
5. Dudenbostel T, Siddiqui M, Oparil Set al. Refractory hypertension: a novel phenotype of antihypertensive treatment failure. Hypertension. 2016;67(6):1085-92.
6. Noubiap JJ, Nansseu JR, Nyaga UF, et al. Global prevalence of resistant hypertension: a meta-analysis of data from 3.2 million patients. Heart. 2019;105(2):98-105.
7. Patel KV, Li X, Kondamudi N, et al. Prevalence of apparent treatment-resistant hypertension in the United States according to the 2017 high blood pressure guideline. Mayo Clin Proc. 2019;94(4):776-82.
8. Carey RM, Calhoun DA, Bakris GL, et al. Resistant hypertension: detection, evaluation, and management: a scientific statement from the American Heart Association. Hypertension. 2018;72(5):e53-90.
9. Carey RM, Sakhuja S, Calhoun DA, et al. Prevalence of apparent treatment-resistant hypertension in the United States. Hypertension. 2019;73(2):424-31.
10. Vongpatanasin W. Resistant hypertension: a review of diagnosis and management. JAMA. 2014;311(21):2216-24.
11. Oparil S, Acelajado MC, Bakris GL, et al. Hypertension. Nat Rev Dis Primers. 2018;4:18014.
12. Fountain JH, Lappin SL. Physiology, renin-angiotensin system. Treasure Island (FL): StatPearls Publishing; 2022.
13. Townsend RR. Pathogenesis of drug-resistant hypertension. Semin Nephrol. 2014;34(5):506-11.
14. Bangash A, Wajid F, Poolacherla R, et al. Obstructive sleep apnea and hypertension: a review of the relationship and pathogenic association. Cureus. 2020;12(5):e8241.
15. Acelajado MC, Hughes ZH, Oparil S, et al. Treatment of resistant and refractory hypertension. Circ Res. 2019;124(7):1061-70.
16. Morris RC Jr, Schmidlin O, Sebastian A, et al. Vasodysfunction that involves renal vasodysfunction, not abnormally increased renal retention of sodium, accounts for the initiation of salt-induced hypertension. Circulation. 2016;133(9):881-93.
17. Calhoun DA. Hyperaldosteronism as a common cause of resistant hypertension. Annu Rev Med. 2013;64:233-47.
18. Landsberg L, Aronne LJ, Beilin LJ, et al. Obesity-related hypertension: pathogenesis, cardiovascular risk, and treatment: a position paper of the Obesity Society and the American Society of Hypertension. J Clin Hypertens (Greenwich). 2013;15(1):14-33.
19. Schiffrin EL. Role of endothelin-1 in hypertension and vascular disease. Am J Hypertens. 2001;14(6 Pt 2):83S-9S.
20. Williams B, MacDonald TM, Morant SV, et al. PATHWAY Study Group. Endocrine and haemodynamic changes in resistant hypertension, and blood pressure responses to spironolactone or amiloride: the PATHWAY-2 mechanisms substudies. Lancet Diabetes Endocrinol. 2018;6(6):464-75.
21. Mancia G, Kreutz R, Brunstrom M, et al. 2023 ESH guidelines for the management of arterial hypertension: Task Force for the management of arterial hypertension of the European Society of Hypertension, endorsed by the International Society of Hypertension and the European Renal Association. J Hypertens. 2023;41(10):1874-2071.
22. Doroszko A, Janus A, Szahidewicz-Krupska E, et al. Resistant hypertension. Adv Clin Exp Med. 2016;25(1):173-83.
23. Aboyans V, Ricco JB, Bartelink MEL, et al. 2017 ESC guidelines on the diagnosis and treatment of peripheral arterial diseases, in collaboration with the ESVS: document covering atherosclerotic disease of extracranial carotid and vertebral, mesenteric, renal, upper and lower extremity arteries. Eur Heart J. 2018;39(9):763-816.
24. Durand H, Hayes P, Morrissey EC, et al. Medication adherence among patients with apparent treatment-resistant hypertension: systematic review and meta-analysis. J Hypertens. 2017;35(12):2346-57.
25. Bakris GL, Agarwal R, Anker SD, et al. Effect of finerenone on chronic kidney disease outcomes in type 2 diabetes. N Engl J Med. 2020;383(23):2219-29.
26. Pitt B, Filippatos G, Agarwal R, et al. FIGARO-DKD Investigators. Cardiovascular events with finerenone in kidney disease and type 2 diabetes. N Engl J Med. 2021;385(24):2252-63.
27. Saneei P, Salehi-Abargouei A, Esmaillzadeh A, et al. Influence of Dietary Approaches to Stop Hypertension (DASH) diet on blood pressure: a systematic review and meta-analysis of randomized controlled trials. Nutr Metab Cardiovasc Dis. 2014;24(12):1253-61.
28. Gay HC, Rao SG, Vaccarino V, et al. Effects of different dietary interventions on blood pressure: systematic review and meta-analysis of randomized controlled trials. Hypertension. 2016;67(4):733-39.
29. Jones DW, Ferdinand KC, Taler SJ, et al. AHA/ACC guideline for the prevention, detection, evaluation, and management of high blood pressure in adults: report of the American College of Cardiology/American Heart Association Joint Committee on Clinical Practice Guidelines. J Am Coll Cardiol. 2025;85(2):e1-e120.
30. McEvoy JW, McCarthy CP, Bruno RM, et al. 2024 ESC Guidelines on arterial hypertension. Eur Heart J. 2024;45(44):3912-4018.
31. Blumenthal JA, Smith PJ, Mabe S, et al. Effects of lifestyle modification on psychosocial function in patients with resistant hypertension: secondary outcomes from the TRIUMPH randomized clinical trial. J Cardiopulm Rehabil Prev. 2024;44(2):64-70.
32. Lopes S, Mesquita-Bastos J, Garcia C, et al. Effect of exercise training on ambulatory blood pressure among patients with resistant hypertension: a randomized clinical trial. JAMA Cardiol. 2021;6(11):1317-23.
33. Schiavon CA, Ikeoka D, Santucci EV, et al. Effects of bariatric surgery versus medical therapy on 24-hour ambulatory blood pressure and the prevalence of resistant hypertension. Hypertension. 2019;73(3):571-77.
34. Agarwal R, Sinha AD, Cramer AE, et al. Chlorthalidone for hypertension in advanced chronic kidney disease. N Engl J Med. 2021;385(27):2507-19.
35. Williams B, MacDonald TM, Morant S, et al. Spironolactone versus placebo, bisoprolol, and doxazosin to determine the optimal treatment for drug-resistant hypertension (PATHWAY-2): a randomised, double-blind, crossover trial. Lancet. 2015;386(10008):2059-68.

36. Krieger EM, Drager LF, Giorgi DMA, et al. Spironolactone versus clonidine as a fourth-drug therapy for resistant hypertension: the ReHOT randomized study (Resistant Hypertension Optimal Treatment). Hypertension. 2018;71(4):681-90.
37. Mcinnes GT. ALLHAT Officers and Coordinators for the ALLHAT Collaborative Research Group. Major outcomes in high-risk hypertensive patients randomized to ACE inhibitor or calcium channel blocker vs diuretic: the ALLHAT trial. JAMA. 2002;288(23):2981-97.
38. Solomon SD, McMurray JJV, Anand IS, et al. PARAGON-HF Investigators and Committees. Angiotensin–neprilysin inhibition in heart failure with preserved ejection fraction. N Engl J Med. 2019;381(17):1609-20.
39. Freeman MW, Halvorsen YD, Marshall W, et al. Phase 2 trial of baxdrostat for treatment-resistant hypertension. N Engl J Med. 2023;388(5):395-405.
40. Ferreira JP, Fitchett D, Ofstad AP, et al. Empagliflozin for patients with presumed resistant hypertension: a post hoc analysis of the EMPA-REG OUTCOME trial. Am J Hypertens. 2020;33(12): 1092-101.
41. Laffin LJ, Rodman D, Luther JM, et al. Aldosterone synthase inhibition with lorundrostat for uncontrolled hypertension: the Target-HTN randomized clinical trial. JAMA. 2023;330(12):1138-39.
42. Zinman B, Wanner C, Lachin JM, et al. Empagliflozin, cardiovascular outcomes, and mortality in type 2 diabetes. N Engl J Med. 2015;373(22):2117-28.
43. Perkovic V, Jardine MJJ, Neal B, et al. Canagliflozin and renal outcomes in type 2 diabetes and nephropathy. N Engl J Med. 2019;380(24):2295-306.
44. Ye N, Jardine MJ, Oshima M, et al. Blood pressure effects of canagliflozin and clinical outcomes in type 2 diabetes and chronic kidney disease: insights from the CREDENCE trial. Circulation. 2021;143(17):1735-49.
45. Bakris GL, Blacher J, Ferdinand KC et al. Top-line results of the first-in-class aminopeptidase-A inhibitor firibastat in treatment-resistant hypertension (FRESH) study. American Heart Association Scientific Sessions; 2022;5-7.
46. Dey SK, Saini M, Prabhakar P, et al. Dopamine β-hydroxylase as a potential drug target to combat hypertension. Expert Opin Investig Drugs. 2020;29(9):1043-57.
47. Schlaich MP, Bellet M, Weber MA, et al. Dual endothelin antagonist aprocitentan for resistant hypertension (PRECISION): a multicentre, blinded, randomised, parallel-group, phase 3 trial. Lancet. 2022;400(10367):1927-37.
48. Kohagura K, Tana T, Higa A, et al. Effects of xanthine oxidase inhibitors on renal function and blood pressure in hypertensive patients with hyperuricemia. Hypertens Res. 2016;39(8):593-7.
49. Bakris GL, Saxena M, Gupta A, et al. RNA interference with zilebesiran for mild to moderate hypertension: the KARDIA-1 randomized clinical trial. JAMA. 2024;331(9):740-9.
50. Desai AS, Karns AD, Badariene J, et al. Add-on treatment with zilebesiran for inadequately controlled hypertension: the KARDIA-2 randomized clinical trial. JAMA. 2025;334(1):46-55.
51. Havasi A, Pagidipati N, Bakris GL, et al. KARDIA-3 study design: zilebesiran as add-on therapy in patients with high cardiovascular risk and hypertension inadequately controlled by standard of care antihypertensives. J Hypertens. 2024;42(Suppl 1):e120.
52. Nakagami H, Morishita R. Recent advances in therapeutic vaccines to treat hypertension. Hypertension. 2018;72(5):1031-6.
53. Krum H, Schlaich MP, Sobotka PA, et al. Percutaneous renal denervation in patients with treatment-resistant hypertension: final 3-year report of the SYMPLICITY HTN-1 study. Lancet. 2014;383(9917):622-9.
54. Bhatt DL, Vaduganathan M, Kandzari DE, et al. Long-term outcomes after catheter-based renal artery denervation for resistant hypertension: final follow-up of the randomized SYMPLICITY HTN-3 Trial. Lancet. 2022;400(10364):1405-16.
55. Böhm M, Kario K, Kandzari DE, et al. Efficacy of catheter-based renal denervation in the absence of antihypertensive medications (SPYRAL HTN-OFF MED Pivotal): a multicentre, randomised, sham-controlled trial. Lancet. 2020;395(10234):1444-51.
56. Mahfoud F, Kandzari DE, Kario K, et al. Long-term efficacy and safety of renal denervation in the presence of antihypertensive drugs (SPYRAL HTN-ON MED): a randomised, sham-controlled trial. Lancet. 2022;399(10333):1401-10.
57. Azizi M, Schmieder RE, Mahfoud F, et al. Endovascular ultrasound renal denervation to treat hypertension (RADIANCE-HTN SOLO): a multicentre, international, single-blind, randomised, sham-controlled trial. Lancet. 2018;391(10137):2335-45.
58. Azizi M, Mahfoud F, Pathak A, et al. Endovascular ultrasound renal denervation in patients with treatment-resistant hypertension (RADIANCE-HTN TRIO): a randomised, multicentre, single-blind, sham-controlled trial. Lancet. 2021;397(10293):2476-86.
59. Mahfoud F, Böhm M, Schmieder R, et al. Effects of renal denervation on kidney function and long-term outcomes: 3-year follow-up from the Global SYMPLICITY Registry. Eur Heart J. 2019;40(42):3474-82.
60. Victor RG. Carotid baroreflex activation therapy for resistant hypertension. Nat Rev Cardiol. 2015;12(8):451-63.
61. Scheffers IJ, Kroon AA, Schmidli J, et al. Novel baroreflex activation therapy in resistant hypertension: results of a European multi-center feasibility study. J Am Coll Cardiol. 2010;56:1254-8.
62. Bisognano JD, Bakris G, Nadim MK, et al. Baroreflex activation therapy lowers blood pressure in patients with resistant hypertension: results from the double-blind, randomized, placebo-controlled Rheos pivotal trial. J Am Coll Cardiol. 2011;58(7):765-73.
63. Hoppe UC, Brandt MC, Wachter R, et al. Minimally invasive system for baroreflex activation therapy chronically lowers blood pressure with pacemaker-like safety profile: results from the Barostim Neo trial. J Am Soc Hypertens. 2012;6:270-6.
64. Bhatt DL, Kristensen AMD, Pareek M, et al. Baroreflex activation therapy for resistant hypertension and heart failure. US Cardiol Rev. 2019;13(2):83-87.
65. Acelajado MC, Pisoni R, Dudenbostel T, et al. Refractory hypertension: definition, prevalence, and patient characteristics. J Clin Hypertens (Greenwich). 2012;14:7-12.
66. Velasco A, Siddiqui M, Kreps E, et al. Refractory hypertension is not attributable to intravascular fluid retention as determined by intracardiac volumes. Hypertension. 2018;72:343-9.
67. Cao G, Chen C, Lin Q, et al. Prevalence, clinical characteristics and echocardiography parameters of non-resistant, resistant and refractory hypertension in Chinese. Postgrad Med. 2017;129: 187-92.

SECTION

3

Cardiometabolic

Section Outline

11. **Slowing Cardiovascular Aging by Promoting Cardiometabolic Health**
Bhabatosh Biswas, Pankaj Sharma, Tapas K Kundu

12. **Obesity and Cardiovascular Diseases**
Amit Malviya, Md Amish Shikoh, Aman Asthana, Animesh Mishra

13. **Myocardial Abnormalities Across the AHA-ACC Heart Failure Spectrum in Diabetic Patients**
Umeshwar Pandey, Kumar Himanshu

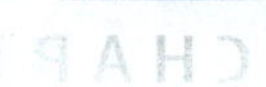

CHAPTER 11

Slowing Cardiovascular Aging by Promoting Cardiometabolic Health

Bhabatosh Biswas, Pankaj Sharma, Tapas K Kundu

ABSTRACT

Cardiovascular aging is a major driver of morbidity and mortality worldwide. It results from cumulative biological insults, lifestyle-dependent exposures, and genetic predispositions that progressively impair vascular integrity and metabolic resilience. The cellular and systemic hallmarks of aging translate into gradual arterial stiffening, endothelial dysfunction, and fibrosis, raising the risk of major adverse cardiovascular events (MACE). Understanding the modulation of these complex interrelated processes and integrating them with clinical interventions is important to lead a long and healthy life. This review brings together evidences from molecular biology, genetics, clinical epidemiology and preventive cardiology to gain mechanistic insights toward slowing cardiovascular aging. Genetic determinants of cardiovascular aging such as *FOXO3, APOE, CETP, IGFBP3, TERT* gene variants, and mosaic loss of Y chromosome (mLOY), reactive oxygen species (ROS), epigenetic effectors such as EZH2, DOT1L, and LSD1, and environmental drivers such as exposure to air pollutants, sedentary lifestyle, sleep disruption, and unhealthy dietary patterns, are discussed. Clinical and translational strategies, including lifestyle modifications, pharmaco-surgical interventions, and digital health innovations, were systematically examined.

Converging evidences highlight cardiometabolic health as the primary lever to slow vascular aging. Lifestyle interventions such as adopting dietary approaches to stop hypertension (DASH), such as the Mediterranean diet, structured physical activity, weight management, tobacco cessation, and restorative sleep, demonstrate cardiovascular protective effects. Similarly, pharmacological strategies such as inhibitors of cholesterol biosynthesis, angiotensin converting enzyme (ACE) inhibitors, angiotensin II receptor blockers (ARBs), sodium-glucose cotransporter-2 (SGLT-2) inhibitors, glucagon-like peptide 1 (GLP-1) receptor agonists, and modulators of epigenetic effectors mitigate cardiometabolic decline. Cardiovascular aging is not an inevitable consequence of chronological age, but a rather dynamic process that could be modified by genetic, environmental and lifestyle factors. An integrated multidomain program anchored in lifestyle optimization, monitoring tools and targeted therapy, may thus be designed to maintain or decelerate cardiovascular aging, extend health span and promote independence in older adults.

Keywords: Cardiovascular aging, cardiometabolic health, hallmarks of aging, genetic and epigenetic determinants, lifestyle interventions, pharmacological therapies, endothelial dysfunction, arterial stiffness, digital health, artificial intelligence, health span.

INTRODUCTION

"Teach us to number our days, that we get a heart of wisdom" (Psalm 90:12), a poetic reminder to the finite lifespan, necessitates a constant endeavor to spend time with purpose and grace. In clinical terms, this ethos translates to preserving the quality of later life years by safeguarding the heart and vasculature health. Cardiovascular aging is a dominant contributor to morbidity and mortality across the globe. As populations age, the prevalence of cardiovascular disease (CVD) rises steeply, driven by cumulative exposure to elevated blood pressure, nicotine, atherogenic lipids, hepatorenal comorbidities, insulin resistance, physical inactivity, unhealthy diet, and environmental stressors. Aging remodels the cardiovascular system through structural and molecular decline that predisposes subject to major adverse cardiovascular events (MACE) such as arrhythmia, heart failure, and stroke. Cardiometabolic disease is a set of non-communicable diseases, including obesity, renal disease, diabetes, and cardiovascular disease that enhance each other with aging.[1] Aging is an intrinsic, and variable multisystem physiological decline in cognition, metabolism and mobility owing to decreased cellular health and intermodular communication, heightened metabolic syndrome and muscular weakness. Frailty, a complex age-associated decline in multi-system reserve, captures such heterogeneity in aging trajectories. Clinicians often use a 30-point or similar index incorporating gait speed, grip strength, comorbid conditions, and social interactions to assess frailty. However, composite scores obscure domain specific impairments. Combining clinical manifestations with polygenic risk scores and biomarker panels offer a path toward precise domain targeted recommendations and earlier intervention.[2] In this chapter, we discuss the mechanisms of cardiovascular aging, specify important genetic and epigenetic contributors, detail clinical expression of cardiometabolic decline, and suggest practical interventions spanning lifestyle, pharmacology, and systems level approaches toward resetting the aging clock. The goal is translational—to provide a coherent framework for clinicians and researchers to slow cardiovascular aging and elevate health span in late life years. Converging geroscientific and preventive cardiology evidence indicates cardiometabolic health as the principal lever to slow down the cardiovascular clock. Though aging is inevitable, its cardiovascular phenotypes, including arrhythmias and lack of heart rate variation (HRV) in elderly under stress, are modifiable in tempo and severity.

HALLMARKS OF AGING AND CARDIOVASCULAR IMPLICATIONS

The hallmarks of aging describe recurrent biological failure modes that accumulate with time. These include genomic instability, telomere attrition, epigenetic changes, loss of proteostasis, mitochondrial dysfunction, deregulated nutrient sensing, cellular senescence, altered intercellular communication, and stem cell exhaustion **(Table 1)**. Genomic instability and telomere shortening foster endothelial cell apoptosis and reduce regenerative capacity, thereby accelerating vascular aging. Mitochondrial dysfunction reduces availability of the energy currency while increasing reactive oxygen species (ROS) levels, thus damaging cardiomyocytes and vascular smooth-muscle cells. Senescent cells adopt a proinflammatory senescence associated secretory phenotype (SASP) that amplifies local inflammation, degrades extracellular matrix, and promotes fibrosis-changes linked to diastolic dysfunction, i.e., heart failure with preserved ejection fraction (HFpEF). Nutrient sensing pathways such as insulin/insulin growth factor (IGF)-1, mechanistic target of rapamycin kinase complex 1 (mTOR-1), sirtuins, and AMP-activated protein kinase (AMPK) modulate metabolism and stress resistance, positioning metabolic reprogramming as a therapeutic handle **(Fig. 1)**.

TABLE 1: Hallmarks of aging and cardiovascular effects.

Hallmark of aging	Cardiovascular effect
Genomic instability	DNA damage in endothelium; cardiomyopathy risk
Telomere attrition	Early vascular aging; endothelial dysfunction
Epigenetic alterations	Vascular gene expression drift; plaque vulnerability
Loss of proteostasis	Protein aggregates; impaired contractility
Mitochondrial dysfunction	Reduced ATP; increased reactive oxygen species (ROS); heart failure
Deregulated nutrient sensing	Insulin resistance; dyslipidemia; mTOR-driven hypertrophy
Cellular senescence and senescence associated secretory phenotype (SASP)	Inflammation; matrix degradation; fibrosis
Altered intercellular communication	Autonomic imbalance; prothrombotic milieu
Stem cell exhaustion	Diminished reparative angiogenesis

CLINICAL EXPRESSION OF CARDIOMETABOLIC DECLINE

Cardiovascular aging and consequent disease vulnerability do not progress uniformly. Many individuals are asymptomatic until a physiological stressor such as infection, dehydration, or exertion, reveals limited reserve. Initial symptoms manifest as weakness, anxiety, fatigue, nausea, dyspnea, dizziness, palpitations, reduced exertion tolerance, and rapid or irregular heartbeats. Arrythmias and lack of HRV, common in old age, may be attributed to arterial stiffening, endothelial dysfunction, microvascular rarefaction, myocardial fibrosis, cardiomegaly, autonomic imbalance, and impaired energetic flexibility. Sustained hypertension or blood pressure (BP) increases left ventricular wall thickness and arterial stiffness, elevates pulse pressure and accelerates damage in brain, kidney, and retina. Aging increases atherogenesis or narrowing of arterial lumen due to chronic buildup of stable or unstable plaque in vascular walls, the main culprit of high BP.[3] Overtime, concentric remodeling and interstitial fibrosis impair diastolic filling and may culminate in HFpEF. In advanced disease, reduced forward flow and congestion lead to cognitive decline and vascular dementia; in the kidney, it advances chronic kidney disease (CKD); and in the eye it produces hypertensive retinopathy with visual impairment. Limited cardiac output or a leaking heart also restricts blood supply to the target organ, causing a lack of oxygen or ischemia. A myocardial ischemia due to insufficient coronary supply manifests as angina, whereas a cerebral ischemia may cause a transient ischemic attack. Atherosclerosis in carotid and intracranial

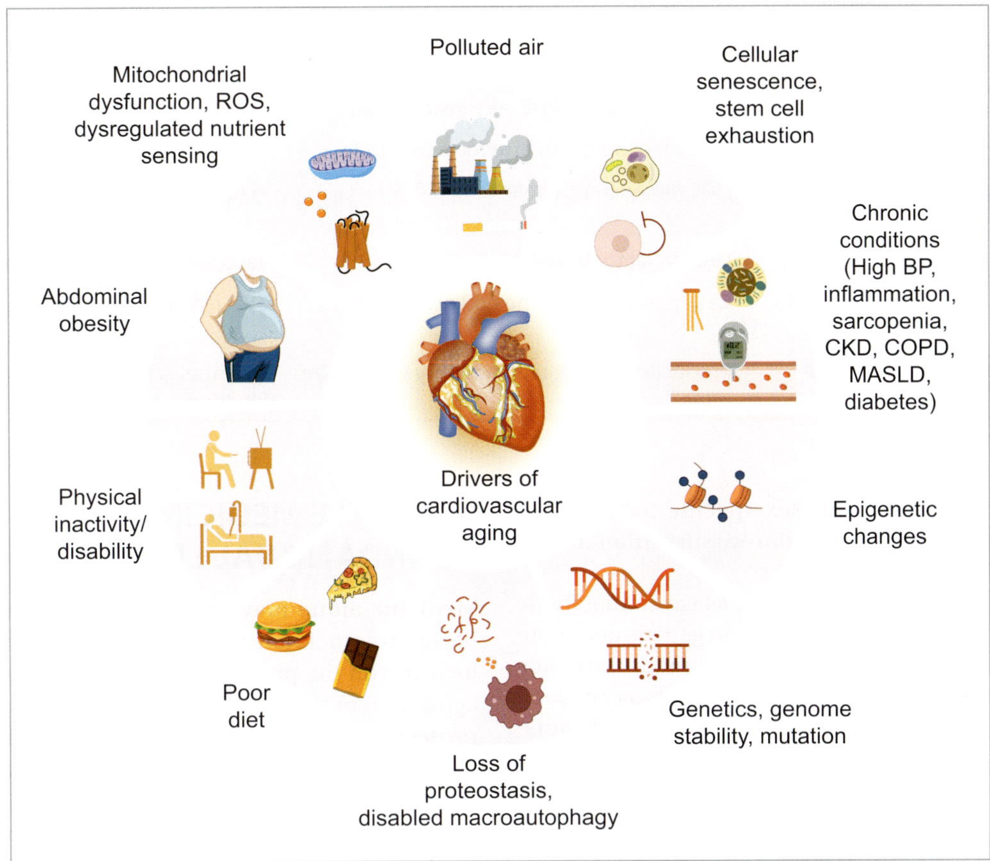

FIG. 1: Drivers of cardiovascular aging.
(CKD: chronic kidney disease; COPD: chronic obstructive pulmonary disease; MASLD: metabolic dysfunction associated steatotic liver disease; ROS: reactive oxygen species)

vessels raises stroke risk. However, a clot or thrombotic plaque-mediated infarction or a complete block of a cerebral or coronary artery may cause a life-threatening stroke or heart attack, respectively. The elderly are also prone to varicose veins, enlarged, twisted veins in the lower limbs that fail to keep efficient blood flow back to the heart, suggesting chronic venous insufficiency caused by damaged valves. Similarly, peripheral arterial disease may manifest as muscular pain or claudication. Besides, the vulnerability to comorbidities, underlying neurohormonal overdrive, inflammatory activation, oxidative stress, and endothelial dysfunction may rise proportionally to cardiometabolic decline.

GENETIC AND EPIGENETIC DETERMINANTS OF CARDIOVASCULAR AGING

Genetic architecture is known to shape resilience and vulnerability to cardiovascular aging. Genome wide association studies (GWAS) implicate hundreds of loci in frailty and longevity including variants of telomerase reverse transcriptase (TERT), endothelial nitric oxide synthase (eNOS3), insulin-like growth factor binding protein 3 (IGFBP-3), cholesteryl ester transfer protein (CETP), apolipoprotein E (ApoE) and forkhead box O3 (*FOXO3*) genes **(Table 2)**. The single nucleotide polymorphism rs2802292 in G allele of FOXO3a, a transcription factor regulating insulin pathway and genetic mechanisms that protect cell against free radical damage, shows strong association with exceptional longevity and negatively correlates with heart disease.[4] Similarly, the ε2 allele of apolipoprotein E (ApoE), a glycoprotein important in lipid transport between body organs, shows a favorable lipid profile relative to ε4, and is enriched in centenarians. CETP (I405V) impacts longevity moderately by modulating HDL and reducing atherosclerosis. Middle-aged men are more prone to coronary heart disease mortality than age-matched women, but the difference reduces during old age. Interestingly, a sex-specific age-related phenomenon, the mosaic loss of Y chromosome (mLOY) in a significant number of immune cells correlates with heightened inflammation, vascular injury, myocardial fibrosis, and increased risk of MACE.[5] These observations highlight an extensive age and genotype associated crosstalk between systems involved in intermediary metabolism, nutrient transport and utilization, and mitochondrial stress

TABLE 2: Longevity-associated gene variants and their cardiovascular relevance.

Gene/Variant	Putative mechanism	Cardiovascular relevance
FOXO (rs2802292/G allele)	Stress resistance; PI3K-Akt, insulin signaling	Lower burden of age-related CVD
APOE (ε2 allele)	Lipid transport; anti-atherogenic profile	Reduced risk of atherogenesis
Cholesteryl ester transfer protein (CETP) (functional variants)	HDL remodeling; cholesterol efflux	Plaque progression
IGFBP3 (promoter and coding variants)	Growth factor bioavailability	Vascular remodeling, inflammatory response
Telomerase reverse transcriptase (TERT) (polymorphisms)	Catalyzes chromosome end protection	CVD risk stratification in aging populations
NOS3 (promoter and coding variants)	Production of anti-inflammatory vasodilator, nitric oxide	Endothelial tone and anti-thrombotic function

alleviation and immunity, with sex-specific pathological trajectories that may require tailored surveillance and therapy.

For complex human disorders such as cardiometabolic disease, making a clear distinction between genetic and more complex, epigenetic regulation at the chromatin interface remains difficult. Epigenetic modulators such as readers, writers, and erasers—of modifications on DNA, and its histone and non-histone binding complement—form a landscape of effectors for molecular memory of environmental exposures.[6] Chromatin regulators such as sirtuins (SIRTs), the class III histone deacetylases (HDACs), DNA methyl transferases (DNMTs) and genes encoding products involved in RNA processing exhibit disease associated aberrant expression profile without an identified DNA mutation. With age, endothelial, and smooth muscle cells acquire epigenetic marks that favor proinflammatory and profibrotic transcripts. An age-related decline in the fat mass and obesity associated protein (FTO), a NAD+ and α-ketoglutarate dependent m^6A demethylase, impairs mitochondrial biogenesis in cardiac tissue and shifts energy source from fatty acid oxidation to glycolysis, causing toxic metabolite accumulation and cardiovascular rigidity, an effect countered by METTL3, methyltransferase like-3, the core catalytic subunit of m^6A-RNA methyltransferase complex. Similar age-related decline in expression of enhancer of zeste homolog 2 (EZH2), a histone methyltransferase with repressive H3K27me3 activity that regulates vascular smooth muscle cell gene expression, causes vascular sclerosis, atherogenesis, and aortic aneurysms. Concomitant hypermethylation of eNOS promoter reduces NO production, promoting hypertension whereas hypomethylation of inflammatory genes in aged endothelial cells leads to chronic low-grade inflammation, a key driver of vascular stiffening and HFpEF. Pharmacological inhibition of chromatin readers such as bromodomain and extraterminal domain containing (BET) proteins is known to reduce inflammatory response by macrophages while inhibition of lysine specific demethylase 1 (LSD1) reduces the extent of atherosclerotic lesions.

LIFESTYLE MEDICINE: FOUNDATIONAL LEVERS

Medicine alone may not permanently cure a deregulated lifestyle-associated CVD in aging populations. However, focusing on the preventive aspect, considering the ability of aging system to adjust its intrinsic homeostatic balance with respect to developing senile background, may contribute to a long and healthy lifespan. Therefore, updating and enhancing lifestyle by including longevity promoting dietary patterns, physical activity, reducing abdominal fat, cessation of nicotine consumption, appropriate sleep and stress relief could counter aging related decline in cardiovascular health **(Table 3)**.

Dietary pattern: A minimally processed, plant-forward eating pattern-akin to Mediterranean or DASH-improves blood pressure, serum lipid profile, insulin sensitivity, and inflammatory tone. Recommendations for elderly emphasize fibrous-cereal, polyphenol and mineral-rich fruits and vegetables, and ω3 unsaturated fatty acid-rich nuts and fish; suggest olive oil, red wine and dairy in moderation; limit refined carbohydrate, high sodium, and saturated- and trans-fat containing ultra-processed food.[7-11] Practical targets include sodium <2 g/day (~5 g salt), fiber ≥25-30 g/day, and regular consumption of nuts and legumes, with intermittent fasting. For individuals with insulin resistance or non-alcoholic fatty liver disease (NAFLD), recently renamed as metabolic dysfunction-associated steatotic liver disease (MASLD), reducing added sugars and sweetened beverages is particularly beneficial in reducing the risk of MACE.[12] Moreover, gut microbiota also influences host serum lipid levels, CVD, Alzheimer's and longevity.[13]

Physical activity: Older adults (≥65 years) may take up at least 150 minutes of moderate intensity aerobics activity per week or aim for a ≥75–150 minutes of vigorous activity per week, in addition to resistance training at least two times a week. Furthermore, in older adults, balance and mobility

TABLE 3: Lifestyle targets with expected cardiometabolic benefits.

Domain	Target/Prescription	Expected benefit
Diet	Mediterranean/DASH; sodium <2 g/day; fiber ≥25–30 g/day	↓ BP, ↑ HDL, ↓ TG, ↓ inflammation
Activity	≥150–300 min/week moderate with 2 days resistance training	↓ BP, ↓ insulin resistance, ↑ VO_2
Weight	5–10% loss over 6–12 months	↓ BP, ↓ TG, ↓ liver fat, ↓ OSA
Sleep	7–9 h/night; treat OSA	↓ BP, ↓ arrhythmia risk, ↑ glycemic control
Tobacco	Complete cessation; counseling and medication	Rapid ↓ CV risk; ↓ stroke and myocardial infarction (MI)
Environment	Indoor filtration on AQI >300	↓ BP-spikes; ↓ inflammatory load

exercises such as yoga and tai chi reduce falls and support autonomy. Even brief activity breaks during prolonged sitting improve glycemic index and oxygen uptake (VO_2).

Digital health, biomarkers, and artificial intelligence: Digitized self-monitoring extends prevention beyond the walls of clinic. Home-based BP, weight, heart rate variability, sleep data, and step count provide a continuous context for long-term analysis. Coupled with periodic laboratory biomarkers such as liver and kidney function test, fasting lipids, A1C for average glucose (mg/dL), apoB, high sensitivity CRP, and natriuretic peptides can give early clinical insights into decompensation.[14] Machine learning-based analysis of multilayered time series clinical variables may be used to generate personalized health care recommendations without burdening clinicians or patients.

Healthy weight and adiposity management: High body mass index (BMI), waist circumference and visceral or ectopic fat collectively capture CDV disease risk, better guiding counseling and intervention. Monitoring fitness data such as BMI, systolic and diastolic BP, heart rate, cholesterol, triglycerides, glucose, and uric acid at regular intervals and reassessing metrics every 3–6 months should be aligned with anti-obesity prescriptions. Intentional weight reduction of 5–10% over a 6–12-month period enhances insulin sensitivity, lowers blood pressure, and triglycerides, reduces liver fat and improves sleep apnea-factors contributing to vascular aging.

Stress and lack of sleep: Consistent sleep-wake timing and 7–9 hours of restorative sleep should be prioritized in the elderly. As obstructive sleep apnea (OSA) elevates blood pressure and sympathetic drive, appropriate screening, and intervention should be implemented in the high-risk patients. Stress relief practices such as mindfulness, meditation, breath work, social connection, and support are known to counter maladaptive neurohumoral activation and should be incorporated in regular routine.[15]

Nicotine consumption and air pollution: Complete nicotine cessation remains one of the most powerful anti-aging interventions for vasculature. Behavioral counseling, pharmacotherapy, and adherence to a relapse prevention plan may contribute to deaddiction. Beyond, one should avoid secondhand smoke and consider air-quality index (AQI) strategies during high pollution episodes.[16]

PHARMACOLOGICAL STRATEGIES WITH VASCULAR ANTI-AGING POTENTIAL

Emerging pharmacological strategies not only aim to manage symptoms of cardiovascular aging but to delay or even reverse them, thereby rejuvenating endothelial and cardiac function. These include strategies to reduce hypertension, activate autophagy, epigenetic modulation, metabolic reprogramming, and senolytic and anti-inflammatory therapies **(Table 4)**.[17] CVD treatment strategies may also utilize drugs such as antiplatelets, anticoagulants, vasodilators, nucleic acid-based drugs and surgery such as bypass grafting or angioplasty.

Blood pressure control: Achieving guideline-directed blood pressure targets reduces arterial stiffness, left ventricular hypertrophy, and stroke risk. First-line drug classes—ACE inhibitors, ARBs, calcium channel blockers, and thiazide diuretics—are frequently combined to regain BP control by acting on renin–angiotensin aldosterone system (RAAS). BP-lowering drug valsartan is an ARB that acts by reducing fluid and sodium retention in heart and kidney, alleviating organ damage. Long-term fixed-dose combinations and home BP monitoring improve adherence and outcomes.

Atherogenic lipid control: Increased circulating levels of low-density lipoproteins (LDL) due to dysfunctional clearance mediated by apo-B100 receptors in clathrin coated pits of hepatocytes cause atherosclerosis. Early and sustained lowering of LDL by inhibiting HMG-CoA reductase, enzyme essential for cholesterol biosynthesis, is achieved by statins. For high-risk patients, stepwise addition of ezetimibe, an inhibitor of enzyme PCSK9 that degrades LDL receptors, or bempedoic acid, an inhibitor of ATP citrate lyase (ACL), an enzyme upstream of HMG-CoA reductase in cholesterol biosynthesis, reduces cumulative exposure and event risk.

TABLE 4: Pharmacotherapies, their vascular aging rationale, and representative outcomes.

Therapy	Vascular aging rationale	Representative outcomes
ACEi/ARB (angiotensin II receptor blockers)	↓ Renin–angiotensin aldosterone system (RAAS) activation; antifibrotic	↓ Stroke/MI; ↓ LV mass
Thiazide/CCB	BP control; ↓ arterial stiffness	↓ MACE with control
High intensity statin	↓ ApoB burden; plaque stabilization	↓ MI/stroke/mortality
Ezetimibe/bempedoic acid	Additional LDL-C reduction	Further event reduction in high-risk group
SGLT-2 inhibitors	Natriuresis; renal-cardiac protection	↓ HF hospitalization; renal benefit
GLP-1 receptor agonists	Weight loss; anti-inflammatory	↓ MACE in high-risk/obesity
Metformin	AMPK–SIRT activation; mitochondrial support	Broad metabolic and vascular benefits
Polyphenols/resveratrol	Antioxidant; sirtuins (SIRT)/forkhead box O (FOXO) pathways	Improved endothelial function in studies
GSK2879552	Epigenetic reprogramming	Reduces plaques
Spermidine	Autophagy induction	Lower MACE

Glycemia and weight control therapy: GLP-1 from intestine activates GLP-1 receptor in atrial cardiac myocytes, stimulating secretion of atrial natriuretic peptide (ANP), which induces hypoxia inducible factor 1 alpha (HIF-1α) expression and ROS, and induces cGMP-mediated smooth muscle relaxation and natriuresis. GLP-1 receptor agonists, semaglutide, and orforglipron, provided health benefits beyond glucose lowering and weight loss, by lowering MACE in obesity with diabetes mellitus and obesity without diabetes, respectively.[18] Likewise, gliflozins, the SGLT-2 inhibitors, developed to treat type 2 diabetes also showed cardiorenal protection in patients with heart failure and CKD by promoting mild natriuresis.

Senolytic and anti-inflammatory therapies: Senescence constrains age-related waste accumulation by halting the progression of damaged or dysfunctional cells, accompanied by a proinflammatory SASP. Cell cycle inhibitors p16Ink4a and p21CIP increase senescence by cell cycle arrest. Accumulation of p16Ink4a showed premature aging phenotype, which could be reversed in mouse by gene inactivation.[19] Accumulation of senescent cells in cardiovascular system causes premature aging and has been targeted in mouse models using senolytic compounds like quercetin.[20]

Epigenetic therapies: Tazemetostat, the first FDA approved EZH2 inhibitor for lymphoma, slows atherosclerotic plaque progression and protects against ischemic brain injury. GSK2879552, a GlaxoSmithKline drug used for small cell lung carcinoma, acts by selective inhibition of LSD1, reducing extent of atherosclerotic lesions. Metformin, a drug for diabetes, is a 5'-AMP activated protein kinase activator that increases H3K79me3 via AMPK-SIRT1-DOT1L axis, enhancing SIRT3 expression and mitochondrial function, delaying endothelial senescence and vascular aging. Besides, NAD+ repletion, BET inhibitors, and FTO activators are also emerging as strategies to restore metabolic flexibility and counter cardiac decline with aging.

GAPS IN KNOWLEDGE TRANSLATION TO PATIENT OUTCOMES

Despite rapid progress, uncertainties remain. The translation of epigenetic modulators and nucleic acid-based therapeutics from experimental models to clinical endpoints requires the development of site-specific delivery modules, rigorous trials with long-term safety monitoring to avoid off-target effects and efficacy considerations. Similarly, the relative contribution of specific longevity variants to actionable endpoints in diverse populations requires further research. Also, tools for measuring biological age of the vasculature such as arterial stiffness metrics, and methylation clocks are promising, yet they need to be standardized for point of care implementation. Equity considerations, such as socioeconomic determinants that shape diet quality, physical activity, access, sleep, and environmental exposures, are paramount. Therefore, interventions for healthy cardiovascular aging must be culturally tailored, scalable, and affordable to produce population level benefits.

CONCLUSION

Aging is not purely a function of chronological time; it rather reflects cumulative biological insults that can be blunted by elevating cardiometabolic health. Improving dietary quality, regular physical activity, restorative sleep, elimination of tobacco, tight control of blood pressure and atherogenic lipids, and judicious use of agents with cardiorenal benefits may bend the trajectory of vascular aging. Moreover, integrating genetic and epigenetic insights from large data sets and digital monitoring enable earlier, more personalized prescription. A multidomain action plan anchored in lifestyle modifications, risk-factor optimization, and pharmacology considering all noncardiac diseases and related medications may thus decelerate cardiovascular aging, compress morbidity, and extend healthy span with a heart that matches the wisdom of a life well numbered.

REFERENCES

1. Bestermann WH Jr. The ADMA-Metformin Hypothesis: Linking the Cardiovascular Consequences of the Metabolic Syndrome and Type 2 Diabetes. Cardiorenal Med. 2011;1(4):211-9.
2. D'Agostino RB, Vasan RS, Pencina MJ, et al. General Cardiovascular Risk Profile for Use in Primary Care. Circulation. 2008;117(6):743-53.
3. Alradwan I, Al Fayez N, Alomary MN, et al. Emerging Trends and Innovations in the Treatment and Diagnosis of Atherosclerosis and Cardiovascular Disease: A Comprehensive Review towards Healthier Aging. Pharmaceutics. 2024;16(8):1037.
4. Klinpudtan N, Allsopp RC, Kabayama M, et al. The Association Between Longevity-Associated FOXO3 Allele and Heart Disease in Septuagenarians and Octogenarians: The SONIC Study. J Gerontol A Biol Sci Med Sci. 2022;77(8):1542-8.
5. Thel MC, Cochran JD, Teruya S, et al. Mosaic Loss of the Y Chromosome Is Enriched in Patients with Wild-Type Transthyretin Cardiac Amyloidosis and Associated with Increased Mortality. Circ Heart Fail. 2024;17(8):e011681.
6. Liu J, Yang M, Zhou B. Epigenetic and epitranscriptomic regulation of cardiac metabolism in aging and disease. J Cardiovasc Aging. 2025;5(3).
7. Bošković M, Živković M, Koričanac G, et al. Walnut Supplementation Restores the SIRT1-FoxO3a-MnSOD/Catalase Axis in the Heart, Promotes an Anti-Inflammatory Fatty Acid Profile in Plasma, and Lowers Blood Pressure on Fructose-Rich Diet. Oxid Med Cell Longev. 2021;5543025.
8. Liu K, Zhu Y, Gao W, et al. Resveratrol alleviates heart failure by activating foxo3a to counteract oxidative stress and apoptosis. Biomed Pharmacother. 2024;181:117716.
9. Mozaffarian D, Kumanyika SK, Lemaitre RN, et al. Cereal, Fruit, and Vegetable Fiber Intake and the Risk of Cardiovascular Disease in Elderly Individuals. JAMA. 2003;289(13):1659-66.
10. Petyaev IM. Lycopene Deficiency in Ageing and Cardiovascular Disease. Oxid Med Cell Longev. 2016;2016:3218605.
11. Xu B, Xu Z, Xu D, et al. Effect of n-3 polyunsaturated fatty acids on ischemic heart disease and cardiometabolic risk factors: a two-sample Mendelian randomization study. BMC Cardiovasc Disord. 2021;21(1):532.
12. Jenkins DJA, Dehghan M, Mente A, et al. Glycemic Index, Glycemic Load, and Cardiovascular Disease and Mortality. N Engl J Med. 2021;384(14):1312-22.
13. Tang WHW, Kitai T, Hazen SL. Gut microbiota in cardiovascular health and disease. Circ Res. 2017;120(7):1183-96.
14. Savonnet M, Rolland T, Cubizolles M, et al. Recent advances in cardiac biomarkers detection: From commercial devices to emerging technologies. J Pharm Biomed Anal. 2021;194:113777.
15. Boehm JK, Kubzansky LD. The heart's content: The association between positive psychological well-being and cardiovascular health. Psychol Bull. 2012;138(4):655-91.
16. Fuller R, Landrigan PJ, Balakrishnan K, et al. Pollution and health: a progress update. Lancet Planet Health. 2022;6(6):e535-47.
17. Abdellatif M, Schmid ST, Fuerlinger A, et al. Anti-ageing interventions for the treatment of cardiovascular disease. Cardiovasc Res. 2025;121(10):1524-36.
18. Lincoff AM, Brown-Frandsen K, Colhoun HM, et al. Semaglutide and Cardiovascular Outcomes in Obesity without Diabetes. N Engl J Med. 2023;389(24):2221-32.
19. Baker JD, Childs BG, Van De Sluis B, et al. Clearance of p16Ink4a-positive senescent cells delays ageing-associated disorders. Nature. 2011;479(7372):232-6.
20. Grootaert MOJ. Cell senescence in cardiometabolic diseases. NPJ Aging. 2024;10(1):46.

CHAPTER 12

Obesity and Cardiovascular Diseases

Amit Malviya, Md Amish Shikoh, Aman Asthana, Animesh Mishra

ABSTRACT

Obesity is a global epidemic in present time worldwide. It affects the entire spectrum of population from children to adults and males as well as females. It is now well recognized as a major health issue among the policy makers, treating physicians, and people themselves. It is directly related to development of cardiovascular diseases as various cardiovascular risk factors such as insulin resistance, diabetes, hypertension, dyslipidemia, obstructive sleep apnea, endothelial dysfunction, vascular resistance, and prothrombotic states. It increases both morbidity and mortality among individuals. Obesity, particularly abdominal/visceral obesity, is an indicator development of cardiovascular diseases and other risk factors which lead to cardiovascular diseases. It is underrecognized modifiable risk factor. Timely identification of obesity should be considered important. Preventing weight gain in people who are prone to weight gain and promoting weight loss among obese via lifestyle modifications, drugs or surgery should be addressed. Our aim should be to identify obesity as a major public health problem and implementing measures to prevent cardiovascular risk factors and diseases arising as a consequence of obesity.

Keywords: Obesity, cardiovascular risk, abdominal/visceral obesity, insulin resistance, hypertension, dyslipidemia, lifestyle modification.

INTRODUCTION

Obesity is a multifactorial disease with a complex pathophysiology. It is recognized as a major risk factor for cardiovascular disease. It is defined as excess body fat accumulation leading to increased mortality and morbidity. Obesity has been declared a disease by WHO and it is a major cause of cardiovascular disease-related deaths. It is a relapsing and progressive condition that has to be addressed on time. It is both preventable and treatable.[1] Although increased body weight contributes to cardiovascular risk factors such as diabetes, hypertension, obstructive sleep apnea, and dyslipidemia, and it also causes structural and functional changes in cardiovascular system leading to cardiovascular diseases both atherosclerotic and nonatherosclerotic but there exists variation in appearance of these risk factors and diseases.[2,3] So now comes the question whether some obese or overweight are metabolically healthy. This has put in forth the discussion the distribution of body fat within body, which determines the appearance of risk factors obesity has not caused health issues but also put forth a financial crisis as a large cost entitled to manage these risk factors as well as diseases.[4] This has put a strain on the economy both at an individual and a social level. Obesity is both preventable and treatable. It is important to prevent weight gain through lifestyle interventions as well as treating people who are obese through drugs and interventions.[5]

What is obesity and overweight?

- Over weight is defined as excess fat deposits.
- Obesity is a chronic complex disease which is characterized by excess fat deposits that can impair health.
- Diagnosis of overweight or obesity is done by body mass index (BMI) also known as Quetelet index which is calculated by dividing a person's weight in kilograms by height in squared in meters (kg/m^2).
- Body mass index categories for diagnosis of obesity varies among adolescent, children, and infants.
- *Children under 5 years of age:*
    - Overweight is defined as weight-for-height >2 standard deviations above WHO Child Growth Standards median.

    - Obesity is defined as weight-for-height >3 standard deviations above the WHO Child Growth Standards median.
- *Children aged between 5 and 19 years:*
    - Overweight is defined as BMI for age >1 standard deviation above the WHO Growth Reference median.
    - Obesity is defined as BMI for age >2 standard deviations above the WHO Growth Reference median.
- *Adults:*
    - Overweight is defined as a BMI ≥ 25 kg/m^2.
    - Obesity is defined as a BMI ≥ 30 kg/m^2.

According to NFHS-5 (2019–2021) in India, overweight is defined as BMI of 23–24.9 kg/m^2 and obesity is defined as BMI of >25 kg/m^2 and higher.

Though BMI has been used for assessment of obesity there, it does not mean that every obese or overweight does develop health complications. From this fact, we come to conclusion that distribution of fat also plays an important role which has been confirmed by advent of imaging techniques. Visceral obesity is far more deleterious than peripheral obesity. So, it is now suggested to measure waist circumference in addition to BMI. Waist circumference is measured with a tape around the iliac crest in standing position. A person with increased waist circumference for a given BMI with risk factors means high visceral obesity. Waist circumference and BMI strongly correlate, therefore, raised waist circumference means total adiposity **(Table 1)**.[1,4,5]

TABLE 1: Waist circumference cutoff (cm).[4,6]

BMI category	Women	Men
Normal weight (18.5–24.9)	80 or more	90 or more
Overweight (25–29.9)	90 or more	100 or more
Obese I (30–34)	105 or more	110 or more
Obese II (35 or more)	115 or more	125 or more

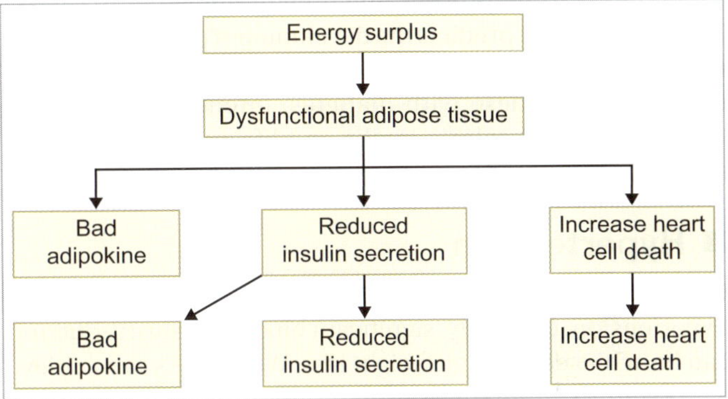

FLOWCHART 1: Complications of high calorie consumption.[7,8]

ETIOLOGY

The cause of obesity is complex and multifactorial which is due to individual and environmental factors. An imbalance between energy intake and energy expenditure is one of the key causal factors leading to obesity and overweight and is related to environmental, social, and societal factors. For instance, changes in food production, food processing, food availability and consumption of high calorie, and low-energy content food contribute to obesity and overweight **(Flowchart 1)**. Sedentary lifestyle contributes to overweight and obesity.[2,3] In return, overweight and obesity further reduces physical activity either due direct effects or due to consequences further perpetuating the vicious cycle of obesity and overweight.[9]

Age and sex also contribute to obesity, prior to menopause women have 50% less visceral fat as compared to men. As there is decline in sex steroids there is a change in distribution body fats ultimately leading to visceral obesity.

Sex hormones play a crucial role in visceral fat distribution which has been demonstrated in intervention involving sex hormones in transsexual population. Male to female transsexuals receiving sex hormones show a decline in visceral fat distribution in contrary to female to male transsexuals receiving sex hormones showing increased visceral fat distribution and deterioration in cardiometabolic risk profile.[10]

TABLE 2: Drugs causing weight gain.[12]

Category	Drugs
Antidiabetics	Insulin, SFU, meglitinides, and pioglitazones
Antidepressants	MAO inhibitors, TCAs, and SSRIs
Antipsychotics	Clozapines, reserpines, olanzapines, risperidone, and haloperidol
Anticonvulsants	Carbamazepine and valproate
Antihistaminics	Cyproheptadine and diphenhydramine
Adrenergic blockers	Propranolol and doxazosin
Adrenal steroids	Corticosteroids

Genetic factors also play a crucial role in susceptibility to obesity. Individuals born to parents who are obese are at risk of developing the same pattern of obesity.[11]

It has been observed that Asians have an increased susceptibility to visceral obesity as compared to Caucasians and Americans.

Alteration of hypothalamic-pituitary-adrenal axis and the endocannabinoid system contributes to visceral adiposity. Adipose tissue is a storehouse of endocannabinoid receptors and overactivation of the endocannabinoid system occurs in visceral obesity. Drugs with suppressive action on the endocannabinoid system shows reduction in visceral obesity **(Table 2)**.[13]

OBESITY AND CARDIOVASCULAR RISK FACTORS (FIG. 1)

Diabetes

Obesity and type 2 diabetes mellitus are strongly correlated. Most of the diabetics are obese and people who are obese are at an increased risk of developing diabetes in future. Insulin resistance is a major pathophysiological pathway in diabetics which tends to be present much before onset of diabetes. Insulin resistance predicts the development of cardiovascular diseases even in absence of diabetes. In people who are overweight or obese with diabetes, intensive weight loss through reduced caloric intake and lifestyle modifications should be promoted to improve metabolic health.[14,15]

Hypertension

Overweight and obesity directly related to development of hypertension. Clinically, significant blood pressure reduction can be achieved through weight loss. Weight loss can achieve a maximum blood pressure reduction. Distribution of body fat also determines development of hypertension. In particular, the visceral fat distribution causes development of hypertension more than peripheral fat distribution. Pathophysiology underlying development of hypertension in obese people includes increased blood volume, venous return, increased arterial stiffness due to a proinflammatory state, release of paracrine molecules which act on vascular musculature, renal dysfunction, compression of renal vasculature by retroperitoneal fat causing activation of RAAS system, insulin resistance, and obstructive sleep apnea. So, it is recommended to maintain a stable BMI to maintain blood pressure within normal limits and to initiate blood pressure lowering drugs in individuals where blood pressure remains elevated despite conservative means.[16]

Dyslipidemia

Low-density lipoprotein (LDL) cholesterol is related to development of atherosclerotic cardiovascular heart diseases. The level of LDL cholesterol and overweight and obesity is not linearly related. Obesity is related to rise in levels of atherogenic components of lipids such as triglycerides, LDL, ApoB, and VLDL. LDL is prone to oxidation and accumulation in vessel walls causing atherosclerotic plaques. Loss of weight is associated with lowering of atherogenic lipids. It is essential to consider regular screening of levels of lipids.

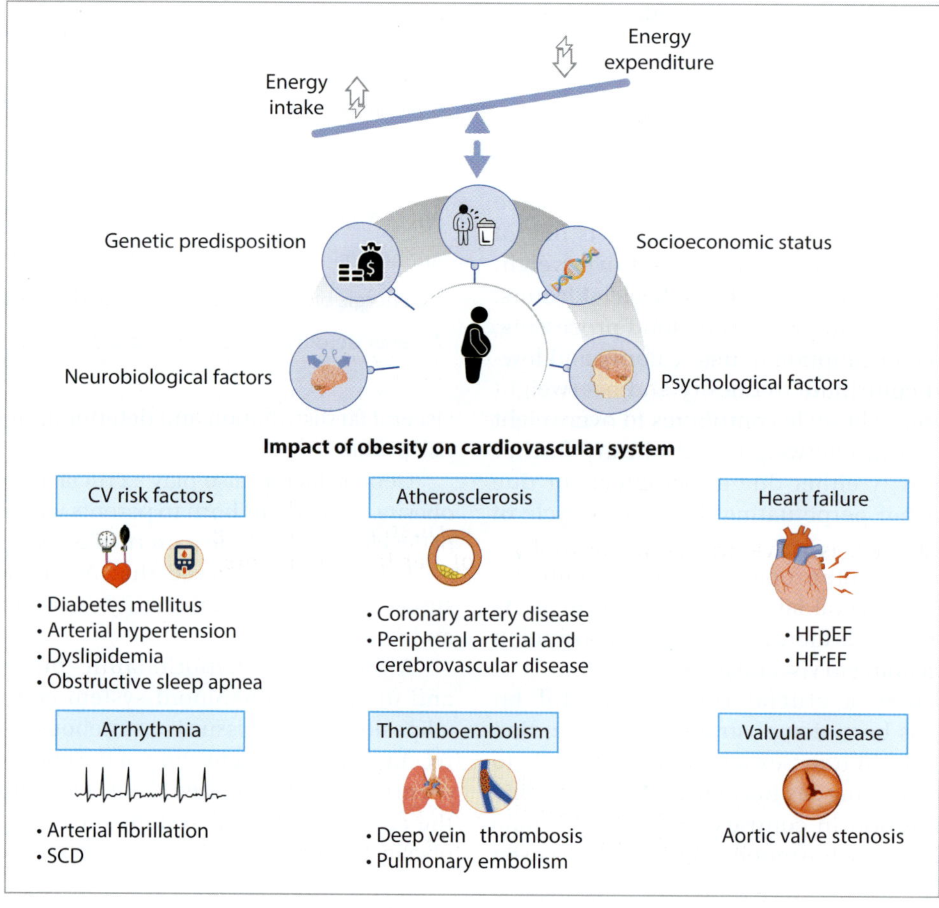

FIG. 1: Obesity and cardiovascular disease.[1]

■ Obstructive Sleep Apnea

Obstructive sleep apnea is a risk factor for hypertension, heart failure, and atrial fibrillation. Obesity is a causal factor for obstructive sleep apnea as well as obstructive sleep apnea increases lethargy, daytime sleepiness which further exacerbates obesity thus setting a vicious cycle. Reduction in body weight is associated with reduction of apnea-hypopnea index and improves the quality of sleep. Obesity increases the amount of neck fat deposits and compression of pharyngeal airway thus increasing the tendency of airways to collapse during sleep. Measurement of neck circumference should be considered an important tool for obese individuals. Weight loss along with continuous positive airway pressure improves obstructive sleep apnea.

OBESITY AND CARDIOVASCULAR DISEASES

■ Obesity and Atherosclerotic Cardiovascular Diseases

Obesity is directly associated with development of atherosclerotic cardiovascular diseases. Obesity itself is a causal agent for cardiovascular diseases and is magnified by the presence of risk factors such as hypertension, diabetes, obstructive sleep apnea, and dyslipidemia. Visceral obesity is more likely to be associated with development of cardiovascular diseases as compared to peripheral obesity. Pathophysiological mechanism underlying this is presence of low-grade inflammation evidenced by circulating levels of proinflammatory cytokines and hsCRP.[17] There have been studies indicating very low BMI which is also a risk factor for cardiovascular diseases setting the debate for obesity paradox. In addition to the development of atherosclerotic cardiovascular diseases, there is also an increased risk of microvascular dysfunction in obese and overweight which has been attributed to oxidative stress, insulin resistance, reduced nitric oxide production, and overactivity of the sympathetic system.[8]

Diagnosis of cardiovascular diseases in obese people is a challenging task. Exercise tests are limiting due to presence of changes in baseline ECG such as left ventricular hypertrophy and ST-segment depression and also due to poor exercise capacity. Noninvasive imaging techniques such as PET and SPECT are challenging due to image distortion, diaphragm, or breast. CT coronary angiography is difficult due to attenuation of signal to noise ratio. Invasive angiography is difficult in terms of vascular access and in obese or overweight radial route is preferred because of difficulty in attaining vascular access via femoral route and need of vascular closure devices. Moreover, radiographic evaluation is challenging due to poor image quality and increased radiation exposure.

Treatment of such patients does not differ much from nonobese individuals. These include antiplatelets, statins, and PCI. Management of cardiovascular risk such as hypertension, diabetes, and dyslipidemia is a key to successful treatment. Care should be taken to look for treatment complications such as contrast-induced nephropathy and vascular complications.[18,19]

■ Obesity and Heart Failure

Obesity is a risk factor for development of atherosclerotic cardiovascular disease which turn leads to heart failure of ischemic origin or HFrEF. Obesity is more strongly associated with development of HFpEF as compared to HFrEF. Pathophysiological mechanisms underlying development of HFpEF include increased blood volume, increased venous return, myopathy, increased filling pressure, cardiovascular remodeling due activation of RAAS system, proinflammatory state, oxidative stress, impaired vasodilatation, uncontrolled hypertension, pericardial restrain due to epicardial fat, loss of ventricular interdependence, and pulmonary hypertension.

Diagnosis of heart failure in obese and overweight is a challenge as there is a poor exercise capacity due to body weight making noninvasive tests like TMT difficult. Moreover, markers like NT-proBNP also cannot be used to predict heart failure as the levels are low in such population either due to reduced production or increased clearance.

For patients with HFrEF, modifying caloric intake may be a treatment option for HFrEF and obesity but a negative caloric balance should be suggested with caution in patients with HFrEF which is already a catabolic state and may in turn predispose the patient to cachexia and increased mortality.

In patients with HFpEF, reduction of body weight either by diet, exercise, pharmacological agents, and interventions is beneficial as it improves exercise capacity, 6-minute walk distance and overcomes insulin resistance as well.[18,20]

■ Obesity and Arrhythmia

There is sufficient data suggesting increased association of obesity and overweight with incidence and progression of atrial fibrillation. Obesity is associated with progression from paroxysmal to permanent atrial fibrillation. Apart from obesity, cardiovascular risk factors such as hypertension and obstructive sleep apnea also increase the risk of atrial fibrillation. Underlying mechanisms include remodeling of cardiac chambers, diastolic dysfunction, chamber enlargement, presence of epicardial fat. Maintenance of a healthy body weight and weight reduction is an important step in primary prevention of atrial fibrillation. In patients with weight loss and treatment of risk factors ensure reducing the burden of atrial fibrillation and maintenance of sinus rhythm. Patients with atrial fibrillation should receive anticoagulation.[21]

■ Obesity and Sudden Cardiac Death

Association between obesity and sudden cardiac death has been established long ago. Most of the cases of sudden cardiac death is caused by nonischemic cardiomyopathy.

Underlying mechanisms include cardiac remodeling, myocardial fibrosis, chamber enlargement, epicardial and intramyocardial fat deposits, electrophysiological changes such as QT prolongation, premature ventricular complexes, and increased QRS interval. Maintenance of body weight helps to reduce substrate for sudden cardiac death by improving cardiac remodeling, decreased mean heart rate and improving ventricular repolarization and conduction, and QT interval.[18]

Obesity and Venous Thromboembolism

Venous thromboembolism including deep vein thrombosis and pulmonary embolism is associated with obesity along with traditional risk factors. In patients who are critically ill, prolonged immobilization, with fracture, active cancer, smoking, and cancer, the risk of thromboembolism is increased several times. It has been suggested that obese patients who are undergoing elective hip or knee arthroplasty or prolonged immobilization, NOACs should be given for prevention and treatment of venous thromboembolism.

Obesity and Valvular Heart Diseases

Patients who are adults and obese are at an increased risk of aortic valve stenosis as compared to general population. Underlying mechanisms include dyslipidemia and a chronic inflammatory state. Maintaining a normal weight has reduced incidence and associated mortality with aortic stenosis. Transcatheter aortic valve replacement can be offered to patients with aortic stenosis.[22]

MANAGEMENT OF OBESITY

Basis of management lies in the fact in identifying people who are at risk of developing obesity such as those born to parents who are obese or have risk factors such as diabetes and hypertension. Obesity is a state of chronic positive energy balance, so our aim is to balance the expenditure against intake. Treatment requires comprehensive approach in terms of dietary, behavioral, psychological, pharmacological, and surgical. Educating people regarding benefits maintaining a healthy lifestyle and maintaining an optimal weight.

Dietary Interventions

Dietary needs of each and every individual should be individualized and tailored according to needs. Calorie restriction should be promoted, and a calorie deficit of 500–750 kcal should be maintained. Exclusion of ultra processed foods, sweetened beverages, and intake of lots of fruits and vegetables, low carbohydrate, and Mediterranean diets. Target weight loss of 5–10% should be achieved.

Physical Activity

Apart from achieving weight loss, physical activity helps to improve cardiometabolic health and is prescribed for treatment of cardiovascular risk factors. According to the current ESC guidelines, current recommendation for an adult is 150–300 minutes per week of moderate intensity or 75–150 minutes of high intensity exercise to reduce all-cause mortality and cardiovascular mortality and morbidity.[23] Barriers to physical activity in obese and overweight should be taken into account and they should be encouraged to stay as active as possible that is switching to nonsedentary behavior such as walking 2 minutes every hour and using stairs. Use of electronic devices such smartwatches and mobile phones to assess physical activity should be promoted.[21]

Psychological Interventions

Stigma associated with obesity should be reduced. Even among healthcare professionals, obesity is stigmatized leading to people not being able to express themselves. This can be achieved by examination tables and chairs to accommodate people of all sizes. Communicating with people is a nonjudgmental and supportive manner. Food is a mechanism to cope with negative emotions and emotional breakdowns. A supportive environment in such situations helps to break vicious cycle. Maintaining a proper duration and quality of sleep to maintain energy balance and metabolism. Patients with disturbed sleep are those with sleep apnea which is commonly seen among obese and overweight. Patients with obesity and sleep apnea have a poor quality of sleep which increases fatigue and inactivity and in turn sets in a vicious cycle of inactivity and further weight gain.[9]

Pharmacological Interventions for Weight Loss

- *Phentermine*: Sympathomimetic
- *Orlistat:* It acts in the intestinal lumen to inhibit pancreatic lipase and gastric lipase to prevent absorption of fats thus causing modest weight loss. Side effects include gastrointestinal such as bloating, flatulence, chronic diarrhea, steatorrhea, increased frequency of defecation, and risk of cholestasis are increased especially in pregnancy and causes malabsorption.
- *Naltrexone:* Opioid receptor antagonist to stimulate POMC secretion which suppresses craving for food and increases satiety. It causes side effects such as constipation, symptoms of opioid withdrawal, headache, dizziness, and seizures.
- *Bupropion:* Dopamine and norepinephrine reuptake inhibitor which leads to stimulation of POMC secretion causing suppression of craving of food and increases satiety. Side effects include constipation, uncontrolled hypertension, chronic diarrhea, headache, sleep disorders, and insomnia.[18,24]
- *Liraglutide and semaglutide:* GLP-1 receptor agonists which stimulate insulin secretion, suppress gastric motility, gastric emptying, have incretin effect, and thus suppress food craving. Initially, they were approved

for diabetes but later on approved for weight loss and metabolism associated with liver disease. Side effects include constipation, dyspepsia, pancreatitis, gastroparesis, and intestinal obstruction. There is increased risk of medullary thyroid carcinoma and multiple endocrine neoplasia in people who have family history.[22,25]

- *Tirzepatide:* It has a dual mode of action causing stimulation of both GLP-1 and GIP thus in turn leading to decreased gastric emptying and increasing satiety. Side effects include dyspepsia, constipation, abdominal fullness, and nausea. There is increased risk of medullary carcinoma of thyroid and multiple endocrine neoplasia.
- *Setmelanotide:* It is a melanocortin-4 (MC4) receptor agonist used for patients with genetic absence of MC4 receptor and it reduces appetite and suppresses satiety. Side effects include hypersensitivity reaction.[26,27]
- *Mazdutide:* Incretin-based polyagonists combining GLP-1R with glucagon receptor agonism are in pipeline.[28,29]
- *Cagrilintide:* Amylin analog is also in study.[30]

Surgical Approach

Intragastric approach: These include endoscopic procedures such as gastric ballooning and sleeve gastroplasty. Intragastric balloons restrict the space available for food and thus promote satiety. Side effects include satiety, nausea, flatulence, mucosal ulceration, perforation, and spontaneous deflation of balloon. Sleeve gastrostomy is an approach to reduce the gastric volume. Endoscopic procedures are indicated in patients with BMI > 30 kg/m^2, <40 kg/m^2, or BMI > 27 kg/m^2 with one or more obesity associated with comorbidities.

Bariatric surgery: It is the most effective weight loss measure, and is indicated individuals with BMI ≥ 40 kg/m^2 and BMI > 35 kg/m^2 with at least one obesity condition. It includes two procedures: Laparoscopic sleeve gastrectomy in which most of stomach along the greater curvature is removed and the other procedure is Roux-en-Y gastric bypass in which a small gastric pouch is directly connected to jejunum. Prominent side effects include leaks, bleeding, perforation, internal hernia, malabsorption, and nutritional deficiencies.[31-34]

CONCLUSION

It is important to identify people with at risk of obesity and overweight with the help of simple parameters. It should be routine for people in community and to identify high-risk population. Evaluation should include BMI, waist circumference, diet, sleep, drugs, level of physical activity, occupation, and family history. Obesity-related risk factors and cardiovascular diseases should be treated to prevent the risk of complications. After risk factors have been detected, patients and family should be educated about the present and future risk of obesity and overweight, then initiation of timely intervention in terms of psychological support, exercise, diet, and control of other risk factors. In people with obesity, drugs and surgery can be considered.

REFERENCES

1. World Health Organization. (2025). Obesity and Overweight. [online] Available from https://www.who.int/news-room/fact-sheets/detail/obesity-and-overweight [Last accessed October, 2025].
2. Volpe M, Gallo G. Obesity and cardiovascular disease: An executive document on pathophysiological and clinical links promoted by the Italian Society of Cardiovascular Prevention (SIPREC). Front Cardiovasc Med. 2023;10:1136340.
3. Tutor AW, Lavie CJ, Kachur S, et al. Updates on obesity and the obesity paradox in cardiovascular diseases. Prog Cardiovasc Dis. 2023;78:2-10.
4. Powell-Wiley TM, Poirier P, Burke LE, et al. Obesity and Cardiovascular Disease: A Scientific Statement From the American Heart Association. Circulation. 2021;143(21):e984-e1010.
5. Koskinas KC, Van Craenenbroeck EM, Antoniades C, et al. Obesity and cardiovascular disease: an ESC clinical consensus statement. Eur Heart J. 2024;45(38):4063-98. Erratum in: Eur Heart J. 2025;46(9):876.
6. The Surveillance of Risk Factors Report Series (SuRF). World Health Organization. 2005. p. 22.
7. Timmis A, Vardas P, Townsend N, et al. European Society of Cardiology: cardiovascular disease statistics 2021. Eur Heart J. 2022;43:799.
8. Battineni G, Sagaro GG, Chintalapudi N, et al. Impact of Obesity-Induced Inflammation on Cardiovascular Diseases (CVD). Int J Mol Sci. 2021;22(9):4798.
9. Hanssen H, Moholdt T, Bahls M, et al. Lifestyle interventions to change trajectories of obesity-related cardiovascular risk from childhood onset to manifestation in adulthood: a joint scientific statement of the task force for childhood health of the European Association of Preventive Cardiology and the European Childhood Obesity Group. Eur J Prev Cardiol. 2023;30(14):1462-72.
10. Lopez-Jimenez F, Almahmeed W, Bays H, et al. Obesity and cardiovascular disease: mechanistic insights and management strategies. A joint position paper by the World Heart Federation and World Obesity Federation. Eur J Prev Cardiol. 2022;29(17):2218-37.
11. Perone F, Spadafora L, Pratesi A, et al. Obesity and cardiovascular disease: Risk assessment, physical activity, and management of complications. Int J Cardiol Cardiovasc Risk Prev. 2024;23:200331.
12. Anekwe CV, Ahn YJ, Bajaj SS, Stanford FC. Pharmacotherapy causing weight gain and metabolic alteration in those with obesity and obesity-related conditions: A review. Ann NY Acad Sci. 2024;1533(1):145-55.
13. Wu YK, Berry DC, Schwartz TA. Weight Stigmatization and Binge Eating in Asian Americans with Overweight and Obesity. Int J Environ Res Public Health. 2020;17(12):4319.
14. Marx N, Federici M, Schütt K, et al. 2023 ESC Guidelines for the management of cardiovascular disease in patients with diabetes. Eur Heart J. 2023;44(39):4043-140. Erratum in: Eur Heart J. 2023;44(48):5060. Erratum in: Eur Heart J. 2024;45(7):518.

15. Larsson J, Auscher S, Shamoun A, et al. Insulin resistance is associated with high-risk coronary artery plaque composition in asymptomatic men between 65 and 75 years and no diabetes: A DANCAVAS cross-sectional sub-study. Atherosclerosis. 2023;385:117328.
16. McEvoy JW, McCarthy CP, Bruno RM, et al. 2024 ESC Guidelines for the management of elevated blood pressure and hypertension. Eur Heart J. 2024;45(38):3912-4018. Erratum in: Eur Heart J. 2025;46(14):1300.
17. Rossello X, Fuster V, Oliva B, et al. Association Between Body Size Phenotypes and Subclinical Atherosclerosis. J Clin Endocrinol Metab. 2020;105(12):3734-44.
18. Sung CW, Huang CH, Chen WJ, et al. Obese cardiogenic arrest survivors with significant coronary artery disease had worse in-hospital mortality and neurological outcomes. Sci Rep. 2020;10(1):18638.
19. Masi S, Rizzoni D, Taddei S, et al. Assessment and pathophysiology of microvascular disease: recent progress and clinical implications. Eur Heart J. 2021;42(26):2590-604.
20. Borlaug BA, Jensen MD, Kitzman DW, et al. Obesity and heart failure with preserved ejection fraction: new insights and pathophysiological targets. Cardiovasc Res. 2023;118(18):3434-50.
21. Gawałko M, Saljic A, Li N, et al. Adiposity-associated atrial fibrillation: molecular determinants, mechanisms, and clinical significance. Cardiovasc Res. 2023;119(3):614-30.
22. Kaltoft M, Langsted A, Nordestgaard BG. Obesity as a Causal Risk Factor for Aortic Valve Stenosis. J Am Coll Cardiol. 2020;75(2):163-76.
23. Burki T. European Commission classifies obesity as a chronic disease. Lancet Diabetes Endocrinol. 2021;9:418.
24. Chen X, He H, Xie K et al. Impact of various exercise types on visceral adipose tissue in individuals with obesity and overweight: a systemic review and network meta analysis of randomised controlled trials Scientific Reports. 2024;14:12137.
25. Butler J, Shah SJ, Petrie MC, et al. Semaglutide versus placebo in people with obesity-related heart failure with preserved ejection fraction: a pooled analysis of the STEP-HFpEF and STEP-HFpEF DM randomised trials. Lancet. 2024;403(10437):1635-48.
26. Finan B, Yang B, Ottaway N, et al. A rationally designed monomeric peptide triagonist corrects obesity and diabetes in rodents. Nat Med. 2015;21(1):27-36.
27. Ji L, Jiang H, Cheng Z, et al. A phase 2 randomised controlled trial of mazdutide in Chinese overweight adults or adults with obesity. Nat Commun. 2023;14:8289.
28. Frías JP, Davies MJ, Rosenstock J, et al. Tirzepatide versus Semaglutide Once Weekly in Patients with Type 2 Diabetes. N Engl J Med. 2021;385(6):503-15.
29. Onakpoya IJ, Lee JJ, Mahtani KR, et al. Naltrexone-bupropion (Mysimba) in management of obesity: A systematic review and meta-analysis of unpublished clinical study reports. Br J Clin Pharmacol. 2020;86(4):646-67. Erratum in: Br J Clin Pharmacol. 2024;90(6):1531-3.
30. Wabitsch M, Farooqi S, Flück CE, et al. Natural History of Obesity Due to POMC, PCSK1, and LEPR Deficiency and the Impact of Setmelanotide. J Endocr Soc. 2022;6(6):bvac057.
31. Pereira JPS, Calafatti M, Martinino A, et al. Epicardial Adipose Tissue Changes After Bariatric and Metabolic Surgery: a Systematic Review and Meta-analysis. Obes Surg. 2023;33(11):3636-48.
32. Sorimachi H, Obokata M, Omote K, et al. Long-Term Changes in Cardiac Structure and Function Following Bariatric Surgery. J Am Coll Cardiol. 2022;80(16):1501-12.
33. Mingrone G, Panunzi S, De Gaetano A, et al. Metabolic surgery versus conventional medical therapy in patients with type 2 diabetes: 10-year follow-up of an open-label, single-centre, randomised controlled trial. Lancet. 2021;397(10271):293-304.
34. Enebo LB, Berthelsen KK, Kankam M, et al. Safety, tolerability, pharmacokinetics, and pharmacodynamics of concomitant administration of multiple doses of cagrilintide with semaglutide 2·4 mg for weight management: a randomised, controlled, phase 1b trial. Lancet. 2021;397(10286):1736-48.

CHAPTER 13

Myocardial Abnormalities Across the AHA-ACC Heart Failure Spectrum in Diabetic Patients

Umeshwar Pandey, Kumar Himanshu

ABSTRACT

Diabetes mellitus has become an epidemic among the growing population and with its increasing prevalence the complications arising from it are also becoming a major source of morbidity. Foremost among these is heart failure, a dreaded complication yet treatable to a large extend if identified properly. The challenge now is not diagnosing heart failure but identifying it early enough to prevent its progression. Identification of myocardial abnormalities using various tools before the dysfunction sets in is the way to go in future.

Keywords: Diabetes mellitus, heart failure, myocardial abnormalities, MRI.

INTRODUCTION

Diabetes mellitus is a major health concern especially in India with the incidence rising over 60% in the past two decades.[1-3] It is worrisome that India now accounts for nearly a quarter of the diabetic burden, and this is only likely to grow. Diabetes is not merely a disease of the pancreas it affects all the organs in the body and leads to end-organ damage. With the various micro- and microvasculature changes that diabetes causes, the heart becomes an epicenter of its effect. It is well recognized that diabetes causes accelerated atherosclerosis which in turn leads to cardiac dysfunction.[1] Over the last two decades, nonatherosclerotic cardiac dysfunction has also been identified, often termed as diabetic cardiomyopathy.[4] Whether associated with atherosclerosis or not, it is now a consensus that cardiac dysfunction associated with diabetes had a poorer prognosis and rapid downhill course. Therefore, it is imperative that diabetic patients are screened regularly for the onset of cardiac dysfunction as early initiation of therapy has been shown to delay the onset and even reverse the disease.

In a large collection of data from an Indian registry of heart failure carried out by Rajesh et al., it was found that more than half of the patients of diabetes without overt cardiac illness had asymptomatic ventricular dysfunction.[2] Identification of this subgroup could help us improve the future outcomes. This finding is not confined to few registries, in fact, it is increasing being reported across the globe.

STAGES OF HEART FAILURE

The ACC classifies any heart failure into four different stages. In the context of diabetes mellitus, these four stages should be seen as described in **Box 1**.[5]

BOX 1: Various stages and relevant features.

Satge A—Risk factors + no structural heart disease

- Only the presence of diabetes mellitus in itself becomes a risk factor and hence every patient of diabetes should be considerd in this stage

Satge B—Structural heart disease present, no symptoms

- Presence of left ventricular hypertrophy or diastolic dysfunction or impaired strain pattern
- The patient however shows no symptoms

Satge C—Symptomatic heart failure

- Symptoms of heart failure seen such as exertional dysnea or fatigue and reduced exercise capacity

Satge D—Advanced heart failure

- Features of advanced heart failure such as orthopnea, resting dysnea, systemic congestion, etc., seen often requiring inpatient therapy

CARDIOMYOPATHY IN DIABETES

Ischemic Cardiomyopathy

- It is well known that diabetes promotes atherosclerosis. Hyperglycemia damages endothelium and impairs nitric oxide availability. The endothelium becomes inflamed and prothrombotic.
- Hyperglycemia also leads to formation of advanced glycation end-products which deposit in vessel wall leading to it stiffening.
- At the same time, diabetes also promotes dyslipidemia contributing to plaque deposition and further inflammation.
- The atherosclerosis in diabetes is thus diffuse and progressive, affecting multiple vessels often throughout their course.
- The pattern of involvement makes treatment difficult and often results in ventricular dysfunction.

Diabetic Cardiomyopathy—Nonischemic

- It is now recognized as a distinct myocardial disease which develops independence of coronary artery disease or valvular disease or hypertension. It results in initial diastolic dysfunction followed by systolic dysfunction.

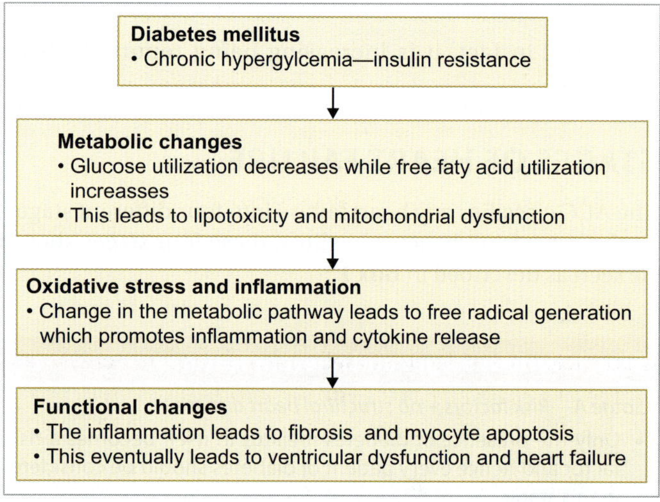

FLOWCHART 1: Mechanism of development of diabetic cardiomyopathy.

- **Flowchart 1** shows the mechanism for development of diabetic cardiomyopathy.[4]

DIAGNOSING IT EARLY

How much does diagnosing heart failure in early stages affect the outcomes? Various meta-analyses have been carried out, using the Kaplan–Meier curves, they suggest that diagnosing it early delays the onset of heart failure and thereby provides mortality benefits.[5]

With the availability of newer drugs specifically SGLT-2 inhibitors and ARNI, there has been a paradigm shift on our outlook toward heart failure. It is no longer seen as a terminal illness. While the shift in the treatment of established heart failure has now percolated across the physicians, much is still desired about preventing the onset of heart failure.

We currently employ three tools to diagnose it early, cardiac biomarkers, strain and stress echocardiography and cardiac MRI as seen in **Figure 1**.

Cardiac Biomarkers

- Their role in diagnosing heart failure in stages C and D has been well validated. They have a higher negative predictive value than positive predictive value.
- The most commonly used biomarkers are high sensitivity troponins and N-terminal pro-B-type natriuretic peptide.
- While their levels may be affected by presence of factors such as anemia, sepsis, and chronic kidney disease, the mere presence of diabetes does not impact their levels.
- The challenge remains on utilizing them in stages A and B. Many small studies have used these biomarkers done serially over a course of 3–6 months. Higher baseline levels or a significant rise in titer may suggest a higher likelihood of progression to high stages.

Echocardiography

- Traditionally echocardiography has been used to diagnose heart failure. It is used to identify the structural abnormalities, chamber sizes, and estimating the ejection fraction (EF). Based on the calculation of EF, heart failure has been classified into heart failure with reduced ejection fraction (HFrEF) if EF is <40%, heart failure with

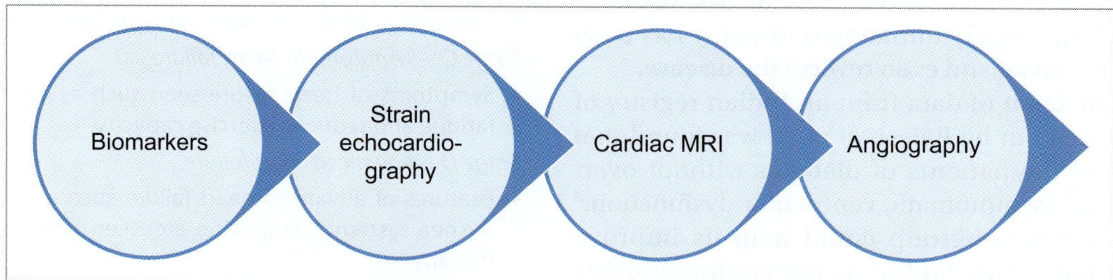

FIG. 1: Tools to diagnose heart failure early.

mid-range ejection fraction (HFmEF) if EF is 40–50%, and heart failure with preserved ejection fraction (HFpEF) if EF is >50–55%.

- During stages A and B, the EF is usually preserved, and structural abnormalities are usually absent. In these stages, impaired diastolic function, presence of ventricular hypertrophy, and atrial enlargement are of prime importance. When present, these factors help to diagnose early heart failure in ACC stages A and B.
- Many a times even these factors are not present, and the routine echocardiogram may appear to be normal. In such cases, stress and strain echocardiography may prove to be useful.[6]

Stress and Strain Echocardiography

- Subjecting patients with an apparently normal echocardiogram to some form of stress such as a treadmill or bicycle ergometry while performing echocardiography simultaneously may help to identify impaired diastolic function or raised pulmonary pressures during exercise. Such patients are likely to develop heart failure soon.
- Strain echocardiography is based on utilizing tissue Doppler imaging to identify the impaired strain which pints toward impaired ventricular relaxation. This precedes structural abnormalities detected on routine echocardiography and hence may help in early identification.

Cardiac Magnetic Resonance Imaging

- It is emerging as the preferred alternative modality of imaging.
- Yang et al.[1] reported that global early diastolic longitudinal strain rate, as measured by MRI, significantly distinguished diabetic individuals in stage A HF from healthy controls.
- The study also showed that myocardial fibrosis plays an important part in the development of heart failure in diabetics.
- While screening the patients, the presence of fibrosis could easily be detected by MRI. Patterns of fibrosis detected on the variations of gadolinium enhancement enhance the accuracy.
- Cardiac MRI can also be used to calculate global longitudinal strain (GLS) and early diastolic strain rate (DSR). The values derived from MRI have been consistently found to be superior to echocardiography.
- In the same study, the diabetic patients were found to have lower GLS and DSRs.

BOX 2: Various changes in cardiac MRI corresponding to the various stages of heart failure.

Stage A:
- Impaired GLS and early diastolic strain rate
- Myocardial fibrosis may be detected

Stage B:
- Further decrease in GLS and DSR
- Extracellular volume fraction increases
- Ventricular ejection fraction is normal

Stages C and D:
- Along with the above changes which increase in quantity
- There is impairment of ejection fraction

(DSR: early diastolic strain rate; GLS: global longitudinal strain)

- A summary of the various cardiac MRI findings can be found in **Box 2**.

Role of Computed Tomography and Invasive Angiography

- When ischemia is likely to be the cause of ventricular dysfunction invasive angiography still continues to be the gold standard and must be advised. It also enables planning the treatment.
- On the other hand, when ischemia is unlikely and the etiology of dysfunction is uncertain, then CT angiography is a valuable tool to establish the diagnosis.
- It avoids the invasive nature of conventional angiography and provides added information about the ventricular and valvular morphology. It may thus be considered a primary tool to establish the etiology of heart failure and rule out ischemia.

CONCLUSION

As the incidence of diabetes mellitus continues to increase, so will the incidence of heart failure. Heart failure is inevitable in diabetics considering the very nature of the disease and its systemic effects. However much can be done to delay the onset of heart failure and atherosclerosis thereby providing long-term morbidity and mortality benefits. The challenge is to identify the onset of the process early; tools such as MRI and advanced echocardiography are of prime importance in it. The benefit of identifying the process early cannot be overstated. Constituting therapies that delay myocardial fibrosis and stabilize the endothelium will definitely slow the disease process.

REFERENCES

1. Yang W, Zhu L, Wu W, et al. Myocardial abnormalities across the AHA/ACC stages of heart failure in patients with diabetes. JACC Asia. 2024;4(12):940-52.
2. Rajput R, Mohan JC, Sawhney JPS, et al. Prevalence of cardiac abnormalities and heart failure in unselected out-patients with type 2 diabetes mellitus and associated clinical factors: Real-world evidence from an Indian registry. Indian Heart J. 2023;75(6): 436-42.
3. Saeedi P, Petersohn I, Salpea P, et al. Global and regional diabetes prevalence estimates for 2019 and projections for 2030 and 2045: Results from the International Diabetes Federation Diabetes Atlas, 9th edition. Diabetes Res Clin Pract. 2019;157:107843.
4. Jia G, Whaley-Connell A, Sowers JR. Diabetic cardiomyopathy: a hyperglycaemia-and insulin-resistance-induced heart disease. Diabetologia. 2018;61(1):21-8.
5. McLellan J, Bankhead CR, Oke JL, et al. Natriuretic peptide-guided treatment for heart failure: a systematic review and meta-analysis. BMJ evidence-based medicine. 2020;25(1):33-7.
6. McDonagh TA, Metra M, Adamo M, et al. 2021 ESC Guidelines for the diagnosis and treatment of acute and chronic heart failure: Developed by the Task Force for the diagnosis and treatment of acute and chronic heart failure of the European Society of Cardiology (ESC) With the special contribution of the Heart Failure Association (HFA) of the ESC. Eur Heart J. 2021;42(36):3599-726.

SECTION

4

Dyslipidemia Management

Section Outline

14. **Implications of Lipid-lowering Therapy for Premature Coronary Artery Disease**
AK Pancholia

15. **The Challenges in Reducing Non-high-density Lipoprotein Cholesterol**
Arvind Kumar, Vipin Kumar

16. **Particle Number and Characteristics of Lipoprotein(a), Low-density Lipoprotein, and ApoB: Perspectives on Contributions to Atherosclerotic Cardiovascular Disease**
JPS Sawhney, Rohan Patel

17. **Childhood LDL Cholesterol, Non-HDL Cholesterol and Adult Atherosclerotic Cardiovascular Events**
Rajeev Gupta, Sonali Sharma

Dyslipidemia Management

CHAPTER 14

Implications of Lipid-lowering Therapy for Premature Coronary Artery Disease

AK Pancholia

ABSTRACT

Premature coronary artery disease (PCAD) is defined as coronary artery disease (CAD) that develops at a younger age than is typically expected, means CAD occurring in men before the age of 55 years and in women before the age of 65 years. CAD before the age of 45 years is defined as "CAD in young". There is a need to identify high-risk features that predict early-onset atherosclerotic cardiovascular disease (ASCVD). While CAD is more common in older individuals, PCAD represents a significant public health concern due to its impact on younger populations. The high-risk conditions in the 20- to 39-year age range (young adults) include tobacco use, elevated blood pressure/hypertension, family history of premature ASCVD, primary severe hypercholesterolemia such as familial hypercholesterolemia, diabetes with diabetes-specific risk enhancing factors, or the presence of multiple other risk-enhancing factors, including females, a history of preeclampsia or menopause under the age 40 years. The current thinking on lipid risk factors such as triglycerides, nonhigh-density lipoprotein cholesterol, apolipoprotein B, or lipoprotein(a) [Lp(a)] is useful in understanding an individual's long-term ASCVD risk. Lp(a) was found to be 10 times more atherogenic than LDL and is found in higher levels in black patients. Furthermore, in patients hospitalized for an acute MI, Lp(a) levels > 80 mg/dL are associated with an increased CAD burden. For halting the disease progression and cardiovascular outcomes in premature CAD, lipid-lowering therapy (LLT) plays a crucial role. Effective lipid management, particularly reducing low-density lipoprotein cholesterol (LDL-C), can halt atherosclerosis, stabilize plaques, and prevent future events. However, underutilization of LLT in younger patients with premature CAD is a concern, hence there is a need for improved screening and proper optimization of treatment strategies.

Keywords: Premature coronary artery disease, lipid-lowering therapy, low-density lipoprotein, LP(a), statin.

INTRODUCTION

First clinical manifestation of coronary artery disease (CAD) in women < 60 years and men < 55 years is defined as premature CAD.[1] Evidences suggest that it is highly prevalent in India.[2,3] According to Global Burden of Diseases study in developing countries, ischemic heart disease (IHD) is one of the important causes of morbidity and mortality in young.[4,5] There are more annual deaths due to IHD in the age group of 20–54 years in India compared to USA, China, and countries in Europe and Central Asia.[6] Even among hospital admissions (both government and private), there are significant proportion of patients with premature CAD.[7] This early onset of CAD is predominantly due to adverse lifestyles among the young.[8,9] Traditional risk factors [hypercholesterolemia, low-density lipoprotein cholesterol (LDL-C), smoking, hypertension, obesity, etc.], as well as emerging risk factors [lipoprotein(a) (Lp(a)), metabolic syndrome, and social determinants] are important causes.[10-14]

PREVALENCE OF DYSLIPIDEMIA IS HIGH IN YOUNG ADULTS

Measurement of cholesterol early in the life is very important to prevent the development and progression of atherosclerosis and subsequent long-term atherosclerotic cardiovascular disease (ASCVD) risk.[15] For managing lipid-related risk, appropriate screening is the first critical step.[16] Unfortunately only one-half of youths aged 6–19 years have ideal levels for standard lipids and apolipoprotein B (ApoB), and only 25% of adolescents have their at least one component of lipid profile in an adverse range.[17] Further evaluation and intensive control are required in those with the highest values **(Table 1)**.

TABLE 1: Reference ranges for pediatric and adolescent lipid and lipoprotein concentrations.

Parameter	Acceptable	Borderline	High
Total cholesterol	<170 mg/dL	170–199 mg/dL	≥200 mg/dL
LDL-C	<110 mg/dL	110–129 mg/dL	≥130 mg/dL
HDL-C	>45 mg/dL	40–45 mg/dL	<40 mg/dL
Non-HDL-C	<120 mg/dL	120–144 mg/dL	≥145 mg/dL
Triglycerides			
0–9 years old	<75 mg/dL	75–99 mg/dL	≥100 mg/dL
10–19 years old	<90 mg/dL	90–129 mg/dL	≥130 mg/dL
Apolipoprotein B	<90 mg/dL	90–109 mg/dL	≥110 mg/dL
Apolipoprotein A-I	<120 mg/dL	115–120 mg/dL	≥115 mg/dL

Source: Adapted from Schefelker JM, Peterson AL. Screening and Management of Dyslipidemia in Children and Adolescents. J Clin Med. 2022;11:6479.

ASCVD RISK RELATES TO DURATION OF EXPOSURE

Research from multiple observational cohort studies has shown that risk of ASCVD increases with increased exposure to elevated LDL-C, independent of other risk factors, in a dose-dependent fashion.[18] In the CARDIA (Coronary Artery Risk Development in Young Adults) study, with a median 16-year follow-up, adults aged 18–30 years, long exposure to high LDL is directly related to increased cardiovascular disease (CVD) risk even after adjusting for other risk factors.[19]

SCREENING GUIDELINES FOR DYSLIPIDEMIA AMONG YOUNG ADULTS

Due to the asymptomatic nature of dyslipidemia, its identification before the development of signs or symptoms of CVD is of paramount importance. Screening may be of particular benefit in identifying young adults with markedly elevated lipid levels due to unrecognized familial hypercholesterolemia (FH). The ESC 2019 guidelines recommend that risk factor screening including the lipid profile should be considered in men > 40 years old, and women > 50 years of age or postmenopausal.[20]

IMPROVING LIPID CONTROL IN YOUNG ADULTS

There is a strong impact of high LDL-C and ApoB in younger individuals compared with older individuals. The association between lipid levels and MI attenuated with increasing age as seen in the INTERHEART (Effect of Potentially Modifiable Risk Factors Associated with Myocardial Infarction) study.[21] Although large cardiovascular outcomes trials of statins have not enrolled young adults, but data from trials of children and adolescents with FH support the safety and efficacy of statins in younger age groups. Long-term follow-up data from WOSCOPS (West of Scotland Study) indicate legacy effect of early initiation of statin therapy as benefit persists even after therapy is discontinued.[22]

FAMILIAL HYPERCHOLESTEROLEMIA

Young adults with FH are at very high risk of CVD and are recommended to initiate high-intensity statin therapy. Although FH is rare, the prevalence of FH is higher in adults with premature ASCVD.[23-25] Individuals with FH often require more aggressive lipid-lowering therapy (LLT), including high-dose statins, ezetimibe, or PCSK9 inhibitors, to manage their extremely high LDL cholesterol levels.[26] There is a need to improving identification and effective therapy of FH. Many adults with FH are not on intensive statin or having suboptimal adherence because of physician inertia or patient concerns about statin associated muscle symptoms. There is a need to overcome these issues. In 2023, EAS (European Atherosclerosis Society) has come out with consensus statement on FH **(Flowchart 1)**.

OTHER TARGETS FOR ASSESSING AND LOWERING LIPID-RELATED RISK

■ Apolipoprotein B

In most of the lab, ApoB is not a part of a standard lipid panel. A standard lipid panel comprises measurement of total cholesterol, HDL-C, and triglycerides, and calculates LDL-C and non-HDL-C. ApoB is often, but not always correlated with LDL-C measurements. Some of the patients with premature CAD have lower than average levels of LDL-C and higher than average ApoB levels what is called as LDL-C and ApoB discordant. This phenomenon was observed in the CARDIA study, where individuals with discordantly high ApoB/low LDL-C had 1.5- to 2.3-fold higher risk of developing

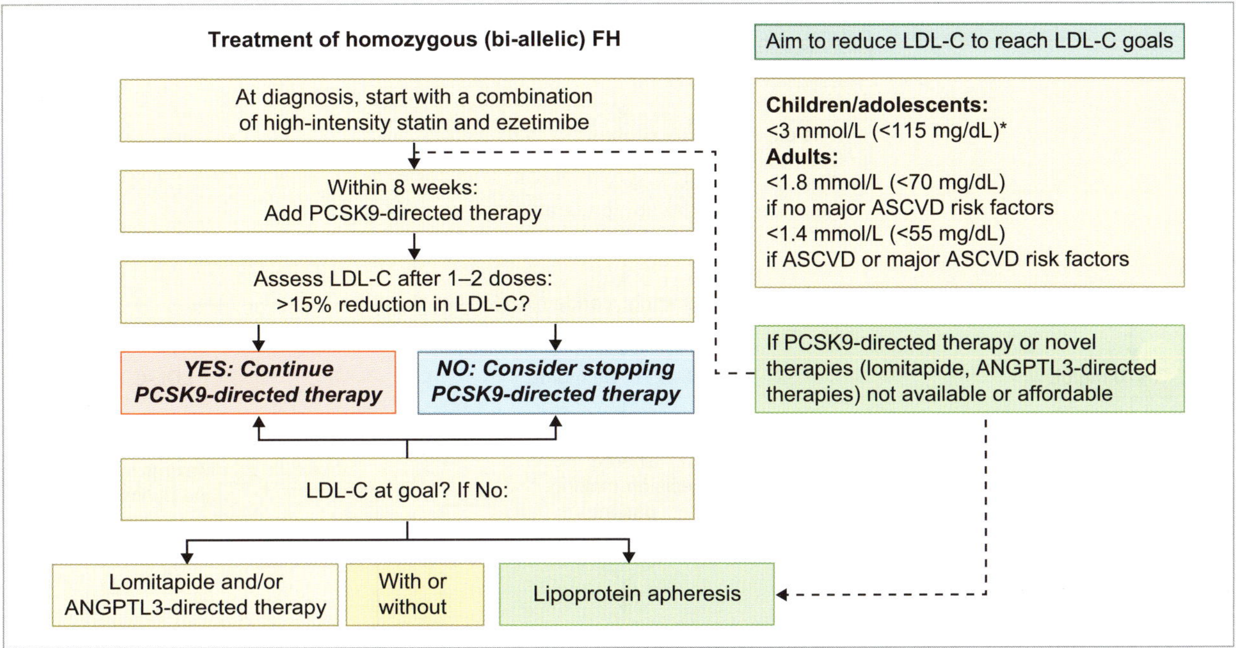

*Lower goals require.

FLOWCHART 1: 2023 Update on EAS consensus statement on homozygous FH.

CAC 25 years later.[27] Treatment for ApoB in premature CAD primarily focuses on lowering ApoB levels through lifestyle modifications and lipid-lowering medications. This includes statins as a cornerstone treatment, along with other therapies such as PCSK9 inhibitors, ezetimibe, and niacin, depending on individual patient needs. The target for Apo B levels is recommended in 2019 ESC guideline, shown in the **Box 1**.

BOX 1: 2019 ESC guideline for ApoB target.

Target ApoB:

- <65 mg/dL—very high risk
- <80 mg/dL—high risk
- <100 mg/dL—moderate CV risk

Source: With permission from Mach F, et al. (2020).[20]

Triglycerides

Elevated triglycerides are associated with increased risk of ASCVD, but it is less clear whether triglycerides are causally associated or whether triglycerides are a marker of another atherogenic moiety of the triglyceride-rich lipoproteins. In a large meta-analysis of randomized trials, triglyceride lowering was associated with lower ASCVD risk, which was somewhat lower than seen for LDL-C, but after excluding REDUCE-IT (Reduction of Cardiovascular Events With Icosapent EthylIntervention Trial), this risk reduction was attenuated. Whether or not triglycerides are causal for ASCVD, persistent hypertriglyceridemia serves as an important marker for young adults at higher risk of events.[28] Plasma triglycerides are usually mildly to moderately elevated in patients with insulin resistance, abdominal obesity, and poor health behaviors. Severe elevation in triglycerides is often due to the combination of unhealthful diet and inadequate physical activity on a background susceptibility of multiple genetic defects. Persistent hypertriglyceridemia is a signal for young adults to improve metabolic fitness. Even mild elevation in triglycerides (>150 mg/dL) was associated with twofold to threefold higher risk of premature MI. In a global systematic review and meta-analysis of risk factors for premature MI, mild elevation in triglycerides (>150 mg/dL) was associated with twofold to threefold higher risk of premature MI. The "2021 ACC Expert Consensus Decision Pathway on the Management of ASCVD Risk Reduction in Patients With Persistent Hypertriglyceridemia" provides indispensable algorithms for the clinician who sees young adults with hypertriglyceridemia **(Flowchart 2)**.[29]

Treatment for high triglycerides in focuses on lifestyle modifications and, when necessary, medications to lower triglyceride levels and reduce cardiovascular risk. Lifestyle changes include dietary adjustments, increased physical activity, and weight management. If lifestyle changes are insufficient, medications such as fibrates, omega-3 fatty acids, and niacin may be considered, often in conjunction with statins.

Lipoprotein(a)

Lp(a) is a genetically modified form of LDL-C particle and has greater propensity than LDL-C, to bind to oxidized lipoproteins. In the context of PCAD, Lp(a) refers to

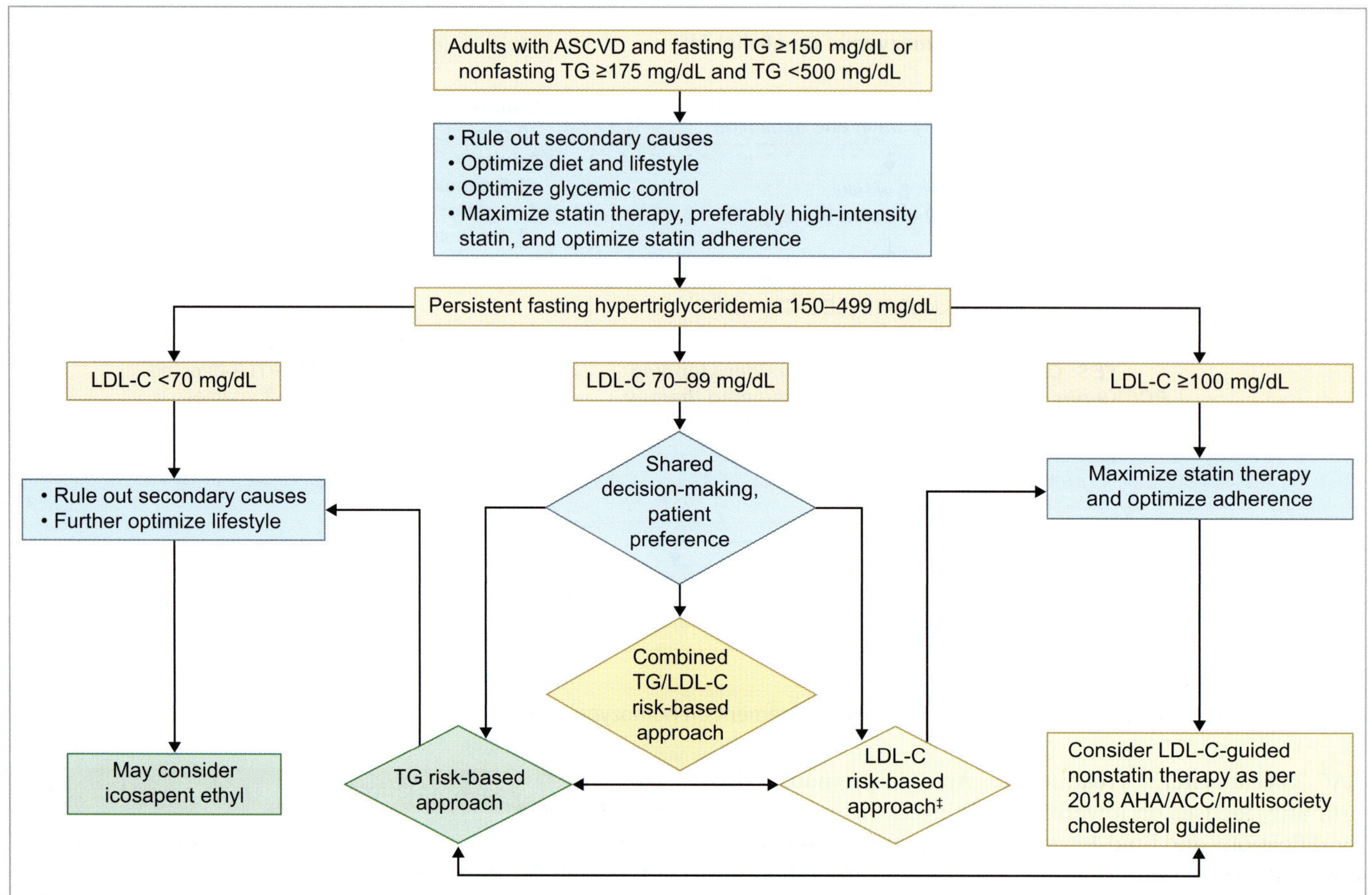

‡High-risk patients can be put on intensive statin along with non-statin LDL-lowering drugs.

FLOWCHART 2: Management of ASCVD risk reduction in patients with persistent hypertriglyceridemia.
Source: With permission from Virani SS, et al. (2021).[29]

lipoprotein(a), a type of LDL that is a strong, genetically determined risk factor for developing the disease, particularly at a young age. Elevated Lp(a) levels are associated with an increased risk of both early and advanced stages of atherosclerosis. Lp(a) appears to be a particularly important ASCVD risk factor for Indians as Indians tend to have high prevalence of elevated Lp(a).[30] Based on these evidences, estimation of Lp(a) levels is strongly recommended for ASCVD risk stratification in Indian subjects, particularly in those who have family history or premature CAD. High Lp(a) concentrations > 30 mg/dL indicate increased risk for incident myocardial infarction,[31] although European Atherosclerosis Society (EAS) consensus statement has proposed 50 mg/dL concentration threshold for an increased risk.[31] Methods recommended for measurement are different in Europe compared to India. Fasting is not required for Lp(a) testing.

Impact of Lipoprotein(a) Levels on the Premature Coronary Event

Study[32] showed a higher prevalence of high Lp(a) level in premature acute coronary syndrome (ACS) patients compared to the general population. According to some studies, there a greater risk for ACS when LDL-C is also elevated. Association with premature ACS becomes even stronger when using a cutoff of 70 mg/dL. Those with Lp(a) levels > 70 mg/dL experienced an event 1.75 years earlier compared to those with levels below this threshold.[33] Treatment of high Lp(a) in premature CAD focuses on managing risk factors and exploring emerging therapies. While lifestyle changes like a healthy diet and exercise are recommended, they don't significantly lower Lp(a) levels. Current treatments are focused on reducing overall cardiovascular risk and include aggressive risk factor management, potential use of niacin, and lipoprotein apheresis. Emerging therapies such as antisense oligonucleotides and siRNA hold promise for future Lp(a) reduction.

LIPID-LOWERING THERAPY FOR PREVENTION OF PREMATURE ASCVD

Rates of ASCVD in middle-aged and older adults are declining largely due to more effective preventive interventions such as LLT,[34] while there is no change in younger individuals. To achieve the WHO's 25 × 25 target of reducing premature

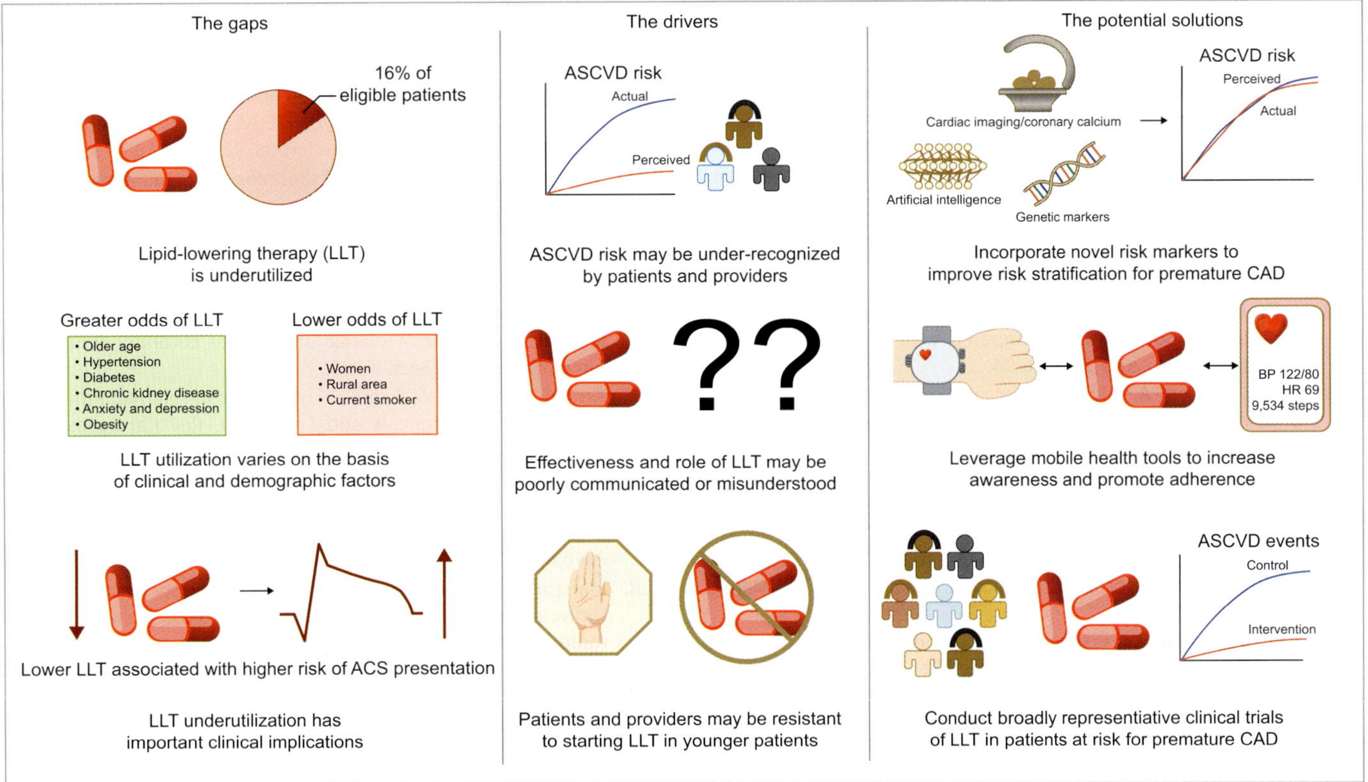

FIG. 1: Challenges and opportunities for prevention in premature coronary artery disease.

Source: Adapted from Khurshid S, Kany S. An Ounce of Prevention for a Pound of Cure?: Lipid-Lowering Therapy for Premature Coronary Disease. JACC Adv. 2024;4(1):101315.

death by 25% by 2025, reduction of death due to premature CAD is very important.[35] Statins are the cornerstone of LLT, possesses a favorable side effect profile and consistently reduces clinical ASCVD events by 20–40% among high-risk individuals,[36] but recent data demonstrate that LLT is underutilized among individuals with premature CAD. Overall LLT utilization was only 14.8%, more among women, smokers, and in rural areas. Good adherence was achieved in only 40% in those who are on LLT **(Fig. 1)**.

Other factors such as rely only on lifestyle modification, cost of drugs, and fear about side effects also contribute to a lack of understanding of the importance of LLT. All these factors also responsible for therapeutic inertia by physicians. There is higher willingness to accept LLT in those with other comorbidities such as hypertension, and diabetes de novo as a sole medication.

CONCLUSION

Majority of patients do not receive LLT before their presentation with the disease. Identifying young adults at risk for premature CAD, and implementation of primary prevention therapy when indicated is the need of the hour. Poor understanding of the role of LLT, along with wrong belief that lifestyle modification alone may be sufficient, drug cost or fear of side effects are other factors. Some of these factors may contribute to therapeutic inertia also by physicians. Even not achieving the guideline recommended LDL levels is another issue. Randomized trials targeting diverse groups at risk for premature CAD are needed to identify optimal therapies including optimization of LLT uptake to prevent ASCVD in young.

REFERENCES

1. Michos E, Choi AD. Coronary artery disease in young adults: a hard lesson but a good teacher. J Am Coll Cardiol. 2019;74:1879-82.
2. Ke C, Gupta R, Xavier D, et al. Divergent trends in ischemic heart disease and stroke mortality in India from 2000 to 2015: a nationally representative mortality survey. Lancet Global Health. 2018;6:914-23.
3. Gupta R, Gaur K. Epidemiology of ischemic heart disease and diabetes in India: an overview of the twin epidemic. Curr Diabetes Rev. 2020;100620186664.
4. Roth GA, Johnson C, Abajobir A, et al. Global, regional, and national cardiovascular disease prevalence, mortality, and disability-adjusted life-years for 10 causes of cardiovascular mortality, 1990

to 2015: a systematic analysis for the Global Burden of Disease Study. J Am Coll Cardiol. 2017;70:1-25.
5. Global Burden of Disease Study 2019 Diseases and Injuries Collaborators. Global burden of 369 diseases and injuries in 204 countries and territories, 1990-2019: a systematic analysis for the Global Burden of Disease Study 2019. Lancet. 2020;396:1204-22.
6. IHME. (2019). Global Burden of Disease Study 2019 Data Resources. [online] Available from http://ghdx.healthdata.org/gbd-2019 [Last accessed October, 2022].
7. Siwach SB. Profile of young acute myocardial infarction in Haryana. J Assoc Phys India. 1998;46:424-6.
8. Joshi PP, Islam S, Pais P, et al. Risk factors for early myocardial infarction in South Asians compared with individuals in other countries. JAMA. 2007;297:286-94.
9. Gupta R, Misra A, Vikram NK, et al. Younger age of escalation of cardiovascular risk factors in Asian Indian subjects. BMC Cardiovasc Disord. 2009;9:28.
10. Enas EA, Mehta J. Malignant coronary artery disease in young Asian Indians: thoughts on pathogenesis, prevention and therapy. Clin Cardiol. 1995;18:131-5.
11. Sharma M, Ganguly NK. Premature coronary artery disease in Indians and its associated risk factors. Vasc Health Risk Manag. 2005;1:217-25.
12. Kaul U, Bhatia V. Perspective on coronary interventions and cardiac surgeries in India. Indian J Med Res. 2010;132:543-8.
13. Gupta MD, Gupta P, Girish MP, et al. Risk factors for myocardial infarction in very young South Asians. Curr Opin Endocrinol Diabetes Obes. 2020;27:87-94.
14. Gupta R, Wood DA. Primary prevention of ischemic heart disease: populations, individuals and healthcare professionals. Lancet. 2019;394:685-96.
15. de Ferranti SD, Steinberger J, Ameduri R, et al. Cardiovascular risk reduction in high-risk pediatric patients: a scientific statement from the American Heart Association. Circulation. 2019;139:e603-34.
16. Grundy SM, Stone NJ, Bailey AL, et al. 2018 AHA/ACC/AACVPR/AAPA/ABC/ACPM/ADA/AGS/ APhA/ASPC/NLA/PCNA guideline on the management of blood cholesterol: a report of the American College of Cardiology/American Heart Association Task Force on Clinical Practice Guidelines. J Am Coll Cardiol. 2019;73:285-350.
17. Perak AM, Ning H, Kit BK, et al. Trends in levels of lipids and apolipoprotein B in US youths aged 6 to 19 years, 1999-2016. JAMA. 2019;321:1895-905.
18. Boron J, Chapman MJ, Krauss RM, et al. Low-density lipoproteins cause atherosclerotic cardiovascular disease: pathophysiological, genetic, and therapeutic insights: a consensus statement from the European Atherosclerosis Society Consensus Panel. Eur Heart J. 2020;41:2313-30.
19. Domanski MJ, Tian X, Wu CO, et al. Time course of LDL cholesterol exposure and cardiovascular disease event risk. J Am Coll Cardiol. 2020;76(13):1507-16.
20. Mach F, Baigent C, Catapano AL, et al. ESC/EAS Guidelines for the management of dyslipidaemias: lipid modification to reduce cardiovascular risk. Eur Heart J. 2019;41 (1):111-88.
21. Sniderman AD, Islam S, McQueen M, et al. Age and cardiovascular risk attributable to apolipoprotein b, low-density lipoprotein cholesterol or non-high-density lipoprotein cholesterol. J Am Heart Assoc. 2016;5:003665.
22. Ford I, Murray H, McCowan C, et al. Long-term safety and efficacy of lowering lowdensity lipoprotein cholesterol with statin therapy: 20-year follow-up of West of Scotland Coronary Prevention Study. Circulation. 2016;133(11):1073-80.
23. De Backer G, Besseling J, Chapman J, et al. Prevalence and management of familial hypercholesterolaemia in coronary patients: an analysis of EUROASPIRE IV, a study of the European Society of Cardiology. Atherosclerosis. 2015;241:169-75.
24. Rallidis LS, Triantafyllis AS, Tsirebolos G, et al. Prevalence of heterozygous familial hypercholesterolaemia and its impact on long-term prognosis in patients with very early ST-segment elevation myocardial infarction in the era of statins. Atherosclerosis. 2016;249:17-21.
25. Nanchen D, Gencer B, Muller O, et al. Prognosis of patients with familial hypercholesterolemia after acute coronary syndromes. Circulation. 2016;134:698-709.
26. Arnold N, Koenig W. Familial Hypercholesterolemia: Pitfalls and Challenges in Diagnosis and Treatment. Rev Cardiovasc Med. 2023;24(8):236.
27. Wilkins JT, Li RC, Sniderman A, et al. Discordance between apolipoprotein B and LDL-cholesterol in young adults predicts coronary artery calcification: the CARDIA study. J Am Coll Cardiol. 2016;67:193-201.
28. Marston NA, Giugliano RP, Im K, et al. Association between triglyceride lowering and reduction of cardiovascular risk across multiple lipid-lowering therapeutic classes: a systematic review and metaregression analysis of randomized controlled trials. Circulation. 2019;140:1308-17.
29. Virani SS, Morris PB, Agarwala A, et al. 2021 ACC expert consensus decision pathway on the management of ASCVD risk reduction in patients with persistent hypertriglyceridemia: a report of the American College of Cardiology Solution Set Oversight Committee. J Am Coll Cardiol. 2021;78(9):960-93.
30. Enas EA, Varkey B, Dharmarajan TS, et al. Lipoprotein(a): an underrecognized genetic risk factor for malignant coronary artery disease in young Indians. Indian Heart J. 2019;71:184-98.
31. Hegele RA, Borén J, Ginsberg HN, et al. Rare dyslipidaemias, from phenotype to genotype to management: a European Atherosclerosis Society task force consensus statement. Lancet DM Endocrinol. 2020;8:50-67.
32. Afshar M, Pilote L, Dufresne L, et al. Lipoprotein(a) interactions with low-density lipoprotein cholesterol and other cardiovascular risk factors in premature acute coronary syndrome (ACS). J Am Heart Assoc 2016;5(4):e003012.
33. Cesaro A, Acerbo V, Scialla F, et al. Role of LipoprotEin(a) in CardiovascuLar diseases and premature acute coronary syndromes (RELACS study): Impact of Lipoprotein(a) levels on the premature coronary event and the severity of coronary artery disease. Nutr Metab Cardiovasc Dis. 2025;35(5):103843.
34. Li Z, Yang Y, Wang X, et al. Comparative analysis of atherosclerotic cardiovascular disease burden between ages 20-54 and over 55 years: insights from the Global Burden of Disease Study 2019. BMC Med. 2024;22:303.
35. Stringhini S, Carmeli C, Jokela M, et al. Socioeconomic status and the 25 x 25 risk factors as determinants of premature mortality: a multicohort study and meta-analysis of 1$7 million men and women. Lancet. 2017;389:1229-37.
36. Naci H, Brugts JJ, Fleurence R, et al. Comparative benefits of statins in the primary and secondary prevention of major coronary events and all-cause mortality: a network meta-analysis of placebo-controlled and active comparator trials. Eur J Prev Cardiol. 2013;20:641-57.

CHAPTER 15

The Challenges in Reducing Non-high-density Lipoprotein Cholesterol

Arvind Kumar, Vipin Kumar

ABSTRACT

Non-high-density lipoprotein cholesterol (non-HDL-C) includes all atherogenic lipoproteins that contain apolipoprotein B, such as low-density lipoprotein cholesterol (LDL-C), very low-density lipoprotein (VLDL), intermediate density lipoprotein (IDL), remnants of chylomicrons, and lipoprotein(a) [Lp(a)]. It serves as a cost effective, non-fasting marker which predicts atherosclerotic cardiovascular disease (ASCVD) risk better than LDL-C alone. Efforts to lower non-HDL-C are limited by pharmacological limitations, inter-individual variability in drug response, incomplete efficacy of combination therapies, and challenges in addressing remnant cholesterol. Managing these limitations requires refined lipid profiling techniques, personalized pharmacogenomic strategies, emerging ribonucleic acid (RNA)-based therapies, and AI-enabled digital health solutions, alongside policy reforms mandating non-HDL-C reporting. Health care providers should also be educated about comprehensive risk prediction advantages of non-HDL-C and its use in improving cardiovascular outcomes.

Keywords: Non-HDL-C, cardiovascular risk, atherogenic lipoproteins, statin therapy, dyslipidemia, residual risk.

INTRODUCTION

Non-high-density lipoprotein cholesterol (non-HDL-C) includes all atherogenic lipoproteins that contain apolipoprotein B (ApoB), such as low-density lipoprotein cholesterol (LDL-C), very low-density lipoprotein (VLDL), intermediate density lipoprotein (IDL), remnants of chylomicrons, and lipoprotein(a) [Lp(a)].[1-3] It is obtained by a simple subtraction of high density lipoprotein cholesterol (HDL-C) from total cholesterol, making it both cost-effective and accessible for widespread clinical use.[1-3] This makes non-HDL-C especially relevant for patients with diabetes, obesity, and metabolic disorders, where residual cardiovascular risk often persists despite optimal LDL-C control.[4]

Accumulating evidence has positioned non-HDL-C as a superior predictor of atherosclerotic cardiovascular disease (ASCVD) risk.[5] Major international guidelines now recommend it as a secondary, or even coprimary therapeutic target.[6,7] Nevertheless, despite its robust clinical value and guideline endorsements, reducing non-HDL-C present diverse challenges.[8-10] This review analyses challenges in achieving optimal non-HDL-C goals, summarizes current guideline recommendations, and explores future opportunities for effective interventions.

THE COMPOSITION AND ROLE OF NON-HIGH-DENSITY LIPOPROTEIN CHOLESTEROL

Non-HDL-C reflects the amount of cholesterol carried by all atherogenic lipoproteins that contain ApoB. These particles, including LDL-C, VLDL, IDL, remnant lipoproteins, and Lp(a), play a critical role in the development and progression of atherosclerosis. Unlike LDL-C, non-HDL-C encompasses triglyceride rich lipoproteins, which are of heightened significance in metabolic syndrome, type 2 diabetes, and obesity.

The calculation is straightforward:

$$\text{Non-HDL-C} = \text{Total cholesterol} - \text{HDL-C}$$

This non-fasting measurement is not affected by postprandial triglyceride excursions as much as LDL-C, making it robust in real world clinical practice.[1-3]

SUPERIOR RISK PREDICTION

Significant residual risk persists among patients who achieve LDL-C targets but have elevated non-HDL-C.[11-13] Particles containing ApoB enter the arterial intima, initiating immune

TABLE 1: Recommended non-HDL-C thresholds for different risk populations.

Risk level	ACC/AHA 2018	ESC/EAS 2019	CS' India 2024	LAI 2023
Extreme risk	N/A	N/A	<70 mg/dL	<80 (category A)/≤60 (category B)/40–45 [mg/dL (category C)]
Very high risk	<85 mg/dL	<85 mg/dL	<85 mg/dL	<100 mg/dL
High risk	<100 mg/dL	<100 mg/dL	<100 mg/dL	<130 mg/dL
Moderate risk	<130 mg/dL	<130 mg/dL	<130 mg/dL	<130 mg/dL

reactions, accumulating cholesterol, causing inflammation, forming foam cells, and leading to unstable plaques; an essential sequence in the development of atherosclerosis.[14,15] Triglyceride rich remnants, as part of this spectrum carry more cholesterol per particle than LDL and have independent proinflammatory and procoagulant properties.[15,16]

Clinical trials and meta-analyses substantiate the clinical superiority of non-HDL-C.[17,18] A meta-analysis of more than 1,30,000 statin treated individuals revealed that non-HDL-C had a stronger association with cardiovascular events than LDL-C or even ApoB.[5] Additionally, studies such as JUPITER,[19] FIELD,[20] CHART-2,[21] and JELIS[22] have underscored the predictive value of non-HDL-C for myocardial infarction (MI) recurrence and all-cause mortality, regardless of whether LDL-C is at goal. Achieving larger and earlier reductions in non-HDL-C post MI is associated with substantial long-term reductions in major adverse cardiovascular events (MACE), all-cause mortality, and nonfatal MI. Patients who reached the guideline target (<2.2 mmol/L) within 2 months and maintained it at 1 year experienced the greatest benefit.[9]

Notably, an approximate 20% reduction in ASCVD risk accompanies each 1 mmol/L reduction in non-HDL-C.[23,24] This has spurred a paradigm shift, with non-HDL-C increasingly viewed as a more clinically relevant measure of atherogenic burden.

ADVANTAGES IN CLINICAL PRACTICE

Non-HDL-C offers several practical advantages over traditional lipid parameters:

- *Non-fasting measurement*: Unlike LDL-C calculations, non-HDL-C can be reliably measured in non-fasting samples, improving patient convenience and clinical workflow.[25-27]
- *Accuracy in hypertriglyceridemia*: When triglyceride levels exceed 400 mg/dL, LDL calculations become unreliable, but non-HDL-C remains relatively accurate.[28,29]
- *Indirect ApoB measurement*: Non-HDL-C correlates strongly with ApoB, reflecting total atherogenic particle number.[27]

GUIDELINES AND RISK STRATIFICATION

International consensus guidelines broadly support the use of non-HDL-C as a secondary or coprimary target. Most set the non-HDL-C goal at 30 mg/dL (0.8 mmol/L) higher than the corresponding LDL-C goal, although this is based more on convention than on solid evidence for all populations.[23,30-33]

Recommended thresholds[6,7,30,31] for different risk populations are shown in **Table 1**.

Recent research indicates that ratios such as non-HDL-C/HDL-C and non-HDL-C/ApoB may be useful for enhanced risk assessment; however, more studies are needed to confirm their effectiveness.[34,35]

TARGETS AFTER MYOCARDIAL INFARCTION

For patients, who have experienced a MI achieving and keeping non-HDL-C below 2.2 mmol/L (85 mg/dL) within 2 months and sustaining that level for 1 year is strongly associated with significant reductions in recurrent MI and overall mortality.[9] These findings suggest that a proactive, intensive approach to lowering non-HDL-C soon after MI rather than a gradual, stepwise up-titration results in greater long-term benefits and challenges current guidelines that recommend incremental adjustments.

MANAGEMENT STRATEGIES AND CHALLENGES

Lifestyle modification remains foundational in dyslipidemia management including non-HDL-C reduction. Diets rich in monounsaturated and polyunsaturated fats, fibers, and plant sterols specifically the Mediterranean diet are effective. Regular aerobic exercise (≥120 minutes/week) alongside dietary changes decrease non-HDL-C.

Pharmacologic therapy mainly centers on statins, with high intensity therapy with agents like rosuvastatin and atorvastatin providing the most significant improvements. Combination therapies such as adding ezetimibe, PCSK9 inhibitors, or bempedoic acid are indicated for high-risk patients or those intolerant of statins. Fibrates, omega-3 fatty acids, and bile acid sequestrants are among the other therapeutic options used primarily in selected patients to effectively lower high triglyceride levels and reduce cardiovascular risk.

The REDUCE-IT trial showed that icosapent ethyl significantly reduced MACE, with these reductions closely tied to decreases in non-HDL-C.[36] In contrast, the PROMINENT trial, which lowered triglycerides using pemafibrate, did not demonstrate improvements in cardiovascular outcomes.[37] This contrast underlines the pivotal role of non-HDL-C as a central predictor and therapeutic target for cardiovascular risk, emphasizing that targeting non-HDL-C yields greater benefits than focusing on triglycerides alone.

MANAGEMENT CHALLENGES

Management of non-HDL-C faces significant challenges from both providers and patients. Providers often have knowledge gaps, with low awareness of non-HDL-C as a secondary treatment target, correct calculation methods, and treatment goals, hindered by unfamiliarity with guidelines.[38] Patient-related challenges mainly involve poor medication adherence, with nonadherence rates exceeding 70% in dyslipidemia patients[39,40] and influenced by side effect concerns, treatment duration, and polypharmacy. Adherence is lower among women, non-white populations, those with low socioeconomic status, and high-intensity statin users, compounded by patients' negative beliefs about medication safety and necessity.[39]

CHALLENGES TO REDUCTION OF NON-HIGH-DENSITY LIPOPROTEIN CHOLESTEROL

Pharmacological and Pathophysiological Complexity

Multiple Lipoprotein Components

Non-HDL-C includes a wide range of lipoprotein particles with different metabolic behaviors and responses to treatments. Statins primarily affect LDL-C, with limited impact on triglyceride rich remnants and other components leading to only moderate reductions in overall non-HDL-C, especially in patients with atherogenic dyslipidemias.[41,42]

Variable Individual Response

Clinical trials often report mean statin effectiveness,[43] masking broad inter-individual variability.[10] Genetics influence drug metabolism and cholesterol biosynthesis, resulting in up to 10% of patients showing minimal LDL-C/non-HDL-C lowering even with intensive statin regimens.[44]

Genome wide association studies have identified single nucleotide polymorphisms (SNPs) associated with statin responsiveness, but practical pharmacogenomic integration into clinical care is still in its infancy.[45]

Incomplete Success with Combination Therapy

Numerous combination regimens (e.g., adding fibrates or niacin) have produced disappointing cardiovascular outcomes despite improving lipid profiles.[42] For example, AIM-HIGH[46] and HPS2-THRIVE (niacin)[47] and FIELD[20]/ACCORD[48] (fibrates) failed to deliver significant reduction in MACE. Only therapies that effect true reduction in atherogenic particle cholesterol, as captured by non-HDL-C, translate to improved outcomes.

Remnant Cholesterol Challenge

PCSK9 inhibitors and other novel agents have yet to demonstrate equally potent effects on remnant cholesterol fractions as on LDL, limiting their absolute benefit for non-HDL-C reduction in some groups.

Diagnostic and Monitoring Issues

Measurement Variability

The accuracy of non-HDL-C measurement depends on precise and reliable assessments of total cholesterol and HDL-C levels, as non-HDL-C is calculated by subtracting HDL-C from total cholesterol. Most direct HDL-C assays do not meet the National Cholesterol Education Program (NCEP) performance goals, leading to significant aggregate error (up to 36.3%). This is exacerbated in patients with hypertriglyceridemia or mixed dyslipidemias, where standard methods are more error prone.

Arbitrary Target Setting

The "30 mg/dL above LDL-C" rule presumes a universal triglyceride-to-cholesterol ratio (5:1) in VLDL, which does not apply across diverse populations or metabolic states. This can cause underestimation or overtreatment in certain individuals, underscoring an urgent need for validated, individualized non-HDL-C targets.

Fasting versus Non-fasting State

Although non-HDL-C provides a convenient non-fasting measurement, lipid levels can still fluctuate after meals, with Asian populations showing particularly notable postprandial decreases in LDL-C and non-HDL-C, further influenced by ethnic differences in lipid metabolism.[44]

Patient-related Barriers

Poor Adherence to Therapy

Medication nonadherence is common among dyslipidemia patients driven by side effect fears, regimen complexity (especially with combination therapies), cultural beliefs, and lack of perceived benefit from preventive medications.[42] Nonadherence is more pronounced in women, non-white populations, low socioeconomic groups, and patients on high-intensity therapies.

Healthy Adherer Effect

"Healthy adherers" are individuals who tend to follow medication regimens properly as well as engage in overall healthier lifestyle behaviors, which can create confounding effects when comparing medication outcomes between real world settings and controlled clinical trials.[10]

Regimen Complexity and Cost

Combination therapy, required in many high-risk cases, increases pill burden and out of pocket expense, creating a substantial barrier to sustained compliance.

■ Implementation and Systemic Barriers

Provider Knowledge Gaps

Many providers have limited familiarity with non-HDL-C as a target, its calculation, and target thresholds partly due to historical focus on LDL-C and incomplete guideline integration.

Laboratory Limitations

Lipid panels may not report non-HDL-C explicitly, or may omit guideline-based targets; limiting clinical follow-up and therapeutic intensification.

Healthcare System Constraints

Resource limitations can restrict access to advanced therapies (like PCSK9 inhibitors), frequent monitoring, and specialist referral, especially in low resource and primary care settings.

■ Special Population Challenges

Diabetes and Metabolic Syndrome

Diabetic patients display "atherogenic dyslipidemia," with raised triglycerides, low HDL-C, and small dense LDL particles. Simply normalizing LDL-C is insufficient; non-HDL-C offers a more encompassing risk metric. Nonenzymatic glycation and oxidative stress further complicate risk.[49]

Chronic Kidney Disease

Chronic kidney disease (CKD) alters hepatic and renal handling of lipoproteins, raising levels of atherogenic remnants and making statins less effective. Systemic inflammation, increased oxidative stress, and disordered mineral metabolism exacerbate vascular disease, necessitating nuanced lipid management.[50]

Pediatric Populations

Children with familial hypercholesterolemia or obesity-related metabolic syndrome frequently have high non-HDL-C with normal LDL-C.[51,52] However, concerns regarding the long-term safety of aggressive pharmacotherapy, limited approved agents, and a need for sustainable lifestyle changes make management complex.

Ethnic and Genetic Variability

Ethnic differences in lipid metabolism and drug response mandate tailored approaches. Asian, African, and European populations display significant differences in both baseline non-HDL-C and responses to intervention.

■ Broader Geographic and Demographic Disparities

Large-scale studies demonstrate notable variations in non-HDL-C levels and associated cardiovascular outcomes between countries and regions, with nations experiencing increasing non-HDL-C levels facing heightened ASCVD burdens.

FUTURE DIRECTIONS AND INNOVATIONS

■ Refined Measurement and Targeting

Advanced lipoprotein profiling using nuclear magnetic resonance spectroscopy or mass spectrometry techniques may enable more precise characterization of individual lipid profiles, allowing for targeted interventions based on specific lipoprotein subclass patterns.

Personalized medicine approaches, which consider individual genetic profiles, metabolic characteristics, and risk factors promise better prediction of statin responsiveness and optimal therapeutic combinations. Pharmacogenetic testing to predict statin responsiveness and guide therapy selection represents an important area for development.

■ Emerging Therapeutics

Ribonucleic acid (RNA)-based therapies[53] and metabolic modulators, such as small interfering RNA and antisense oligonucleotides, are being developed to target specific components of lipid metabolism.

Volanesorsen is an antisense oligonucleotide that binds specifically to the mRNA of apolipoprotein CIII (apoC III), causing its degradation and thereby preventing the production of apoC III protein, which normally hinders triglyceride metabolism and the liver's clearance of chylomicrons, leading to enhanced breakdown and removal of triglycerides.[54,55]

Evinacumab is a fully human monoclonal antibody that is an inhibitor of angiopoietin-like 3 (ANGPTL3), which is an inhibitor of lipoprotein and endothelial lipase.[55] Pemafibrate is a new selective PPARα modulator that activates PPARα with greater potency and selectivity compared to fenofibrate.[56] These highly specialized therapies are expensive, require careful patient selection, and may have limited applicability to the broader population requiring non-HDL-C reduction.

Anti-inflammatory agents aimed at pathways intersecting with atherogenesis (e.g., IL-1β inhibitors)[57] may offer adjunctive risk reduction independent of traditional lipid lowering modalities.

Digital Health and System Solutions

Artificial intelligence (AI) and machine learning can facilitate risk stratification, predict adherence challenges, and support remote monitoring via telemedicine and mobile health applications. Integrating automated reminders and standardized protocols into EHRs can overcome many present clinical workflow hurdles.

Health Policy and Systemic Reforms

Efforts are needed to:

- Mandate inclusion of non-HDL-C values and guideline-based targets in all laboratory lipid reports.
- Promote provider education, ongoing clinical audit, and use of decision support tools to flag high-risk patients.
- Advocate for health system investment in effective, accessible therapies and coordinated care models that prioritize secondary prevention in cardiovascular medicine.

CONCLUSION

Non-HDL-C offers superior predictive value by encompassing all atherogenic lipoproteins, particularly valuable in patients with complex lipid profiles, diabetes, and metabolic syndrome. Reducing non-HDL-C presents complex challenges beyond traditional lipid management due to the involvement of multiple lipoprotein species, limited impact of current therapies on non-LDL components, significant variability in individual drug responses, and ongoing issues with patient adherence. Despite biochemical improvements seen with some combination therapies targeting triglyceride rich lipoproteins, consistent cardiovascular benefits remain elusive. Additional obstacles include difficulties in measurement, arbitrary target definitions, and insufficient guideline integration, which complicate effective clinical implementation. Addressing these issues requires a multifaceted strategy involving personalized medicine, novel therapeutics specifically targeting remnant cholesterol and other non-LDL fractions, healthcare system improvements, and consideration of global lipid pattern disparities.

REFERENCES

1. Brunner FJ, Waldeyer C, Ojeda F, et al. Application of non-HDL cholesterol for population-based cardiovascular risk stratification: results from the Multinational Cardiovascular Risk Consortium. Lancet. 2019;394(10215):2173-83.
2. Verbeek R, Hovingh GK, Boekholdt SM. Non-high-density lipoprotein cholesterol: current status as cardiovascular marker. Curr Opin Lipidol. 2015;26(6):502-10.
3. Stürzebecher PE, Katzmann JL, Laufs U. What is 'remnant cholesterol'? Eur Heart J. 2023;44(16):1446-8.
4. Yun YM. Apolipoprotein B, Non-HDL Cholesterol, and LDL Cholesterol as Markers for Atherosclerotic Cardiovascular Disease Risk Assessment. Ann Lab Med. 2023;43(3):221-2.
5. Johannesen CDL, Mortensen MB, Langsted A, et al. Apolipoprotein B and Non-HDL Cholesterol Better Reflect Residual Risk than LDL Cholesterol in Statin-treated Patients. J Am Coll Cardiol. 2021;77(11):1439-50.
6. Puri R, Bansal M, Mehta V, et al. Lipid Association of India 2023 update on cardiovascular risk assessment and lipid management in Indian patients: Consensus statement IV. J Clin Lipidol. 2024; 18(3):e351-73.
7. Sawhney JPS, Ramakrishnan S, Madan K, et al. CSI clinical practice guidelines for dyslipidemia management: Executive summary. Indian Heart J. 2024;76:S6-19.
8. Katsi V, Argyriou N, Fragoulis C, et al. The Role of Non-HDL Cholesterol and Apolipoprotein B in Cardiovascular Disease: A Comprehensive Review. J Cardiovasc Dev Dis. 2025;12(7):256.
9. Schubert J, Leosdottir M, Lindahl B, et al. Intensive early and sustained lowering of non-high-density lipoprotein cholesterol after myocardial infarction and prognosis: the SWEDEHEART registry. Eur Heart J. 2024;45(39):4204-15.
10. De Geest B, Van Linthout S. Non-HDL-cholesterol reduction: the challenges of applying clinical trial results in the real world. Eur Heart J. 2024;45(39):4216-8.
11. Aguiar C, Alegria E, Bonadonna RC, et al. A review of the evidence on reducing macrovascular risk in patients with atherogenic dyslipidaemia: A report from an expert consensus meeting on the role of fenofibrate–statin combination therapy. Atheroscler Suppl. 2015;19:1-12.
12. Boekholdt SM, Arsenault BJ, Mora S, et al. Association of LDL Cholesterol, Non–HDL Cholesterol, and Apolipoprotein B Levels with Risk of Cardiovascular Events among Patients Treated with Statins: A Meta-analysis. JAMA. 2012;307(12):1302-9.
13. Suzuki K, Oikawa T, Nochioka K, et al. Elevated Serum Non-HDL (High-density Lipoprotein) Cholesterol and Triglyceride Levels as Residual Risks for Myocardial Infarction Recurrence Under Statin Treatment. Arterioscler Thromb Vasc Biol. 2019;39(5):934-44.
14. Jebari-Benslaiman S, Galicia-García U, Larrea-Sebal A, et al. Pathophysiology of Atherosclerosis. Int J Mol Sci. 2022;23(6): 3346.
15. Tabas I, García-Cardeña G, Owens GK. Recent insights into the cellular biology of atherosclerosis. J Cell Biol. 2015;209(1):13-22.
16. Borén J, Packard CJ. Keeping remnants in perspective. Eur Heart J. 2021;42(42):4333-5.
17. Nordestgaard BG. Triglyceride-rich Lipoproteins and Atherosclerotic Cardiovascular Disease: New Insights from Epidemiology, Genetics, and Biology. Circ Res. 2016;118(4):547-63.
18. Burnett JR, Hooper AJ, Hegele RA. Remnant Cholesterol and Atherosclerotic Cardiovascular Disease Risk. J Am Coll Cardiol. 2020;76(23):2736-9.
19. Lawler PR, Akinkuolie AO, Harada P, et al. Residual Risk of Atherosclerotic Cardiovascular Events in Relation to Reductions in Very-low-density Lipoproteins. J Am Heart Assoc. 2017;6(12): e007402.
20. A Keech, R J Simes, P Barter, et al. Effects of long-term fenofibrate therapy on cardiovascular events in 9795 people with type 2 diabetes mellitus (the FIELD study): randomised controlled trial. Lancet. 2005;366(9500):1849-61.
21. Oikawa T, Sakata Y, Nochioka K, et al. Prognostic Impact of Statin Intensity in Heart Failure Patients with Ischemic Heart Disease: A Report from the CHART-2 (Chronic Heart Failure Registry

and Analysis in the Tohoku District 2) Study. J Am Heart Assoc. 2018;7(6):e007524.

22. Oikawa S, Yokoyama M, Origasa H, et al. Suppressive effect of EPA on the incidence of coronary events in hypercholesterolemia with impaired glucose metabolism: Sub-analysis of the Japan EPA Lipid Intervention Study (JELIS). Atherosclerosis. 2009;206(2):535-9.
23. Mach F, Baigent C, Catapano AL, et al. 2019 ESC/EAS Guidelines for the management of dyslipidaemias: lipid modification to reduce cardiovascular risk: The Task Force for the management of dyslipidaemias of the European Society of Cardiology (ESC) and European Atherosclerosis Society (EAS). Eur Heart J. 2020;41(1):111-88.
24. Stein EA, Raal FJ. Lipid-lowering Drug Therapy for CVD Prevention: Looking into the Future. Curr Cardiol Rep. 2015;17(11):104.
25. Darras P, Mattman A, Francis GA. Nonfasting lipid testing: the new standard for cardiovascular risk assessment. CMAJ Can Med Assoc J. 2018;190(45):E1317-8.
26. Guo LL, Chen YQ, Lin QZ, et al. Non-HDL-C is More Stable Than LDL-C in Assessing the Percent Attainment of Non-fasting Lipid for Coronary Heart Disease Patients. Front Cardiovasc Med. 2021;8:649181.
27. Baker RA, Forbes RA. Non-HDL Cholesterol: A New Endpoint in Cardiometabolic Health Monitoring. Prim Care Companion J Clin Psychiatry. 2010;12(5):PCC.09l00940.
28. Virani SS. Non-HDL Cholesterol as a Metric of Good Quality of Care. Tex Heart Inst J. 2011;38(2):160-2.
29. Packard CJ, Saito Y. Non-HDL cholesterol as a measure of atherosclerotic risk. J Atheroscler Thromb. 2004;11(1):6-14.
30. Mach F, Koskinas KC, Roeters van Lennep JE, et al. 2025 Focused Update of the 2019 ESC/EAS Guidelines for the management of dyslipidaemias. Atherosclerosis. 2025:120479.
31. Grundy SM, Stone NJ, Bailey AL, et al. 2018 AHA/ACC/AACVPR/AAPA/ABC/ACPM/ADA/AGS/APhA/ASPC/NLA/PCNA Guideline on the Management of Blood Cholesterol: Executive Summary: A Report of the American College of Cardiology/American Heart Association Task Force on Clinical Practice Guidelines. Circulation. 2019;139(25):e1082-143.
32. Nordestgaard BG, Langlois MR, Langsted A, et al. Quantifying atherogenic lipoproteins for lipid-lowering strategies: Consensus-based recommendations from EAS and EFLM. Atherosclerosis. 2020;294:46-61.
33. Levinson SS. Non-high-density Lipoprotein Cholesterol and Guidelines for Cholesterol Lowering in Recent History. Lab Med. 2020;51(1):14-23.
34. Millán J, Pintó X, Muñoz A, et al. Lipoprotein ratios: Physiological significance and clinical usefulness in cardiovascular prevention. Vasc Health Risk Manag. 2009;5:757-65.
35. Huang A, Qi X, Wei L, et al. Non-HDL-c/TC: A Novel Lipid-related Marker in the Assessment of Severity of Coronary Artery Lesions and Cardiovascular Outcomes. Cardiol Res Pract. 2019;2019:5931975.
36. Sayah N, Bhatt DL, Miller M, et al. Icosapent ethyl following acute coronary syndrome: the REDUCE-IT trial. Eur Heart J. 2024;45(13):1173-6.
37. Pradhan AD, Glynn RJ, Fruchart JC, et al. Triglyceride Lowering with Pemafibrate to Reduce Cardiovascular Risk. N Engl J Med. 2022;387(21):1923-34.
38. Virani SS, Steinberg L, Murray T, et al. Barriers to non-HDL cholesterol goal attainment by providers. Am J Med. 2011;124(9):876-880.e2.
39. Alefishat E, Jarab AS, Al-Qerem W, et al. Factors Associated with Medication Non-adherence in Patients with Dyslipidemia. Healthcare. 2021;9(7):813.
40. Naqvi TZ. Statin Adherence and Effects on Outcome in Premature Coronary Artery Disease. JACC Adv. 2023;2(10):100700.
41. Nayor M, Murthy VL, Shah RV. For Non-HDL Cholesterol, "Lower is Better" but "Lower for Longer" May Be Best. Circ Res. 2020;126(7):836-8.
42. Hansen MK, Mortensen MB, Olesen KKW, et al. Non-HDL cholesterol and residual risk of cardiovascular events in patients with ischemic heart disease and well-controlled LDL cholesterol: a cohort study. Lancet Reg Health Eur. 2023;36:100774.
43. Langlois MR, Sniderman AD. Non-HDL Cholesterol or apoB: Which to Prefer as a Target for the Prevention of Atherosclerotic Cardiovascular Disease? Curr Cardiol Rep. 2020;22(8):67.
44. Raja V, Aguiar C, Alsayed N, et al. Non-HDL-cholesterol in dyslipidemia: Review of the state-of-the-art literature and outlook. Atherosclerosis. 2023;383:117312.
45. Dabiri H, Mortezaei Z. Genome-wide association study of therapeutic response to statin drugs in cardiovascular disease. Sci Rep. 2024;14(1):18005.
46. AIM-HIGH Investigators; Boden WE, Probstfield JL, et al. Niacin in Patients with Low HDL Cholesterol Levels Receiving Intensive Statin Therapy. N Engl J Med. 2011;365(24):2255-67.
47. HPS2-THRIVE Collaborative Group; Landray MJ, Haynes R, et al. Effects of Extended-release Niacin with Laropiprant in High-risk Patients. N Engl J Med. 2014;371(3):203-12.
48. ACCORD Study Group; Ginsberg HN, Elam MB, et al. Effects of Combination Lipid Therapy in Type 2 Diabetes Mellitus. N Engl J Med. 2010;362(17):1563-74.
49. Gillard BK, Rosales C, Xu B, et al. Rethinking reverse cholesterol transport and dysfunctional high-density lipoproteins. J Clin Lipidol. 2018;12(4):849-56.
50. Stenvinkel P, Heimbürger O, Paultre F, et al. Strong association between malnutrition, inflammation, and atherosclerosis in chronic renal failure. Kidney Int. 1999;55(5):1899-911.
51. Khoury M, Bigras JL, Cummings EA, et al. The Detection, Evaluation, and Management of Dyslipidemia in Children and Adolescents: A Canadian Cardiovascular Society/Canadian Pediatric Cardiology Association Clinical Practice Update. Can J Cardiol. 2022;38(8):1168-79.
52. Strong JP, Malcom GT, McMahan CA, et al. Prevalence and Extent of Atherosclerosis in Adolescents and Young Adults Implications for Prevention from the Pathobiological Determinants of Atherosclerosis in Youth Study. JAMA. 1999;281(8):727-35.
53. Huang HYR, Badar S, Said M, et al. The advent of RNA-based therapeutics for metabolic syndrome and associated conditions: a comprehensive review of the literature. Mol Biol Rep. 2024;51(1):493.
54. Gouni-Berthold I, Schwarz J, Berthold HK. Updates in Drug Treatment of Severe Hypertriglyceridemia. Curr Atheroscler Rep. 2023;25(10):701-9.
55. Moura JMDSPD, Mendes PFAPP, Reigota CP, et al. New drugs coming up in the field of lipid control. e-J Cardiol Pract. 2020;19:8-16.
56. Yamashita S, Masuda D, Matsuzawa Y. Pemafibrate, a New Selective PPARα Modulator: Drug Concept and its Clinical Applications for Dyslipidemia and Metabolic Diseases. Curr Atheroscler Rep. 2020;22(1):5.
57. Peiró C, Lorenzo Ó, Carraro R, et al. IL-1β Inhibition in Cardiovascular Complications Associated to Diabetes Mellitus. Front Pharmacol. 2017;8:363.

CHAPTER 16

Particle Number and Characteristics of Lipoprotein(a), Low-density Lipoprotein, and ApoB: Perspectives on Contributions to Atherosclerotic Cardiovascular Disease

JPS Sawhney, Rohan Patel

ABSTRACT

There are multiple modifiable risk factors leading to atherosclerotic cardiovascular disease. One of them is dyslipidemia. Elevated LDL-cholesterol has an established role in ASCVD. Reduction of LDL-C by pharmacological means has shown significant reduction in ASCVD events. However, there is still residual ASCVD risk which can be contributed to elevated lipoprotein (a) level. Due to its unique composition, Lp(a) has high atherogenicity than LDL particles on a per particle basis. This has been proven in some studies, which has shown that the risk of ASCVD events is around six times higher with Lp(a)–ApoB than LDL–ApoB for similar increment in their levels in terms of molar concentration. However, in any individual, usually total particles of LDL are much more than Lp(a) leading to higher overall ASCVD risk contribution by LDL particles. Therapeutic options to reduce Lp(a) levels are limited. PCSK 9 inhibitors can reduce Lp(a) levels by 20–25% and exploratory analysis of their trials has shown greater cardiovascular benefit with reduction of Lp(a) level beyond target LDL-C level. Novel Lp(a) reduction therapies such as Pelacarsen, Olpasiran, and Lepodisiran have shown to reduce Lp(a) levels by >90%. However, their cardiovascular outcome trials are still undergoing which will provide further insight into cardiovascular benefits of reducing Lp(a) levels.

Keywords: Lipoprotein(a), atherogenicity, per particle risk.

INTRODUCTION

Lipoprotein(a) [Lp(a)] is a genetically determined, highly atherogenic lipoprotein contributing to residual cardiovascular risk despite optimal LDL-C control. Its unique structure, rich in oxidized phospholipids, enhances inflammation and plaque formation. Emerging therapies targeting Lp(a) may significantly reduce atherosclerotic cardiovascular disease beyond current lipid-lowering strategies.

DYSLIPIDEMIA AND ATHEROSCLEROTIC CARDIOVASCULAR DISEASE RISK

Atherosclerotic cardiovascular disease is the leading cause of morbidity and mortality worldwide. There are multiple risk factors which are responsible for ASCVD that can be modified. One of the major risk factors is dyslipidemia with elevated LDL-cholesterol (LDL-C) and apolipoprotein B (ApoB) level. LDL is the most abundant ApoB containing molecules in plasma which deliver cholesterol to the various tissue including intima of the arteries susceptible to atherosclerosis. Various epidemiological, genetic, and clinical studies have confirmed the role of elevated LDL-C level in initiation and progression of atherosclerosis.[1] Multiple randomized studies have shown that lowering LDL-C significantly reduces risk of atherosclerotic cardiovascular disease and major adverse cardiovascular events. Cholesterol Treatment Trialists metanalysis of multiple randomized controlled trials of statin therapy showed that every 1 mmol/L (39 mg/dL) reduction in LDL-C was associated with 21% reduction in major adverse cardiovascular events over median follow up of 4.9 years.[2]

RESIDUAL ATHEROSCLEROTIC CARDIOVASCULAR DISEASE RISK

Despite lifestyle and multiple pharmacological interventions to reduce risk of developing ASCVD and cardiovascular events, a huge "residual risk" remains despite adequate control of LDL-C level. This residual risk could be related to elevated ApoB containing triglyceride rich lipoprotein (TRLs) which can contribute to atherogenesis, elevated Lp(a) level, persistent systemic inflammation as detected by elevated high sensitivity CRP levels or residual prothrombotic state.[3]

APOLIPOPROTEIN B AND ATHEROSCLEROTIC CARDIOVASCULAR DISEASE RISK

Apolipoprotein B is a hydrophobic protein which is present in LDL, Lp(a), and TRL particles including chylomicrons, very low-density lipoproteins (VLDL), intermediate density lipoproteins (IDL). From atherogenesis point, ApoB level is likely superior to LDL-C level in predicting ASCVD risk as it reflects total atherogenic particles in circulation rather than just cholesterol content of lipoproteins. This is particularly true in conditions with hypertriglyceridemia (metabolic syndrome, obesity, and diabetes mellitus) in which there is increased small dense LDL particles with relatively high triglyceride component and low cholesterol component. In these conditions, measuring cholesterol content of LDL only will likely underestimate ASCVD risk.[4] This issue has been clinically validated in multiple studies such as INTERHEART study[5] and Framingham Heart Study[6] which showed that, when discordant ASCVD risk is closely related to atherogenic lipoprotein particles (ApoB particles) rather than cholesterol content of specific lipoproteins.

However, despite growing evidence suggesting possible superiority of ApoB level in predicting ASCVD risk, its measurement is not included in routine lipid profile and ApoB specific assays are costly. Moreover, large, randomized control trials using ApoB as therapeutic targets are lacking.[7] Some studies have suggested that non-HDL cholesterol, which can be derived from routine lipid profile, can be used instead of ApoB level to determine additional ASCVD risk particularly when ApoB assays are not readily available.[8] The European and Canadian guidelines have provided treatment target values for both non-HDL-C and ApoB which may lead to better prediction and management of residual ASCVD risk.[4]

LIPOPROTEIN (A) AND ATHEROSCLEROTIC CARDIOVASCULAR DISEASE RISK

Elevated Lp(a) levels are an important factor contributing to residual ASCVD risk even after correcting for LDL-C and ApoB levels. Lp(a) is similar to LDL but contains a unique protein known as apolipoprotein(a). Synthesis of apolipoprotein(a) is regulated by *LPA* gene. Thus, serum concentration of Lp(a) level is influenced by activity of *LPA* gene which encodes apo(A). There is significant difference between metabolism of Lp(a) and other lipoprotein molecules including LDL. The LDL receptor mediated reuptake plays only a minor role in regulating Lp(a) levels. Hence, Lp(a) levels are regulated at genetic level by the production of apolipoprotein(a) in the liver.[9]

Nonetheless, significant differences can be seen in Lp(a) levels within the population. Genetic determination of Lp(a) level alone cannot explain these variations. Numerous nongenetic factors can affect serum Lp(a) levels. Dietary modification such as replacement of dietary saturated fat with carbohydrates or unsaturated fat can increase Lp(a) levels modestly. During pregnancy, Lp(a) levels tend to increase particularly during second and third trimesters; however, exogenous administration of hormones such as estrogen (i.e., hormone replacement therapy) can modestly reduce Lp(a) levels. Endocrine disorders such as hypothyroidism elevates Lp(a) levels and hyperthyroidism lowers Lp(a) levels modestly. In CKD, there is mild elevation in Lp(a) levels which depends upon the stages of CKD.[10]

Numerous epidemiological studies have shown a significant causal association between Lp(a) levels and ASCVD as well as calcific aortic stenosis.[11] In India, around 25% population has elevated Lp(a) level and a study has shown that higher Lp(a) levels were found more commonly among young ACS patients and were more commonly associated with multivessel disease.[12] According to CSI clinical practice guidelines for management of dyslipidemia, elevated Lp(a) level >50 mg/dL is considered as a risk enhancing factor and along with heterozygous familial hypercholesterolemia and ASCVD is considered as extremely high-risk group where target LDL-C level should be <40 mg/dL.[13]

Similar to LDL, Lp(a) contains ApoB. Apolipoprotein B is considered as a common feature among different atherogenic lipoprotein particles. However, various studies have shown that atherogenicity of Lp(a) is not completely explained by ApoB alone. An analysis done by Trinder et al.[14] showed that the odds ratios for CAD were 1.78 for 50 mg/dL increase in LDL-C levels (95% CI 1.63–1.94; $p < 0.001$) and 1.33 for 50 mg/dL increase in Lp(a) mass (95% CI 1.30–1.36; $p < 0.001$) on univariate Mendelian randomization. For 120 nmol/L increase in Lp(a) was 1.51 (95% CI 1.45–1.57). In multivariate analysis with ApoB, the OR of CAD with 50 mg/dL increase in LDL-C was markedly attenuated [OR 1.00 (0.91–1.09 with 95% CI)], while the OR for a 50 mg/dL increase in Lp (a) mass remained unchanged. These findings suggest that ApoB is sufficient to explain the risk of CAD associated with LDL-C but not with Lp(a).

INDIVIDUAL CONTRIBUTION OF LDL-C, ApoB, AND LP(a) TO ASCVD RISK

Lp(a) is a causal factor for ASCVD. However, its atherogenicity relative to LDL-C on a per particle base is not known. To evaluate the atherogenicity of individual atherogenic particles, a unique analysis was performed in the UK Biobank by quantitating LDL-C and Lp(a) associated ASCVD risk.

Study used genome-wide association studies and identified two clusters of single nucleotide polymorphisms—

one comprising 107 variants linked to Lp(a) [Lp(a)-ApoB] concentration, the other with 143 variants linked to LDL (LDL-ApoB) concentration. LDL-ApoB and Lp(a)-ApoB levels were converted to molar concentration and the relationship of this genetically predicted Lp(a)-ApoB and LDL-ApoB clusters with CHD risk was assessed. The Mendelian randomization-derived OR for CHD for a 50 nmol/L higher Lp(a)-ApoB was 1.28 (95% CI 1.24–1.33) compared with only 1.04 (95% CI 1.03–1.05) for the same increment in LDL-ApoB. Likewise, use of polygenic scores to rank subjects according to difference in Lp(a)-apoB versus difference in LDL-ApoB revealed a greater HR for CHD per 50 nmol/L increase in the Lp(a) cluster (1.47; 95% CI 1.36–1.58) compared with the LDL cluster (1.04; 95% CI 1.02–1.05). This analysis showed that atherogenicity of Lp(a) particle is approximately six times (point estimate of 6.6; 95% CI 5.1–8.8) more than that of LDL particle on a per-particle basis. There were some limitations of this study such as inclusion of both primary and secondary prevention population, majority of population being Caucasian, inadequate lipid lowering and antiplatelet therapy. However, this study concluded that even if ApoB concentration is similar in an isolated LDL and Lp(a) particle, risk of atherogenesis is more with Lp(a)-ApoB as compared to LDL-ApoB particle.[15] This observation is similar to previous study which showed that total ApoB level is not able to explain whole ASCVD risk of Lp(a).[13] This approach helps in better estimation and control of ASCVD risk as compared to LDL-C alone as LDL-C only measures cholesterol in LDL particle in determining ASCVD risk and ignores other components which may be contributing to ASCVD.[15]

Marsten et al.[16] performed similar analysis from UK Biobank data. They included patients without ASCVD (primary prevention cohort) and calculated Lp(a) ApoB level and non-Lp(a) ApoB levels. During a median follow-up of 12 years, the HR for cardiovascular events per 100 nmol/L of Lp(a)-ApoB was 1.24, whereas for non-Lp(a) ApoB it was 1.05. These results are similar to previous analysis depiction that Lp(a) may have more atherogenicity than other lipoprotein particles.

MECHANISM OF HIGH ATHEROGENICITY OF LIPOPROTEIN (A) PARTICLE

There are multiple possible explanation of high atherogenicity associated with Lp(a) particle than LDL-C. One, Lp(a) particles are smaller and denser than LDL due to their low triglyceride component allowing them to easily accumulate and get modified in the intima of artery leading to initiation of atherogenesis. Second, Lp(a) contains proinflammatory oxidized phospholipids which increases local inflammation and promotes atherosclerosis. Third, some proteomes present in Lp(a) also act as a proinflammatory compounds and promote atherogenesis **(Fig. 1)**.[17]

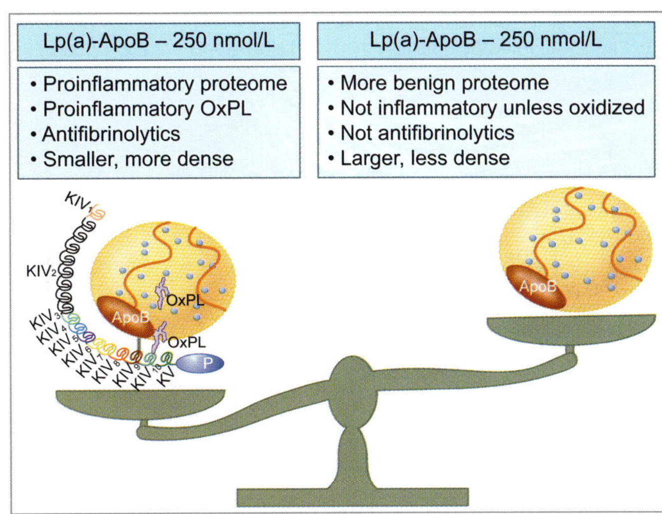

FIG. 1: Mechanism of high atherogenicity of Lp (a) and per particle ASCVD risk.

Source: Adapted from Tsimikas S, et al. (2024).[17]

LIMITATIONS OF PER PARTICLE ASCVD RISK APPROACH

In majority individuals, number of LDL particles are higher than Lp(a) particles. For example, Lp(a) levels are usually <75 nmol/L (<30 mg/dL) and considered as highly elevated when they are approximately 250 nmol/L (~100 mg/dL). In contrast, untreated LDL-C levels are usually 130 mg/dL or 2,360,000–3,320,000 nmol/L and ApoB levels are approximately 100 mg/dL or 1,949 nmol/L. Thus, even though individual Lp(a) particles may have more atherogenicity at the per-particle level, the relative excess of ApoB and cholesterol molecules on LDL particles contributes to a higher risk of ASCVD **(Fig. 2)**.[16]

CLINICAL IMPLICATION OF HIGHER ATHEROGENICITY OF LP(A) ON PER PARTICLE BASIS

One important clinical implication is that to determine more accurate and residual ASCVD risk, Lp(a) level must be considered, and all adults should undergo Lp(a) measurement at least once in a life. Another important implication is that lowering Lp(a) levels could reduce cardiovascular events rate beyond target LDL-C and ApoB levels. However, lipid lowering therapies which are approved do not have similar efficacy in reducing Lp(a) levels. Statins, Ezetimibe, and Bempedoic acid do not reduce Lp(a) levels. PCSK 9 inhibitors reduce Lp(a) levels by 20–25%. Exploratory analysis of FOURIER trial showed that higher Lp(a) levels were associated with higher rates of MACE irrespective of LDL levels. In this trial, Evolocumab significantly reduced Lp(a) level and those patients with higher baseline Lp(a) level derive greater reduction in cardiovascular events.[18]

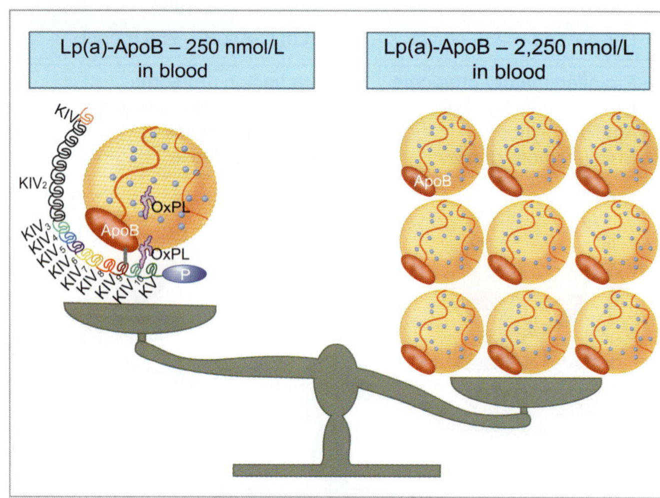

FIG. 2: Total particle ASCVD risk.
Source: Adapted from Tsimikas S, et al. (2024).[17]

Novel Lp(a) reduction therapies such as Pelacarsen (anti sense oligonucleotide), Olpasiran, and lepodisiran (Si RNA) have shown to reduce Lp(a) level by >90%. Randomized trials showing their cardiovascular benefits are ongoing. Results of these randomized trials will provide further insights in possible cardiovascular benefits seen with Lp(a) reduction. Lp(a) level could well become an important therapeutic target to reduce residual ASCVD risk beyond LDL and ApoB levels.[19]

CONCLUSION

All these analysis shows that Lp(a) has significant more atherogenicity than LDL on a per particle basis. However, as total number of LDL particles are more than Lp(a) particles, overall contribution of LDL is more to ASCVD risk. Targeting Lp(a) with specific drugs might help in reducing residual ASCVD risk.

REFERENCES

1. Du Z, Qin Y. Dyslipidemia and Cardiovascular Disease: Current Knowledge, Existing Challenges, and New Opportunities for Management Strategies. J Clin Med. 2023;12(1):363.
2. Tokgozoglu L, Libby P. The dawn of a new era of targeted lipid-lowering therapies. Eur Heart J. 2022;43:3198-208.
3. Noothi SK, Ahmed MR, Agrawal DK. Residual risks and evolving atherosclerotic plaques. Mol Cell Biochem. 2023;478(12):2629-43.
4. Cole J, Zubirán R, Wolska A, et al. Use of Apolipoprotein B in the Era of Precision Medicine: Time for a Paradigm Change? J Clin Med. 2023;12(17):5737.
5. Sniderman AD, Islam S, Yusuf S, et al. Discordance analysis of apolipoprotein B and non-high density lipoprotein cholesterol as markers of cardiovascular risk in the INTERHEART study. Atherosclerosis. 2012;225:444-9.
6. Pencina MJ, D'Agostino RB, Zdrojewski T, et al. Apolipoprotein B improves risk assessment of future coronary heart disease in the Framingham Heart Study beyond LDL-C and non-HDL-C. Eur J Prev Cardiol. 2015;22:1321-7.
7. Kohli-Lynch CN, Thanassoulis G, Moran AE, et al. The clinical utility of apoB versus LDL-C/non-HDL-C. Clin Chim Acta. 2020;508:103-8.
8. Welsh C, Celis-Morales CA, Brown R, et al. Comparison of Conventional Lipoprotein Tests and Apolipoproteins in the Prediction of Cardiovascular Disease. Circulation. 2019;140(7):542-52.
9. Boffa MB, Koschinsky ML. Lipoprotein(a) and cardiovascular disease. Biochem J. 2024;481(19):1277-96.
10. Enkhmaa B, Berglund L. Non-genetic influences on lipoprotein(a) concentrations. Atherosclerosis. 2022;349:53-62.
11. Maloberti A, Fabbri S, Colombo V, et al. Lipoprotein(a): Cardiovascular Disease, Aortic Stenosis and New Therapeutic Option. Int J Mol Sci. 2022;24(1):170.
12. Sawhney JP, Kumar A, Tyagi K, et al. Prevalence of Lp (a) in acute coronary syndrome and its association with severity of disease among patients admitted to a tertiary care hospital. Atherosclerosis. 2023;379:S52.
13. Sawhney JP, Ramakrishnan S, Madan K, et al. CSI clinical practice guidelines for dyslipidemia management: executive summary. Indian Heart J. 2024;76:S6-19.
14. Trinder M, Zekavat SM, Uddin MM, et al. Apolipoprotein B is an insufficient explanation for the risk of coronary disease associated with lipoprotein(a). Cardiovasc Res. 2021;117(5):1245-7.
15. Björnson E, Adiels M, Taskinen M-R, et al. Lipoprotein(A) is markedly more atherogenic than LDL: an apolipoprotein B-based genetic analysis. J Am Coll Cardiol. 2024;83:385-95.
16. Marston NA, Melloni GEM, Murphy SA, et al. Per-particle cardiovascular risk of lipoprotein(a) vs. non-Lp(a) apolipoprotein B containing lipoproteins. J Am Coll Cardiol. 2024;83(3):470-2.
17. Tsimikas S, Bittner V. Particle Number and Characteristics of Lipoprotein(a), LDL, and apoB: Perspectives on Contributions to ASCVD. J Am Coll Cardiol. 2024;83(3):396-400.
18. O'Donoghue ML, Fazio S, Giugliano RP, et al. Lipoprotein (a), PCSK9 inhibition, and cardiovascular risk: insights from the FOURIER trial. Circulation. 2019;139(12):1483-92.
19. Rader DJ. Targeting Lipoprotein (a)—the Next Frontier in Cardiovascular Disease. New England Journal of Medicine. 2025;392(17):1740-2.

CHAPTER

17

Childhood LDL Cholesterol, Non-HDL Cholesterol and Adult Atherosclerotic Cardiovascular Events

Rajeev Gupta, Sonali Sharma

ABSTRACT

Coronary artery disease (CAD) has assumed epidemic proportions in India, with the country leading in premature deaths from this condition. The process of coronary atherosclerosis starts in early childhood and progresses episodically over the life course. Low-density lipoprotein cholesterol (LDL-C) and other pro-atherogenic lipoproteins are clubbed as non-high-density lipoprotein cholesterol (non-HDL-C) as markers of apolipoprotein B (apoB). Epidemiological studies have reported that raised LDL-C and non-HDL-C levels in childhood are markers of adult atherosclerotic cardiovascular disease (CVD). Multiple observational studies have reported that they track into adulthood and persistently raised levels are associated with a hazard ratio of 5.17 per unit increase in z-score for non-fatal and fatal cardiovascular events in single- and multi-country cohorts. No similar studies exist in India. LDL-C years (LDL-C × age) and non-HDL-C years could be proxy indicators for age-related tracking of these cholesterol subtypes. In the India Heart Watch study (n = 5,816 participants, 11 urban locations), we reported a significant correlation of LDL-C years and non-HDL-C years with QRISK2 risk algorithm, suggesting the importance of these lipid parameters in childhood. The importance of childhood LDL-C and non-HDL-C needs to be confirmed using large prospective randomized lifestyle or drug trials beginning in childhood and evaluation of CVD outcomes decades later, for the generation of high-quality evidence and guideline development.

Keywords: Atherosclerosis, cardiovascular disease, childhood lipids, cholesterol lipoproteins, coronary artery disease, LDL cholesterol, non-HDL cholesterol, preventive cardiology.

INTRODUCTION

Low-density lipoprotein cholesterol (LDL-C) and non-high-density lipoprotein cholesterol (non-HDL-C) are important lipid markers associated with increased cardiovascular disease (CVD) risk.[1] LDL-C is the most important atherosclerotic coronary artery disease (CAD) risk factor and there is humongous experimental, pathophysiological, epidemiological, clinical and randomized trial evidence to support the importance of LDL-C as a risk factor for all types of CAD and at all ages.[2,3] Elevated LDL-C levels promote cholesterol deposition in arterial walls, triggering inflammation and plaque instability.[2] Non-HDL-C has also emerged as an important CAD risk factor.[4] Non-HDL-C includes LDL-C and other atherogenic lipoproteins such as very-low-density lipoprotein (VLDL) and intermediate-density lipoproteins (IDL), providing a broader measure of cardiovascular risk.[5,6] It captures all cholesterol carried by apolipoprotein B-containing lipoproteins, which are directly implicated in atherogenesis. Non-HDL-C is particularly valuable when triglycerides are elevated, as it accounts for remnant lipoproteins that LDL-C alone may miss,[6] especially in patients with metabolic syndrome or diabetes. Both markers are used to assess and manage CVD risk.[6]

Childhood LDL cholesterol levels play a pivotal role in the development of adult CVD, as atherosclerosis often begins early in life.[7] Elevated LDL-C in youth promotes endothelial dysfunction and plaque formation, which track into adulthood, increasing the risk of atherosclerotic CVD events.[2] Prospective cohort studies demonstrate that childhood LDL-C is associated with adult atherosclerotic CVD, with a hazard ratio (HR) of 1.27 per unit increase in z-score for fatal events.[7] Non-HDL-C shows even stronger predictive value, highlighting its utility for risk assessment **(Table 1)**.[7,8]

Persistent dyslipidemia from childhood to adulthood markedly elevates CVD risk (HR 5.17), independent of adult levels **(Table 1)**. However, resolution of elevated childhood non-HDL-C by adulthood normalizes risk (HR 1.13),

TABLE 1: Predictive value of childhood LDL-C and non-HDL-C for prediction of adult atherosclerotic CVD events in i3C consortium (C-index).[7]

	LDL-cholesterol	Non-HDL-cholesterol
Fatal CVD events	0.74 (0.70–0.78)	0.75 (0.70–0.79)
Fatal/Non-fatal CVD events	0.72 (0.69–0.75)	0.72 (0.69–0.75)

(CVD: cardiovascular disease; LDL-C: low-density lipoprotein cholesterol; non-HDL-C: non-high density lipoprotein cholesterol)

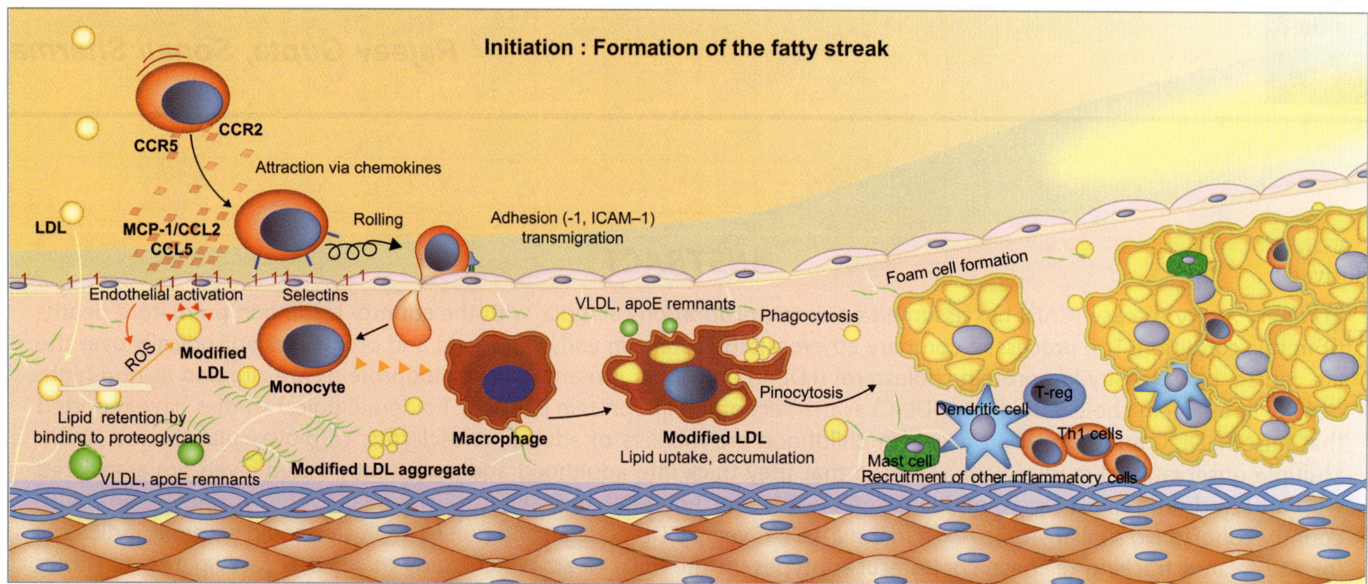

FIG. 1: Importance of low-density lipoproteins in atherosclerosis initiation and progression.

Source: Linton MRF, Yancey PG, Davies SS, et al. The Role of Lipids and Lipoproteins in Atherosclerosis. In: Feingold KR, Ahmed SF, Anawalt B, et al. (Eds). Endotext. South Dartmouth (MA): MDText.com, Inc.; 2000.

underscoring the benefits of early interventions such as lifestyle modifications or statins.[7] In this review, we focus on the impact of childhood LDL-C and non-HDL-C on cardiovascular events over the life course and provide data relevant to India.

BIOCHEMISTRY AND PATHOPHYSIOLOGY OF LOW-DENSITY LIPOPROTEIN CHOLESTEROL

Molecular structure and biochemistry: LDLs are derived from very low-density lipoproteins (VLDL) and intermediate-density lipoproteins (IDL), and they are further enriched in cholesterol.[2] LDL is responsible for transporting the majority of cholesterol present in the bloodstream. The principal apolipoprotein associated with LDL is B-100, with each LDL particle containing a single apoB-100 molecule. Small, dense LDL particles exhibit a greater propensity for atherogenesis compared to their larger counterparts. They demonstrate diminished affinity for the LDL receptor, resulting in prolonged circulation time, readily infiltrate arterial walls and bind strongly to intra-arterial proteoglycans, leading to entrapment. Additionally, small, dense LDL particles are more susceptible to oxidation, enhancing macrophage uptake **(Fig. 1)**.[2,9]

Low-density lipoproteins kinetics: More than 70% of circulating LDL is cleared via hepatocyte LDL receptor-mediated endocytosis, with the remainder taken up by extrahepatic tissues. An increase in hepatic LDL receptors increases LDL clearance, decreasing plasma LDL-C levels. Conversely, decreased hepatic LDL receptors slow LDL clearance, raising plasma LDL levels. LDL receptor levels in the liver are regulated by hepatocyte cholesterol content. As cellular cholesterol levels decrease, inactive sterol regulatory element binding proteins (SREBPs) are transported from the endoplasmic reticulum to the Golgi where proteases cleave the SREBPs into active transcription factors. Active SREBPs enter the nucleus to stimulate LDL receptor transcription and cholesterol synthesis enzymes, including HMG-CoA reductase. When cellular cholesterol is high, SREBPs remain inactive in the endoplasmic reticulum. Cholesterol oxidation activates LXR, which stimulates E3 ubiquitin ligase transcription for LDL receptor degradation (IDOL). The cell regulates LDL receptor activity based on cholesterol availability. Low cellular cholesterol increases LDL receptor activity for enhanced uptake, while high cholesterol decreases receptor activity and LDL uptake. PCSK9, a secreted protein, targets LDL receptors for lysosomal degradation. PCSK9 loss-of-function mutations and inhibitors increase LDL receptor activity and lower LDL, while gain-of-function mutations decrease receptor activity and raise LDL levels.[2,9,10]

Low-density lipoproteins pathophysiology: The pathogenesis of atherosclerotic plaque is widely recognized to involve a complex interplay of processes, including endothelial cell activation, monocyte infiltration, LDL particles internalization by macrophages, foam cell formation, local inflammation, and modifications to the extracellular matrix (R).[2] Disturbed laminar flow causes endothelial dysfunction enabling LDL particles to cross the endothelial layer and accumulate within the intima. After oxidation caused by myeloperoxidase derived from inflammatory cells, LDL particles activate CD36 receptors on macrophages, which form complexes with TLR4 and TLR6 receptors and transduce signals leading to NF-B activation and chemokine expression. The chemokines stimulate immune cell infiltration into the intima, initiating the atherosclerotic plaque development. Macrophages phagocytize more and more LDL particles and evolve into foam cells, which are susceptible to apoptosis and, finally, necrosis.[2,9,10]

BIOCHEMISTRY AND PATHOPHYSIOLOGY OF NON-HDL CHOLESTEROL

Definition: Non-HDL-C is a composite measure of cholesterol in LDL, TRL, triglyceride-rich lipoproteins (TRLs), TRL remnants, and Lp(a)-excluding HDL.[6,11] It is calculated by deducting HDL-C from TC in the lipid panel and represents serum cholesterol of apoB-carrying lipoproteins.[11]

Very low-density lipoproteins, IDL and remnants, kinetics and pathophysiology: VLDL particles are produced by the liver and are triglyceride-rich.[12] They contain apolipoprotein B-100, C-I, C-II, C-III, and E. apoB-100 is the core structural protein and each VLDL particle contains one apoB-100 molecule. The size of the VLDL particles can vary depending on the quantity of triglyceride carried in the particle. The catabolism of triglycerides from VLDL by muscle and adipose tissue leads to the generation of intermediate-density lipoprotein (IDL) particles, which are enriched in cholesterol. These IDL particles contain apolipoproteins B-100 and E and are considered pro-atherogenic.[13]

Triglyceride, kinetics, and pathophysiology: TRLs and their remnants with long-term retention in the arterial wall are proinflammatory after oxidative, enzymatic or nonenzymatic cleavage modifications, and directly activate vascular endothelium to secrete chemokines and express adhesion molecules, leading to monocytes recruitment.[14,15] Subsequently, monocytes differentiate into macrophages in vascular subendothelial space, co-phagocytizing lipoproteins with macrophages directly activated by pro-inflammatory TRLs to form foam cells. Moreover, pro-inflammatory TRLs induce VSMCs to convert to macrophage-like cells, exacerbating the wall's pre-existing inflammatory response through secreting a variety of proinflammatory cytokines, thereby promoting atherosclerosis **(Fig. 2)**.

CHILDHOOD LDL-CHOLESTEROL AND NON-HDL-CHOLESTEROL

■ Low-density Lipoprotein Cholesterol

The harmful effects of raised LDL cholesterol emerge in early childhood and amplify over the life course.[2,10] Studies in the United States and elsewhere have highlighted the varying prevalence and patterns of LDL cholesterol levels in children, which are influenced by genetic, lifestyle, and environmental factors.[16] A 2024 study from the Strong Heart Family Study found that 40% of Native American youth aged 15–39 had high LDL-C levels (≥100 mg/dL), with 2.8% showing very high levels (≥160 mg/dL).[17] A US-Centers for Disease Control study reported that 7–10% of US children have elevated LDL (≥130 mg/dL), often linked to obesity or familial hypercholesterolemia (FH).[18] In Europe, similar trends are noted, with studies like the Copenhagen General Population Study indicating LDL levels in children averaging 90–110 mg/dL, though FH prevalence (1:200–1:500) increases high LDL cases.[19] In Asia, particularly Japan, studies (e.g., Osawa et al., 2022)[20] show lower LDL levels (80–100 mg/dL) in children, with declines during puberty due to hormonal changes. Globally, the rising childhood adiposity is increasing the LDL-C levels.

In India, data on childhood dyslipidemia are limited but indicate rising concerns.[21,22] A Jaipur study of 237 children aged 13–17 reported borderline hypercholesterolemia (170–199 mg/dL) in 33% and definite hypercholesterolemia in 6.8%.[23] A Delhi study of 1,236 adolescents found high LDL (>95th percentile) in 12–13%, with hypertriglyceridemia and low HDL more prevalent.[24] Other studies from Delhi and South India indicate 12–13% of adolescents have high LDL (>95th percentile), with urban populations showing higher levels (up to 130 mg/dL) associated with dietary shifts and sedentary lifestyles.[25] FH prevalence in India is notably high (1:125–1:450), contributing to elevated LDL. The ICMR-INDIAB study noted regional variations, with higher dyslipidemia in Northern States and urban areas, driven by dietary habits and increasing obesity.[26] India faces challenges with low awareness and limited pediatric lipid studies, necessitating further research.[22] Cross-country comparisons are challenging due to inconsistent screening ages and methods. Although a universal lipid screening is recommended in the US, it is not well implemented in Asia and India, where targeted screening for high-risk groups prevails.

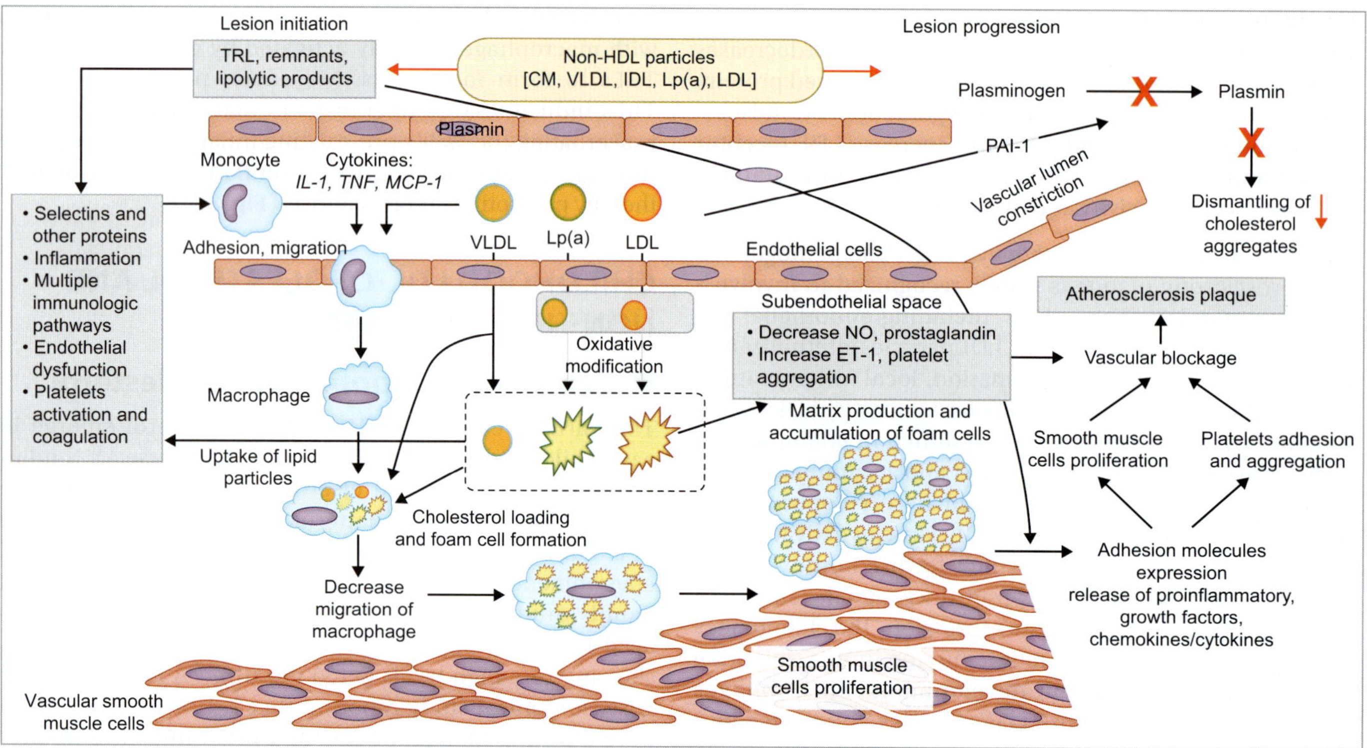

FIG. 2: Importance of non-HDL cholesterol in atherosclerosis.

Source: Raja V, Aguiar C, Alsayed N, et al. Non-HDL cholesterol in dyslipidemia: review of the state-of-the-art literature and outlook. Atherosclerosis. 2023;383:117312.

Non-high-density Lipoprotein Cholesterol

Non-HDL cholesterol, a measure of all atherogenic lipoproteins (LDL, VLDL, and others), is increasingly used to assess cardiovascular risk in children. Data on non-HDL cholesterol levels in childhood across the United States, Europe, Asia, and India show large variations, which could be influenced by genetics, diet, physical activity, and socioeconomic factors. There are no harmonized global studies.[11] In the US, the American Academy of Pediatrics recommends non-HDL-C levels below 145 mg/dL for children aged 2-19.[8] Studies, such as those from the National Health and Nutrition Examination Survey (NHANES), report average non-HDL-C levels of 100–120 mg/dL in US children, with 8–12% exceeding 145 mg/dL, often linked to obesity, diabetes, FH. Higher levels are noted in adolescents.[27] In Europe, data from studies such as the IDEFICS study (covering multiple countries) indicate non-HDL-C levels averaging 95–115 mg/dL in children aged 2–10, with 5–10% exceeding thresholds.[28] FH prevalence contributes to the elevated levels, particularly in Northern Europe. European guidelines emphasize non-HDL as a screening tool, with cutoffs similar to US.[1,3] In Asia, particularly Japan and China, studies report lower non-HDL-C levels (80–110 mg/dL) in children, however, urban regions show higher levels (up to 130 mg/dL).[6,29]

In India, studies from urban centers such as Delhi report non-HDL levels of 110–135 mg/dL in adolescents, with 15–20% exceeding 145 mg/dL, driven by high FH prevalence.[30] Rural Indian children often have lower levels (90–110 mg/dL).[31,25] Cross-country comparisons are limited by inconsistent screening protocols and age groups. The US and Europe advocate universal lipid screening (ages 9–11, 17–21), while Asia and India focus on high-risk groups.[32] Rising obesity globally underscores the need for standardized non-HDL monitoring in childhood.[32,33]

TRACKING OF LDL AND NON-HDL CHOLESTEROL INTO ADULTHOOD AND CAD

Childhood LDL-C levels play a critical role in the development of atherosclerotic cardiovascular diseases (ASCVD) in adulthood, as they tend to track over the life course and contribute to cumulative vascular damage.[4,7,8,34] Atherosclerosis begins early in life, with elevated LDL-C promoting plaque formation that progresses into clinical events such as myocardial infarction or stroke.[10] Longitudinal studies demonstrate that maintaining low LDL-C from youth can significantly mitigate lifelong risk.[35]

Tracking of LDL-C from childhood to adulthood shows moderate stability.[7,8] In the Busselton study (Australia), involving 1,764 children followed for up to 27 years, the correlation coefficients for cholesterol levels ranged from 0.35 to 0.55, with stronger tracking over shorter intervals.[34] Approximately 55–60% of children in the highest quartile remained there in mid-life, adjusting to 80% after accounting for regression to the mean. The KiGGS cohort, tracking 1,716 German youth from prepuberty to young adulthood (mean follow-up 15 years), reported correlations of 0.60 for non-HDL-C (encompassing LDL-C) and 0.56 for total cholesterol, higher in men (0.67 vs. 0.53 in women).[36] Factors such as BMI increase and oral contraceptive use in females influenced higher adult levels, explaining up to 62% of variance in men. In healthy children, normal LDL-C stabilizes early, with high year-to-year tracking. Sex differences emerge—girls have higher LDL-C in childhood, but levels may equalize or reverse post-puberty **(Fig. 3)**.

Elevated childhood total cholesterol levels have a linear relationship to hazard ratio of adult fatal and/or non-fatal cardiovascular events in the i3C consortium study of >20,000 children followed for 35 years **(Fig. 3)**. The relationship is similar for fatal cardiovascular events.[8] Elevated childhood LDL-C and non-HDL-C levels correlate directly with adult ASCVD. In the i3C Consortium (21,126 participants, 35-year follow-up), each z-score increase in childhood cholesterol raised fatal ASCVD risk (HR 1.27; 95% CI 1.14–1.41) and fatal/nonfatal events (HR 1.35; 95% CI 1.13–1.60) **(Fig. 4)**.[8] Non-HDL-C performed better for prediction (C-index difference 0.0054, **Table 1**). Another i3C analysis of 10,634 individuals confirmed childhood LDL-C's direct effect on mid-life CVD independent of adult factors.[37] In 5,121 adolescents from multiple cohorts, persistent dyslipidemic non-HDL-C from childhood yielded HR 5.17 for CVD events, while resolution by adulthood normalized risk (HR 1.13).[38] Life-course trajectories in the Bogalusa Heart Study, USA (1,201 participants) linked high-stable or rapidly increasing LDL-C patterns to greater carotid intima-media thickness (mean difference up to 0.104 mm), indicating subclinical atherosclerosis **(Fig. 4)**.[7]

Non-HDL-C also emerges as a robust predictor of atherosclerotic CVD when tracked from childhood to adulthood. Longitudinal data from the International Childhood Cardiovascular Cohort (i3C) consortium reveal moderate tracking of non-HDL-C levels, with a correlation coefficient of 0.587 between childhood (ages 3–19) and adult (ages 20–40) z-scores in a pooled analysis of 5,121 participants.[8] In this cohort, followed for a mean of 8.9 years post-age 40, childhood non-HDL-C was linked to increased adult CVD events (HR 1.42; 95% CI 1.18–1.70 per 1-unit z-score increase), though attenuated after adjusting for adult levels (HR 1.12; 95% CI 0.89–1.41). Resolution of dyslipidemic non-HDL-C by adulthood normalizes risk, akin to persistently normal levels (HR 1.13; 95% CI 0.50–2.56), while persistent dyslipidemia elevates it substantially (HR 5.17; 95% CI 2.80–9.56), and incident adult dyslipidemia doubles it (HR 2.17; 95% CI 1.00–4.69).

The i3C study of 21,126 participants, with 35-year follow-up,[39] confirmed childhood non-HDL-C and LDL-C associations with fatal/nonfatal ASCVD (HRs 1.27–1.35 per z-score), but non-HDL-C outperformed LDL-C in discrimination (C-index difference 0.0038–0.0054). Discordantly elevated non-HDL-C with normal LDL-C heightened risk (HR 1.90–1.94). Other research supports tracking, with childhood non-HDL-C explaining 41% variance in adult levels.[35] Early screening, non-fasting non-HDL-C measurement, and interventions such as lifestyle changes could mitigate lifelong CVD burden, emphasizing a life-course approach to lipid management.[32,33,40]

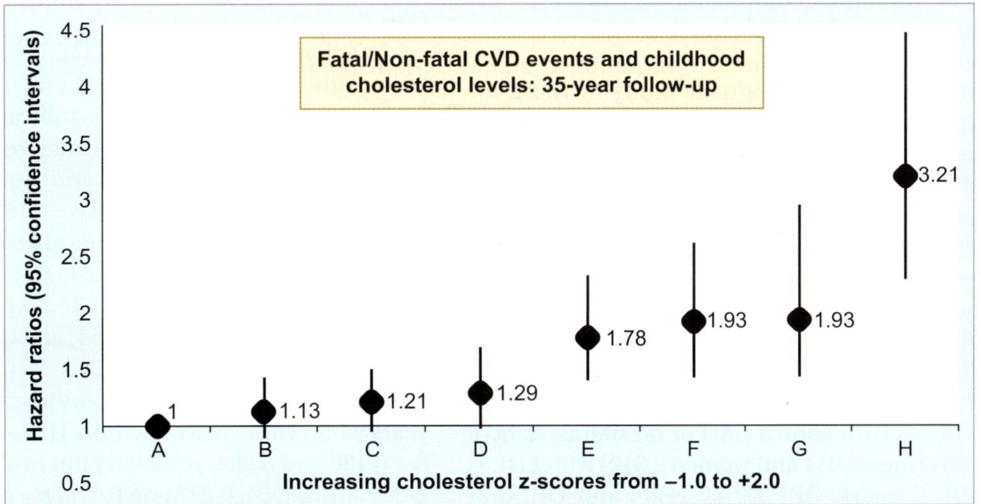

FIG. 3: Increasing cholesterol z-scores at childhood and association with adult fatal/non-fatal cardiovascular disease—data source i3C consortium.[8]

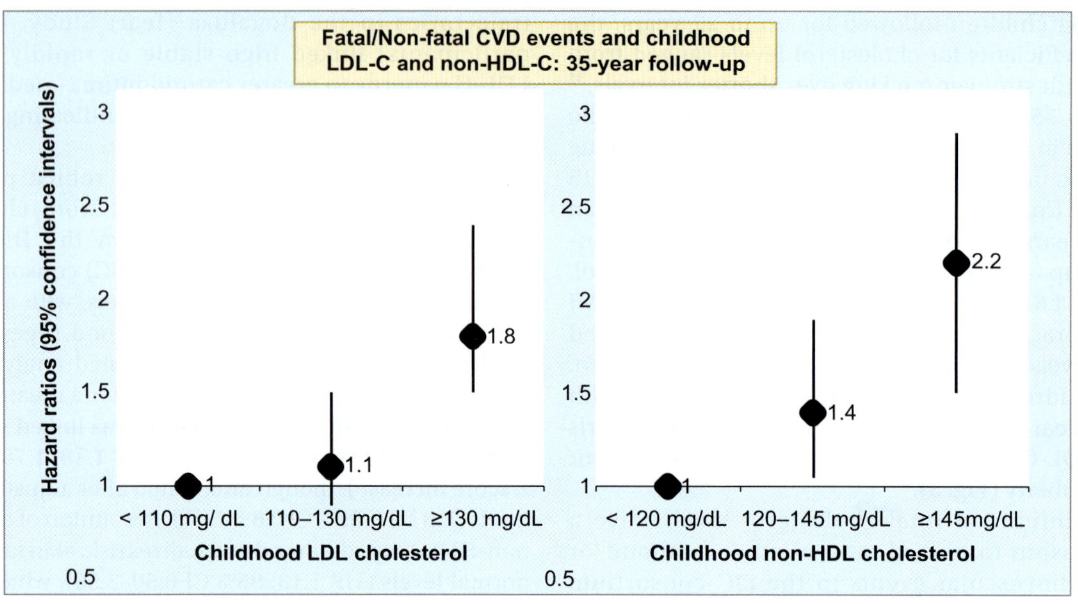

FIG. 4: Childhood LDL-C and non-HDL-C and association with adult fatal/non-fatal cardiovascular disease—data source i3C consortium.[8]

LDL-CHOLESTEROL AND NON-HDL CHOLESTEROL YEARS IN INDIA HEART WATCH

Low-density lipoprotein cholesterol years (LDLCY), which is age multiplied by LDL cholesterol (mg/dL) in statin-naïve individuals, is considered an important atherosclerosis risk factor.[41,42] There are no studies of the predictive importance of non-HDL cholesterol years (NHDLCY). It has been reported that an LDLCY of >5,000 predicts a high risk of future CAD events.[43] Accordingly, children with FH (LDL-C $\geq$200 mg/dL) have a very high risk of early CVD events by the age of 25 years. Studies in developed countries have confirmed the prognostic importance of LDLCY,[43] but there are no studies from developing countries.

India Heart Watch was a multisite study in India for the identification of important socioeconomic, lifestyle, physiological and metabolic coronary risk factors at multiple urban sites across the country.[44,45] Details of various lipoprotein lipids have been reported earlier.[46] We performed a study to evaluate the correlation of LDL-C years and non-HD-C years with 10-year and lifetime QRISK2 scores in India using data from the India Heart Watch. The study was conducted among adults at 11 urban sites. Community-based data on sociodemographic, anthropometric, and biochemical CAD risk factors were obtained in 6,198 individuals. We excluded individuals with known CAD or on statins; data of 5,816 participants (men 3,034 and women 2,510) with LDL-C years, non-HDL-C years, QRISK2-10 years and QRISK2-lifetime (LT) scores were analyzed. Correlations of LDL-C years and non-HDL-C years with QRISK2 (10 years, LT) in IHW were performed using subgroup-analyses (LDL-C years were grouped into <5,000, 5,000–7,500, and >7,500 and non-HDL-C years into <8,000, 8,000–10,500, and >10,500 years) using univariate correlation and multivariate regression **(Fig. 5)**.

We also found that the increasing QRISK2-10 years and QRISK2-LT correlated with LDL-C years and non-HDL-C years subgroups ($p < 0.01$) **(Fig. 5)**. Increasing LDLCY and NHDLCY groups correlated significantly with QRISK2-10 years ($R^2 = 0.276$ and 0.350) and QRISK-2-LT ($R^2 = 0.024$ and 0.053), respectively ($p < 0.001$). Increasing LDLCY and NHDLCY also correlated significantly with age, body mass index, hypertension, diabetes, and tobacco use ($p < 0.001$) **(Fig. 5)**.

Pearson's correlation of LDL-C years and non-HDL-C years with QRISK2-10 (r = 0.541 and 0.601) and QRISK2-LT (r = 0.000 and 0.000) was also significant ($p < 0.001$) **(Fig. 6)**. Risk-factor adjusted regression analyzes showed a significant association of LDL-C years and non-HDL-C years with QRISK2-10 years (standardized $\beta = 0.188$ and 0.284, $p < 0.001$) but not with QRISK2-LT (standardized $\beta = 0.027$ and 0.019, p = ns). Significant correlation of LDL-C years with QRISK2-10 ($R^2 = 0.276$) and QRISK-2-LT ($R^2 = 0.024$), and non-HDL-C years with QRISK2-10 ($R^2 = 0.350$) and QRISK2-LT ($R^2 = 0.053$) was also observed ($p < 0.001$). Risk-factor adjusted regression analyses confirmed a significant association of QRISK2-10 years with LDL-C years and non-HDL-C years (standardized $\beta = 0.188$ and 0.284, $p < 0.001$) but not with QRISK2-lifetime (standardized $\beta = 0.027$ and 0.019, p = ns).

Thus, in a population-based study in India, we found that both LDL-C years and non-HDL-C years correlate

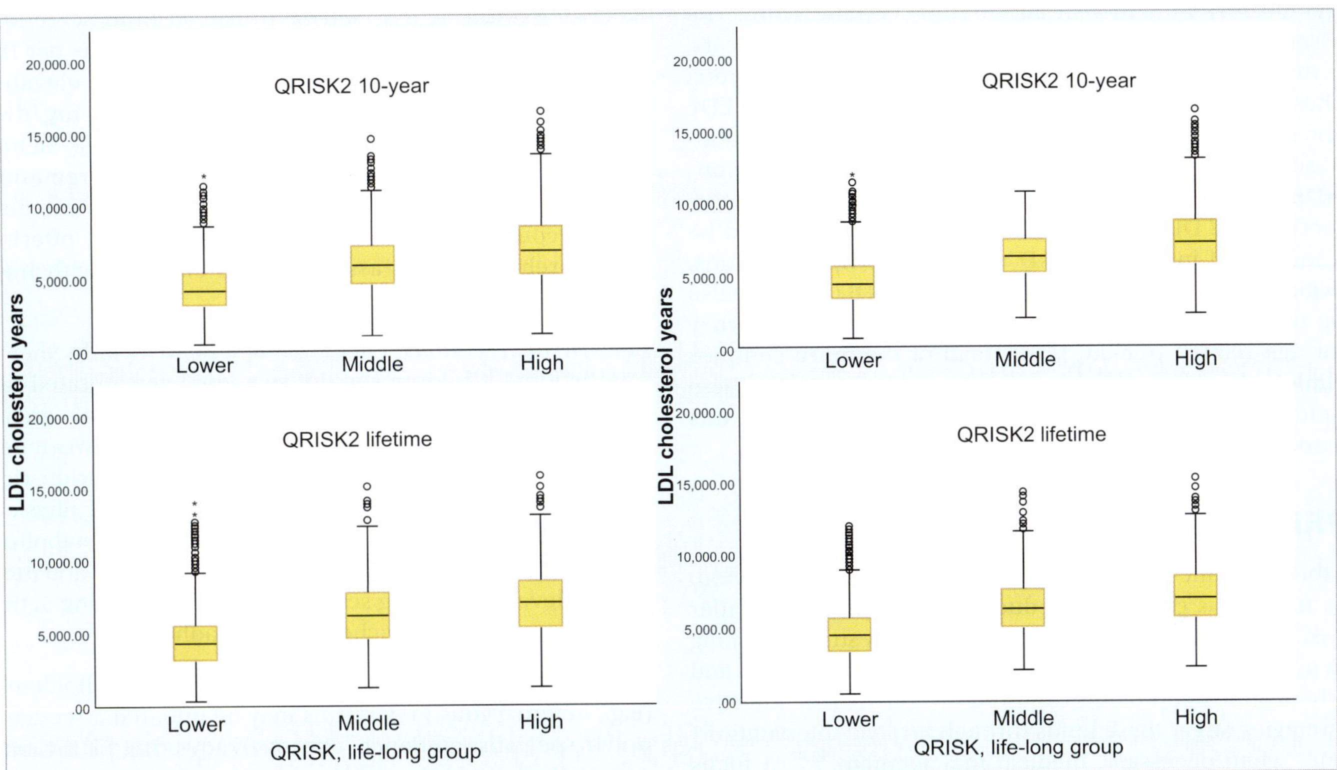

FIG. 5: Box plots of mean LDL-C and non-HDL-C years with low, middle, and high 10-year QRISK2 and lifetime QRISK2 scores in the India Heart Watch (*p* <0.001).

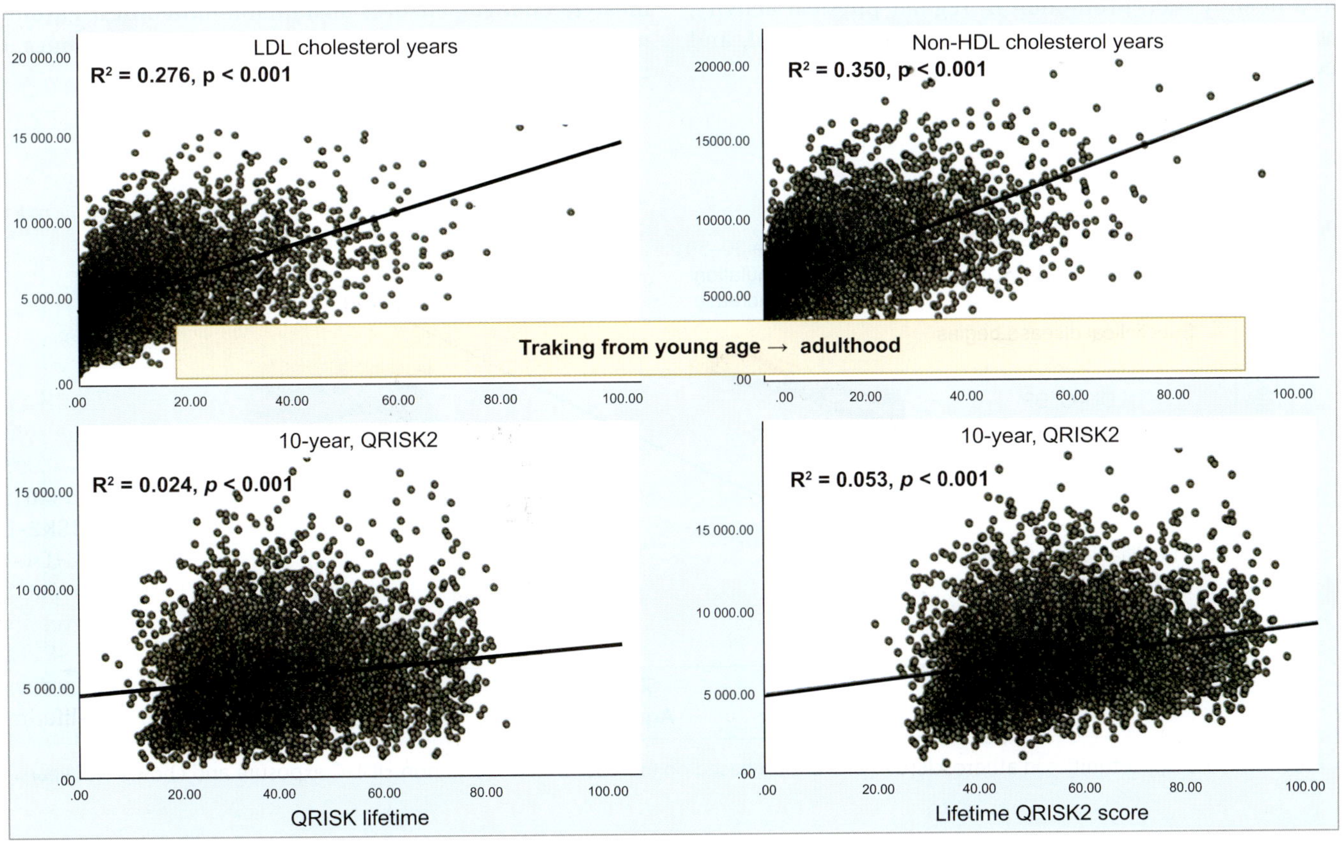

FIG. 6: Correlation of LDL-C years and non-NHDL-C years with 10-year QRISK2-10 years and lifetime QRISK2-scores. An example of age-associated tracking of these cholesterol lipoproteins.

significantly with 10-year and lifetime QRISK2 score. The association with QRISK2-lifetime, but not QRISK2-10 years, is attenuated following adjustment for other risk factors. These findings highlight the importance of increasing LDL cholesterol as well as non-HDL cholesterol in a population-based study in India. As the LDL cholesterol and non-HDL cholesterol levels track from childhood to adulthood, increasing LDL-C years and non-HDL-C years would be a marker of increasing CAD risk of these lipid fractions, beginning from childhood to adulthood. LDLCY could also be used as a cardiovascular risk assessment tool (proxy for age-related tracking),[48] instead of the more complex clinical algorithms.[49,50] A prospective study that tracks these lipid fractions from childhood is required to confirm this association using large and long-term studies **(Fig. 7)**.

PREVENTION STRATEGIES

Atherosclerotic CVD prevention should begin in childhood, as this age is critical for reducing lifelong cardiovascular risk.[51] Atherosclerosis begins early, with fatty streaks forming in arteries during childhood, driven by elevated LDL-C and atherogenic lipoproteins captured by non-HDL-C. Effective strategies target these lipids through lifestyle interventions and, when necessary, medical management.[32,47] A focus on managing low-density lipoprotein cholesterol (LDL-C) and non-high-density lipoprotein cholesterol (non-HDL-C) **(Fig. 6)**. The interventions should be holistic and also focus on a healthy diet, promotion of regular physical activity, avoidance of addictions to tobacco, vaping, alcohol, and recreational drugs.[53]

Screening and risk assessment: Universal lipid screening is recommended between ages 9–11 and 17–21, as per the American Academy of Paediatrics, to identify elevated LDL-C (>130 mg/dL) or non-HDL-C (>145 mg/dL). Targeted screening is advised for children with risk factors such as obesity, diabetes, or family history of premature cardiovascular disease. Non-HDL-C is particularly valuable as it accounts for all atherogenic lipoproteins, offering a comprehensive risk assessment in children with high triglycerides.

Lifestyle interventions: Encouraging a heart-healthy diet is foundational. Children should consume low-saturated-fat, high-fiber diets rich in fruits, vegetables, and whole grains to lower LDL-C and non-HDL-C. Limiting sugar-sweetened beverages and processed foods reduce triglyceride-rich lipoproteins, a component of non-HDL-C. Regular physical activity, at least 60 minutes daily, promotes lipid metabolism and weight management, further decreasing LDL-C and non-HDL-C levels. Reducing screen time and promoting active play are practical approaches to ensure adherence.[52]

Medical management: For children with severe dyslipidemia (e.g., heterozygous FH), statins may be initiated after age 8 under specialist guidance, effectively lowering LDL-C and non-HDL-C. Early intervention prevents the progression of subclinical atherosclerosis.

Education and family involvement: Engaging families in lifestyle changes ensures sustainable outcomes. Parental modeling of healthy behaviors reinforces adherence in children **(Table 2)**.

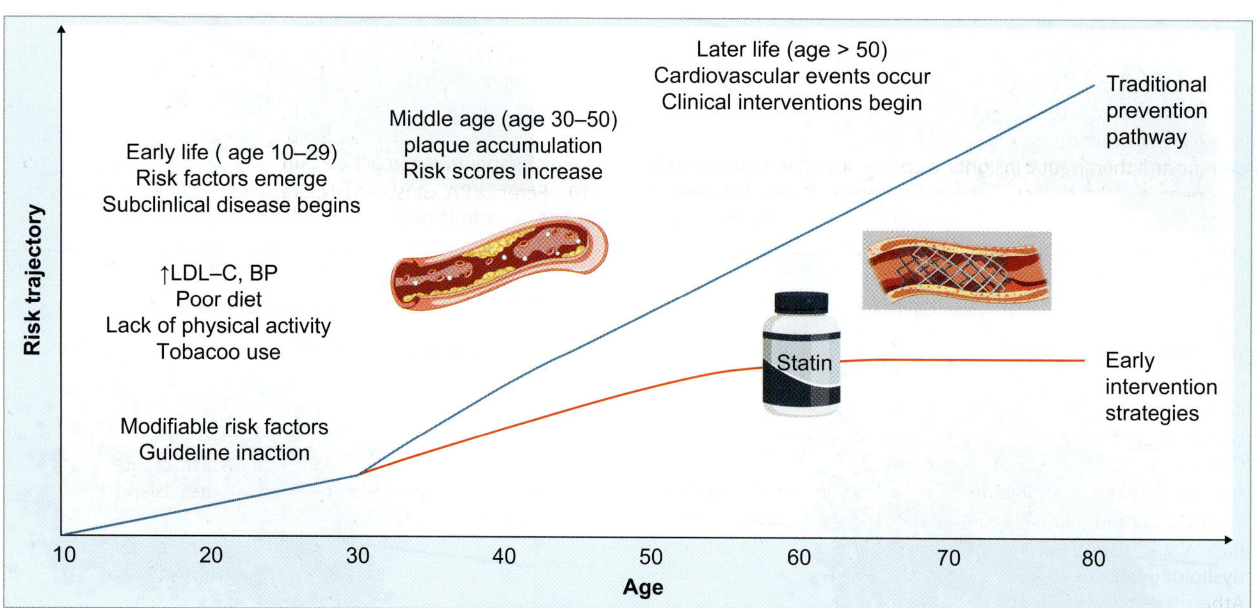

FIG. 7: Missed opportunities in atherosclerosis prevention based on life-course LDL-C and non-HDL-C exposure and cholesterol years.

TABLE 2: Prevention strategies in childhood for adult atherosclerotic cardiovascular disease.

Strategy	Description	Mechanism of action
Physical activity	Encourage at least 60 minutes of moderate-to-vigorous activity daily (e.g., sports, cycling)	Improves lipid profiles, reduces blood pressure, and enhances insulin sensitivity
Weight management	Monitor BMI and promote a healthy weight through a balanced diet and exercise	Prevents obesity-related dyslipidemia and early atherosclerotic changes
Avoid tobacco exposure	Prevent exposure to second-hand smoke and discourage smoking initiation	Reduces endothelial damage and inflammation linked to atherosclerosis
Blood pressure control	Screen and manage hypertension through lifestyle or medication if needed	Decreases vascular stress and prevents early arterial stiffness
Diabetes prevention	Promote a healthy lifestyle to prevent type 2 diabetes; screen high-risk children	Reduces hyperglycemia-related vascular damage and dyslipidemia
Lipid screening	Universal lipid screening between ages 9–11 and 17–21	Early identification and management of dyslipidemia to reduce long-term risk

CONCLUSION

Low-density lipoprotein-C and non-HDL-C are markers of atherogenic apolipoprotein B and have roots in early childhood and adolescence. The present review shows that the levels of these cholesterol lipoproteins track into adulthood and raised childhood levels are associated with increased risk of fatal and non-fatal CVD events in adulthood, depending on the childhood values. There are small studies from India that have reported levels of these cholesterol lipoproteins in children and adolescents. Large prospective outcome studies similar to those in the USA, Europe, Australia, and East Asian countries are required (e.g., Bogalusa study, i3C Consortium Prospective Study, etc.) in India. A small statin trial in children with familial hypercholesterolemia reported a significant reduction in the progression of carotid intima-media thickness and a reduction in the risk of CVD in adulthood associated with a 32% decline in LDL-C levels.[54] The importance of childhood LDL-C and non-HDL-C needs to be confirmed using large prospective randomized lifestyle or drug trials beginning in childhood and evaluation of CVD outcomes decades later, for the generation of high-quality evidence and guideline development.

REFERENCES

1. Mach F, Baigent C, Catapano AL, et al. 2019 ESC/EAS guidelines for the management of dyslipidemia: lipid modification to reduce cardiovascular risk. Eur Heart J. 2020;41:111-88.
2. Boren J, Chapman MJ, Krauss RM, et al. Low-density lipoproteins cause atherosclerotic cardiovascular disease: pathophysiological, genetic and therapeutic insights: a consensus statement from the European Atherosclerosis Society Consensus Panel. Eur Heart J. 2020; 41:2313-30.
3. Grundy SM, Stone NJ, Bailey AL, et al. 2018 AHA/ACC/AACVPR/AAPA/ABC/ACPM/ADA/AGS/APhA /ASPC/ NLA/PCNA guideline on the management of blood cholesterol: a report of the American College of Cardiology/American Heart Association Task Force on clinical practice guidelines. Circulation. 2019;139: e1082-e1143.
4. Ference BA, Graham I, Tokgozoglu L, et al. Impact of lipids on cardiovascular health: JACC health promotion series. J Am Coll Cardiol. 2018;72:1141-56.
5. Ray KK, Ference BA, Severin T, et al. World Heart Federation cholesterol roadmap 2022. Global Heart. 2022;17:75.
6. Raja V, Aguiar C, Alsayed N, et al. Non-HDL cholesterol in dyslipidemia: review of the state-of-the-art literature and outlook. Atherosclerosis. 2023;383:117312.
7. Wu F, Jacobs DR, Daniels SR, et al. Non-HDL-C levels from childhood to adulthood and CVD events. JAMA. 2024;331: 1834-44.
8. Wu F, Jounala M, David J, et al. Childhood non-HDL cholesterol and LDL cholesterol and adult atherosclerotic cardiovascular events. Circulation. 2024; 149:217-26.
9. Akram MA, Khodja A, Dalibalta S, et al. The role of lipids in atherosclerosis: focus on molecular biology and mechanisms and therapeutic approaches. Curr Med Chem. 2024;32:3044-68.
10. Ference BA, Ginsberg HN, Graham I, et al. Low-density lipoproteins cause atherosclerotic cardiovascular disease. 1. Evidence from genetic, epidemiological, and clinical studies. A consensus statement from the European Atherosclerosis Society Consensus Panel. Eur Heart J. 2017;38:2459-72.
11. Blaha MJ, Blumenthal RS, Brinton EA, et al. The importance of non-HDL cholesterol reporting in lipid management. J Clin Lipidol. 2008;2:267-73.
12. Casso FMJ, Farzam K. Biochemistry: very low density lipoprotein. In: StatPearls. Treasure Island (FL): StatPearls Publishing; 2025.
13. Narang D, Al-Horani RA. Biochemistry: intermediate density lipoprotein. In: StatPearls. Treasure Island (FL): StatPearls Publishing; 2025.
14. Xu D, Xie L, Cheng C, et al. Triglyceride-rich lipoproteins and cardiovascular diseases. Front Endocrinol. (Lausanne). 2024;15: 1409653.
15. Akivis Y, Alkaissi H, McFarlane SI, et al. The role of triglycerides in atherosclerosis: recent pathophysiologic insights and therapeutic implications. Curr Cardiol Rev. 2024;20:39-49.

16. Guirguis-Blake JM, Evans CV, Coppola EL, et al. Screening for lipid disorders in children and adolescents. JAMA. 2023; 330:261-74.
17. Miao G, Pechlaner R, Fiehn O, et al. Longitudinal lipidomic signature or coronary heart disease in American Indian people. J Am Heart Assoc. 2024;13:e031825.
18. Centres for Disease Control and Prevention (CDC). Prevalence of abnormal lipid levels among youth- United States 1999-2006. MMWR. 2010;59:29.
19. Christensen JJ, Ulven SM, Retterstol K, et al. Comprehensive lipid and metabolite profiling of children with and without familial hypercholesterolemia: a cross-sectional study. Atherosclerosis. 2017; 266:48-97.
20. Osawa E, Asakura K, Okamura T, et al. Tracking pattern of total cholesterol levels from childhood to adolescence in Japan. J Atheroscler Thromb. 2022;29:38-49.
21. Gupta R, Rao RS, Misra A. Recent trends in epidemiology of dyslipidemias in India. Indian Heart J. 2017;69:382-92.
22. Sharma S, Gaur K, Gupta R. trends in epidemiology of dyslipidemias in India. Indian Heart J. 2024;76(Suppl 1):S20-S28.
23. Gupta R, Goyle A, Kashyap S, et al. Prevalence of atherosclerosis risk factors in adolescent school children. Indian Heart J. 1998;50:511-5.
24. Arora M, Mathur C, Rawal T, et al. Socioeconomic differences in prevalence of biochemical, physiological, and metabolic risk factors for non-communicable diseases among urban youth in Delhi, India. Prev Med Rep. 2018;12:33-9.
25. Kirti K, Singh SK. Quantifying the burden of lipid anomalies among adolescents in India. BMC Cardiovasc Disord. 2022; 22:385.
26. Anjana RM, Unnikrishnan R, Deepa M, et al. Metabolic non-communicable disease health report of India: the ICMR-INDIAB national cross-sectional study. Lancet Diab Endocrinol. 2023;11: 474-89.
27. US Preventive Services Task Force. Screening for lipid disorders in children and adolescents. JAMA. 2016;316:625-53.
28. Henauw SD, Michels N, Vyncke K, et al. Blood lipids among young children in Europe: results from the European IDEFICS study. Int J Obesity. 2014;38:S67-S75.
29. Kelishadi R, Haghdoost A, Moosazadeh M, et al. A systematic review and meta-analysis on screening lipid disorders in pediatric age-group. J Res Med Sciences. 2015;20:1191-9.
30. Khalil A, Gupta S, Madan A, et al. Lipid profile norms in children. Indian Ped. 1995;1177-80.
31. Dhok A, Dubey Y. Status of serum lipid profile in the young population in rural areas. Int J Med Sci Public Health. 2018;7: 121-25.
32. NCEP Expert Panel on Blood Cholesterol Levels in Children and Adolescents. National Cholesterol Education Program (NCEP): Highlights of the Report of the Expert Panel on Blood Cholesterol Levels in Children and Adolescents. Pediatrics 1992;89(3):495-501.
33. Barlow SE. Expert committee recommendations regarding the prevention, assessment, and treatment of child and adolescent overweight and obesity: Summary report. Pediatrics. 2007;120: S164-92.
34. Adams C, Burke V, Beilin LJ, Cholesterol tracking from childhood to adult mid-life in children from the Busselton study. Acta Ped. 2007;94:275-80.
35. Zhang Y, Pletcher MJ, Vittinghof E, et al. Association between cumulative low-density lipoprotein cholesterol exposure during young adulthood and middle age and risk of cardiovascular events. JAMA Cardiol. 2021;6:1406-13.
36. Konigstein K, Buschges JC, Schmidt-Truckass A, et al. Cardiovascular risk in childhood is associated with carotid intima-media thickness and stiffness in adolescents and young adults: The KiGGS cohort. J Adolescent Health. 2024;74:123-9.
37. Jacobs DR, Woo JG, Sinaiko AR, et al. Childhood cardiovascular risk factors and adult cardiovascular events. N Engl J Med. 2022;386:1877-88.
38. Dai Y, Sheng Y, Zheng Z, Di W. Cumulative remnant cholesterol exposure during young adulthood and middle age and risk of cardiovascular events: A 30-year population-based cohort study. Int J Cardiol. 2024;414:132435.
39. Dwyer T, Jacobs DR, Woo JG, et al. Childhood risk factors and cardiovascular disease outcomes in adulthood. Preliminary findings from the International Childhood Cardiovascular Cohort (i3C) Consortium. Eur Heart J. 2019; 40:ehz748.0082
40. Schmitt C, Yohannan TM. Transitioning adolescents and young adults with lipid disorders to adult health care. Curr Atheroscl Rep. 2024; 26:693-700.
41. Ference BA, Yoo W, Alech I, et al. Effect of long-term exposure to lower low-density lipoprotein cholesterol beginning early in life on the risk of coronary heart disease. J Am Coll Cardiol. 2012;60:2631-9.
42. Shapiro MD, Bhatt DL. Cholesterol years for ASCVD risk prediction and treatment. J Am Coll Cardiol. 2020;76:1517-20
43. Ference BA, Braunwald E, Catapano AL. The LDL cumulative exposure hypothesis: evidence and practical implications. Nature Rev Cardiol. 2024;21:701-16.
44. Gupta R, Deedwania PC, Sharma KK, et al. Association of education, occupation and socioeconomic status with cardiovascular risk factors in Asian Indians: A cross-sectional study. PLoS One. 2012; 7:e044098.
45. Gupta R, Sharma KK, Gupta BK, et al. Geographic epidemiology of cardiometabolic risk factors in urban middle-class residents in India: A cross-sectional study. J Global Health. 2015; 5:10411.
46. Guptha S, Gupta R, Deedwania P, et al. Cholesterol lipoproteins, triglycerides and prevalence of dyslipidemias among urban Asian Indian subjects: a cross-sectional study. Indian Heart J. 2014; 66:280-8.
47. Braunwald E. How to live to 100 before developing coronary artery disease: a suggestion. Eur Heart J. 2022;43:249-50.
48. Wilkins JT, Ning H, Allen NB, et al. Prediction of cumulative exposure to atherogenic lipids during early adulthood. J Am Coll Cardiol. 2024;84:961-73.
49. Khan SS, Coresh J, Pencina MJ, et al. Novel prediction equations for absolute risk assessment of total cardiovascular disease incorporating cardiovascular-kidney-metabolic health: a scientific statement from the American Heart Association. Circulation. 2023;148:1982-2004.
50. Grant JK, Ndumele CE, Martin SS. The evolving landscape of cardiovascular risk assessment. JAMA. 2024;332:967-9.
51. Raitakari O, Pahkala K, Magnussen CG. Prevention of atherosclerosis from childhood. Nature Rev Cardiol. 2022;19:543-54.
52. Morton K, Heindl B, Clarkson S, et al. Primordial prevention of atherosclerotic cardiovascular disease. J Cardiopulm Rehab Prev. 2022;42:389-96.
53. Gupta R, Wood DA. Primary prevention of ischemic heart disease: populations, individuals, and healthcare professionals. Lancet. 2019;394:685-96.
54. Luirink IK, Wiegman A, Kusters M, et al. 20-year follow-up of statins in children with familial hypercholesterolemia. N Engl J Med. 2019;381:1547-56.

SECTION

5

Heart Failure

Section Outline

18. **Worsening Heart Failure: Definition and Management**
Dhiman Kahali, Debdatta Kar, Padma Madhab Bisoi

19. **Pulmonary Hypertension in Heart Failure: The Good, the Bad, and the Ugly**
A Purnanand

20. **Progression from Pre-heart Failure, Heart Stress to Subclinical Heart Failure**
Arpita Katheria, Ankit Kumar Sahu, Aditya Kapoor

21. **Immunology of Heart Failure: Deconstructing Inflammatory Risk**
Amal Kumar Khan, Anish Kumar Khan, Amartya Khan

22. **Iron Deficiency States and Effective Iron Repletion Strategies in Chronic Heart Failure**
Ankit Kumar Sahu, Arshad Nazir, Pranjal Raparia

23. **Risk Scores in the Management of Heart Failure**
Ashish Jha, Abhijit Bharali

24. **Issues in Reversing Advanced Heart Failure**
Awadhesh K Sharma, Sayar Ahmad Pandit

25. **Early Initiation of GDMT in HFrEF: Accelerating Outcomes with Timely Evidence-based Titration**
Dikshit Byomakesh, Behera Soumen Prasad

26. **Mixed Cardiogenic-vasodilatory Shock**
Biswajit Majumder, Somnath Maji, Suvadeep Biswas, Ratul Ghosh

27. **Chronic Right-sided Heart Failure and Tricuspid Regurgitation: "No Longer a Forgotten Entity"**
Chandrakanta Mishra

28. **Neuromodulation Interventions in the Management of Heart Failure**
Manoj Bansal

29. **Congestion and Diuretic Resistance in Worsening Heart Failure**
HK Chopra

30. **Role of Imaging in Heart Failure Risk Stratification**
Haresh Mehta, Raghav R Nagpal, Kayan Siodia

31. **Can Left Ventricular Wall Strain Predict Heart Failure?**
Jagdish Chander Mohan, Madhu Shukla

32. **Medical Therapy of Cardiogenic Shock: Contemporary Use of Inotropes and Vasopressors**
Kashinath Ghosh Hazra, Ahitagni Banerjee

33. **Continuum of Preshock to Classic Cardiogenic Shock**
MU Rabbani

34. **Triaging of Patients of Acute Decompensated Heart Failure**
Pranab Jyoti Bhattacharyya, Maitreyee Bhattacharyya

35. **Gut Hypothesis of Heart Failure: Role of Gut Microbiota–Derived Metabolites**
Puneet Rastogi

36. **Diuretic Potentiation Strategies in Acute Heart Failure**
SK Dwivedi, Somil Verma

37. **Approaches in Heart Failure with Mildly Reduced and Preserved Ejection Fraction**
Vidyut Jain, Avani Jain

38. **Characteristics and Outcomes of Patients with Valvular Cardiogenic Shock**
Sumanyu Suresh, Harikrishnan Sivadasanpillai

39. **Hemodynamic Assessment by Right Heart Catheterization in Management of Heart Failure**
Bijay Prakash Pandey, Rajat Kar

CHAPTER 18

Worsening Heart Failure: Definition and Management

Dhiman Kahali, Debdatta Kar, Padma Madhab Bisoi

ABSTRACT

Worsening heart failure (WHF) marks clinical deterioration in patients with chronic heart failure despite stable therapy. It includes both hospitalized and outpatient cases requiring IV or intensified diuretic therapy. Current definitions often overlook subclinical worsening detected by biomarkers such as NT-proBNP or troponin. Emerging pharmacologic options—vericiguat, sotagliflozin, omecamtiv mecarbil, digitoxin, and levosimendan—along with remote monitoring and device-based therapies such as CardioMEMS and cardiac contractility modulation, have expanded management strategies. A precision-based, proactive approach can reduce hospitalizations and improve patient outcomes.

Keywords: Worsening heart failure, NT-proBNP, diuretic therapy, levosimendan, digitoxin, vericiguat, sotagliflozin, omecamtiv mecarbil, remote monitoring, CardioMEMS, cardiac contractility modulation.

INTRODUCTION

Worsening heart failure (WHF) is defined by escalating signs and symptoms of heart failure (HF) in patients with chronic HF despite previously stable therapy. This definition also requires the need for a hospitalization for HF, treatment of HF in the emergency department, or receipt of intravenous (IV) diuretic therapy in the outpatient setting **(Fig. 1)**.[1,2]

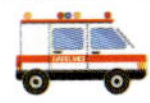

FIG. 1: Worsening heart failure (WHF) in patients (diagnosis to treatment).

TRADITIONAL DEFINITIONS OF WORSENING HEART FAILURE

Hospitalization for Heart Failure

The definition of WHF has evolved over time. For decades, WHF has been equated with the deterioration of HF signs and symptoms requiring hospitalization.

Worsening Heart Failure without Hospitalization

There are at least three potential scenarios in which a patient may present with WHF and receive treatment without hospitalization—outpatient IV diuretic administration, escalation of outpatient oral diuretic therapy, and ED visit and discharge without hospitalization.

LIMITATIONS AND UNCERTAINTIES OF THE CURRENT DEFINITION

Despite increasing recognition of WHF in trials and guidelines, the current definition has limitations and associated areas of uncertainty (Central Illustration) **(Table 1)**.[1]

Subclinical Worsening

A limitation of the current WHF definition is that absence of overtly worsening signs and symptoms is not always an indication of lower risk. Biomarker levels are powerful predictors of morbidity and mortality. This "silent worsening" can be unrecognized and undertreated, particularly as patients with worsening HF decrease their activity levels which can potentially mask the development of overt symptoms.

Routinely available parameters, such as ejection fraction, blood pressure, and heart rate have limitations and are not very accurate in defining WHF. In the future, these may be refined by more comprehensive assessment of changes in biological characteristics using biomarker or omics profiling.

Asymptomatic increases in N-terminal pro-B-type natriuretic peptide (NT-proBNP) (e.g., >30%) or new-onset troponin elevation (without acute coronary syndrome) have shown prognostic value.

DEFINING CRITERIA FOR ESCALATED ORAL THERAPY

In the Danish cohort study, intensification was defined as:

- Newly prescribed oral loop diuretic of minimum 80 mg/day furosemide equivalent;
- Doubled dosage of loop diuretic to minimum 160 mg/day furosemide equivalent;
- Newly prescribed thiazide diuretic in addition to 160 mg/day furosemide equivalent.

The CHAMP-HF study utilized a definition as either **(Table 2)**:

- Any change in total daily dose higher than previous dose;
- Addition of metolazone; or
- Switch from any dose of furosemide

NOVEL THERAPIES AND FUTURE DIRECTIONS

Novel therapies are shown in **Figure 2** and **Table 3**.

TABLE 1: Definition of worsening heart failure.

Central illustration: Considering the definition of worsening heart failure	
Current definition: • Deterioration of HF signs and symptoms in a patient with chronic HF, despite previous stable background therapy • Requires urgent escalation of therapy, including hospitalization, ED visit, or outpatient IV diuretic therapy, ± outpatient oral therapy*	
Limitations and uncertainties with the current definition	**Potential future directions**
• Inability to detect asymptomatic but clinically meaningful worsening • Definition anchored to treatment provided rather than biology • Uncertain time horizon following WHF event to distinguish WHF vs. return to "stable" persistent HF • Unclear level of required background therapy to differentiate WHF from "untreated" HF • No consensus on definition of escalated oral therapy	• Continue efforts to establish an objective, reproducible, biologic definition of WHF (e.g., biomarkers, omics, risk models, implantable hemodynamic monitoring) • Perform clinical trials to inform management of WHF, including optimal escalation of existing therapies for chronic HF and use of novel therapies • Consider routine inclusion of WHF across various locations of care (i.e., inpatient and outpatient) within clinical trial eligibility criteria and endpoints

*Traditional definition focused on the receipt of intravenous (IV) diuretic therapy. Further data may be needed to operationalize outpatient escalation of oral therapies within a worsening heart failure (WHF) definition.

(ED: emergency department; HF: heart failure)

Source: Greene SJ, Bauersachs J, Brugts JJ, et al. Worsening Heart Failure: Nomenclature, Epidemiology, and Future Directions: JACC Review Topic of the Week. J Am Coll Cardiol. 2023;81(4):413-24.

TABLE 2: Recent clinical trials inclusive of patients with worsening heart failure (WHF).

Clinical trial	Study drugs	Inclusion criteria	Primary endpoint and duration	Primary endpoint result	Select secondary or exploratory endpoint results
PIONEER-HF	Sacubitril–valsartan vs. enalapril	Patients with HFrEF who were hospitalized for ADHF ($n = 881$)	Change in NT-proBNP from baseline through weeks 4 and 8	*Percent change in NT-proBNP concentration with sacubitril/valsartan*: −46.7% *Percent change with enalapril*: −25.3% • *Ratio of change*: 0.71 (95% CI 0.63–0.81); $p < 0.001$	*Cardiovascular death or HF hospitalization over 8 weeks*: • *Sacubitril/valsartan event rate*: 9.2% • *Enalapril event rate*: 15.2% • *HR 0.58 (95% CI 0.39–0.87)*; $p = 0.007$
AFFIRM-AHF	Ferric carboxymaltose (up to 24 weeks) vs. placebo	Patients with iron deficiency, LVEF <50%, and who were stabilized after an episode of AHF requiring hospitalization ($n = 1,110$)	Total hospitalizations for HF and CV death up to 52 weeks	*Ferric carboxymaltose event rate*: 57.2/100 patient-years *Placebo event rate*: 72.5/100 patient-years • *Rate ratio*: 0.79 (95% CI 0.62–1.01); $p = 0.059$	*Total HF hospitalizations*: • Ferric carboxymaltose: 217 *Placebo*: 294 • *Rate ratio*: 0.74 (95% CI 0.58–0.94); $p = 0.013$ cardiovascular death: • *Ferric carboxymaltose event rate*: 14% *Placebo event rate*: 14% • *HR* 0.96 (95% CI 0.70–1.32); $p = 0.81$
VICTORIA	Vericiguat vs. placebo	Patients with CHF (NYHA functional class II, III, or IV), EF <45%, and evidence of WHF ($n = 5,050$). WHF was defined as HF hospitalization within the prior 6 months, or receipt of IV diuretic therapy without hospitalization within the prior 3 months	Composite of CV death or first hospitalization for HF, over a median follow-up of 10.8 months	*Vericiguat event rate*: 33.6/100 patient-years *Placebo event rate*: 37.8/100 patient-years • *HR* 0.90 (95% CI 0.82–0.98); $p = 0.02$	*Hospitalization for HF*: • *Vericiguat event rate*: 25.9/100 patient-years *Placebo event rate*: 29.1/100 patient-years • *HR* 0.90 (95% CI 0.81–1.00) *Cardiovascular death*: • *Vericiguat event rate*: 12.9/100 patient-years *Placebo event rate*: 13.9/100 patient-years • *HR* 0.93 (95% CI 0.81–1.06) *Total HF hospitalizations*: • *Vericiguat*: 1,223 – *Placebo*: 1,336 • *HR* 0.91 (95% CI 0.84–0.99); $p = 0.02$
GALACTIC-HF	Omecamtiv mecarbil vs. placebo	Inpatients and outpatients with symptomatic CHF and an EF ≤35% ($n = 8,256$)	Composite of a first heart-failure event (hospitalization or urgent visit for HF) or CV death, over a median follow-up of 21.8 months	*Omecamtiv mecarbil event rate*: 24.2/100 patient-years *Placebo event rate*: 26.3/100 patient-years *HR* 0.92 (95% CI 0.86–0.99); $p = 0.03$	*WHF event*: • *Omecamtiv mecarbil event rate*: 18.7/100 patient-years *Placebo event rate*: 20.3/100 patient-years • *HR* 0.92 (95% CI 0.86–1.00) *Cardiovascular death*: • *Omecamtiv mecarbil event rate*: 10.9/100 patient-years *Placebo event rate*: 10.8/100 patient-years • *HR* 1.01 (95% CI 0.92–1.11); $p = 0.86$

Continued

Continued

Clinical trial	Study drugs	Inclusion criteria	Primary endpoint and duration	Primary endpoint result	Select secondary or exploratory endpoint results
SOLOIST-WHF	Sotagliflozin vs. placebo	Patients with type 2 diabetes mellitus who were recently hospitalized for WHF ($n = 1,222$)	Total CV deaths, hospitalizations for HF, and urgent visits for HF, over a median follow-up of 9 months	*Sotagliflozin event rate*: 51.0/100 patient-years *Placebo event rate*: 76.3/100 patient-years • HR 0.67 (95% CI 0.52–0.85); $p < 0.001$	Hospitalizations or urgent visits for HF: • *Sotagliflozin*: 194 • *Placebo*: 297 • Rate ratio: 0.64 (95% CI 0.49–0.83); $p <0.001$ *Cardiovascular death*: • *Sotagliflozin*: 51 • *Placebo*: 58 *HR* 0.84 (95% CI 0.58–1.22); $p = 0.36$
EMPULSE	Empagliflozin vs. placebo	Patients hospitalized for acute de novo or decompensated chronic HF ($n = 530$)	Composite of all-cause death, HF events, and ≥5-point change from baseline in KCCQ-TSS using a win ratio, at 90 days	Win ratio favored empagliflozin (1.36, 95% CI 1.09–1.68); $p = 0.005$	*Cardiovascular death or HF event*: • *Empagliflozin event rate*: 55.0/100 patient-years *Placebo event rate*: 80.45/100 patient-years • *HR* 0.69 (95% CI 0.45–1.08) Change from baseline in KCCQ-TSS • *Empagliflozin*: 36.19 • – *Placebo*: 31.73 – • *Adjusted mean difference*: 4.45 (95% CI 0.32–8.59)

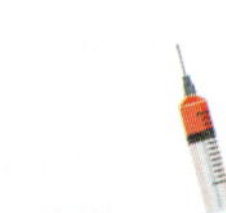

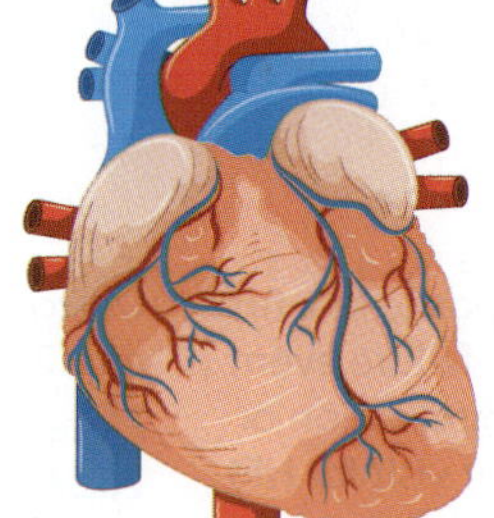

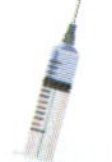

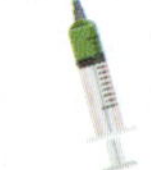

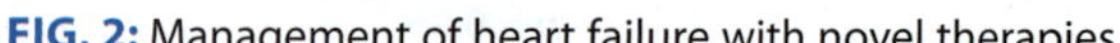

FIG. 2: Management of heart failure with novel therapies.

TABLE 3: Novel drug therapies with trials and findings.

Drug	Trials and main findings
Levosimendan	*LevoRep trial*: Intermittent levosimendan infusion did not significantly improve patients' functional capacity and quality of life *LION-HEART trial*: Intermittent levosimendan administration was effective in decreasing the serum concentration of NT-proBNP and was associated with improvement in clinical symptoms *LAICA study*: Repetitive levosimendan infusion is effective in reducing the HF hospitalization rate and HF worsening in patients with advanced HF *LeoDOR trial:* Repetitive levosimendan administration in patients with a recent HF hospitalization did not result in post-hospitalization clinical stability
Vericiguat	*VICTORIA trial*: The primary composite of death from cardiovascular causes or first hospitalization for HF was lower in those who received vericiguat
Omecamtiv mecarbil	*GALACTIC-HF trial*: The primary composite endpoint of hospitalization or urgent visit for HF and death from cardiovascular causes is reduced in patients treated with OM *METEORIC-HF trial*: OM did not increase exercise capacity after 20 weeks of treatment *COSMIC-HF trial*: Guiding the administration of OM through drug pharmacokinetic is associated with reduction in ventricular diameter and cardiac function improvement
Sotagliflozin	*SOLOIST-WHF trial*: The primary endpoint, a combination of total number of cardiovascular deaths, hospitalizations and urgent visits for HF, resulted lower, and the benefits of an early initiation of sotagliflozin, before or immediately after hospital discharge, was highlighted *SCORED trial*: Sotagliflozin reduced the composite endpoint of HF hospitalization, urgent ambulatory visit and cardiovascular death, along with major incidence of adverse events

ROLE OF DIGOXIN

- *What DIG (1997) did—and did not—show*:
    - *Population*: Chronic HFrEF in sinus rhythm, on background ACEi/diuretics (pre-beta-blocker era).
    - *Result*: No mortality benefit, but fewer HF hospitalizations with digoxin versus placebo.
- *What DIGIT-HF adds (digitoxin, ESC 2025)*:
    - *Population:* Symptomatic HFrEF (NYHA II–IV, LVEF ≤40%) on contemporary GDMT (ARNI/ACEi/ARB, β-blocker, MRA, SGLT-2i as used).
    - *Primary outcome (all-cause death or first HF hospitalization):* Reduced with digitoxin versus placebo (e.g., HR ~0.82; $p \approx 0.03$; absolute risk reduction ~4–5%).
    - A PubMed record (2025) likewise concludes that digitoxin lowered the combined risk of death or HF hospitalization versus placebo on top of GDMT.
- *Practical positioning (today)*:
    - *With DIGIT-HF*: Digitoxin now has randomized evidence suggesting improvement in a hard composite (death or first HF hospitalization) on top of modern GDMT, which is a step beyond the hospitalization-only signal from DIG. Guideline updates are pending; early expert coverage emphasizes that digitoxin could be a useful add-on in advanced HFrEF when further neurohormonal up-titration is limited (e.g., low BP, CKD), provided therapeutic monitoring and toxicity vigilance.

REPETITIVE LEVOSIMENDAN INFUSION IN WORSENING HEART FAILURE: THE ACHIEVEMENT OF HEMODYNAMIC STABILIZATION[3-6]

Mechanism of Action

- *Class*: Inodilator; calcium sensitizer with pleiotropic effects.
- *Active metabolite*: OR-1896
    - Produced via hepatic acetylation.
    - Plasma protein binding ~40%, half-life 75–80 hours.
    - Explains persistence of effects for 7–9 days post-infusion.

Molecular Actions

- *Inotropic effect*:
    - Sensitizes cardiac troponin C (cTnC) to Ca^{2+} binding.
    - Enhances systolic contractility without impairing diastolic relaxation.
    - Avoids excess intracellular Ca^{2+}, thus reducing risk of arrhythmias.
- *Vasodilatory effect*:
    - Opens ATP-dependent K^+ channels (K-ATP) in vascular smooth muscle.
    - Causes vasodilation (pulmonary, coronary, and systemic).

- Interaction with endothelial NO pathway contributes to vasodilation.
- *Phosphodiesterase-3 (PDE3) inhibition*:
  - Selective PDE3 inhibition → moderate rise in cAMP and intracellular Ca^{2+}.
  - Additional positive inotropic effect, depending on PDE localization.
- *Other organ benefits*:
  - Improves renal function and peripheral organ perfusion.
  - Key role in critically ill and advanced HF patients.

Key Clinical Trials of Intermittent Levosimendan in Worsening Heart Failure

LEVOREP (2013, Altenberger et al.)[7]

- *Design*: Multicenter, randomized, and double-blind ($n = 120$).
- *Population*: NYHA III–IV, LVEF ≤35%, poor 6 MWT.
- *Intervention*: Repetitive outpatient infusions.
- *Endpoints*: Composite of ≥20% improvement in 6MWT + ≥15% KCCQ improvement.
- *Results*:
  - No significant improvement in functional capacity or QoL.
  - Similar adverse events in both groups (tachycardia, arrhythmias).
  - More drop in SBP in Levosimendan group.
- *Conclusion*: Neutral trial.

LION-HEART (2016, Comín-Colet et al.)[8]

- *Design*: Multicenter, randomized, and double-blind ($n = 69$, 2:1).
- *Intervention*: 6-hour IV infusion every 2 weeks × 12 weeks.
- *Primary outcome*: NT-proBNP reduction.
- *Results*:
  - Significant reduction in NT-proBNP
  - Clinical symptom improvement
- *Conclusion*: Positive biochemical and symptomatic effects.

LAICA (2017, García-González et al.)[9]

- *Design*: Multicenter, randomized ($n = 213$, 3:1).
- *Intervention*: 24-hour infusion once monthly × 12 months.
- *Endpoints*: HF rehospitalization, death, NYHA class, NT-proBNP, QoL.
- *Results*:
  - Reduced HF hospitalization and worsening events.
  - Suggested safety and benefit in advanced HF.
- *Conclusion*: Favorable for reducing decompensation.

LeoDOR (2021)[10]

- *Design*: Multicenter, randomized ($n = 264$, 2:1).
- *Intervention*: 6-hour versus 24-hour infusion every 2 weeks × 12 weeks.
- *Primary endpoint*: Composite (death, urgent transplant/VAD, non-fatal HF events, and NT-proBNP).
- *Results*: Did not show significant post-hospitalization stability benefit.
- *Conclusion*: Neutral trial.

Other Uses

Bridge-to-optimization: May allow initiation/titration of guideline-directed HF therapies in patients previously intolerant (Masarone et al.).

INNOVATIVE PHARMACOLOGICAL TARGETS IN WORSENING HEART FAILURE

Vericiguat

- *Mechanism*: Stimulates soluble guanylate cyclase (sGC), enhancing the NO–sGC–cGMP pathway.
- *Effect*: Improves vasodilation, reduces fibrosis, hypertrophy, and cardiac remodeling.
- *VICTORIA trial (2020):*[11]
  - Enrolled 5050 patients with LVEF <45% and recent WHF.
  - 10% reduction in CV death or first HF hospitalization versus placebo.
  - Most effective in patients with moderate NT-proBNP levels.

Omecamtiv Mecarbil

- *Mechanism*: Direct cardiac myosin activator improves systolic function without increasing Ca^{2+} or O_2 demand.
- *GALACTIC-HF trial:*[12] Reduced composite of CV death or HF events.
- *Cosmic-HF and meteoric-HF trials:*[13,14]
  - Improved systolic function but no effect on exercise capacity.
  - Safe in patients with cardiorenal syndrome.

Sotagliflozin

- *Mechanism*: Dual SGLT-1 and SGLT-2 inhibitor.
- Lowers glucose, reduces inflammation, and improves cardiac metabolism.
- *SOLOIST-WHF trial:*[15] Reduced CV deaths, hospitalizations, and urgent visits in T2DM patients with recent WHF.
- *SCORED trial:*[16] Benefit in T2DM with CKD; reduced adverse CV outcomes.

These emerging therapies offer *targeted benefits* in WHF, especially in high-risk, symptomatic patients with limited response to conventional therapy **(Fig. 3)**.

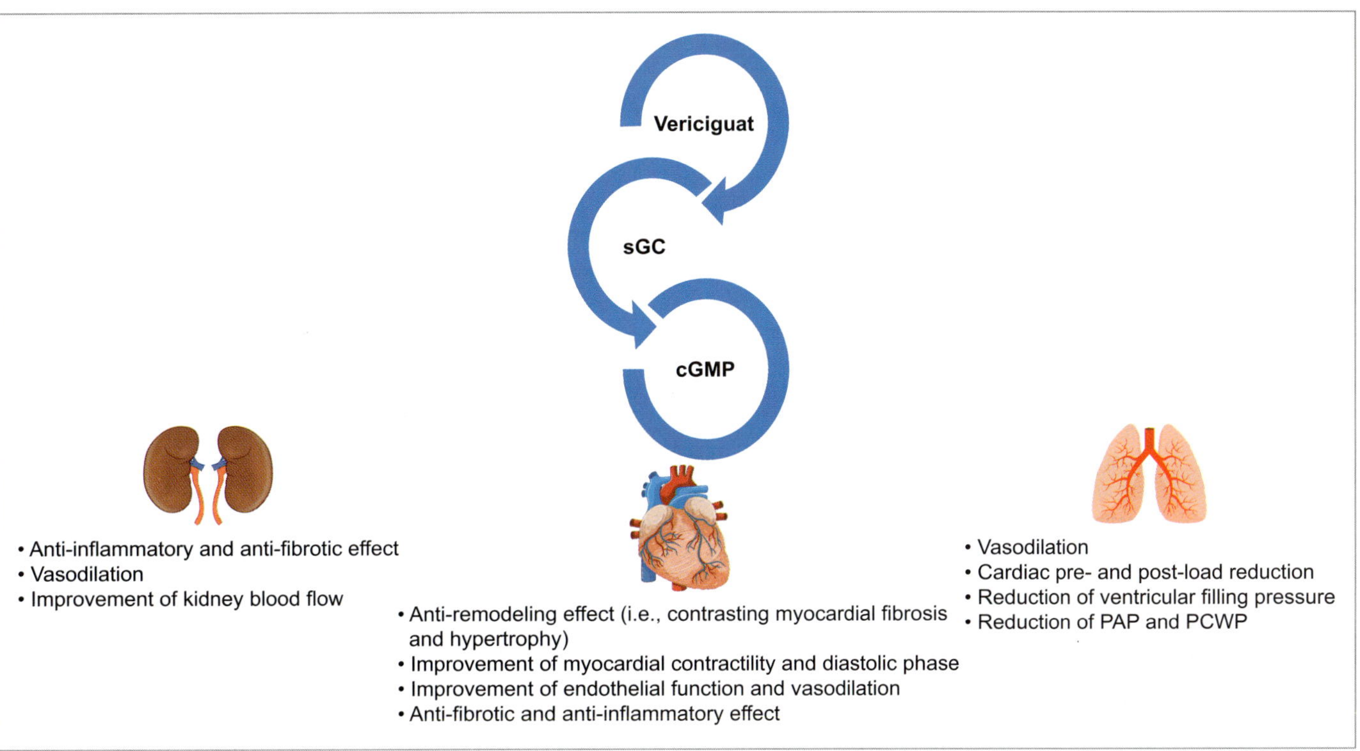

FIG. 3: Therapies for management of congestion in heart failure.

MANAGEMENT OF CONGESTION IN HEART FAILURE: DIURETICS AND INNOVATIVE STRATEGIES

Persistent congestion in WHF is strongly associated with early readmission and poor prognosis. Loop diuretics remain the first-line therapy, inhibiting Na^+-K^+-$2Cl^-$ transport in the loop of Henle. The *DOSE trial* recommended IV loop diuretics at 2.5× the oral dose for better symptom relief, though it did not meet its primary endpoints. The *TRANSFORM-HF trial* found no mortality difference between torsemide and furosemide, suggesting the dose may matter more than the agent.

Emerging therapies such as *SGLT-2 inhibitors* (e.g., empagliflozin and dapagliflozin) have shown promise. Trials such as *EMPAG-HF, EMPA-RESPONSE-AHF*, and *EMPULSE* demonstrated increased urine output and reduced NT-proBNP without worsening renal function. *DAPA-RESPONSE-AHF* echoed these benefits with dapagliflozin **(Table 4)**.

Acetazolamide, a proximal tubule diuretic, enhanced decongestion when combined with loop diuretics in the *ADVOR trial*, though its combination with SGLT-2i is still unstudied. *Hydrochlorothiazide (HCTZ)* also improved urinary output and weight loss in the *CLOROTIC trial* but increased renal impairment risk.

Finerenone, a novel non-steroidal MRA, showed cardiovascular and renal benefits in patients with diabetes and CKD in *FIDELIO-DKD* and *FIGARO-DKD* trials. The *ARTS-HF trial* reported its safety and efficacy in WHF patients with CKD or diabetes.

These findings underscore the evolving landscape of *diuretic optimization* and *combination strategies* in HF management.

ADVANCES IN REMOTE MONITORING TECHNOLOGIES FOR HEART FAILURE MANAGEMENT

Remote hemodynamic monitoring is transforming HF management, allowing earlier detection of decompensation and timely therapeutic adjustments. One of the most established technologies in this field is *CardioMEMS*, an implantable sensor placed in the pulmonary artery that transmits *real-time pulmonary artery pressure (PAP)* data to healthcare providers.

The *CHAMPION trial* demonstrated that daily PAP-guided therapy using CardioMEMS significantly reduced HF hospitalizations in NYHA class III patients with a recent HF admission, with excellent safety outcomes—98.6% freedom from complications and 100% sensor reliability.

The *MONITOR-HF trial* conducted in the era of optimized medical therapy, confirmed the added value of CardioMEMS in improving *quality of life*, as shown by significant improvements in *KCCQ-12 scores*, even in patients receiving quadruple HF therapy.

TABLE 4: Therapies for management of congestion in heart failure.

Drug	Trials and main findings
SGLT-2i	*EMPAG-HF*: In patients with acute decompensated HF, the early initiation of empagliflozin on top of standard diuretic improves urinary output *EMPA-RESPONSE-AHF*: In acute HF patients, the use of empagliflozin is associated with reduction in WHF, death and rehospitalization, and increased urinary output *EMPULSE trial*: Starting empagliflozin in patients admitted for AHF is associated with early and effective decongestion *DAPA-RESPONSE-AHF*: In patients with acute HF, dapagliflozin is associated with diuresis and symptoms improvement
Acetazolamide	*ADVOR trial*: In patients with acute decompensated HF, the addition of acetazolamide on top of furosemide is associated with increased rate of decongestion
HCTZ	*CLOROTIC trial*: Patients treated with HCTZ on top of intravenous furosemide show significant weight loss and better 24 hours urinary output, but no difference in terms of dyspnea
Finerenone	*FIDELIO-DKD*: Finerenone reduces the risk of kidney disease progression and cardiovascular events, including HF hospitalization, in patients with diabetes mellitus and chronic kidney disease *FIGARO-DKD*: Finerenone reduces the incidence of new HF and improved HF outcomes in patients with diabetes mellitus and chronic kidney disease, regardless of HF presence *ARTS-HF*: Finerenone determines a significant reduction in NT-proBNP levels in patients with WHF and diabetes mellitus and/or chronic kidney disease

TABLE 5: Devices with trials and findings.

Device	Trials and main findings
CardioMEMS	*CHAMPION trial*: Significant reduction in HF hospital admissions in patients with daily PAP monitoring through CardioMEMS was observed *MONITOR-HF trial*: CardioMEMS improves the QoL of HF patients with a significant increase in KCCQ-12 score *EMBRACE-HF trial*: A prompt reduction in PAP in patients treated with empagliflozin and monitored with CardioMEMS was observed
V-LAP	*VECTOR-HF study*: A significant correlation was found between the mean LA pressure and mean PCWP
CCM	*FIX-HF-4 study and FIX-HF-5*: CCM is safe and effective in improving exercise tolerance and QoL, while reducing HF hospitalizations
BAT	*BeAT-HF study and HOPE4HF study*: BAT therapy significantly improves QoL, exercise capacity and reduces NT-proBNP levels

The *EMBRACE-HF trial* explored CardioMEMS in conjunction with empagliflozin, showing a *rapid reduction in pulmonary pressures*, confirming its decongestive effect.

Beyond CardioMEMS, *left atrial pressure monitoring* with devices such as *V-LAP* is gaining interest, particularly in HFpEF. The *VECTOR-HF study* showed a strong correlation between V-LAP measurements and invasive pressure readings, with improvements in NYHA class and QoL.

Emerging devices such as the *FIRE1 system*, which monitors the *inferior vena cava* for fluid overload, are still in early stages, with ongoing animal studies.

These innovations highlight the shift toward precision, proactive HF care, leveraging continuous data to optimize therapy and prevent hospitalizations.

WHEN PHARMACOLOGICAL THERAPY IS NOT ENOUGH: CARDIAC CONTRACTILITY MODULATION AND BAROREFLEX ACTIVATION THERAPY

For heart failure patients who remain symptomatic despite optimal medical therapy (OMT), particularly those with LVEF between 25 and 45% and non-LBBB QRS morphology, cardiac contractility modulation (CCM) offers a novel device-based option.

Unlike CRT or pacemakers, CCM delivers non-excitatory electrical impulses during the absolute refractory period, improving intracellular calcium handling and myocardial contractility without increasing oxygen demand.

The FIX-HF-4 trial demonstrated that CCM significantly improved exercise tolerance and quality of life in patients with HFrEF, with no significant difference in adverse events. Similarly, the FIX-HF-5 trial confirmed that CCM, when added to OMT, reduced HF hospitalizations and enhanced functional capacity **(Table 5)**.

Despite promising results, limitations such as short follow-up and a predominantly younger, male cohort suggest the need for further large-scale studies to assess long-term outcomes and mortality benefits.

Meanwhile, baroreflex activation therapy (BAT) targets the autonomic imbalance in HF by stimulating baroreceptors, leading to reduced sympathetic tone and increased parasympathetic activity.

The Barostim Neo™ system has shown efficacy in reducing NT-proBNP, improving NYHA class, and enhancing exercise capacity, as supported by both the HOPE4HF and BeAT-HF trials.

Together, CCM and BAT expand the therapeutic toolbox for patients with advanced HF who are not candidates for CRT, offering symptom relief and potential reductions in hospitalization.

CONCLUSION

Worsening heart failure remains a turning point that signals increased vulnerability and adverse outcomes. The current hospitalization-based definitions are inadequate, as many patients deteriorate silently or in outpatient care. Incorporating biomarkers, remote monitoring, and individualized diuretic strategies can help us identify decompensation earlier. Novel therapies such as vericiguat, sotagliflozin, and digitoxin, along with device-based options such as CardioMEMS and CCM, provide us with valuable additions when conventional therapy is exhausted. Going forward, a proactive, precision-driven approach is essential to reduce readmissions and improve survival in this high-risk group.

REFERENCES

1. Greene SJ, Bauersachs J, Brugts JJ, et al. Worsening Heart Failure: Nomenclature, Epidemiology, and Future Directions: JACC Review Topic of the Week. J Am Coll Cardiol. 2023;81(4):413-24.
2. Metra M, Tomasoni D, Adamo M, et al. Worsening of chronic heart failure: Definition, epidemiology, management and prevention. A clinical consensus statement by the Heart Failure Association of the European Society of Cardiology. Eur J Heart Fail. 2023;25: 776-91.
3. Antoniades C, Tousoulis D, Koumallos N, et al. Levosimendan: Beyond its simple inotropic effect in heart failure. Pharmacol Ther. 2007;114:184-97.
4. Papp Z, Édes I, Fruhwald S, et al. Levosimendan: Molecular mechanisms and clinical implications: Consensus of experts on the mechanisms of action of levosimendan. Int J Cardiol. 2012;159:82-7.
5. Yilmaz MB, Grossini E, Silva Cardoso JC, et al. Renal effects of levosimendan: A consensus report. Cardiovasc Drugs Ther. 2013;27:581-90.
6. Heringlake M, Alvarez J, Bettex D, et al. An update on levosimendan in acute cardiac care: Applications and recommendations for optimal efficacy and safety. Expert Rev Cardiovasc Ther. 2021;19:325-35.
7. Altenberger J, Parissis JT, Costard-Jaeckle A, et al. Efficacy and safety of the pulsed infusions of levosimendan in outpatients with advanced heart failure (LevoRep) study: A multicentre randomized trial. Eur J Heart Fail. 2014;16:898-906.
8. Comín-Colet J, Manito N, Segovia-Cubero J, et al. Efficacy and safety of intermittent intravenous outpatient administration of levosimendan in patients with advanced heart failure: The LION-HEART multicentre randomised trial. Eur J Heart Fail. 2018;20:1128-36.
9. García-González MJ, de Mora-Martín M, López-Fernández S, et al. Rationale and design of a randomized, double-blind, placebo controlled multicenter trial to study efficacy, security, and long term effects of intermittent repeated levosimendan administration in patients with advanced heart failure: LAICA study. Cardiovasc Drugs Ther. 2013;27:573-9.
10. Pölzl G, Altenberger J, Comín-Colet J, et al. Repetitive levosimendan infusions for patients with advanced chronic heart failure in the vulnerable post-discharge period: The multinational randomized LeoDOR trial. Eur J Heart Fail. 2023;25:2007-17.
11. Planelles-Herrero VJ, Hartman JJ, Robert-Paganin J, et al. Mechanistic and structural basis for activation of cardiac myosin force production by omecamtiv mecarbil. Nat Commun. 2017;8:190.
12. Teerlink JR, Felker GM, McMurray JJ, et al. Chronic Oral Study of Myosin Activation to Increase Contractility in Heart Failure (COSMIC-HF): A phase 2, pharmacokinetic, randomised, placebo-controlled trial. Lancet. 2016;388:2895-903.
13. Teerlink JR, Diaz R, Felker GM, et al. Omecamtiv Mecarbil in Chronic Heart Failure with Reduced Ejection Fraction: Rationale and Design of GALACTIC-HF. JACC Heart Fail. 2020;8:329-40.
14. Lewis GD, Voors AA, Cohen-Solal A, et al. Effect of Omecamtiv Mecarbil on Exercise Capacity in Chronic Heart Failure with Reduced Ejection Fraction: The METEORIC-HF Randomized Clinical Trial. JAMA. 2022;328:259-69.
15. Bhatt DL, Szarek M, Steg PG, et al. Sotagliflozin in Patients with Diabetes and Recent Worsening Heart Failure. N Engl J Med. 2021;384:117-28.
16. Bhatt DL, Szarek M, Pitt B, et al. Sotagliflozin in Patients with Diabetes and Chronic Kidney Disease. N Engl J Med. 2021;384: 129-39.

CHAPTER 19

Pulmonary Hypertension in Heart Failure: The Good, the Bad, and the Ugly

A Purnanand

ABSTRACT

Pulmonary hypertension (PH) is a common and prognostically significant complication of heart failure (HF). This chapter reviews the hemodynamic classification of PH in HF—distinguishing isolated postcapillary PH (IpcPH) from combined post- and precapillary PH (CpcPH)—and the clinical implications of these phenotypes. We discuss the recent lowering of hemodynamic thresholds for defining PH, which has increased the recognized prevalence of PH in HF and improved risk stratification. IpcPH and CpcPH are contrasted in terms of pathophysiology and prognosis, with CpcPH "the ugly" portending worse outcomes than IpcPH "the bad", and the absence of PH "the good" being associated with the most favorable prognosis. Current clinical management focuses on optimizing HF therapy and addressing underlying causes, as dedicated pulmonary vasodilators have not shown benefit in PH due to left heart disease. We highlight recent trials and guideline updates, including the 2022 ESC/ERS guidelines that incorporate new hemodynamic definitions and emphasize treating the HF rather than adding PAH-specific drugs. Emerging approaches—such as implantable hemodynamic monitors, novel pharmacotherapies under investigation, and interventional strategies—are discussed, along with a roadmap for future research.

Keywords: Heart failure, pulmonary hypertension, hemodynamic classification, postcapillary PH, right ventricular dysfunction, HFpEF.

INTRODUCTION

Pulmonary hypertension (PH) is a common complication of heart failure (HF), seen in up to 80% of advanced cases and affecting both HFrEF and heart failure with preserved ejection fraction (HFpEF). Elevated left-heart filling pressures cause postcapillary PH, which may progress to combined PH due to pulmonary vascular remodeling.[1] This results in right ventricular dysfunction and systemic complications. Recent updates from the ESC/ERS redefine PH with lower hemodynamic thresholds and distinguish isolated postcapillary PH (IpcPH) from combined post- and precapillary PH (CpcPH). These classifications reflect a continuum of risk. This chapter examines the evolving understanding of PH in HF and reviews prognostic, diagnostic, and management strategies based on current evidence.[2]

HEMODYNAMIC CLASSIFICATION IN HEART FAILURE-ASSOCIATED PULMONARY HYPERTENSION

Definition and updated criteria: Pulmonary hypertension due to left HF (classified as group 2 PH) is defined hemodynamically by an elevated mean pulmonary arterial pressure (mPAP) *>20 mm Hg* (at rest) in the presence of high left-sided filling pressure [pulmonary artery wedge pressure (PAWP) *>15 mm Hg*].[2,3] This definition was revised from the older threshold of mPAP ≥25 mm Hg, based on data indicating that even mPAP 21–24 mm Hg is above normal and is associated with worse outcomes.[4-6] In addition, the 2022 ESC/ERS guidelines lowered the cutoff for abnormal pulmonary vascular resistance (PVR) from >3 wood units (WUs) to *>2 WUs* to identify cases with a significant precapillary component. Within PH-HF, two hemodynamic phenotypes are recognized:

- *IpcPH:* mPAP >20 mm Hg with PAWP >15 mm Hg, and a PVR ≤2 WUs. This reflects PH purely due to elevated left heart pressures (a "passive" backward transmission of pressure) without significant intrinsic pulmonary arteriolar disease.
- *CpcPH:* mPAP >20 mm Hg, PAWP >15 mm Hg, and PVR >2 WUs. This denotes a mixed picture where, in addition to left-sided pressure elevation, there is increased PVR, implicating pulmonary vascular remodeling, and reactive vasoconstriction. CpcPH was previously defined by PVR >3 WUs; lowering the threshold to >2 WUs has substantially increased the recognized prevalence of CpcPH in HF.

PREVALENCE AND IMPACT OF THE NEW DEFINITION

The 2022 ESC/ERS guidelines introduced significant changes in the hemodynamic criteria used to define PH in HF, notably lowering the mPAP threshold from ≥25 mm Hg to >20 mm Hg and reducing the PVR cutoff from >3 to >2 WUs. Applying these updated definitions has substantially increased the proportion of HF patients identified with PH, particularly those reclassified as having CpcPH.[1,4]

In the 2024 PH-HF multicenter study involving 662 HF patients undergoing right heart catheterization (RHC), the prevalence of postcapillary PH increased from 83.8 to 91.5% with the revised mPAP threshold. More strikingly, the prevalence of CpcPH rose from 42.0 to 67.2% after applying the lower PVR cutoff—a relative increase of 60%. These newly reclassified patients, previously diagnosed with IpcPH, were found to have significantly worse event-free survival. Even mild elevations of mPAP (21–24 mm Hg) or PVR (2–3 WUs) were associated with adverse outcomes. The optimal PVR threshold for predicting HF-related events was ~2.2 WUs, confirming the validity of the new definition.[2,5]

These findings are consistent with data from other international cohorts. For instance, a UK registry study demonstrated that patients with mPAP >20 mm Hg or PVR >2 WUs had reduced survival compared to those below these thresholds. This reinforces the importance of early identification and classification of PH severity in HF populations.[6]

Ultimately, the revised criteria enhance prognostication, reclassify high-risk patients more accurately, and emphasize that even modest elevations in pulmonary pressure or resistance should prompt closer monitoring and more aggressive HF management.[6,7]

CLINICAL ASSESSMENT AND DIAGNOSTIC APPROACH

Identifying PH in a patient with HF requires a high index of suspicion and careful hemodynamic assessment. Many signs and symptoms of PH overlap with those of HF (e.g., dyspnea, fatigue, and edema), making it challenging to distinguish whether a patient's limitations are due to HF alone or HF with significant PH. The clinical evaluation should integrate history, physical examination, and noninvasive testing to estimate the probability of PH-LHD, followed by confirmation with invasive hemodynamic monitoring when indicated.[1-4]

Screening and noninvasive evaluation: Transthoracic *echocardiography* is the best screening tool for PH in HF. Echocardiography can estimate pulmonary artery systolic pressure (PASP) from tricuspid regurgitant velocity and assess signs of RV pressure overload (such as RV dilation or interventricular septal flattening). Elevated PASP on echo (e.g., >40–50 mm Hg) in a patient with known HF raises suspicion for PH, although echo estimates can be imprecise. The 2022 ESC/ERS guidelines outline a structured three-step diagnostic algorithm: (1) *Clinical suspicion*—identify high-risk features for PH-HF such as long-standing HF symptoms, atrial fibrillation (AF), older age, obesity, or left atrial enlargement; (2) *Detection by echocardiography*—assess the probability of PH based on TR jet velocity and other echo signs; (3) *Confirmation by RHC*—in patients with intermediate or high PH probability, especially if PH severity could influence management. Patients with HF and signs of significant PH or RV dysfunction should be referred to a specialized PH center for comprehensive evaluation, including invasive assessment **(Flowchart 1)**.[5-7]

Pulmonary function tests and high-resolution CT may be done to evaluate coexisting lung disease if suspicion for combined group 2+3 PH (HF + pulmonary disease) exists.

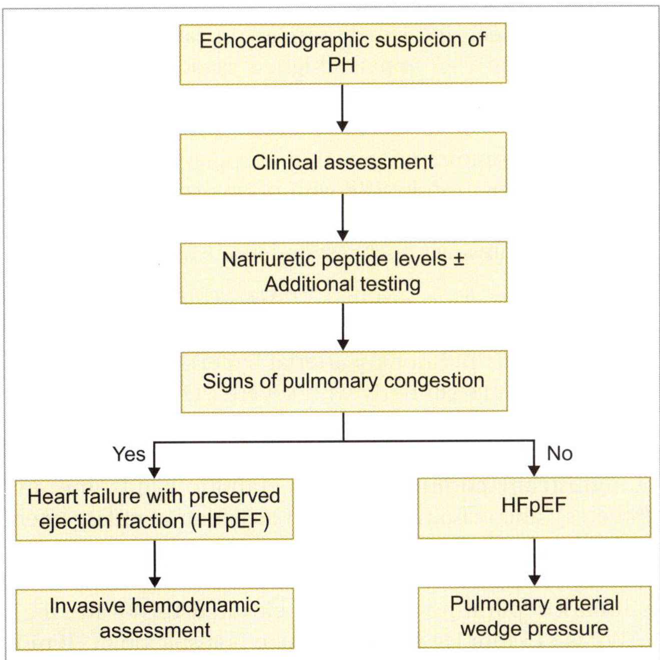

FLOWCHART 1: Diagnostic pathway for PH in HF (based on ESC/ERS guidelines).
(HF: heart failure; PH: pulmonary hypertension)

Ventilation/perfusion (V/Q) scan is recommended in all PH evaluations to screen for chronic thromboembolic PH (CTEPH); in an HF patient, an abnormal V/Q might suggest an alternative or coexisting cause of PH.[1,4]

Hemodynamic confirmation with RHC: Right heart catheterization is required to definitively diagnose PH and classify it as IpcPH versus CpcPH. RHC directly measures PA pressures, PAWP, and cardiac output, allowing calculation of PVR. In HF patients, careful attention must be paid to accurate PAWP measurement (properly timed at end-expiration) to avoid misclassification. If PAWP is borderline (in the 13–15 mm Hg range) and the clinical picture suggests HF (e.g., history of hypertension, AF, and LV hypertrophy on echo), additional provocative testing can unmask occult HF. Two commonly used maneuvers are: *Fluid challenge*—administering 500 mL of IV saline over 5 minutes during RHC. In normal subjects, PAWP rises only slightly; in HFpEF, PAWP will often rise above 18 mm Hg with this preload stress. An abnormal PAWP response to fluid (≥18–20 mm Hg) indicates left heart disease as the cause of PH. *Exercise challenge*—having the patient perform supine leg exercise during RHC while measuring pressures. A PAWP ≥25 mm Hg during exercise is suggestive of HFpEF rather than primary pulmonary vascular disease. Exercise hemodynamics can be technically challenging, so fluid loading is an easier alternative in many laboratories.[6-8]

If the RHC reveals PH with elevated PAWP, then by definition it is PH-LHD (group 2). The next step is to calculate PVR to subtype into IpcPH or CpcPH as discussed. It is also a good practice to measure directly the left ventricular end-diastolic pressure (LVEDP) if possible (by crossing into the left ventricle), when PAWP is high, to corroborate that the wedge accurately reflects left-sided pressure. In cases where PAWP is elevated and PVR appears high, a vasodilator challenge (e.g., inhaled nitric oxide or intravenous nitroprusside) can sometimes be tried to see if PVR drops significantly—though this is more commonly done in precapillary PH. In PH due to HF, a drastic drop in PVR with normalizing PAWP might indicate a large reversible vasoconstrictive component **Flowchart 2** (however, such responders are rare in practice).[7,8]

Differentiating from group 1 (PAH): One of the critical challenges is distinguishing advanced HFpEF + CpcPH from idiopathic pulmonary arterial hypertension (PAH), as they can present similarly with severe PH and RV failure. Clues favoring HF as the cause of PH include older age (>60 years), history of hypertension or AF, presence of significant comorbidities (metabolic syndrome and diabetes), and echo findings such as left atrial enlargement or LV hypertrophy. In PAH, patients are often younger and lack overt left-heart disease signs. The hemodynamic hallmark separating them is an elevated PAWP in HF. If PAWP is ≤15 mm Hg at rest but there is suspicion of HFpEF, the aforementioned fluid or exercise challenge can reveal latent elevation in left-sided pressures. Current guidelines emphasize the importance of invasive testing in any patient

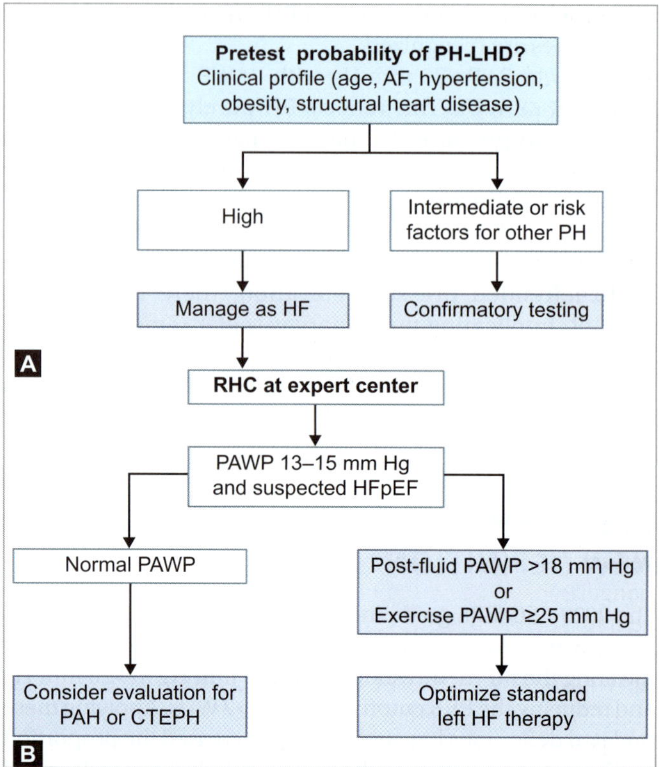

FLOWCHARTS 2A AND B: Hemodynamic diagnostic algorithm for PH due to HFpEF. (A) Determine the pretest probability of PH-LHD based on clinical profile (age, AF, hypertension, obesity, and structural heart disease). If probability is high, manage as HF; if intermediate or risk factors for other PH present, proceed to confirmatory testing. (B) Perform RHC at an expert center for definitive diagnosis. If PAWP is borderline (13–15 mm Hg) in a patient with suspected HFpEF, perform a provocative test (exercise or volume challenge) to detect occult elevation of left-sided filling pressures. A post-fluid PAWP >18 mm Hg or exercise PAWP ≥25 mm Hg confirms HF as the driver of PH. Standard left HF therapy should be optimized in all cases. Only if hemodynamics clearly indicates a precapillary profile (normal PAWP) should one consider evaluation for PAH or CTEPH causes.

(AF: atrial fibrillation; HF: heart failure; HFpEF: heart failure with preserved ejection fraction; PAH: pulmonary arterial hypertension; PAWP: pulmonary artery wedge pressure; PH: pulmonary hypertension)

Source: Adapted from the 6th World Symposium recommendations.

with suspected PH and risk factors for HFpEF, to avoid mistakenly diagnosing PAH and exposing the patient to inappropriate therapy.[8,9]

CLINICAL MANAGEMENT STRATEGIES

The cornerstone of managing PH in the setting of HF is optimal treatment of the underlying cardiac dysfunction. Unlike pulmonary arterial hypertension (PAH, group 1), where targeted pulmonary vasodilators are a mainstay, there is no approved therapy specifically aimed at reducing pulmonary pressure in PH due to HF (group 2), independent of treating the underlying HF. Current international guidelines explicitly discourage the use of PAH-targeted drugs (e.g., endothelin receptor antagonists, phosphodiesterase-5 inhibitors, and prostacyclin analogs) in PH-HF patients outside clinical trials, primarily due to lack of efficacy and potential harm. The clinical focus, therefore, is firmly on aggressive HF management, which in many cases can improve or even resolve PH if it is largely passive and postcapillary in nature (IpcPH).[1,2]

GUIDELINE-DIRECTED HEART FAILURE THERAPY

All patients with HF-associated PH should be placed on guideline-directed heart failure therapy (GDMT) tailored to their HF phenotype. For patients with reduced ejection fraction (HFrEF), therapy includes ACE inhibitors or angiotensin receptor–neprilysin inhibitors (ARNIs), β-blockers, mineralocorticoid receptor antagonists (MRAs), and SGLT-2 inhibitors. These agents not only improve survival but also reduce left-sided filling pressures and pulmonary venous congestion, which in turn lowers mPAP. In HFpEF, diuretics remain the cornerstone for symptom relief through volume control, while management of comorbid conditions—such as hypertension, diabetes, and obesity—is crucial due to the lack of robust HFpEF-targeted medications.[3,4]

The emergence of *SGLT-2 inhibitors* as a therapeutic breakthrough in HFpEF is particularly promising. The EMBRACE-HF trial demonstrated that empagliflozin significantly reduced pulmonary artery diastolic pressure (PADP) by approximately 1.5–2 mm Hg over 12 weeks in patients with HF and implanted pulmonary artery pressure (PAP) sensors. Other studies have linked SGLT-2 inhibitors to reductions in pulmonary capillary wedge pressure (PCWP) both at rest and during exercise, likely due to their natriuretic, osmotic, and vascular effects.[4-6]

Management must also include meticulous volume optimization using diuretics and dietary sodium restriction, as well as addressing rhythm disturbances. Rate or rhythm control of AF, which is common in HFpEF, may improve left ventricular diastolic function and reduce left atrial pressures, indirectly lowering pulmonary pressures.

INTERVENTIONS FOR CORRECTABLE CAUSES

In cases where PH is driven by a specific cardiac lesion such as mitral regurgitation or aortic stenosis, *early intervention* is essential. Surgical or transcatheter correction—such as mitral valve repair or transcatheter aortic valve replacement (TAVR)—can substantially reduce left atrial pressure and potentially reverse pulmonary venous hypertension. However, if pulmonary vascular remodeling has already occurred (CpcPH), PH may persist despite correction of the underlying lesion.[4,7]

Recent data from patients undergoing mitral clip repair indicate that the presence of preprocedural PH is associated with higher rates of postprocedure mortality and recurrent HF hospitalization, emphasizing the value of timely referral before PH becomes irreversible.[7-9]

MONITORING AND FOLLOW-UP

Given the prognostic significance of PAP in HF, *hemodynamic-guided therapy* has gained traction. Remote monitoring using implantable wireless PAP sensors (e.g., CardioMEMS) allows clinicians to track pulmonary pressures and adjust therapy proactively. Both clinical trials and real-world evidence (e.g., CHAMPION and MEMS-HF) have demonstrated that PAP-guided management reduces HF-related hospitalizations in both HFrEF and HFpEF patients. These benefits extend across PH phenotypes, including both IpcPH and CpcPH. In the MEMS-HF subanalysis, SGLT-2 inhibitors were shown to significantly lower PAP in monitored patients, suggesting a synergistic role for these agents in targeted HF-PH management.[10,11]

PULMONARY VASODILATOR THERAPIES—TRIALS AND GUIDELINES

Despite their theoretical appeal, *PAH-specific pulmonary vasodilators* have not shown consistent benefit in PH due to HF:

- *PDE-5 inhibitors* (e.g., sildenafil and tadalafil) have failed to demonstrate improved outcomes in large trials. The RELAX trial showed no benefit in exercise capacity, and the more recent PASSION trial of tadalafil in CpcPH was terminated early. Alarmingly, a higher mortality rate was observed in the treatment arm (15% vs. 3%), raising significant safety concerns. The SioVAC trial similarly showed harm with sildenafil after valvular surgery. Consequently, guidelines recommend against PDE-5 inhibitors in IpcPH and caution against their use in CpcPH outside research settings.
- *Soluble guanylate cyclase stimulators* (e.g., riociguat) showed modest hemodynamic benefit in early studies but were associated with hypotension and have not progressed to approval for group 2 PH.
- *Endothelin receptor antagonists* (e.g., bosentan and macitentan) have either failed to show benefit or led to adverse effects like fluid retention, as seen in the MELODY-1 trial.
- *Prostacyclin analogs* are contraindicated in PH-HF due to the risk of precipitating pulmonary edema. Their only use may be as a temporary bridge to transplant in inpatient settings for selected patients.

ADVANCED HEART FAILURE THERAPIES

For patients with *refractory HF and severe PH, heart transplantation* or *mechanical circulatory support* is considered. However, elevated PVR poses a major challenge for isolated heart transplant, as it increases the risk of right ventricular failure in the allograft. Pretransplant strategies to lower PVR—such as intravenous inotropes, vasodilators, or *left ventricular assist device (LVAD)* implantation—can improve transplant eligibility.

Left ventricular assist devices reduce left-sided filling pressures, often resulting in partial reversal of PH over several weeks. Patients with initially contraindicating PVR may become transplant-eligible post-LVAD. In rare, end-stage cases with fixed PH unresponsive to LV unloading, *heart-lung transplantation* may be considered, though limited by organ availability and surgical risk.[9,10]

INVESTIGATIONAL INTERVENTIONAL THERAPIES

Innovative device-based interventions are under investigation. *Interatrial shunt devices* (e.g., IASD) create a controlled communication between the left and right atria to decompress the left atrium and lower PAWP. Trials such as REDUCE LAP-HF II and RELIEVE-HF have shown hemodynamic improvements, but results on clinical endpoints have been mixed. In some studies, shunt recipients had higher event rates, possibly due to increased right heart volume load.

These devices are not yet approved, and future research is needed to identify suitable subgroups—such as patients with markedly elevated PAWP and preserved RV function. Additionally, treating comorbidities such as obstructive sleep apnea (OSA) and obesity in HFpEF may offer ancillary PH benefits by lowering pulmonary vascular load.[8,9]

EMERGING THERAPIES AND FUTURE DIRECTIONS

Given the unsatisfactory results of pulmonary vasodilators so far, there is a strong impetus for *new approaches* to PH in HF. Recent consensus statements provide a roadmap for future research. The Heart Failure Association (HFA) of the ESC in 2024 published a comprehensive roadmap highlighting strategies to discover effective therapies for PH-HF. Key directions include:

- *Phenotype-driven trials:* Recognizing that HFpEF with PH is a heterogeneous population, future studies may target specific phenotypes (e.g., CpcPH with PVR >5 WUs, or those with certain biomarker profiles). Enriching trials with patients who have more "active" pulmonary vascular disease might increase the chance of detecting a drug effect, as they have room for pulmonary vascular improvement.v
- *Combination therapies and novel targets:* Researchers are exploring drugs beyond the traditional PAH classes. Some novel agents under investigation include pulmonary vasodilators that also have antifibrotic or antiremodeling properties, and drugs that improve RV function (since RV failure is a key driver of outcomes in PH-HF). One promising avenue is the inhibition of pathways such as TGF-β or galectin-3 that contribute to both cardiac fibrosis and vascular remodeling. These are still in preclinical or early-phase trials.
- *Inflammation and endothelial dysfunction modulation:* HFpEF with PH often involves systemic inflammation and endothelial activation. Therapies that address these (such as anti-inflammatory agents or drugs improving endothelial function) could indirectly benefit the pulmonary vasculature. For instance, systemic IL-1 or IL-6 blockers are being considered in HFpEF trials and may have downstream effects on PH if they improve overall cardiovascular function.
- *Gene and cell therapies:* Though still experimental, cell-based therapies (like mesenchymal stem cells) are being tested in advanced HF to improve ventricular function and may have ancillary benefits on the pulmonary circulation. Likewise, gene therapy targeting the RV or pulmonary vessels could be a future approach for end-stage cases.[10,11]

Importantly, future trials will likely incorporate the refined hemodynamic definitions and use sophisticated endpoints. Beyond traditional outcomes, *hemodynamic endpoints* (like change in PVR or PAWP) and *RV function metrics* (e.g., MRI-derived RV volumes or strain) are being used to gauge if a therapy is making a meaningful impact on the cardiopulmonary unit. There is also interest in *adaptive trial designs* that can weed out ineffective therapies faster and focus on those showing signals of benefit.[3,11]

On the *guideline front*, expect to see updates as evidence accumulates. The 2022 ESC/ERS guidelines acknowledged the lack of approved treatments for PH-HF and remained conservative in recommendations. If a new therapy demonstrates clear benefit in a well-defined PH-HF population, future guidelines would incorporate that. Additionally, as noninvasive technologies improve, we may see more guidance on using imaging or biomarker tools to monitor PH severity in HF (for example, serial echocardiographic measurement of tricuspid regurgitation gradient or RV function as a surrogate to track PH).[12,13]

CONCLUSION

Pulmonary hypertension in HF reflects both disease severity and progression. Using the lens of "the good, the bad, and the ugly," HF patients can be stratified—those without PH fare best "good", those with IpcPH have intermediate risk "bad", and those with CpcPH face the worst prognosis "ugly" due to pulmonary vascular remodeling and right heart dysfunction. Early recognition and preventing progression from IpcPH to CpcPH are critical. Management hinges on optimal HF care—volume control, neurohormonal therapies, and correction of structural issues. PAH-targeted drugs have not shown benefit and are not recommended. Advanced cases may require invasive monitoring or devices like LVADs. As research evolves, future therapies may better address CpcPH. Until then, timely diagnosis, accurate classification, and guideline-based HF management remain key to improving outcomes in this high-risk population.

REFERENCES

1. McLaughlin VV, Archer SL, Badesch DB, et al. Pulmonary Hypertension Treatment & Management. Medscape. [Online] Available from: https://emedicine.medscape.com/article/2500055-guidelines [Updated on January 9, 2024].
2. Inampudi C, Silverman D, Simon MA, et al. Pulmonary Hypertension in the Context of Heart Failure with Preserved Ejection Fraction. Chest. 2021;160(6):2232-46.
3. Hoeper MM, Oerke B, Wissmüller M, et al. Tadalafil for Treatment of Combined Postcapillary and Precapillary Pulmonary Hypertension in Patients with Heart Failure and Preserved Ejection Fraction: A Randomized Controlled Phase 3 Study. Circulation. 2024;150(8):600-10. Erratum in: Circulation. 2025;151(11):e763.
4. Guimaraes L, Lindenfeld J, Sandoval J, et al. Interatrial shunting for heart failure: Current evidence and future perspectives. *EuroIntervention*. 2019;15(2):164-71.
5. Humbert M, Kovacs G, Hoeper MM, et al. 2022 ESC/ERS Guidelines for the diagnosis and treatment of pulmonary hypertension. Eur Heart J. 2022;43(38):3618-731.
6. Rosenkranz S, Hoeper MM, Maron BA. Pulmonary hypertension in heart failure: the good, the bad, and the ugly. Eur Heart J. 2024;45(35):3289-291.
7. Fauvel C, Damy T, Berthelot E, et al. Post-capillary pulmonary hypertension in heart failure: impact of current definition in the PH-HF multicentre study. Eur Heart J. 2024;45(35):3274-88.
8. Karia N, Howard L, Johnson MK, et al. Predictors of outcomes in mild pulmonary hypertension according to 2022 ESC/ERS guidelines: the EVIDENCE-PAH UK study. Eur Heart J. 2023;44(49):4678-91.
9. Omote K, Sorimachi H, Obokata M, et al. Pulmonary vascular disease in pulmonary hypertension due to left heart disease: pathophysiologic implications. Eur Heart J. 2022;43(36):3417-31.
10. Assmus B, Angermann CE, Anker SD, et al. Effects of remote haemodynamic-guided heart failure management in patients with different subtypes of pulmonary hypertension: insights from the MEMS-HF study. Eur J Heart Fail. 2022;24(12):2320-30.
11. Nassif ME, Qintar M, Windsor SL, et al. Empagliflozin effects on pulmonary artery pressure in patients with heart failure: results from the EMBRACE-HF trial. Circulation. 2021;143(17): 1673-86.
12. Ameri P, Pollesello P, Mercurio V, et al. A roadmap for therapeutic discovery in pulmonary hypertension associated with heart failure: consensus statement from the Translational Research Committee of the Heart Failure Association (HFA). Eur J Heart Fail. 2024;26(5):707-29.
13. Maron BA, Brittain EL, Hess E, et al. Pulmonary vascular resistance and clinical outcomes in patients with pulmonary hypertension: a retrospective cohort study. Lancet Respir Med. 2020;8: 873-84.

CHAPTER 20

Progression from Pre-heart Failure, Heart Stress to Subclinical Heart Failure

Arpita Katheria, Ankit Kumar Sahu, Aditya Kapoor

ABSTRACT

Heart failure is estimated to be present in 64 million people around the world (1–3% of general adult population) with incidence of 1–20 cases per thousand person years, and leads to significant morbidity and mortality.[1] Patients of heart failure are routinely diagnosed once they become symptomatic, by which time the heart has already undergone significant irreversible damage. It is now known that the progression from a healthy heart toward heart failure in most of the cases is a continuous spectrum, rather than a sudden occurrence.[2] This has led to enormous interest in identification of a subset of patients at high risk for heart failure, without overt signs and symptoms of heart failure. Newer terminologies have been introduced to classify these high-risk patients, in order to ensure timely diagnosis, and early introduction of disease-modifying therapy, before the onset of irreversible damage.

Keywords: Heart failure, pre-heart failure, asymptomatic left ventricular dysfunction, heart stress, subclinical heart failure, natriuretic peptides, biomarkers, screening, early diagnosis, disease-modifying therapy.

INTRODUCTION

Pre-heart failure is a term used to denote early stages of heart failure, before the development of clinical symptoms. Since the patient is asymptomatic at this time, it is difficult to diagnose this condition.[3] ACC/AHA have identified four stages of heart failure, with progressively poorer outcomes with advancing stages—stage A includes patients at risk for heart failure, stage B includes pre-heart failure, stage C includes symptomatic heart failure, while stage D includes advanced heart failure **(Table 1)**.[4] Prevalence of pre-heart failure has been reported from 11 to 42.7% in general population in various studies, 5–10 times greater than prevalence of symptomatic heart failure.[5]

The universal definition of heart failure enumerates three subsets of patients in stage B (pre-heart failure):[3]

1. *Structural heart disease:* Valvular heart disease, cardiac chamber enlargement, ventricular wall motion abnormality, left ventricular hypertrophy, and myocardial tissue abnormality.
2. *Abnormal cardiac function:* Left or right ventricular systolic dysfunction, increased filling pressures, and abnormal diastolic dysfunction.
3. *Elevated natriuretic peptide or cardiac troponin levels,* especially postexposure to cardiotoxins.

HEART STRESS

The term heart stress was used for the first time in a consensus document of the Heart Failure Association of the European Society of Cardiology, for asymptomatic patients with risk factors for heart failure, and raised natriuretic peptide levels, with or without structural heart disease or cardiac dysfunction. *NT-proBNP ≤50 pg/mL was used to rule out heart stress in asymptomatic patients* with diabetes or other risk factors, while age-adjusted cutoff values of NT-proBNP levels were used to rule in heart stress **(Table 2)**.[6]

SUBCLINICAL HEART FAILURE

Subclinical heart failure is the stage immediately preceding overt symptomatic heart failure. This condition includes structural and/or functional dysfunction of myocardium along with deranged cardiac biomarkers.[2] Although patients remain asymptomatic, this condition is not benign. There

TABLE 1: Stages of heart failure (HF).

Stages of HF	Definition	Examples
Stage A: At risk for HF	At risk for HF, but without symptoms, structural heart disease, or cardiac biomarkers of stretch or injury	*Patients with*: • Hypertension • Diabetes • Metabolic syndrome and obesity • Exposure to cardiotoxic agents
Stage B: Pre-heart failure	No symptoms or signs of HF and evidence of one of the following: • Structural heart disease • Evidence of increased filling pressures • Patients with risk factors and raised biomarkers	*Structural heart disease*: • Reduced LV or RV systolic function • Ventricular hypertrophy • Chamber enlargement • Valvular heart disease *Evidence of increased filling pressures*: • By invasive hemodynamic measurements • By noninvasive imaging (e.g., Doppler echocardiography) *Patients with risk factors and raised biomarkers*: • Increased levels of BNPs • Persistently elevated cardiac troponin
Stage C: Symptomatic HF	Structural heart disease with current or previous symptoms of HF	
Stage D: advanced HF	Marked HF symptoms that interfere with daily life with recurrent hospitalizations despite optimizing GDMT	

Source: Modified from Heidenreich PA, Bozkurt B, Aguilar D, et al. 2022 AHA/ACC/HFSA guideline for the management of heart failure: a report of the American College of Cardiology/American Heart Association Joint Committee on Clinical Practice Guidelines. J Am Coll Cardiol. 2022;79(17):e263-e421.

TABLE 2: Screening of asymptomatic patients with CV risk factors (heart stress).[6]

	Rule out	Gray zone	Rule in
NT-proBNP level	≤50 pg/mL		• <50 years: ≥75 pg/mL • 50–74 years: ≥150 pg/mL • ≥75 years: ≥300 pg/mL
Impression of heart stress	Very unlikely	Not likely	Likely
Advice	Repeat NT-proBNP in 1 year	Repeat NT-proBNP in 6 months	Echocardiography (Refer to heart failure expert if dysfunction detected)

is high risk of cardiovascular events and development of symptomatic heart failure in near future.

CLASSIFICATION AND CONTINUUM OF PRE-HEART FAILURE

A new classification of pre-heart failure has been proposed, based on structural and functional changes of heart and abnormal cardiac biomarkers **(Fig. 1)**.[2]

Pre-heart failure type 1: This includes patients with cardiac structural or functional derangements along with normal serum natriuretic peptide levels. Structural abnormalities include valvular heart disease, cardiac chamber enlargement, ventricular wall motion abnormality, left ventricular hypertrophy, and myocardial tissue abnormality, while functional abnormalities include left or right ventricular systolic dysfunction, or abnormal diastolic function. The prognosis in such patients depends on the magnitude of structural or functional abnormality of the heart.

In a substudy of the Framingham Heart Study Offspring cohort with baseline echocardiography data available, the prevalence of asymptomatic LV systolic dysfunction (LVEF ≤50%) was 3.0%. During a follow-up period of up to 12 years, rates of CHF were significantly higher in patients with ALVD as compared to normal LV systolic function (HR 4.7, 95% CI 2.7–4.8). Moreover, worsening LV systolic dysfunction was associated with poorer outcomes.[7]

Pre-heart failure type 2: This includes patients with *heart stress*, i.e., abnormal cardiac biomarkers, in the absence of structural or functional derangements of the heart. This category includes patients at risk for heart failure, for example, diabetes mellitus, hypertension, obesity, coronary artery disease, with structurally and functionally normal hearts. NT-proBNP is the most commonly used cardiac biomarker for

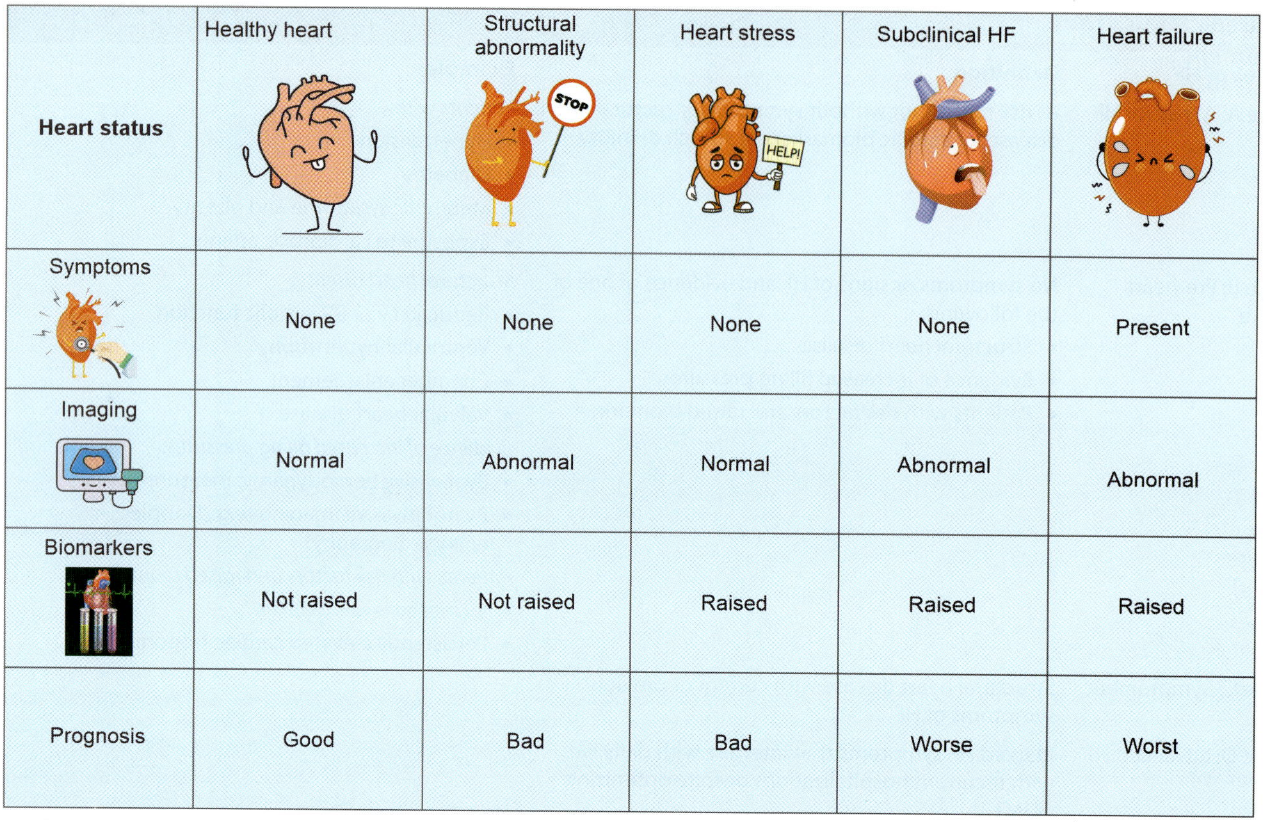

Heart status	Healthy heart	Structural abnormality	Heart stress	Subclinical HF	Heart failure
Symptoms	None	None	None	None	Present
Imaging	Normal	Abnormal	Normal	Abnormal	Abnormal
Biomarkers	Not raised	Not raised	Raised	Raised	Raised
Prognosis	Good	Bad	Bad	Worse	Worst

FIG. 1: Progression from healthy heart to heart failure.

Source: Adapted from Bayes-Genis A, Bozkurt B. Pre-Heart Failure, Heart Stress, and Subclinical Heart Failure: Bridging Heart Health and Heart Failure. JACC Heart Fail. 2024;12(6):1115-8.

heart failure, and as discussed in **Table 2**, NT-proBNP cutoff values have been proposed to rule out heart stress.

Pre-heart failure type 3: This category includes patients with *subclinical heart failure*, i.e., structural and/or functional dysfunction of myocardium along with deranged cardiac biomarkers.

A study showed that asymptomatic high-risk patients with diastolic dysfunction and raised natriuretic peptides had a significantly worse prognosis (event rate 7.9 per 100 person-years) when compared to control group (normal diastolic function and normal natriuretic peptides—event rate 1.7 per 100 person-years), diastolic dysfunction and normal natriuretic peptides (event rate 3.2 per 100 person-years), and normal diastolic function and raised natriuretic peptides (event rate 4.2 per 100 person-years).[8] This study supported the observation that subclinical heart failure is associated with poorer outcomes.

Progression from pre-heart failure to symptomatic heart failure: Pre-heart failure, if left untreated gradually progresses to symptomatic heart failure. There is scarce data on this progression from asymptomatic to symptomatic heart failure. Few observational studies have reported the need for hospitalization for heart failure in previously asymptomatic patients from 1.1 to 9.8% and mortality of 0.6 to 1.6%.[5]

SCREENING FOR PRE-HEART FAILURE

Since at this stage, the patients do not show classical signs and symptoms of heart failure, it is difficult to diagnose pre-heart failure in patients at risk, e.g., those with diabetes, hypertension, and obesity.

In these high-risk patients, Heart Failure Association has proposed the acronym FIND-HF (*F*atigue, *I*ncreased water accumulation, *N*atriuretic Peptide testing, *D*yspnea-*H*eart *F*ailure) to remind healthcare professionals to suspect heart failure in these patients, and to have low threshold for natriuretic peptide testing.[6]

The STOP-HF trial randomized over 1,300 participants with one or more cardiovascular risk factors (hypertension, diabetes mellitus, hypercholesterolemia, obesity, arrhythmia requiring therapy, moderate to severe valvular heart disease, and vascular disease) to usual care (control group) or screening with BNP (intervention group). Among the intervention group, echocardiography and collaborative care with primary care physician and cardiovascular specialist was done in those with raised BNP (≥50 pg/mL). There were more cardiovascular investigations and higher usage of RAAS blockers in the intervention group, which resulted in lower incidence of LV dysfunction with or without heart failure in the intervention group as compared to control group (odds ratio, 0.55; 95% CI 0.37–0.82; $p = 0.003$).[9]

Based on this and similar other studies,[10] experts have recommended that apart from having a high degree of clinical suspicion, routine screening in at-risk patients with annual natriuretic peptides or cardiac troponins (in case of exposure to cardiotoxins), and urine albumin:creatinine ratio in diabetics should be done for early identification of pre-heart failure **(Flowchart 1)**.[11]

TREATMENT

All patients found to have pre-heart failure during routine screening should be educated regarding self-monitoring, adopting heart-healthy habits, regular follow-up, and adherence to prescribed medication.

- *Optimized treatment of preexisting risk factors:* First step in treatment of pre-heart failure includes optimized treatment of preexisting risk factors, like diabetes, hypertension, CAD, obesity, and valvular heart disease. Tight glycemic control, optimal blood pressure control, managing cholesterol levels, adherence to medication and weight loss helps in delaying the progression to overt heart failure.
- *Lifestyle modification:* Lifestyle modification plays an important role in pre-heart failure patients. Healthy diet with focus on Mediterranean, plant-based, whole grain, and DASH diet, regular physical activity, smoking cessation, and weight loss aid in controlling the risk factors and may protect from development of heart failure.[4]
- *Management of asymptomatic LV dysfunction:* Preexisting comorbidities such as diabetes, hypertension, and obesity are found to be associated with asymptomatic LV dysfunction. In patients with symptomatic heart failure with reduced ejection fraction (HFrEF), four pillars of therapy [angiotensin-converting enzyme (ACE) inhibitor/ARNI/ARB, β-blockers, mineralocorticoid receptor antagonist, and SGLT-2 inhibitor] are considered the standard of care. Though, in asymptomatic LV dysfunction, data on role of these drugs remains scanty.

Angiotensin-converting enzyme inhibitors are known to inhibit the adverse cardiac remodeling after ACS with reduced LV systolic function. Studies of ACE inhibitors in asymptomatic LV dysfunction have also shown decreased heart failure hospitalizations and mortality.[12] Study of valsartan in postmyocardial infarction patients with LV dysfunction (25% of these patients were asymptomatic) showed it to be comparable to captopril in terms of MACE.[3,13] ACC/AHA guidelines recommend ACE inhibitors [ARBs if intolerance to ACE inhibitor in case of recent myocardial infarction (MI)] as class I indication for asymptomatic patients with LVEF ≤40% to prevent heart failure and reduce mortality.[4] Due to insufficient data, ARNI is not indicated in asymptomatic LV dysfunction.

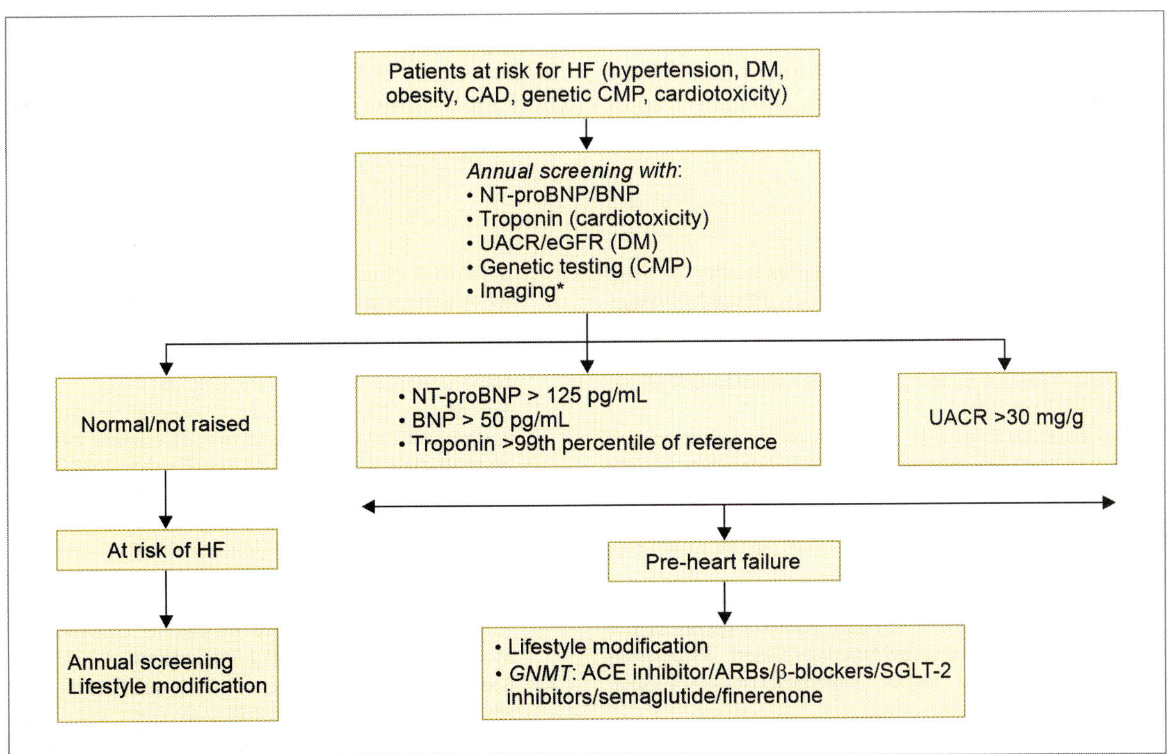

*Imaging (echocardiography/cardiac MRI) should be done in selected patients, e.g., patients with CAD, abnormal ECG or biomarkers, exposure to cardiotoxins, hereditary/genetic CMP, arrhythmia.

FLOWCHART 1: Screening of patients "at risk for heart failure (HF)".[11]

(CMP: cardiomyopathy; DM: diabetes mellitus; HF: heart failure; UACR: urine albumin to creatinine ratio)

Beta-blockers also prevent adverse remodeling of heart and have been shown to improve outcomes in asymptomatic LV dysfunction. In the SOLVD prevention trial, they were found to have synergistic action with enalapril to reduce mortality.[14]ACC/AHA guidelines recommend β-blockers as class I indication for asymptomatic patients with LVEF ≤ 40% to prevent symptomatic heart failure.[4]

Mineralocorticoid receptor antagonists and SGLT-2 inhibitors are not routinely indicated in asymptomatic LV dysfunction in nondiabetic patients.[15]

MANAGEMENT OF DIABETES AND CHRONIC KIDNEY DISEASE/ALBUMINURIA WITH PRE-HEART FAILURE

The cardiovascular outcome trials of SGLT-2 inhibitors in diabetics with high risk for or established cardiovascular disease (CVD) have shown reduction in risk for heart failure hospitalization.[16,17] Majority of patients in these trials did not have symptomatic heart failure at baseline, suggesting benefit in pre-heart failure as well.[15] Based on these findings the ACC/AHA guidelines recommend SGLT-2 inhibitors as class I indication for type 2 diabetes patients with established CVD or those who are at high risk for CVD, to prevent HF hospitalizations.[4]

In patients of diabetic nephropathy, SGLT-2 inhibitors have been shown to prevent heart failure hospitalizations and worsening renal function[18] and are recommended in this patient population. In chronic kidney disease (CKD) patients, dapagliflozin was shown to reduce heart failure hospitalizations and death from cardiovascular causes apart from decreased worsening of renal function and mortality.[19] This effect was shown irrespective of diabetic status. These studies suggest SGLT-2 inhibitors may have a role in certain subsets of pre-heart failure patients (diabetes and chronic kidney disease).[15]

A selective, nonsteroidal mineralocorticoid receptor antagonist, finerenone has also shown improved cardiorenal outcomes in recent studies in diabetic patients with CKD. In particular, it was seen to reduce incident heart failure and heart failure hospitalizations.[20,21] ACE inhibitors and ARBs have also been shown to reduce heart failure in diabetic nephropathy.[15]

ROLE OF DEVICE THERAPY IN PRE-HEART FAILURE

In patients with asymptomatic LV dysfunction, at least 40 days after MI, with LVEF ≤ 30% with expected survival of >1 year, implantable cardioverter defibrillator (ICD) implantation is considered a class I indication to prevent sudden cardiac death.[4]

CONCLUSION

As pre-heart failure is asymptomatic, it is imperative that high-risk patients such as those suffering from diabetes, hypertension, and obesity, CKD should be screened periodically for pre-heart failure. In those who are diagnosed as pre-heart failure, early institution of disease-modifying therapy along with optimal control of risk factors and reinforcement of lifestyle modification are mandatory to check the progression to overt heart failure and decrease the morbidity and mortality associated with it.

REFERENCES

1. Savarese G, Becher PM, Lund LH, et al. Global burden of heart failure: a comprehensive and updated review of epidemiology. Cardiovasc Res. 2023;118(17):3272-87.
2. Bayes-Genis A, Bozkurt B. Pre-Heart Failure, Heart Stress, and Subclinical Heart Failure: Bridging Heart Health and Heart Failure. JACC Heart Fail. 2024;12(6):1115-8.
3. Bozkurt B, Coats AJ, Tsutsui H, et al. Universal definition and classification of heart failure: a report of the Heart Failure Society of America, Heart Failure Association of the European Society of Cardiology, Japanese Heart Failure Society and Writing Committee of the Universal Definition of Heart Failure. J Card Fail. 2021;27(4):387-413.
4. Heidenreich PA, Bozkurt B, Aguilar D, et al. 2022 AHA/ACC/HFSA guideline for the management of heart failure: a report of the American College of Cardiology/American Heart Association Joint Committee on Clinical Practice Guidelines. J Am Coll Cardiol. 2022;79(17):e263-e421.
5. Bergamasco A, Luyet-Déruaz A, Gollop ND, et al. Epidemiology of Asymptomatic Pre-heart Failure: a Systematic Review. Curr Heart Fail Rep. 2022;19(3):146-56.
6. Bayes-Genis A, Docherty KF, Petrie MC, et al. Practical algorithms for early diagnosis of heart failure and heart stress using NT-proBNP: A clinical consensus statement from the Heart Failure Association of the ESC. Eur J Heart Fail. 2023;25(11):1891-8.
7. Wang TJ, Evans JC, Benjamin EJ, et al. Natural history of asymptomatic left ventricular systolic dysfunction in the community. Circulation. 2003;108(8):977-82.
8. Gori M, Lam CSP, D'Elia E, et al. Integrating natriuretic peptides and diastolic dysfunction to predict adverse events in high-risk asymptomatic subjects. Eur J Prev Cardiol. 2021;28(9):937-45.
9. Ledwidge M, Gallagher J, Conlon C, et al. Natriuretic peptide-based screening and collaborative care for heart failure: the STOP-HF randomized trial. JAMA. 2013;310(1):66-74.
10. Huelsmann M, Neuhold S, Resl M, et al. PONTIAC (NT-proBNP Selected Prevention of Cardiac Events in a Population of Diabetic Patients Without a History of Cardiac Disease): a prospective randomized controlled trial. J Am Coll Cardiol. 2013;62(15):1365-72.
11. Bozkurt B. It Is Time to Screen for Heart Failure: Why and How? JACC Heart Fail. 2022;10(8):598-600.
12. Jong P, Yusuf S, Rousseau MF, et al. Effect of enalapril on 12-year survival and life expectancy in patients with left ventricular systolic dysfunction: a follow-up study. Lancet. 2003;361(9372):1843-8.
13. Pfeffer MA, McMurray JJ, Velazquez EJ, et al. Valsartan, captopril, or both in myocardial infarction complicated by heart failure,

left ventricular dysfunction, or both. N Engl J Med. 2003;349(20): 1893-906.

14. Exner DV, Dries DL, Waclawiw MA, et al. Beta-adrenergic blocking agent use and mortality in patients with asymptomatic and symptomatic left ventricular systolic dysfunction: a post hoc analysis of the Studies of Left Ventricular Dysfunction. J Am Coll Cardiol. 1999;33(4):916-23.
15. Bozkurt B. Pre-Heart Failure: An Important Opportunity to Prevent a Deadly Disease. JACC Heart Fail. 2023;11(8 Pt 1):1027-31.
16. Wiviott SD, Raz I, Bonaca MP, et al. Dapagliflozin and cardiovascular outcomes in type 2 diabetes. N Engl J Med. 2019;380:347-57.
17. Zinman B, Wanner C, Lachin JM, et al. Empagliflozin, cardiovascular outcomes, and mortality in type 2 diabetes. N Engl J Med. 2015;373:2117-28.
18. Perkovic V, Jardine MJ, Neal B, et al. Canagliflozin and renal outcomes in type 2 diabetes and nephropathy. N Engl J Med. 2019;380(24):2295-306.
19. Heerspink HJL, Stefansson BV, Correa-Rotter R, et al. Dapagliflozin in patients with chronic kidney disease. N Engl J Med.2020;383(15):1436-46.
20. Filippatos G, Anker SD, Agarwal R, et al. Finerenone reduces risk of incident heart failure in patients with chronic kidney disease and type 2 diabetes: analyses from the FIGARO-DKD Trial. Circulation. 2022;145(6):437-47.
21. Filippatos G, Anker SD, Pitt B, et al. Finerenone and heart failure outcomes by kidney function/albuminuria in chronic kidney disease and diabetes. J Am Coll Cardiol HF. 2022;10(11): 860-70.

CHAPTER 21

Immunology of Heart Failure: Deconstructing Inflammatory Risk

Amal Kumar Khan, Anish Kumar Khan, Amartya Khan

ABSTRACT

The etiology and pathogenesis of heart failure (HF) are still not clear; the persistent inflammation of myocardium is believed to play a key role in the pathogenesis across all spectrum of HF subtypes in different ways. There is a significant correlation between inflammation and HF with preserved ejection fraction (HFpEF). Inflammatory biomarkers, including tumor necrosis factor-alpha (TNF-α) and its receptors (TNFR1 and TNFR2), interleukins like IL-1, IL-6, and IL-10, are often elevated in patients with HFpEF. Chronic, low-grade systemic inflammation leading to the production of several inflammatory cytokines and immune cells might have detrimental effects on myocardial structure and function.

Keywords: HFpEF, inflammatory biomarkers, TNF-α, interleukins, systemic inflammation.

INTRODUCTION

Heart failure (HF) is a clinical syndrome characterized by symptoms and signs induced by the structural and/or functional compromise of the heart, presenting as dyspnea, fatigue, and fluid retention, and so on. HF can be categorized into three types: (1) HF with midrange ejection fraction, (2) HF with reduced ejection fraction (HFrEF), and (3) HF with preserved ejection fraction (HFpEF).[1] This syndrome arises from the intricate interplay of myocardial injury, neurohormonal activation, inflammatory response, and renal impairment.[2,3] Although the pathophysiology and causation of heart failure are still unclear, the ongoing myocardial inflammation is thought to be crucial to the pathophysiology of all range of HF subtypes in various ways.[4] In the BIOSTAT CHF (Biology Study to Tailored Treatment in Chronic Heart Failure) trial,[5] a significant correlation between inflammation and HFpEF was demonstrated. This may be partially attributed to the noncardiac comorbidities present in HFpEF patients, including diabetes mellitus, hypertension, obesity, anemia, chronic obstructive pulmonary disease, and chronic kidney disease, all of which are susceptible to a systemic inflammatory state that can exacerbate HFpEF.[6] We require a more comprehensive understanding of how specific inflammatory cytokines, immune cells, and extracardiac organs interact and affect cardiac function to provide a foundational basis for disease intervention and drug development. Tumor necrosis factor-alpha (TNF-α) and its receptors (TNFR1 and TNFR2), inflammatory cytokines like interleukins, IL-1, patients with HFpEF frequently have higher levels of IL-6 and IL-10. Myocardial structure and function may be negatively impacted by persistent, low-grade systemic inflammation that produces a number of inflammatory cytokines and immune cells. **(Figs. 1A and B)**.[7]

ROLE OF INFLAMMATORY CYTOKINES IN HEART FAILURE

The levels of several inflammatory mediators, including TNF-α, interleukin-6 (IL-6), IL-1, IL-18, and immunological antigens, were validated to be increased in the plasma of HF patients.[3] The "cytokine hypothesis" states that inflammation contributes to the pathogenesis of HF.[8] Till date, various functions of cytokines in HF have been revealed **(Table 1)**.

Tumor Necrosis Factor

Tumor necrosis factor is the first cytokine found to be increased in the peripheral blood of HF cases. Elevated serum TNF position indicated impaired cardiac function and poor prognosis.[9] TNF exerts its function through binding to the receptors. It is unprotected with TNFR1 whereas protected with TNFR2.[10] Constantly increased TNF decreases β1-adrenergic responsiveness, induces cell apoptosis, and destroys the balance between matrix metalloproteinases (MMPs) and tissue inhibitor of metalloproteinase, resulting

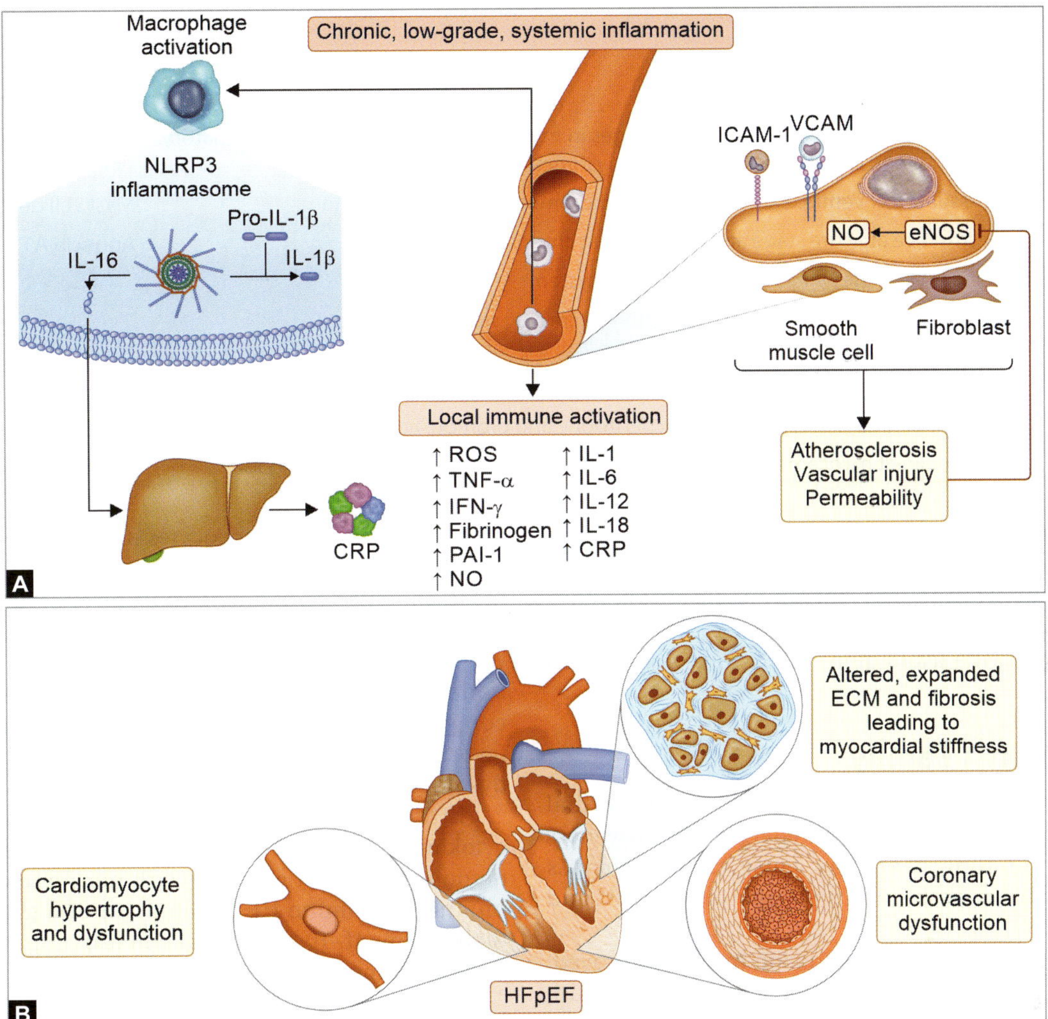

FIGS. 1A AND B: (A) Inflammatory pathways. Chronic, low-grade systemic inflammation activates nucleotide oligomerization domain-like receptor family, pyrin domain-containing (NLRP3) inflammasome, leading to the cleavage and activation of proinflammatory cytokines. Inflammation also promotes endothelial dysfunction, atherosclerosis, and vascular injury. (B) All these alterations may contribute to the development of heart failure with preserved ejection fraction (HFpEF).

(CMD: coronary microvascular dysfunction; eNOS: endothelial nitric oxide synthase; ICAM-1: intercellular adhesion molecule-1; IL-1β: interleukin-1β; IL-6: interleukin-6; NO: nitric oxide; PAI-1: plasminogen activator inhibitor-1; TNF-α: tumor necrosis factor-α; VCAM: vascular cell adhesion molecule; VSMC: vascular smooth muscle cell)

TABLE 1: Cytokines in heart failure.

Cytokines	Functions
TNF-α✱★◆■	Induce inflammatory genes expression and apoptosis, release proinflammatory cytokines, and promote adverse remodeling
Fas✱★◆	Trigger programmed cell death
IL-1✱★◆■	Induce negative inotropic effect through impairing-adrenergic responsiveness and disturbing calcium handling
ST2✱★◆⊙	Negatively modulate TLR signaling, inhibit nuclear factor kappa B (NF-κB) activation
IL-6✱★◆■	Pleiotropic proinflammatory responses
IL-10✱◆	Inhibits proinflammatory cytokines secretion, blocks ROS release, and modulates TNF-α-mediated responses

✱ Participate in pathogenesis.
★ Prognostic value.
◆ Identify high-risk patients.
■ Potential therapeutic target.
⊙ Diagnostic value.

(Fas: factor associated suicide; IL-1: interleukin-1; IL-6: interleukin-6; IL-10: interleukin-10; ROS: reactive oxygen species; ST2: suppression of tumorigenicity 2; TLR: toll-like receptor; TNF: tumor necrosis factor)

TABLE 2: Main immune cells in heart failure.

Immune cells	Functions	Potential therapeutic targets from animal studies
Macrophages	Elevated CCR2MHCII^{high}Ly6c macrophages in myocardium could secrete inflammatory cytokines and contribute to ventricular dysfunction	CCR2–CCL2 signaling axis
Mast cells	Attenuate left ventricular remodeling and promote cardiac dysfunction	Mast cell depletion
Neutrophils	Destructive at acute stage and protective at chronic stage	Annexin A1
Natural killer cells	Release cytokines and modulate immune system	
Dendritic cells	Protective at acute stage and destructive at chronic stage	
CD4 T cells	• TH1 cells are mainly proinflammatory • TH2 cells are mainly profibrosis • TH17 cells contribute to cardiac hypertrophy and promote adverse cardiac remodeling	
B cells	Induce direct myocardial injury, produce inflammatory cytokines, and antibodies	B-cell depletion

in ventricular hypertrophy, dilatation, and diminished ejection fraction.[11] However, the trials targeting TNF with infliximab [ATTACH (Anti-TNF Therapy Against Congestive Heart Failure) trial] or etanercept [RENEWAL (Randomized Etanercept Worldwide Evaluation) trial][12] gave poor results **(Table 2)**.

Interleukin-1 Family

According to one report, IL-1 is a "soluble myocardial depressant factor."[13] By affecting adrenergic responsiveness and calcium handling, IL-1 may cause cardiomyocytes to have reversible negative inotropic effects in vitro[14] and in vivo.[15]

By blocking IL-1, cardiac dysfunction may be improved, inflammatory infiltration may be decreased, and calcium homeostasis may be restored.[16]

Canakinumab is a human monoclonal antibody targeting IL-1β, approved for treating many autoimmune diseases, and in the prespecified subanalysis of the Canakinumab Anti-inflammatory Thrombosis Outcome Study (CANTOS), it demonstrated that canakinumab successfully decreased HF-related hospitalization and all-cause mortality in patients with a history of MI and raised high-sensitivity C-reactive protein (hs-CRP) in a dose-dependent manner.[17] Recombinant IL-1 receptor antagonist anakinra was created as a rheumatoid arthritis disease-modifying treatment.

Anakinra decreased hs-CRP when compared to a placebo in the VCU-ART-3 trial, which included 99 patients with a mean left ventricular ejection fraction (LVEF) of 51% who were hospitalized for ST-elevation MI.[18] Twelve patients with HFpEF (median BNP 32 pg/mL) and hs-CRP > 2 mg/L were included in the D-HART study and were given anakinra instead of a matching placebo. After 2 weeks, patients assigned to anakinra had reduced hs-CRP and higher peak VO_2.[19]

Suppression of tumorigenicity 2 (ST2), a decoy receptor of IL-33, is another member of IL-1 cytokine superfamily, IL-33 which is a member of interleukin cytokine super family and secreted by cardiomyocytes under mechanical stress is independently and positively associated with poor outcomes in HF patients and might be valuable to predict prognosis.[20]

Although clinical trials specifically targeted at the therapeutic effects of anti-IL-6 on HF have not been undertaken, elevated circulating IL-6 was identified in congestive HF patients, and this showed a significantly favorable link with increasing cardiac symptoms and renal dysfunction.[21]

Interleukin-10 prevents many proinflammatory cytokines, including TNF-α, from being secreted.[22] It has been demonstrated that giving growth hormone or intravenous immunoglobulin to HF patients causes a significant rise in their plasma IL-10 levels, which in turn improves their heart contractile function.[23]

ROLE OF IMMUNE CELLS IN HEART FAILURE

The heart harbors all of the major immune cell types in the steady state, including monocytes, macrophages, T cells, neutrophils, B cells, dendritic cells (DCs), natural killer (NK) cells, and mast cells.[24]

Macrophages

At healthy status, heart macrophages were dominated by CCR2 macrophages, which could further divide into two categories by MHCII expression (CCR2MHCII^{high} macrophage and CCR2MHCII^{low} macrophage). CCR2 macrophages originate from embryonic precursors and mainly function in coronary system development, angiogenesis, and immune quiescence.[25] The increased CCR2 macrophages could produce inflammatory cytokines and chemokines, which in turn causes cardiac T-cell expansion and contributes to cardiomyocyte damage, cardiac remodeling, and pathological hypertrophy.[26] Clinically, the abundance of CCR2 macrophages was positively associated with adverse left ventricular remodeling and persistent left ventricular dysfunction in HF patients.[27] So far, no CCR2 modulating therapy has been approved for clinical indications. CCR2-targeted lipid nanoparticle-encapsulated small interfering RNA[28] had obtained therapeutic benefits in both ischemic and nonischemic HF by decreasing the proinflammatory monocyte infiltration in the myocardium **(Table 3)**.

Mast Cells

Originally, mast cells were thought to be responsible for allergic and anaphylactic reactions. However, new studies have confirmed that cardiac mast cells also have a role in other physiological processes, such as angiogenesis and vascular homeostasis.[29] According to studies, patients with end-stage cardiomyopathy had a markedly higher number of mast cells in their hearts, which triggered MMPs and the breakdown of myocardial fibrillar collagen, promoting unfavorable cardiac remodeling.[30] In animal models, either mast cell elimination or suppression of their degranulation could reduce left ventricular remodeling and cardiac dysfunction and increase survival rates.[31]

TABLE 3: Clinical trials investigating anti-inflammatory agents in heart failure.

Trial (year)	Setting	Treatment groups	Number of patients	Follow-up	Primary endpoint	Results	Study limitations
Anti-TNF-α ATTACH (2003)	Chronic HF (NYHA III–IV, LVEF ≤35%)	Infliximab vs. placebo	150	6	Change in clinical status at 14 weeks	No difference	Only HFrEF
RENAISSANCE, RECOVER, RENEWAL (2004)	Chronic HF (NYHA II–IV, LVEF ≤30%)	Etanercept vs. placebo	2,048	6	RENAISSANCE and RECOVER: Clinical status at 24 weeks. RENEWAL: CVM or HF hospitalization from RENAISSANCE and RECOVER	All neutrals. Safety: more infections with etanercept	Only HFrEF
Colchicine							
COPS (2020)	ACS and evidence of CAD managed with PCI or medical therapy	Colchicine vs. placebo	795	12	All-cause mortality, ACS, urgent revascularization, or ischemic CVA	No difference. Safety concern: ↑ACM (8 vs. 1, $p = 0.017$) and non-CVM with colchicine (5 vs. 0, $p = 0.024$)	History of HF not reported
Phospholipase A2 inhibitors							
SOLID-TIMI 52 (2014)	Recent ACS (NYHA III–IV HF excluded)	Darapladib vs. placebo	13,026	30	CAD-related death, MI, or urgent revascularization	No difference	History of HF not reported. No data on LVEF
STABILITY (2014)	Chronic CAD (NYHA III–IV HF excluded)	Darapladib vs. placebo	15,828	444	CVM, MI, or CVA	No difference	History of HF not reported. No LVEF data
VISTA-16 (2014)	ACS; HF: 17.8%	Varespladib vs. placebo	5,145	6	CVM, MI, CVA, or UA	No difference	Termination of the trial for futility and possible harm. No LVEF data

(ACM: all-cause mortality; ACS: acute coronary syndrome; ASA: acetylsalicylic acid; AUC: area under the curve; CAD: coronary artery disease; CI: confidence interval; CK-MB: creatine kinase-muscle brain; CMR: cardiac magnetic resonance; CVA: cerebrovascular accident; CVM: cardiovascular mortality; EF: ejection fraction; HDL-C: high-density lipoprotein-cholesterol; HF: heart failure; HR: hazard ratio; hs-CRP: high-sensitivity C-reactive protein; IL-6: interleukin-6; Lp-PLA2: lipoprotein-associated phospholipase A2; LVEF: left ventricular ejection fraction; LVESV: left ventricular end-systolic volume; MACE: major adverse cardiovascular events; MI: myocardial infarction; NSTE: non-ST elevation; PCI: percutaneous coronary intervention; PROBE: prospective randomized observer-blinded endpoint; RCA: resuscitated cardiac arrest; sPLA2: soluble phospholipase A2; STEMI: ST-elevation myocardial infarction; SVG: saphenous vein graft; T2DM: type 2 diabetes mellitus; TnI: troponin I; UA: unstable angina)

Neutrophils

Neutrophils participate in various cardiovascular diseases via releasing degranulation products, delivering microvesicles and cytokines.[32] Neutrophil/lymphocyte ratio could predict acute HF patients with a higher risk of vascular events.[33] In patients with AMI who developed congestive HF, 92.5% had relative neutrophilia (neutrophil > 65%), whereas in patients with AMI who did not develop into congestive HF, the incidence of neutrophilia was 45%.[34] Recently, researchers found that in infarct healing process, neutrophils could promote macrophage polarization toward a proreparative and proangiogenesis phenotype through releasing neutrophil gelatinase-associated lipocalin (NGAL) and annexin A1.[35]

Natural Killer Cells

Circulating NK cells were dramatically reduced in number with diminished cytolytic function in HF patients, as well as coronary heart disease patients and ischemic heart disease patients.[36] By preventing inflammatory cell accumulation and limiting collagen production from cardiac fibroblasts, NK cells could suppress the development of cardiac fibrosis.[37]

Dendritic Cells

In AMI, the migration and accumulation of DCs to the infarction point were elevated and DC depletion resulted in worsening post-MI remodeling.[38] DC infiltration was decreased in the cardiac tissue of symptomatic DCM patients, which indicated a reduced ejection fraction.[39] Hence, the function of DCs may not be the same in acute and chronic HF.

T Cells

T cells that participated in the pathogenesis of HF came from the elevated T cell-generated cytokines, IL-2 and IL-10, in the plasma of HF patients.[40] CD4 and CD8 T cells, as well as CD4 subsets (TH1, TH2, TH17, and Treg cells), were also infiltrated in the failing heart.[41]

B Cells

B cells could produce proinflammatory cytokines including TNF-α, lymphotoxin, IL-1, and IL-6 after acquiring cytokine secretion capability. These cytokines were reported to attenuate left ventricular function and promote cardiac remodeling.[42]

Extracardiac Organs

As a systemic disease, HF causes multiorgan damage through various mechanisms. Similarly, remote organ-related inflammatory responses would further deteriorate cardiac function **(Figs. 2 and 3)**.[43]

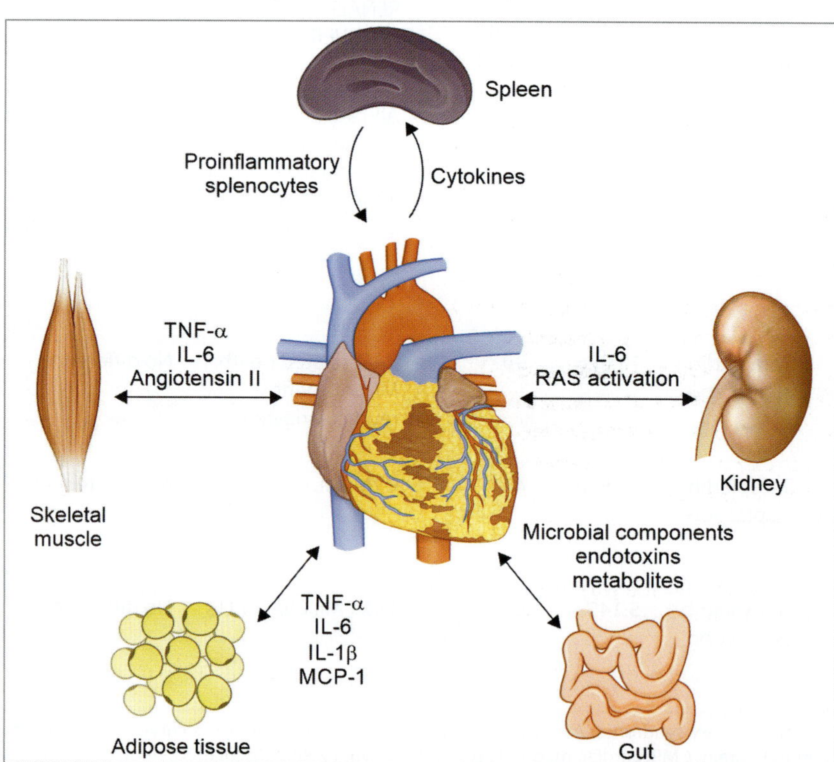

FIG. 2: There is an interaction between heart and extracardiac organs. Heart failure and inflammatory responses will influence each other. After an injury, splenic monocytes can mobilize and accumulate in myocardium to induce cardiac injury. In systemic inflammation, elevated circulating inflammatory cytokines, adipokines, and peripheral organ hypoperfusion could induce renal dysfunction, gut microbiota disorder, and skeletal muscle catabolism, which will further aggravate cardiac dysfunction.

(IL: interleukin; TNF: tumor necrosis factor)

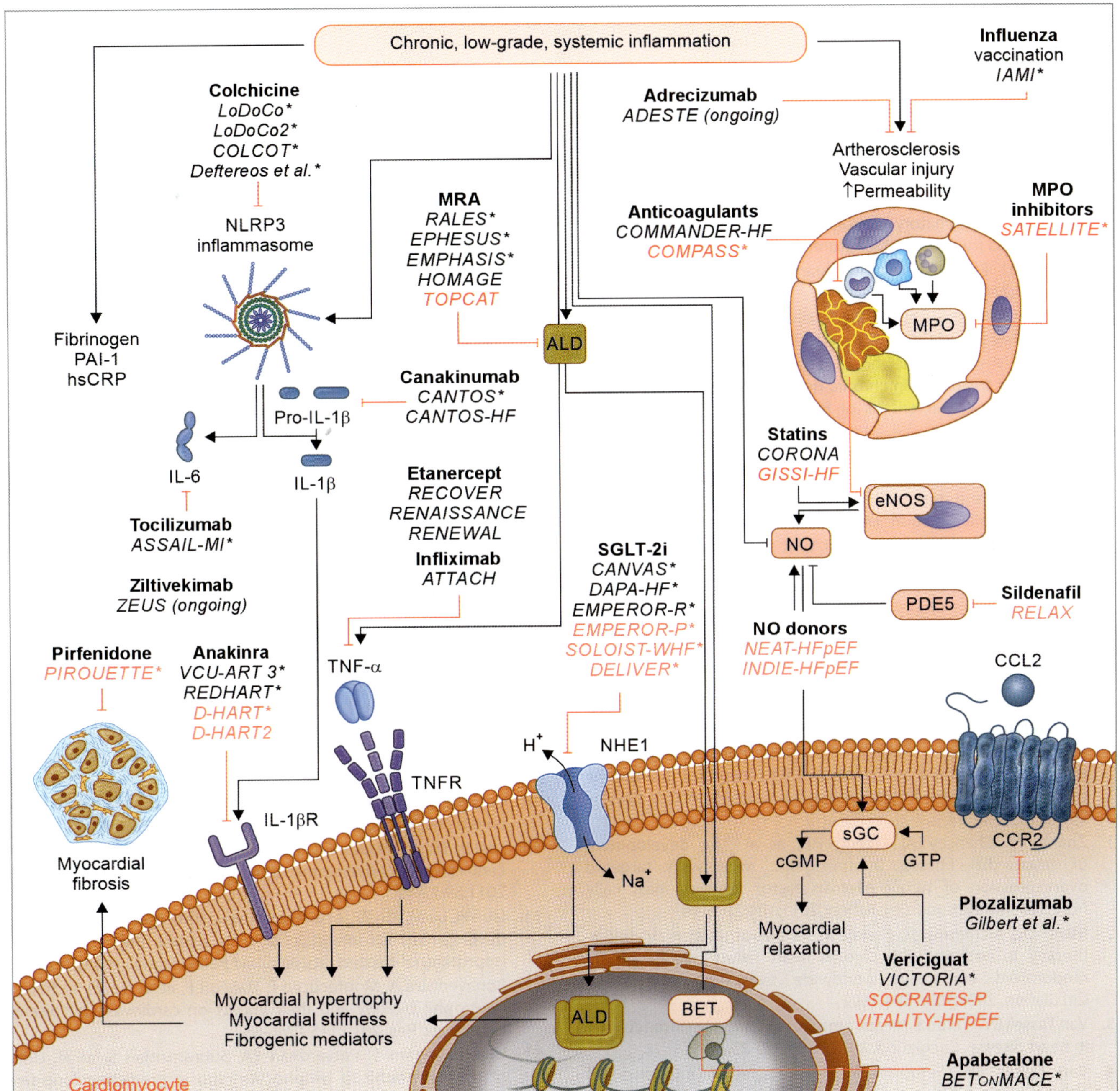

*Trials/studies that met their primary endpoint.

FIG. 3: Clinical trials targeting inflammatory pathways in patients with heart failure. Many different biochemical pathways are involved in inflammation-driven heart injury and can be targeted at different levels. Drugs are in bold, while clinical trials are in italics.

(BET: bromodomain and extra-terminal motif; CCL2: C–C chemokine ligand 2; CCR2: C–C chemokine receptor type 2; cGMP: cyclic guanosine monophosphate; ECM: extracellular matrix; eNOS: endothelial nitric oxide synthase; GTP: guanosine triphosphate; HFpEF: heart failure with preserved ejection fraction; IL-1β-R: interleukin-1β receptor; MPO: myeloperoxidase; NLRP3: nucleotide oligomerization domain-like receptor family, pyrin domain-containing; NO: nitric oxide; PDE5: phosphodiesterase-5; sGC: soluble guanylate cyclase; TNFR: tumor necrosis factor receptor)

CONCLUSION

Inflammation plays a crucial role in the development and progression of HF. While clinical trials have shown variable results, ongoing research continues to explore the role of targeted immunomodulatory therapy. Regular evaluation of inflammatory status and a personalized approach to management may help refine risk assessment and improve long-term outcomes.

REFERENCES

1. Ponikowski P, Voors AA, Anker SD, et al. ESC guidelines for the diagnosis and treatment of acute and chronic heart failure: the Task Force for the diagnosis and treatment of acute and chronic heart failure of the European Society of Cardiology (ESC). Developed with the special contribution of the Heart Failure Association (HFA) of the ESC. Eur J Heart Fail. 2016;18: 891-975.
2. Mann DL. Inflammatory mediators and the failing heart: past, present, and the foreseeable future. Circ Res. 2002;91:988-98.
3. Braunwald E. Biomarkers in heart failure. N Engl J Med. 2008;358:2148-59.
4. Dick SA, Epelman S. Chronic heart failure and inflammation: what do we really know? Circ Res. 2016;119:159-76.
5. Voors AA, Anker SD, Cleland JG, et al. A systems BIOlogy study to TAilored treatment in chronic heart failure: rationale, design, and baseline characteristics of BIOSTAT-CHF. Eur J Heart Fail. 2016;18:716-26.
6. Paulus WJ, Tschope C. A novel paradigm for heart failure with preserved ejection fraction: comorbidities drive myocardial dysfunction and remodeling through coronary microvascular endothelial inflammation. J Am Coll Cardiol. 2013;62:263-71.
7. Matsubara J, Sugiyama S, Nozaki T, et al. Pentraxin 3 is a new inflammatory marker correlated with left ventricular diastolic dysfunction and heart failure with normal ejection fraction. J Am Coll Cardiol. 2011;57:861-9.
8. Mann DL. Innate immunity and the failing heart: the cytokine hypothesis revisited. Circ Res. 2015;116:1254-68.
9. Rauchhaus M, Doehner W, Francis DP, et al. Plasma cytokine parameters and mortality in patients with chronic heart failure. Circulation. 2000;102:3060-7.
10. Monden Y, Kubota T, Inoue T, et al. Tumor necrosis factor-alpha is toxic via receptor 1 and protective via receptor 2 in a murine model of myocardial infarction. Am J Physiol Heart Circ Physiol. 2007;293:H743-53.
11. Zhang W, Chancey AL, Tzeng HP, et al. The development of myocardial fibrosis in transgenic mice with targeted overexpression of tumor necrosis factor requires mast cell–fibroblast interactions. Circulation. 2011;124:2106-16.
12. Mann DL, McMurray JJ, Packer M, et al. Targeted anticytokine therapy in patients with chronic heart failure: results of the randomized etanercept worldwide evaluation (RENEWAL). Circulation. 2004;109:1594-1602.
13. Van Tassell BW, Toldo S, Mezzaroma E, et al. Targeting interleukin-1 in heart disease. Circulation. 2013;128:1910-23.
14. Van Tassell BW, Seropian IM, Toldo S, et al. Interleukin-1β induces a reversible cardiomyopathy in the mouse. Inflamm Res. 2013;62:637-40.
15. Buckley LF, Abbate A. Interleukin-1 blockade in cardiovascular diseases: a clinical update. Eur Heart J. 2018;39:2063-9.
16. Sager HB, Heidt T, Hulsmans M, et al. Targeting interleukin-1β reduces leukocyte production after acute myocardial infarction. Circulation. 2015;132:1880-90.
17. Everett BM, Cornel JH, Lainscak M, et al. Anti-inflammatory therapy with canakinumab for the prevention of hospitalization for heart failure. Circulation. 2019;139:1289-99.
18. Abbate A, Trankle CR, Buckley LF, et al. Interleukin-1 blockade inhibits the acute inflammatory response in patients with ST-segment-elevation myocardial infarction. J Am Heart Assoc. 2020;9:e014941.
19. Van Tassell BW, Arena R, Biondi-Zoccai G, et al. Effects of interleukin-1 blockade with anakinra on aerobic exercise capacity in patients with heart failure and preserved ejection fraction (from the D-HART pilot study). Am J Cardiol. 2014;113:321-7.
20. Anand IS, Rector TS, Kuskowski M, et al. Prognostic value of soluble ST2 in the valsartan heart failure trial. Circ Heart Fail. 2014;7:418-26.
21. Hanberg JS, Rao VS, Ahmad T, et al. Inflammation and cardio-renal interactions in heart failure: a potential role for interleukin-6. Eur J Heart Fail. 2018;20:933-4.
22. Ouyang W, Rutz S, Crellin NK, et al. Regulation and functions of the IL-10 family of cytokines in inflammation and disease. Annu Rev Immunol. 2011;29:71-109.
23. Adamopoulos S. Effects of growth hormone on circulating cytokine network, and left ventricular contractile performance and geometry in patients with idiopathic dilated cardiomyopathy. Eur Heart J. 2003;24:2186-96.
24. Pinto AR, Ilinykh A, Ivey MJ, et al. Revisiting cardiac cellular composition. Circ Res. 2016;118:400-9.
25. Lavine KJ, Epelman S, Uchida K, et al. Distinct macrophage lineages contribute to disparate patterns of cardiac recovery and remodeling in the neonatal and adult heart. Proc Natl Acad Sci U S A. 2014;111:16029-34.
26. Patel B, Bansal SS, Ismahil MA, et al. CCR2+ monocyte-derived infiltrating macrophages are required for adverse cardiac remodeling during pressure overload. JACC Basic Transl Sci. 2018;3:230-44.
27. Bajpai G, Schneider C, Wong N, et al. The human heart contains distinct macrophage subsets with divergent origins and functions. Nat Med. 2018;24:1234-45.
28. Gordon S. Targeting a monocyte subset to reduce inflammation. Circ Res. 2012;110:1546-8.
29. da Silva EZ, Jamur MC, Oliver C. Mast cell function: a new vision of an old cell. J Histochem Cytochem. 2014;62:698-738.
30. Levick SP, Melendez GC, Plante E, et al. Cardiac mast cells: the centrepiece in adverse myocardial remodelling. Cardiovasc Res. 2011;89:12-19.
31. Liu YH, Lu M, Xie ZZ, et al. Hydrogen sulfide prevents heart failure development via inhibition of renin release from mast cells in isoproterenol-treated rats. Antioxid Redox Signal. 2014;20:759-69.
32. Bonaventura A, Montecucco F, Dallegri F, et al. Novel findings in neutrophil biology and their impact on cardiovascular disease. Cardiovasc Res. 2019;115:1266-85.
33. Uthamalingam S, Patvardhan EA, Subramanian S, et al. Utility of the neutrophil to lymphocyte ratio in predicting long-term outcomes in acute decompensated heart failure. Am J Cardiol. 2011;107:433-8.
34. Kyne L, Hausdorff JM, Knight E, et al. Neutrophilia and congestive heart failure after acute myocardial infarction. Am Heart J. 2000;139:94-100.
35. Ferraro B, Leoni G, Hinkel R, et al. Pro-angiogenic macrophage phenotype to promote myocardial repair. J Am Coll Cardiol. 2019;73:2990-3002.
36. Backteman K, Ernerudh J, Jonasson L. Natural killer (NK) cell deficit in coronary artery disease: no aberrations in phenotype but sustained reduction of NK cells is associated with low-grade inflammation. Clin Exp Immunol. 2014;175:104-12.
37. Ong S, Rose NR, Cihakova D. Natural killer cells in inflammatory heart disease. Clin Immunol. 2017;175:26-33.

38. Anzai A, Anzai T, Nagai S, et al. Regulatory role of dendritic cells in postinfarction healing and left ventricular remodeling. Circulation. 2012;125:1234-45.
39. Pistulli R, Konig S, Drobnik S, et al. Decrease in dendritic cells in endomyocardial biopsies of human dilated cardiomyopathy. Eur J Heart Fail. 2013;15:974-85.
40. Marriott JB, Goldman JH, Keeling PJ, et al. Abnormal cytokine profiles in patients with idiopathic dilated cardiomyopathy and their asymptomatic relatives. Heart. 1996;75:287-90.
41. Nevers T, Salvador AM, Grodecki-Pena A, et al. Left ventricular T-cell recruitment contributes to the pathogenesis of heart failure. Circ Heart Fail. 2015;8:776-87.
42. Vazquez MI, Catalan-Dibene J, Zlotnik A. B cells responses and cytokine production are regulated by their immune microenvironment. Cytokine. 2015;74:318-26.
43. Li H, Chen C, Wang DW. Inflammatory cytokines, immune cells, and organ interactions in heart failure. Front Physiol. 2021;12:695047.

CHAPTER

22

Iron Deficiency States and Effective Iron Repletion Strategies in Chronic Heart Failure

Ankit Kumar Sahu, Arshad Nazir, Pranjal Raparia

ABSTRACT

Iron deficiency is increasingly recognized as a prevalent and clinically significant comorbidity in patients with heart failure, irrespective of the presence of anemia. Nearly half of all patients with chronic heart failure and up to 80% of those with acute decompensation demonstrate evidence of absolute or functional iron deficiency. The pathophysiology is multifactorial, involving chronic inflammation, increased hepcidin levels, reduced intestinal absorption, and impaired mobilization of stored iron, ultimately leading to mitochondrial dysfunction, reduced exercise capacity, and worsening symptoms. Conventional markers such as serum iron and total iron-binding capacity are unreliable in this context, and diagnosis relies on ferritin and transferrin saturation thresholds validated in major clinical trials. Multiple randomized controlled trials have shown that intravenous iron therapy, particularly ferric carboxymaltose and ferric derisomaltose, improves exercise capacity and quality of life and reduces recurrent heart failure hospitalizations. Conversely, oral iron supplementation has proven largely ineffective due to poor absorption and tolerability. International guidelines now recommend routine screening for iron deficiency in heart failure and intravenous iron replacement in selected patients. Correction of iron deficiency is a safe and evidence-based strategy that enhances functional capacity and reduces the burden of heart failure.

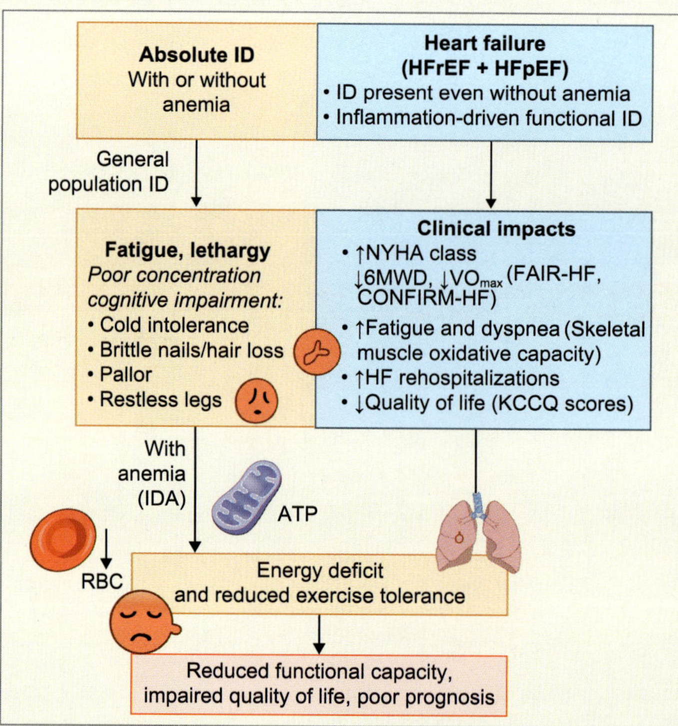

Keywords: Iron deficiency, heart failure with reduced ejection fraction, iron supplementation, heart failure with reduced ejection fraction.

INTRODUCTION

Heart failure (HF), characterized by the heart's inability to maintain adequate cardiac output for tissue perfusion or to do so only at elevated filling pressures, remains a major public health burden worldwide. Among the myriad comorbidities that complicate HF management, iron deficiency (ID)—both with and without anemia—has emerged as a clinically significant and modifiable factor influencing prognosis, exercise tolerance, quality of life, and even mortality.

Contemporary research has firmly established ID as more than a hematologic disorder in HF; it represents a systemic condition with implications for mitochondrial bioenergetics, skeletal muscle metabolism, and neurohormonal modulation. Notably, these pathophysiologic alterations occur independent of hemoglobin levels, and iron replacement in HF patients with isolated ID (i.e., nonanemic ID) has demonstrated robust therapeutic benefit in randomized controlled trials (e.g., FAIR-HF, CONFIRM-HF, and AFFIRM-AHF).[1-3]

Consequently, major cardiology societies, including the European Society of Cardiology (ESC, 2021) and American College of Cardiology/American Heart Association/Heart Failure Society of America (ACC/AHA/HFSA, 2022), have incorporated screening and management of ID into standard guidelines for chronic heart failure care.[4,5]

GLOBAL BURDEN OF IRON DEFICIENCY IN HEART FAILURE

Iron deficiency is the most common nutritional deficiency worldwide, affecting an estimated 2 billion people, per World Health Organization (WHO) estimate.[6] In the context of HF, multiple large-scale observational studies and registries have demonstrated a prevalence of 30–60% depending on the population, disease stage, and whether absolute or functional ID is considered **(Table 1)**.

EPIDEMIOLOGY IN CHRONIC HEART FAILURE

In the FAIR-HF trial, which enrolled 459 patients with NYHA class II–III HFrEF, approximately 50% had laboratory-confirmed ID, with or without anemia.[1] Similarly, the CONFIRM-HF study, which followed patients over 52 weeks, reinforced this prevalence across broader geographic cohorts.[2] A large registry analysis by Comin-Colet et al.[7] involving 1,506 stable CHF patients in Europe identified ID in 54% of individuals, with functional ID comprising the majority (ferritin 100–299 ng/mL, TSAT <20%). Importantly, even in nonanemic patients, ID was independently associated with worse 6-minute walk distance, lower peak oxygen consumption (VO_2 max), and higher NYHA class.

PREVALENCE IN ACUTE DECOMPENSATED HEART FAILURE

The AFFIRM-AHF trial evaluated patients recently hospitalized for acute decompensated HF and reported ID in up to 80% of participants. Notably, ID at the time of discharge was associated with higher risk of rehospitalization and persistent symptoms.[3]

PREVALENCE IN HEART FAILURE WITH PRESERVED EJECTION FRACTION

While historically underexplored, recent studies have demonstrated a similarly high prevalence of ID in HFpEF. The prevalence of ID in patients with HFpEF (PREFER-HFpEF) study found that up to 60% of patients with LVEF ≥50% met criteria for ID, suggesting a pathophysiological overlap between HF phenotypes.[8]

TABLE 1: Prevalence of iron deficiency in major heart failure studies.

Study	Year	HF phenotype	Study population (*n*)	ID prevalence
FERRIC-HF	2008	HFrEF (NYHA II–III)	35	~45–50%
FAIR-HF	2009	HFrEF (NYHA II–III)	459	~50%
IRON-HF	2013	HFrEF (NYHA II–III)	18	100%
CONFIRM-HF	2015	HFrEF (NYHA II–III)	304	~50%
IRONOUT-HF	2017	HFrEF (NYHA II–III)	225	100%
EFFECT-HF	2017	HFrEF (NYHA II–III)	174	~55%
PREFER-HFpEF	2019	HFpEF	350	~60%
AFFIRM-AHF	2020	ADHF	1108	~80%
IRONMAN	2022	HFrEF (NYHA II–III)	1820	70%

(ADHF: acute decompensated heart failure; HFpEF: heart failure with preserved ejection fraction; HFrEF: heart failure with reduced ejection fraction; ID: iron deficiency)

Definition and Diagnostic Criteria

Iron deficiency in HF can be categorized into two principal phenotypes **(Table 2)**:

- *Absolute ID*: It is characterized by depleted total body iron stores, most commonly due to nutritional inadequacy, gastrointestinal losses, or malabsorption.[6,9] It is defined by serum ferritin <100 ng/mL.
- *Functional ID*: It refers to inadequate bioavailability of iron for metabolic processes despite normal or elevated stores. It typically results from inflammation-induced sequestration of iron within the reticuloendothelial system.[10] It is defined by ferritin 100–299 ng/mL with transferrin saturation (TSAT) <20%.

Transferrin saturation is considered the most sensitive indicator of biologically available iron in circulation.[1] It reflects the proportion of transferrin-bound iron capable of tissue delivery, and low TSAT levels are strongly predictive of impaired oxygen transport and utilization.[10]

Etiology

Iron deficiency in HF is multifactorial.[1,10,11] Instead, it represents a complex interplay of factors including chronic inflammation, impaired iron absorption, poor dietary intake, gastrointestinal blood loss, renal dysfunction, and pharmacological influences.[4,5,9,12] These mechanisms may act in isolation or, more commonly, in tandem, resulting in both absolute and functional ID.[7,10]

Chronic Inflammation and Hepcidin Regulation

One of the central contributors to functional ID in HF is chronic low-grade inflammation.[10,11] HF is increasingly recognized as a proinflammatory state, characterized by elevated cytokines such as interleukin-6 (IL-6) and tumor necrosis factor-alpha (TNF-α).[11] These cytokines stimulate hepatic production of hepcidin, a key regulatory peptide that inhibits iron absorption and release by binding to and degrading ferroportin, the only known cellular iron exporter.[11,12] Increased hepcidin levels reduce iron egress from enterocytes, macrophages, and hepatocytes, thereby limiting iron availability despite normal or elevated stores—a hallmark of functional ID.[10,11] This hepcidin–ferroportin axis is thus a pivotal mediator of iron restriction in HF patients and a target of interest in evolving therapeutic strategies.[11]

TABLE 2: Diagnostic criteria for iron deficiency in heart failure.

Parameter	Absolute ID	Functional ID
Ferritin	<100 ng/mL	100–299 ng/mL
Transferrin saturation (TSAT)	<20%	<20%
Hemoglobin	May be normal	May be normal

$[TSAT = \frac{\text{Serum iron}}{\text{TIBC}} \times 100]$

(ID: iron deficiency; TIBC: total iron binding capacity)

Gastrointestinal Malabsorption

Patients with HF commonly exhibit gut edema due to elevated venous pressures and splanchnic congestion.[9] These alterations impair nutrient absorption, including that of iron **(Flowchart 1)**. The intestinal mucosa, particularly in the duodenum where iron absorption primarily occurs, may suffer from reduced perfusion and barrier dysfunction.[11] Proton pump inhibitors (PPIs), frequently used in HF for gastrointestinal prophylaxis, further inhibit gastric acid secretion—an essential factor for solubilizing dietary non-heme iron and facilitating its uptake.[11]

Nutritional Deficiencies and Anorexia

In advanced HF, patients often experience cachexia, anorexia, and restricted intake due to early satiety or fatigue.[9] This leads to suboptimal consumption of iron-rich foods, particularly heme iron sources such as red meat. Additionally, dietary habits in some populations may inherently lack sufficient iron bioavailability due to high phytate content (e.g., cereals, legumes) which chelates and inhibits iron absorption.[6,9]

Occult Blood Loss and Gastrointestinal Comorbidities

Chronic blood loss, often insidious can contribute significantly to absolute ID.[9] This may arise from angiodysplasias, peptic ulcers, gastritis, or the use of antiplatelet and anticoagulant therapies.[9,11] Studies suggest that up to 30% of HF patients may harbor occult gastrointestinal bleeding, especially in the elderly or those with concomitant chronic kidney disease (CKD).[9]

Renal Dysfunction and Erythropoiesis-impaired Iron Utilization

Renal impairment, a common comorbidity in HF, further compounds ID. Reduced erythropoietin synthesis, uremic toxin accumulation, and elevated inflammatory mediators

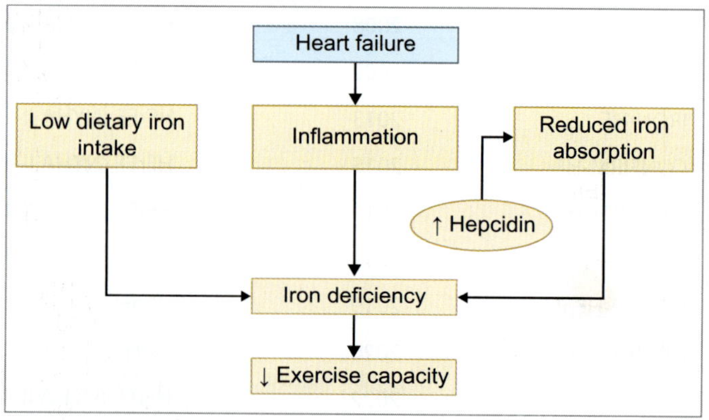

FLOWCHART 1: Mechanism of iron deficiency in heart failure.

contribute to blunted erythropoiesis and inefficient iron utilization. This is particularly relevant in the cardiorenal syndrome spectrum.[12]

Drug Induced

Several commonly used HF medications contribute to ID:

- *Antiplatelets/anticoagulants:* Increase risk of gastrointestinal bleeding.
- *PPIs:* Reduce gastric acid required for nonheme iron solubilization.
- *ACE inhibitors/ARBs:* Associated with suppression of erythropoiesis and potential gastrointestinal side effects.

Pathogenesis

The pathogenesis of ID in HF is multifaceted and spans molecular, cellular, and systemic domains **(Flowchart 2)**. It involves disrupted iron homeostasis, altered regulatory protein expression, impaired absorption, sequestration mechanisms, and dysfunction across critical organ systems such as the heart, liver, kidney, and gastrointestinal tract. These derangements cumulatively impact oxygen transport, mitochondrial function, skeletal muscle metabolism, and inflammatory signaling.[10,11]

Molecular Pathways: Hepcidin–Ferroportin Axis

The cornerstone of iron regulation lies in the hepcidin–ferroprotein pathway. Hepcidin, a peptide hormone synthesized in the liver, is the master regulator of systemic iron metabolism. It binds to ferroportin, the only known iron exporter expressed on enterocytes, hepatocytes, and macrophages, triggering its internalization and degradation.

- *High hepcidin levels:* Induced by inflammation (IL-6 and TNF-α), result in ferroportin degradation and reduced iron efflux
- *Low hepcidin levels:* Stimulated by hypoxia or erythropoietic drive, promote increased iron absorption and release

In HF, persistent inflammation sustains elevated hepcidin levels, particularly in functional ID. This causes iron trapping within the reticuloendothelial system and limits its bioavailability for erythropoiesis and mitochondrial use, even if total body iron stores are adequate.[11]

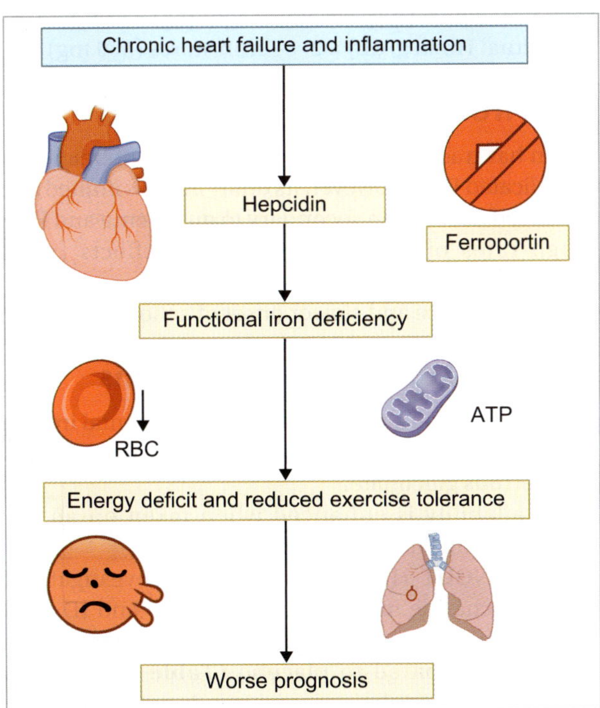

FLOWCHART 2: Pathogenesis of heart failure in iron deficiency.

Iron's Role in Cellular and Mitochondrial Physiology

Iron is vital for the function of multiple enzymes, particularly those involved in oxidative phosphorylation and cellular respiration:

- *Cytochromes complexes I–IV:* Iron–Sulphur clusters and heme groups are essential components of mitochondrial electron transport.
- *Ribonucleotide reductase:* Iron-dependent enzyme crucial for DNA synthesis.
- *Catalase and peroxidase:* Iron-based enzymes in oxidative stress defense.

In HF, systemic ID leads to impaired mitochondrial ATP generation, particularly in cardiac and skeletal myocytes, resulting in fatigue, dyspnea, and reduced exercise tolerance.[10,11]

Organ-level Dysfunction

Heart

Reduced myocardial iron content in failing hearts has been confirmed via biopsy and imaging studies. Iron is necessary for cardiomyocyte energy metabolism, contractility, and calcium handling. ID leads to decreased force generation, worsened systolic/diastolic function, and arrhythmogenic potential. Studies have shown that even in nonanemic HF patients, low myocardial iron correlates with worse NYHA class and exercise parameters.[12]

Liver

Liver is central to iron storage and hepcidin production. In congestive hepatopathy due to right HF, iron metabolism may be disrupted through altered hepcidin synthesis or venous congestion.[11] Hepatic iron sequestration without systemic availability is common in functional ID.

Gastrointestinal Tract

Splanchnic congestion and gut edema impair nutrient and iron absorption.[9,11] Ischemia-reperfusion injury due to low cardiac output may reduce mucosal barrier integrity and expression of iron transporters (e.g., DMT1 and DCYTB).

PPIs reduce ferric to ferrous conversion, further limiting uptake.

Kidney

Chronic kidney disease, often comorbid in HF, reduces erythropoietin production and impairs iron handling.[12] Elevated fibroblast growth factor-23 (FGF-23) in CKD-HF syndromes may further interfere with iron metabolism.[12]

Clinical Presentation and Classification

Iron deficiency, whether absolute or functional, produces a spectrum of clinical manifestations in patients with or without HF. In the general population, ID may remain subclinical until anemia sets in. However, in the setting of HF—both reduced ejection fraction (HFrEF) and preserved ejection fraction (HFpEF)—ID independently contributes to symptom burden, exercise intolerance, and poor outcomes, even in the absence of anemia.[12]

Symptoms of Iron Deficiency in the General Population

Standalone ID typically presents with nonspecific and gradually progressing symptoms such as fatigue, lethargy, impaired cognitive function, poor concentration, restless legs syndrome, cold intolerance, brittle nails, hair loss, pallor of the skin, and conjunctivae. When progressing to iron deficiency anemia (IDA), symptoms may worsen to include exertional dyspnea, palpitations, light-headedness, and signs of cardiovascular compensation (tachycardia and systolic murmurs).[13]

CLASSIFICATION OF ANEMIA IN HEART FAILURE

Anemia in HF is defined as:
- Hemoglobin <13 g/dL in men
- Hemoglobin <12 g/dL in women

Prevalence of anemia in HF ranges from 20 to 40%, depending on population and HF phenotype. It is often multifactorial, with ID, CKD, inflammation, and medication effects contributing.[14]

Staging of Iron Deficiency

Staging helps guide the clinical evaluation and timing of intervention:
- *Stage I:* Depleted iron stores—low ferritin and normal TSAT
- *Stage II:* Iron-deficient erythropoiesis—low TSAT and rising soluble transferrin receptor (sTfR)
- *Stage III:* ID anemia—low Hb, MCV, ferritin, TSAT, and increased sTfR

This staged approach provides a pathophysiologic continuum from early iron depletion to overt anemia.[13,15]

RATIONALE FOR IRON SUPPLEMENTATION IN HEART FAILURE

Iron deficiency is not merely a bystander but a therapeutic target in HF. Independent of anemia, ID has been linked to adverse outcomes, including reduced exercise capacity, worsened quality of life, and increased risk of hospitalization.[1,5,6,8] Correction of ID, particularly via intravenous (IV) iron, has demonstrated significant clinical benefit in randomized controlled trials. This therapeutic strategy is now endorsed in guideline-directed HF management.[10,16]

Therapeutic Endpoints

Management of ID in HF is aimed at achieving two sets of endpoints:
1. *Biochemical endpoints*:
   - Normalization of serum ferritin and TSAT levels[1]
   - Improvement in hemoglobin if IDA is present[13]
2. *Clinical endpoints*:
   - Improved NYHA class and exercise tolerance (6MWD and VO_2 max)
   - Reduced fatigue and dyspnea
   - Decreased HF hospitalizations and emergency visits
   - Improved health-related quality of life (KCCQ scores)

Intravenous Iron Therapy

Intravenous iron circumvents issues of poor GI absorption and rapidly replenishes iron stores **(Table 3)**. It is now the preferred route for managing ID in patients with symptomatic HF.[1,3,5,6] Dose calculation (Ganzoni formula):

Total iron deficit (mg) = Body weight (kg) × (Target Hb – actual Hb in g/dL) × 2.4 + Iron stores (500 mg)

Oral Iron Therapy

Oral iron has traditionally been the mainstay of treatment for uncomplicated IDA. However, its utility in HF is limited due to:
- Reduced absorption secondary to gut edema and PPI use
- High rates of gastrointestinal side effects (nausea, constipation, and abdominal pain)
- Poor adherence and slower onset of action

Dose Calculation and Regimens

- *Typical oral iron dosing:* 100–200 mg elemental iron daily.
- Preparations include ferrous sulphate, ferrous fumarate, and ferrous gluconate.
- Bioavailability is enhanced when taken on an empty stomach with vitamin C.

The IRONOUT-HF trial[11] specifically investigated oral iron polysaccharide in patients with HFrEF and ID, finding no significant improvement in exercise capacity or iron parameters compared to placebo **(Table 4)**. Given poor outcomes in HF populations, oral iron is not recommended in symptomatic HF with ID per ESC 2021 and ACC/AHA/HFSA 2022 guidelines.[10,16]

Monitoring and Follow-up

Patients receiving IV iron should be monitored for:

- *Clinical response:* NYHA class, 6MWD, and symptom burden
- *Laboratory reassessment at 4–12 weeks posttherapy:*
    - Ferritin
    - TSAT
    - Hemoglobin
- Repeat dosing if ID recurs or persists

Routine monitoring for hypersensitivity or iron overload is recommended, especially for those with comorbid CKD or hepatic disease.

TABLE 3: Commonly available intravenous iron formulations and their key pharmacological features.

Formulation	Dose administered in a single sitting	Total duration of dose administration	Hypersensitivity testing required	Comments
Ferric carboxymaltose	750–1,000 mg in 15–250 mL	Slow intravenous push or infusion over 15 minutes	No	Preferred due to safety and efficacy
Iron sucrose	100–200 mg in 100 mL	Slow intravenous push or infusion over 30 minutes	No	Requires multiple administrations
Ferric derisomaltose	1,000 mg (20 mg/kg) in 100–500 mL	20 minutes	No	Newest formulation; higher single-dose option
Ferric gluconate	125–250 mg in 110–250 mL	1–2 hours	No	Better safety profile
Ferumoxytol	510 mg in 50–200 mL	15 minutes	No	Used for IDA in CKD; potential for use as vascular MRI contrast agent when gadolinium is contraindicated
Iron dextran complex	100–1,000 mg in 250–1,000 mL	3–5 minutes for test dose followed by 1-hour observation period; 2–6 hours for rest of dose	Yes	More prone to cause severe hypersensitivity reactions

(CKD: chronic kidney disease; IDA: iron deficiency anemia; MRI: magnetic resonance imaging)

TABLE 4: Randomized controlled trials of oral iron in heart failure.

Trial	Year	Trial design and population	Oral intervention (dose/duration)	Comparator	No. of patients (analyzed)	Follow-up	Primary outcome	Key finding
IRON-HF	2013	Multicenter, randomized, double-blind RCT in anemic HF patients	Ferrous sulfate 200 mg TID PO for 8 weeks	IV iron sucrose 200 mg weekly ×5 weeks, and placebo arms (three-arm)	23 randomized (18 with full follow-up)	3 months (primary peak VO_2 change)	Change in peak VO_2	IV iron increased peak VO_2 (~+3.5 mL/kg/min); oral iron group had no increment in peak VO_2. Ferritin and TSAT rose in both iron groups; hemoglobin rose similarly. Study small/underpowered
IRONOUT-HF	2017	Multicenter, double-blind RCT in patients with HFrEF (LVEF ≤40%) and iron deficiency	Oral iron polysaccharide 150 mg twice daily	Placebo	225 randomized (analyzed set ~98–225 depending on outcome)	16 weeks	Change in peak VO_2 (exercise capacity)	No significant improvement in peak VO_2 vs. placebo; minimal biochemical repletion; oral iron did not improve clinical exercise capacity

Continued

Continued

Trial	Year	Trial design and population	Oral intervention (dose/duration)	Comparator	No. of patients (analyzed)	Follow-up	Primary outcome	Key finding
Zdravković et al. (Effects of 6 months of oral ferrous and ferric supplement therapy in patients who were hospitalized for decompensated CHF)	2019	RCT (two-arm) in patients hospitalized for ADHF	Ferrous fumarate (oral) vs. ferric hydroxide-polymaltose complex (oral)	Active oral comparator (two oral formulations)	201 randomized (100 vs. 101)	6 months	6-minute walk distance (6MWD), hemoglobin, NYHA class	Both oral preparations improved Hb, 6MWD and NYHA class at 6 months; the trial compared two oral forms. Results supportive for oral repletion in this setting, but this was not a placebo-controlled trial
Suryani et al. (Oral ferrous sulphate improves functional capacity in HF patients with IDA)	2022	Double-blind RCT in HF patients with iron-deficiency anemia	Oral ferrous sulphate for 12 weeks	Placebo (double-blind)	(See paper)—single-center randomized cohort; numbers reported in article	~12 weeks	Functional capacity (6MWD), NYHA class, iron indices	Reported significant improvement in functional capacity and iron parameters vs. placebo after 12 weeks. This positive result was in an IDA (anemic) HF cohort in Indonesia; generalizability may differ

(6MWD: 6-minute walk distance; ADHF: acute decompensated heart failure; CHF: congestive heart failure; HFrEF: heart failure with reduced ejection fraction; IDA: iron deficiency anemia; LVEF: left ventricular ejection fraction; NYHA: New York Heart Association; RCT: randomized controlled trial; TSAT: transferrin saturation; VO_2: oxygen consumption)

Clinical Implications

Functional Capacity and Symptoms

Iron deficiency in HF correlates with reduced exercise tolerance, independent of anemia.[1,2] It contributes to decreased mitochondrial oxidative capacity and impaired oxygen utilization in peripheral tissues, particularly skeletal muscle.[15] Multiple studies (e.g., CONFIRM-HF and EFFECT-HF) have shown that correcting ID leads to measurable improvements in 6MWD and peak VO_2, directly translating to enhanced daily functioning and symptom burden relief **(Table 5)**.

Prognosis

Iron deficiency in HF has been linked with increased risk of hospitalization and mortality. A meta-analysis of 10,565 patients from 10 studies revealed that ID was associated with a 52% increase in all-cause mortality and 43% increase in HF hospitalizations, independent of hemoglobin levels.[10]

Health Economics

The economic burden of HF is amplified by comorbid ID. Increased hospitalization rates, prolonged rehabilitation, and reduced productivity due to fatigue and dyspnea translate into substantial direct and indirect costs. In a German cost-utility analysis, IV iron therapy with ferric carboxymaltose was found to be cost-effective in reducing rehospitalizations and improving quality-adjusted life years (QALYs) in CHF patients with ID.[16]

Guideline Recommendations

Based on this compelling evidence base, both ESC 2021 and ACC/AHA/HFSA 2022 guidelines now recommend routine screening and treatment of ID in patients with HF:

- *ESC (2021):*[4] In all patients with HF and suspected or confirmed ID (ferritin <100 ng/mL or 100–299 ng/mL with TSAT <20%), IV iron therapy with ferric carboxymaltose is recommended to improve symptoms and quality of life (Class IIa, Level A).

TABLE 5: Randomized control trials of intravenous iron supplementation in heart failure.

Study	Year	Design and population	Intervention (dose)	Comparator	No. of patients (randomized)	Follow-up	Primary outcome	Key findings/ results
FERRIC-HF	2008	Single-blind RCT; symptomatic chronic HF (HFrEF) with ID ± anemia	Iron sucrose (200 mg IV weekly ×5)	Standard care/placebo (observer-blinded)	35	2–3 months	Change in exercise tolerance (peak VO_2/6MWD)	IV iron improved exercise tolerance and symptoms vs. control in this small trial
FAIR-HF	2009	Multicenter, double-blind RCT; ambulatory HFrEF (NYHA II–III) with ID ± anemia	Ferric carboxymaltose (200–1,000 mg IV per protocol; initial correction + maintenance)	Placebo (saline)	459	24 weeks	Patient global assessment and NYHA class	FCM significantly improved patient global assessment, NYHA class and 6MWD vs. placebo; benefit in anemic and nonanemic patients
CONFIRM-HF	2015	Double-blind, placebo-controlled RCT; symptomatic ambulatory HF with ID	Ferric carboxymaltose (dosing per body weight, up to 1,000 mg)	Placebo	304	52 weeks	Change in 6MWD at 24 weeks (maintained to 52 weeks)	FCM produced sustained and clinically meaningful improvement in 6MWD, QoL, and reduced fatigue over 52 weeks
EFFECT-HF	2017	Randomized trial in HFrEF patients with ID	Ferric carboxymaltose (500–1,000 mg per protocol)	Standard care	174	24 weeks	Change in peak VO_2 on CPET	FCM preserved or improved peak VO_2 compared with standard care; favorable effect on exercise capacity
AFFIRM-AHF	2020	Multicenter, double-blind RCT; ADHF with ID, stabilized at discharge	Ferric carboxymaltose: 1,000 mg (± additional dosing) near discharge	Placebo	1,108	52 weeks	Composite of total HF hospitaliza-tions and CV death	No significant reduction in primary composite endpoint, but reduced recurrent HF hospitalizations and improved QoL
IRONMAN	2022	Large pragmatic RCT; HFrEF and ID in real-world setting	Ferric derisomaltose (single high-dose infusions up to 1,500 mg as needed)	Standard care	1,820	Median 2.7 years	*Primary composite*: Recurrent HF hospitaliza-tions and CV death	Numerical reduction (~18% relative) but not statistically significant; signals of benefit in secondary analyses
HEART-FID	2023	Multicenter, double-blind, placebo-controlled RCT; HFrEF (LVEF ≤45%), NYHA II–IV with ID	Ferric carboxymaltose (dosing per Ganzoni formula)	Placebo	3,065	Median 1.9 years	*Hierarchical composite*: Death, HF hospitaliza-tions, 6MWD	Primary outcome not met, but fewer deaths (8.6% vs. 10.3%), fewer HF hospitalizations, modest 6MWD gain

(6MWD: 6-minute walk distance; ADHF: acute decompensated heart failure; FCM: ferric carboxymaltose; HFrEF: heart failure with reduced ejection fraction; IDA: iron deficiency anemia; LVEF: left ventricular ejection fraction; NYHA: New York Heart Association; QoL: quality of life; RCT: randomized controlled trial; VO_2: oxygen consumption)

- *ACC/AHA/HFSA (2022):*[5] In symptomatic HFrEF (NYHA II–III), screening for ID is reasonable, and treatment with IV iron may be considered to improve functional status and QoL (Class IIb, Level B-R).

Future Frontiers

Iron Deficiency in Heart Failure with Preserved Ejection Fraction

Historically underrepresented in clinical trials,[14,17] patients with HFpEF also exhibit a high prevalence of ID (~40–60%), similar to those with HFrEF. Given the growing burden of HFpEF in the aging population, there is significant interest in extending iron repletion strategies to this cohort.

Iron Therapy in Ischemic Cardiomyopathy

Emerging observational studies suggest that ID is associated with worse myocardial remodeling and LV function in ischemic cardiomyopathy (ICMP). Iron repletion may contribute to improved myocardial energetics and mitochondrial function and reduce arrhythmogenic burden post-MI.[9] Proposed mechanisms include modulation of oxidative stress, mitochondrial repair, and endothelial

TABLE 6: Ongoing trials for intravenous iron supplementation in heart failure.

Trial	Design and enrollment	Study population	Active treatment group	Control group	Outcomes	Follow-up period
FAIR-HF2 (NCT03036462)	Phase 4, triple blinding, randomized controlled trial; *n* = 1,200	Chronic HF (≥3 months) with LVEF<45%; NYHA II–III or HF hospitalization past 12 months or elevated NP; ID: ferritin<100 or ferritin 100–299 + TSAT <20%; Hb 9.5–14.0	Ferric carboxymaltose 1,000 mg bolus + 500–1,000 mg within 4 weeks (max 2,000 mg induction); maintenance 500 mg q4mo unless Hb>16 or ferritin>800	Placebo	*Primary*: Composite of recurrent HF hospitalizations and CV death	≥6 months, mean follow-up >2 years
Effect of IV iron replacement on exercise capacity in individuals with HF (NCT05816265)	Phase 4, open-label, randomized controlled trial; *n* = 40	NYHA II or I, LVEF ≤40%, not admitted; ID: ferritin <100 or ferritin 100–300 + TSAT <20%	Ferric carboxymaltose per physician discretion; dose at 1 week post-enrollment	No placebo	• *Primary*: Exercise capacity (peak VO_2 via CPET), KCCQ score • *Secondary*: 6MWD in improved NYHA class	2 months
INERTIA trial (NCT04786769)	Phase 4, quadruple blinding, randomized controlled trial; *n* = 2,500	Severe AS for TAVR/SAVR; Hb 8–15; ID: ferritin <100 or ferritin 100–299 + TSAT <20%	Ferric carboxymaltose per BW/Hb; repeat at 12 weeks if ID persists	Placebo	• *Primary*: Time to first HF hospitalization or CV death • *Secondary*: 6MWD, KCCQ score	Up to 52 weeks
COREVIVE-HFpEF (NCT05991128)	Phase 4, double blinding, randomized controlled trial; *n* = 170	HFpEF (LVEF ≥50%) hospitalized for AHF, stable post-GDMT; ID: ferritin <100 or ferritin 100–299 + TSAT <20%; Hb 9–13.5 (women) or 9–14.5 (men)	Ferric derisomaltose per BW/Hb (max 1,500–2,000 mg)	Placebo	• *Primary*: 6MWD change baseline–day 3 • *Secondary*: 6MWD change at 2 and 4 weeks; KCCQ change	Up to 4 weeks

Continued

Continued

Trial	Design and enrollment	Study population	Active treatment group	Control group	Outcomes	Follow-up period
COREVIVE-HFrEF (NCT05971732)	Phase 4, double blinding, randomized controlled trial; *n* = 146	HF (LVEF <50%) hospitalized for AHF, stable post-GDMT; ID: ferritin <100 or ferritin 100–299 + TSAT <20%; Hb 9–13.5 (women) or 9–14.5 (men)	Ferric derisomaltose as per body weight/Hb (max 1,500–2,000 mg)	Placebo	• *Primary*: 6MWD change baseline–day 3 • *Secondary*: 6MWD change at 2 and 4 weeks; KCCQ change	Up to 4 weeks
IRONMET-HFpEF (NCT04945707)	Phase 4, quadruple blinding, randomized controlled trial; *n* = 66	Outpatient HFpEF (LVEF ≥50%, NYHA II–IV), elevated NP; Hb >9 and <15; ID: ferritin <100 or ferritin 100–300 + TSAT <20%; Peak VO_2 ≤75% predicted by CPET	Ferric derisomaltose 1,000 mg once (BW<50 kg: 20 mg/kg)	Placebo	*Primary*: Peak VO_2 via CPET	12 weeks
RESAFE (NCT04974021)	Single-arm prospective cohort study; *n* = 106	Outpatient HFrEF (LVEF ≤40%) with implanted cardiac device ≥3 months	Ferric carboxymaltose (per clinical routine)	Not applicable	• *Primary*: Hb ≥12, ferritin ≥50, TSAT >20% • *Secondary*: VT events on device	6–12 months
INFERRCT (NCT05759078)	Phase 4, triple blinding, randomized controlled trial; *n* = 2,000	STEMI/NSTEMI ≤4 weeks prerandomization; ID: TSAT <20% and/or ferritin<100; ≥3 of: LVEF ≤50%, NP elevated, congestion needing IV diuretics, DM, AF, CAD, incomplete revascularization, prior MI, age ≥70, eGFR <60	Ferric carboxymaltose 1,000 mg on day of randomization; repeat at 4 and 8 months if ID persists	Placebo	• *Primary*: Hierarchical—1. CV death; 2. HF events; 3. Time to first HF event; 4. QoL change • *Secondary*: HF events, QoL change	52 weeks, QoL EQ-5D at 32 weeks

(6MWD: 6 minute walk distance; ADHF: acute decompensated heart failure; AF: atrial fibrillation; AS: aortic stenosis; CAD: coronary artery disease; CPET: cardiopulmonary exercise testing; DM: diabetes mellitus; FCM: ferric carboxymaltose; GDMT: guideline directed medical therapy; HFrEF: heart failure with reduced ejection fraction; IDA: iron deficiency anemia; KCCQ: Kansas city cardiomyopathy questionnaire; LVEF: left ventricular ejection fraction; NP: natriuretic peptide; NYHA: New York Heart Association; QoL: quality of life; RCT: randomized controlled trial; SAVR: surgical aortic valve replacement; TAVR: transcatheter aortic valve replacement; TSAT: transferrin saturation; VO_2: oxygen consumption; VT: ventricular tachycardia)

function enhancement. Small-scale studies show improved GLS and LVEF after FCM in ICMP cohorts **(Table 6)**.

Role of Iron Supplementation Post-PCI and CABG

Patients undergoing revascularization procedures (PCI or CABG) often exhibit ID, which may impair tissue repair, prolong rehabilitation, and worsen outcomes. Anemia and ID are associated with higher periprocedural complications and longer ICU/hospital stay. Small pilot studies (e.g., FERICABG) have shown improvement in functional status and shorter time to ambulation with perioperative IV iron.[9] However, larger trials are needed to validate these findings.

Guideline Evolution and Research Gaps

As data accumulates, future updates to HF management guidelines are expected to extend IV iron recommendations to include HFpEF, clarify role of IV iron in post-ACS, post-

CABG, and primary prevention, define optimal biomarkers (e.g., sTfR and hepcidin) for monitoring iron status and explore combination therapy with erythropoietin stimulating agents (ESA) in CKD-HF overlap patients.

CONCLUSION

Iron deficiency is a highly prevalent and modifiable comorbidity in patients with both chronic and acute HF irrespective of ejection fraction status. Increasing clinical and mechanistic evidence demonstrates that ID has detrimental effects beyond hematologic compromise, affecting cellular energetics, myocardial performance, skeletal muscle metabolism, and neurohormonal homeostasis. As a result, the presence of ID represents a critical therapeutic opportunity to improve functional capacity, reduce hospitalizations, and potentially enhance survival. In the Indian context, with an exceptionally high background prevalence of ID and ID anemia, implementation of iron therapy is particularly vital. National cardiology societies and health systems should aim to integrate ID screening into routine HF care, scale access to IV iron formulations, and improve patient awareness. Identification and targeted correction of ID—particularly through intravenous iron supplementation—should be considered a cornerstone of modern HF therapy.

REFERENCES

1. Anker SD, Comin Colet J, Filippatos G, et al. Ferric carboxymaltose in patients with heart failure and iron deficiency. N Engl J Med. 2009;361(25):2436-48.
2. Ponikowski P, van Veldhuisen DJ, Comin-Colet J, et al. Beneficial effects of long-term intravenous iron therapy with ferric carboxymaltose in patients with symptomatic heart failure and iron deficiency. Eur Heart J. 2015;36(11):657-68.
3. Ponikowski P, Kirwan BA, Anker SD, et al. Ferric carboxymaltose for iron deficiency at discharge after acute heart failure: a multicenter, double-blind, randomized, controlled trial. Lancet. 2020;396(10266):1895-904.
4. McDonagh TA, Metra M, Adamo M, et al. 2021 ESC Guidelines for the diagnosis and treatment of acute and chronic heart failure. Eur Heart J. 2021;42(36):3599-726.
5. Heidenreich PA, Bozkurt B, Aguilar D, et al. 2022 AHA/ACC/HFSA guideline for the management of heart failure. J Am Coll Cardiol. 2022;79(17):e263-421.
6. World Health Organization. Worldwide prevalence of anaemia 1993–2005: WHO Global Database on Anaemia. Geneva: WHO; 2008.
7. Comin–Colet J, Enjuanes C, González G, et al. Iron deficiency is a key determinant of health-related quality of life in patients with chronic heart failure regardless of anaemia status. Eur J Heart Fail. 2013;15(10):1164-72.
8. Bekfani T, Pellicori P, Morris DA, et al. Prevalence of iron deficiency in patients with HFpEF and its relation to functional capacity and quality of life. ESC Heart Fail. 2019;6(5):940-8.
9. Pratibha V, Kumar P, Bansal S, et al. Iron deficiency in Indian heart failure patients: a prospective observational study. Indian Heart J. 2021;73(5):601-7.
10. Jankowska EA, Rozentryt P, Witkowska A, et al. Iron deficiency: an ominous sign in patients with systolic chronic heart failure. Eur Heart J. 2010;31(15):1872-80.
11. Macdougall IC, Ponikowski P, Dignass AU. Intravenous iron therapy in patients with chronic heart failure: review of recent evidence and future directions. Heart Fail Rev. 2022;27(5):1455-69.
12. Klip IT, Comin-Colet J, Voors AA, et al. The failing heart and the kidney: the cardiorenal syndrome. Cardiorenal Med. 2013;3(2):87-98.
13. Lewis GD, Malhotra R, Hernandez AF, et al. Effect of oral iron repletion on exercise capacity in patients with heart failure with reduced ejection fraction and iron deficiency: the IRONOUT HF randomized clinical trial. J Am Med Assoc. 2017;317(19):1958-66.
14. Ministry of Health and Family Welfare. National Family Health Survey (NFHS-5), India Fact Sheet. Government of India; 2021.
15. Martens P, Dupont M, Mullens W. Iron deficiency as therapeutic target in heart failure with preserved ejection fraction. J Am Coll Cardiol Heart Fail. 2021;9(10):813-21.
16. Wolff G, Kropff J, Schaller S, et al. Cost-effectiveness of ferric carboxymaltose in patients with chronic heart failure and iron deficiency in Germany. Clinicoecon Outcomes Res. 2013;5:437-47.
17. Yancy CW, Jessup M, Bozkurt B, et al. 2013 ACCF/AHA guideline for the management of heart failure: a report of the American College of Cardiology Foundation/American Heart Association Task Force on Practice Guidelines. J Am Coll Cardiol. 2013;62(16):e147-239.

CHAPTER

23

Risk Scores in the Management of Heart Failure

Ashish Jha, Abhijit Bharali

ABSTRACT

Heart failure (HF) affects over 64 million people worldwide, with high morbidity and mortality despite therapeutic advances. Risk stratification is essential for identifying high-risk patients, guiding management, and optimizing resources. This chapter summarizes HF risk scores across the disease spectrum. Diagnostic tools (Framingham, ARIC, and PCP-HF) enable early detection; prognostic models (SHFM, MAGGIC, GWTG-HF, CORONA, and BIOSTAT-CHF) estimate long-term outcomes; and acute HF scores (ADHERE, EHMRG, MEESSI, OTTAWA, OPTIMIZE-HF, STRATIFY, and PROTECT) aid triage and discharge planning. Advanced HF scores (INTERMACS, HFSS, MECKI, and CHARM) inform device or transplant timing. Integrating multiple models with clinical judgment supports personalized, precision HF management.

Keywords: Heart failure, risk scores for acute heart failure, risk scores for prognosis in heart failure.

INTRODUCTION

Heart failure (HF) is a clinical syndrome in which the heart cannot meet the metabolic demands of the body. HF affects >64 million people worldwide and is associated with high morbidity, frequent hospitalizations, and considerable mortality. Despite advances in guideline-directed therapies, mortality after a hospitalization for HF remains high, with 30-day and 1-year mortality rates ranging from 4 to 12% and 20 to 30%.[1] Risk stratification is therefore essential to differentiate patients at high risk of adverse outcomes who may benefit from intensive management from those at low risk who might be managed safely as outpatients. Over the past two decades, numerous risk scores have been developed for patients with acute, chronic, and advanced HF, but their integration into clinical decisionmaking remains limited. This chapter summarizes contemporary risk models, highlights their strengths and limitations, and proposes a pragmatic algorithm for incorporating risk scores into HF management.

WHY RISK STRATIFICATION MATTERS?

Heart failure encompasses a heterogeneous population in which prognoses range from near normal survival to very poor survival. Accurate risk stratification helps clinicians counsel patients regarding prognosis, prioritize resources such as mechanical circulatory support (MCS) or transplantation, and tailor follow-up intensity. Moreover, risk scores can inform decisions about hospital disposition; e.g., emergency departments need tools to identify patients suitable for safe outpatient management. However, an editorial commentary from the Journal of the American College of Cardiology noted that despite the proliferation of risk scores, very few are routinely used in practice because guidelines seldom link treatment recommendations to risk assessments and because risk-based alerts alone do not change clinician behavior.[2] The authors emphasized that for risk scores to be useful, they must be embedded within evidence-based care pathways and evaluated in randomized trials. They also highlighted the need for artificial intelligence (AI) and electronic health record integration to manage large volumes of data generated by wearable devices and monitoring systems.

Diagnostic Scores for Acute Heart Failure

In the preclinical and early symptomatic stages of HF, timely identification of at-risk individuals is paramount. Diagnostic risk scores serve as screening tools, enabling stratification of individuals according to their likelihood of developing HF and guiding decisions regarding further evaluation or preventive therapy.

The *Framingham Heart Failure Risk Score (FHS-HF)*, developed from the landmark Framingham Heart Study, is a sex-specific model estimating the 10-year risk of incident heart failure in asymptomatic adults.[3] It uses readily obtainable variables—age, BMI, systolic blood pressure (SBP), electrocardiographic left ventricular hypertrophy, history of valvular heart disease, diabetes, prior myocardial infarction, and smoking status. It is particularly useful for primary prevention, enabling early identification of high-risk individuals, guiding lifestyle counseling, and prompting timely initiation of antihypertensive, lipid-lowering, or glucose-lowering therapy.

The *Atherosclerosis Risk in Communities (ARIC) Heart Failure Risk Score* extends this approach to a large, multiethnic population.[4] It incorporates many FHS-HF variables but addition of NT-proBNP and race markedly enhances its predictive accuracy and reclassification. Optional inclusion of electrocardiographic abnormalities further refines risk estimation.

The *Primary Care Partner–Heart Failure (PCP-HF) Score* was designed for practicality in primary care.[5] It includes fasting glucose, BMI, total and HDL cholesterol, SBP, smoking status, antihypertensive medication, diabetes medication, QRS duration, and age-race interactions to predict 10-year absolute risk for incident HF.

Collectively, these diagnostic scores form the first step in the heart failure risk continuum, supporting early, structured detection of vulnerable individuals and providing a foundation for ongoing risk surveillance as the disease evolves.

Prognostic Scores (Long-term Mortality/Outcome Prediction)

Prognostic scores in HF, such as *SHFM, MAGGIC, GWTG-HF, CORONA, and BIOSTAT-CHF*, integrate clinical, laboratory, and demographic variables to estimate long-term mortality and adverse outcomes. They help stratify patients into risk categories, guiding personalized treatment intensity, follow-up frequency, and advanced therapy consideration.

The *Seattle Heart Failure Model (SHFM)* is a validated multivariable prognostic system designed to estimate 1-, 2-, and 3-year survival in chronic HF.[6] It incorporates demographic factors (age and sex), clinical variables [New York Heart Association (NYHA) class, body weight, SBP, left ventricular ejection fraction], laboratory parameters (serum sodium, hemoglobin, lymphocyte percentage, uric acid, and total cholesterol), treatment details (ACE inhibitors/ARBs, beta-blockers, statins, diuretics, and allopurinol), and device therapy status (ICD and CRT). Each parameter contributes a weighted coefficient, and the total score aligns with predicted survival, facilitating individualized prognostic discussions and guiding long-term management.

The *MAGGIC Risk Score* (Meta-analysis Global Group in Chronic Heart Failure) was derived from pooled data of over 39,000 patients and predicts 1- and 3-year all-cause mortality.[6] It uses 13 common clinical parameters—age, sex, SBP, BMI, left ventricular ejection fraction, serum creatinine, smoking, diabetes, COPD, NYHA class, time since diagnosis, and use of beta-blockers and ACEIs/ARBs. Each factor is assigned points based on mortality association, with the total score categorizing patients into low-, intermediate-, or high-risk groups.

Get with the Guidelines–Heart Failure Risk Score

The score developed by the American Heart Association from data on over 39,000 hospitalized patients predicts in-hospital mortality using seven readily available variables: Age, SBP, heart rate, BUN, serum sodium, presence of COPD, and race (Black vs. non-Black).[7] Each variable is assigned a certain number of points, resulting in a total score ranging from 0 to 100. Risk categories are often defined as low (≤43), intermediate (44–53), and high (≥54). While the score does not dictate specific treatment pathways, it is valuable for identifying low-risk patients who might be suitable for early discharge and high-risk patients who may benefit from intensive monitoring, advanced therapies, or early palliative care involvement. It has been validated in diverse patient populations and shown to predict both in-hospital and 30-day mortality **(Table 1)**.

The original study did not specify a particular treatment strategy based on the GWTG-HF score. Nevertheless, the score can help identify patients at low risk of inhospital death who might be candidates for early discharge or observation unit care. Conversely, patients with high scores may warrant intensive monitoring, early initiation of advanced therapies and discussion with palliative care. Subsequent studies have validated the score in diverse populations and compared it with laboratory based risk models such as the Intermountain Risk Score. A rural hospital analysis showed that the GWTG-HF score independently predicted 30 days mortality, with higher tertiles associated with increased odds of death **(Table 2)**.

Acute Heart Failure Admission or In-hospital Risk Scores

Risk models for acute heart failure (AHF)—such as *ADHERE, EHMRG, MEESSI, OTTAWA, OPTIMIZE-HF, STRATIFY, PROTECT, etc.*, are designed to estimate in-hospital mortality, early complications, or likelihood of readmission. By guiding clinical priorities, informing safe discharge timing, and focusing follow-up resources, these scores help improve short-term outcomes and risk stratification in emergency or hospital settings.

Among AHF risk prediction tools, the *ADHERE Risk Tree* is a straightforward bedside model from the Acute Decompensated Heart Failure National Registry, designed to predict in-hospital mortality using only three admission parameters: BUN, SBP, and serum creatinine. Sequential cutoffs—BUN >43 mg/dL, SBP <115 mm Hg,

TABLE 1: Components and scoring of the GWTG-HF risk score.

Variable	Categories	Approximate points	Commentary
Blood urea nitrogen	<30 mg/dL; 30–43 mg/dL; >43 mg/dL	0; 11; up to 22 points	BUN is the strongest predictor; levels >43 mg/dL contribute up to 22 points
Systolic blood pressure	>140 mm Hg; 115–140 mm Hg; <115 mm Hg	0; 8; up to 15 points	Lower blood pressure indicates poor perfusion; SBP <115 mm Hg adds up to 15 points
Age	<50; 50–59; 60–69; 70–79; ≥80 years	0; 5; 9; 11; up to 13 points	Age contributes progressively more points; patients ≥80 years receive ~13 points
Heart rate	<75; 75–99; ≥100 beats/min	0; 5; up to 7 points	Tachycardia reflects sympathetic activation and worse prognosis
Serum sodium	>140; 135–140; <135 mmol/L	0; 3; up to 6 points	Hyponatremia is associated with neurohormonal activation and poor outcomes
Chronic obstructive pulmonary disease	No; Yes	0; ~3 points	Presence of COPD adds a modest increment due to comorbidity
Race	Black; non-Black	0; up to 4 points	Non-Black race adds points reflecting disparities observed in the derivation cohort

TABLE 2: Comparative summary of prognostic scores.[6]

Score name	Primary purpose	Key variables	Risk stratification	Significance
Seattle Heart Failure Model (SHFM) (2006)	Predict survival in chronic HF and guide therapy decisions	Age, sex, LVEF, NYHA class, SBP, weight, medications, laboratory values, and device therapy	Predicts 1, 2 and 3year survival; widely used for selecting candidates for device therapy; *Cstatistic ~0.73*	Widely validated; integrates clinical, lab, and therapy data
MAGGIC Risk Score (2018)	Estimate mortality risk using pooled chronic HF data	Age, sex, LVEF, NYHA class, BMI, creatinine, diabetes, COPD, and HF etiology	Total score 0–49; higher scores correlate with increased 1 and 3 year mortality; *Cstatistic ~0.76–0.82*	Large-pooled dataset enhances generalizability
GWTG-HF Risk Score (2018)	Predict in-hospital mortality in acute HF admissions	Age, SBP, HR, sodium, BUN, race, and weight, medical history	Score range; higher score predicts higher in-hospital death risk, *AUC ~0.80*	Used in quality improvement and benchmarking
CORONA Risk Score	Predict outcomes in elderly ischemic HF patients	Age, NYHA class, LVEF, creatinine, BMI, prior MI, diabetes, and atrial fibrillation	Categorized into low, medium, and high-risk groups	Tailored for elderly ischemic HF, guiding targeted care
BIOSTAT-CHF Risk Tool	Predict mortality and HF hospitalization in chronic HF	Age, LVEF, NT-proBNP, hemoglobin, eGFR, HF duration, and signs/symptoms	Continuous and categorical; predicts 2-year outcomes	Integrates biomarkers and clinical data for personalized care

creatinine >2.75 mg/dL—enable rapid classification into low-, intermediate-, or high-risk groups without complex scoring, making it highly practical for early decision-making.[6] The *EHMRG (Emergency Heart Failure Mortality Risk Grade)* estimates 7-day mortality in ED presentations of AHF, incorporating age, arrival mode, SBP, heart rate, oxygen saturation, potassium, creatinine, troponin, active cancer and prior metolazone use.[8] The *MEESSI-AHF (Multiple Estimation of risk based on the Spanish Society of Emergency Medicine-Acute Heart Failure)* predicts 30-day all-cause mortality using 13 ED-based variables including demographics, vitals, labs, NYHA class, functional status (Barthel index), prior HF visits, arrival mode, and active cancer, stratifying patients into four risk levels.[8] The *Ottawa Heart Failure Risk Score* focuses on predicting short-term serious adverse events using 10 variables—such as cerebrovascular disease, active cancer, metolazone use, ambulance arrival, SBP, oxygen saturation, heart rate, potassium, creatinine, and troponin—to guide admission versus safe discharge decisions.[8]

The *OPTIMIZE-HF score*, derived from the Organized Program to Initiate Lifesaving Treatment in Hospitalized Patients with Heart Failure registry, estimates in-hospital mortality using admission data such as age, SBP, BUN, sodium, heart rate, and history of COPD.[9] *The STRATIFY Decision Tool* identifies patients at low risk for serious 30-day postdischarge adverse events by evaluating SBP, heart rate, oxygen saturation, sodium, creatinine, troponin, recent hospitalizations, and comorbidities like COPD and diabetes; abnormal values increase risk, aiding safe discharge planning and follow-up scheduling.[8] The *PROTECT Risk Score* predicts 60-day mortality or cardiovascular/renal rehospitalization after acute decompensation, incorporating SBP, heart rate, sodium, BUN, creatinine, prior HF admissions, and comorbidities, with hypotension, renal dysfunction, hyponatremia, and frequent admissions strongly impacting risk.[10] Collectively, these models, relying on routine clinical and laboratory parameters, support evidence-based, personalized management of AHF patients from admission through postdischarge care **(Table 3)**.

Advanced Heart Failure/Device Therapy Selection Scores

Advanced heart failure and device therapy selection scores are essential for determining the timing and appropriateness of interventions such as implantable cardioverter-defibrillators (ICD), cardiac resynchronization therapy (CRT), left ventricular assist devices (LVAD), and heart transplantation. These tools integrate functional capacity, prognostic markers, and comorbidity burden to identify patients most likely to benefit from advanced therapies.

The *INTERMACS* Profiles offer a standardized framework for classifying advanced heart failure, initially designed for patients under consideration for MCS. In ambulatory patients, profiles 4–7 range from severe resting symptoms to stable advanced NYHA class III status, reflecting variations in functional limitation, symptom burden, and recent clinical instability. Lower profiles correspond to higher short-term mortality, and a greater likelihood of requiring MCS or transplantation, as shown in the this classification, assists in determining optimal referral timing for advanced therapies while weighing survival prospects against quality-of-life goals.[12] The *Heart Failure Survival Score (HFSS)* is a validated prognostic tool for transplant evaluation, incorporating resting heart rate, mean blood pressure, LVEF, serum sodium, ischemic etiology, intraventricular conduction defect, and peak VO_2.[13] It stratifies patients into low-, medium-, and high-risk groups, offering superior prognostic accuracy compared to peak VO_2 alone. When combined with INTERMACS, HFSS enhances decision-making for MCS or transplant timing.

TABLE 3: Comparative summary of acute heart failure risk scores.[11]

Score name	Primary purpose	Key variables	Risk stratification	Significance
ADHERE Risk Tree (2005)	Predict in-hospital mortality in acute decompensated HF	BUN, systolic BP, and serum creatinine	Tree-based classification into low, intermediate, high mortality risk, *AUC ~0.80*	Rapid bedside tool to guide early triage and management
EHMRG (Emergency Heart Failure Mortality Risk Grade) (2012/2019)	Predict 7-day mortality for ED patients with acute HF	Age, SBP, HR, O_2 saturation, creatinine, potassium, troponin, and comorbidities	Point-based score; higher points = higher short-term mortality, *Cstatistic 0.80*	Supports ED disposition decisions and early intervention
MEESSI (2019)	Predict 30-day mortality in acute HF in ED settings	Age, SBP, HR, oxygen saturation, potassium, creatinine, NT-proBNP, and comorbidities	Points-based; stratifies into very low, low, intermediate, high risk, *Cstatistic 0.83*	Valid in diverse populations; aids safe discharge or admission decisions
OTTAWA (2013/2017)	Predict 14-day serious adverse events post-ED discharge in acute HF	Age, SBP, HR, O_2 saturation, creatinine, potassium, and ED therapy response	Categorizes into low, intermediate, high event risk, *CStatistic 0.78*	Identifies patients safe for discharge vs. needing observation
OPTIMIZE-HF Score (2008)	Predict in-hospital and postdischarge mortality in hospitalized HF	Demographics, vitals, labs, comorbidities, and LVEF	Risk groups based on composite clinical data, *Cstatistic 0.72*	Facilitates benchmarking, quality improvement, and discharge planning
STRATIFY Decision Tool (2015)	Predict risk of adverse events in hospitalized HF patients	Demographics, comorbidities, vital signs, and laboratories	Points-based risk groups, *Cstatistic 0.68*	Guides monitoring intensity and discharge readiness
PROTECT Risk Score (2012)	Predict 30-day readmission in decompensated HF	Demographics, prior admissions, vitals, labs, comorbidities	Higher scores = higher readmission probability	Enables targeted interventions to reduce readmissions

The *MECKI Score* merges functional, cardiac, and renal metrics—peak VO_2, VE/VCO_2 slope, hemoglobin, sodium, ejection fraction, and eGFR—to estimate 2-year risk of cardiovascular death or urgent transplant. The *CHARM risk score* (Colorado Heart Failure Acuity Risk Model) score is a validated tool to predict short- and long-term mortality in patients waitlisted for heart transplantation.[14] It incorporates clinical and serological parameters, stratifies candidates into six tiers, and demonstrates high predictive accuracy, thereby improving objectivity and fairness in organ allocation **(Table 4)**.

Heart Failure with Preserved Ejection Fraction Score

The heart failure with preserved ejection fraction (HFpEF) score is a diagnostic tool designed to estimate the probability of HFpEF in patients presenting with unexplained dyspnea. One widely used model is the H_2FPEF score, which incorporates six weighted variables: Heavy (BMI), hypertensive, atrial fibrillation, pulmonary hypertension, elderly, and filling pressure elevated. The total score ranges from 0–9, with higher scores indicating a greater likelihood of HFpEF **(Table 5)**.[15]

Total possible score: 0–9 points. *0–1 points:* Low probability of HFpEF (<20%), *2–5 points:* Intermediate probability (~41–80%), *6–9 points:* High probability (>90%).

This scoring system streamlines diagnosis, reducing reliance on invasive testing. Its significance lies in facilitating early identification, guiding targeted therapy, and differentiating HFpEF from noncardiac causes of dyspnea. Integrated with functional tests and natriuretic peptide levels, it strengthens clinical decision-making and ensures timely, tailored management in suspected HFpEF cases.

PROPOSED ALGORITHM FOR RISK-BASED MANAGEMENT

Flowchart 1 presents a simplified algorithm for incorporating risk scores into HF management. Upon presentation with AHF, clinicians should assess vital signs, biomarkers, and

TABLE 4: Comparative summary of Advanced Heart Failure Risk Scores.

Score name	Primary purpose	Key variables	Risk stratification	Significance
INTERMACS Profiles (2009)	Profile advanced HF patients for mechanical support or transplant timing	Functional status, symptom burden, and recent clinical events (Profiles 1–7)	Categorizes patients into seven profiles; used to time mechanical circulatory support; discrimination moderate *CStatistic ~0.65*	Guides timing for MCS referral, aligning treatment with prognosis
Heart Failure Survival Score (HFSS)	Prognosis and transplant candidate selection in chronic HF	Resting HR, BP, LVEF, sodium, ischemic etiology, conduction defect, and peak VO_2	Designed to predict survival in ambulatory patients evaluated for transplant; low (<8.1), medium and high-risk categories	Improves accuracy of transplant listing and timing
MECKI Score (2013)	Prognosis in chronic HF integrating exercise, cardiac, and renal parameters	Peak VO_2, VE/VCO_2 slope, hemoglobin, sodium, LVEF, and eGFR	Predicts cardiovascular death, urgent transplantation or left ventricular assist device implantation within 2 years; *Cstatistic ~0.80*	Combines functional capacity and organ status for precise risk assessment
CHARM Risk Score (2023)	Predict all-cause mortality in chronic HF	Age, sex, NYHA class, LVEF, BP, HR, BMI, creatinine, diabetes, MI, and HF hospitalization	AUCs *0.83* for 90 day and *0.80* for 180 day mortality among heart transplant wait list patients	Enhances mortality prediction, aiding individualized management

TABLE 5: Components of the HFpEF score.

Parameter	Criteria	Points
Heavy (BMI >30 kg/m^2)	Yes	2
Hypertensive (≥2 antihypertensive drugs)	Yes	1
Atrial fibrillation (paroxysmal or persistent)	Yes	3
Pulmonary artery systolic pressure >35 mm Hg (echo)	Yes	1
Elder (age >60 years)	Yes	1
Filling pressure (E/e' >9 on echo)	Yes	1

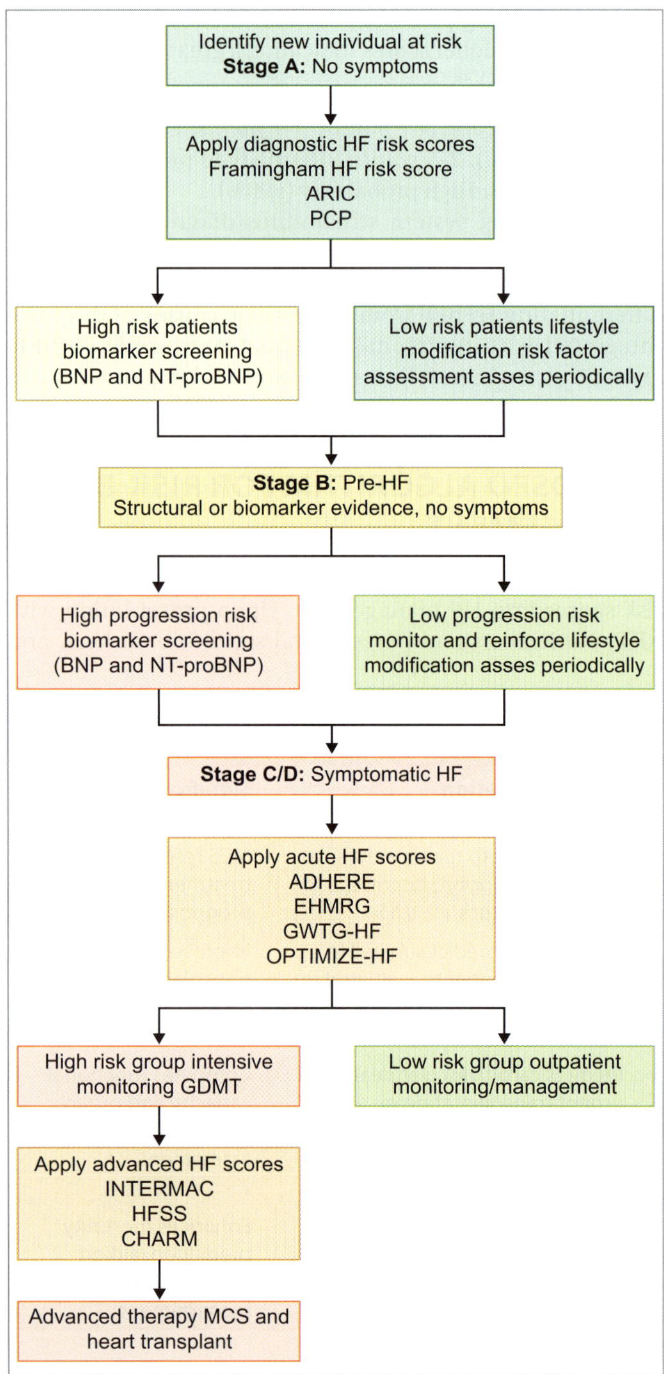

FLOWCHART 1: Risk-guided management of heart failure.

comorbidities to calculate a validated AHF score, such as MESSI-AHF or EHMRG. Low-risk patients may be considered for early discharge with outpatient follow-up, whereas high-risk patients should be admitted to monitored settings and receive guideline-directed therapy. During hospitalization, calculation of the GWTG-HF or ADHERE score can help determine the need for intensive monitoring and inform discussions about palliative care. At discharge, chronic HF models such as MAGGIC or SHFM may guide follow-up intervals and identify candidates for advanced therapies or cardiac rehabilitation. Patients with advanced HF should undergo assessment using models such as CHARM and PREDICTHF and be referred to transplant or ventricular assist device programs as appropriate. Throughout, simplified scores and comorbidity-focused models can aid in tailoring care to individual patient characteristics.

FUTURE DIRECTIONS IN RISK SCORE INTEGRATION

Advances in *machine learning (ML)* and *artificial intelligence (AI)* offer opportunities to enhance HF risk prediction beyond conventional regression-based scores. AI models can process vast, multidimensional datasets—including echocardiographic parameters, wearable sensor data, and high-resolution hemodynamic signals—to generate real-time, adaptive risk estimates. Integration of *omics-based biomarkers* (genomics, proteomics, and metabolomics) may allow identification of molecular phenotypes with distinct prognostic and therapeutic profiles.

The future of HF risk stratification lies in *continuous, dynamic risk monitoring*. Wearable devices and implantable sensors can capture daily fluctuations in heart rate variability, pulmonary artery pressures, or activity levels, feeding into cloud-based predictive algorithms. These systems could provide automated alerts for impending decompensation, enabling preemptive interventions such as diuretic titration or early clinic visits—potentially averting hospitalizations.

Finally, future research should focus on *validating integrated scoring frameworks* in diverse populations, incorporating patient-reported outcomes, and assessing the impact of score-guided management in randomized controlled trials. Such efforts will be essential to bridge the gap between predictive analytics and tangible improvements in patient survival, functional capacity, and quality of life.

CONCLUSION

The combination of multiple HF risk scores offers distinct advantages over relying on a single model. First, it allows *cross-validation of risk estimates*, enhancing confidence in clinical decisions. Discordance between scores can prompt deeper diagnostic evaluation or closer follow-up. Second, different scores capture *complementary dimensions of risk*: For example, a diagnostic score may flag an asymptomatic hypertensive patient for early echocardiography, while a prognostic score later quantifies postdiagnosis survival, and an advanced HF score guides transplant timing. Third, integrated use facilitates *resource prioritization*, ensuring that high-risk patients receive earlier access to advanced therapies, while lower-risk patients avoid unnecessary interventions.

Nevertheless, challenges remain. Many scores are derived from specific cohorts and may require *local recalibration* before widespread implementation. Variability in data availability—such as absence of NT-proBNP in some settings—can limit applicability. Overreliance on numerical scores without clinical context risks inappropriate decisions, particularly in patients with atypical presentations or comorbidities not captured by the model.

The integration of multiple risk scores—complemented by clinical judgment—should be viewed not as an academic exercise but as a cornerstone of modern HF care. Future developments in AI-driven dynamic risk modeling, coupled with real-time data from wearables and remote monitoring, promise to further enhance predictive accuracy and care personalization. By embedding integrated risk assessment into clinical workflows, the cardiology community can advance toward *precision heart failure management*, optimizing outcomes for patients across all stages of the disease.

REFERENCES

1. Ran J, Zhou P, Wang J, et al. Global, regional, and national burden of heart failure and its underlying causes, 1990–2021: results from the Global Burden of Disease Study 2021. Biomark Res. 2025;13:16.
2. Heidenreich PA, Bozkurt B, Aguilar D, et al. 2022 AHA/ACC/HFSA guideline for the management of heart failure: executive summary. J Am Coll Cardiol. 2022;79(17):1757-80.
3. Vasan RS, Enserro DM, Beiser AS, et al. Lifetime risk of heart failure among participants in the Framingham Study. J Am Coll Cardiol. 2022;79(3):250-63.
4. Bavishi A, Bruce M, Ning H, et al. Predictive accuracy of heart failure-specific risk equations in an electronic health record-based cohort. Circ Heart Fail. 2020;13(11):e007462.
5. Agarwal SK, Chambless LE, Ballantyne CM, et al. Prediction of incident heart failure in general practice. Circ Heart Fail. 2012;5(4):422-9.
6. Bo X, Zhang Y, Liu Y, et al. Performance of the heart failure risk scores in predicting 1-year mortality and short-term readmission of patients. ESC Heart Fail. 2023;10(1):502-17.
7. İlhan B, Bozdereli Berikol G, Doğan H, et al. The prognostic accuracy of Get With The Guidelines-Heart Failure score alone and with lactate among acute symptomatic heart failure patients: a retrospective cohort study. Anatol J Cardiol. 2024;28(6):305-11.
8. Collins SP, Pang PS. Acute heart failure risk stratification. Circulation. 2019;139(9):1157-61.
9. Wang Y, Wang Y, Zhang W. The utility of the adjusted-OPTIMIZE-HF risk model for predicting in-hospital length of stay in the Chinese population. Ann Palliat Med. 2021;10(2):1445-55.
10. O'Connor CM, Abraham WT, Albert NM, et al. The PROTECT in-hospital risk model: 7-day outcome in patients hospitalized with acute heart failure and renal dysfunction. Eur J Heart Fail. 2012;14(6):605-12.
11. Miró Ò, Rossello X, Platz E, et al. Risk stratification scores for patients with acute heart failure in the emergency department: a systematic review. Eur Heart J Acute Cardiovasc Care. 2020;9(5):375-98.
12. Stevenson LW, Pagani FD, Young JB, et al. INTERMACS profiling identifies ambulatory patients at high risk on medical therapy after hospitalizations for heart failure. Circ Heart Fail. 2017;10(4):e003032.
13. Goda A, Williams P, Mancini D, et al. Selecting patients for heart transplantation: comparison of the Heart Failure Survival Score (HFSS) and the Seattle Heart Failure Model (SHFM). J Heart Lung Transplant. 2011;30(11):1236-43.
14. Stansfield BK, Givertz MM, Patel CB, et al. The Colorado Heart Failure Acuity Risk Model: a mortality model for waitlisted cardiac transplant patients. JACC Adv. 2024;3(14):101449.
15. Pieske B, Tschöpe C, De Boer RA, et al. How to diagnose heart failure with preserved ejection fraction: the HFA–PEFF diagnostic algorithm: a consensus recommendation from the Heart Failure Association (HFA) of the European Society of Cardiology (ESC). Eur Heart J. 2019;40(40):3297-317.

CHAPTER

24

Issues in Reversing Advanced Heart Failure

Awadhesh K Sharma, Sayar Ahmad Pandit

ABSTRACT

Advanced heart failure is marked by persistent, severe symptoms that greatly reduce a patient's quality of life and often lead to repeated hospital stays. This highlights the importance of maximizing both medical management and supportive care. Evaluating the pumping ability of the left ventricle—both its contraction (systolic) and relaxation (diastolic) phases—is crucial for tracking disease progression, assessing the effectiveness of standard treatments, and determining when more intensive therapies are needed. Treatment options for advanced heart failure include heart transplantation, long-term use of mechanical circulatory support devices, or, in some cases, palliative care. In recent years, various transcatheter procedures have been developed and are being explored as innovative treatment strategies. These emerging devices may provide valuable new options for patients with left ventricular dysfunction by promoting structural improvements and potentially enhancing clinical outcomes.

Keywords: Advanced heart failure, reverse remodeling therapies, mechanical circulatory support.

INTRODUCTION

Heart failure (HF) is a clinical condition that arises from structural or functional impairments in the heart, leading to inadequate ventricular filling or ejection of blood. When patients continue to experience significant symptoms and limitations in physical activity despite adherence to optimal medical therapy, they are considered to have advanced, refractory, or end-stage HF. This condition is associated with frequent hospitalizations and substantial deterioration in quality of life, highlighting the necessity for optimized pharmacological and supportive care. Treatment strategies for advanced heart failure (AHF) include heart transplantation (HTx), durable mechanical circulatory support (MCS), and palliative care options **(Table 1)**.[1]

As per the 2018 consensus endorsed by the European Society of Cardiology (ESC) and American Heart Association (AHA), a diagnosis of AHF should be made when all the following are observed despite maximum GDMT:

- *Persistent and severe symptoms:* Symptoms aligning with NYHA class III (advanced) or IV.
- *Severe cardiac abnormalities:* Presence of at least one of the following:
  - Left ventricular ejection fraction (LVEF) ≤ 30%
  - Isolated right ventricular dysfunction
  - Severe valvular or congenital abnormalities not amenable to surgical repair
  - Preserved LVEF (≥40%) with:
    - Elevated BNP or NT-proBNP, or
    - Moderate-to-severe diastolic dysfunction
- *Recent clinical deterioration:* At least one episode in the past year of hospitalization or unscheduled visit requiring:
  - High-dose intravenous (IV) diuretics or multiple agent diuretic therapy for fluid overload
  - Inotropic or vasopressor support for low cardiac output
  - Malignant ventricular arrhythmias
- *Impaired exercise capacity demonstrated by:*
  - Inability to perform physical activity
  - 6-minute walk distance <300 m
  - Peak VO_2 <12–14 mL/kg/min attributed to cardiac dysfunction

PATHOPHYSIOLOGY OF ADVANCED HEART FAILURE

A detailed assessment of left ventricular systolic and diastolic performance is vital for understanding HF progression, evaluating responses to medical therapy, and determining the need for escalation to advanced therapies.

TABLE 1: Criterion for advanced heart failure.

Criteria	HFA (ESC)	ACC/AHA
NYHA class	III (advanced)/IV	III–IV
Peak VO_2 (pVO_2)	<12–14 mL/kg/min	<14 mL/kg/min or <50% predicted
6-minute walk test (6MWT)	<300 m	<300 m
Hospitalizations	>1 unplanned visit or hospitalization in past 12 months: • Congestion needing high-dose IV diuretics or combination • Low output needing inotropes/vasoactive drugs • Malignant arrhythmias	• ≥2 HF admissions in 12 months • ≥2 unscheduled visits (ED/clinic)
Arrhythmias	>1 ventricular arrhythmia	• Recurrent refractory VT • Frequent ICD shocks
Echocardiography	LVEF ≤ 30%, isolated RV failure, nonoperable valve or congenital abnormalities, or severe diastolic dysfunction	LVEF < 30%
BNP/NT-proBNP	Persistently high or rising levels	Persistently elevated levels
End-organ damage	Liver or kidney dysfunction, or cardiac cachexia	• Progressive hepatic/renal dysfunction • Cardiac cachexia
Pulmonary hypertension	Type 2 PH (secondary to left heart disease)	Pulmonary hypertension
Medical therapy tolerance	Intolerant of optimal dose of any HF drug	• Intolerance to RAAS inhibitor due to hypotension/renal dysfunction • Intolerance to β-blockers from worsening HF or hypotension
Diuretics	Increasing requirement	Escalation to >160 mg furosemide/day or use of metolazone
Hypotension	SBP < 90 mm Hg	Frequent SBP < 90 mm Hg
Hyponatremia	Present	Serum sodium < 134 mEq/L
1-year mortality prediction	MAGGIC or SHFM predicted survival ≤80%	>20% 1-year mortality by MAGGIC or SHFM

(HF: heart failure; SHFM: Seattle Heart Failure Model)

Progression of HF based on ACC/AHA staging:

- Stage B involves reduced LVEF due to increasing end-diastolic volume (EDV), while stroke volume (SV) is relatively preserved. Treatment with agents such as ACE inhibitors, β-blockers, and mineralocorticoid receptor antagonists aims to limit EDV expansion and reverse remodeling.
- Stage C is characterized by significant elevations in EDV and end-diastolic pressure (EDP), resulting in pulmonary hypertension and subsequent right heart involvement. Volume management relies on diuretics, with requirement of vasodilators, inotropes, or ultrafiltration during acute exacerbations. Chronic management includes four pillar drug treatment including ARNI/ACE inhibitors/ARBs, β-blockers, SGLT-2 inhibitors, and mineralocorticoid antagonists. ARNI has been shown to decrease LV filling pressure and causes reduction of PCWP.[2] SGLT-2 inhibitors also have been found to reduce PCWP in HF patients.[3]
- Stage D reflects end-stage HF with worsening SV and progressive LV dilation, often associated with mitral regurgitation and poor response to conventional therapies. These patients may require inotropes, MCS devices, or HTx.

REFERRAL AND RISK STRATIFICATION[1]

Patients with NYHA class II symptoms accompanied by warning signs or those in class III/IV who are unresponsive to current guideline recommended therapy should be promptly referred to specialized AHF centers. Delayed referrals may result in irreversible complications, including severe pulmonary hypertension, right ventricular failure, or cardiac cachexia.

There are various prognostic tools devised for assessment and referral for advanced treatment. These include:

- Seattle Heart Failure Model (SHFM)
- Metabolic Exercise Cardiac Kidney Index (MECKI)
- Heart Failure Survival Score (HFSS)
- MAGGIC risk score—predicts 1-year mortality above 20%
- INTERMACS profiles—widely used for assessing MCS candidacy and timing

REVERSE REMODELING THERAPIES

Therapies aimed at inducing reverse remodeling play a central role in AHF management. These include both biologic and structural interventions. The aim of these therapeutic options is to enhance myocardial contractility, reduce vascular resistance and wall stress, lower filling pressure, and decrease myocardial fibrosis.

Biologic Interventions

These therapies modulate molecular pathways and neurohormonal activation to facilitate structural improvements.

- *RAAS inhibition:*
  - *Agents:* ACE inhibitors, ARBs, and ARNI
  - *Effects:* Reduce afterload, wall stress, and interstitial fibrosis
- *Neurohormonal modulators:*
  - *Agents:* β-blockers
  - *Effects:* Lower filling pressures and inhibit fibrotic pathways
- *Congestion and diuretic resistance:* Cardiorenal syndrome and diuretic resistance are common in AHF. It needs multiagent diuretic therapy including uptitration of loop diuretics, ambulatory or home IV diuretic therapy, adjuvant thiazides/metolazone with caution for risk of electrolyte imbalance. ADVOR trial has demonstrated role of acetazolamide with loop diuretics for enhanced decongestion. In refractory cases, ultrafiltration and peritoneal dialysis are viable alternatives offering improved fluid management with hemodynamic and inflammatory advantages.
- *Inotropes:* Inotropes enhance cardiac output and reduce filling pressures. Though their long-term benefits remain unclear, selected patients may benefit from IV inotropes as a bridge to MCS or HTx, or as palliative therapy.
- *Other agents:*
  - *Cardiac myosin activator:* Omecamtiv mecarbil, a cardiac myosin activator, showed reduced HF events or CV death in the GALACTIC-HF trial. LeoDOR trial of levosimendan is aimed to clarify its role in AHF. Pecavaptan, a dual vasopressin V1a/V2 antagonist, has shown superior hemodynamic effects in preclinical models of advanced HF.

Device-based therapies also promote biological reverse remodeling by modifying loading conditions. For example:

- *Mechanical support devices:*
  - *Devices:* Left ventricular assist device (LVAD) and CRT
  - *Effect*: ↓ wall stress and ↑ contractility
- *Functional mitral regurgitation (fMR) treatments:*
  - *Types:* Surgical (MVr or MVR) and percutaneous (e.g., MitraClip)
  - *Effect*: ↓ filling pressures and ↓ wall stress

Physical Interventions

Physical reverse remodeling, aims at direct anatomical modification of the heart—like reducing LV mass or altering its geometry through direct structural intervention.[4-6] This concept initially emerged with surgical techniques such as:

- *Dor procedure:* Removal of dyskinetic aneurysmal myocardium.
- *Batista procedure:* Resection of viable but hypokinetic myocardium.

Outcomes varied considerably. The Dor procedure showed benefit by excluding nonfunctional myocardium, while the Batista procedure often led to restrictive physiology and poor outcomes. Although these surgical techniques are no longer favored, emerging transcatheter devices now offer new promise for physical remodeling.

The various physical interventions for reversing AHF include:

- *Surgical exclusion:*
  - *Techniques*: Batista and Dor procedures, aneurysmectomy, and Revivent TC
  - *Effect*: ↓ LV volume and ↓ wall stress
- *Constraint devices:*
  - *Examples*: Acorn and Paracor
  - *Effect*: ↓ wall stress
- *Partitioning devices:*
  - *Examples*: Parachute and Eucardia
  - *Effect*: ↓ LV volume and segmental unloading
- *Reshaping devices:*
  - *Examples*: Myocor, AccuCinch, Cardiac Success, and MIRTH
  - *Effect*: Structural reverse remodeling

RECENT ADVANCES FOR REVERSING REMODELING

With the introduction of percutaneous intervention devices for mitral valve repair/replacement[7] and aortic valve replacement, the cohort of advanced HF patients has got a remarkable improvement both in terms of symptomatic benefit as well as favorable effects on mortality. Some of the mitral valve devices include Tendyne valve by Abbott, Intrepid by Medtronic, and SAPIEN M3 by Edwards Lifesciences—along with other transcatheter mitral repair technologies like the Half-Moon posterior mitral leaflet repair system (Half-Moon Medical) and NeoChord (NeoChord Inc.). These devices represent a promising frontier for patients with left ventricular systolic dysfunction and have potential for structural remodeling in advanced HF. Also cardiac magnetic resonance (CMR)—based studies have demonstrated that transcatheter aortic valve replacement (TAVR) can regress diffuse myocardial fibrosis and reduce myocyte hypertrophy.[8] Evidence from the PARTNER (Placement of Aortic Transcatheter Valves) trials—including PARTNER I, II, and S3—revealed that in aortic stenosis patients, TAVR results in a 14.5% reduction in LV mass index at 1 year, across a range of patients from intermediate to inoperable surgical risk.[9] These findings underscore the emerging role of structural interventions[4] in mediating reverse remodeling, not only mechanically improving valvular hemodynamics but also due to favorable myocardial effects at the tissue level.

TEMPORARY MECHANICAL CIRCULATORY SUPPORT

Temporary mechanical circulatory support (T-MCS) devices serve as bridges to recovery, decision, or heart replacement therapy, with selection based on the etiology of cardiogenic shock (CS), patient physiology, and required cardiac output augmentation. The various devices for T-MCS are as mentioned below.

Intra-aortic Balloon Pump (IABP)

Intra-aortic balloon pump (IABP) is a catheter-based balloon placed between the left subclavian artery and renal arteries. It inflates during diastole and deflates during systole, enhancing coronary perfusion and reducing LV afterload. It contributes ~0.5 L/min to cardiac output. The Altshock-2 trial will assess clinical outcome of early IABP in acute decompensated HF-CS (NCT04369573).

Impella Ventricular Support Systems

Impella, a microaxial flow device, is inserted across the aortic valve and unloads the LV while increasing coronary flow and reducing pulmonary capillary wedge pressure. It has models delivering up to 5 L/min. While clinical evidence remains inconclusive, Impella is valuable for RV support and LV unloading during extracorporeal membrane oxygenation (ECMO).[10,11]

Extracorporeal Membrane Oxygenation

Venoarterial extracorporeal membrane oxygenation provides full circulatory and respiratory support up to 6 L/min. Used in refractory CS, it restores perfusion but may increase LV afterload and preload, leading to pulmonary congestion. LV unloading may be achieved with IABP, Impella, or surgical vents. Common complications include bleeding, stroke, limb ischemia, and infection. A recent meta-analysis found that ECMO was associated with improved survival outcomes in patients with CS compared to IABP, whereas no significant survival benefit was noted when ECMO was compared with Impella or TandemHeart devices.[12]

Tandem Heart

TandemHeart includes a transseptal left atrial inflow and femoral artery outflow via an extracorporeal pump, delivering up to 4 L/min. It reduces LV filling pressures and oxygen demand. However, implantation is complex and survival benefit[13] is unproven.

LONG-TERM MANAGEMENT OF ADVANCED HEART FAILURE

- *HTx:* HTx remains the gold standard in AHF, offering substantial improvements in survival[14] (>12 years median) and quality of life. However, it is associated with risks such as rejection, infection, vasculopathy, and long-term complications of immunosuppression.
- *LVAD:* LVADs, especially HeartMate 3, offer durable MCS with improved hemocompatibility and survival (80% at 1 year, 70% at 2 years).[1] INTERMACS profiles guide surgical timing. Trials like Early-VAD and SweVAD aim to better define appropriate timing for LVAD therapy.
- *Total artificial heart:* CARMAT-TAH is a novel invention that is a pneumatically powered artificial heart. It is biocompatible, pulsatile with systole as well as diastolic phases and adapts to physiological demand of patient. Though initial studies suggest its high rate of complication[15] than LVADs, trials are ongoing to fully explore its role.

ISSUES IN REVERSING HEART FAILURE, IS LEFT VENTRICULAR ASSIST DEVICE EXPLANTATION POSSIBLE?

There is paucity of data available at addressing the reverse remodeling in advanced HF patients. Many patients with advanced HF are not suitable for HTx due to factors such as advanced age, comorbidities, obesity, psychosocial issues, or chronic HF-related complications such as pulmonary hypertension and renal dysfunction. The current availability of centrifugal pumps which offer significantly improve durability need to be appraised for excellent outcomes in advanced HF patients and long-term studies are required to study their role in reverse remodeling of these patients.

A retrospective cohort study (2005-2020) by Itagaki et al.[16] using the United Network for Organ Sharing (UNOS) registry revealed that out of 15,728 continuous-flow LVADs implanted as a bridge to transplantation, only 126 devices (0.7%) were explanted due to myocardial recovery within 2 years. In select cohorts—especially patients under 40 years of age, those with nonischemic cardiomyopathy (NICM), no prior implantable cardioverter-defibrillator, and implanted with the HeartMate II device—the cumulative incidence of myocardial recovery reached 8.7%, and further increased to 10.7% in nonobese female patients. A key point here is that these findings may significantly underestimate true recovery rates since the registry excludes patients implanted with LVADs as destination therapy, bridge to candidacy, or bridge to recovery—groups that make up about 50% of all LVAD recipients.

A prospective multicenter trial, RESTAGE-HF,[17] conducted at six US centers employing aggressive recovery protocols (maximally tolerated guideline-directed medical therapy and scheduled testing), showed a high rate of 40% successful explantation in 40 NICM patients within 18 months.

The patients maintained freedom from transplantation, LVAD support, or death at 12 months postexplantation. This trial highlights that registries do not capture the true potential of myocardial recovery and that proactive strategies could lead to much higher success rates.

Historically, US transplant systems have discouraged recovery-focused strategies due to potential reductions in transplant volume and financial implications. Also, changes in the UNOS transplant allocation system now favor temporary MCS devices for higher transplant priority, thereby reducing durable LVAD use and, consequently, recovery opportunities.[18] Even when explantation is considered, many centers list patients for transplantation postexplant "just in case," which may not accurately reflect actual recovery success. Such strategies further weaken the enthusiasm for holding studies on reverse remodeling of refractory HF.

GUIDELINE RECOMMENDATION

The latest International Society of Heart and Lung Transplantation (ISHLT) guidelines recommend:

- All patients on LVAD support should be evaluated for myocardial recovery before listing for transplantation.
- Maximal guideline-directed medical therapy should be optimized during LVAD support, as this is associated with improved recovery rates and patient outcomes.

CONCLUSION

Reverse remodeling in advanced HF is possible with the latest armamentarium of biological and physical remodeling strategies. Interestingly most of these are transcatheter interventions that avoid the surgical morbidity of previously advised surgical interventions. With such great advances, it is possible that advanced HF may recover its function completely or partially and thus avoid need for HTx. Younger NICM patients are particularly promising candidates for recovery. LVAD explantation strategies may extend life expectancy significantly—by combining LVAD-supported time with postexplant recovery period before eventual transplantation if needed. Even if a patient later requires transplant, the extended timeline could provide long-term survival advantages. This evolving evidence base suggests that expanding recovery-focused protocols and overcoming systemic barriers could revolutionize advanced HF treatment by reducing dependence on transplantation and improving patient-centered outcomes.

Disclaimer: No conflict of interests.

REFERENCES

1. Crespo-Leiro MG, Metra M, Lund LH, et al. Advanced heart failure: a position statement of the Heart Failure Association of the European Society of Cardiology. Eur J Heart Fail. 2018;20:1505-35.
2. Gentile P, Cantone R, Perna E, et al. Haemodynamic effects of sacubitril/valsartan in advanced heart failure. ESC Heart Fail. 2022;9:894-904.
3. Omar M, Jensen J, Frederiksen PH, et al. Effect of empagliflozin on hemodynamics in patients with heart failure and reduced ejection fraction. J Am Coll Cardiol. 2020;76:2740-51.
4. Brener MI, Uriel N, Burkhoff D. Left ventricular volume reduction and reshaping as a treatment option for heart failure. Struct Heart. 2020;4(4):264-83.
5. Alkhunaizi FA, Brener MI, Burkhoff D. Device-based ventricular reverse remodeling: a multimechanistic therapeutic strategy. J Am Coll Cardiol Basic Transl Sci. 2023;8(1):51-4.
6. Artrip JH, Oz MC, Burkhoff D. Left ventricular volume reduction surgery for heart failure: a physiologic perspective. J Thorac Cardiovasc Surg. 2001;122(4):775-82.
7. Lander MM, Brener MI, Goel K, et al. Mitral interventions in heart failure. JACC Heart Fail. 2023;11(8 Pt 2):1055-69.
8. Treibel TA, Kozor R, Schofield R, et al. Reverse myocardial remodeling following valve replacement in patients with aortic stenosis. J Am Coll Cardiol. 2018;71(8):860-71.
9. Chau KH, Douglas PS, Pibarot P, et al. Regression of left ventricular mass after transcatheter aortic valve replacement: the PARTNER trials and registries. J Am Coll Cardiol. 2020;75(19):2446-58.
10. Schrage B, Ibrahim K, Loehn T, et al. Impella support for acute myocardial infarction complicated by cardiogenic shock. Circulation. 2019;139:1249-58.
11. Pappalardo F, Schulte C, Pieri M, et al. Concomitant implantation of Impella® on top of veno-arterial extracorporeal membrane oxygenation may improve survival of patients with cardiogenic shock. Eur J Heart Fail. 2017;19:404-12.
12. Ouweneel DM, Schotborgh JV, Limpens J, et al. Extracorporeal life support during cardiac arrest and cardiogenic shock: a systematic review and meta-analysis. Intensive Care Med. 2016;42:1922-34.
13. Burkhoff D, Cohen H, Brunckhorst C, et al. A randomized multicenter clinical study to evaluate the safety and efficacy of the TandemHeart percutaneous ventricular assist device versus conventional therapy with intra-aortic balloon pumping for treatment of cardiogenic shock. Am Heart J. 2006;152:469.e1-8.
14. Mehra MR, Canter CE, Hannan MM, et al. The 2016 International Society for Heart Lung Transplantation listing criteria for heart transplantation: a 10-year update. J Heart Lung Transplant. 2016;35:1-23.
15. Arabía FA, Cantor RS, Koehl DA, et al. Interagency registry for mechanically assisted circulatory support report on the total artificial heart. J Heart Lung Transplant. 2018;37:1304-12.
16. Itagaki S, Moss N, Toyoda N, et al. Incidence, outcomes, and opportunity for left ventricular assist device weaning for myocardial recovery. JACC Heart Fail. 2024;12(5):893-901.
17. Birks EJ, Rame JE, Cunningham C, et al. Response by Birks et al to Letters Regarding Article, "Prospective Multicenter Study of Myocardial Recovery Using Left Ventricular Assist Devices (RESTAGE-HF [Remission from Stage D Heart Failure]): Medium-term and Primary End Point Results". Circulation. 2021;143(22):e1017-e1018.
18. Topkara VK, Sayer GT, Clerkin KJ, et al. Recovery with Temporary Mechanical Circulatory Support while Waitlisted for Heart Transplantation. J Am Coll Cardiol. 2022;79(9):900-13.

CHAPTER 25

Early Initiation of GDMT in HFrEF: Accelerating Outcomes with Timely Evidence-based Titration

Dikshit Byomakesh, Behera Soumen Prasad

ABSTRACT

Heart failure with reduced ejection fraction (HFrEF) continues to be a major global health issue, with high hospitalization rates, reduced quality of life, and increased mortality. Guideline-directed medical therapy (GDMT) is a proven method for improving these outcomes. This therapeutic regimen includes four key drug classes: sodium-glucose cotransporter-2 (SGLT-2) inhibitors, angiotensin receptor–neprilysin inhibitors (ARNIs), β-blockers, and mineralocorticoid receptor antagonists (MRAs), which modify disease progression by targeting essential neurohormonal pathways. Empirical evidence strongly supports the early initiation of all four drug classes, particularly during hospitalization or shortly thereafter. Prompt initiation of therapy can lower mortality, reduce readmissions, and enhance patient functionality within weeks. However, delays in initiation are common because of safety concerns, clinical inertia, and monitoring constraints. Hospital settings offer an ideal environment for initiating therapy under controlled supervision. The "4 × 4" strategy—initiating all four drugs within 4 weeks—is both practical and effective, allowing for rapid titration to target doses while ensuring safety. Clinical stability is crucial before starting GDMT, with regular monitoring of blood pressure, renal function, heart rate, and electrolyte levels. Adjustments are carefully made to prevent hypotension, bradycardia, and electrolyte imbalance. Practical adaptations are necessary in diverse contexts, such as India, where underuse and underdosing are common. Patient-specific protocols enhance implementation without compromising the safety. Contemporary models incorporate telemonitoring to support remote follow-ups and adherence. In conclusion, the early, structured, and comprehensive application of GDMT changes the course of HFrEF. Each dose and week is critical. Clinicians are encouraged to act decisively by initiating therapy early, titrating safely, and personalizing therapy. Such actions translate evidence into practice and practice into survival.

Keywords: HFrEF, GDMT, early initiation, mortality reduction, heart failure management.

INTRODUCTION

Heart failure with reduced ejection fraction (HFrEF) remains a major global health challenge affecting morbidity, mortality, and healthcare utilization despite advances in treatment.[1] Treatment has evolved from symptom management to evidence-based strategies targeting the neurohormonal pathways.[2] Current guideline-directed medical therapy (GDMT) for HFrEF comprises four key pharmacological categories: angiotensin receptor–neprilysin inhibitors (ARNIs) or renin–angiotensin system inhibitors (RAS inhibitors), β-blockers (BBs), mineralocorticoid receptor antagonists (MRAs), and sodium-glucose cotransporter-2 inhibitors (SGLT-2 inhibitors), known as the "four pillars" of HFrEF treatment.[3]

Evidence supports their combined use to decrease mortality, reduce hospitalizations, and enhance quality of life.[4] HFrEF is characterized by heart failure symptoms with a left ventricular ejection fraction of 40% or less, owing to myocardial impairment that limits effective blood pumping.[1,3] It causes high morbidity and mortality, frequent hospitalizations, impaired quality of life, and substantial healthcare costs.[4] The pathophysiology involves neurohormonal activation, including the renin–angiotensin–aldosterone and sympathetic nervous systems, leading to cardiac remodeling and dysfunction.[5] The early initiation of GDMT in HFrEF is crucial for improving outcomes across healthcare settings.[1] These four drug classes offer complementary mechanisms that reduce mortality and hospitalizations when combined.[2,3] Despite these benefits, therapy initiation is often delayed due to therapeutic inertia and safety concerns.[4,5]

Acute heart failure hospitalization provides an opportunity to assess the outcomes of GDMT by improved monitoring.[6] Research shows that early prescription of all four drugs within 48 hours of hospital admission reduces mortality and readmissions.[7] Rapid initiation protocols, such as the "4 × 4" strategy, have shown feasibility and improved survival.[8]

Despite the benefits shown in large randomized controlled trials, real-world implementation remains inadequate, with gaps in initiation, optimization, and dosing.[5] In-hospital initiation and early postdischarge titration are critical opportunities to bridge these gaps, using clinical monitoring to enhance safety and adherence.[6] Data suggest that early prescription of quadruple therapy during acute decompensated heart failure admissions improves outcomes, including reduced mortality, lower 30-day readmissions, and shortened hospital stays.[7] Thus rapid initiation with the "4 × 4" approach has shown feasibility in patients, translating at bedside, into improved patient survival.[8]

What is guideline-directed medical therapy?
Guideline-directed medical therapy is essential for managing HFrEF due to significant short- and long-term risks, which can only be effectively mitigated through early and comprehensive neurohormonal blockade rather than by mere addressing of symptoms.[1]

The concept of GDMT emerged from pivotal randomized controlled trials conducted in the late 20th century. It began with the introduction of ACE inhibitors and BBs during the 1980s and the 1990s, followed by the development of MRAs in the early 2000s and, more recently, SGLT-2 inhibitors in the 2010s. The widely endorsed "four-pillar" framework is the outcome of this progressive accumulation of evidence over the years. Recent guidelines have shifted the focus from the gradual, step-by-step addition of medications to a more rapid or concurrent initiation, aiming to reduce the time required to achieve the full therapeutic benefits.[2,3]

Rationale behind use of four drug classes in GDMT:
The rationale is twofold: First, the four distinct drug classes, when used together, provide additive, disease-modifying effects on remodeling and events; second, clinical benefits begin to appear within weeks of starting treatment, so any delay results in missed opportunities for improvement.[2-4]

However, there is widespread underuse and insufficient dosing across healthcare settings, which is why hospitalization is now viewed as a strategic opportunity to initiate and increase the dosage of all four agents while closely monitoring blood pressure, renal function, potassium levels, and patient tolerance.[5,6]

Recent registry studies have confirmed that the earlier in-hospital prescription of all four drugs is associated with lower in-hospital mortality, fewer readmissions within 30 days, and shorter hospital stays, while also enhancing continuation at discharge.[7] Practical implementation models, such as a "4 × 4" pathway that aims to establish all four treatment pillars within 4 weeks, have shown safety and improved event-free survival when adapted and adopted to individual contraindications, such as bradycardia, hypotension, or renal dysfunction.[8] Consensus frameworks have been developed for specific health systems (e.g., India), highlighting pragmatic, profile-based sequencing and monitoring algorithms to increase uptake and adherence in various resource settings without compromising evidence standards.[9] A recent open-access systematic review and network meta-analysis supports this strategy, ranking combinations that include the core triad (ACE inhibitor/ARNI + BB + MRA) and demonstrating additional benefits with SGLT-2 inhibitor, thereby affirming the "four-pillar" foundation for reducing mortality and hospitalizations.[10]

PRIMARY GOALS OF GUIDELINE-DIRECTED MEDICAL THERAPY

The primary goals of GDMT for HFrEF are to lower mortality, reduce the frequency of hospitalizations, and improve the patient's quality of life and functional capacity. Evidence shows that timely initiation, particularly during hospitalization or soon after, maximizes the early benefits, prevents clinical deterioration, and enhances long-term outcomes. The consensus is that GDMTs success depends on both the completeness of the regimen and the speed at which it is established, with benefits validated across randomized trials, studies and meta-analyses from diverse healthcare setups **(Table 1)**.

EVIDENCE-BASED STEPWISE INITIATION OF GUIDELINE-DIRECTED MEDICAL THERAPY

To initiate GDMT effectively, the process must be structured, timely, and safe, which can be achieved through two key steps: (1) assessing clinical stability and (2) starting therapy once stability is confirmed. Before therapy begins, clinical stability should be evaluated, ensuring that the patient is euvolemic, without signs of congestion, hypotension, or bradycardia, and with adequate renal function.[11,12] Stability must be confirmed prior to initiating GDMT.

An SGLT-2 inhibitor is prescribed when the estimated glomerular filtration rate (eGFR)[13,14] is above 20–30 mL/min/1.73 m² and should be considered for nearly all eligible patients with CAD. Sacubitril/valsartan (ARNI) is preferred over ACE inhibitor/ARB in patients new to renin–angiotensin–aldosterone system (RAAS) blockade because of stronger supporting evidence. A BB is introduced once volume status is stable and perfusion is adequate. An MRA is added unless the serum potassium level exceeds 5.0 mmol/L or the eGFR is below 30 mL/min/1.73 m², necessitating frequent monitoring.

Blood pressure, heart rate, potassium levels, renal function, and volume status should be assessed at each step. Doses are adjusted every 1–2 weeks, aiming for target or maximally tolerated levels within 4–6 weeks of treatment

TABLE 1: Findings of GDMT across studies.

Authors	Study type/design	Findings
Patolia et al., Duke University[3]	Review	Guideline-directed medical therapy (GDMT) has efficacy in saving lives and reducing hospitalizations. However, a significant number of patients do not receive the complete regimen of medications. Initiating the full spectrum of pharmacological interventions promptly, even during the hospital stay, can effectively address this deficiency
Schwann et al., American College of Cardiology[6]	Expert analysis	GDMT during hospitalization is effective because of the ability of healthcare professionals to closely monitor patients. This close supervision facilitates adherence to the prescribed medications and enables patients to achieve optimal dosages more rapidly
Echeverría et al., Fundación Cardiovascular de Colombia[7]	Retrospective cohort	The administration of all four GDMT drugs within 48 hours of hospital admission significantly decreased mortality rates, reduced hospital readmissions, and shortened the duration of hospital stays
Sze et al., University of Leicester[8]	Prospective study	The study evaluated a "4 × 4" regimen, which involves administering all four drugs over a 4-week period, and demonstrated that this approach is safe, feasible, and associated with improved survival outcomes without complications
Ponde et al., PD Hinduja National Hospital[9]	Expert consensus	GDMT should be adapted according to the specific condition of each patient and the resources available, thereby enhancing accessibility and continuity of treatment for a greater number of individuals
Tang et al., University of Florida[10]	Systematic review and network meta-analysis	Many drug combinations were compared, and it was found that using all four main GDMT drugs together works best to lower deaths and hospitalizations

TABLE 2: The four pharmacological agents/classes of GDMT and their rationale for use in early initiation.

Drug class (examples)	Priority for early start*	Core rationale for usage	Effects on progression and remodeling
SGLT-2 inhibitors (dapagliflozin and empagliflozin)	1	Fast, hemodynamically gentle, no titration, broad eligibility; early event reduction even in hospital or within weeks[3,6-8,10]	↓ CV death/HF hospitalization; early symptom gains; favorable diuretic-sparing natriuresis; signals of reverse remodeling and NP reduction; benefits additive to ARNI/BB/MRA[3,4,6-8,10] (India: Underuse has been documented; rapid-start is urged)[11,12]
ARNI (sacubitril/valsartan)	2	Superior to ACE inhibitor for hard outcomes; rapid benefit and reverse-remodeling effects; can be started in-hospital with monitoring[3,4,6,7,10]	↓ Mortality and HF hospitalization; reverse remodeling (↓ LV volumes, ↑ LVEF), ↓ NT-proBNP; improves QoL early; facilitates device deferral while optimizing meds[3,4,6,10] (For India: Eligibility for protocol is high but uptake is modest)[11,12]
β-blockers (BB) (carvedilol, metoprolol succinate, and bisoprolol)	3	Antiadrenergic disease modification; arrhythmic death reduction; start after clinical stabilization (euvolemic and adequate BP) and titrate upwards[3,6]	↓ Mortality (including sudden death), ↓ hospitalizations; reverse remodeling over months; improves LVEF and HR control; target doses ideal[3,4,6] (India context: Under-dosing common; once started, continuation improves)[11,12]
MRA (spironolactone and eplerenone)	4	Antifibrotic RAAS blockade "beyond ACE inhibitor/ARB/ARNI;" powerful add-on with low BP impact; early start feasible if K^+/eGFR parameters allow[3,6,10]	↓ Mortality and HF hospitalization; antifibrotic reverse remodeling; watch K^+/creatinine; substantial additive benefit in quadruple regimens[3,4,6,10] (For India: Monitoring access can limit use; profile-based clinical decision making is recommended)[9,11,12]

*Priority reflects *practical early-start sequencing* widely supported in recent papers—SGLT-2 inhibitor (no titration, fast benefit) and ARNI early; β-blocker once stable; MRA as soon as laboratories permit—while recognizing that all four are equal "foundational" pillars and should be established rapidly (e.g., in-hospital or "4 × 4" within 4 weeks) for maximal benefit.[3,6-8,10]

Indian context: National and regional registries show high mortality with *under-utilization and under-dosing* of GDMT; consensus frameworks advocate *patient-profile-based* initiation and monitoring to raise uptake and adherence.[9,11,12]

(ARNI: angiotensin receptor–neprilysin inhibitor; eGFR: estimated glomerular filtration rate; GDMT: guideline-directed medical therapy; MRA: mineralocorticoid receptor antagonist; RAAS: renin–angiotensin–aldosterone system; SGLT-2: sodium-glucose cotransporter-2)

initiation. Minor changes in creatinine or blood pressure are managed through diuretic adjustments. Therapy should be discontinued only when clinically essential. This evidence-based approach facilitates early disease modification and enhances the likelihood of reverse remodeling in the heart **(Table 2)**.

FOLLOW-UP AND MONITORING POSTINITIATION OF GUIDELINE-DIRECTED MEDICAL THERAPY

Clinicians should monitor patients every 1–2 weeks during GDMT titration, as the initial treatment phase poses the greatest risk of hypotension, bradycardia, and electrolyte imbalance.[3,9,13] Regular assessments allow for the early detection of adverse changes, ensuring the safe continuation of therapy.[12,15] At each visit, blood pressure and heart rate are evaluated; a sustained systolic blood pressure below 90 mm Hg or heart rate below 50 bpm often requires dose adjustment.[4,7] Electrolyte levels, especially potassium, are measured because both hyperkalemia (>5.5 mmol/L) and hypokalemia (<3.5 mmol/L) can increase the risk of arrhythmias and limit the use of MRAs or RAAS blockers.[3,9]

Monitoring creatinine and eGFR helps to identify any decline in renal function; an increase in creatinine exceeding 30% from baseline may necessitate therapeutic modification.[13] If symptoms such as dizziness, fatigue, or presyncope occur, drug dosages are typically reduced by half or titration is paused for one cycle.[11,12] When renal markers show mild deterioration without accompanying symptoms, diuretics are adjusted before altering the dosage. Additionally, digital and telehealth methods may be employed to collect interim data on blood pressure, heart rate, and symptoms, facilitating timely decision-making without the need for continuous in-person visits **(Table 3)**.[15]

Initiating and titrating GDMT for HFrEF has special considerations owing to patient comorbidities, physiological reserve, and drug-specific risks.[3,5,7,10,12,14] Elderly patients or those exhibiting frailty may require a more gradual titration process to prevent hypotension or renal impairment.[5,12] In patients with borderline blood pressure, it may be prudent to commence treatment with SGLT-2 inhibitors and MRAs—agents with minimal impact on blood pressure—before introducing ARNIs or BBs.[10,14] Renal dysfunction necessitates vigilant monitoring of creatinine and potassium levels, particularly when initiating MRAs or ARNIs, as both can elevate potassium levels and decrease the glomerular filtration rate (GFR).[5,12]

Patients with bradycardia or conduction disorders may exhibit poor tolerance to BBs; thus, dose selection and pacing support should be tailored to the individual.[3,7] Patients with diabetes may benefit from the early use of SGLT-2 inhibitors for glycemic control and cardiorenal protection.[10,14] Volume status is critical; BBs in patients with congestion can exacerbate symptoms, whereas excessive diuresis poses risks of hypotension and prerenal azotemia.[3,5] These adjustments not only enhance safety but also minimize treatment interruptions while maintaining progress toward full-dose therapy adherence, which is strongly correlated with reverse remodeling and improved clinical outcomes.[7,12,14]

The adverse effects of GDMT in HFrEF can be categorized into early- and late-onset reactions, reflecting both pharmacologic onset and cumulative exposure risks. Early reactions typically manifest within days to weeks of treatment initiation or dose escalation. ARNIs, ACE inhibitors, and ARBs frequently induce symptomatic hypotension, particularly in elderly or volume-depleted patients, along with transient increases in serum creatinine levels.[3,5,6,12] BBs may precipitate bradycardia, atrioventricular block, or transient fatigue if administered before achieving euvolemia.[7,10] SGLT-2 inhibitors occasionally result in mild volume depletion, hypotension, or genital mycotic infections shortly after initiation.[14,15] MRAs and RAAS-acting agents are associated with an early risk of hyperkalemia, particularly in individuals with a baseline eGFR < 60 mL/min/1.73 m^2 or elevated serum potassium levels.[5,12]

Late adverse effects are typically associated with chronic exposure. Spironolactone may cause gynecomastia and menstrual irregularities due to its antiandrogenic effects, while long-term RAAS inhibition occasionally results in progressive hyperkalemia in patients with deteriorating renal function.[5,12] Rarely, ARNIs and ACE inhibitors induce late-onset angioedema, sometimes occurring months after therapy initiation.[3,6] Prolonged BB use in predisposed individuals may unmask conduction disease or exacerbate

TABLE 3: Clinical pearls for GDMT—week 1–6.

Week	Intervention	Clinical pearls
0–1	*Start ARNI* (sacubitril/valsartan)[3,4,6] ± *SGLT-2 inhibitor* (dapagliflozin/empagliflozin)[4,6,9]	Early dual start gives rapid neurohormonal and metabolic benefit.[3,4,6,9] Begin ARNI if SBP ≥100 mm Hg, eGFR ≥ 30 mL/min/1.73 m^2. SGLT-2 inhibitor safe if eGFR > 20–30 mL/min/1.73 m^2. Recheck BP, HR, creatinine, potassium after 1 week
2–3	Add β-blocker (carvedilol, bisoprolol, and metoprolol succinate)[1,3,7]	Only add when euvolemic and no symptomatic bradycardia.[1,7] Avoid if HR < 50 bpm or SBP < 90 mm Hg. Start low, double every 2 weeks if tolerated. Watch for fatigue or HF worsening
4–5	Add mineralocorticoid receptor antagonist (spironolactone/eplerenone)[5,12]	Start if $K^+ \leq 5.0$ mmol/L, eGFR ≥ 30 mL/min/1.73 m^2.[5,12] Check K^+/creatinine at 3–7 days, then 1 month. Hyperkalemia risk higher in elderly and diabetics
6+	Titrate all agents to target or maximally tolerated doses[10]	Increase doses every 1–2 weeks.[10,13] Accept mild creatinine rise (<30%). Adjust diuretics first if BP low. Keep BP, HR, renal function, and K^+ under regular review

(ARNI: angiotensin receptor–neprilysin inhibitor; eGFR: estimated glomerular filtration rate; GDMT: guideline-directed medical therapy; SGLT-2: sodium-glucose cotransporter-2)

depressive symptoms.[7,10] In patients using SGLT-2 inhibitors, recurrent genital infections or rare instances of euglycemic ketoacidosis may emerge over extended therapy.[14] Also, it is imperative that timely reporting of ADRs be done, which safeguards patients while ensuring continuous and judicious implementation of GDMT.

CONCLUSION

Heart failure with reduced ejection fraction changes lives, but GDMT can change the story. Evidence shows that starting all four pillars early, titrating with intent, and monitoring with precision transforms prognosis. Each week is significant, and every administered dose is crucial. Clinicians who make prompt and decisive interventions foster progress toward recovery rather than deterioration. The course of action is evident: initiate, escalate, and personalize while maintaining a balance between safety and effectiveness. Each timely and well-monitored GDMT intervention represents a progression away from hospitalization and a movement toward the restoration of quality of life.

REFERENCES

1. Biegus J, Moayedi Y, Saldarriaga C, et al. Getting ahead of the game: in-hospital initiation of HFrEF therapies. Eur Heart J Suppl. 2022;24(Suppl L):L38-L44.
2. Bozkurt B. What to and not to monitor for uptitration of GDMT in patients with heart failure. JACC Heart Fail. 2022;10(11): 881-4.
3. Patolia H, Khan MS, Fonarow GC, et al. Implementing guideline-directed medical therapy for heart failure: JACC focus seminar 1/3. J Am Coll Cardiol. 2023;82(6):529-43.
4. Carrizales-Sepúlveda EF, Ordaz-Farías A, Vargas-Mendoza JA, et al. Initiation and up-titration of guideline-directed medical therapy for patients with heart failure: better, faster, stronger! Card Fail Rev. 2024;10:e03.
5. Schwann AN, Jaffe LM, Givertz MM, et al. Early initiation of guideline-directed medical therapy for heart failure after cardiac surgery. Ann Thorac Surg. 2024;118(4):792-800.
6. Schwann AN, Riello R, Ahmad T. (2022). Inpatient initiation of HFrEF therapies. [online] Available from https://www.acc.org/Latest-in-Cardiology/Articles/2022/06/01/12/11/Inpatient-Initiation-of-HFrEF-Therapies [Last accessed October, 2025].
7. Echeverría LE, Rojas LZ, Serrano-García AY, et al. Early prescription of quadruple therapy in acute decompensated heart failure with reduced ejection fraction: A propensity score-matched analysis. ESC Heart Fail. 2025;12(4):2814-26.
8. Sze S, Thaitirarot C, Krishnan S, et al. Early and rapid initiation of quadruple therapy for heart failure with reduced ejection fraction: a real-world experience. Clin Med. 2025;25:100296.
9. Ponde CK, Mohan JC, Oomman A, et al. An Indian Expert Consensus on Patient-profile-based Implementation of Guideline-directed Medical Therapy in the Management of Heart Failure With Reduced Ejection Fraction: APPROACH-HF. J Card Fail. 2025:S1071-9164(25)00294-5.
10. Tang H, Germinal K, Milfort A, et al. The most effective combination of pharmacological therapy for heart failure with reduced ejection fraction: a network meta-analysis of randomized controlled trials. BMC Cardiovasc Disord. 2024;24:666.
11. Chaturvedi V, Parashar A, Jha RK, et al. Guideline-directed medical therapy use and outcomes in Indian patients with heart failure with reduced ejection fraction: insights from the National Heart Failure Registry. Indian Heart J. 2023;75(5):291-8.
12. Mishra S, Yadav R, Gupta A, et al. Implementation of quadruple therapy for heart failure with reduced ejection fraction in a tertiary care center in India: feasibility, safety, and early outcomes. J Pract Cardiovasc Sci. 2024;10(2):85-93.
13. McDonagh TA, Metra M, Adamo M, et al. 2021 ESC Guidelines for the Diagnosis and Treatment of Acute and Chronic Heart Failure. *Eur Heart J*. 2021;42(36):3599-726.
14. Heidenreich PA, Bozkurt B, Aguilar D, et al. 2022 AHA/ACC/HFSA Guideline for the Management of Heart Failure. J Am Coll Cardiol. 2022;79(17):e263-e421.
15. Spethmann S, Hindricks G, Koehler K, et al. Telemonitoring for chronic heart failure: narrative review of the 20-year journey from concept to standard care in Germany. J Med Internet Res. 2024;26:e63391.

CHAPTER 26

Mixed Cardiogenic-vasodilatory Shock

Biswajit Majumder, Somnath Maji, Suvadeep Biswas, Ratul Ghosh

ABSTRACT

A severe and complex condition occurs when cardiogenic shock is compounded by abnormal blood vessel dilation, disrupting the body's natural response mechanisms and exacerbating the shock. Conversely, shock caused by blood vessel dilation can be further complicated by myocardial dysfunction, leading to inadequate blood circulation. Systemic issues can trigger both heart muscle dysfunction and abnormal blood vessel relaxation, resulting in a mixed shock state. Effective management requires identifying and treating both the initial and complicating conditions, as well as close monitoring of hemodynamic changes. Treatment typically involves medications to support heart function and blood pressure. Due to the lack of a standardized definition, research on mixed shock is limited, highlighting the need for further studies. Effective management requires judicious use of vasopressors and inotropes may need invasive hemodynamic monitoring, and consideration of mechanical circulatory support (MCS) in refractory cases.

Keywords: Mixed shock, cardiogenic shock, vasodilatory shock, hemodynamic monitoring, inotropes, vasopressors, mechanical circulatory support.

INTRODUCTION

Circulatory shock patients are categorized into three main types—hypovolemic, vasodilatory/distributive, and cardiogenic.[1] Cardiogenic shock is a complex condition where the heart fails to pump enough blood, causing inadequate organ perfusion. Traditional models predict compensation through blood vessel constriction to maintain blood pressure. However, some cardiogenic shock patients exhibit low blood vessel resistance, leading to a mixed shock state with both cardiogenic and vasodilatory features.[2,3] This condition is heterogeneous, with various underlying causes and clinical outcomes. This high-risk, understudied subgroup of cardiogenic shock patients will be briefly described in this chapter.

DEFINITION

Mixed shock is a complex condition lacking a uniform definition, but it can be conceptually defined as hypotension with end-organ hypoperfusion due to acute cardiac insufficiency and systemic vasodilation. Characterized by low cardiac output, low systemic vascular resistance, and normal or elevated ventricular filling pressures, mixed shock diagnosis relies on invasive hemodynamic monitoring, with pulmonary artery catheterization as the gold standard. Clinically relevant thresholds remain ill-defined, but a cardiac index <2.2 L/min/m^2 is a commonly used diagnostic threshold, and a low systemic vascular resistance is defined as <800 dyn/cm/s-5.[4,5]

PROPOSED PHENOTYPES OF MIXED CARDIOGENIC SHOCK[6]

Mixed shock can occur through various pathways; often involving a primary insult followed by secondary mechanisms or disease processes. A conceptual model categorizes mixed shock into three groups:

1. *Cardiogenic-vasodilatory shock:* Initial cardiac insult (e.g., acute myocardial infarction) followed by pathological vasodilation.
2. *Vasodilatory-cardiogenic shock*: Initial vasodilatory shock (e.g., septic shock) followed by cardiac compromise and low output.
3. *Primary mixed shock:* Single primary insult (e.g., postcardiac arrest syndrome) causing both cardiac and vascular dysfunction.

These groups may overlap, and distinctions can be challenging to determine in clinical practice **(Fig. 1)**.

CARDIOGENIC-VASODILATORY SHOCK

Cardiogenic-vasodilatory shock occurs when a primary cardiac condition leads to low cardiac output and cardiogenic shock, followed by a sudden drop in vascular tone, resulting in mixed shock. This condition is marked by the initial development of pure cardiogenic shock, which then progresses to inappropriate vasodilation counteracts the body's natural response to shock, leading to a maladaptive decrease in systemic vascular resistance and worsening hypotension.[7]

Various conditions can trigger cardiogenic shock, which may then progress to mixed cardiogenic-vasodilatory shock due to secondary infections, inflammatory responses, or medication side effects. For instance, severe heart attacks can lead to pump failure, sparking a systemic inflammatory response that causes blood vessels to dilate excessively. Similarly, heart failure and acute myocarditis can also trigger this type of shock, highlighting the connection between inflammation, cardiac dysfunction, and vascular impairment.[8]

INFECTION IN PATIENTS WITH ACUTE CARDIOVASCULAR DISEASE

In patients with acute cardiovascular disease, infections can trigger a severe systemic inflammatory response, exacerbating outcomes. This response, known as systemic inflammatory response syndrome (SIRS), can occur with or without a documented infection. Critically ill cardiac patients are more susceptible to infections, and those with cardiogenic shock often exhibit elevated inflammation markers, making it challenging to distinguish between infected and uninfected

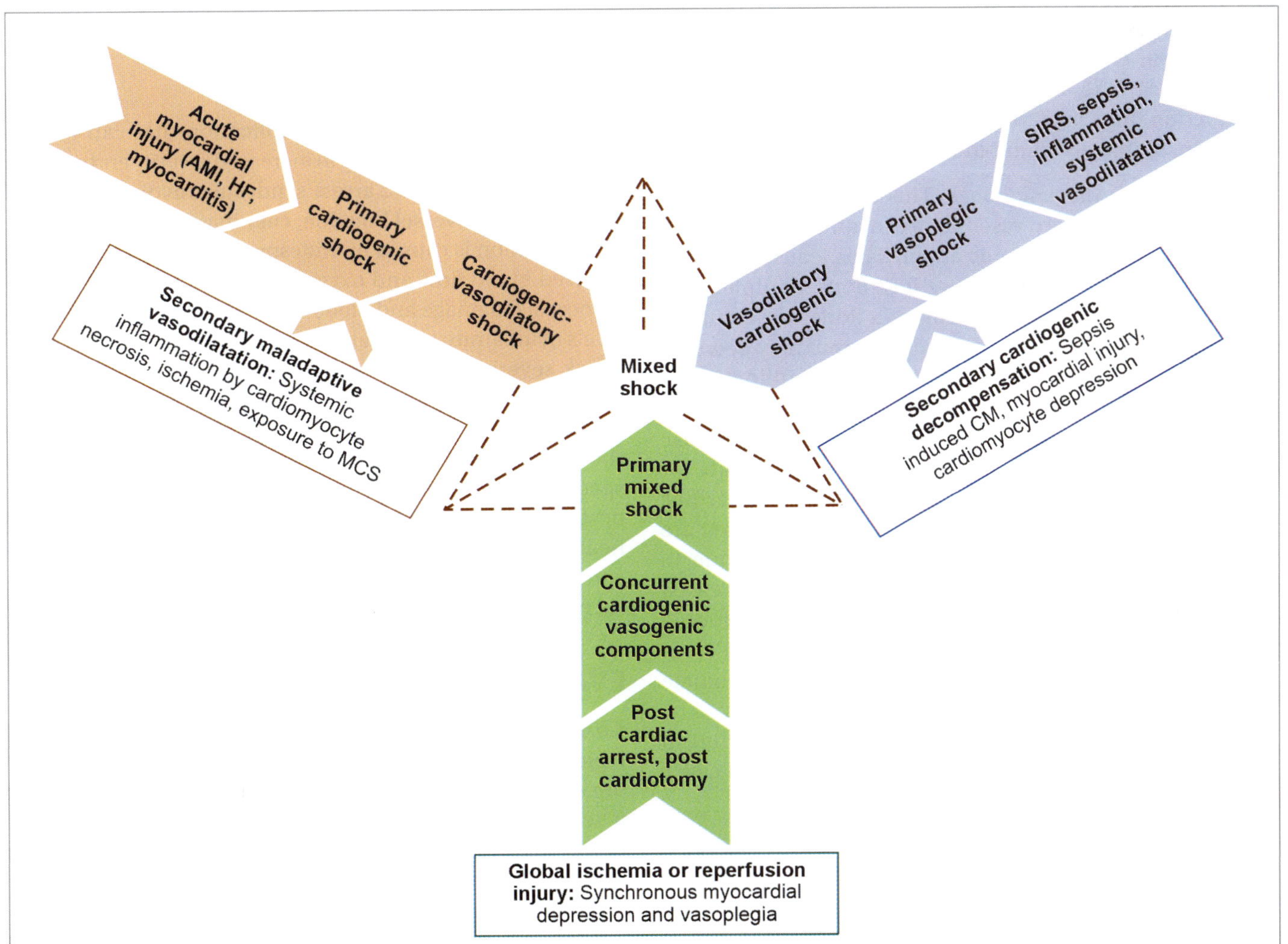

FIG. 1: Different phenotypes of mixed shock.
Source: With permission from Jentzer JC, et al. (2024).[6]

individuals.[9] The co-occurrence of cardiogenic shock and sepsis is associated with higher mortality rates, worse shock, and poorer survival outcomes.[10]

INFLAMMATION AND VASODILATION IN CARDIOGENIC SHOCK

Cardiogenic shock (CS) occurs when the heart's pumping ability fails, resulting in reduced cardiac output, systemic hypoperfusion, and hypotension. In response, the body activates the sympathetic nervous system, inducing compensatory tachycardia and peripheral vasoconstriction. However, this compensatory mechanism can eventually fail, leading to maladaptive vasodilation and the development of mixed cardiogenic-vasodilatory shock.[11] Systemic inflammation plays a pivotal role in the development of mixed shock, triggered by factors such as infection, cardiac injury, and tissue ischemia. This inflammatory response is characterized by elevated levels of cytokines, including interleukins, tumor necrosis factor-alpha (TNF-α), and C-reactive protein, which contribute to uncontrolled vasodilation, endothelial dysfunction, and microvascular dysfunction. The resulting vasoplegia, microvascular dysfunction, and oxidative stress can compromise organ perfusion, ultimately contributing to adverse outcomes.

Vasodilatory-cardiogenic shock: This complex shock state occurs when a primary vasodilatory insult, often triggered by systemic inflammation or anaphylaxis, converges with acute cardiac dysfunction. Severe infections, noninfectious inflammation, and adverse drug reactions are common precipitating factors. In sepsis, cardiac output may decrease due to various mechanisms, leading to a combination of vasodilation and cardiac dysfunction. Initially, patients experience systemic vasodilation, followed by signs of cardiac impairment due to the heart's inability to compensate for increased demand.[12] Patients with pre-existing cardiac conditions, such as cardiomyopathy or valve disease, are more susceptible to deterioration during sepsis due to fluid overload and systemic stress, resulting in decreased cardiac output. New cardiac issues may arise, including stress-induced cardiomyopathy, demand ischemia, or valve damage. In rare instances, sepsis itself can culminate in mixed vasodilatory-cardiogenic shock, characterized by both low cardiac output and vasodilation, often occurring in severe infections where multiple factors converge to cause cardiac and vascular dysfunction.[13]

Cardiac dysfunction in vasodilatory shock: It is precipitated by a plethora of pro-inflammatory cytokines, including TNF-α, nitric oxide (NO), and reactive oxygen species. These molecules exert a deleterious effect on myocardial function by reducing intracellular calcium, thereby inducing direct myocardial depression. Stress-induced cardiomyopathy, encompassing takotsubo syndrome, can manifest during acute illnesses, culminating in ventricular systolic dysfunction.[14]

A sympathetic surge, coupled with excessive beta-adrenergic receptor activation, can elicit direct myocardial toxicity. Furthermore, demand myocardial ischemia and infarction can compromise cardiac function, ultimately contributing to the development of mixed shock. Elevated levels of dipeptidyl dipeptidase-3 and adrenomedullin are associated with impaired cardiac contractility and adverse outcomes. These intricate mechanisms collectively contribute to the emergence of mixed shock in patients with vasodilatory shock.[15,16]

Primary mixed shock: It occurs when a single underlying condition triggers both cardiogenic and vasodilatory shock components. This can happen simultaneously or in sequence, resulting in a combination of low cardiac output and vasoplegia. In some cases, the shock phenotype may shift from one type to another, with mixed shock being a transitional state **(Fig. 2)**.

POSTCARDIAC ARREST AND POSTCARDIOTOMY SHOCK

Cardiac arrest is a serious complication that can lead to cardiogenic shock, resulting in increased severity and a poorer prognosis. Postcardiac arrest syndrome involves impaired heart and blood vessel function, culminating in mixed shock. This condition is caused by widespread injury resulting from reduced blood flow and oxygenation, leading to temporary myocardial damage and blood vessel dysfunction.[17] Elevated levels of inflammatory markers are associated with increased shock severity and worse outcomes. The condition often progresses through stages, commencing with cardiogenic shock, followed by mixed shock, and eventually vasodilatory shock. A shock-like state can occur following heart surgery specifically postcardiotomy cases, exhibiting parallels with postresuscitation syndrome.[18] Key features include impaired heart muscle function, widespread inflammation, and cardiac impairment, typically marked by weakened right-sided heart function.

EVALUATION OF MIXED SHOCK

Clinical features: Patients presented with mixed shock typically have severe hypotension and evidence of inadequate organ perfusion, necessitating vasopressor support. At first it seems that symptoms may align with either cardiogenic or vasodilatory shock, but later conflicting findings often emerge. Reversal of anticipated clinical and hemodynamic findings is a hallmark of mixed shock.

Systemic inflammation is a common occurrence, but its presence is not exclusive to infection. As such, a thorough evaluation and empiric antimicrobial therapy may be warranted.

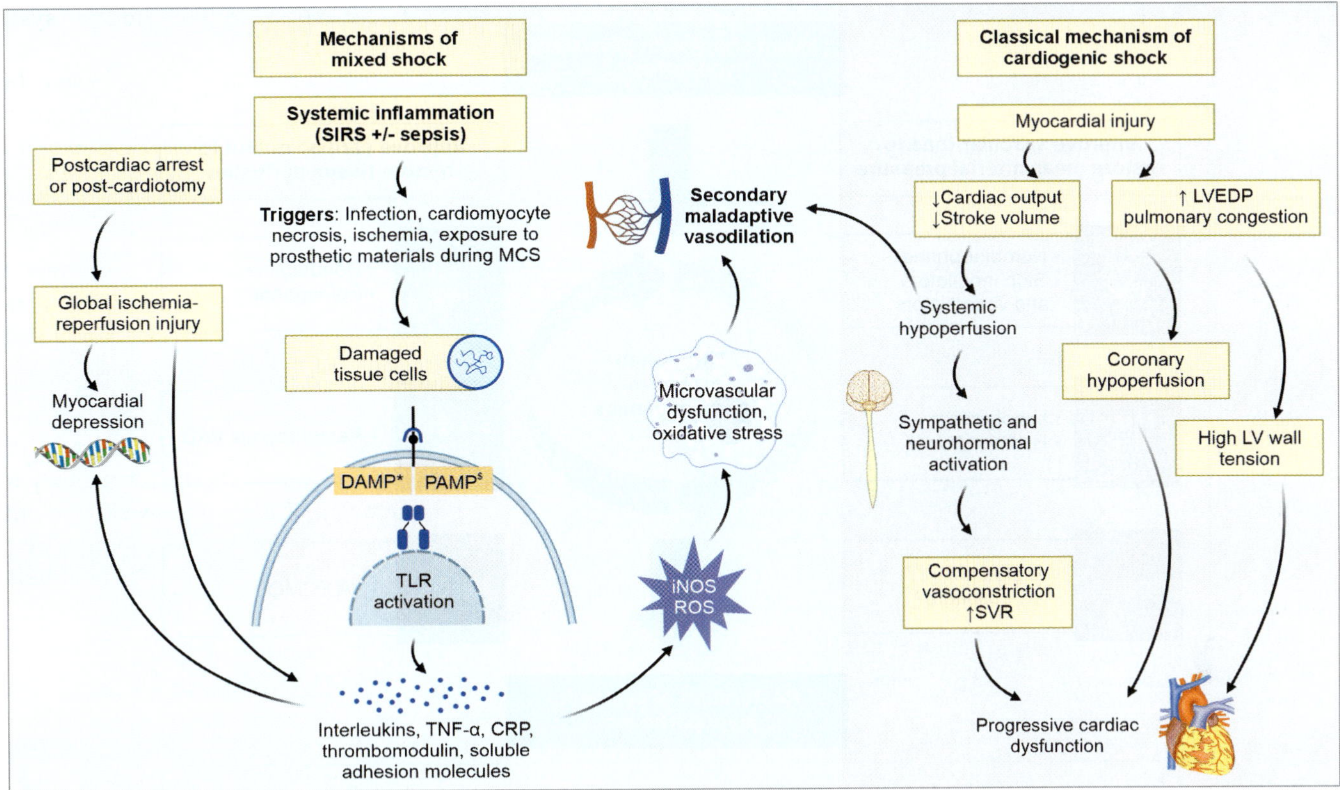

*Damage-associated molecule pattern molecules
$Pathogen-associated molecular pattern molecules.

FIG. 2: Different pathophysiological mechanisms of mixed shock.
Source: With permission from Jentzer JC, et al. (2024).[6]

Hemodynamic assessment in mixed shock: Accurate diagnosis relies on invasive hemodynamic monitoring to measure cardiac output and systemic vascular resistance. While a pulmonary artery catheter is considered the gold standard, alternative methods can estimate cardiac output when it is unavailable. Evaluating cardiac function is crucial, particularly in cases with vasodilatory components. This involves assessing myocardial ischemia through cardiac biomarkers, electrocardiography, and bedside echocardiography, with coronary angiography potentially necessary if acute myocardial ischemia is suspected.[19]

MANAGEMENT

Fluid Management in Mixed Shock

Patients with mixed shock require careful fluid management. Small amount of crystalloid bolus may be given with caution to assess preload-responsiveness, though static filling pressures alone are not a reliable marker of volume response. Restrictive fluid therapy is commonly advantageous following initial stabilization.[20]

Vasoactive Medications in Mixed Shock

Vasoactive medications are employed to stabilize hemodynamics in mixed shock, though there is no randomized control trial till date to back up the data. Invasive hemodynamic monitoring informs treatment decisions, enabling tailored adjustments of inotropes and vasopressors to optimize cardiac output and blood pressure.[21]

Mechanical Circulatory Support in Cardiogenic Shock

Mechanical circulatory support devices, such as intra-aortic balloon pumps, percutaneous ventricular assist devices, and veno-arterial extracorporeal membrane oxygenation (VA-ECMO), can improve systemic and coronary perfusion, reduce cardiac filling pressures, and facilitate revascularization in CS patients. The efficacy of these interventions may be hindered by vasoplegia in mixed shock.[22]

Selection of mechanical circulatory support (MCS) devices should consider the underlying cause and hemodynamic profile, ideally informed by pulmonary artery catheter (PAC) data. MCS is typically better suited for patients with primary cardiogenic shock that progresses to mixed shock. VA-ECMO is commonly used for refractory mixed shock, but its use is associated with substantial risks and should be reserved for patients with refractory shock **(Fig. 3)**.

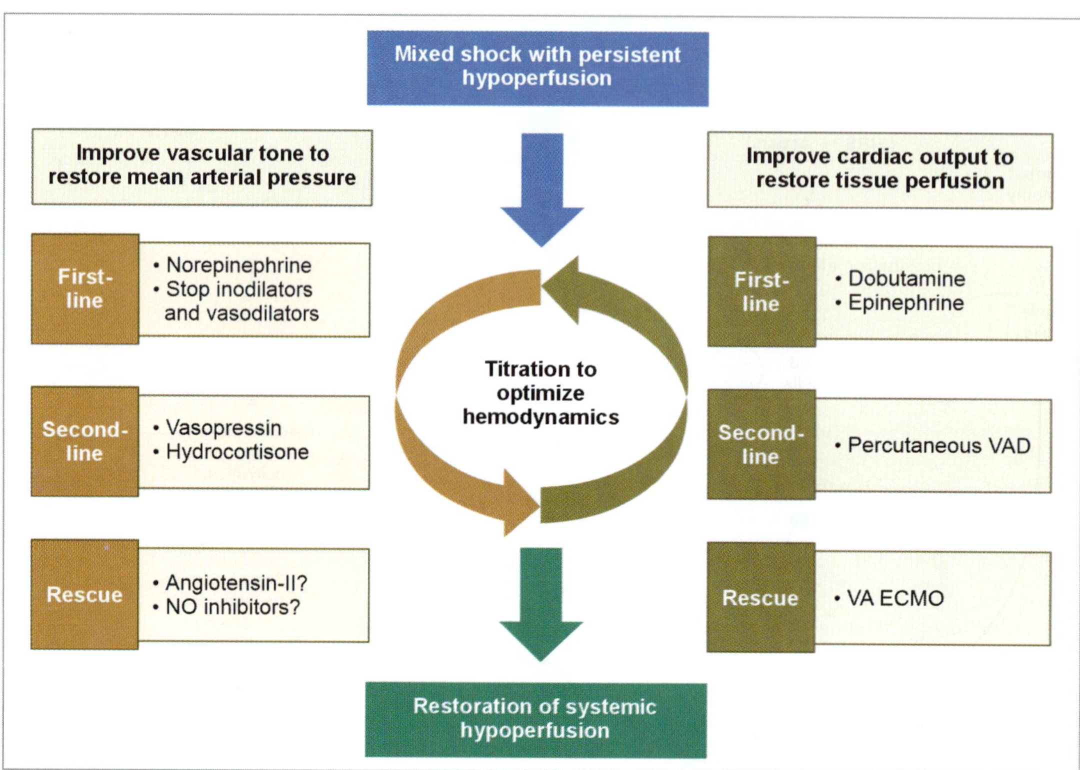

FIG. 3: Overview of management of mixed shock.
Source: With permission from Jentzer JC, et al. (2024).[6]

CONCLUSION

Mixed shock represents a complex and multifaceted clinical entity that defies a standardized definition yet can be conceptually characterized by hypotension and end-organ hypoperfusion resulting from the synergistic effects of acute cardiac insufficiency and systemic vasodilation. Cardiogenic-vasodilatory shock is a severe and complex condition occurs when cardiogenic shock is associated with or complicated by abnormal blood vessel dilation, disrupting the body's natural response mechanisms. Conversely, vasodilatory shock from septicemia can be further complicated by myocardial dysfunction, leading to inadequate blood circulation. Systemic issues can trigger both heart muscle dysfunction and abnormal blood vessel relaxation, resulting in a mixed shock state. Optimal management of this complex condition necessitates a multifaceted approach, wherein the primary objective is meticulously prioritized. If augmenting mean arterial pressure is the initial imperative, then vasopressors such as noradrenaline or vasopressin are judiciously employed as first-line agents, complemented by rigorous modulation of the inflammatory response. Conversely, if optimizing tissue perfusion is the paramount concern, then inotropes such as dobutamine or noradrenaline are initially utilized, potentially followed by mechanical circulatory support via VA-ECMO for refractory cases. Effective hemodynamic stabilization requires discerning use of vasopressors and inotropes, often necessitating invasive hemodynamic monitoring and thoughtful consideration of MCS in recalcitrant cases.

REFERENCES

1. Waksman R, Pahuja M, van Diepen S, et al. Standardized definitions for cardiogenic shock research and mechanical circulatory support devices: scientific expert panel from the Shock Academic Research Consortium (SHARC). Circulation. 2023;148:1113-26.
2. Menon V, Slater JN, White HD, et al. Acute myocardial infarction complicated by systemic hypoperfusion without hypotension: report of the SHOCK trial registry. Am J Med. 2000;108:374-80.
3. Berg DD, Kaur G, Bohula EA, et al. Prognostic significance of haemodynamic parameters in patients with cardiogenic shock. Eur Heart J Acute Cardiovasc Care. 2023;12:651-60.
4. van Diepen S, Katz JN, Albert NM, et al. Contemporary management of cardiogenic shock: a scientific statement from the American heart association. Circulation. 2017;136:e232-68.
5. Hochman JS. Cardiogenic shock complicating acute myocardial infarction: expanding the paradigm. Circulation. 2003;107:2998-3002.
6. Jentzer JC, Berg DD, Chonde MD, et al. Mixed Cardiogenic-Vasodilatory Shock: Current Insights and Future Directions. JACC Adv. 2024;4(1):101432.

7. Krychtiuk KA, Vrints C, Wojta J, et al. Basic mechanisms in cardiogenic shock: part 1-definition and pathophysiology. Eur Heart J Acute Cardiovasc Care. 2022;11:356-65.
8. van Diepen S, Vavalle JP, Newby LK, et al. The systemic inflammatory response syndrome in patients with ST-segment elevation myocardial infarction. Crit Care Med. 2013;41:2080-7.
9. Jentzer JC, Lawler PR, van Diepen S, et al. Systemic inflammatory response syndrome is associated with increased mortality across the spectrum of shock severity in cardiac intensive care patients. Circ Cardiovasc Qual Outcomes. 2020;13(12):e006956.
10. Jentzer JC, Ahmed AM, Vallabhajosyula S, et al. Shock in the cardiac intensive care unit: changes in epidemiology and prognosis over time. Am Heart J. 2021;232:94-104.
11. Ceglarek U, Schellong P, Rosolowski M, et al. The novel cystatin C, lactate, interleukin-6, and N-terminal pro-B-type natriuretic peptide (CLIP)-based mortality risk score in cardiogenic shock after acute myocardial infarction. Eur Heart J. 2021;42:2344-52.
12. Shvilkina T, Shapiro N. Sepsis-Induced myocardial dysfunction: heterogeneity of functional effects and clinical significance. Front Cardiovasc Med. 2023;10:1200441.
13. Vallabhajosyula S, Pruthi S, Shah S, et al. Basic and advanced echocardiographic evaluation of myocardial dysfunction in sepsis and septic shock. Anaesth Intensive Care. 2018;46:13-24.
14. Singh T, Khan H, Gamble DT, et al. Takotsubo syndrome: pathophysiology, emerging concepts, and clinical implications. Circulation. 2022;145:1002-19.
15. Takagi K, Blet A, Levy B, et al. Circulating dipeptidyl peptidase 3 and alteration in haemodynamics in cardiogenic shock: results from the OptimaCC trial. Eur J Heart Fail. 2020;22:279-86.
16. Tolppanen H, Rivas-Lasarte M, Lassus J, et al. Adrenomedullin: a marker of impaired hemodynamics, organ dysfunction, and poor prognosis in cardiogenic shock. Ann Intensive Care. 2017;7:6.
17. Vallabhajosyula S, Verghese D, Henry TD, et al. Contemporary management of concomitant cardiac arrest and cardiogenic shock complicating myocardial infarction. Mayo Clin Proc. 2022;97:2333-54.
18. Jentzer JC, Chonde MD, Dezfulian C. Myocardial dysfunction and shock after cardiac arrest. BioMed Res Int. 2015;2015:314796.
19. Kadosh BS, Berg DD, Bohula EA, et al. Pulmonary artery catheter use and mortality in the cardiac intensive care unit. JACC Heart Fail. 2023;11:903-14.
20. Silversides JA, Major E, Ferguson AJ, et al. Conservative fluid management or deresuscitation for patients with sepsis or acute respiratory distress syndrome following the resuscitation phase of critical illness: a systematic review and meta-analysis. Intensive Care Med. 2017;43:155-70.
21. Jentzer JC, Hollenberg SM. Vasopressor and inotrope therapy in cardiac critical care. J Intensive Care Med. 2021;36:843-56.
22. Henry TD, Tomey MI, Tamis-Holland JE, et al. Invasive management of acute myocardial infarction complicated by cardiogenic shock: a scientific statement from the American heart association. Circulation. 2021;143:e815-29.

CHAPTER 27

Chronic Right-sided Heart Failure and Tricuspid Regurgitation: "No Longer a Forgotten Entity"

Chandrakanta Mishra

ABSTRACT

The tricuspid valve (TV) and right ventricle (RV), once relegated to a secondary role in cardiac pathology, are now recognized as crucial structures with profound and independent prognostic importance. Right-sided heart failure (RHF) and tricuspid regurgitation (TR) are intrinsically linked to severely diminished quality of life (QoL), frequent hospitalizations for heart failure, and increased mortality if not addressed in a timely manner. Early identification of distinct RHF and TR phenotypes and their severity is paramount for guiding appropriate and timely therapy, including isolated TV surgery or transcatheter tricuspid valve intervention (TTVI). The objective of such interventions is not merely to improve survival or reduce hospitalization rates but to halt the progression of RHF and enhance the QoL. This review provides clinicians with a framework to identify the right patient at the right time, intervening before the cascade of RV dysfunction and systemic congestion leads to irreversible end-organ damage. This approach reframes the central clinical challenge from managing end-stage RHF to preventing its progression, integrating palliative strategies alongside curative care as an essential component of comprehensive management.

Keywords: Tricuspid regurgitation, right heart failure, RV dysfunction, tricuspid valve repair, tricuspid valve replacement.

INTRODUCTION: A PARADIGM SHIFT IN UNDERSTANDING THE RIGHT HEART

Right-sided heart failure (RHF) and tricuspid regurgitation (TR) are associated with a significant burden of morbidity and mortality, leading to a severely reduced quality of life (QoL) and frequent hospitalizations.[1,2] The prevalence of this condition disproportionately affects older women, particularly those with atrial fibrillation (AF) and heart failure with preserved ejection fraction (HFpEF). While mild TR is a common echocardiographic finding, but clinically significant (greater than moderate) TR prevalence increases sharply with age, affecting 3–6% of individuals over 75 years old.[3,4] Importantly, significant TR is independently associated with a 40–70% increase in all-cause mortality over 1–4 years, even after adjusting for comorbidities.[5] Despite these statistics, the condition remains frequently undertreated, with referrals for intervention often occurring late, after the onset of fixed right-sided failure.

Historically, the tricuspid valve (TV) and right ventricle (RV) were dismissed as the "forgotten valve and ventricle," with the prevailing view being that treating the left heart would consequently resolve TR. This perspective has yielded to a modern paradigm in which the right heart and TV are understood as a dynamic, load-sensitive system. In this updated model, the right heart's function is an integration of:

- Intrinsic RV contractility and geometry
- Pericardial constraints
- Venous return and right atrial (RA) pressure-volume dynamics
- Pulmonary afterload
- The competence of the entire tricuspid apparatus, including its leaflets, chordae, papillary muscles, and highly distensible annulus.

Within this framework, TR is not merely a marker of disease but an *active amplifier* of RV volume and pressure overload. This establishes a self-perpetuating pathophysiological loop of annular dilatation, worsening leaflet malcoaptation, and progressive systemic venous hypertension **(Flowchart 1)**.

Advances in multimodality imaging and more nuanced grading systems have catalyzed earlier identification and facilitated the shift from late, high-risk surgery to staged, and phenotype-guided interventions. The primary clinical goal has thus been reframed from managing end-stage RHF to preventing its progression by intervening before irreversible end-organ damage occurs.

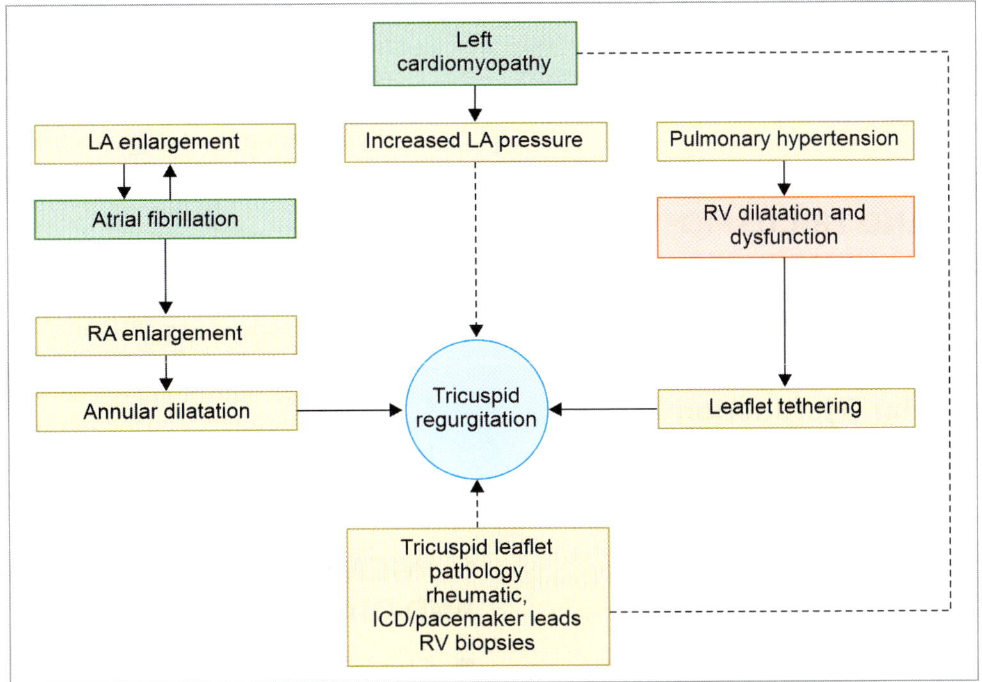

FLOWCHART 1: Pathophysiology of tricuspid regurgitation and heart failure.
(ICD: implantable cardioverter-defibrillator; LA: left atrium; RA: right atrium; RV: right ventricle)

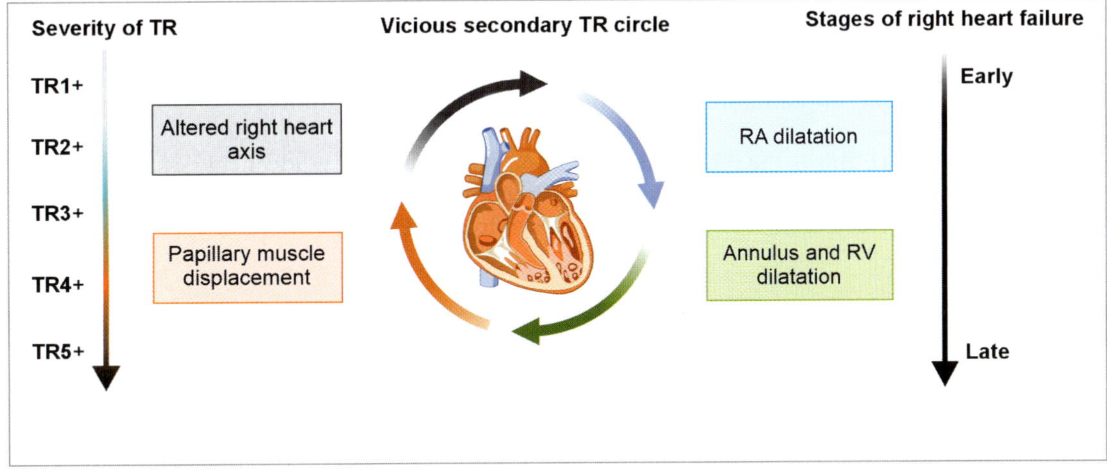

FIG. 1: Detrimental effects of TR on the progression of heart failure.
(RA: right atrium; RV: right ventricle; TR: tricuspid regurgitation)

INTERWOVEN PATHOPHYSIOLOGY OF RIGHT-SIDED HEART FAILURE AND TRICUSPID REGURGITATION

A detailed understanding of the complex pathophysiological relationship between the RV, RA, and TV is essential for accurate diagnosis and effective therapy. The 2024 HFA/EAPCI consensus statement[6] clarifies that *right ventricular dysfunction (RVD)* is an impairment of RV function, whereas *RHF* is the clinical syndrome of signs and symptoms that results from RVD. This distinction is critical, as asymptomatic RVD can precede the development of overt RHF. Furthermore, RHF with significant TR can occur even without severe intrinsic RVD, highlighting *the primary role the TV* can play.

The progression of RHF and TR is often a vicious cycle **(Fig. 1)**. It typically begins with an initiating insult, such as increased RV afterload from left-sided heart disease or pulmonary hypertension (PH). The RV undergoes maladaptive remodeling to maintain forward flow, leading to progressive dilatation and dysfunction. This ventricular remodeling, in turn, causes or exacerbates secondary TR by distorting the TV annulus and tethering the leaflets. The resultant volume overload from TR imposes further strain on the RV, promoting more dilatation and dysfunction, which further worsens the TR. This cycle culminates in progressive RHF and systemic venous congestion.

CLASSIFICATION OF RIGHT VENTRICULAR DYSFUNCTION AND TRICUSPID REGURGITATION PHENOTYPES

An updated classification of RVD and TR is vital, as it directly informs etiology-specific treatment strategies.

Right Ventricular Dysfunction

Chronic RHF due to RVD is broadly classified into two categories:

1. *Primary RVD:* It is caused by a primary decrease in RV function (contractility and/or lusitropy).
2. *Secondary RVD:* Resulting from RV pressure or volume overload, or right atrial remodeling **(Table 1)**.

Tricuspid Regurgitation

Tricuspid regurgitation can be both a cause and a consequence of RVD. The mechanistic classification of TR extends beyond a simple primary/secondary distinction **(Figs. 2 and 3)**.

- *Primary TR (5–10% of cases):* It arises from an intrinsic structural abnormality of the valvular or subvalvular apparatus, including cardiac implantable electronic device (CIED)-related TR.
- *Secondary TR (~85% of cases):* This is the most common phenotype and results from either atrial or ventricular pathology. It is further subdivided into:
  - *Atrial-secondary TR (A-STR):* It is driven by atrial remodeling, often from long-standing AF, with a relatively preserved RV size and function.[7,8] A-STR carries a better prognosis than V-STR. An aggressive rhythm-control strategy, such as catheter ablation, may be an effective first-line therapy, as restoring sinus rhythm can lead to reverse remodeling of the RA and tricuspid annulus.
  - *Ventricular-secondary TR (V-STR):* It is driven by ventricular pathology from chronic pressure or volume overload (e.g., PH). In V-STR, rhythm control is unlikely to be sufficient, and the therapeutic focus must be on addressing the elevated RV afterload or intervening directly on the valve.

It is important to note that different phenotypes of RHF and TR frequently coexist in the same patient.

CLINICAL PRESENTATION, TRAJECTORY, AND DIAGNOSIS

Clinical Course

Right-sided heart failure and TR manifest as a multiorgan syndrome involving both cardiac and extracardiac structures, including the liver, kidneys, gastrointestinal tract, and brain. The clinical course is often insidious. Early symptoms are frequently nonspecific—such as fatigue, dyspepsia, or minor edema—even in the presence of severe TR. This subtlety often leads to a significant delay in diagnosis, allowing for unchecked disease progression.

As the condition advances, systemic venous congestion becomes the dominant driver of a debilitating multiorgan syndrome **(Fig. 4)**.[9,10]

TABLE 1: Causes of right-sided heart failure.

	Primary RV dysfunction	Secondary RV dysfunction	
Right atrial remodeling	**Primary decrease in RV function (contractility or lusitropy)**	**RV pressure overload**	**RV volume overload**
Atrial fibrillation	Amyloidosis	Congenital heart disease	Extracardiac arteriovenous shunt
Atrial myopathy (i.e., associated with HFpEF)	Cardiotoxicity	Precapillary or postcapillary pulmonary hypertension*	High-output states, including concomitant LV volume overload
Tricuspid regurgitation	Constrictive pericarditis	Pulmonary artery stenosis	Intracardiac left-to-right shunt
	Myocarditis	Pulmonary valve stenosis	Post-LVAD
	Postcardiac surgery or post-LVAD		Pulmonary regurgitation
	RV cardiomyopathy		Tricuspid regurgitation
	RV myocardial infarction		
	Sarcoidosis		
	Systemic sclerosis		

*Pulmonary arterial hypertension, left-sided heart disease (including left-sided valvular heart disease, HFrEF, HFmrEF and HFpEF), lung disease and/or hypoxia, chronic thromboembolic pulmonary hypertension, or other mechanisms.

(HFmrEF: heart failure with mildly reduced ejection fraction; HFpEF: heart failure with preserved ejection fraction; HFrEF: heart failure with reduced ejection fraction; LV: left ventricular; LVAD: left ventricular assist device; RV: right ventricular)

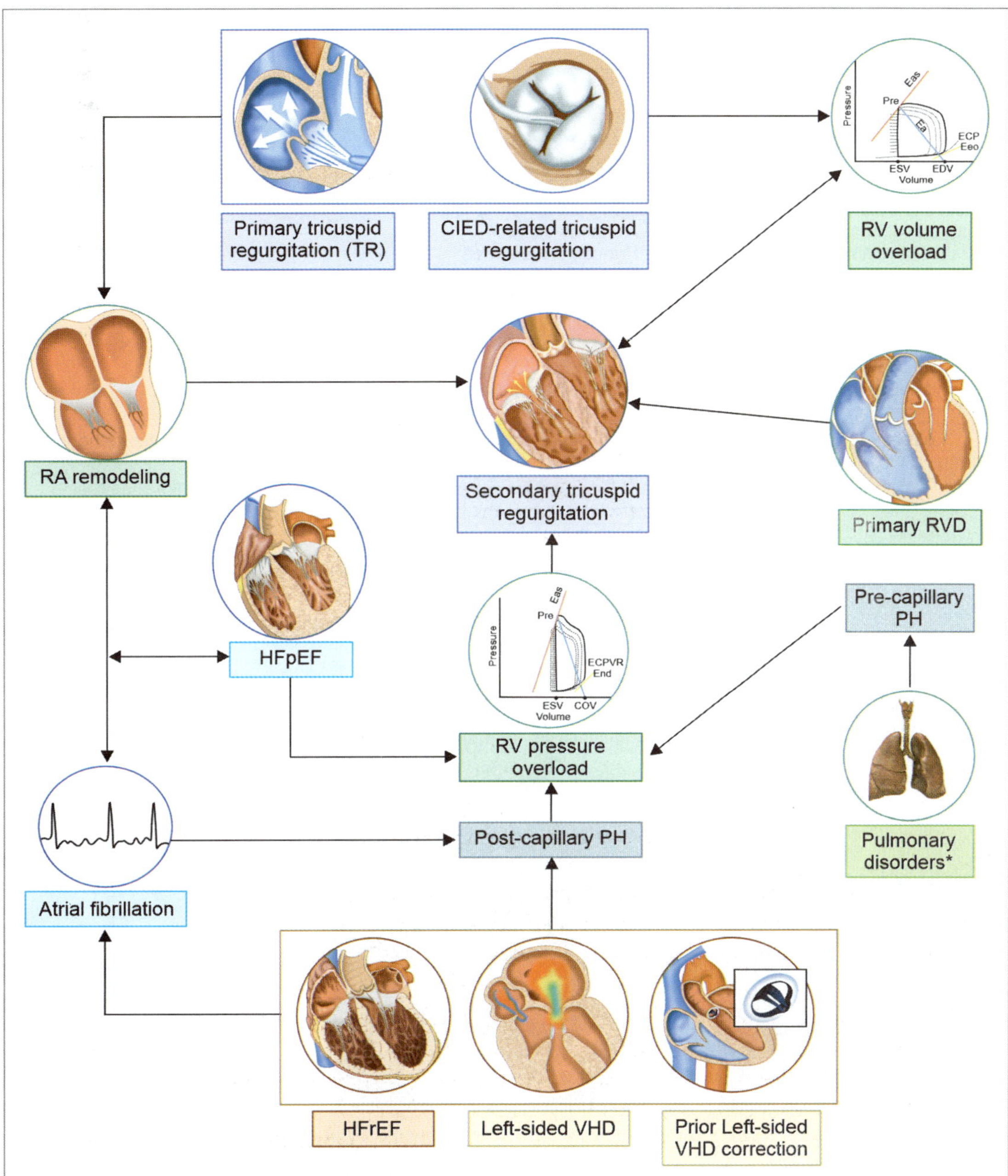

*COPD: Interstitial lung diseases, etc. leading to cor pulmonale

FIG. 2: Etiopathogenesis and mechanisms of RHF and TR.

(CIED: cardiovascular implantable electronic device; HFpEF: heart failure with preserved ejection fraction; HFrEF: heart failure with reduced ejection fraction; PH: pulmonary hypertension; RA: right atrium; RHF: right-sided heart failure; RV: right ventricle; RVD: right ventricular dysfunction)

- *Hepatosplanchnic congestion* causes abdominal distension, anorexia, early satiety, and nutrient malabsorption. Chronic passive congestion of the liver can lead to "cardiac cirrhosis," characterized by hepatic dysfunction.
- *Renal congestion* from increased central venous pressure leads to *cardiorenal syndrome*, marked by worsening renal function, and diuretic resistance.
- *Pulmonary congestion* results from increased ventricular interdependence

Diagnostic Workup and Staging

Given the silent nature of early disease, a high index of clinical suspicion is necessary. "Red flag" indicators should prompt a timely diagnostic workup **(Table 2)**.

Accurate phenotyping, risk stratification, and procedural planning require an integrated, multimodality diagnostic pathway **(Flowchart 2)**.

A key advance in staging is the expanded *five-tiered grading system for TR severity*: mild, moderate, severe, massive, and

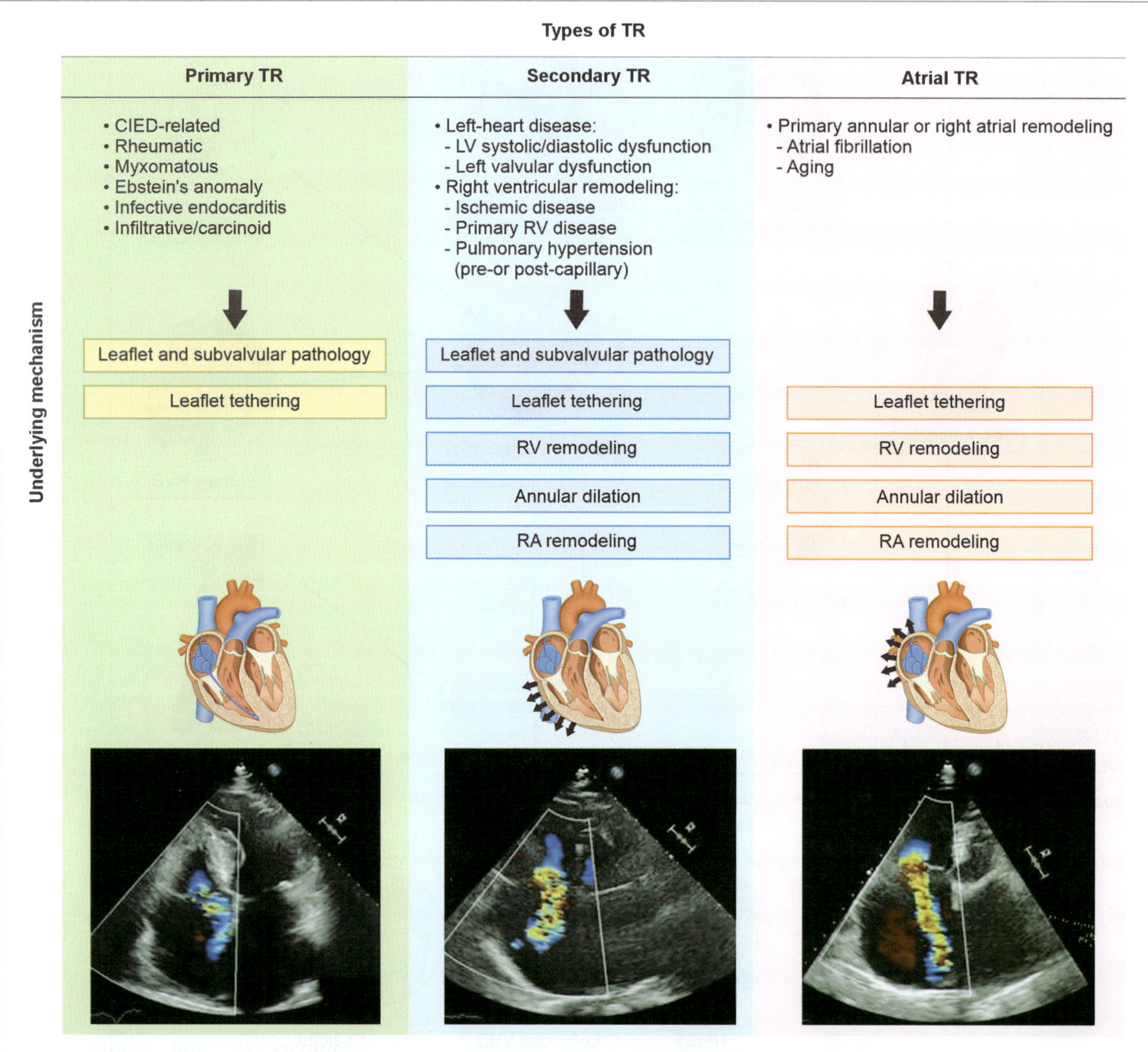

FIG. 3: Etiopathogenesis and classification of tricuspid regurgitation. The three main types of TR are associated with different mechanisms of disease, which may overlap.

(CIED: cardiovascular implantable electronic device; LV: left ventricle; RA: right atrium; RV: right ventricle; TR: tricuspid regurgitation)

Source: Leone PP, Chiarito M, Regazzoli D, et al. Prognostic value of tricuspid regurgitation. Rev Cardiovasc Med. 2022;23(2):76.

torrential **(Fig. 5)**. This new scale is prognostically significant, as it captures the incremental risk associated with the most extreme degrees of regurgitation that were previously grouped under the broad "severe" category.

Right heart catheterization (RHC) is an indispensable component of the preinterventional workup. It overcomes the limitations of Doppler echocardiography, which can underestimate pulmonary artery pressures in severe TR, and it allows for the precise differentiation of precapillary versus postcapillary PH. This distinction is vital, as severe precapillary PH is a strong predictor of poor outcomes and may be a relative contraindication to transcatheter tricuspid valve intervention (TTVI).

A discordance between echocardiographic and invasive hemodynamic assessments is a potent negative prognostic marker. In massive or torrential TR, the low-velocity regurgitant jet can lead to a deceptively low estimation of systolic pulmonary artery pressure by echo. RHC, however,

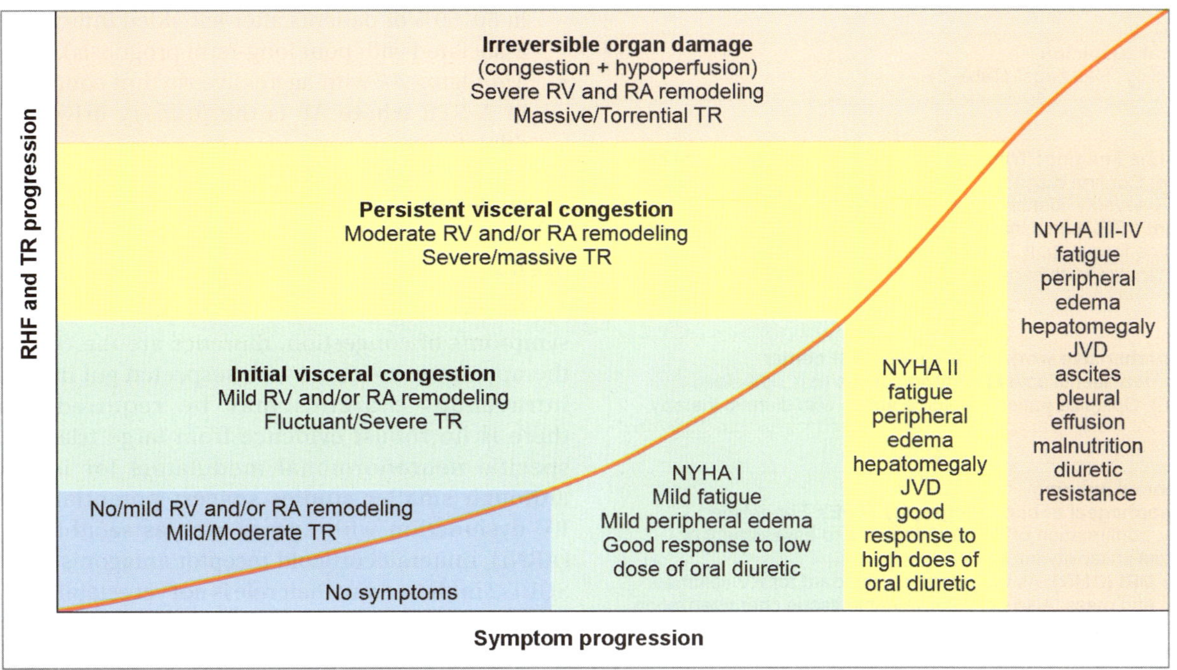

FIG. 4: Clinical course and progression of right-sided heart failure and TR.
(RA: right atrium; RHF: right-sided heart failure; RV: right ventricle; TR: tricuspid regurgitation)

TABLE 2: Red flags for the early identification of RHF and/or significant TR.

Category	Red flag indicators
Clinical history	History of left-sided VHD, HF (any EF), long-standing AF, COPD/pulmonary disease, CIED implantation
Symptoms	Unexplained or worsening peripheral edema, new-onset ascites, persistent fatigue, exertional dyspnea, and abdominal bloating/early satiety
Physical examination signs	Elevated jugular venous pressure (JVP), positive abdominojugular reflux, pulsatile hepatomegaly, and holosystolic murmur at the left sternal border
Laboratory findings	Worsening renal function (rising creatinine/BUN), new or worsening cholestatic liver profile (↑GGT, ALP, and bilirubin), elevated NT-pro-BNP, elevated CA-125 (as a marker of systemic congestion)

(AF: atrial fibrillation; CIED: cardiovascular implantable electronic device; RHF: right-sided heart failure; TR: tricuspid regurgitation)

will unmask the severely elevated mean pulmonary and RV diastolic pressures. This discordance is not a measurement error but a *hemodynamic signature* of advanced disease and should be considered a significant negative prognostic factor during heart team discussions.

A STRUCTURED AND MULTIDISCIPLINARY MANAGEMENT FRAMEWORK

Identifying the "Therapeutic Window"

The timing of intervention is critical and framed by the concept of a "therapeutic window" to avoid clinical futility. Predictors of poor outcomes after TV intervention include severe RVD,[11] massive/torrential TR,[12] established end-organ damage,[13] severe precapillary PH,[14] and high discordance between echo and RHC findings.[15] Intervening too late, after the onset of these factors, renders the procedure futile; the valve may be repaired, but the patient's clinical trajectory is unlikely to improve. Isolated TV surgery in late-stage disease carries an operative mortality as high as 16%.

Conversely, the landmark *TRILUMINATE Pivotal trial*[16] demonstrated that in a low-risk population with severe symptomatic TR, i.e., TTVI (TEER with TriClip) led to significant improvements in QoL but not in mortality or heart failure hospitalizations compared to medical therapy. This evidence collectively suggests that intervening too early may expose patients to procedural risk for a primarily symptomatic benefit, while intervening too late is futile **(Fig. 6)**.[17] The central question for the heart team must shift from, *"Can we technically fix the valve?"* to *"Is the patient*

1. Clinical suspicion
Triggered by "Red flags" (Table 2)

↓

2. First-line imaging: Transthoracic echocardiography (TTE)
Purpose: Confirm diagnosis, assess RV/RA size and function, grade TR severity, identify potential etiology.
Decision: If TR is less than severe, pursue medical management and routine follow-up. If TR is severe or greater, proceed to comprehensive evaluation.

↓

3. Comprehensive work-up at a specialist center
Action: Treat identifiable underlying causes (e.g., left-sided VHD, AF). Optimize patient's volume status with diuretic therapy.

↓

4. Advanced imaging
Transesophageal echocardiography (TOE): For detailed TV anatomy, confirmation of TR mechanism, and assessment of anatomical suitability for TTVI
Cardiac MRI (CMR): As the reference standard for RV volumes, function, and mass. Also provides valuable tissue characterization.
Cardiac CT (CCT): For detailed 3D anatomy of the TV annulus, surrounding structures (e.g., right coronary artery), and vascular access, crucial for preprocedural planning of TTVI.

↓

5. Mandatory hemodynamic assessment: Right heart catheterization
Purpose: To be performed in all patients considered for intervention after volume optimization. Crucial for confirming or excluding pulmonary hypertension (PH), differentiating precapillary vs. postcapillary PH, measuring pulmonary vascular resistance (PVR), and assessing cardiac output (Fick method preferred over thermodilution is severe TR).

↓

6. Data integration for multidisciplinary heart team decision

FLOWCHART 2: Diagnostic algorithm for suspected RHF and/or significant TR.
(AF: atrial fibrillation; RA: right atrium; RV: right ventricle; TR: tricuspid regurgitation; TTVI: transcatheter tricuspid valve intervention; TV: tricuspid valve)

beyond the point where fixing the valve will meaningfully alter their clinical course?".

Stepwise Management

The ESC 2024 consensus statement outlines a structured management plan **(Flowchart 3)**.

Step 1

Treat the underlying etiology: The first-line approach is to address the primary driver of the RHF and TR **(Fig. 7)**. This includes:

- *Optimizing guideline-directed medical therapy (GDMT)* for HFrEF or HFpEF
- *Addressing left-sided valvular disease* via surgical or transcatheter intervention. (*Note:* Significant TR persists in 50–60% of patients after left-sided intervention and is associated with poor long-term prognosis).
- *Managing AF* with aggressive rhythm control, especially in A-STR where AF is the primary driver of annular dilatation.
- *Treating PH* with specific therapies according to guidelines

Step 2

Medical management of RHF: For patients with persistent symptoms of congestion, diuretics are the cornerstone of therapy. In severe cases with suspected gut malabsorption, intravenous diuretics may be required. Currently, there is no robust evidence from large trials to support specific neurohormonal modulators for isolated RHF, although smaller studies suggest potential benefits for RV dysfunction with agents such as sacubitril/valsartan (ARNI), mineralocorticoid receptor antagonist (MRAs), and SGLT-2 inhibitor, but their role is not yet established. Medical therapy should not unduly delay referral for intervention in appropriate candidates.

Step 3

Tricuspid valve interventions, when significant TR persists despite optimal medical management, valve-directed intervention may be considered in the absence of precapillary PH, severe RV dysfunction, and end-organ damage **(Fig. 8)**.

- *Surgery: Isolated TV surgery* is effective in *early-stage of primary severe TR* (*class I recommendation*) but has high mortality in patients with advanced RHF and end-organ dysfunction. *Concomitant TV repair* should be considered in patients with *moderate primary or secondary TR* undergoing left-sided valve surgery to avoid progression of TR and RV remodeling (*class IIa*).
- *Transcatheter tricuspid valve intervention:* TTVI is a critical option for symptomatic patients with *severe TR at high surgical risk*. Based on trials like TRILUMINATE[16] and TRISCEND-II,[18] TTVI is best understood, not as a lifesaving intervention but as a powerful palliative therapy to improve QoL. The ideal candidate *is highly symptomatic severe TR, i.e., primary (class IIa) and secondary V-STR* (*class I*) undergoing left-sided valve surgery. Patient counseling must center on the realistic expectation of symptomatic improvement rather than a survival benefit **(Table 3, Flowchart 4, and Fig. 9)**.

INTEGRATED CARE PATHWAY: FROM HEART TEAM TO LIFETIME MANAGEMENT

The complex management of RHF and TR necessitates a coordinated, longitudinal care model delivered by a specialized, multidisciplinary *heart team* within a high-volume heart valve center. This team should include a heart failure specialist, an interventional cardiologist, a cardiac

Parameters	Mild	Moderate	Severe	Massive	Torrential
Qualitative • Color doppler • CW doppler					
Semiquantitative • Vena contracta (mm²) • PISA radius (mm) • Backflow in hepatic veins	< 3 ≤ 5 Systolic dominance	3–6.9 6–9 Systolic flattening	7–13.9 >9 Systolic flow reversal	14–20 - Systolic flow reversal	> 21 - Systolic flow reversal
Quantitative • EROA (mm²) by PISA • Reg. vol (mL) by PISA	< 2 < 30	2–3.9 30–44	4.0–5.9 45–59	6.0–7.9 60–74	> 8.0 > 75

FIG. 5: Echocardiographic evaluation and grading of tricuspid regurgitation (TR).

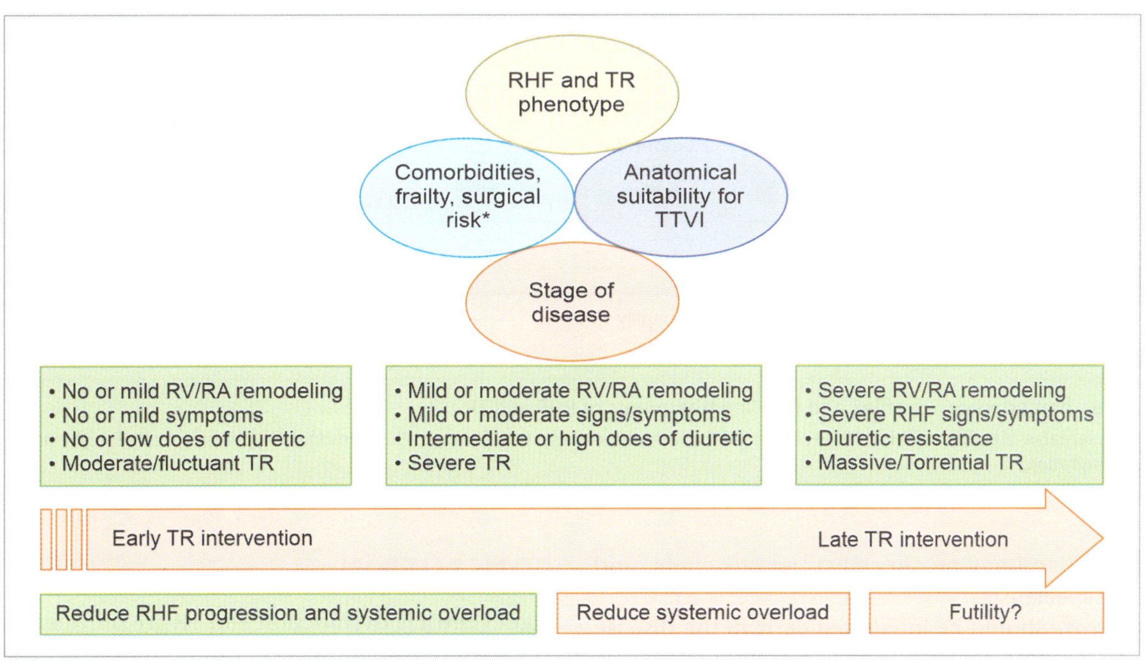

*TRI-SCORE.

FIG. 6: Comprehensive evaluation of patients with RHF and TR for possible intervention.[17]

(RHF: right-sided heart failure; TR: tricuspid regurgitation; TTVI: transcatheter tricuspid valve intervention)

Source: With permission from Dreyfus J, et al. (2022).[17]

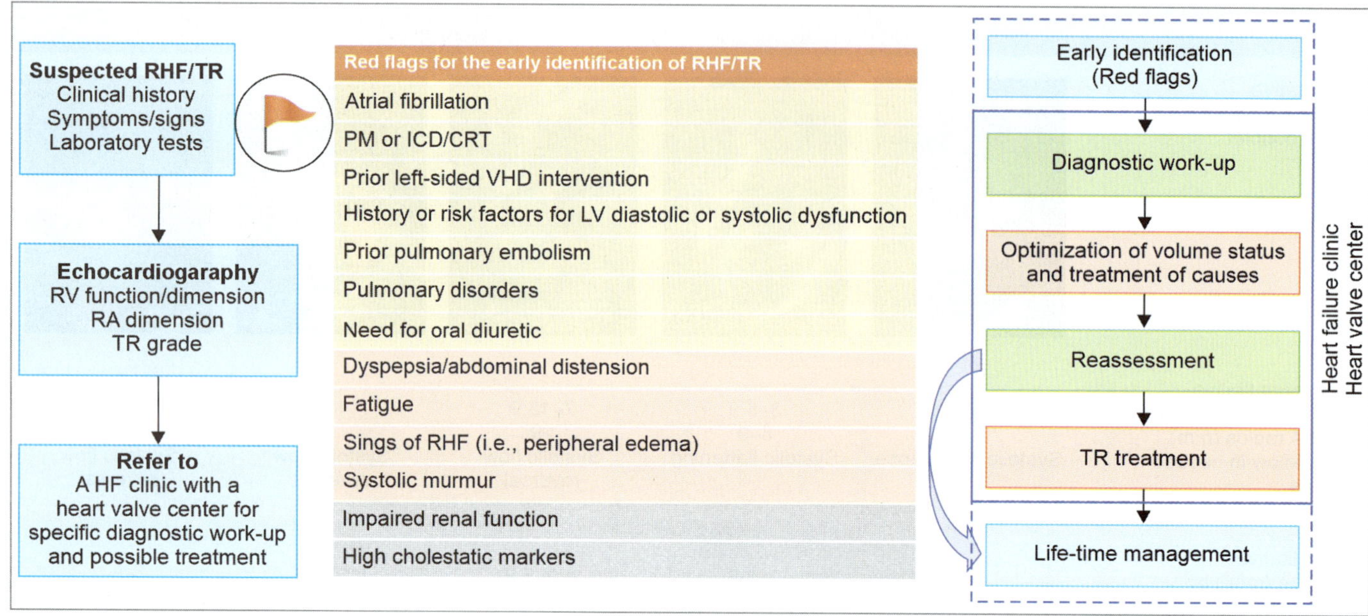

FLOWCHART 3: Step-by-step management of patients with RHF and TR.

(LV: left ventricle; PH: pulmonary hypertension; RA: right atrium; RV: right ventricle; RHF: right-sided heart failure; TR: tricuspid regurgitation)

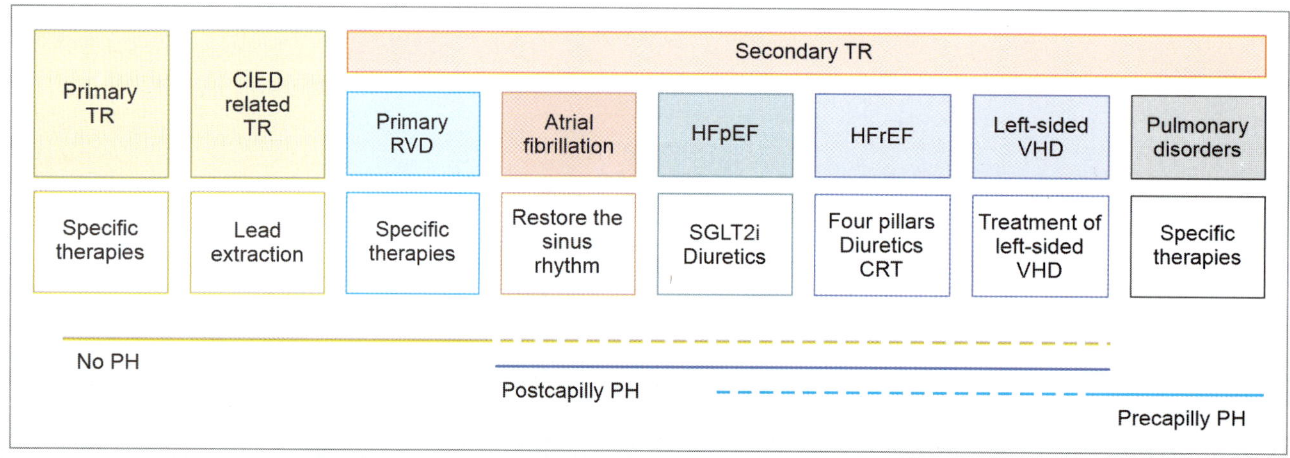

FIG. 7: Etiologies, hemodynamic profiles, and first-line treatments of RHF and TR.

(CIED: cardiac implantable electronic device; HFrEF: heart failure with reduced ejection fraction; PH: pulmonary hypertension; RHF: right-sided heart failure; TR: tricuspid regurgitation)

surgeon, a cardiac imaging specialist, geriatricians, and palliative care specialists.

Palliative care should be integrated early in the disease course for all patients with advanced symptoms. It should coexist with curative therapies rather than being reserved as a last resort, aligning perfectly with the QoL-focused goals of modern interventions like TTVI. For symptomatic patients who are not candidates for intervention, a direct pivot to formal palliative care services is an evidence-aligned step.

CONCLUSION

Right ventricle dysfunction and TR are prevalent conditions, associated with poor outcomes that require a targeted therapeutic strategy to mitigate the risk of RHF progression. Therapeutic decisions must be tailored to the underlying etiology. Significant knowledge gaps remain, particularly regarding the optimal timing and modality of intervention for severe TR. Furthermore, the lack of evidence-based

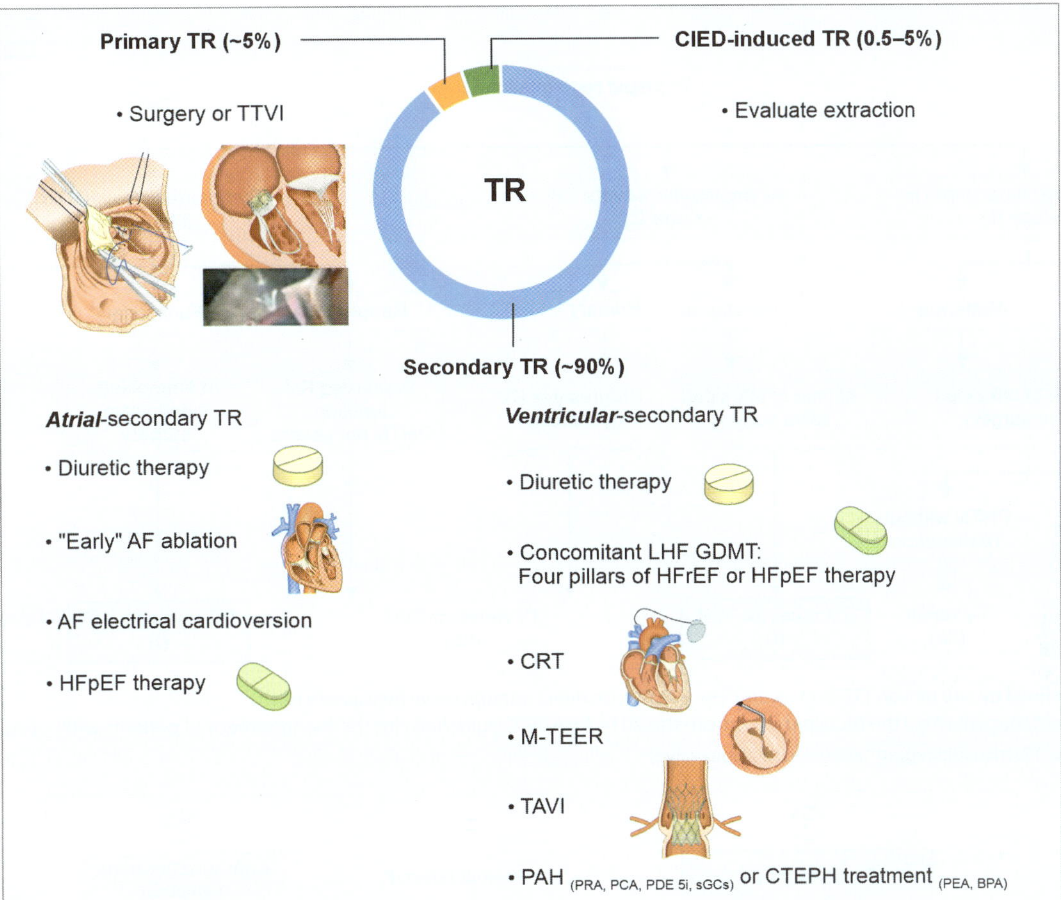

FIG. 8: Decision-making treatment of TR according to the etiology.[2]

(AF: atrial fibrillation; CIED: cardiac implantable electronic device; GDMT: guideline-directed medical therapy; HFpEF: heart failure with preserved ejection fraction; HFrEF: heart failure with reduced ejection fraction; TR: tricuspid regurgitation; TTVI: transcatheter tricuspid valve intervention)

TABLE 3: ESC Congress 2025 recommendations for management of patients with TR.

Recommendations	Class	level
Careful evaluation of TR etiology, stage of the disease (i.e., degree of TR severity, RV and LV dysfunction, and PH), patient operative risk, and likelihood of recovery by a multidisciplinary Heart Team is recommended in patients with severe TR prior to intervention (New)	I	C
Patients with TR and left-sided valvular heart disease requiring surgery		
Concomitant TV repair should be considered in patients with moderate primary or secondary TR, to avoid progression of TR and RV remodeling (REV.)	IIa	B
Concomitant TV repair may be considered in selected patients with mild secondary TR and tricuspid annulus dilatation (≥40 mm or >21 mm/m^2), to avoid progression of TR and RV remodeling (REV.)	IIb	B
Patients with severe TR without left-sided valvular heart disease requiring surgery		
Transcatheter TV treatment should be considered to improve quality of life and RV remodeling in high-risk patients with symptomatic severe TR despite optimal medical therapy in the absence of severe RV dysfunction or precapillary PH (REV.)	IIa	A

(LV: left ventricle; PH: pulmonary hypertension; RV: right ventricle; TR: tricuspid regurgitation; TV: tricuspid valve)

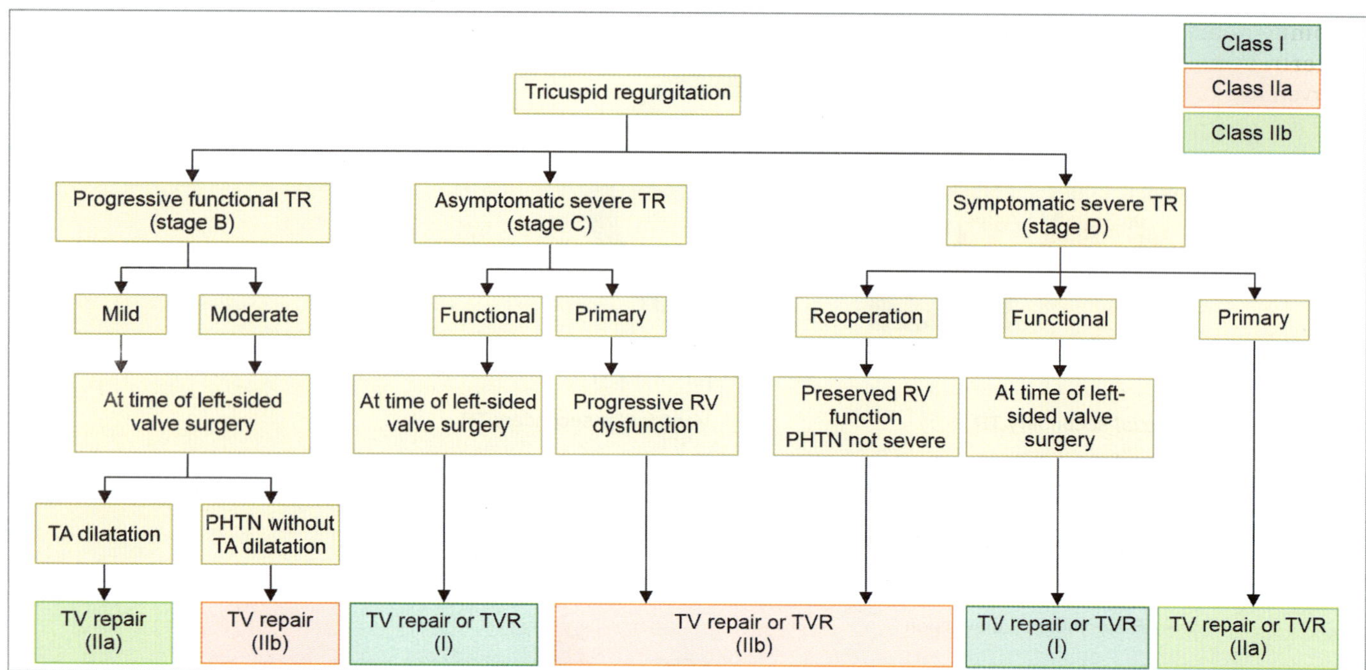

*TA dilatation is defined by >40 mm on TTE (>21 mm/m^2) or >70 mm on direct intraoperative measurement.

FLOWCHART 4: Management of the tricuspid valve from the 2014 AHA/ACC guidelines for the management of patients with valvular heart disease.
(RV: right ventricle; TR: tricuspid regurgitation; TV: tricuspid valve)

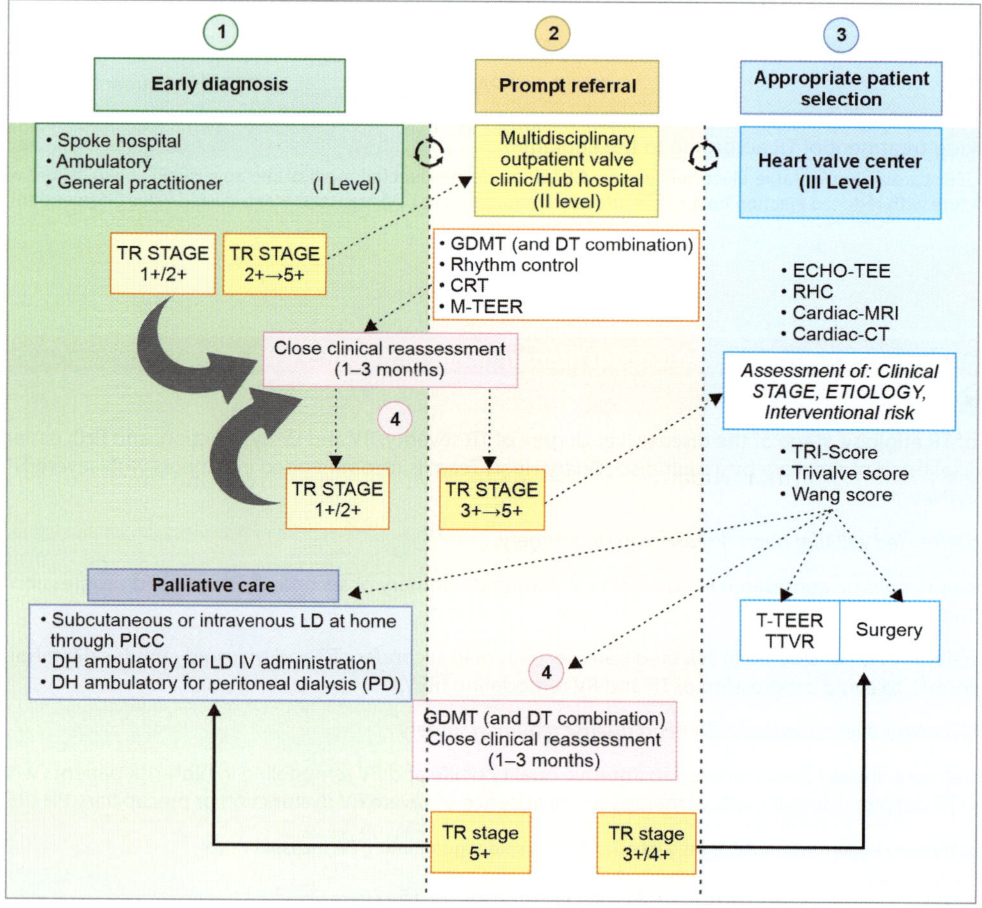

FIG. 9: Clinical management algorithm for TR.
(GDMT: guideline-directed medical therapy; TR: tricuspid regurgitation)

recommendations for medical therapy contributes to undertreatment and disease progression. Delaying intervention until the late stages results in excessive morbidity and mortality. Therefore, all patients with significant symptomatic TR should be referred to a specialized heart valve center for comprehensive evaluation by a multidisciplinary heart team. This collaborative assessment is mandatory to determine risks, weigh the expected benefits against potential harms, and identify the most appropriate treatment strategy for each individual patient.

REFERENCES

1. Iglesias-Garriz I, Olalla-Gomez C, Garrote C, et al. Contribution of right ventricular dysfunction to heart failure mortality: A meta-analysis. Rev Cardiovasc Med. 2012;13:e62-9.
2. Edward J, Banchs J, Parker H, et al. Right ventricular function across the spectrum of health and disease. Heart. 2023;109:349-55.
3. d'Arcy JL, Coffey S, Loudon MA, et al. Large-scale community echocardiographic screening reveals a major burden of undiagnosed valvular heart disease in older people: The OxVALVE population cohort study. Eur Heart J. 2016;37:3515-22.
4. Vieitez JM, Monteagudo JM, Mahia P, et al. New insights of tricuspid regurgitation: A large-scale prospective cohort study. Eur Heart J Cardiovasc Imaging. 2021;22:196-202.
5. Prihad E. Tricuspid valve regurgitation: no longer the "forgotten valve". Eur J Cardiol Pract. 2018;16:13.
6. Adamo M, Chioncel O, Pagnesi M, et al. Epidemiology, pathophysiology, diagnosis and management of chronic right-sided heart failure and tricuspid regurgitation. A clinical consensus statement of the Heart Failure Association (HFA) and the European Association of Percutaneous Cardiovascular Interventions (EAPCI) of the ESC. Eur J Heart Fail. 2024;26(1):18-33.
7. Galloo X, Dietz MF, Fortuni F, et al. Prognostic implications of atrial vs. ventricular functional tricuspid regurgitation. Eur Heart J Cardiovasc Imaging. 2023;24:733-41.
8. Schlotter F, Dietz MF, Stolz L, et al. Atrial functional tricuspid regurgitation: Novel definition and impact on prognosis. Circ Cardiovasc Interv. 2022;15:e011958.
9. Konstam MA, Kiernan MS, Bernstein D, et al. American Heart Association Council on Clinical Cardiology; Council on Cardiovascular Disease in the Young; and Council on Cardiovascular Surgery and Anesthesia. Evaluation and management of right-sided heart failure: A scientific statement from the American Heart Association. Circulation. 2018;137:e578-e622.
10. Arrigo M, Huber LC, Winnik S, et al. Right ventricular failure: Pathophysiology, diagnosis and treatment. Card Fail Rev. 2019;5:140-6.
11. Kresoja KP, Rommel KP, Lucke C, et al. Right ventricular contraction patterns in patients undergoing transcatheter tricuspid valve repair for severe tricuspid regurgitation. JACC Cardiovasc Interv. 2021;14:1551-61.
12. Miura M, Alessandrini H, Alkhodair A, et al. Impact of massive or torrential tricuspid regurgitation in patients undergoing transcatheter tricuspid valve intervention. JACC Cardiovasc Interv 2020;13:1999-2009.
13. Muntane-Carol G, Taramasso M, Miura M, et al. Transcatheter tricuspid valve intervention in patients with right ventricular dysfunction or pulmonary hypertension: Insights from the TriValve Registry. Circ Cardiovasc Interv. 2021;14:e009685.
14. Stocker TJ, Hertell H, Orban M, et al. Cardiopulmonary hemodynamic profile predicts mortality after transcatheter tricuspid valve repair in chronic heart failure. JACC Cardiovasc Interv. 2021;14:29-38.
15. Lurz P, Orban M, Besler C, et al. Clinical characteristics, diagnosis, and risk stratification of pulmonary hypertension in severe tricuspid regurgitation and implications for transcatheter tricuspid valve repair. Eur Heart J. 2020;41:2785-95.
16. Sorajja P, Whisenant B, Hamid N, et al. Transcatheter Repair for Patients with Tricuspid Regurgitation. N Engl J Med. 2023;388(20):1833-42.
17. Dreyfus J, Audureau E, Bohbot Y, et al. TRI-SCORE: A new risk score for in-hospital mortality prediction after isolated tricuspid valve surgery. Eur Heart J. 2022;43:654-62.
18. Hahn RT, Makkar R, Thourani VH, et al. Transcatheter Valve Replacement in Severe Tricuspid Regurgitation. N Engl J Med. 2025;392(2):115-26.

CHAPTER 28

Neuromodulation Interventions in the Management of Heart Failure

Manoj Bansal

ABSTRACT

Heart failure (HF) remains a growing global health concern. With its prevalence continuing to rise unabated, this condition places a considerable burden on healthcare systems globally. The dysregulation of the autonomic nervous system, as evident in heightened sympathetic activity, serves as an attractive pathophysiological target for newer therapies and HF. The degree of neurohormonal activation has been found to correlate to the severity of symptoms, decline in functional capacity, and mortality.[4] Nonpharmacological interventions targeting this neurohormonal activation act by restoring the balance between sympathetic nervous system and parasympathetic nervous system and may alter the renin–angiotensin–aldosterone system (RAAS) levels and potentially benefit various HF syndromes. Such neuromodulation will reduce the systemic inflammation and complement the existing pharmacological and device-based therapies.

Keywords: Neuromodulation, heart failure, renal denervation, vagal nerve stimulation, baroreceptor activation therapy.

INTRODUCTION

Heart failure (HF) remains a growing global health concern. With its prevalence continuing to rise unabated, this condition places a considerable burden on healthcare systems globally. This burden is more in societies with aging populations. Even after remarkable evolution in its management, mortality associated with HF is high and is 6–7% per year in patients with stable HF and approximately 25% per year in patients with acute HF.[1] In patients with heart failure and reduced ejection fraction (HFrEF) guideline-directed medical therapy (GDMT) advocates use of the "four pillars" of HF management. These are four classes of disease-modifying medications: Angiotensin receptor-neprilysin inhibitors (ARNIs) or ACE inhibitors/angiotensin II receptor blockers (ARBs), beta-blockers, mineralocorticoid receptor antagonists (MRAs), and sodium-glucose cotransporter-2 inhibitors (SGLT-2i). Despite robust evidence from randomized controlled trials and strong guideline recommendations, the real-world implementation of GDMT in patients with HFrEF remains suboptimal. Heart failure with preserved ejection fraction (HFpEF) is a clinical condition where apart from comorbidity management only few effective treatments like therapy with SGLT-2i are available to improve long-term outcomes, including quality of life, physical performance, and survival. So, identifying new therapeutic targets and exploring additional treatment strategies continues to be crucial for relieving symptoms and potentially enhancing prognosis in HF.

Among these, excessive activation of the sympathetic nervous system and the renin–angiotensin–aldosterone system (RAAS) leads to sodium and water retention, vasoconstriction, myocardial inflammation, as well as interstitial and myocyte remodeling.[2,3] The dysregulation of the autonomic nervous system, as evident in heightened sympathetic activity, serves as an attractive pathophysiological target for newer therapies and HF. The degree of neurohormonal activation has been found to correlate to the severity of symptoms, decline in functional capacity, and mortality.[4] Nonpharmacological interventions targeting this neurohormonal activation act by restoring the balance between sympathetic nervous system and parasympathetic nervous system and may alter the RAAS levels and potentially benefit various HF syndromes. Such neuromodulation will reduce the systemic inflammation and complement the existing pharmacological and device-based therapies. Neuromodulation interventions in the management of HF include renal sympathetic nerve denervation, direct and indirect vagal nerve stimulation, spinal cord stimulation, baroreflex activation therapy (BAT), carotid sinus stimulation, aortic arch stimulation, splanchnic nerve modulation, and cardiopulmonary nerve stimulation.

RENAL DENERVATION

Renal denervation (RDN) is an interventional approach that targets the sympathetic nervous system with the goal of modulating the renal sensory afferent and sympathetic efferent nerve fiber activity, leading to reduced plasma renin activity and aldosterone concentrations. There is lowering of central sympathetic activity, an important contributor to the pathogenesis of many cardiovascular and metabolic diseases.[5] RDN finds place as an adjunct therapy for select patients in European guidelines and has also been endorsed by other cardiovascular and hypertension societies. RDN has an emerging role for neuromodulation in chronic HF.

Renal Denervation in Heart Failure with Reduced Ejection Fraction

Renal denervation reduces the renal sympathetic activity. This will reduce renin release, sodium, water retention, and lead to an improvement in renal function and renal blood flow. This improvement will be augmented by the attenuation of RAAS activation. Preclinical data showed that the modulation of renal sympathetic nerve activity by RDN can decrease neprilysin activity, leading to increased levels of cardioprotective natriuretic peptide.[6,7] This may reduce end-systolic volume and restore left ventricular (LV) function.[7] When compared with sham controls, RDN in hypertensive patients was associated with reduced plasma renin activity and aldosterone levels, both of which are key targets in the management of HF patients.[8]

The first-in-human study investigating the utility of RDN in HF was Renal Artery Denervation in Chronic Heart Failure (REACH)-Pilot study, representing a proof-of-concept study.[9] This uncontrolled study included only seven patients. These patients had a mean left ventricular ejection fraction (LVEF) of 43%. Both symptoms and exercise capacity as measured by a 6-minute walk distance were evaluated. 6 months post-therapy both revealed with no adverse events. This study was followed by the SYMPLICITY-HF (RDN in patients with chronic HF and impaired renal function) study,[10] in which 39 patients with symptomatic HFrEF underwent RDN. N-terminal pro-B-type natriuretic peptide (NT-proBNP) levels, LVEF, and 6-minute walk distance were evaluated 12 months post-therapy. NT-proBNP levels reduced significantly, but the other two parameters did not improve. The IMPROVE-HF-I study randomly assigned 50 patients with a LVEF ≤ 35% and New York Heart Association (NYHA) class ≥ II, in a 1:1 ratio, to either RDN and optimal medical therapy (OMT) or OMT alone. The primary safety endpoint was the occurrence of a combined endpoint of cardiovascular death, rehospitalization for HF, and acute kidney injury at 6 months. The primary efficacy endpoint was the change in iodine-123 meta-iodobenzylguanidine (^{123}I-MIBG) heart-to-mediastinum ratio (HMR) at 6 months.[11] After 6 months, no significant changes in cardiac sympathetic nerve activity at 6 months as measured using ^{123}I-MIBG were found. The IMPROVE-HF-I study, however, used Vessix RDN System, which failed to prove its efficacy in patients with hypertension[12] and thus challenges the interpretation of these results.

The ongoing Prospective, Multicenter, Randomized, Blinded, Sham-controlled, Feasibility Study of Renal Denervation in Patients With Chronic Heart Failure (RE-ADAPT-HF, NCT04947670) trial will recruit up to 144 symptomatic HF patients with an LVEF < 45% despite GDMT to undergo ultrasound RDN or sham procedure. Change in 6-minute walk distance at 6-month follow-up between groups is the primary outcome of study.

Renal Denervation in Heart Failure with Preserved Ejection Fraction

Heart failure with preserved ejection fraction is a growing health care concern affecting millions of people worldwide. This debilitating chronic disease with high morbidity and mortality, unlike HFrEF, has limited evidence-based pharmacological treatments. Comorbidities like hypertension, diabetes, and central obesity pathologically activate the sympathetic nervous system. This sympathetic nervous system overactivation contributes to HFpEF pathology. Interest has grown in RDN as potential therapy for HFpEF because of paucity for effective pharmacotherapies and the role of sympathetic nervous system overactivation in HFpEF pathology.

The ongoing single-center, randomized, double-blind, sham-controlled Renal Denervation to Treat Heart Failure with Preserved Ejection Fraction (UNLOAD-HFpEF, NCT05030987) study is randomizing symptomatic HFpEF patients with hypertension and elevated cardiac filling pressures (LV end-diastolic pressure ≥ 16 mm Hg and PCWP ≥ 15 mm Hg at rest or ≥25 mm Hg during exercise) to receive either ultrasound RDN or a sham procedure. The primary outcome is PCWP at 20 W workload, which will be measured at 6 months between the groups as the primary outcome.

Along with the ongoing trials, future randomized trials are needed to further evaluate this therapy for HFpEF patients, particularly in the presence of hypertension.

VAGAL NERVE STIMULATION

Cervical Vagal Nerve Stimulation

Vagus nerve stimulation (VNS) aims to restore autonomic balance by upregulating vagal activity.[13] Refractory depression and epilepsy have been successfully treated by VNS.[14,15] Increased sympathetic activity is associated with worse outcomes in patients with HF. Autonomic modulation via VNS is associated with improvement in hemodynamics, reduction in plasma norepinephrine, restoration of baroreflex sensitivity, and improved survival in animal models. Increasing parasympathetic tone by cervical vagus nerve stimulation (cVNS) showed a beneficial effect on cardiac function and improved long-term survival in rats with HF.[16] VNS reduces proinflammatory cytokines and favorably affects systemic inflammation. VNS increases nitric oxide levels in cardiac myocytes, which in turn increases ventricular contractility. VNS significantly reduces SNS activity from left stellate ganglion leading to a reduction in frequency of atrial arrhythmias in HF patients.

CardioFit device (BioControl Medical) was implanted in eight patients with advanced HF for cVNS as an initial human study. This device stimulated the cervical vagus nerve approximately 3 cm below the bifurcation of the carotid artery via low current electrical impulses. After 6 months, cVNS improved NYHA class and 6-minute walk distance and reduced LV end-systolic volume.[17]

This study was extended by a phase II study, the European multicentre CardioFit study, in 32 patients with symptomatic NYHA class II to IV HF (LVEF < 35%).[18] Right closed loop cervical VNS (preferentially efferent stimulation to maximize B-type fiber recruitment while minimizing A-type fiber recruitment) was performed to assess tolerability and safety at 1 year. No major safety concerns were noted in the study. Autonomic modulation via VNS has been evaluated in three pivotal clinical trials: Autonomic Neural Regulation Therapy of Enhance Myocardial Function in Heart Failure (ANTHEM-HF), Neural Cardiac Therapy for Heart Failure, and Increase of Vagal Tone in Congestive Heart Failure (INOVATE-HF).[19-21]

The ANTHEM-HF was an open-label phase II trial in 60 patients with NYHA Class II to III HF (LVEF < 40%). In this trial, the patients were randomized in 1:1 fashion and they underwent either right or left cervical vagal nerve stimulation using a bipolar vagal electrode without preferential efferent stimulation at 10 Hz frequency.[20] In the study, pooled analysis revealed a slightly favorable profile with right VNS with an increase in LVEF, QoL, and NYHA symptoms.[20]

The Increase of Vagal Tone in Heart Failure (INOVATE-HF) trial was the largest randomized trial on cVNS in HF involving 707 HFrEF patients. These patients were randomized 3:2 to cVNS (CardioFit, BioControl Medical) plus GDMT or GDMT alone. The trial failed to meet its primary efficacy endpoint of mortality or HF hospitalization, which was not significantly different between groups after a mean follow-up of 16 months (30.3% vs. 25.8%, $p = 0.37$).[21]

The ANTHEM-HFrEF study was originally planned for up to 800 participants but was stopped early after enrolling 500 patients. The participants were randomized to cVNS plus GDMT or GDMT alone.[22] After the second interim analysis, the Company stopped enrolment, beginning the process to close the clinical study and winding down the HF program. The analysis of data did not reveal a sufficiently strong positive impact on functional or mortality endpoints.

To summarize, and based on the available evidence, the long-term effects of cVS on HF outcomes remain uncertain.

Aortic Vagal Nerve Stimulation

Aortic vagal nerve stimulation is also being evaluated as a potential therapeutic intervention for improving cardiac function and alleviating clinical symptoms in HF patients by modulating autonomic nervous system equilibrium. These studies base themselves on the fact that ventricular-arterial coupling and aortic compliance are controlled by aortic endothelial cells and neural parasympathetic transmission.[23,24] In addition, the vagal aortic afferent nerves, located in the upper part of the thoracic aorta, mediate parasympathetic neuronal transmission to the brain.[23-25] Device-based aortic vagal nerve stimulation regulate parasympathetic tone via chronic stimulation of vagal afferents in the descending aorta. The Endovascular NeuromoDulation Treatment for Heart Failure Patients (ENDO-HF, NCT02633644) feasibility study evaluates the safety and feasibility of percutaneous neuromodulation of aortic wall via Harmony aortic stimulation system in the treatment of up to 20 patients with HF over 5 years of follow-up. The patients were treated with Harmony System via implantation and activation of the Harmony endovascular neurostimulator.

However, according to the United States Clinical Trials Registry, the ENDO-HF trial has been terminated.[26]

SPINAL CORD STIMULATION

Spinal cord stimulation, done by electrode placement in the upper thoracic segments of the spinal cord, reduces cardiac sympathetic nerve activity. This is done by diminution of the signaling through the spinal cord and the dorsal root ganglia and the preganglionic sympathetic efferents.[27,28] IN animal models with HF, the sympatholytic effects of SCS have shown to reverse remodeling and exhibit antiarrhythmic effects.[29,30]

Two randomized clinical trials, SCS HEART and DEFEAT-HF, have done to evaluate this therapy in HF.[31,32] The Thoracic Spinal Cord Stimulation for Heart Failure as a Restorative Treatment (SCS HEART) study was a prospective, multicenter pilot trial in patients with NYHA class III HF, LVEF 20–35%, and implanted defibrillator device who were prescribed stable OMT. Dual thoracic SCS leads were used at the T1-T3 level. The device was programmed to provide SCS for 24 h/day (50 Hz at pulse width 200 μs). At 6 months, SCS improved symptoms (NYHA class −1, $p = 0.002$) and LVEF (+5%, $p < 0.001$). However, the Determining the Feasibility of Spinal Cord Neuromodulation for the Treatment of Chronic Heart Failure (DEFEAT-HF) study failed to document significant changes in clinical outcomes in patients with HF who received SCS.[32] The discordant results of these two studies are related to differences in both electrode positioning, and duration of stimulation could be the reason for discordant results of these two studies.

BAROREFLEX ACTIVATION THERAPY

Baroreflex activation therapy is done by application of electrical impulses and stimulation of baroreceptors located in the carotid sinus region. A technique initially developed and clinically used in resistant hypertension, BAT may cause decrease in blood pressure and heart rate. This effect is achieved by stimulation of afferent nerves through the dorsal medulla, resulting in sympathetic attenuation and increased vagal tone.[33,34]

Chronic BAT was initially in 11 patients with advanced HF (NYHA class III) on GDMT.[34] All patients underwent unilateral BAT and showed improvement in HF symptoms, 6-minute walk distance, and LVEF at 6 months.[35] These improvements persisted through 2 years of follow-up.[36] HOPE4HF was the randomized controlled trial conducted. In this randomized controlled trial, 146 symptomatic HFrEF patients were randomized to receive GDMT alone or GDMT plus BAT. At 6 months, there was a significant improvement in NYHA functional class, quality of life (QoL), and 6-minute walk distance.[37]

Baroreflex Activation Therapy for Heart Failure (BeAT-HF) study included 408 symptomatic HFrEF patients with LVEF ≤ 35% on GDMT who were ineligible for cardiac resynchronization therapy (CRT).[38] Patients were randomized 1:1 to receive either GDMT alone or GDMT plus unilateral BAT. This trial had an adaptive design and divided into two phases, i.e., the premarket ($n = 264$) and postmarket phase. After 6 months of follow-up, BAT was safe and significantly improved QoL.[38]

Heart failure reduced ejection fraction patients were randomized in the postmarket phase of the BeAT-HF study and evaluated the potential of this therapy to reduce mortality and hospitalizations in HFrEF patients.[38,39] The patients were randomized into two groups, treatment with BAT plus GDMT versus GDMT alone to evaluate the effect of BAT on reducing mortality and hospitalizations. 323 HFrEF patients underwent the study with a median follow-up of 3.7 years. Although the study did not meet its primary endpoint demonstrating a neutral effect on CV death and HF hospitalizations, but there was a long-term durability in symptomatic improvement (QoL, 6-minute walking distance, and NYHA class). This trial confirmed the safety of this approach to neuromodulation in HFrEF patients.[39]

The Effect of the MobiusHD system in Patients With Heart Failure (HF-FIM, NCT04590001) study is an ongoing, open-label, single-arm study with the primary objective of evaluating the safety and effectiveness of the endovascular, device-based baroreceptor enhancement system. Initially investigated in patients with resistant hypertension, this system causes passive activation of the baroreceptors in carotid body, thereby increasing carotid artery wall stretch while maintaining pulsatility.[40,41] This causes attenuation of sympathetic activity and increased parasympathetic activity.

In patients who remain symptomatic even after application of all guideline-recommended HF therapies, BAT could represent an adjunctive device-based approach. However, until further evidence on the safety and efficacy of BAT in HF patients becomes available, careful patient selection for BAT is recommended.

SPLANCHNIC NERVE MODULATION

The splanchnic venous compartment contains about 30% of the total blood volume and is heavily innervated by sympathetic nerves.[42] Splanchnic vein stimulation leads to vasoconstriction. Around 25% of the total blood volume from the splanchnic blood pool can be made available into the central venous system via this mechanism, thereby rapidly increasing cardiac preload and cardiac index.[42,43]

This first-in-human study of splanchnic nerve modulation included 11 patients with HFpEF and showed both the safety of the procedure over 12 months of follow-up and sustained improvement in NT-proBNP, health status, and 6-minute walk distance compared to this time window.[44] The REBALANCE-HF trial randomized 116 patients with HFpEF to greater right splanchnic nerve ablation with the Satera™ Ablation System or a sham procedure (Fudim M, unpublished data presented at the Heart Failure Society of America 2023 Annual Scientific Meeting).

These favorable outcomes in HFpEF patients are promising but larger, powered trials are needed to assess the safety and efficacy of splanchnic nerve modulation in HF management.

CONCLUSION AND FUTURE DIRECTION

Pharmacological and device therapies have significantly improved for the management of HF; however, there is still a big need for additional therapeutic strategies to further improve symptoms and prognosis in both HFrEF and HFpEF. Given the important role of autonomic nervous system in the pathophysiology of HF, there is considerable work going on therapeutic interventions that reverse autonomic imbalance. Still larger studies are required to finally evaluate their potential role; GDMT and wherever needed CRT should be done. The right patients for neuromodulation therapy and the device that will benefit that particular patient need to be identified very early.[45]

Ongoing and future studies will increase our understanding into the potential benefits of neuromodulation interventions in HF.

REFERENCES

1. McClellan M, Brown N, Califf RM, et al. Call to action: Urgent challenges in cardiovascular disease: A presidential advisory from the American Heart Association. Circulation. 2019;139:e44-e54.
2. Kemp CD, Conte JV. The pathophysiology of heart failure. Cardiovasc Pathol. 2012;21:365-71.
3. Mentz RJ, O'Connor CM. Pathophysiology and clinical evaluation of acute heart failure. Nat Rev Cardiol. 2016;13:28-35.
4. Pahuja M, Akhtar K, Krishan S, et al. Neuromodulation therapies in heart failure: A state-of-the-art review. JSCAI. 2023;2(6):1-12.
5. Lauder L, Fisher NDL, Bohm M, et. al. Renal denervation in hypertension and chronic heart failure. JACC Cardiovasc Interv. 2025;18(15):1833-47.
6. Böhm M, Ewen S, Wolf M. Renal denervation halts left ventricular remodeling and dysfunction in heart failure: New shores ahead. J Am Coll Cardiol. 2018;72:2622-4.
7. Sharp TE 3rd, Polhemus DJ, Li Z, et al. Renal denervation prevents heart failure progression via inhibition of the renin-angiotensin system. J Am Coll Cardiol. 2018;72:2609-21.
8. Mahfoud F, Townsend RR, Kandzari DE, et al. Changes in plasma renin activity after renal artery sympathetic denervation. J Am Coll Cardiol. 2021;77:2909-19.
9. Davies JE, Manisty CH, Petraco R, et al. First-in-man safety evaluation of renal denervation for chronic systolic heart failure: Primary outcome from REACH-Pilot study. Int J Cardiol. 2013;162:189-92.
10. Hopper I, Gronda E, Hoppe UC, et al. Sympathetic response and outcomes following renal denervation in patients with chronic heart failure: 12-month outcomes from the Symplicity HF feasibility study. J Card Fail. 2017;23:702-7.
11. Feyz L, Nannan Panday R, Henneman M, et al. Endovascular renal sympathetic denervation to improve heart failure with reduced ejection fraction: The IMPROVE-HF-I study. Neth Heart J. 2022;30:1490-59.
12. Weber MA, Kirtane AJ, Weir MR, et al. The REDUCE HTN: REINFORCE: Randomized, sham-controlled trial of bipolar radiofrequency renal denervation for the treatment of hypertension. JACC Cardiovasc Interv. 2020;13:461-70.
13. Guzik M, Urban S, Iwanek G, et al. Novel therapeutic devices in heart failure. J Clin Med. 2022;11(15):4303.
14. González HFJ, Yengo-Kahn A, Englot DJ. Vagus nerve stimulation for the treatment of epilepsy. Neurosurg Clin N Am. 2019;30(2):219-30.
15. Hilz MJ. Transcutaneous vagus nerve stimulation – a brief introduction and overview. Auton Neurosci. 2022;243:103038.
16. Li M, Zheng C, Sato T, et al. Vagal nerve stimulation markedly improves long-term survival after chronic heart failure in rats. Circulation. 2004;109(1):120-4.
17. Schwartz PJ, De Ferrari GM, Sanzo A, et al. Long term vagal stimulation in patients with advanced heart failure: First experience in man. Eur J Heart Fail. 2008;10:884-91.
18. De Ferrari GM, Crijns HJGM, Borggrefe M, et al. Chronic vagus nerve stimulation: a new and promising therapeutic approach for chronic heart failure. Eur Heart J. 2011;32(7):847-55.
19. Zannad F, De Ferrari GM, Tuinenburg AE, et al. Chronic vagal stimulation for the treatment of low ejection fraction heart failure: results of the NEural Cardiac TherApy foR Heart Failure (NECTAR-HF) randomized controlled trial. Eur Heart J. 2015;36(7):425-33.
20. Premchand RK, Sharma K, Mittal S, et al. Autonomic regulation therapy via left or right cervical vagus nerve stimulation in patients with chronic heart failure: results of the ANTHEM-HF trial. J Card Fail. 2014;20(11):808-16.
21. Gold MR, Van Veldhuisen DJ, Hauptman PJ, et al. Vagus nerve stimulation for the treatment of heart failure: the INOVATE-HF trial. J Am Coll Cardiol. 2016;68(2):149-58.
22. Konstam MA, Udelson JE, Butler J, et al.; ANTHEM-HFrEF Investigators and Coordinators. Impact of autonomic regulation therapy in patients with heart failure: ANTHEM-HFrEF pivotal study design. Circ Heart Fail. 2019;12:e005879.
23. Li L, Huang C, Ai J, et al. Structural re-modeling of vagal afferent innervation of aortic arch and nucleus ambiguous (NA) projections to cardiac ganglia in a transgenic mouse model of type 1 diabetes (OVE26). J Comp Neurol. 2010;518:2771-93.
24. Min S, Chang RB, Prescott SL, et al. Arterial baroreceptors sense blood pressure through decorated aortic claws. Cell Rep. 2019;29:2192-201.
25. Paolisso P, Dagan A, Gallinoro E, et al. Aortic thoracic neuromodulation in heart failure with preserved ejection fraction. ESC Heart Fail. 2023;10:699-704.
26. ClinicalTrials.gov. (2023). Endovascular NeuromoDulation Treatment fOr Heart Failure Patients (ENDO-HF). Identifier number NCT02633644. [online] Available from https://www.clinicaltrials.gov/study/NCT02633644?term=AREA%5BSponsorSearch%5D(COVERAGE%5BFullMatch%5DEXPANSION%5BNone%5D(%22Enopace%20Biomedical%22))&rank=1 [Last accessed November, 2025].
27. Ardell JL. Heart failure: Mechanisms of spinal cord neuromodulation for heart disease. Nat Rev Cardiol. 2016;13:127-8.
28. Dusi V, Angelini F, Zile MR, et al. Neuromodulation devices for heart failure. Eur Heart J Suppl. 2022;24:E12-E27.
29. Wang S, Zhou X, Huang B, et al. Spinal cord stimulation protects against ventricular arrhythmias by suppressing left stellate ganglion neural activity in an acute myocardial infarction canine model. Heart Rhythm. 2015;12:1628-35.
30. Lopshire JC, Zhou X, Dusa C, et al. Spinal cord stimulation improves ventricular function and reduces ventricular arrhythmias in a canine postinfarction heart failure model. Circulation. 2009;120:286-94.
31. Tse HF, Turner S, Sanders P, et al. Thoracic Spinal Cord Stimulation for Heart Failure as a Restorative Treatment (SCS HEART study): First-in-man experience. Heart Rhythm. 2015;12:588-95.
32. Zipes DP, Neuzil P, Theres H, et al.; DEFEAT-HF Trial Investigators. Determining the feasibility of spinal cord neuromodulation for the treatment of chronic systolic heart failure: The DEFEAT-HF study. JACC Heart Fail. 2016;4:129-36.
33. Schwartz PJ, La Rovere MT, De Ferrari GM, et al. Autonomic modulation for the management of patients with chronic heart failure. Circ Heart Fail. 2015;8:619-28.
34. Chatterjee NA, Singh JP. Novel interventional therapies to modulate the autonomic tone in heart failure. JACC Heart Fail. 2015;3:786-802.
35. Gronda E, Seravalle G, Brambilla G, et al. Chronic baroreflex activation effects on sympathetic nerve traffic, baroreflex function, and cardiac haemodynamics in heart failure: A proof-of-concept study. Eur J Heart Fail. 2014;16:977-83.
36. Gronda E, Seravalle G, Trevano FQ, et al. Long-term chronic baroreflex activation. J Hypertens. 2015;33:1704-8.
37. Abraham WT, Zile MR, Weaver FA, et al. Baroreflex activation therapy for the treatment of heart failure with a reduced ejection fraction. JACC Heart Fail. 2015;3:487-96.
38. Zile MR, Lindenfeld J, Weaver FA, et al. Baroreflex activation therapy in patients with heart failure with reduced ejection fraction. J Am Coll Cardiol. 2020;76:1-13.

39. CVRx. (2023). CVRx reports preliminary results of the BeAT-HF post-market randomized clinical trial. [online] Available from https://ir.cvrx.com/news-releases/news-release-details/cvrx-reports-preliminary-results-beat-hf-post-market-randomized [Last accessed November, 2025].
40. Salah HM, Fudim M, Burkhoff D. Device interventions for heart failure. JACC Heart Fail. 2023;11:1039-54.
41. Spiering W, Williams B, Van der Heyden J, et al.; CALM-FIM_EUR Investigators. Endovascular baroreflex amplification for resistant hypertension: A safety and proof-of principle clinical study. Lancet. 2017;390:2655-61.
42. Fudim M, Sobotka PA, Dunlap ME. Extracardiac abnormalities of preload reserve. Circ Heart Fail. 2021;14:e007308.
43. Fudim M, Boortz-Marx RL, Ganesh A, et al. Splanchnic nerve block for chronic heart failure. JACC Heart Fail. 2020;8:742-52.
44. Fudim M, Zirakashvili T, Shaburishvili N, et al. Transvenous right greater splanchnic nerve ablation in heart failure and preserved ejection fraction: First-in-human study. JACC Heart Fail. 2022;10:744-52.
45. Abdin A, Lauder L, Fudim M, et al. Neuromodulation interventions in the management of heart failure. Eur J Heart Fail. 2024;26(2): 502-10.

CHAPTER 29

Congestion and Diuretic Resistance in Worsening Heart Failure

HK Chopra

ABSTRACT

Worsening heart failure (WHF) marks a critical phase of heart failure progression, defined by recurrent congestion and frequent hospitalizations. Congestion, rather than ejection fraction, determines symptoms and outcomes across HF phenotypes. Diuretic resistance—driven by neurohormonal activation, tubular remodeling, gut edema, and renal hypoperfusion—remains a major challenge. Loop diuretics are central to therapy, yet up to one-third of patients show inadequate response, requiring sequential nephron blockade, SGLT-2 inhibitors, acetazolamide, or ultrafiltration. The 2023 HFA-ESC guidelines emphasize early sodium-based response assessment, dose titration, and GDMT optimization. Early postdischarge follow-up and volume-guided decongestion remain vital to reducing rehospitalization and mortality.

Keywords: Worsening heart failure, congestion, diuretic resistance, loop diuretics, SGLT-2 inhibitors, ultrafiltration, decongestion, heart failure management.

INTRODUCTION

Heart failure (HF) is a chronic and progressive clinical syndrome marked by periods of relative stability interspersed with episodes of clinical deterioration, often driven by escalating congestion. These episodes signal a critical inflection point in the trajectory of HF and are associated with an increased risk of morbidity, hospitalization, and mortality. This pattern reflects a transition from compensated chronic HF to a decompensated state, now increasingly recognized as "Worsening Heart Failure (WHF)" rather than the most restrictive term "Acute Heart Failure (AHF)".[1] Click or tap here to enter text.The term WHF is gaining acceptance as it more accurately captures the heterogeneous clinical spectrum of HF exacerbations across different care settings including urgent outpatient visits, emergency department presentations, and inpatient admissions.[2,3]

Emerging evidence, including data from implantable hemodynamic monitors, indicates that so-called "acute" HF events are often preceded by weeks of progressive subclinical congestion, challenging the conventional notion of AHF as an abrupt event. This paradigm shift supports the use of WHF as a more accurate descriptor, particularly in patients with chronic HF who experience incremental symptom burden and require escalation of therapy. Notably, WHF accounts for approximately 80–90% of HF-related hospitalizations, highlighting its dominant role in the clinical and economic burden of HF management.[2,3]

DE NOVO VERSUS WORSENING HF: CONTRASTING CLINICAL PROFILES

Patients presenting with de novo HF, those without a prior diagnosis or history of chronic HF typically exhibit a distinct clinical phenotype. These individuals are often younger with fewer comorbidities such as diabetes, chronic kidney disease, or atrial fibrillation, and demonstrate a lower burden of structural heart disease, particularly coronary artery disease. Due to these characteristics, de novo HF is frequently associated with more favorable short-term outcomes and a higher potential for partial or complete recovery of myocardial function. Nevertheless, the occurrence of hospitalization for HF, even in de novo presentations, is a critical prognostic marker. Data indicate that patients hospitalized for HF, regardless of chronicity, experience a threefold increase in mortality compared to those managed exclusively in the outpatient setting.[4,5]

Evolving perspectives in HF classification have shifted away from viewing AHF as an isolated syndrome. It is now more accurately conceptualized as a clinical event within the broader HF continuum. Presentations may range from subacute ambulatory congestion requiring outpatient intensification of therapy to abrupt hemodynamic collapse necessitating intensive care unit admission. In this context, the term *WHF* offers a more inclusive and pathophysiologically consistent descriptor. WHF encompasses the full clinical spectrum of HF decompensation, irrespective of care setting and reflects the underlying progression of disease often driven by unrecognized or subclinical congestion.[6] **Box 1** illustrates the clinical profile of de novo HF and its role in the HF continuum.

CONGESTION: THE UNIVERSAL MARKER ACROSS EJECTION FRACTION PHENOTYPES

Congestion, not ejection fraction, is the hallmark of WHF. Despite similar hemodynamic presentations in HF with reduced ejection fraction (HFrEF) and HF with preserved ejection fraction (HFpEF), distinct pathophysiologies exist. HFpEF patients often have *interstitial congestion* without overt fluid overload due to altered venous compliance and increased arterial stiffness. This results in elevated filling pressures even when volume appears normal.[7,8]

Hospitalization, whether for de novo HF or WHF, is a sentinel event. The ESC-HF Long-Term Registry documented *1-year mortality rates of 23.6%* in hospitalized patients versus just *6.4%* in those with stable HF.[9] These findings are echoed in recent real-world data from Asia and India, which underscore the substantial burden of mortality and readmissions following discharge.[10]

BOX 1: Clinical profile of de novo HF and its role within the HF continuum.

- *De novo HF patients:* Younger, fewer comorbidities, lower CAD burden, and potential recovery
- *Hospitalization impact:* Three times higher mortality than outpatient care
- *HF continuum:* Not isolated, spans from mild congestion to ICU collapse
- *WHF:* Inclusive term for all decompensations

Despite significant therapeutic advances including pharmacologic and device-based interventions, no *single intervention* reliably reduces mortality or readmission in WHF. Nonetheless, evidence indicates that up to 70% of early rehospitalizations may be preventable through timely initiation or re-optimization of guideline-directed medical therapy (GDMT), structured follow-up, and enhanced patient engagement strategies **(Flowchart 1)**.[11]

THE HEMODYNAMIC PROFILE: CLINICAL RELEVANCE OF CONGESTION

Congestion drives hospitalization, dyspnea, and outcomes in HF. Clinically, patients are stratified into four hemodynamic profiles based on congestion ("wet" vs. "dry") and perfusion ("warm" vs. "cold"), detailed in **Table 1**. The *"cold and wet"* profile, marked by hypoperfusion and fluid overload, has the worst prognosis. The "wet and warm" phenotype characterized by fluid overload with preserved perfusion is the most common, whereas the "cold and wet" profile, denoting both congestion and hypoperfusion, carries the worst prognosis.[11]

Signs of hypoperfusion such as cool extremities, oliguria, and mental confusion, and overt congestion (e.g., raised

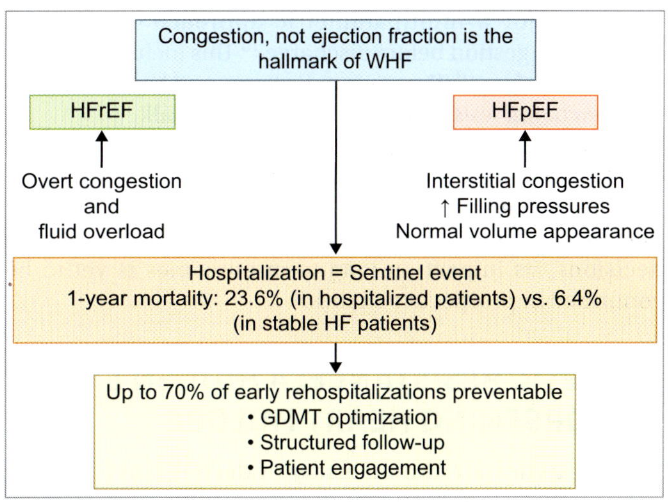

FLOWCHART 1: Pathophysiology and clinical impact of worsening heart failure (WHF).

TABLE 1: Clinical profiles of patients with acute heart failure (AHF).

Profile	Congestion status	Perfusion status	Clinical features	Prognosis
Warm and dry	Absent	Preserved	Stable chronic HF	Best
Warm and wet	Present	Preserved	Dyspnea, edema, and elevated JVP	Moderate
Cold and dry	Absent	Impaired	Hypotension, fatigue, and cool extremities	Poor
Cold and wet	Present	Impaired	Hypoperfusion + congestion and mental confusion	Worst

(JVP: jugular venous pressure)

JVP, rales, and edema) guide bedside assessment. Notably, hemodynamic congestion often precedes fluid overload, underscoring the importance of subclinical detection.[7,11]

Although acute pulmonary edema is dramatic, most WHF cases involve gradual fluid accumulation, often missed until symptoms escalate.[11,12] Implantable monitors now reveal a subacute worsening phase spanning days to weeks, challenging the notion of AHF as a "sudden" event.

THE CHALLENGE OF EUVOLEMIA: MORE THAN SYMPTOM RESOLUTION

Achieving true decongestion is central to WHF management, yet assessing euvolemia remains a clinical challenge. Many patients may appear clinically stable yet harbor significant *subclinical congestion*, complicating decisions on decongestive therapy.[13] Clinical signs and symptom relief such as weight loss or dyspnea improvement often *do not correlate* with actual hemodynamic status.[14,15]

Given these limitations, emerging tools are gaining traction. Lung ultrasound, a sensitive method for detecting pulmonary congestion, outperforms chest X-rays in identifying interstitial edema and pleural effusion.[16,17] It is now increasingly integrated into HF assessment pathways.

The Heart Failure Association (HFA) of the ESC now advocates for a multiparametric approach to evaluate residual congestion before discharge.[18] This includes:

- *Clinical signs:* JVP, peripheral edema, and hepatomegaly.
- *Functional tests:* For example, 6-minute walk
- *Imaging:* Chest X-ray, lung ultrasound, IVC diameter
- *Biomarkers:* Natriuretic peptides

While this comprehensive assessment may improve detection of unresolved congestion and aid therapeutic decisions, its impact on long-term outcomes is yet to be confirmed in prospective studies.

DIURETIC RESISTANCE: A HIDDEN ENEMY IN WORSENING HEART FAILURE

Loop diuretics are the mainstay of decongestive therapy in patients hospitalized with WHF, used in >90% of cases requiring their use for symptomatic relief and volume management.[2,3] However, their effectiveness is often attenuated by diuretic resistance—a frequent and under-recognized barrier to achieving euvolemia. Diuretic resistance is broadly defined as an inadequate natriuretic or diuretic response despite high-dose loop diuretic administration.

Clinically, resistance may be suspected when there is failure to relieve congestion or achieve weight reduction despite the administration of ≥80 mg/day of oral furosemide or its intravenous equivalent.[11,19] Alternatively, a poor diuretic response may be quantified as reduced weight loss per 40 mg of furosemide administered with lower values indicating impaired efficacy.[20] In the Spanish RICA (Registro de Insuficiencia Cardiaca) registry, diuretic resistance was observed in approximately 21% of hospitalized HF patients. These patients exhibited significantly worse baseline profiles, including lower blood pressure, estimated glomerular filtration rate (eGFR), serum sodium, and hemoglobin, along with elevated serum uric acid levels. Notably, diuretic resistance was associated with a 37% increase in 1-year mortality.[21]

The pathophysiology of diuretic resistance in WHF is multifactorial and complex **(Table 2)**. Mechanisms include impaired oral absorption due to gut edema, reduced drug delivery from hypoalbuminemia, adaptive nephron remodeling (e.g., distal tubular hypertrophy), neurohormonal activation leading to sodium and water retention, and diminished renal perfusion from elevated central venous pressures.[22]

Another critical clinical challenge is the development of worsening renal function (WRF) during diuretic therapy. Traditionally, even transient elevations in serum creatinine prompted clinicians to reduce or withhold diuretics out of concern for renal injury. However, this cautious approach may be counterproductive. Accumulating evidence suggests that transient WRF in the context of aggressive diuresis may reflect favorable hemodynamic shifts, namely, effective decongestion rather than intrinsic renal injury.[19,20]

In patients with HF, elevated central venous and intra-abdominal pressures are major contributors to renal congestion, exerting a greater influence on renal function than reduced cardiac output alone.[11,23] Importantly, robust diuresis within the first 24–48 hours of hospitalization has been associated with a lower incidence of persistent WRF,

TABLE 2: Mechanisms of diuretic resistance in WHF.

Contributing factors	Mechanism
Gut edema	↓ Oral diuretic absorption
Hypoalbuminemia	↓ Diuretic transport to nephron due to reduced protein binding
Distal tubular hypertrophy	↑ Sodium reabsorption (adaptive response)
Neurohormonal activation	Vasoconstriction, sodium/water retention
Chronic loop diuretic exposure	Nephron remodeling and loss of responsiveness
Reduced renal perfusion	↓ GFR and ↓ delivery of drug to active site

(GFR: glomerular filtration rate)

greater symptomatic improvement, and better long-term outcomes.[24,25]

Thus, transient increases in serum creatinine should not automatically prompt therapeutic de-escalation. Instead, clinicians should adopt a congestion-guided decongestion strategy, evaluating renal function in the context of volume status, urine output, hemodynamic markers, and overall clinical presentation rather than relying solely on serum-creatinine trajectories.

BREAKING THROUGH RESISTANCE: EVIDENCE-BASED INTERVENTIONS

Loop diuretics remain the cornerstone of decongestive therapy in patients with WHF, however, diuretic resistance poses a significant barrier to achieving therapeutic goals. While furosemide is widely used, torsemide offers superior bioavailability (80–90%) and a longer half-life.[26] Nevertheless, findings from the TRANSFORM-HF trial revealed no significant difference between torsemide and furosemide in terms of 12-month mortality or HF rehospitalizations.[27,28] Thus, choice of loop diuretic should be guided by clinical response rather than agent preference.

In cases where standard or even high-dose loop diuretics fail to achieve effective decongestion, an intensified diuretic strategy becomes necessary. The DOSE-AHF trial demonstrated that high-dose intravenous (IV) loop diuretics (2.5 times the patient's oral home dose) were associated with improved fluid and weight loss compared to standard dosing.[29] However, traditional markers such as weight change and net fluid loss often correlate poorly with true volume status. The European Society of Cardiology (ESC) now endorses spot urinary sodium and chloride measurements (1–2 hours postdiuretic dose) as more reliable markers of diuretic efficacy.

When escalating doses of loop diuretics fail to achieve adequate diuresis, *sequential nephron blockade* becomes the next logical step. This approach typically includes the addition of a thiazide-like diuretic (e.g., metolazone and hydrochlorothiazide) or a proximal tubule agent such as acetazolamide to enhance distal sodium delivery and overcome compensatory sodium reabsorption. These strategies have shown improved natriuresis and symptomatic relief in patients with diuretic resistance. Pharmacological adjunctive therapies with their mechanism of action and key trials supporting their role are summarized in **Table 3**.

Although *ultrafiltration (UF)* offers theoretical advantages such as controlled fluid removal and reduced neurohormonal activation but trials such as CARRESS-HF showed no benefit over diuretics and even reported worse renal function.[36] Similarly, the AVOID-HF[37] and PURE-HF[38] trials provided limited evidence to support widespread use. Accordingly, UF should be reserved for patients with true refractory congestion despite maximal pharmacotherapy.

THE EUROPEAN SOCIETY OF CARDIOLOGY 2023 HFA ALGORITHM: A PRAGMATIC STEPWISE STRATEGY

The 2023 HFA of the ESC outlines a systematic algorithm to guide clinicians through the escalating management of diuretic resistance. The key clinical actions are summarized in **Table 4**.

BEYOND DISCHARGE: LONG-TERM STRATEGY AND MONITORING

Following discharge after a WHF episode, patients remain at heightened risk for early rehospitalization and mortality. Structured follow-up, ideally within 7–14 days, is critical to reassess fluid status, renal function, and serum electrolytes, and to titrate GDMT.

Loop diuretic therapy should be progressively reduced to the lowest effective dose once euvolemia is achieved to minimize the risks of renal dysfunction, neurohormonal

TABLE 3: Pharmacological adjunctive therapies in diuretic resistance.

Strategy	Mechanism	Key trials/Evidence	Clinical notes
Sequential nephron blockade	Adds thiazide-type diuretics/MRAs to loop diuretics	ADVOR[30] ESC 2023[31]	Effective but risk of electrolyte disturbances; monitor closely
Acetazolamide	Proximal tubular sodium inhibition	ADVOR[30]	↑ Decongestion, ↓ hospital stay; low risk of renal harm
MRAs (e.g., spironolactone)	Potassium-sparing natriuresis	ATHENA[32]	No clear benefit in WHF setting
SGLT-2 inhibitors	Osmotic diuresis and improved sodium handling	DAPA-HF,[33] EMPEROR,[34] and SOLOIST-WHF[35]	Reduce HF hospitalization; emerging role in acute settings
Vasodilators (e.g., nitrates)	Reduce preload/afterload; improve renal perfusion	Limited RCTs	Useful in hypertensive and congested patients
Ultrafiltration (UF)	Mechanical removal of fluid and sodium	CARRESS-HF[36] and AVOID-HF[37]	Reserved for refractory cases; mixed results on outcomes

(ESC: European Society of Cardiology; MRAs: mineralocorticoid receptor antagonists; SGLT-2: sodium-glucose cotransporter-2 inhibitors)

TABLE 4: Practical guide to navigating the challenges of diuretic resistance in WHF.

Step	Strategy	Remarks
1. Prompt IV loop diuretic initiation	20–40 mg IV furosemide for naïve patients; 1–2 × home dose for chronic users	Start promptly; consider torsemide/bumetanide if oral bioavailability is a concern
2. Monitor early response	Spot urinary sodium/chloride at 1–2 hours post-dose	Sodium <50–70 mmol/L suggests inadequate response
3. Dose escalation	Increase IV loop dose or switch to continuous infusion	Reassess response within 6–12 hours; monitor electrolytes and renal function
4. Pharmacologic adjuncts	Metolazone (2.5–5 mg/day), acetazolamide (500 mg IV), consider MRA	Use cautiously with renal dysfunction; monitor closely for electrolyte imbalance
5. Ultrafiltration (selective use)	For refractory fluid overload unresponsive to pharmacologic therapy	Invasive; limited data supporting long-term benefit
6. Vasodilators (selective use)	Nitrates, hydralazine for hypertensive patients or high SVR	Useful to reduce preload/afterload; limited trial evidence
7. Transition to GDMT	Start or optimize β-blockers, ARNi, MRAs, and SGLT-2 inhibitors prior to discharge	Ensures long-term disease modification and reduces future hospitalizations

(SVR: systemic vascular resistance; GDMT: guideline-directed medical therapy)

TABLE 5: Diuretic titration strategy following WHF discharge.

Patient profile	Recommended postdischarge strategy
Diuretic-naïve before WHF	Initiate low-dose loop diuretic (e.g., furosemide 20–40 mg/day)
Chronic diuretic use prior to WHF	Resume or increase dose; taper based on volume status and renal function
Euvolemic and stable at discharge	Taper to minimum effective dose; closely monitor for recurrence of congestion
Residual congestion at discharge	Maintain higher dose with frequent outpatient follow-up

activation, and electrolyte derangements. This tapering process must be individualized: patients previously on chronic diuretics may require higher maintenance doses, whereas diuretic-naïve individuals may be initiated on low-dose therapy.

Meta-analytic evidence suggests that loop diuretics may reduce the composite endpoint of death or WHF in chronic HF.[22] However, high outpatient doses have also been associated with increased mortality, potentially reflecting both disease severity and adverse hemodynamic effects of over-diuresis.

Newer pharmacological agents offer the potential to reduce diuretic dependence. ARNi therapies promote reverse remodeling and natriuresis, enabling diuretic dose reduction.[39,40] Likewise, SGLT-2 inhibitors produce modest natriuresis and reduce interstitial congestion without activating the RAAS axis, making them valuable for long-term fluid management.

While natriuretic peptide-guided therapy has not shown consistent benefit, remote hemodynamic monitoring via pulmonary artery pressure sensors (e.g., CHAMPION trial) has demonstrated reductions in HF hospitalizations in selected patients.[41]

Crucially, hospitalization offers a unique window for the initiation and optimization of GDMT. Data suggest that initiating evidence-based therapies during admission significantly improves long-term adherence and clinical outcomes. β-blockers, ARNi, MRAs, and SGLT-2 inhibitors should be introduced or uptitrated before discharge in hemodynamically stable patients.

Additionally, evaluation and management of comorbidities and precipitating factors such as atrial fibrillation, uncontrolled hypertension, diabetes, infection, or myocardial ischemia are essential to preventing recurrent decompensation. Practical diuretic titration strategy post-AHF discharge is summarized in **Table 5**.

RED FLAGS NOT TO MISS IN WORSENING HEART FAILURE MANAGEMENT

Early identification of subtle clinical signs can prevent progression to refractory HF. Clinicians should maintain a high index of suspicion for the following indicators:

- Incomplete decongestion at discharge
- Rising creatinine misinterpreted as injury rather than hemodynamic shift
- Poor diuretic response despite escalation
- Delayed or missed initiation of GDMT
- Lack of structured postdischarge follow-up
- Symptom-based management without objective volume assessment

A vigilant, proactive, and patient-centric approach integrating clinical judgment, diagnostic tools, and evidence-based therapies is essential for improving outcomes in patients with WHF.

CONCLUSION: REFRAMING WORSENING HEART FAILURE MANAGEMENT FOR IMPROVED CLINICAL OUTCOMES

Worsening heart failure, predominantly precipitated by progressive congestion and often complicated by diuretic resistance, remains a major driver of hospitalizations, morbidity, and healthcare resource utilization. Despite the ubiquitous use of loop diuretics, a substantial proportion of patients are discharged with residual congestion, a potent predictor of early readmission and adverse outcomes. This highlights the urgent need for more accurate assessment tools and a tailored and pathophysiology-based therapeutic approach.

Emerging strategies including sequential nephron blockade, early incorporation of SGLT-2 inhibitors, and remote hemodynamic monitoring offer promising avenues to enhance decongestion efficacy, improve volume control, and prevent recurrent hospitalizations. Nonetheless, these tools must be integrated within a broader clinical framework that prioritizes early recognition of therapeutic non-responder, timely escalation of decongestive interventions, and prompt initiation or optimization of GDMT.

Effective WHF management necessitates a paradigm shift, from reactive, symptom-driven care to a proactive, evidence-guided strategy focused on aggressive yet safe volume removal. This approach must be coupled with vigilant postdischarge follow-up, structured titration of therapies, and comprehensive management of comorbid conditions.

Ultimately, the therapeutic goal in WHF must extend beyond transient decongestion to meaningful transformation of long-term outcomes through early intervention, precision-guided therapy, and sustained clinical vigilance.

"The objective is no longer just decongestion,
it is the transformation of prognosis."

REFERENCES

1. Kristjánsdóttir I, Thorvaldsen T, Lund LH. Congestion and Diuretic Resistance in Acute or Worsening Heart Failure. Card Fail Rev. 2020;6:e25.
2. Bayes-Genis A, Aimo A, Jhund P, et al. Biomarkers in heart failure clinical trials. A review from the Biomarkers Working Group of the Heart Failure Association of the European Society of Cardiology. Eur J Heart Fail. 2022;24(10):1767-77.
3. McDonagh TA, Metra M, Adamo M, et al.; ESC Scientific Document Group. 2021 ESC Guidelines for the diagnosis and treatment of acute and chronic heart failure. Eur Heart J. 2021;42(36):3599-726.
4. Triposkiadis F, Xanthopoulos A, Parissis J, et al. Pathogenesis of chronic heart failure: cardiovascular aging, risk factors, comorbidities, and disease modifiers. Heart Fail Rev. 2022;27(1):337-44.
5. Lee KS, Moser DK, Dracup K. The association between comorbidities and self-care of heart failure: a cross-sectional study. BMC Cardiovasc Disord. 2023;23(1):157.
6. Heidenreich PA, Bozkurt B, Aguilar D, et al.; ACC/AHA Joint Committee Members. 2022 AHA/ACC/HFSA Guideline for the Management of Heart Failure: A Report of the American College of Cardiology/American Heart Association Joint Committee on Clinical Practice Guidelines. Circulation. 2022;145(18):e895-e1032.
7. Verbrugge FH, Martens P, Dauw J, et al. Natriuretic Response to Acetazolamide in Patients With Acute Heart Failure and Volume Overload. J Am Coll Cardiol. 2023;81(20):2013-24.
8. Ponikowski P, Mentz RJ, Hernandez AF, et al. Efficacy of ferric carboxymaltose in heart failure with iron deficiency: an individual patient data meta-analysis. Eur Heart J. 2023;44(48):5077-91.
9. Chioncel O, Parissis J, Mebazaa A, et al. Epidemiology, pathophysiology and contemporary management of cardiogenic shock - a position statement from the Heart Failure Association of the European Society of Cardiology. Eur J Heart Fail. 2020;22(8):1315-41.
10. Harikrishnan S, Bahl A, Roy A, et al.; NHFR investigators. Clinical profile and 90-day outcomes of 10,851 heart failure patients across India: National Heart Failure Registry. ESC Heart Fail. 2022;9(6):3898-908.
11. Mullens W, Martens P, Testani JM, et al. Renal effects of guideline-directed medical therapies in heart failure: a consensus document from the Heart Failure Association of the European Society of Cardiology. Eur J Heart Fail. 2022;24(4):603-19.
12. Angermann CE, Assmus B, Anker SD, et al.; MEMS-HF Investigators. Pulmonary artery pressure-guided therapy in ambulatory patients with symptomatic heart failure: the CardioMEMS European Monitoring Study for Heart Failure (MEMS-HF). Eur J Heart Fail. 2020;22(10):1891-901.
13. Ambrosy AP, Pang PS, Khan S, et al.; EVEREST Trial Investigators. Clinical course and predictive value of congestion during hospitalization in patients admitted for worsening signs and symptoms of heart failure with reduced ejection fraction: findings from the EVEREST trial. Eur Heart J. 2013;34(11):835-43.
14. Lala A, McNulty SE, Mentz RJ, et al. Relief and Recurrence of Congestion During and After Hospitalization for Acute Heart Failure: Insights From Diuretic Optimization Strategy Evaluation in Acute Decompensated Heart Failure (DOSE-AHF) and Cardiorenal Rescue Study in Acute Decompensated Heart Failure (CARESS-HF). Circ Heart Fail. 2015;8(4):741-8.
15. Testani JM, Brisco MA, Kociol RD, et al. Substantial Discrepancy Between Fluid and Weight Loss During Acute Decompensated Heart Failure Treatment. Am J Med. 2015;128(7):776-83.e4.
16. Maw AM, Hassanin A, Ho PM, et al. Diagnostic Accuracy of Point-of-Care Lung Ultrasonography and Chest Radiography in Adults With Symptoms Suggestive of Acute Decompensated Heart Failure: A Systematic Review and Meta-analysis. JAMA Netw Open. 2019;2(3):e190703.
17. Platz E, Merz AA, Jhund PS, et al. Dynamic changes and prognostic value of pulmonary congestion by lung ultrasound in acute and chronic heart failure: a systematic review. Eur J Heart Fail. 2017;19(9):1154-63.
18. Mullens W, Damman K, Harjola VP, et al. The use of diuretics in heart failure with congestion—a position statement from the Heart Failure Association of the European Society of Cardiology. Eur J Heart Fail. 2019;21(2):137-55.

19. Damman K, Gori M, Claggett B, et al. Renal Effects and Associated Outcomes During Angiotensin-Neprilysin Inhibition in Heart Failure. JACC Heart Fail. 2018;6(6):489-98.
20. Greene SJ, Butler J, Fonarow GC. Contextualizing Risk Among Patients With Heart Failure. JAMA. 2021;326(22):2261-2.
21. Trullàs JC, Casado J, Morales-Rull JL, et al. Prevalence and outcome of diuretic resistance in heart failure. Intern Emerg Med. 2019;14(4):529-37.
22. Cox ZL, Hung R, Lenihan DJ, et al. Diuretic Strategies for Loop Diuretic Resistance in Acute Heart Failure: The 3T Trial. JACC Heart Fail. 2020;8(3):157-68.
23. Verbrugge FH, Dupont M, Steels P, et al. The kidney in congestive heart failure: 'are natriuresis, sodium, and diuretics really the good, the bad and the ugly?'. Eur J Heart Fail. 2014;16(2):133-42.
24. Goldsmith SR, Bart BA, Burnett J. Decongestive therapy and renal function in acute heart failure: time for a new approach? Circ Heart Fail. 2014;7(3):531-5.
25. Joles JA, Bongartz LG, Gaillard CA, et al. Renal venous congestion and renal function in congestive heart failure. J Am Coll Cardiol. 2009;54(17):1632; author reply 1632-3.
26. Martens P, Dauw J, Verbrugge FH, et al. Decongestion With Acetazolamide in Acute Decompensated Heart Failure Across the Spectrum of Left Ventricular Ejection Fraction: A Prespecified Analysis From the ADVOR Trial. Circulation. 2023;147(3):201-11.
27. Kapelios CJ, Greene SJ, Mentz RJ, et al.; TRANSFORM-HF Investigators. Torsemide Versus Furosemide After Discharge in Patients Hospitalized With Heart Failure Across the Spectrum of Ejection Fraction: Findings From TRANSFORM-HF. Circ Heart Fail. 2024;17(3):e011246.
28. Greene SJ, Velazquez EJ, Anstrom KJ, et al.; TRANSFORM-HF Investigators. Effect of Torsemide Versus Furosemide on Symptoms and Quality of Life Among Patients Hospitalized for Heart Failure: The TRANSFORM-HF Randomized Clinical Trial. Circulation. 2023;148(2):124-34.
29. Wilson BJ, Bates D. Diuretic Strategies in Acute Decompensated Heart Failure: A Narrative Review. Can J Hosp Pharm. 2024; 77(1):e3323.
30. Mullens W, Dauw J, Martens P, et al.; ADVOR Study Group. Acetazolamide in Acute Decompensated Heart Failure with Volume Overload. N Engl J Med. 2022;387(13):1185-95.
31. McDonagh TA, Metra M, Adamo M, et al.; ESC Scientific Document Group. 2023 Focused Update of the 2021 ESC Guidelines for the diagnosis and treatment of acute and chronic heart failure: Developed by the task force for the diagnosis and treatment of acute and chronic heart failure of the European Society of Cardiology (ESC) With the special contribution of the Heart Failure Association (HFA) of the ESC. Eur J Heart Fail. 2024;26(1): 5-17.
32. Butler J, Anstrom KJ, Felker GM, et al.; National Heart Lung and Blood Institute Heart Failure Clinical Research Network. Efficacy and Safety of Spironolactone in Acute Heart Failure: The ATHENA-HF Randomized Clinical Trial. JAMA Cardiol. 2017;2(9):950-8.
33. Martinez FA, Serenelli M, Nicolau JC, et al. Efficacy and Safety of Dapagliflozin in Heart Failure With Reduced Ejection Fraction According to Age: Insights From DAPA-HF. Circulation. 2020;141(2):100-11.
34. Anker SD, Butler J, Filippatos G, et al.; EMPEROR-Preserved Trial Investigators. Empagliflozin in Heart Failure with a Preserved Ejection Fraction. N Engl J Med. 2021;385(16):1451-61.
35. Bhatt DL, Szarek M, Steg PG, et al.; SOLOIST-WHF Trial Investigators. Sotagliflozin in Patients with Diabetes and Recent Worsening Heart Failure. N Engl J Med. 2021;384(2):117-28.
36. Bart BA, Goldsmith SR, Lee KL, et al. Cardiorenal rescue study in acute decompensated heart failure: rationale and design of CARRESS-HF, for the Heart Failure Clinical Research Network. J Card Fail. 2012;18(3):176-82.
37. Costanzo MR, Negoianu D, Jaski BE, et al. Aquapheresis Versus Intravenous Diuretics and Hospitalizations for Heart Failure. JACC Heart Fail. 2016;4(2):95-105.
38. ESC 365. (2018). Peripheral ultrafiltration: the PURE-HF trial and first insights from the prospective Gentle-UF registry. [online] Available from https://esc365.escardio.org/presentation/171699 [Last accessed Oct., 2025].
39. Murakami Y, Kiuchi S, Hisatake S, et al. Combination of SGLT2 Inhibitors and Loop Diuretics in the Treatment of Heart Failure. J Pers Med. 2025;15(3):99.
40. Vardeny O, Claggett B, Kachadourian J, et al. Reduced loop diuretic use in patients taking sacubitril/valsartan compared with enalapril: the PARADIGM-HF trial. Eur J Heart Fail. 2019;21(3): 337-41.
41. Givertz MM, Stevenson LW, Costanzo MR, et al.; CHAMPION Trial Investigators. Pulmonary Artery Pressure-Guided Management of Patients With Heart Failure and Reduced Ejection Fraction. J Am Coll Cardiol. 2017;70(15):1875-86.

CHAPTER

30

Role of Imaging in Heart Failure Risk Stratification

Haresh Mehta, Raghav R Nagpal, Kayan Siodia

ABSTRACT

Imaging is central to the diagnosis, phenotyping, and risk stratification of heart failure (HF). Modern modalities, such as echocardiography (including strain), cardiac magnetic resonance (CMR) with late gadolinium enhancement (LGE), T1/extracellular volume (ECV) mapping, nuclear techniques [single-photon emission computed tomography (SPECT)/positron emission tomography (PET)/metaiodobenzylguanidine (MIBG)], and cardiac CT, provide complementary prognostic information.

A stepwise multimodal approach [baseline transthoracic echocardiography (TTE) → targeted CMR/nuclear/CT when indicated] improves patient selection for device therapy, revascularization, and advanced HF referral for transplantation. Standardized imaging thresholds and integration with biomarkers can enhance prognostic discrimination.

Keywords: Heart failure, risk stratification, device therapy, nuclear imaging, electrophysiologic virtual heart.

INTRODUCTION

Imaging is indispensable for diagnosing and staging HF, determining its etiology, and guiding treatment decisions [including implantable cardioverter-defibrillator (ICD), cardiac resynchronization therapy (CRT), revascularization, and advanced therapies]. Major society guidelines recommend a multimodality approach: transthoracic echocardiography (TTE) as first line in all patients, with cardiac magnetic resonance (CMR), nuclear imaging, and CT used for problem-solving, tissue characterization, viability assessment, or when echo is nondiagnostic.

OVERVIEW OF MODALITIES: STRENGTHS AND LIMITATIONS

Transthoracic echocardiography (TTE) (2D/3D + Doppler + strain): First line; left ventricular ejection fraction (LVEF), left ventricular end-diastolic diameter (LVEDD), diastolic indices, right ventricular (RV) function, pulmonary pressures; strain [global longitudinal strain (GLS)] provides incremental prognostic information.

- *CMR:* Gold standard volumes/ejection fraction (EF); tissue characterization [late gadolinium enhancement (LGE) for focal fibrosis/scar; T1 mapping/extracellular volume (ECV) for diffuse interstitial disease]; excellent for myocarditis, infiltrative disease, and scar quantification.
- *Nuclear [single-photon emission computed tomography (SPECT)/positron emission tomography (PET), metaiodobenzylguanidine (MIBG), bone scintigraphy/amyloid tracers):* Perfusion/viability (SPECT/PET); sympathetic innervation (123I-MIBG/C11-HED) associated with arrhythmic risk; bone scintigraphy (99mTc-PYP) for transthyretin amyloidosis (ATTR) amyloid detection.
- *Cardiac CT:* Best for coronary anatomy when CMR contraindicated or computed tomography angiography (CTA) preferred; can provide additional structural information.

KEY PROGNOSTIC IMAGING MARKERS (TABLES 1 AND 2)

Left Ventricular Ejection Fraction

Central in classification [heat failure with reduced ejection fraction (HFrEF), heart failure with mid-range ejection fraction (HFmrEF), and heart failure with preserved ejection fraction (HFpEF)] and device decisions. Major guidelines use LVEF ≤ 35% as a pivotal threshold for consideration of ICD/CRT therapy in selected patients with symptomatic HFrEF, despite optimal medical therapy.[1]

TABLE 1: Imaging markers, thresholds, and representative prognostic impact.

Imaging marker	Typical threshold(s)	Representative prognostic impact
LVEF	≤35%	Guideline threshold for ICD/CRT consideration in selected symptomatic HFrEF patients
LV dilatation	LVEDD: Moderate dilatation (men: 64–68 mm; women: 58 to 61 mm), severe dilatation (men: ≥69 mm; women: ≥62 mm)	Independent predictor of SCD
LACI	>34.7%	Higher HF hospitalization and MACE
GLS (echo)	GLS less negative than –16% (i.e., –15%, –14%, etc.)	GLS provides incremental prognostic value vs. LVEF; each 1% worsening associated with increased risk (meta-analytic findings)
LGE (CMR)—ischemic scar	Infarct size ≥15% LV mass	Larger scar size associated with higher mortality and ventricular arrhythmia risk; infarct size ~15–20% reported in numerous cohorts
LGE (CMR)—nonischemic mid-wall	Presence vs. absence	Mid-wall LGE in DCM: HR ≈2.4 for death/SCD in cohort study (Gulati et al.)
ECV (CMR T1 mapping)	ECV >28–30% (laboratory-dependent)	Higher ECV independently associated with HF hospitalization/death (HR increases per % unit)
RV dysfunction (echo/CMR)	TAPSE <16 mm; RVEF <45%, RVGLS <19%	RV dysfunction predicts mortality and HF outcomes independently
Nuclear rest/stress perfusion—thallium/tetrofosmin	Global burden of inducible ischemia >15%	Higher risk of MACE
123I-MIBG (sympathetic)	Low heart-to-mediastinum ratio	Predicts arrhythmic events and SCD risk
C11-HED	High denervation to perfusion mismatch	Predicts arrhythmic events and SCD risk
99mTc-PYP bone scan	Perugini grade ≥2	Diagnostic for ATTR cardiac amyloid in appropriate context; impacts prognosis and therapy

(ATTR: transthyretin amyloidosis; CMR: cardiac magnetic resonance; CRT: cardiac resynchronization therapy; DCM: dilated cardiomyopathy; ECV: extracellular volume; GLS: global longitudinal strain; HED: hydroxyephedrine; HF: heart failure; HFrEF: heat failure with reduced ejection fraction; HR: hazard ratio; ICD: implantable cardioverter-defibrillator; LACI: left atrioventricular coupling index; LGE: late gadolinium enhancement; LV: left ventricular; LVEDD: left ventricular end-diastolic diameter; LVEF: left ventricular ejection fraction; MACE: major adverse cardiovascular event; MIBG: metaiodobenzylguanidine; PYP: pyrophosphate; RV: right ventricular; RVGLS: right ventricle global longitudinal strain; SCD: sudden cardiac death; TAPSE: tricuspid annular peak systolic excursion)

Left Ventricular Dilatation

- *The American Society of Echocardiography criteria:* LVEDD—moderate dilatation (men: 64–68 mm; women: 58–61 mm), severe dilatation (men: ≥69 mm; women: ≥62 mm).
- Left ventricular (LV) dilatation is an independent predictor of overall mortality and sudden cardiac death (SCD).[2]
- Moderate or severe LV dilation in patients with low EF is associated with significantly higher odds of SCD than in those with low EF with nondilated or mildly dilated LVs.[2]
- A study evaluating concordance in linear and volumetric definitions of LV dilatation in HFrEF patients found that the worst outcomes were in those with concordant LV dilatation by both criteria of left ventricular end-diastolic diameter index (LVEDDi) and left ventricular end-diastolic volume index (LVEDVi), than in those with discordant LV dilatation.[3]

Secondary Mitral Regurgitation

- The increasing severity of secondary mitral regurgitation (SMR), as assessed using quantitative methods, has been correlated with increasing rates of death and heart failure hospitalization (HFH), irrespective of the etiology of the underlying cardiomyopathy (ischemic or nonischemic).[4]
- Its volumetric quantification and etiology, carpentier IIIb versus atrial functional mitral regurgitation (AFMR), needs to be accurately defined using imaging.

Strain Including Global Longitudinal Strain and Other Myocardial Deformation Indices

- Can be assessed by speckle-tracking echocardiography (STE) or by feature tracking cardiac magnetic resonance imaging (FT-CMR)
- LV GLS ≤ –16% (some laboratories use ≤ –15% to –18% cutoffs) is commonly cited as abnormal. Several meta-analyses and studies have shown that GLS adds incremental prognostic value beyond LVEF in predicting mortality and HF hospitalization/major adverse cardiovascular event (MACE).[5,6]
- In stage D heart failure (HF), right ventricular free wall strain (RVFWS) is a useful predictor of RV failure in

TABLE 2A AND B: Comparison of imaging modalities.

Table 2A

Modality	Sequences	Characteristics studied	Evaluation of structure	Evaluation of function	Tissue characterization	Cost
Echocardiography	2D, 3D, Doppler, STE	LVEF, strain, volumetric/ pressure	++	++	+	Low
CMR	LGE, T2, T1/ECV	Strain, scar, diffuse fibrosis	+++	+++	+++	Moderate
SPECT	123I-MIBG, TC99m tetrofosmin, 201-thallium	Viability, perfusion, innervation	+	+	++	High
PET	F-18 FDG, C11-HED	Scar, viability, innervation	++	+	++	High

Table 2B

	Measurement	Scar identification/ quantification	Scar density estimation	Quantification of scar border zone	Identification of diffuse fibrosis	Evidence for use as a decision aid for risk stratification
Late gadolinium enhancement	Semiquantitative	+++	-	++	-	+++
T1 mapping	Quantitative	+	+	-	+	+
Extracellular volume mapping	Quantitative	++	+++	+	+++	+/-

(CMR: cardiac magnetic resonance; HED: hydroxyephedrine; PET: positron emission tomography; SPECT: single-photon emission computed tomography; STE: speckle-tracking echocardiography)

those undergoing left ventricular assist device (LVAD) implantation. A peak longitudinal RV strain cutoff of –9.6% predicts RV failure with 68% sensitivity and 76% specificity.[7]

- LV rotational indices may be used to distinguish between cardiomyopathies and aid in diagnosis. Their role in prognostication independent of other traditional parameters is unclear at present.[8]
- Peak LV twist and peak LV untwist rates are significantly impaired in patients with cardiac amyloidosis (CA) whereas peak LV twist rate is significantly increased in patients with hypertrophic cardiomyopathy (HCM). In HCM, peak LV untwist rate remains normal. Time to peak LV untwist rate is significantly prolonged in both CA and HCM.[8]
- Left atrial (LA) strain can further refine the grading of diastolic dysfunction, increase detection and has an incremental role over LA volume index in patients at risk or with established HF. Abnormal LA reservoir strain is associated with worse functional status and incident HFHs at 2 years (adjusted odds ratio 6.6; 95% CI 2.6–16.6).[9]

Atrioventricular Coupling Index

- Left atrioventricular coupling index (LACI), right atrioventricular coupling index (RACI) and their combined index—combined atrioventricular coupling index, are independent predictors of adverse events in dilated cardiomyopathy (DCM) and provide additional prognostic information beyond conventional risk factors.[10]
- The Youden index identified 34.7% as the ideal LACI threshold to identify patients at higher risk.[10]
- Pezel et al. demonstrated novel prognostic utility of stress CMR-derived LACI in acute HF. Elevated LACI values, reflected impaired left atrioventricular coupling and independently correlated with increased risk of acute HF hospitalization or cardiovascular mortality in patients with both preserved and impaired myocardial perfusion reserves.[11]
- In HCM, LACI exhibited superior predictive power for determining new-onset atrial fibrillation (AF) compared with conventional LA parameters.[12]

Late Gadolinium Enhancement on Cardiac Magnetic Resonance: Focal Replacement Fibrosis

- *Ischemic infarct scar:* Extent of LGE (percent LV mass) correlates with mortality and arrhythmic risk. Larger infarct size (e.g., mean infarct sizes reported often ~15–20% LV mass in cohorts) is associated with worse outcomes. The ability to detect replacement fibrosis with the presence, extent, and distribution of LGE makes CMR essential in diagnosing and risk-stratifying cardiomyopathies in patients with stage B and C HF.[13]

- *Nonischemic mid-wall fibrosis:* Presence of mid-wall LGE in DCM confers substantially increased risk—Gulati et al. (JAMA 2013) reported mid-wall fibrosis associated with higher all-cause mortality and SCD [hazard ratio (HR) for composite outcomes ~2.4].[14]
- A specific distribution of LGE, namely a ring-like pattern, is independently associated with ventricular arrhythmias in patients with DCM, and proved more robust than multifocal LGE. The lack of linear correlation between LGE and LVEF, might partly explain the discordant results of ICD trials in nonischemic cardiomyopathy.[15]

T1 Mapping/Extracellular Volume Fraction: Diffuse Interstitial Fibrosis

- ECV thresholds vary, but several studies use ECV > 28–30% as abnormal; higher ECV correlates with increased HF hospitalization and mortality. Recent large cohorts show ECV is independently associated with the composite of HF hospitalization and death with HRs reported per unit increase in ECV independent of LGE and LVEF.[16]
- In patients with CAD, native T1 and ECV showed strong predictive association in univariate analyses, and native T1 was the strongest independent predictor among all imaging markers and risk scores for survival, cojoint with LGE extent for MACE. It detects diffuse myocardial disease in non-infarcted myocardium, which is a major driver of poor outcome, and is separate from the regional myocardial damage visualized by LGE.[17]

Right Ventricular Function and Pulmonary Pressures

- RV assessment is an essential part of evaluation and stratification of HFrEF patients to identify patients at higher risk for adverse outcomes.[18]
- Tricuspid annular peak systolic excursion (TAPSE) <16 mm, RV fractional area change (FAC) <35%, RV free-wall strain less negative than ~-20% predict worse outcomes; pulmonary artery systolic pressure (PASP) > 50 mm Hg associated with increased mortality/rehospitalization. Echo and CMR RV parameters are independently prognostic.[18]
- 2D STE has been proposed for better evaluation of RV function by echocardiography. 2D right ventricle global longitudinal strain (RVGLS) and RVFWLS may more accurately reflect RV function, surpassing FAC and TAPSE for predicting overall and CV mortality in various studies. It has the advantage of being an automated user-independent parameter.[19]

Viability and Ischemia (Nuclear/Stress CMR/Stress Echo)

- Presence of substantial viable myocardium (variously defined; many studies use >10–15% dysfunctional but viable myocardium or mismatch segments) identifies patients more likely to improve function after revascularization; viability-guided revascularization may improve outcomes in selected ischemic cardiomyopathy patients.[20]
- Global burden of inducible myocardial ischemia >15% of the LV indicates high risk of cardiac events.[20]

Amyloid and Specific Disease Imaging

- *Bone scintigraphy (99mTc-PYP):* A Perugini grade ≥2 uptake in absence of monoclonal protein effectively diagnoses transthyretin (ATTR) cardiac amyloid noninvasively. Detection changes prognosis and management allowing for use of targeted therapies like tafamidis.[21]
- Delayed ^{18}F-florbetaben cardiac uptake was able to discriminate cardiac amyloidosis caused by light-chain deposition from amyloid transthyretin cardiac amyloidosis and other mimicking conditions.[21]

Cardiac Fibroblastic Activity Assessment

- Profibrotic activity-targeting PET has an incremental value in addition to morphological information obtained by CMR.
- Studies have shown that, after acute MI, the [^{68}Ga]Ga-FAPI04 PET signal exceeded the under-perfused area in the myocardium and was linked to cardiac functional deterioration during follow-up.[22]
- It can aid in assessing the severity of myocardial damage and predict the risk of future HF.
- In HF, fibroblast activation protein inhibitor (FAPi) uptake is higher in the early stages of disease and gradually decreases as fibrosis progresses.[22]

Cardiac Shear Wave Elastography

- Shear wave elastography (SWE) using high-frame rate (HFR) echocardiography is an emerging and noninvasive method for the assessment of myocardial properties.
- Shear waves (SWs) are mechanical waves that can be artificially generated by the radiation force of a focused ultrasound impulse. SW velocities at end diastole have been shown to correlate with the filling pressures of the LV.
- In heart transplant (HT) recipients, SWE has been shown to have a good correlation with CMR markers of diffuse fibrosis and with invasively determined LV filling pressures.[23]
- It has the potential to become a valuable noninvasive method for the assessment of diastolic myocardial properties in follow-up risk stratification of HT recipients.[23]
- Its role in other patient cohorts is under further research.

Epicardial Adipose Tissue

- HFpEF patients exhibit significantly higher epicardial adipose tissue (EAT) volumes and may be used for further

characterizing HFpEF phenotypes and individualizing risk assessment in selected populations. Higher EAT is associated with adverse prognosis.[24]
- In ongoing research, various studies are evaluating models combining clinical and CMR-derived features, especially EAT volume/EAT density, to improve support for HFpEF diagnosis and predict risk/outcomes.

Coronary Microvascular Dysfunction

- Coronary microvascular dysfunction (CMD) coexists in both HFrEF/HFpEF and ischemic/nonischemic cardiomyopathy subtypes. The severity of CMD correlates with the progression of HF and is strongly associated with increased risk of MACE and all-cause mortality.[25]
- Although, the underlying pathophysiology of CMD—structural versus functional may differ between HFpEF and HFrEF groups respectively, both may equally contribute to adverse outcomes.
- Rest/stress myocardial perfusion PET is used for noninvasive quantification of coronary flow reserve (CFR).
- In a study of HFrEF patients, rest/stress myocardial perfusion PET used to quantify CFR found that lower CFR (≤1.65) was associated with a twofold increased risk of MACE compared to those with higher CFR (>1.65).[25]

IMAGING-DRIVEN DECISIONS: WHEN AND HOW IMAGING CHANGES MANAGEMENT?

Implantable Cardioverter–Defibrillator/ Cardiac Resynchronization Therapy Selection

- *LVEF remains central:* LVEF ≤ 35% after ≥3 months of optimized therapy is the guideline-based starting point for primary-prevention ICD consideration in appropriate patients;[1] however, imaging markers such as extensive LGE or abnormal GLS may indicate elevated arrhythmic risk even when LVEF is >35% and can inform shared decision-making (some observational data support this).
- LV dyssynchrony in determining suitability for CRT. Presence of significant mechanical LV dyssynchrony on imaging is a predictor of higher CRT response. Strain dyssynchrony index (SDI) and regional strain pattern index (RSPI) can further help to predict CRT response. Strain imaging can also be used to identify LV electrical activation pattern and segments with latest activation to guide LV lead implantation during CRT.[26]

Revascularization in Ischemic Cardiomyopathy

Viability imaging (PET, SPECT, dobutamine stress echo, and stress CMR) can identify myocardium likely to recover; presence of substantial viability can favor revascularization, though randomized trial data have nuances—integrate viability findings with clinical context.[1]

Identification of Specific and Treatable Etiologies

CMR for myocarditis, sarcoidosis, and infiltrative disease (amyloid) changes prognosis and guides disease-specific therapy (e.g., immunosuppression for active myocarditis and tafamidis for ATTR amyloid). Bone scintigraphy/PET plays an essential role in amyloid diagnosis.

Need for Valve Interventions

- Identifying and quantifying coexistant stenotic/regurgitant valve pathologies which are contributing to HF. Assessing anatomic suitability for mitral/tricuspid transcatheter edge-to-edge repair (TEER) or transcatheter mitral/tricuspid valve replacement (TMVR/TTVR) in cases of severe mitral/tricuspid regurgitation, degenerative MS, etc. Similarly, identifying aortic valve pathologies and need for replacement.
- Early correction of severe SMA is essential in improving long-term outcomes in HFrEF in patients fulfilling the COAPT/RESHAPE2 criteria.
- In patients with left bundle branch block (LBBB), LV dysfunction, and severe secondary MR who are candidates for CRT, CRT should be done first and then to reassess MR severity to determine need for M-TEER. Post-CRT, MR severity may show improvement in some patients, and this may obviate the need for any valve intervention.

PRACTICAL IMAGING PATHWAY (ALGORITHM)

Step 1—all patients with suspected or confirmed HF: Baseline TTE with LVEF, Doppler diastolic indices, GLS (if available), RV assessment, LA volume, PASP estimate, chamber dimensions/volumes, LV dilatation, regurgitant valve pathologies, and dyssynchrony indices.

Step 2—if etiology unclear or further tissue characterization needed: CMR with LGE and T1/ECV mapping (contraindications permitting). CMR is preferred when echo images are suboptimal or to quantify fibrosis/scar.

Step 3—if ischemia suspected or viability informs decision: Stress imaging (stress echo, stress CMR, and PET/SPECT viability).

Step 4—if amyloid suspected (red flags: LV wall thickening with low voltages, HFpEF phenotype, carpal tunnel, and neuropathy): Bone scintigraphy (99mTc-PYP) ± serum/urine testing for monoclonal protein; CMR and PET as adjunct.

Step 5—if coronary anatomy required or CMR contraindicated: CTA.

Step 6—for further arrhythmic risk stratification is required: 123I-MIBG SPECT/11C-HED; electrophysiologic virtual heart model.

SERIAL IMAGING: MONITORING RESPONSE AND SAFETY

- *When to repeat echo:* Clinical deterioration, major therapy change, or pre-/postprocedure/device evaluation. GLS and 3D volumes are sensitive for early detection of change.
- *Repeat CMR:* For reassessment of myocarditis, amyloid progression, or pre-LVAD/transplant planning when clinically indicated.

WHAT ARE ELECTROPHYSIOLOGIC VIRTUAL HEART MODELS?

Electrophysiologic virtual heart models are patient-specific, three-dimensional digital reconstructions of the heart, generated using imaging data (most often from cardiac magnetic resonance—CMR—and multislice CT).[27] These models simulate real-time cardiac electrical activity and arrhythmia mechanisms by incorporating details such as:

- Myocardial geometry
- Tissue heterogeneity (fibrosis and scar)
- Structural remodeling
- Electrophysiologic properties at the cellular and organ level

Advanced imaging is essential for these models:

- *CMR* provides detailed assessment of myocardial scar and fibrosis via LGE and T1 mapping.
- *CT* helps to delineate cardiac geometry and wall thickness.
- *Fusion imaging* combines modalities for comprehensive structural and tissue characterization.

How these advances impact SCD prediction in HF: Enhanced individualized risk stratification?

- *Mechanistic simulation:* Virtual models can simulate how arrhythmic triggers propagate in a specific patient's heart, directly testing vulnerability to malignant ventricular arrhythmias that lead to SCD. This is unlike traditional risk factors (like LVEF alone), which cannot reveal arrhythmia mechanisms.
- *Substrate analysis:* By quantifying the amount, location, and pattern of myocardial fibrosis or scar, models can distinguish patients with high arrhythmogenic risk, even when EF is only mildly reduced.
- *Dynamic reassessment:* The approach allows for periodic updates using repeat imaging, capturing changes in arrhythmia susceptibility as disease progresses or remodels.

Demonstrated Superiority Over Traditional Methods

- Virtual heart models have outperformed conventional clinical metrics [such as LVEF thresholds or New York Heart Association (NYHA) class] in predicting arrhythmic events and SCD, both in ischemic and nonischemic cardiomyopathy cohorts **(Table 3)**.
- These models can identify high-risk patients who fall outside guideline-based ICD criteria, providing precision medicine opportunities to prevent both undertreatment and unnecessary device implantation.

Guiding Therapy

Beyond prediction, imaging-derived virtual heart models have been used prospectively to guide catheter ablation for ventricular arrhythmias by identifying targets, thereby reducing future SCD risk.[27]

LIMITATIONS, GAPS, AND FUTURE DIRECTIONS

- *Harmonization needed:* GLS and ECV thresholds vary with vendor/sequence; standardization efforts are ongoing.
- *Prognostic models:* Need prospective validation of combined imaging + biomarkers + clinical risk tools to inform individual therapy decisions (ICD/CRT selection beyond simple LVEF thresholds).
- *Artificial intelligence (AI) and automation:* Promising for reproducible strain and LGE quantification; requires validation across populations.

TABLE 3: Comparison of virtual heart modeling versus traditional risk metrics.

Feature	Traditional metrics (e.g., LVEF, NYHA)	Electrophysiologic virtual heart models
Arrhythmia mechanism	No	Yes (simulated in silico)
Scar/Fibrosis assessment	Limited (indirect)	Precise (location, pattern, and amount)
Patient-specific	Partially	Fully individualized
Dynamic reassessment	No	Yes (update with new imaging)
Direct arrhythmia testing	No	Yes (simulated triggers and substrate)
Predictive performance	Moderate	Improved (validated in studies)

(LVEF: left ventricular ejection fraction; NYHA: New York Heart Association)

CONCLUSION

- Recent advances in imaging have greatly improved prognostication of different HF phenotypes beyond the simplistic volumetric and flow and pressure characterization.
- Hybrid devices and image processing techniques have allowed fusion of nuclear images with high-resolution morphologic images of cardiac structure and function obtained from other imaging modalities.
- AI and machine learning (ML) have the potential to transform imaging interpretation, workflow optimization, and patient-specific risk calculation.
- Integrate imaging results with biomarkers and clinical context when selecting patients for ICD/CRT, revascularization, or advanced therapies.

REFERENCES

1. McDonagh TA, Metra M, Adamo M, et al. 2021 ESC Guidelines for the diagnosis and treatment of acute and chronic heart failure. Eur Heart J. 2021;42(36):3599-726.
2. Narayanan K, Reinier K, Teodorescu C, et al. Left ventricular diameter and risk stratification for sudden cardiac death. J Am Heart Assoc. 2014;3(5):e001193.
3. Kasa G, Teis A, Juncà G, et al. Clinical and prognostic implications of left ventricular dilatation in heart failure. Eur Heart J Cardiovasc Imaging. 2024;25(6):849-56.
4. Camaj A, Thourani VH, Gillam LD, et al. Heart Failure and Secondary Mitral Regurgitation: A Contemporary Review. J Soc Cardiovasc Angiogr Interv. 2023;2(6Part B):101195.
5. Marschall A, Calva FD, Sánchez IG, et al. Global Longitudinal Strain versus Left Ventricular Ejection Fraction for the Prediction of Short-term Clinical Progression in Asymptomatic Stable Heart Failure Patients. J Cardiovasc Echogr. 2025;35(1):32-6.
6. Wang TKM, Desai MY, Collier P, et al. Determining the thresholds for abnormal left ventricular strains in healthy subjects by echocardiography: a meta-analysis. Cardiovasc Diagn Ther. 2020;10(6):1858-73.
7. Vogel F, Sollie ZW, Kilic A, et al. Prediction of Right Heart Failure in LVAD Candidates: Current Approaches and Future Directions. J Cardiovasc Dev Dis. 2025;12(7):240.
8. Monda E, Palmiero G, Limongelli G. Left ventricular rotational mechanics in cardiac amyloidosis - reply. Int J Cardiol. 2021;345:152.
9. Samiei N, Abbasi F, Shojaeifard M, et al. The Role of Left Atrial Strain in Detecting Left Ventricular Diastolic Dysfunction: Comparison between the 2009 and 2016 Recommendations. J Tehran Heart Cent. 2021;16(2):58-67.
10. Pezel T, Garot P, Toupin S, et al. AI-Based Fully Automated Left Atrioventricular Coupling Index as a Prognostic Marker in Patients Undergoing Stress CMR. JACC Cardiovasc Imaging. 2023;16(10):1288-302.
11. Lange T, Backhaus SJ, Schulz A, et al. Cardiovascular magnetic resonance-derived left atrioventricular coupling index and major adverse cardiac events in patients following acute myocardial infarction. J Cardiovasc Magn Reson. 2023;25:24.
12. Meucci MC, Fortuni F, Galloo X, et al. Left atrioventricular coupling index in hypertrophic cardiomyopathy and risk of new-onset atrial fibrillation. Int J Cardiol. 2022;363:87-93
13. Lahoti N, Jabbour RJ, Ariff B, et al. Cardiac MRI in cardiomyopathies. Future Cardiol. 2022;18(1):51-65.
14. Mandawat A, Chattranukulchai P, Mandawat A, et al. Progression of Myocardial Fibrosis in Nonischemic DCM and Association With Mortality and Heart Failure Outcomes. JACC Cardiovasc Imaging. 2021;14(7):1338-50.
15. Chen W, Qian W, Zhang X, et al. Ring-like late gadolinium enhancement for predicting ventricular tachyarrhythmias in non-ischaemic dilated cardiomyopathy. Eur Heart J Cardiovasc Imaging. 2021;22(10):1130-8.
16. Berdibekov BS, Alexandrova SA, Bulaeva NI, et al. Prognostic value of myocardial tissue characterization by cardiac magnetic resonance imaging using T1 mapping in nonischemic dilated cardiomyopathy: a systematic review and meta-analysis. Clin Radiol. 2025;80:106726.
17. Paiva L, Ferreira MJ, Afonso S, et al. Cardiac T1 mapping in non-ST-segment elevation myocardial infarction: temporal changes in myocardial fibrosis. Front Cardiovasc Med. 2025;12:1563368.
18. Heidenreich PA, Bozkurt B, Aguilar D, et al. 2022 AHA/ACC/HFSA guideline for the management of heart failure. J Am Coll Cardiol. 2022;79(17):e263-e421.
19. Houard L, Benaets MB, de Meester de Ravenstein C, et al. Additional Prognostic Value of 2D Right Ventricular Speckle-Tracking Strain for Prediction of Survival in Heart Failure and Reduced Ejection Fraction: A Comparative Study With Cardiac Magnetic Resonance. JACC Cardiovasc Imaging. 2019;12(12):2373-85.
20. Gimelli A, Lakshmanan S, Della Tommasina V, et al. What Is New in Risk Assessment in Nuclear Cardiology? Heart Fail Clin. 2025;21(3):407-15.
21. Wang SY, Huang YH, Chen YC, et al. 2025 Update Consensus of 99mTc-Pyrophosphate Scintigraphy in the Transthyretin Cardiac Amyloidosis from the Taiwan Society of Cardiology and the Society of Nuclear Medicine of the Republic of China. Acta Cardiol Sin. 2025;41(1):55-71.
22. Diekmann J, Koenig T, Thackeray JT, et al. Cardiac Fibroblast Activation in Patients Early After Acute Myocardial Infarction: Integration with MR Tissue Characterization and Subsequent Functional Outcome. J Nucl Med. 2022;63(9):1415-23.
23. Petrescu A, Bézy S, Cvijic M, et al. Shear Wave Elastography Using High-Frame-Rate Imaging in the Follow-Up of Heart Transplantation Recipients. JACC Cardiovasc Imaging. 2020;13(11):2304-13.
24. Liu J, Yu Q, Li Z, et al. Epicardial adipose tissue density is a better predictor of cardiometabolic risk in HFpEF patients: a prospective cohort study. Cardiovasc Diabetol. 2023;22(1):45.
25. Joh HS, Shin D, Lee JM, et al. Prognostic Impact of Coronary Flow Reserve in Patients With Reduced Left Ventricular Ejection Fraction. J Am Heart Assoc. 2022;11(15):e025841.
26. Galli E, Galand V, Le Rolle V, et al. The saga of dyssynchrony imaging: Are we getting to the point. Front Cardiovasc Med. 2023;10:1111538.
27. Gillette K, Gsell MAF, Strocchi M, et al. A personalized real-time virtual model of whole heart electrophysiology. Front Physiol. 2022;13:907190.

CHAPTER 31

Can Left Ventricular Wall Strain Predict Heart Failure?

Jagdish Chander Mohan, Madhu Shukla

ABSTRACT

Heart failure (HF) is a clinical syndrome of effort intolerance based in cardiovascular system and characterized by variable neurohumoral activation. Underlying the clinical picture, there are morpho-dysfunctional and electrically unstable cardiomyocytes with increased extracellular matrix and probable capillary rarefaction. Diseased myocardium exhibits many pathophysiological phenomena that include inflammation, fibrosis, hypertrophy, apoptosis, necrosis, pyroptosis, and oncosis. Mechanical work or force generation is progressively impaired secondary to these changes. Impaired force generation can be assessed by studying the imaging-based mechanical properties such as left ventricular wall strain, ejection fraction, and mechanical work. Although strain is multidimensional, it can be resolved in any single dimension to reduce complexity and enhance clinical utility. Strain can also be coupled with systemic pressure to provide global mechanical work and work efficiency. Reduced strain, even with other parameters of function being in normal range, is a sensitive marker of left ventricular dysfunction. Earliest evidence of cardiac dysfunction is reduced global longitudinal strain. It has been proposed that reduced longitudinal strain in an apparently asymptomatic subject should be labeled stage B HF. Traditional cardiovascular risk factors such as obesity, smoking, diabetes, hypertension, and dyslipidemia are known to accelerate ventricular and vascular aging and cause subclinical dysfunction (reduced longitudinal strain), which is a precursor to HF. This chapter deals with the role of left ventricular wall strain evaluation in predicting incident clinical HF and hospitalization for HF.

Keywords: Heart failure, myocardial strain, global longitudinal strain, ejection fraction.

INTRODUCTION

The left ventricle is a bidirectional almost synchronous force generator with viscoelastic behavior governed by three-dimensional syncytium.[1] The force generated is used for suction and filling in diastole and for propulsion of blood during systole. The force of the left ventricle for a given load is the surrogate for function. Impaired function when manifest clinically is heart failure (HF). The generated force deforms the myocardial multidimensional geometry during the entire cardiac cycle **(Figs. 1 to 3)**. This deformation is called strain, which can be resolved in three dimensions as a simple force indicator.[2] Strain in simple words expresses stretching, compression, pull, or pressure on an object. Conventionally, imaging provides information about longitudinal, radial, and tangential strain **(Fig. 2)** and rotational or torsional strain can be derived from tangential strain of the opposite poles of the ventricle.[3] Strain assessment replicates myocardial

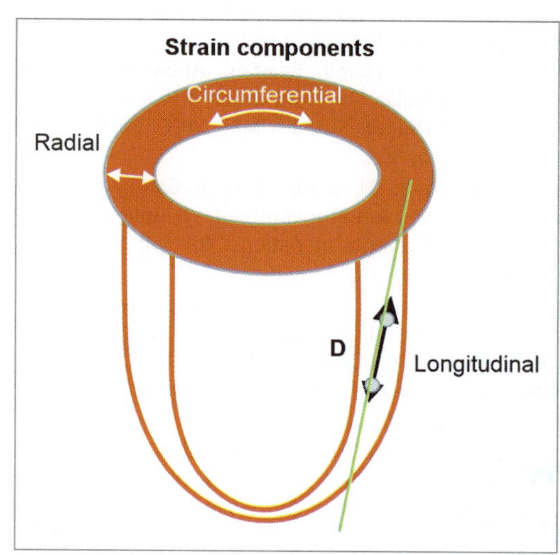

FIG. 1: Vectors of myocardial strain.

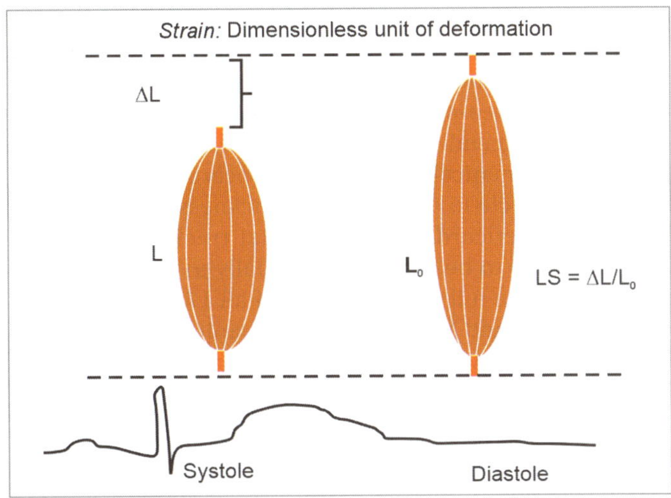

FIG. 2: Longitudinal strain (LS). L_0 is the original end-diastolic length and ΔL is the shortening fraction.

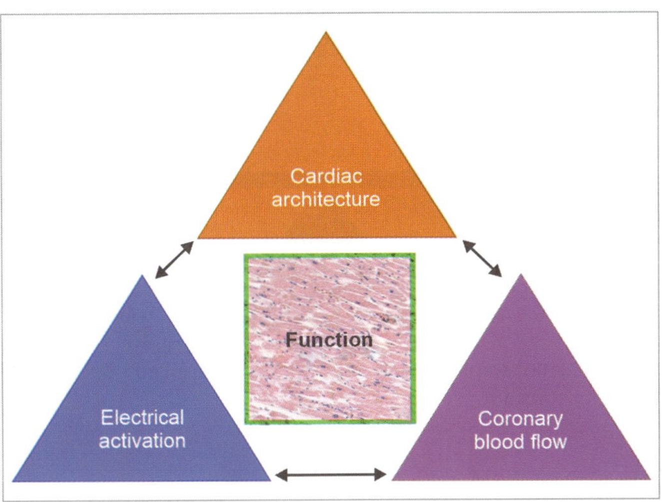

FIG. 4: The intrinsic determinants of myocardial function.

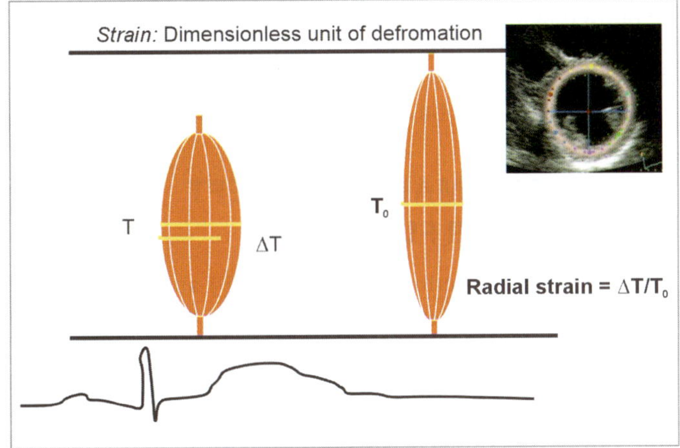

FIG. 3: Radial strain. T_0 denotes original or end-diastolic thickness and ΔT suggests shortening fraction.

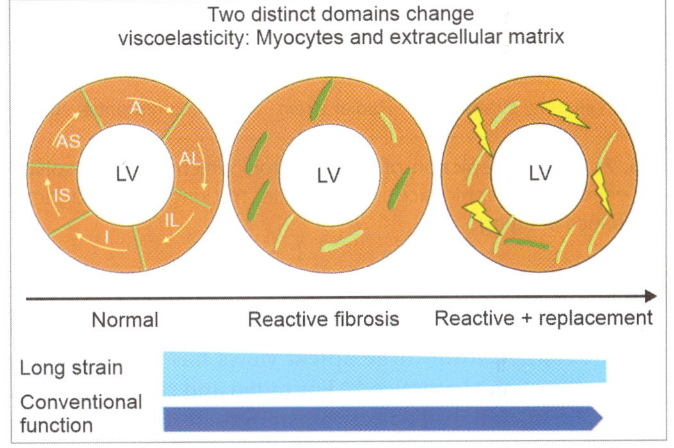

FIG. 5: Myocardial dysfunction is secondary to changes in cardiac myocytes and extracellular matrix. Replacement fibrosis also plays a role.

fiber geometry, which gives an apparent impression of discrete inner longitudinal, radial, and outer tangential muscle bundles.[2] The myocardial force is not an indicator of intrinsic contractile function but a product of contractility, load, and frequency of stimulus. Hence, strain is situational, dynamic, and interdependent. The complex geometry, activation sequence, fiber direction, conduction pattern, vasculature, and shape of the cardiac chambers and their interrelationship with one another make assessment of subclinical dysfunction an arduous task **(Figs. 4 and 5)**.

BIOPHYSICS OF STRAIN

Any time a force is applied to a viscoelastic material, it changes its geometry (gets deformed). Dimensionless fractional change in length, area, or volume of a solid object on applying force compared to original length, area, or volume expresses strain. An elastic material like myocardium undergoes temporary deformation and gets back to normal size or shape as the deforming force is removed. This follows Hooke's law,[4] which states that greater is the force applied, greater is the strain linked by elasticity constant **(Fig. 6)**. This constant of elasticity changes with myocytic hypertrophy, fibrosis, expansion of extracellular matrix, or abnormal protein or lipid or glycogen accumulation.

STRAIN VECTORS

Longitudinal strain defines the function of subendocardial fibers, while radial and circumferential strains represent functioning of the middle layer and subepicardial fibers **(Fig. 7)**. In diseased states, subendocardial fibers get involved

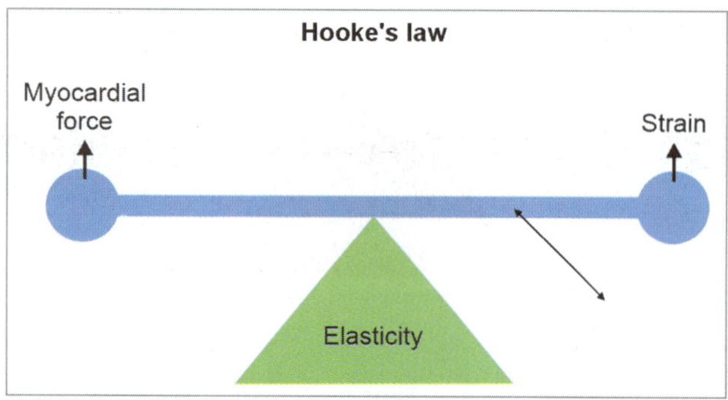

FIG 6: Relationship between strain and force applied governed by elasticity constant.

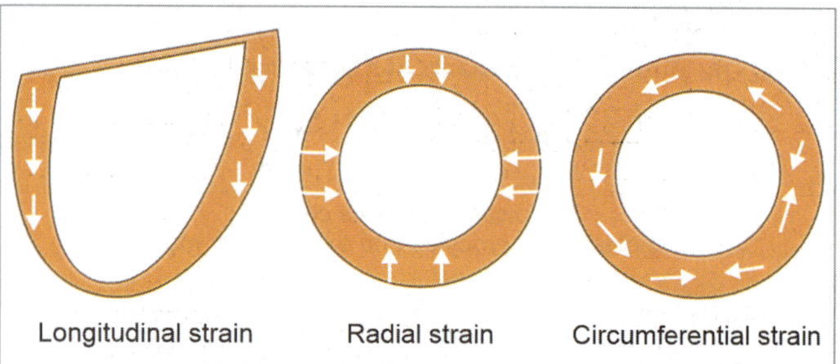

FIG. 7: Graphic depiction of strain vectors which can be resolved by echocardiographic acoustic speckle tracking and magnetic resonance imaging.

early, and hence, left ventricular global longitudinal strain (GLS) obtained from three apical views has found prime-time use in clinical practice.[4-6] For radial and circumferential strains, basal, mid, and apical parasternal short-axis views are needed, which are usually not simultaneously and not easy to obtain with adequate tracking quality in all patients. Also, radial and circumferential strains parallel the trajectory of ejection fraction and do not always predict early dysfunction. Hence, most studies have deployed global peak longitudinal strain as the default deformation index. This is, however, not to belittle the significance of circumferential strain, which has incremental prognostic value.[7] It is possible to obtain all vectors of strain from a single 3D echocardiographic examination, but the latter lacks adequate reproducibility and validity and suffers from limited availability and vendor specificity.

ASSESSMENT OF LEFT VENTRICULAR GLOBAL LONGITUDINAL STRAIN

Left ventricular global longitudinal strain (LV GLS) is the only validated parameter used in routine clinical practice. Although cardiac magnetic resonance imaging provides its accurate assessment, echocardiography is the most often deployed technique. It is derived from three apical views recorded either sequentially or simultaneously by triplane imaging. Semiautomatic or fully automatic algorithm can be used on three-consecutive cardiac cycles by marking three points on end-diastolic and end-systolic frames.[8] The software automatically tracks the myocardium throughout the cardiac cycle to cover the full thickness of the wall but precluding pericardium. Myocardial tracking is verified and may have to be corrected manually to ensure optimal inclusion of the full wall thickness of all 17 segments. Peak strain is obtained by all these three apical views at end-systole defined by aortic valve closure and plotted as bull's eye map **(Figs. 8 and 9)**. Currently, only global mean of peak strain is used in prediction models although one can also assess end-systolic and postsystolic strains as well. Higher is the peak GLS (more negative), better is the heart function. Standard deviation of the peak strain dispersion can also be obtained and has prognostic value **(Fig. 10)**. 3D multidimensional strain from a single beat is feasible but has found limited clinical utility.[9] Peak longitudinal strain can be plotted against cuff blood pressure to obtain myocardial mechanical work **(Fig. 11)** from strain-pressure loops.[10] Regional strain is not recommended for clinical use although pattern reading may be helpful in some cases.

STRAIN AS A MARKER OF LEFT VENTRICULAR FUNCTION

Left ventricular ejection fraction (LVEF) as a predictor of incident HF is an insensitive parameter as the latter can occur at any level of ejection fraction. Ejection fraction is an endocardial measure, while strain is a myocardial phenomenon. In addition, ejection fraction has a larger bias and variation in measurements. Longitudinal strain runs ahead of ejection fraction as a sensitive marker of subtle left ventricular dysfunction.[11] It is robust, objective, and more reproducible. Subclinical myocardial dysfunction that is characterized by impaired LV GLS is often present in patients with asymptomatic cardiovascular disease. Many risk factors such as obesity, diabetes, hypertension, metabolic syndrome, alcoholism, and chronic smoking are all associated with variably reduced global longitudinal function.[12] A large patient-level meta-analysis has proposed a GLS >–16% to be the absolute threshold indicating myocardial dysfunction regardless of vendor or clinical covariates.[13] The addition of GLS to the LV systolic function assessment refines disease classification and improves both prognosis and management. Longitudinal strain gets affected much earlier in diseased states compared to circumferential and radial strains, which largely determine ejection fraction. Compensatory increased radial strain despite impaired longitudinal strain in early disease states maintains normal ejection fraction. Unlike variable ejection fraction in HF, longitudinal strain has a more or less unidirectional

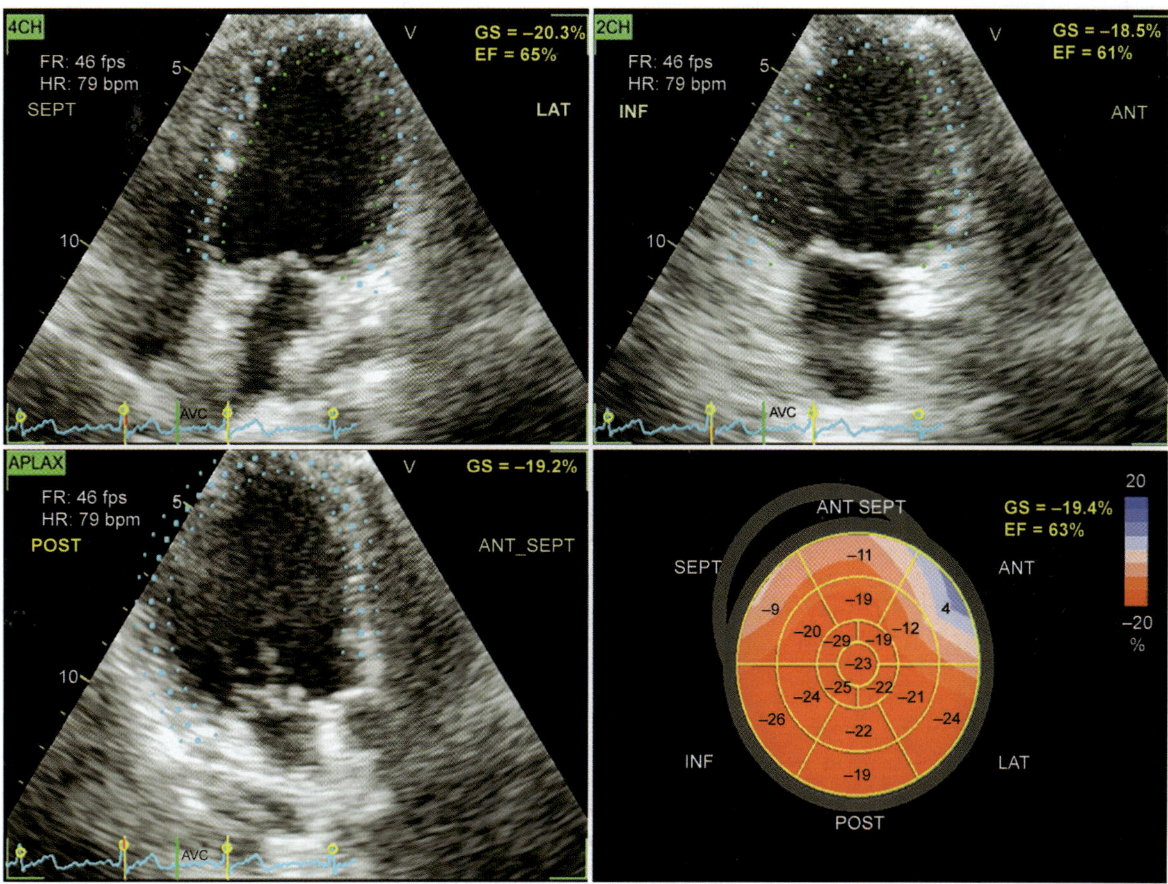

FIG. 8: Left ventricular peak systolic longitudinal strain plotted as Bull's eye map in 17 segments.

relationship in a vast majority of HF **(Figs. 12 and 13)**. It is subnormal in all patients with reduced and mildly reduced ejection fraction and in about two-thirds of patients with HF with preserved ejection fraction. Although more emphasis has been placed on systolic strain, diastolic strain also has a lot of predictive and prognostic significance. Hence, longitudinal strain is a measure of function index rather than systolic index. Strain defines morphofunctional phenotypes of HF better than ejection fraction.

LONGITUDINAL STRAIN AND CONVENTIONAL RISK FACTORS

Ageing impairs GLS, although ejection fraction increases with advancing age.[14] This has implications for higher prevalence of HFpEF in the elderly. Hypertension per say has small effect on GLS, but impairment is more in the presence of increased left ventricular mass.[15] Overweight and obesity both have been implicated for impaired GLS.[16] In a study from India, long-standing diabetes was characterized by low GLS (> –15%) in 70% of the cases.[17] Other studies have not reported such a high frequency of impaired GLS. Subclinical left ventricular systolic dysfunction is prevalent in asymptomatic elderly patients with type 2 diabetes mellitus, and impaired GLS is independent and incremental (×2) in the prediction of incident HF.[18] This association persists even after multivariable adjustment for age, sex, heart rate, systolic blood pressure, LVEF, left ventricular mass index, left ventricular dimension, deceleration time, left atrium dimension, *E*/*e*′, and pro B-type natriuretic peptide. In a recent study, every component of metabolic syndrome was shown to negatively influence myocardial strain and mechano-energetic efficiency.[19] Clearly, left ventricular strain is an early and more sensitive index of impaired systolic function.[20]

STRAIN AS A PREDICTOR OF ADVERSE REMODELING

Global longitudinal strain has proven to be an early and powerful predictor of adverse remodeling following myocardial infarction **(Fig. 14)**. Adverse remodeling is defined as an increase in left ventricular end-diastolic volume with or without fall in ejection fraction. Adverse remodeling

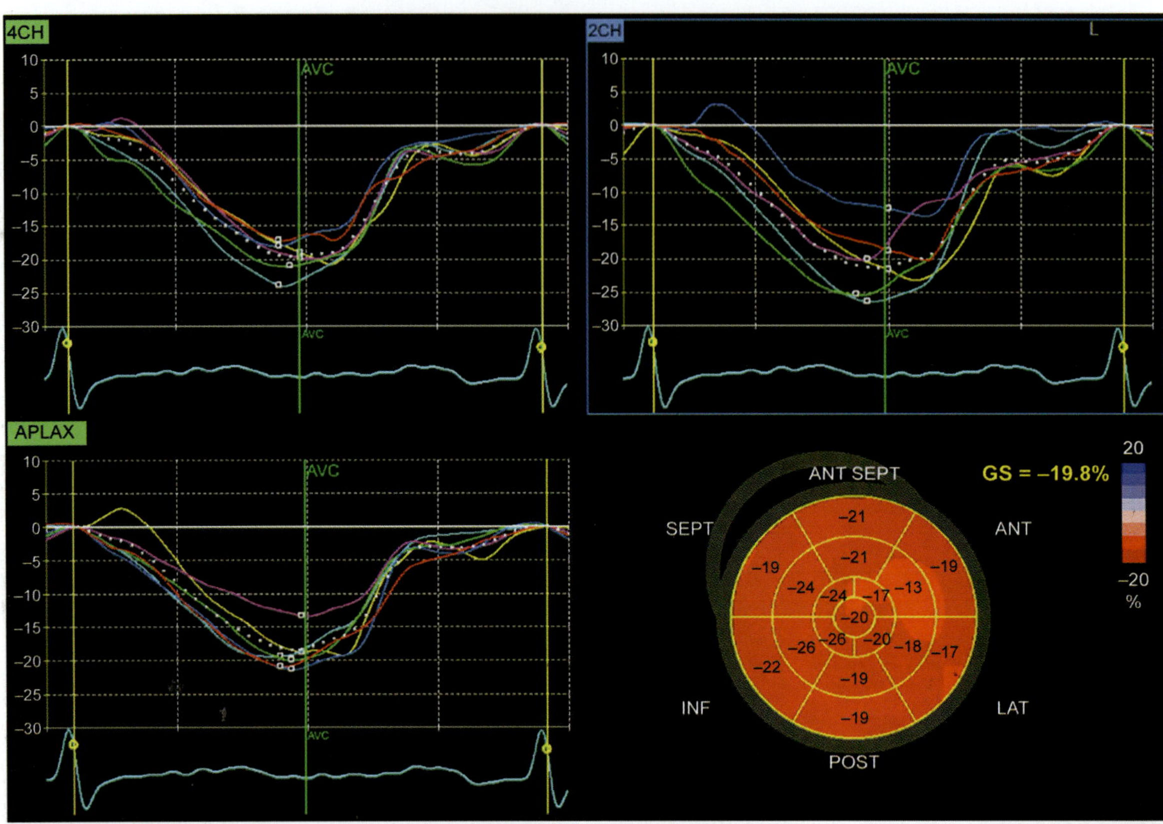

FIG. 9: Individual longitudinal segmental strain (GLS) curves with Bull's eye map in a normal subject. Numerically, GLS < 16% is abnormal, and 16–18% is borderline.

may lead to HF besides increasing risk of sudden death. A meta-analysis of multiple studies has shown that a one percent change (decrease in number) is associated with 20% chance of adverse remodeling with an inflection point being at -10–12%.[21] There are other studies which have correlated impaired GLS with raised natriuretic peptides.[22,23]

STRAIN AS A PREDICTOR OF HEART FAILURE

Biochemical dysfunction precedes mechanical dysfunction, and mechanical dysfunction precedes clinical HF. Ultrastructural and biochemical changes due to abnormal metabolites, proteins, and toxins, weaken the cardiomyocytes and increase extracellular matrix. Studies have shown that common risk factors for HF (diabetes, hypertension, alcoholism, etc.) adversely affect myocardial mechanics even though subjects are asymptomatic and may have normal ejection fraction and other functional parameters.[18,19] The left ventricular GLS predicts incident HF in a variety of patients with coronary artery disease.[22,23] In a single-center study of 410 (patients >65 years of age and with one or more HF risk factors), GLS was impaired in one-third of the population and was an independent predictor of HF along with left ventricular mass.[24] The Copenhagen City Heart Study is a longitudinal cohort study of cardiovascular disease and risk factors in a low-risk general population. In this cohort study, compared with participants in the fourth quartile of GLS, those in the first quartile demonstrated an ≈5-fold higher risk of HF (first quartile vs. fourth quartile HR 4.7; 95% CI 2.0–5.4; $p < 0.001$). GLS was a superior predictor of cardiovascular outcomes in men compared with that in women.[25] In a meta-analysis of studies from the general population (n = 11,744 subjects), GLS predicted new-onset HF although overall cardiovascular outcome were better predicted.[26] In patients with left bundle branch block, GLS independently predicts hospitalization for HF and cardiovascular death.[27]

STRAIN IN CARDIO-ONCOLOGY

Several oncological agents are cardiotoxic and can cause left ventricular dysfunction and HF. It has been proposed to monitor chemotherapy-related cardiotoxicity by periodic echocardiographic examination and biomarker assessment.[28] The left ventricular GLS change (a 15% or more relative decrease) has been suggested as a parameter of subtle left ventricular dysfunction. An early diagnosis

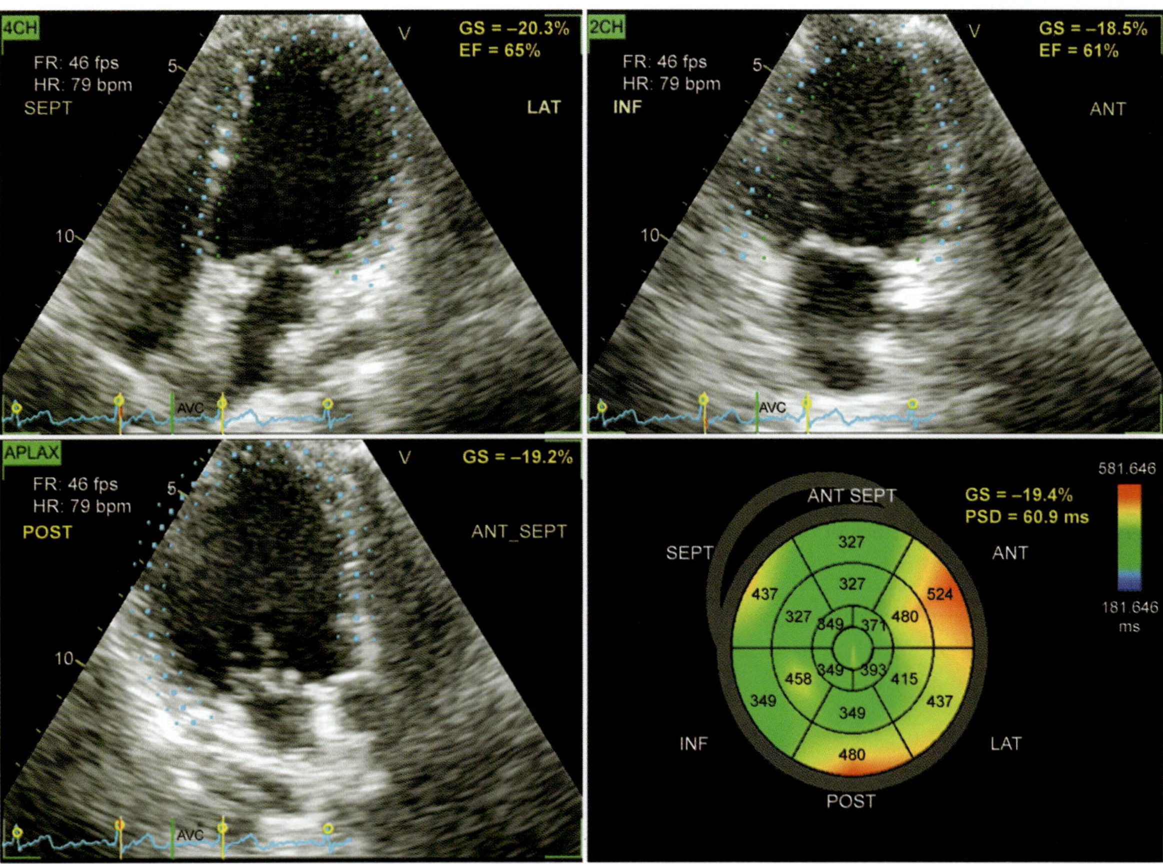

FIG. 10: Depicting global peak systolic longitudinal strain along with standard deviation of strain dispersion. Upper value of this standard deviation is 55 msec.

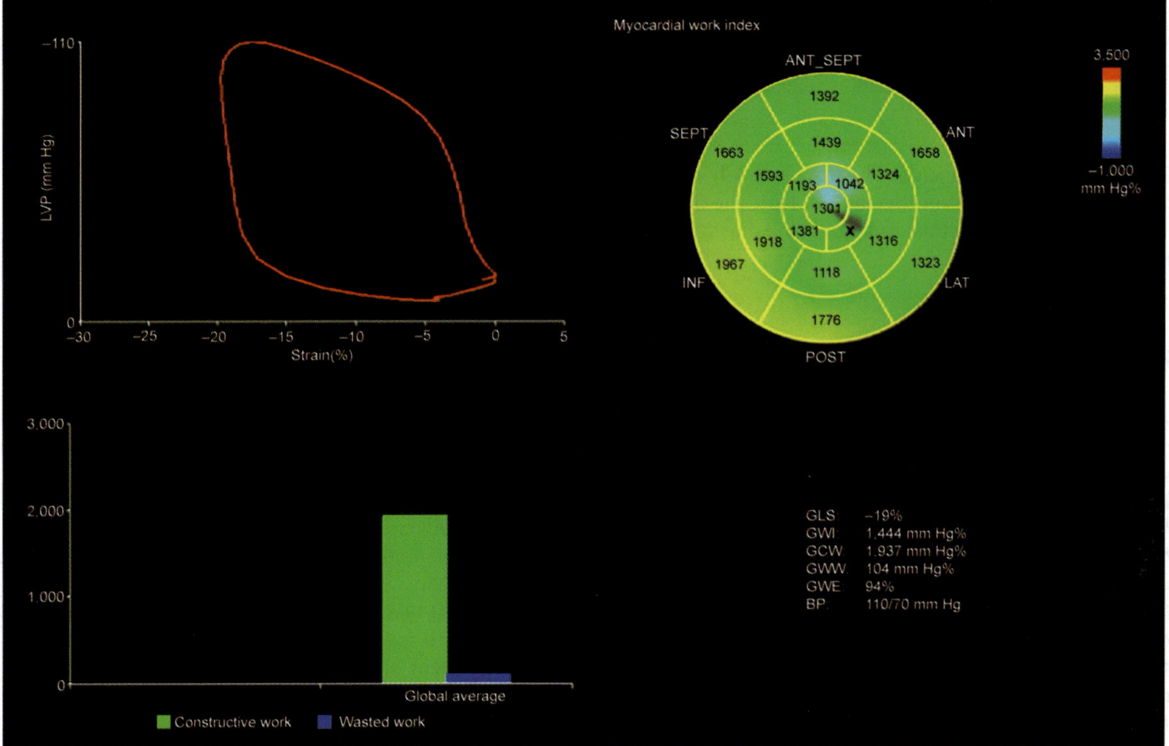

FIG. 11: Pressure-strain loop to depict left ventricular mechanical work in a normal subject.

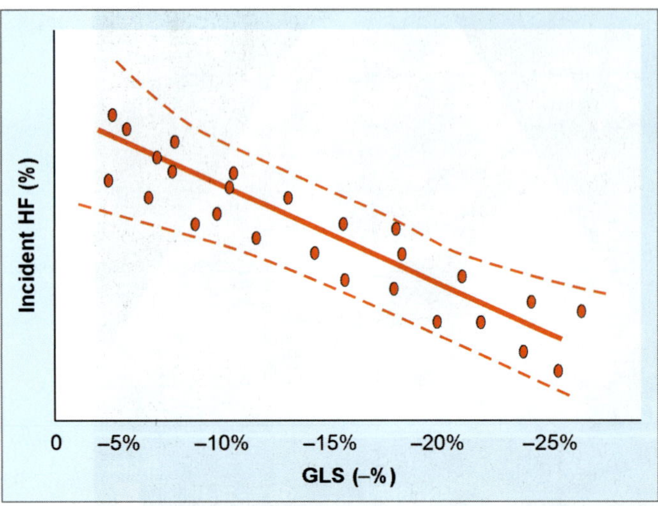

FIG. 12: Inverse relationship between incident heart failure and GLS.

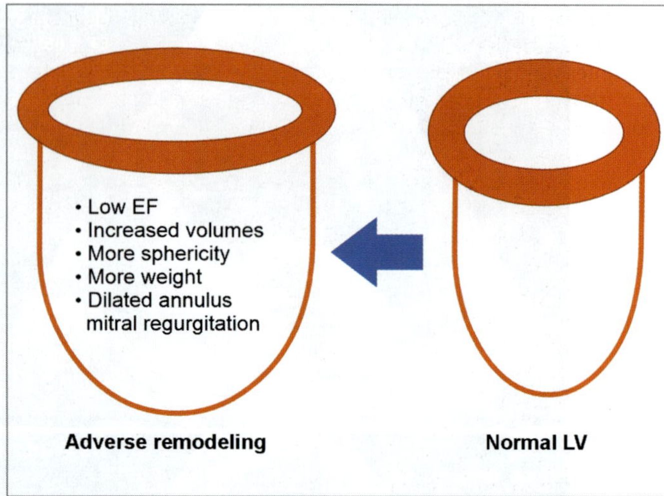

FIG. 14: The concept of adverse remodeling following myocardial infarction.

(EF: ejection fraction)

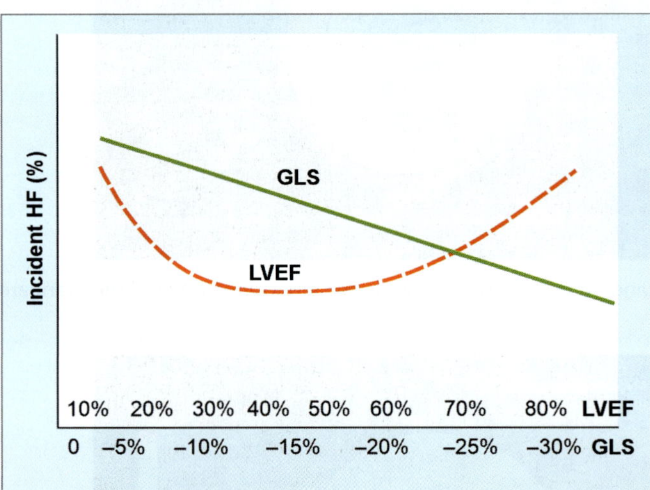

FIG. 13: Relationship between incident heart failure, left ventricular ejection fraction (LVEF), and left ventricular GLS. Note the dichotomy between two parameters of systolic function. LVEF has a U-shaped relationship with incident HF.

of asymptomatic cardiotoxicity allows the initiation of a cardioprotective treatment and potential change in oncology treatment. The results of a randomized study support the use of GLS-guided monitoring of chemotherapeutic toxicity.[29]

CONCLUSION

Strain is a novel way of expressing myocardial function. Long-axis function of the heart measured by GLS is a simple, robust, and more objective parameter of early left ventricular dysfunction. It determines HF trajectory of patients with one or more risk factors and may guide appropriate cardioprotective therapy to prevent serious adverse outcomes. Other vectors of cardiac strain have enhanced our understanding of cardiac mechanics and have some predictive value but not as much as GLS. GLS-based myocardial work efficiency and quantum of wasted work may help in refining the predictive power.

REFERENCES

1. Buckberg G, Hoffman JIE, Mahajan A, et al. Cardiac Mechanics Revisited. Circulation. 2008;118:2571-87.
2. Sengupta PP, Korinek J, Belohlavek M, et al. Left ventricular structure and function: basic science for cardiac imaging. J Am Coll Cardiol. 2006;48:1988-2001.
3. Trivedi SJ, Altman M, Stanton T, et al. Echocardiographic strain in clinical practice. Heart Lung Circ. 2019;28:1320-30.
4. Emig R, Zgierski-Johnston CM, Timmermann V, et al. Passive myocardial mechanical properties: meaning, measurement, models. Biophys Rev. 2021;13:587-610.
5. Marwick TH. Measurement of strain and strain rate by echocardiography: ready for prime time? J Am Coll Cardiol. 2006;47:1313-27.
6. Smiseth OA, Torp H, Opdahl A, et al. Myocardial strain imaging: how useful is it in clinical decision making? Eur Heart J. 2016;37:1196-207.
7. Tolvaj M, Fábián A, Tokodi M, et al. There is more than just longitudinal strain: Prognostic significance of biventricular circumferential mechanics. Front Cardiovasc Med. 2023;10:1082725.
8. Voigt JU, Pedrizzetti G, Lysyansky P, et al. Definitions for a common standard for 2D speckle tracking echocardiography: consensus document of the EACVI/ASE/Industry Task Force to Standardize Deformation Imaging. Eur Heart J Cardiovasc Imaging. 2015;16:1-11.

9. Badano LP, Cucchini U, Muraru D, et al. Use of three-dimensional speckle tracking to assess left ventricular myocardial mechanics: inter-vendor consistency and reproducibility of strain measurements. Eur Heart J Cardiovasc Imaging. 2013;14:285-93.
10. Ilardi F, D'Andrea A, D'Ascenzi F, et al. Myocardial work by echocardiography: principles and applications in clinical practice. J Clin Med. 2021;10:4521.
11. Szymanski C, Levy F, Tribouilloy C. Should LVEF be replaced by global longitudinal strain? Heart. 2014;100:1655-6.
12. Haji K, Huynh Q, Wong C, et al. Improving the Characterization of Stage A and B Heart Failure by Adding Global Longitudinal Strain. J Am Coll Cardiol Img. 2022;8:1380-7.
13. Voigt JU, Cvijic M. 2- and 3-Dimensional myocardial strain in cardiac health and disease. JACC Cardiovasc Imaging. 2019;12:1849-63.
14. Kuznetsova T, Herbots L, Richart T, et al. Left ventricular strain and strain rate in a general population. Eur Heart J. 2008;29:2014-23.
15. Narayanan A, Aurigemma GP, Chinali M, et al. Cardiac mechanics in mild hypertensive heart disease: a speckle-strain imaging study. Circ Cardiovasc Imaging. 2009;2:382-90.
16. Wang Y, Yang H, Huynh Q, et al. Diagnosis of Nonischemic Stage B Heart Failure in Type 2 Diabetes Mellitus: Optimal Parameters for Prediction of Heart Failure. JACC Cardiovasc Imaging. 2018;11: 1390-400.
17. Rajput R, Mohan JC, Sawhney JPS, et al. Prevalence of cardiac abnormalities and heart failure in unselected out-patients with type 2 diabetes mellitus and associated clinical factors: Real-world evidence from an Indian registry. Indian Heart J. 2023;75:436-42.
18. Jiang L, Li Y, Li XM, et al. The adverse effects of metabolic disorder on left ventricular myocardial mechano-energetic efficiency and dysfunction in ischemic cardiomyopathy: insight from a cardiac MRI study. Cardiovasc Diabetol. 2025;24:261-7.
19. Almeida AL, Teixido-Tura G, Choi EY, et al. Metabolic syndrome, strain, and reduced myocardial function: multi-ethnic study of atherosclerosis. Arq Bras Cardiol. 2014;102:327-35.
20. Blomstrand P, Sjöblom P, Nilsson M, et al. Overweight and obesity impair left ventricular systolic function as measured by left ventricular ejection fraction and global longitudinal strain. Cardiovasc Diabetol. 2018;113-24.
21. Huttin O, Coiro S, Selton-Suty C, et al. Prediction of left ventricular remodeling after a myocardial infarction: Role of myocardial deformation: A systematic review and meta-analysis. PLoS ONE. 2016;11:e0168349.
22. Kaufmann D, Szwoch M, Kwiatkowska J, et al. Global longitudinal strain can predict heart failure exacerbation in stable outpatients with ischemic left ventricular systolic dysfunction. PLoS One. 2019;14(12):e0225829.
23. Ersbøll M, Valeur N, Mogensen UM, et al. Relationship between Left Ventricular Longitudinal Deformation and Clinical Heart Failure during Admission for Acute Myocardial Infarction: A Two-Dimensional Speckle-tracking Study. J Am Soc Echocardiog. 2012;25:1280-9.
24. Yang H, Negishi K, Wang Y, et al. Echocardiographic screening for non-ischaemic stage B heart failure in the community. Eur J Heart Fail. 2016;18:1331-9.
25. Biering-Sørensen T, Biering-Sørensen SR, Olsen FJ, et al. Global Longitudinal Strain by Echocardiography Predicts Long-term Risk of Cardiovascular Morbidity and Mortality in a Low-risk General Population: The Copenhagen City Heart Study. Circ Cardiovasc Imaging. 2017;10(3):e005521.
26. Al Saikhan L, Park C, Hardy R, et al. Prognostic implications of left ventricular strain by speckle-tracking echocardiography in the general population: a meta-analysis. Vasc Health Risk Manag. 2019;15:229-51.
27. Hwang IC, Cho GY, Yoon YE, et al. Association between Global Longitudinal Strain and Cardiovascular Events in Patients with Left Bundle Branch Block Assessed Using Two-dimensional Speckle-tracking Echocardiography. J Am Soc Echocardiogr. 2018;31:52-63.
28. Lyon AR, López-Fernández T, Couch LS, et al.; ESC Scientific Document Group. 2022 ESC Guidelines on cardio-oncology developed in collaboration with the European Hematology Association (EHA), the European Society for Therapeutic Radiology and Oncology (ESTRO) and the International Cardio-Oncology Society (IC-OS). Eur Heart J. 2022;43:4229-361.
29. Thavendiranathan P, Negishi T, Somerset E, et al.; SUCCOUR Investigators. Strain-Guided Management of Potentially Cardiotoxic Cancer Therapy. J Am Coll Cardiol. 2021;77(4):392-401.

CHAPTER 32

Medical Therapy of Cardiogenic Shock: Contemporary Use of Inotropes and Vasopressors

Kashinath Ghosh Hazra, Ahitagni Banerjee

ABSTRACT

Cardiogenic shock is a complex heterogenous clinical syndrome due to primary cardiac disorder with tissue hypoperfusion resulting from diminished cardiac output leading to multiorgan failure with high mortality. Inotropes and vasopressors form the cornerstone of therapy bridging patients to recovery, revascularization, or mechanical circulatory support (MCS). Given the diverse cardiogenic shock phenotypes (acute myocardial infraction, acute left ventricular failure, RV shock, biventricular, arrhythmic, mechanical complications, etc.) individualized therapy is necessary. However, their use requires a nuanced understanding of hemodynamic profiles, myocardial oxygen consumption, and arrhythmogenic potential. Evidence till date shows no clear advantage of one agent over the other, reinforcing that these drugs provide only supportive measures rather than definitive cure. Additionally, their beneficial advantages should be balanced with safety concerns. While cardiogenic shock remains one of the most challenging scenarios in cardiology, we are still groping in the dark for an ideal universally acceptable protocol of management although artificial intelligence-based machine learning coupled with phenotype-guided precision medicine may enlighten us in near future. Till then, these drugs provide a pragmatic lifesaving therapy for these critically ill patients.

Keywords: Cardiogenic shock, inotropes, vasopressors, norepinephrine.

INTRODUCTION

Cardiogenic shock (CS) is a serious clinical syndrome caused by a primary cardiac disorder leading to clinical and biochemical evidence of tissue hypoperfusion resulting from diminished cardiac output culminating into multiorgan failure and often death.[1] It is most commonly precipitated by acute myocardial infraction (AMI-CS), but other causes include acute decompensated heart failure, severe valvular lesions, arrhythmias, and myocardial inflammation. Despite modern advances, CS remains highly lethal- short-term mortality is approximately 30–40% and approaches 50% in 1 year.[2,3]

In this background, early recognition of this dreadful condition is essential before prolonged tissue hypoperfusion renders irreversible damage and early stabilization with inotropes and vasopressors is mandatory. The features described in **Table 1** will help in diagnosis of CS.

The *Society for Cardiovascular Angiography and Interventions (SCAI)* stages of CS from early at-risk states (stage A–B) to profound collapse (stage E), based on clinical, hemodynamic, and biochemical parameters **(Box 1)**.

TABLE 1: Features of cardiogenic shock.

Clinical	Hemodynamic	Biochemical
• Cold clammy extremities • Mental confusion • Oliguria • Narrow pulse pressure	• Cardiac index <2.2 L/min/m^2 • Cardiac power output <0.6 W • Pulmonary capillary wedge pressure >18 mm Hg	• Raised serum creatinine • Metabolic acidosis • Serum lactate >2 mmol/L

BOX 1: The Society for Cardiovascular Angiography and Interventions (SCAI) staging of shock.[4]

SCAI staging of CS (2022 Consensus):

- *Stage A ("at risk")*: High-risk ACS/HF without hypoperfusion
- *Stage B ("beginning")*: Hypotension, tachycardia, but preserved perfusion
- *Stage C ("classic")*: Hypotension + hypoperfusion needing support
- *Stage D ("deteriorating")*: Worsening shock despite therapy
- *Stage E ("extremis")*: Circulatory collapse with impending arrest

Management strategy of CS:
Expert consensus:
- Initial stabilization
- Early identification and treatment of underlying cause
- Risk stratification and transfer to intensive care units
- Team-based approaches to correction of end-organ hypoperfusion[1]

Main targets are:
- Restoring systemic perfusion
- Augmenting cardiac output to reverse hypoperfusion
- Minimizing adverse effects
- Serving as a bridge to PCI, surgery, or MCS[5]

HISTORICAL CONTEXT OF PHARMACOTHERAPY

For decades, inotropes and vasopressors have been used; the first use dates back to 1893 when English physician George Oliver assessed sheep glandular extract on his son to check radial arterial vasoreactivity.[6] The term "inotrope" was coined from ancient Greek terms *"is" meaning force/sinew and "tropos" meaning changing.*[7] Catecholamines restore mean arterial pressure (MAP) and contractility but increase myocardial oxygen consumption, while noncatecholamine inotropes provide lusitropic or vasodilatory effects with attendant risk hypotension.

Cardiogenic shock represents the *final common pathway of severe cardiac dysfunction, hallmark being mismatch between cardiac output and tissue oxygen demand, culminating in multiorgan failure.*[8]

Hemodynamic targets for therapy are described in **Table 2**. Pathophysiology of cardiogenic shock **(Flowchart 1)**. Pressure volume loop under normal and CS with alternation by drugs **(Figs. 1A to D)**.

TABLE 2: Hemodynamic targets for therapy.

Parameter	Shock state	Therapeutic goal
MAP	<65 mm Hg	Restore ≥65 mm Hg with vasopressors
Cardiac index	<2.2 L/min/m²	Target >2.2 L/min/m² with inotropes
PCWP	>18 mm Hg	Reduce to 15–18 mm Hg (optimize preload)
Lactate	>2 mmol/L	Normalize (<2 mmol/L)

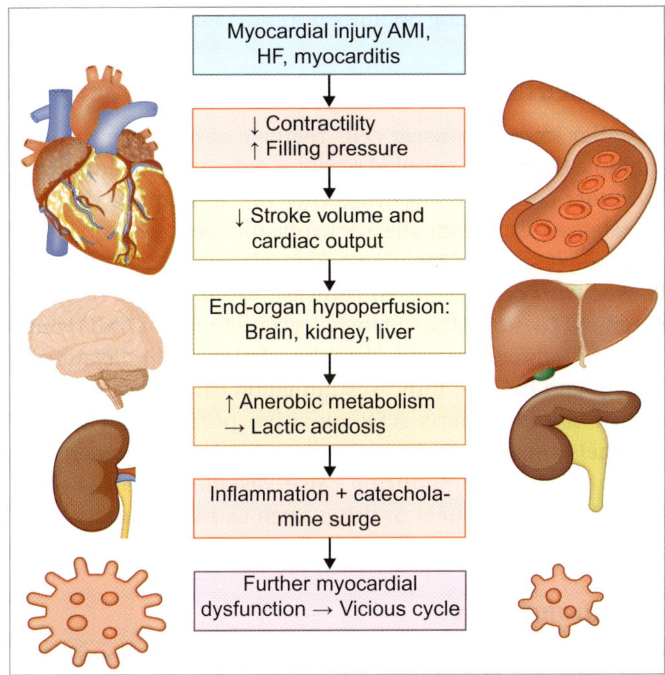

FLOWCHART 1: Pathophysiology of cardiogenic shock.

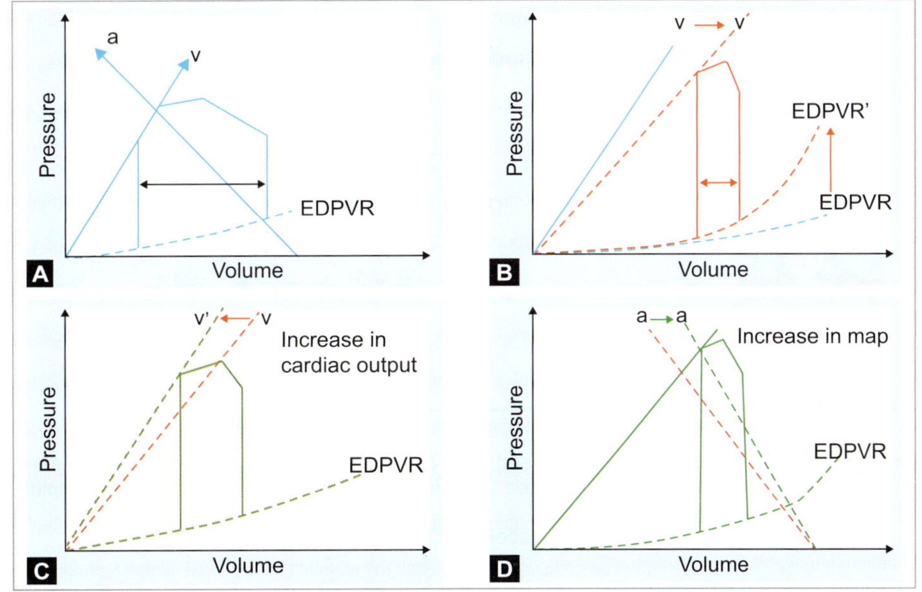

FIGS. 1A TO D: Pressure volume loop: (A) Normal (blue); (B) In cardiogenic shock (red)—there is increase in ventricular volume (V), filling pressures resulting from reduced stroke volume and contractility; (C) *Use of inotropes*—the curve shifts to left *due to increased stroke volume and contractility* (green); (D) *Use of vasopressors* shifts the curve to the right by *increased MAP, and hence, left ventricular afterload* (a) (black).

MECHANISM OF ACTION OF INOTROPES

Cardiac Myocyte

Catecholamines and phosphodiesterase III inhibitors increase intracellular calcium concentration (which paradoxically is responsible for arrhythmia and adverse effects) and hence are also called *calcitropes* **(Flowchart 2)**. To circumvent the limitations of calcium toxicity:

- *Myotropes* acting on sarcomere—calcium sensitizer facilitating actin myosin complex **(Fig. 2)**.
- *Mitotropes*: Acting on mitochondria **(Flowchart 3)**.

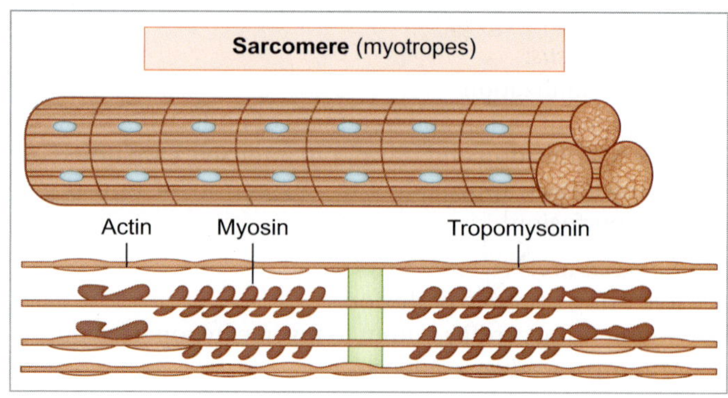

FIG. 2: Myotropes act on actin myosin complex.

Vascular Smooth Muscle (Flowchart 4)

Vascular smooth muscle cells regulate vessel tone through multiple G-protein-coupled receptor pathways. α_1-*Adrenergic receptors* couple to *Gq*, triggering phospholipase C (PLC) to releases $Ca^{2+}$from the sarcoplasmic reticulum, raising cytosolic [Ca^{2+}] and forming a Ca^{2+}calmodulin complex that causes *vasoconstriction*. In contrast, β_2-*adrenergic receptors* couple to *Gs*, activating adenylyl cyclase to raise cAMP which leads to reduced myosin phosphorylation and relaxation of the smooth muscle; thus, β_2 stimulation causes *vasodilation*. *Levosimendan* opens ATP-sensitive potassium (K_ATP) channels, causing arterial and venous dilation. *Norepinephrine* and high-dose epinephrine raise vascular tone, whereas epinephrine's β_2 effect or drugs such as *milrinone* promote vasodilation.

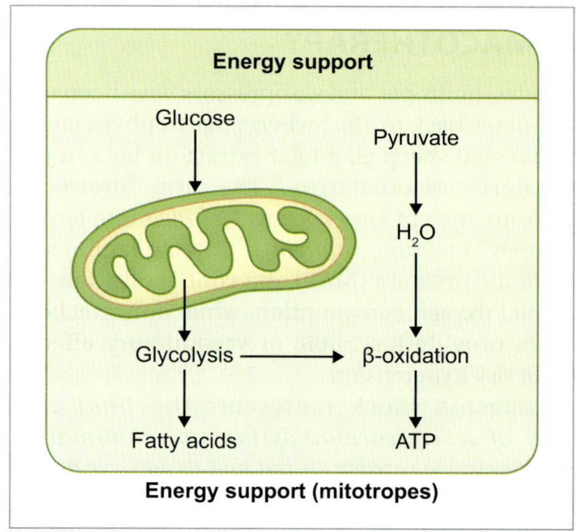

FLOWCHART 3: Mechanism of action of mitotropes, switching fatty acid oxidation to glucose utilization for energy efficiency.

Catecholamines

Catecholamines act via *adrenergic receptor stimulation*, enhancing chronotropy, inotropy, and vascular tone.

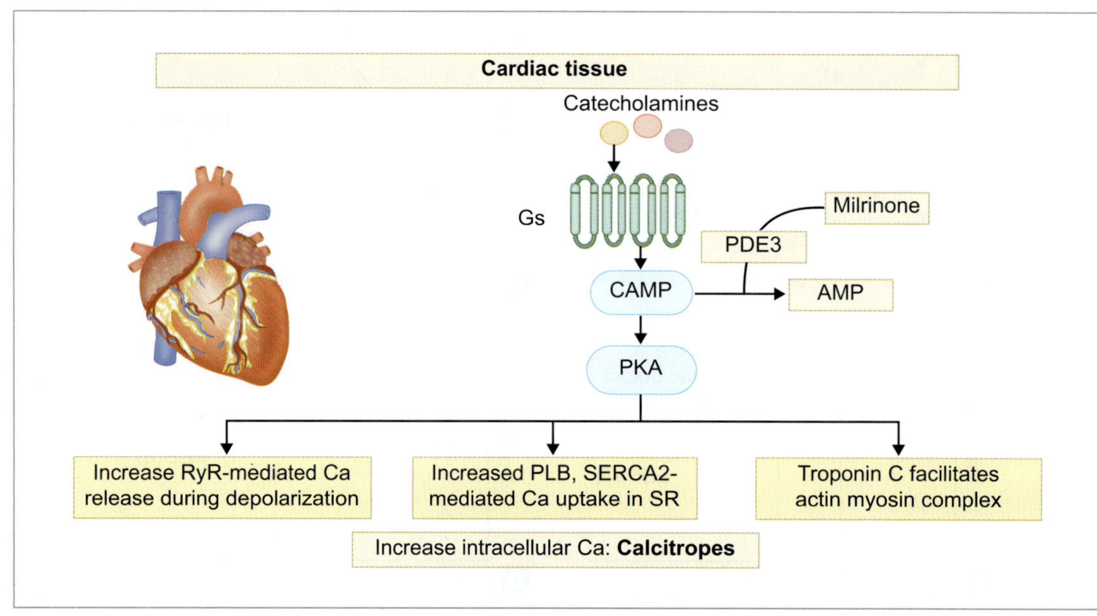

FLOWCHART 2: Mechanism of action of calcitropes.

(Gs: G stimulatory receptor; PDE3: phosphodiesterase 3; PKA: protein kinase A; PLB: phospholamban; RyR: rynadine receptor)

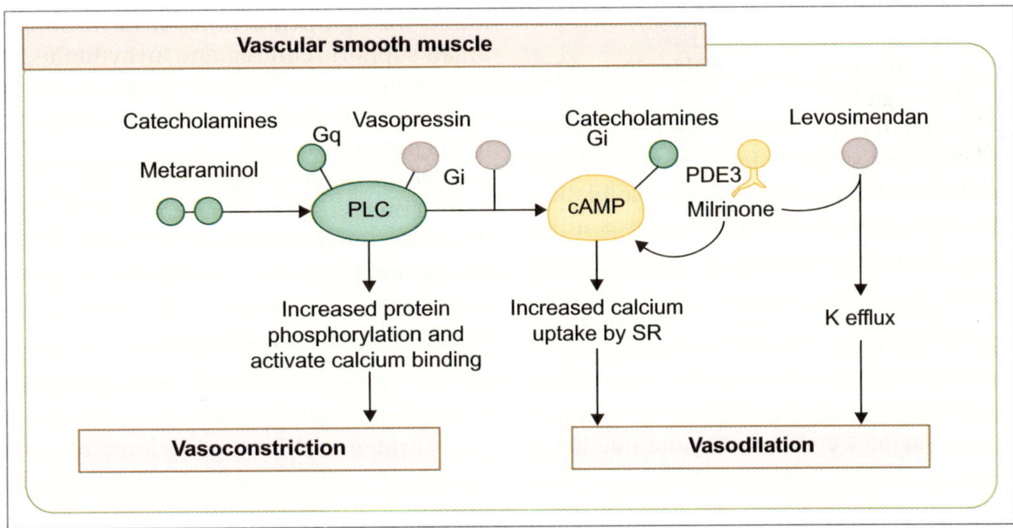

FLOWCHART 4: Mechanism of action of inotropes and vasopressors on vascular smooth.
(Gq: G stimulatory; Gi: G inhibitory; PLC: phospholipokinase C)

Norepinephrine

Norepinephrine is a potent catecholamine vasopressor with predominant α*1*-adrenergic agonism causing peripheral vasoconstriction, thereby increasing MAP and moderate β*1* activity. This causes intense vasoconstriction with mild positive inotropy and chronotropy. Norepinephrine is considered the *vasopressor of choice* in CS based on both clinical experience and comparative studies. By raising MAP through vasoconstriction, NE can improve coronary perfusion pressure and vital organ perfusion. Unlike pure inotropes, it does not directly increase cardiac output in a severely failing heart and may even reduce output if afterload rises excessively. *Main adverse effects are related to its vasoconstrictor potency: Limb ischemia, digital gangrene, mesenteric ischemia, and reflex bradycardia.* NE can precipitate arrhythmias, but less so than dopamine or epinephrine at equivalent pressure targets. *Hemodynamically, norepinephrine increases MAP and vital organ perfusion with only a modest rise in heart rate, avoiding excessive myocardial oxygen demand.*[1] The *chief advantage* of norepinephrine is its robust blood pressure support with relatively lower arrhythmogenicity. Its main limitation is the marked increase in afterload, which can depress cardiac output in severe left ventricular dysfunction; thus, an inotropic agent is often coadministered to maintain forward flow.

Epinephrine

Epinephrine is a potent mixed adrenergic agonist, stimulating β1, β2, and α1 receptors. At lower doses, β1 effects predominate, leading to increased cardiac contractility and heart rate (↑CO), along with β2-mediated vasodilation in skeletal muscle that can reduce afterload. At higher doses, α1-mediated vasoconstriction becomes significant, although epinephrine's concurrent β2 activity may cause a *net neutral effect on blood pressure at certain doses.* Clinically, epinephrine can improve cardiac index, but it *raises myocardial oxygen consumption and lactate levels.* In CS patients, epinephrine has been associated with lactic acidosis (due to β2-stimulated glycolysis), tachyarrhythmias, and splanchnic hypoperfusion. For these reasons, epinephrine is *not recommended as first-line therapy* in CS. It may be considered as a *last-resort or salvage inotrope* in refractory shock, particularly in cardiac arrest or anaphylactic shock scenarios. Many experts prefer adding *low-dose vasopressin* or increasing NE over using epinephrine in CS.

Dopamine

Dopamine is an endogenous catecholamine and precursor of norepinephrine that has dose-dependent pharmacologic profiles. At low infusion rates (2–5 µg/kg/min), dopamine predominantly stimulates D1/D2 dopaminergic receptors causing renal and splanchnic vasodilation. Intermediate doses (5–10 µg/kg/min) activate β1-adrenergic receptors, increasing heart rate and contractility. High doses (10–20 µg/kg/min) principally stimulate α1 receptors, causing peripheral vasoconstriction. *In theory, dopamine can thus act as an "inodilator" at low doses and an "inopressor" at high doses.* It tends to provoke more tachycardia and arrhythmias than other catecholamines. A landmark trial (SOAP-II) in shock (mostly septic and cardiogenic) found *dopamine led to more arrhythmic events and higher mortality in the CS subset* compared to norepinephrine.[9] Dopamine can also interfere with endocrine and immune function (e.g., reducing pituitary prolactin, growth hormone, and causing immunosuppression). Given its *unfavorable risk profile,* current guidelines recommend avoiding dopamine except in bradycardic hypotensive patients where dopamine's chronotropy might help.

Dobutamine

Dobutamine is a synthetic catecholamine with predominantly β1-adrenergic agonist effect (about 3:1 β1 to β2) and minor α1 activity. It is a potent inotrope increasing myocardial contractility and stroke volume, with relatively mild chronotropic effect. Due to balanced β2 vasodilation and weak α1 activation, dobutamine often causes a net *decrease in systemic vascular resistance* or at least avoids further vasoconstriction. Cardiac output typically rises and filling pressures fall with dobutamine. Because it can modestly reduce afterload, dobutamine is particularly useful in *right ventricular (RV) failure*, by lowering pulmonary vascular resistance and augmenting RV contractility, it improves RV output in acute RV shock. Dobutamine has a very short half-life (~2 minutes) and is rapidly titratable, reaching steady state within minute. However, tachyphylaxis can develop within 48–72 hours due to downregulation of cardiac β-receptors. Adverse effects include dose-dependent *tachycardia and arrhythmias*, hypotension (especially if the patient is vasodilated or if dose >10 μg/kg/min), and myocardial ischemia if oxygen demand outstrips supply. High doses (>20 μg/kg/min) are discouraged as they provide little additional output but markedly increase heart rate and risk of arrhythmia. In practice, dobutamine is often started at 2.5–5 μg/kg/min and titrated up to ~10 μg/kg/min as tolerated. It remains the inotrope of choice in low-output CS with preserved BP.[10]

Phosphodiesterase-3 Inhibitors: Milrinone

Milrinone is a phosphodiesterase-3 (PDE3) inhibitor that provides *inotropy and vasodilation* by a nonadrenergic mechanism. By inhibiting the breakdown of cAMP in cardiac myocytes and vascular smooth muscle, milrinone increases intracellular calcium availability and myocardial contractility, while also causing relaxation of vascular smooth muscle (systemic and pulmonary vasodilation). Milrinone also enhances myocardial lusitropy (diastolic relaxation), which can improve ventricular filling in acute heart failure. A key feature is that milrinone's effects *do not depend on β-receptor stimulation*, so it retains efficacy even in the presence of β-blockers. Hemodynamically, milrinone tends to significantly reduce SVR and pulmonary vascular resistance, which can benefit patients with concomitant pulmonary hypertension or RV dysfunction by unloading the RV. The net effect is increased cardiac index with lowered filling pressures. However, because of its vasodilatory action, milrinone frequently causes *hypotension*. It can also provoke arrhythmias (atrial and ventricular) similar to other inotropes. Milrinone has a longer half-life (~2 hours) than catecholamines and is renally excreted, so its effects may linger in renal impairment.

The recent DOREMI trial (2021) compared milrinone versus dobutamine in CS (primarily ADHF patients) and found *no significant differences in outcomes*—mortality, organ support requirement, arrhythmias, and hypotension rates were similar between the two groups.[11] This suggests that *milrinone is an acceptable alternative to dobutamine* as initial inotropic therapy.

Enoximone and *other PDE3 inhibitors* have similar effects; enoximone is used in some countries as an alternative PDE3 inhibitor. The principles of use and side effects mirror those of milrinone.

Calcium Sensitizers

Levosimendan is a unique inotropic agent that *sensitizes troponin C to calcium*, thereby stabilizing the actin-myosin cross-bridge and increasing force of contraction without raising intracellular calcium or myocardial oxygen demand. In addition, levosimendan causes vasodilation via two mechanisms: It opens K_ATP channels in vascular smooth muscle (arterial and venous dilation) and also has a mild PDE3 inhibitory effect. It also *enhances ventriculoarterial coupling* along with anti-inflammatory and antistunning effects. The net result is an *"inodilator" profile*: Increased cardiac output and reduced preload and afterload. Notably, levosimendan's inotropy is maintained even in the presence of β-blockade (under β-blockade it functions more as a PDE3 inhibitor). It has two active metabolites (OR-1896 and OR-1855) that have long half-lives (~80 hours), conferring a sustained hemodynamic effect for up to 7–9 days after a 24-hour infusion. This prolonged action can be advantageous for "bridge" therapy but also means hypotension can persist if it occurs during infusion. Its major benefit is improving contractility without increasing myocardial oxygen consumption.

In clinical trials for acute decompensated HF, levosimendan improved hemodynamics, but large trials did not show a mortality benefit over dobutamine. In CS, small studies and meta-analyses suggest *levosimendan may improve hemodynamics and possibly outcomes in milder forms of shock*. Recent meta-analyses have hinted at a mortality benefit with levosimendan in CS complicating acute MI, although a large trial in acute heart failure (SURVIVE) showed no survival advantage over dobutamine.[12] Many of these patients received levosimendan as an add-on to catecholamines. It has also been used to facilitate weaning of VA-ECMO by improving myocardial function. The main side effect is *hypotension* from vasodilation, headache and reflex tachycardia and arrhythmias (e.g., atrial fibrillation) at higher doses. Given its cost and mixed evidence, current guidelines reserve levosimendan for select scenarios of CS with caution if blood pressure is marginal, often requiring concomitant vasopressor support.

Vasopressin acts on V1a receptors of vascular smooth muscle, causing potent vasoconstriction independent of adrenergic receptors. It also has V1b (pituitary) and V2 (renal) effects that can lead to water retention and cortisol release. In CS, endogenous vasopressin levels may actually be low ("relative vasopressin deficiency" in prolonged shock). Low-dose vasopressin infusions (0.03 units/min) are sometimes added to NE in patients with refractory hypotension, with the goal of raising blood pressure and reducing required NE dose. It is typically reserved for vasoplegic scenarios or as a second-line agent if NE alone is insufficient. Importantly, vasopressin has *no direct inotropic or chronotropic effect.* Adverse effects include digital ischemia, hypertension, and potentially decreased cardiac output if afterload is markedly elevated. Vasopressin does not promote arrhythmias and can be useful when tachyarrhythmias limit adrenergic dosing. In summary, vasopressin is a valuable adjunct vasopressor in CS, particularly when a catecholamine-sparing effect is desired or in mixed shock states.[13]

Istaroxime is a dual Na^+/K^+-ATPase inhibitor and SERCA2a activator leading to increased contractility, improved lusitropy efficacy in acute HF (HORIZON-HF, SEISMiC 2022) causing improved CO, BP, and relaxation.[14] Trials are on for *shock and decompensated HF.*

Table 3 summarizes the pharmacologic profiles of commonly used inotropes and vasopressors in cardiogenic shock, including their primary receptor targets, hemodynamic effects, dosing, and key adverse effects.

Adverse events with inotrope/vasopressors are caused because of increase in myocardial cytosolic calcium and heart rate leading to increased myocardial oxygen demand with concomitant decrease in coronary perfusion pressure (LVEDP—aortic diastolic pressure) and tachycardia induced reduction of diastolic coronary perfusion time.

- *Hypotension: Milrinone > dobutamine*
- *Digital and splanchnic ischemia: Vasopressor > norepinephrine > epinephrine.*
- *Renal dysfunction: Milrinone accumulation*
- *Arrhythmias* are caused because of increased intracellular calcium. *Dopamine > epinephrine > dobutamine > milrinone > NE.*
- *Lactate elevation: Epinephrine >> others.*
- *Mortality: Highest with epinephrine/dopamine; lowest with NE-based regimens*

*Efficacy of vasopressors through stages of cardiogenic shock **(Fig. 3)**:*

A. *Mechanical efficiency* due to increase in systemic vascular resistance (SVR) and MAP
B. *Mechanical inefficiency* due to microcirculatory dysfunction, vasodilatation
C. *Metabolic inefficiency* due desensitization of adrenoreceptors, vasoplegia, MODS, and SIRS

Though there are negative observational studies with:

- *ESCHF long-term registry (increased risk of long-term death)*

TABLE 3: Pharmacologic profiles of commonly used inotropes and vasopressors in cardiogenic shock, including their primary receptor targets, hemodynamic effects, dosing, and key adverse effects.

Drug	Primary receptor activity	Hemodynamic effects	Typical dose range	Key adverse effects
Norepinephrine	α1 (strong), β1 (moderate) agonist	Potent vasoconstriction (↑ SVR, ↑ MAP); modest ↑ inotropy; may ↓ CO if afterload↑ too much	0.1–1 µg/kg/min (titrate to MAP)	Peripheral ischemia, reflex bradycardia; arrhythmias (less than dopamine)
Epinephrine	β1 = β2, α1 (mixed agonist)	Dose-dependent effects: Low dose ↑ CO (β1 inotropy, β2 vasodilation), higher dose ↑ SVR (α1) but also β2 vasodilation can blunt BP effect	0.05–0.5 µg/kg/min	Tachyarrhythmias, lactic acidosis (β2-mediated); increases myocardial O_2 consumption
Dopamine	Dose-dependent: D1/D2 at low dose; β1 at moderate; α1 at high dose	Low (2–5 µg/kg/min): Renal vasodilation (obsolete); Moderate (5–10): ↑ contractility and HR; High (10–20): vasoconstriction (↑ SVR)	2–20 µg/kg/min	Arrhythmias (atrial and ventricular); endocrine effects (e.g., pituitary suppression); Increased mortality in CS vs. NE
Dobutamine	β1 (strong), β2 (moderate), and α1 (weak)	↑ Contractility (inotropy) and mild vasodilation (↓ SVR); modest ↑ HR	2–20 µg/kg/min	Tachyarrhythmias, hypotension at higher doses; tachyphylaxis with prolonged use
Milrinone	Phosphodiesterase-III inhibitor (nonadrenergic)	↑ Contractility and lusitropy; vasodilation (↓ SVR/PVR)	0.25–0.75 µg/kg/min	Hypotension (from vasodilation), arrhythmias; accumulation in renal dysfunction
Levosimendan	Calcium sensitizer (troponin C) + PDE-III inhibition + KATP channel opening	↑ Contractility without ↑ Ca^{2+} or O_2 demand; vasodilation (arterial and venous)	0.05–0.2 µg/kg/min (after loading dose)	Hypotension, headache; long action (active metabolite ~1 week)
Vasopressin	V1a receptor agonist (non-adrenergic)	Intense vasoconstriction (↑ SVR) via smooth muscle V1 receptors; no direct cardiac effects	0.03–0.04 U/min (fixed dose)	Reflex bradycardia; hyponatremia; peripheral ischemia. Primarily used as adjunct to reduce catecholamine dose

- *CardShock study (increased 90-day mortality)*
- *ALARM-HF (more in hospital mortality in acute HF), ESC, and AHA/ACC guidelines recommend norepinephrine as the vasopressor of choice in cardiogenic shock patients with hypotension.*

Box 2 showing different trials, registry data and meta-analysis.

CLINICAL PROTOCOLS AND SPECIAL SCENARIOS: PHENOTYPE-GUIDED THERAPY

Acute myocardial infarction–related CS (AMI-CS):

- *Problem:* Severe LV dysfunction, ischemia-driven contractile failure

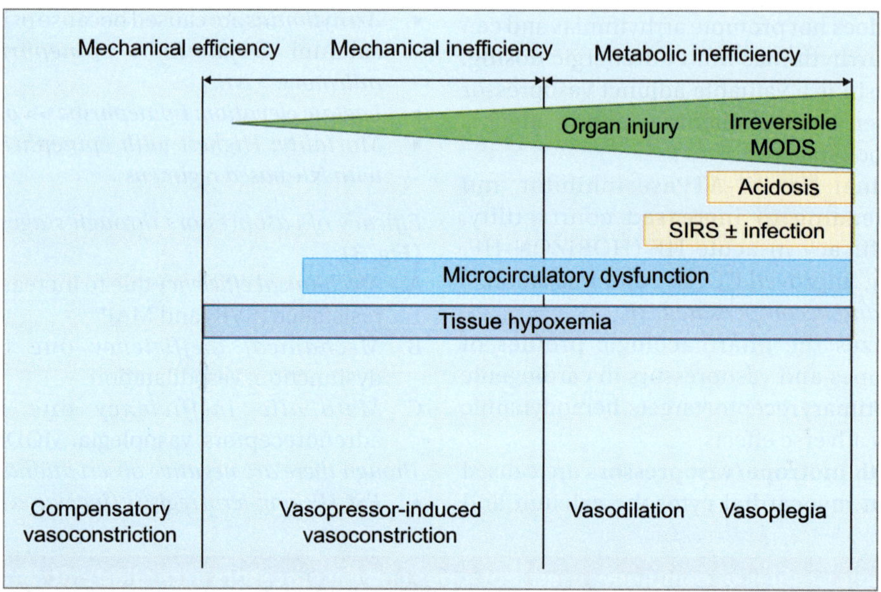

FIG. 3: Efficacy of vasopressors on shock.

BOX 2: Landmark trials, registry data, and meta-analysis.

Landmark trials:

SOAP II (1,679 patients, 2010):

- Compared norepinephrine versus dopamine in shock
- *Result*: Norepinephrine reduced arrhythmias and mortality[9]
- *Clinical takeaway*: Dopamine is no longer recommended

OPTIMA CC (57 patients, 2018):

- Compared epinephrine versus norepinephrine in AMI-CS
- *Result*: Epinephrine caused lactic acidosis, tachyarrhythmias, and worse metabolic profile[10]
- *Clinical takeaway:* Epinephrine should be reserved for refractory CS

DOREMI (192 patients, 2021):

- Dobutamine versus milrinone
- *Result: No significant difference in composite outcome (death, arrest, MCS, and renal replacement.*[11] Milrinone favored in RV shock, nonischemic cardiomyopathy
- *Clinical takeaway:* Inotrope choice should be phenotype driven

Registry data:

- *CCS registry (2022): Norepinephrine* was the most common vasopressor (>70%), associated with better survival vs. dopamine/epinephrine[15]
- *FRENCH-SHOCK (2023): Milrinone* use increased in HF-CS and RV-CS, with better lactate clearance compared to dobutamine[16]
- *CSWG data (2024):* Epinephrine use independently predicted mortality, while norepinephrine + dobutamine combination was common in stage D/E shock[17]

Meta-analyses and systemic reviews (Cochrane reviews):

- *2022 META analysis of 15 RCTs (n = 3,800):* Norepinephrine superior to dopamine/epinephrine in mortality and arrhythmias[18]
- *2023 network meta-analysis:* Levosimendan reduced biomarkers of injury and improved hemodynamics, but no clear mortality benefit[19]
- *2024 review of novel agents:* Omecamtiv and istaroxime promising but not yet guideline endorsed[20,21]

- *Preferred therapy:*
  - Norepinephrine to restore perfusion pressure
  - Dobutamine to augment contractility (if MAP stable)
- *Avoid*: Epinephrine unless refractory; dopamine discouraged
- *Trials*: OPTIMA CC confirmed NE + dobutamine safer than epinephrine[10]

Advanced HF-CS (chronic decompensated):
- *Problem*: Progressive low-output HF with neurohormonal activation
- *Preferred therapy*: Dobutamine or milrinone depending on renal function/BP phenotypes[11]

Right ventricular failure–CS (RV-CS):
- *Problem:* Poor RV contractility, ↑ pulmonary pressures
- *Preferred therapy:*
  - Milrinone (↓ PVR and ↑ RV contractility)
  - Inhaled pulmonary vasodilators as adjunct
- *Evidence:* PDE3 inhibitors provide greatest value.[16]

Takotsubo cardiomyopathy with cardiogenic shock with LVOT obstruction:
- *Catecholamines are contraindicated* (further aggravation of LVOT obstruction)
- *Drug of choice:* Vasopressin and levosimendan

Monitoring, Weaning, and Safety

Monitoring Requirements

Effective therapy in CS requires *intensive hemodynamic and metabolic monitoring* **(Table 4)**.

Weaning strategies:
- *Stabilization phase:* MAP > 65 mm Hg, CI >2.2 L/min/m^2, lactate <2 mmol/L.
- *Stepwise tapering:*
  - Wean vasopressors first (e.g., vasopressin → norepinephrine)
  - Maintain inotrope support until afterload is stable
- *Transition to oral therapy:*
  - In advanced HF-CS, switch to GDMT (ARNI, SGLT-2i, MRA, BB) as tolerated. Some require chronic inotrope infusions (e.g., home milrinone).
  - *Bridge or destination:* Consider LVAD/transplant in refractory HF-CS.

The proposed algorithm for management of cardiogenic shock is shown in **Flowchart 5**.

Weaning-induced Pulmonary Edema

Spontaneous breathing during transition from mechanical ventilation causes negative intrathoracic pressure which

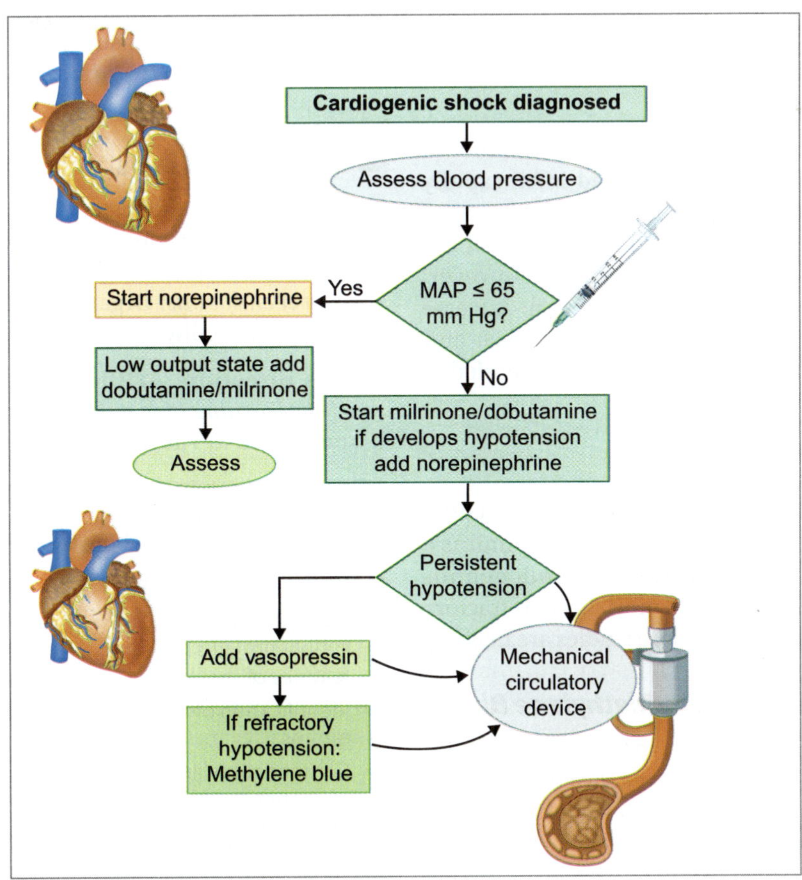

FLOWCHART 5: Proposed algorithm for management of cardiogenic shock.

TABLE 4: Hemodynamic monitoring during cardiogenic shock treatment.

Clinical	Noninvasive	Invasive
• Higher neurological function • Pulse rate and pulse volume • Blood pressure and capillary refilling time • Urine output • Bilateral basal crepts • Hepatomegaly • Gallop rhythm	• ECG monitoring • Chest X-ray • Echocardiogram	• ABG with lactate • Central venous catheter • Pulmonary artery catheter • Pulmonary artery pulsatility index

increases venous return (RV preload) and LV afterload. This leads to acute increase in LV filling pressures (↑ PCWP). If LV is weak (CS, LV dysfunction), this triggers acute pulmonary edema. *Pulmonary artery catheter (PAC) shows* rise in PCWP during spontaneous breathing trial. *Risk factors include LV systolic or diastolic dysfunction, high preload dependence, ischemia. Management includes* optimization of fluid balance with *diuretics* or natriuretic peptides, along with avoidance of excessive preload reduction which can cause atelectasis, thick secretions etc. Inotropes are generally not helpful as they increase O_2 demand, *levosimendan* may help due to vasodilatory and lusitropic effects. It is advisable to delay weaning until patient is stable without vasopressors.

Emerging Novel Molecules

Angiotensin II

Potent vasoconstrictor via AT1 receptors (vascular smooth muscle, adrenal gland). It causes increased MAP rapidly and reduces vasopressor requirements. It has a potential role in refractory vasodilatory shock and some cases of CS, especially RAAS blockade (ARNI overdosage). However, it may increase afterload, worsening LV function. Adverse effects include headache, chest pressure, dyspepsia, and orthostatic hypotension, thus not routinely recommended in CS pending more evidence.

Procizumab

Procizumab is a monoclonal antibody inhibiting CDPP3 (enzyme degrading angiotensin II and enkephalins). It reduces refractory shock by preserving endogenous vasopressors, early trials show reduced mortality in refractory CS. However, it is still experimental, more studies are needed.

Nitric Oxide Synthase Inhibitors/Methylene Blue

Block excessive nitric oxide (NO) production, which contributes to vasoplegia and improves vascular tone in distributive shock (postcardiotomy, septic shock) also may reduce catecholamine requirements.

However, there is risk of paradoxical hypoxemia, hemolysis, methemoglobinemia, and renal dysfunction. It has limited role in CS.

Adjunctive Therapies

- *SGLT-2 inhibitors (dapagliflozin, empagliflozin):* Experimental role in acute HF-CS; pleiotropic effects (natriuresis, metabolic shift)[22]
- *Metabolic modulators:* Agents like *perhexiline, trimetazidine* studied for ischemic metabolic efficiency.
- *Inflammation-targeted therapies:* Anti-IL-6 monoclonals in early testing for cytokine-driven myocardial dysfunction.[23]

Integration with mechanical circulatory support (MCS):

- Drugs alone often insufficient in *SCAI stage D/E*
- *New paradigm: Hybrid strategy* = NE (pressor) + inotrope + early MCS

Research Gaps

Newer studies should foster:

- *Long-term outcomes*: Chronic inotrope dependence, renal outcomes
- *Novel endpoints*: Organ recovery, quality of life, not just 30-day mortality

Future direction: Artificial intelligence in the form of *machine learning* may guide us in future management of CS as mentioned in **Table 5**.

TABLE 5: Incorporation of AI in CS management.

Machine learning in CS	
Unsupervised learning	**Supervised learning**
• Identification of subphenotypes based on features of shock • Identification of treatment groups • Consolidating large datasets of continuous hemodynamic monitoring	• Predicting the likelihood of having CS in a patient • Predicting mortality risk • Predicting response to interventions • Predicting survival in bridge to transplant patients

TABLE 6: Phenotype classification of cardiogenic shock.

Noncongested	Cardiorenal	Cardiometabolic
• Lowest lactate level • Impaired cardiac index	• Higher age, comorbidities • Pulmonary congestion	• Highest lactate • Highest acid base imbalance, highest mortality

Precision medicine: Clustering clinical features, hemodynamic data ECG, ECHO along with biomarker values like BNP, troponin, lactate, etc., helps us to unravel the pathobiology of CS state.[24]

Proposed trials now divide patients into *noncongested, cardiorenal and cardiometabolic subgroups* (Cardiogenic Shock Working Group) *for phenotype tailored management by machine learning algorithms* **(Table 6)**.[25]

CONCLUSION

Medical therapy with vasopressors and inotropes is the cornerstone in initial stabilization of CS. A clear understanding of cardiovascular physiology and careful tailoring of therapy to each patient's needs remain indispensable for prompt restoration of tissue perfusion regardless of underlying etiology, albeit with potential adverse side effects, with norepinephrine emerging as the favored agent. The choice and dosage of agents must account for phenotype differences and anticipate complications. Future research with artificial intelligence, especially machine learning-based phenotyping, promises future triage and prognostication in CS[26]—success will depend on collaborative research, real time integration, and external validation.

REFERENCES

1. Chioncel O, Parissis J, Mebazaa A, et al. Epidemiology, thophysiology and contemporary management of cardiogenic shock – a position statement from the Heart Failure Association of the European Society of Cardiology. Eur J Heart Fail. 2020;22: 1315-41.
2. Riccard M, Pagnesi M. Chioncel O, et al. Medical therapy of cardiogenic shock: Contemporary use of inotropes and vasopressors. ESC. 2024;26(4):411-31.
3. Naidu SS, Baran DA, Jentzer JC, et al. SCAI SHOCK stage classification expert consensus update: a review and incorporation of validation studies. J Am Coll Cardiol. 2022;79:933-46.
4. Harjola VP, Lassus J, Sionis A, J, et al. Contemporary role of inotropes and vasopressors in cardiogenic shock: ESC position paper. Eur Heart J Acute Cardiovasc Care. 2021;10(4): 348-64.
5. Schumann J, Henning A, Bauersachs J, et al. Pathophysiology of cardiogenic shock: recent insights and implications for therapy. Eur Heart J Suppl. 2021;23(Suppl B):B12-9.
6. Zarychanksi R, Ariano RE, Paunovic B, et al. Historical perspectives in critical care medicine:blood transfusion, intravenous fluids, inotropes/vasopressors, and antibiotics. Crit Care Clin. 2009;25;201-20.
7. Psotka MA, Gottlieb SS, Francis GS, et al. Cardiac calcitropes, myotropes and mitotropes outcomes in cardiogenic shock: JACC review topic of the week. J Am Coll Cardiol. 2019;2345-53.
8. Gustafsson F, Metra M, Filippatos G, et al. Inotropic therapy in patients with advanced heart failure: A clinical update. Eur J Heart Fail. 2023;25(4):631-48.
9. De Becker D, Biston P, Devriendt J, et al. Comparison of dopamine and norepinephrine in the treatment of cardiogenic shock. N Engl J Med. 2010;362(9):779-89.
10. Zhang Y, Sun J, Hu J, et al. Vasopressor and inotrope therapy in cardiogenic shock: a systematic review and meta-analysis. Crit Care. 2022;26(1):34.
11. Mathew R, El-SherifN, Van Diepen, et al. Milrinone vs dobutamine in cardiogenic shock: The DOREMI randomized trial. N Engl J Med. 2021;385:516-25.
12. Pollesello P, Parissis J, Bettex D, et al. Levosimendan in cardiogenic shock: updated evidence and expert consensus. Eur Heart J Acute Cardiovasc Care. 2023;12(5):450-63.
13. Kapur NK, Schreiber T, O'Neill W, et al. Future directions in cardiogenic shock management: precision medicine, inotropes, and devices. J Am Coll Cardiol. 2024;84(6):567-80.
14. Teerlink JR, Diaz R, Felker GM, et al. Cardiac myosin activation with omecamtiv mecarbil in systolic heart failure (GALACTIC-HF). N Engl J Med. 2021;384(2):105-16.
15. Vincent JL, Von Lewinski D, Herold L, et al. The CardShock registry: long-term outcomes and therapies in shock patients. Intensive Care Med. 2022;48:112-22.
16. Tarvasmäki T, Lassus J, Sund R, et al. Milrinone in RV failure and pulmonary hypertension: registry experience. Eur Heart J Acute Cardiovasc Care. 2022;11(7):587-95.
17. Kapur NK, Garan AR, Basir MB, et al. Clinical phenotypes and outcomes in cardiogenic shock: The CSWG registry. J Am Coll Cardiol. 2024;83(12):1150-63.
18. Zhou X, Hu Y, Chen R, et al. Comparative efficacy of vasopressors and inotropes in cardiogenic shock: network meta-analysis. Eur Heart J. 2023;44(20):1856-67.
19. Ouweneel DM, Eriksen E, Sjauw KD, et al. Hemodynamic monitoring in cardiogenic shock: contemporary evidence and guidelines. Eur Heart J Acute Cardiovasc Care. 2022;11(5):431-40.
20. Papp Z, Agostoni P, Morelli A, et al. Istaroxime: an emerging inotrope-lusitrope for acute heart failure and cardiogenic shock. Eur Heart J. 2022;43(15):1436-46.
21. Teerlink JR, Diaz R, Felker GM, et al. Cardiac myosin activation with omecantiv mecarbil in systolic heart failure (GALACTIC HF). N Engl J Med. 2021:384(2):105-16.
22. Bhatt AS, Jhund PS, Vaduganathan M, et al. Role of SGLT2 inhibitors in acute HF and shock: emerging evidence. JACC Heart Fail. 2023;11(1):57-67.
23. Anker SD, Butler J, Filippatos G, et al. Inflammatory modulation in heart failure and cardiogenic shock. Eur J Heart Fail. 2023;25(6):879-89.
24. Zwek, Elric, MD K, et al. Clinical Course of patients in Cardiogenic Shock Stratified by phenotype. JACC Heart Fail. 2023;11(10):1304-15.
25. Zweck E, Li S, Burkhoff D, et al. Profiling of Cardiogenic Shock: Incorporating Machine Learning into Bedside Management. JCSCAI. 2025;1(3):102047.
26. Mebazaa A, Soussi S. Precision Medicine in Cardiogenic Shock. JACC Heart Fail. 2023;11(10):1316-9.

CHAPTER 33

Continuum of Preshock to Classic Cardiogenic Shock

MU Rabbani

ABSTRACT

Cardiogenic shock (CS) is a life-threatening condition marked by systemic hypoperfusion with end organ dysfunction due to cardiac dysfunction. CS is a dynamic state that evolves from preshock (a compensated, at-risk phase) to overt CS due to rapidly changing pathophysiology, interplay of compensatory mechanisms, and variable response to treatment. The Society for Cardiovascular Angiography and Interventions (SCAI) classification is widely used for staging the CS. Understanding this dynamic continuum is critical for early recognition, risk stratification, and multidisciplinary assessment to guide effective interventions, such as reperfusion, pharmacological support, and mechanical circulatory support devices.

Keywords: Cardiogenic shock, continuum, preshock, SCAI staging.

INTRODUCTION

Cardiogenic shock (CS) represents a critical state characterized by inadequate cardiac output (CO) leading to systemic hypoperfusion and end-organ dysfunction. Mortality rates despite advances in treatment with revascularization and mechanical circulatory support (MCS) remain high from 35 to 50%.[1,2] CS is not a singular state but a dynamic continuum ranging from preshock states, where patients are at risk but not yet critically compromised, to classic CS, marked by profound hemodynamic instability and multiorgan failure. Understanding this spectrum is crucial for timely intervention to halt progression and improve outcomes. This chapter explores the pathophysiology, clinical presentation, diagnostic strategies, and management approaches across this continuum.

The Society for Cardiovascular Angiography and Interventions (SCAI) shock classification, introduced in 2019 and updated in 2022, provides a structured framework to categorize this continuum from preshock to CS in aiding in risk stratification and management.[3]

EPIDEMIOLOGY

Cardiogenic shock complicates approximately 7–10% of acute myocardial infarction (AMI) cases and 5% of heart failure (HF) admissions. As per CCCTN Registry, HF-related CS, account for over 50% of cases in contemporary cardiac intensive careunits.[4].

The prevalence of CS has decreased in AMI settings due to early revascularization, dropping to 2.8% in recent French registries, but remains a significant challenge in HF due to its complex etiologies.[5]

PATHOPHYSIOLOGY OF THE CONTINUUM

■ Preshock State

The preshock state is an early phase of cardiac dysfunction where CO is reduced but compensatory mechanisms maintain adequate tissue perfusion.[6] This stage often arises from acute insults such as AMI, myocarditis, or with chronic conditions as heart failure with reduced ejection fraction (HFrEF). The pathophysiological features in preshock state include:

- *Reduced CO:* A decline in stroke volume due to impaired myocardial contractility, often triggered by ischemia, inflammation, or mechanical complications (e.g., papillary muscle rupture).
- *Compensatory mechanisms:* Activation of the sympathetic nervous system increases heart rate and contractility, while peripheral vasoconstriction (mediated by catecholamines and the renin-angiotensin-aldosterone system) maintains blood pressure. However, these mechanisms increase myocardial oxygen demand, potentially exacerbating ischemia.
- *Subclinical hypoperfusion:* End-organ perfusion may be preserved, but subtle signs of tissue hypoxia, such as

elevated lactate levels (<2 mmol/L) or mild renal/hepatic dysfunction, may emerge.

Transition to Early Cardiogenic Shock

As cardiac dysfunction worsens, compensatory mechanisms begin to fail, marking the transition to early CS. This phase is characterized by:

- *Worsening hemodynamic compromise:* Cardiac index (CI) typically falls below 2.2 L/min/m^2, with increased left ventricular end-diastolic pressure (LVEDP) or pulmonary capillary wedge pressure (PCWP >15 mm Hg).
- *Systemic inflammation:* Myocardial injury triggers a systemic inflammatory response, releasing cytokines, TNF-α and IL-6 further depressing myocardial function, increasing vasodilation, and reducing systemic vascular resistance (SVR).
- *Development of early end-organ dysfunction:* Signs of hypoperfusion become more evident including oliguria, altered mental status, or lactate levels rising to 2–4 mmol/L.

Classic Cardiogenic Shock

Classic CS represents the end-stage of this continuum, defined by severe hemodynamic instability and overt end-organ failure. Diagnostic criteria include:

- Systolic blood pressure (SBP) <90 mm Hg for >30 minutes (or need for vasopressors to maintain SBP >90 mm Hg).
- CI <1.8 L/min/m^2 (without support) or <2.2 L/min/m^2 (with support)
- Evidence of end-organ hypoperfusion (e.g., lactate >4 mmol/L, acute kidney injury, transaminitis, or altered mentation).[7]

In classic CS, the vicious cycle of myocardial ischemia, reduced CO, and systemic hypoperfusion leads to multiorgan failure. Refractory CS, a subset, is marked by persistent hypotension despite maximal medical and mechanical support, often with mortality approaching 80–90%.[8]

CLINICAL PRESENTATION ACROSS THE CONTINUUM

Preshock

Patients in the preshock state may present with subtle symptoms, often overshadowed by the underlying condition (e.g., AMI). Common symptoms include:

- Fatigue, dyspnea on exertion, or orthopnea
- Tachycardia and mild hypotension with SBP 90–100 mm Hg
- Normal or slightly cool extremities, with preserved urine output
- Echocardiographic evidence of reduced left ventricular ejection fraction (LVEF) or regional wall motion abnormalities

Early Cardiogenic Shock

With progress to early CS the symptoms and signs become more evident:

- Persistent tachycardia and hypotension (SBP 80–90 mm Hg)
- Cool, clammy extremities, and delayed capillary refill
- Reduced urine output (<0.5 mL/kg/h) and rising serum creatinine
- Pulmonary congestion (rales, elevated jugular venous pressure)
- Lactate levels of 2–4 mmol/L, indicating early tissue hypoxia

Classic Cardiogenic Shock

Patients in classic CS exhibit overt signs of hemodynamic collapse:

- Profound hypotension (SBP <80 mm Hg) and weak pulses
- Cyanosis, cold extremities, and mottled skin
- Severe oliguria or anuria, with acute kidney injury
- Altered mental status, ranging from confusion to obtundation
- Lactate >4 mmol/L, reflecting severe hypoperfusion

DIAGNOSTIC STRATEGIES

Early identification of patients along the CS continuum is critical for improving outcomes. Recognition of preshock and early CS prompting early intervention in these patients may offset development of overt CS. The patients may be triaged with the following diagnostic approaches:

Clinical Assessment

- *History and physical examination:* Identifying risk factors such as recent MI, HF history, and hypoperfusion presenting with cool extremities and altered mentation.
- *Vital signs monitoring:* Continuous monitoring of blood pressure, heart rate, and oxygen saturation to detect early hemodynamic changes.

Laboratory Markers

- *Serum lactate:* A key marker of tissue hypoxia, with levels >2 mmol/L indicate progression toward CS.
- *Troponins and BNP:* Elevated cardiac biomarkers suggest myocardial injury or stress.
- *Renal and hepatic panels:* Rising creatinine, transaminases, or bilirubin reflect end-organ dysfunction.

Imaging and Hemodynamic Monitoring

- *Echocardiography:* Assesses LV functions, wall motion abnormalities, and mechanical complications such as papillary muscle rupture or ventricular septal rupture.

TABLE 1: SCAI updated shock stages.

Stage	Description	Mortality (%)
A: At risk	No shock but at risk (e.g., large AMI)	3
B: Beginning (preshock)	Hemodynamic instability. No hypoperfusion	10
C: Classic	Hypoperfusion with or without hypotension	20–30
D: Deteriorating	Severe hypoperfusion requiring multiple vasopressors or mechanical circulatory support	40–50
E: Extremis	Persistent shock despite maximal support	60–80

(AMI: acute myocardial infarction; SCAI: Society for Cardiovascular Angiography and Interventions)

- *Pulmonary artery catheterization:* Provides direct measurement of CI, PCWP, and SVR, particularly in early or classic CS to guide therapy.[9]
- *Noninvasive hemodynamic monitoring:* Devices such as pulse contour analysis or bioreactance can estimate CO in preshock states.[1]

RISK STRATIFYING THE CONTINUUM OF CARDIOGENIC SHOCK

The Society for Cardiovascular Angiography and Interventions shock stages: The SCAI shock classification, updated in 2022, categorizes CS into five stages based on clinical, hemodynamic and laboratory parameters.[3] This framework has been validated across diverse cohorts, demonstrating its utility in risk stratification.[6] Key features are shown in **Table 1**.

CardShock risk score: Incorporates age, lactate, and prior MI to predict mortality risk in CS **(Table 2)**.[10]

TABLE 2: CardShock risk score for in hospital mortality in cardiogenic shock.

Variables	Score
Age > 75	1
Confusion at presentation	1
Previous MI/CABG	1
ACS etiology	1
LVEF < 40%	1
Blood lactate:	
• <2 mmol/L	0
• 2–4 mmol/L	1
• >4 mmol/L	2
eGFR:	
• >60 mL/min/1.73 m^2	0
• 30–60 mL/min/1.73 m^2	1
• <30 mL/min/1.73 m^2	2

Note: Low risk (0–3), mortality 8.7%; intermediate risk (4–5), mortality 36%; high risk (6–9), mortality 77%.

(LVEF: left ventricular ejection fraction; MI: myocardial infarction)

Phenotyping Cardiogenic Shock

The Society for Cardiovascular Angiography and Interventions shock staging is widely used in diagnosis and prognosis of CS. However, patients with CS have distinct phenotypes at presentation. These are associated with unique profiles and in-hospital mortality. Data from two international cohorts, Cardiogenic Shock Working Group Registry (subsets: CSWG-MI, CSWG-HF) and the Danish Retro-shock MI Registry (DRR) were analyzed and validated with machine learning approach. Accordingly, SCAI staging was done. Out of three distinct three phenotypes, the cardioembolic shock phenotype had the highest risk of evolving to further advance stages and mortality compared with other phenotypes of noncongested and cardiorenal.[11]

Further to clarify and categorize phenotypes along the continuum of pre/early CS to conventional Cs (SCAI stage C), CCU admissions (N: 28703) across 47 sites in USA from 2017 to 2023 were enrolled in the Critical Care Cardiology Trials Network Registry (CCCTN).[12] Four phenotypes were identified as detailed in **Table 3**.

The phenotypes in the continuum from preshock to classical CCCTN registry showed stepwise increase in mortality. One-third of patients with isolated hypotension proceeded to overt CS. Higher mortality rates were observed in normotensive CS, a distinct CS phenotype, and those with HF with isolated hypotension in comparison to isolated low CO. Therefore, contrary to standard definitions of CS, the presence of hypoperfusion alone is marker for higher mortality in absence of hypotension. Conversely, patients with low CO with no clinical evidence of hypoperfusion are at substantial risk for clinical deterioration.[12]

SCAI 3-axis Model

The 3-axis model of CS is a multidimensional framework introduced in the 2022 update to the SCAI-SHOCK classification system. It integrates three key dimensions, shock severity (SCAI stages A–E), clinical phenotypes (AMI-CS, HF-CS), and risk modifiers (cardiac arrest with coma, age, lactate, and frailty) to enhance risk stratification, prognostication, and treatment decisions in CS. It is essential

TABLE 3: CS phenotypes in CCCTN registry.

Phenotype	Isolated low CO	HF with isolated hypotension	Normotensive CS	SCAI stages C CS
	• Hemodynamics in <24 hours • CI <2.2 L/min without MCS • No hypoperfusion by laboratory	• Hypotension without shock • Admission diagnosis of heart failure • No hypoperfusion	• MAP >60 mm Hg (or SBP >90 mm Hg) without vasoactive or MCS • Hypoperfusion by laboratories	• Site reported CS • Need for one vasoactive or MCS device • Hypoperfusion by laboratories
Mortality	3.6%	11.0%	17.0%	24.0%
Preshock	←		→	Shock

(CCCTN: Critical Care Cardiology Trials Network; CO: cardiac output; CS: cardiogenic shock; HF: heart failure; MCS: mechanical circulatory support; SBP: systolic blood pressure; SCAI: Society for Cardiovascular Angiography and Interventions)

to differentiate a patient who is "high risk" due to severe shock with poor hemodynamics from a patient who is "high risk" due to nonmodifiable risk factors for mortality.[3] Established and emerging biomarkers may further refine risk stratification. The model was developed to address the heterogeneity of CS patients and improve clinical communication and trial design.

The 2025 ACC Expert Consensus Statement on the Evaluation and Management of Cardiogenic Shock provides comprehensive, evidence-based recommendations for the evaluation and management of CS. This document, endorsed by the American College of Cardiology, integrates the 2022, SCAI-SHOCK classification (Stages A–E), recent data from DanGer Shock trial,[13] and real-world evidence from registries like the CCCTN.[12] It emphasizes early recognition, multidisciplinary care, and tailored interventions across the CS continuum from preshock to classic CS. The guidelines complement the SCAI staging system by providing actionable protocols for clinical practice.[14]

ACC 2025 GUIDELINES FOR EVALUATION AND MANAGEMENT OF CARDIOGENIC SHOCK

The ACC guidance prioritizes rapid and accurate assessment to confirm CS, determines its severity, and identifies the underlying phenotype, AMI-CS, and HF-CS. Key evaluation strategies include:

Point-of-Care Ultrasound

- Recommended within 6 hours of presentation to differentiate CS from other shock types (e.g., hypovolemic and distributive) and identify etiologies (e.g., left ventricular dysfunction, right ventricular failure, and tamponade).
- Assesses left ventricular ejection fraction (LVEF <40% indicates severe dysfunction), RV function, and valvular abnormalities.

Hemodynamic Monitoring

- Pulmonary artery catheters (PACs) are strongly recommended for SCAI stages C–E to measure CI <2.2 L/min/m², PCWP > 15 mm Hg, and central venous pressure (CVP > 12 mm Hg).
- Early PAC use (within 6 hours) is associated with a 10–15% reduction in mortality by guiding therapy optimization.

Biomarkers

- Measure lactate (hypoperfusion >2 mmol/L; severe >4 mmol/L) every 2–4 hours to assess severity and treatment response.
- Additional markers such as NT-proBNP, IL-6, cystatin C, and adrenomedullin enhance prognostication, particularly in HF-CS.

SCAI Staging

- Use the 2022 SCAI classification stages A–E as shown in **Table 1**.
- Reassess every 12–24 hours to detect progression as 42.3% of stage B progress to stage C within 24 hours.

Management Strategies by SCAI Stage

The ACC guidance provides stage-specific recommendations, emphasizing multidisciplinary shock teams, and timely escalation of care.

Stage A (At Risk)

Optimize guideline-directed medical therapy (GDMT) for underlying conditions. There is need to address risk factors (glycemic control and fluid status) to prevent progression. In large AMI, it is imperative to start GDMT and prepare for possible PCI.

Stage B (Beginning/Preshock)

- Administer cautious fluids (e.g., 200 mL saline over 15–30 minutes), if no pulmonary edema
- Initiate low-dose inotropes (e.g., dobutamine 2–5 μg/kg/min), if CI remains low

- Early shock team consultation to plan potential escalation.[1]

Stage C (Classic/Early CS)

- Start norepinephrine (0.05–0.5 μg/kg/min) for hypotension, preferred over dopamine due to lower arrhythmia risk
- Consider early MCS (e.g., Impella CP for AMI-CS), if lactate >2 mmol/L or persistent hypotension after 1–2 hours of vasopressors
- For AMI-CS, prioritize culprit-lesion-only PCI within 90 minutes (38% mortality vs. 63% with delayed/multivessel PCI)[15]
- Use noninvasive ventilation if respiratory distress is present.

Stage D (Deteriorating/Classic CS)

- Escalate to multiple vasopressors (norepinephrine + vasopressin) or MCS (e.g., Impella 5.0, VA-ECMO) based on center expertise
- Transfer to high-volume level ICUs, associated with 15–20% lower mortality
- For HF-CS, consider inotropes (e.g., milrinone) alongside MCS to address congestion
- Mechanical ventilation for 78–88% of patients with respiratory failure

Stage E (Extremis)

- Evaluate for advanced MCS (VA-ECMO, biventricular support) or heart transplantation in eligible patients
- May initiate early palliative care discussions, as given mortality is >80%.
- Need to limit futile interventions in patients with irreversible organ damage.

Multidisciplinary Care

- *Shock teams:* Multidisciplinary shock teams combining cardiologists, intensivists, and surgeons have been shown to improve survival by 10–15% in stage B–E by streamlining decision-making and MCS deployment.
- *Regional systems:* Transfer stage D–E patients to level I ICUs with MCS and transplant capabilities, reducing mortality by 15–20% compared to low-volume centers.
- *Protocolized care:* Use standardized algorithms (e.g., lactate-guided vasopressor titration, PAC-driven MCS decisions) to reduce variability.

Mechanical Circulatory Support

- *Impella:* Preferred for AMI-CS in stages C–D, with a 12.7% mortality reduction at 180 days[13]
- *VA-ECMO:* Considered for stage D–E refractory shock, but no 30-day mortality benefit seen in ECLS-SHOCK, 2023 with increased bleeding risk[16]
- *Intra-aortic balloon pump (IABP):* No survival benefit (IABP-SHOCK II, 2020), but stabilizes pre-PCI patients[17]

EMERGING TRENDS AND FUTURE DIRECTIONS

Recent research emphasizes the importance of early recognition and intervention in the CS continuum. Advances include:

- Ongoing studies such as PACCS (NCT05485376) for PAC efficacy and LevoHeartShock (NCT04020263) for levosimendan are highlighted[18,19]
- *Biomarker-guided therapy:* Novel biomarkers, such as sST2, microRNAs, DPP3, and adrenomedullin may improve risk stratification in preshock states[20]
- *Artificial intelligence:* Machine learning models integrating hemodynamic, laboratory, and imaging data are being developed to predict progression to CS[9]
- *Phenotyping:* Machine learning-based phenotyping (e.g., Zweck's noncongested, cardiorenal, and cardiometabolic) enhances personalized care[11]

CONCLUSION

The continuum from preshock to classic CS represents a spectrum of increasing hemodynamic compromise and end-organ dysfunction. Early recognition of preshock states, guided by clinical assessment, biomarkers, and hemodynamic monitoring, allows for timely interventions that can halt progression. Management strategies must be tailored to the stage of shock, ranging from optimization of preload and revascularization in preshock to advanced MCS and multiorgan support in classic CS. Ongoing research and technological advancements hold to promise for further improving outcomes in this high-risk population. Clinicians must remain vigilant, leveraging both established tools and emerging innovations to navigate this complex and dynamic continuum effectively.

REFERENCES

1. Chioncel O, Parissis J, Mebazaa A, et al. Epidemiology, pathophysiology and contemporary management of cardiogenic shock – a position statement from the Heart Failure Association of the European Society of Cardiology. Eur J Heart Fail. 2020;22(8):1315-41.
2. Shah KS, O'Malley C, Kapur NK, et al. Cardiogenic shock 2025: understanding real world outcomes and contemporary practice to help guide improvements in care. Am Heart J Plus. 2025;53:100493.
3. Naidu SS, Baran DA, Jentzer JC, et al. SCAI SHOCK Stage Classification Expert Consensus Update: A Review and Incorporation of Validation Studies. J Soc Cardiovasc Angiogr Interv. 2022;1(1):100008.

4. Berg DD, Bohula EA, van Diepen S, et al. Epidemiology of Shock in Contemporary Cardiac Intensive Care Units: Data From the Critical Care Cardiology Trials Network Registry. Circ Cardiovasc Qual Outcomes. 2019;12(3):e005618.
5. Aissaoui N, Puymirat E, Delmas C, et al. Trends in cardiogenic shock complicating acute myocardial infarction. Eur J Heart Fail. 2020;22(4):664-72.
6. Jentzer JC, van Diepen S, Barsness GW, et al. Cardiogenic Shock Classification to Predict Mortality in the Cardiac Intensive Care Unit. J Am Coll Cardiol. 2019;74(17):2117-28.
7. Jentzer JC, Kashani KB, Wiley BM, et al. Laboratory markers of acidosis and mortality in cardiogenic shock: developing a definition of hemometabolic shock. Shock. 2022;57(1):31-40.
8. Fisher T, Hill N, Kalakoutas A, et al. Prognostic factors associated with mortality in cardiogenic shock: a systematic review and meta-analysis. Crit Care. 2024;28(1):192.
9. Mehta A, Vavilin I, Nguyen AH, et al. Contemporary approach to cardiogenic shock care: a state-of-the-art review. Front Cardiovasc Med. 2024;11:1354158.
10. Harjola VP, Lassus J, Sionis A, et al. Clinical picture and risk prediction of short-term mortality in cardiogenic shock. Eur J Heart Fail. 2017;17(5):501-9.
11. Zweck E, Thayer KL, Helgestad OKL, et al. Phenotyping cardiogenic shock. J Am Heart Assoc. 2021;10(14):e020085.
12. Patel SM, Berg DD, Bohula EA, et al. Continuum of Preshock to Classic Cardiogenic Shock in the Critical Care Cardiology Trials Network Registry. JACC Heart Fail. 2024;12(9):1553-62.
13. Møller JE, Engstrøm T, Jensen LO, et al. Microaxial flow pump or standard care in infarct-related cardiogenic shock. N Engl J Med. 2024;390(15):1382-93.
14. Sinha SS, Morrow DA, Kapur NK, et al. 2025 Concise clinical guidance: an ACC expert consensus statement on the evaluation and management of cardiogenic shock: a report of the American College of Cardiology Solution Set Oversight Committee. J Am Coll Cardiol. 2025;85(16):1618-41.
15. Jung C, Wernly B, Masyuk M, et al. A Bayesian reanalysis of the CULPRIT-SHOCK trial. Eur Heart J Acute Cardiovasc Care. 2024;13(10):701-8.
16. Thiele H, Zeymer U, Akin I, et al. Extracorporeal life support in infarct-related cardiogenic shock. N Engl J Med. 2023;389(14):1286-97.
17. Thiele H, Zeymer U, Thelemann N, et al. Intra-aortic balloon pump in cardiogenic shock complicating acute myocardial infarction: Long-term 6-year outcome of the randomized IABP-SHOCK II trial. Circulation. 2020;142(20):1886-96.
18. ClinicalTrials.gov. (2025). Pulmonary Artery Catheter in Cardiogenic Shock Trial (PACCS). [online] Available from https://clinicaltrials.gov/study/NCT05485376 [Last accessed October, 2025].
19. ClinicalTrials.gov. (2025). Effect of Early Use of Levosimendan Versus Placebo on Top of a Conventional Strategy of Inotrope Use on a Combined Morbidity-mortality Endpoint in Patients With Cardiogenic Shock (LevoHeartShock). [online] Available from https://clinicaltrials.gov/study/NCT04020263?tab=history [Last accessed October, 2025].
20. Ceglarek U, Schellong P, Thiele H, et al. Biomarker-based mortality risk score in patients with acute myocardial infarction and cardiogenic shock: the CLIP score. Eur Heart J. 2020;41(Suppl_2):ehaa946.

CHAPTER

34

Triaging of Patients of Acute Decompensated Heart Failure

Pranab Jyoti Bhattacharyya, Maitreyee Bhattacharyya

ABSTRACT

Acute decompensated heart failure (ADHF) is one of the most common causes of hospitalization in the elderly and is significantly associated with frequent hospital readmissions along with increased morbidity and mortality. Although guidelines focus on the latest means to diagnose and treat acute and chronic heart failure patients, strategies to triage patients with ADHF presenting to the emergency department (ED) are lacking. This often leads to unnecessary hospital admissions and at times early disposition of the patient, which can lead to frequent readmissions.

Keywords: Triaging, acute decompensated heart failure.

INTRODUCTION

Acute decompensated heart failure (ADHF) is one of the most common causes of hospitalization in patients >65 years of age.[1] It is defined as new onset or recurrence of symptoms and signs of heart failure requiring urgent or emergency therapy resulting in unscheduled care or hospitalization.[2,3] It frequently presents as an acute decompensation of chronic HF and less frequently as the first manifestation of HF.[4] ADHF results in unplanned hospital admissions and is associated with high morbidity and mortality including frequent hospital readmissions.[1]

A variety of overlapping terms have been used to characterize acute heart failure namely "acute heart failure syndromes" (AHFS), "acute decompensated heart failure" (ADHF), "acute decompensation of chronic heart failure" (ADCHF), "worsening heart failure" (WHF), and "hospitalization for heart failure" (HHF).[3]

EPIDEMIOLOGY

The prevalence of HF in India is around 1% of the population;[5] the exact incidence of HF in India is not clear and is estimated to be between 1.3 and 23 million, mostly attributed to coronary artery disease, obesity, diabetes mellitus, and rheumatic heart disease.[6] Posthospitalization events including death and readmission account for 27.3% among HF patients in India.[7] Compliance to guideline-directed medical therapy is low, which frequently leads to acute decompensation and poor outcomes.[8]

In-hospital mortality of ADHF ranges from 4 to 7% in the Western world, with 6-month adverse event rates of around 35%.[9-12] Data from India is scarce. Few Indian studies and trials suggest a 6-month mortality rate of around 10% for patients with ADHF.[13] The AFAR study (Acute Failure Registry Study) that focused on the epidemiology of ADHF in India found high rates of in-hospital and 6-month mortality as well rehospitalization at 6 months (30.8%, 26.3%, and 39.5%, respectively), which reflects the seriousness of this condition and the need for prompt triaging to salvage these patients.[14]

IMPORTANCE OF TRIAGING

Since ADHF has been associated with high morbidity and mortality rates, it is important to triage these patients in order to manage them effectively.

Although numerous advances have been made in the diagnosis and management of patients with chronic HF, strategies for triaging and management of patients with ADHF in the ED are scarce due to lack of well-designed clinical trials. Most of these patients visit hospitals and are subsequently admitted for congestive symptoms, and less commonly for respiratory failure, ventricular tachyarrhythmias, and urgent diagnostic or therapeutic procedures. Despite that fact that over 80–90% of the patients with ADHF are admitted, <10% have acute life-threatening illness.[15] This again highlights the importance of having a strategic plan to effectively triage and manage them.

Triaging should start immediately once the patient comes into medical contact, be it prehospital or in the ED. A brief history taking followed by clinical examination and necessary laboratory investigations along with electrocardiography, chest radiography, and ultrasonography can help in identifying the high-risk patients. This helps in classifying patients into different subgroups, each subgroup having different management algorithm with simultaneous identification and management of potentially reversible causes and triggering events. The greatest challenge lies in admission to an intensive care unit (ICU), or a general hospital ward or home discharge after a short period of monitoring in the ED-dependent observation unit.

A simple way is to triage these patients presenting in the ED into three categories, namely immediate risk (measures of acute severity), intermediate risk (predictors of events through 30 days), and low risk **(Table 1)**.[15,16]

Due to time constraints while working in the ED, identification of certain high-risk features in ADHF patients can also help in swift triaging. These features include low blood pressure, ischemic electrocardiographic changes, impaired renal function, hyponatremia, and elevated cardiac biomarkers (troponin and natriuretic peptides).[17] A common strategy is to identify patients free of these "high-risk" features; such patients can be discharged from the ED after a brief period of observation.[17]

A quick bedside assessment of the patient can help in identification of the hemodynamic profile **(Flowchart 1)**.[3]

Congestion at rest is suggestive of elevated left-sided filling pressures whereas evidence of low perfusion pressure at rest is suggestive of predominant elevation of right-sided filling pressures. The most common hemodynamic profile encountered is the "warm and wet" profile (elevated or normal blood pressure).[3] The cold and wet profile is associated with clinical evidence of hypoperfusion namely reduced mentation, cool extremities, narrow pulse pressure, and reduced urine output.[3] **Flowchart 1** provides a quick and easy way to assess hemodynamic status of patients with ADHF at bedside and triage them accordingly.

Besides the risk categories mentioned above, few other factors should also be considered which further add to the morbidity and mortality in such patients. These include advanced age, frailty, number of previous heart failure hospitalizations, comorbidities (diabetes mellitus, liver disease, cancer, dementia, and chronic obstructive airway disease), known low left ventricular ejection fraction in heart failure with reduced ejection fraction (HFrEF) and associated right ventricular dysfunction.[15]

Addressing the factors that potentially trigger an episode of worsening heart failure is important. These include nonadherence to medical regimen, sodium or fluid restriction, consumption of medications that enhance sodium retention (NSAIDs, steroids, and thiazolidinediones), excessive alcohol intake or illicit drug use, infections, anemia, hypo- or hyperthyroidism, arrhythmias, uncontrolled hypertension, and acute myocardial ischemia.[15]

A risk stratification algorithm for patients with ADHF in the ED is provided in **Flowchart 2**.[3,15]

The "wet and warm" patient typically responds to diuretic and vasodilator therapy.[3] The "dry and warm" patient is managed with adjustment of oral therapy.[3] The "dry and cold" patient is hypoperfused and hypovolemic; fluid challenge followed by ionotropic support should be considered.[3] The "wet and cold" patient should be managed with ionotropic support and vasopressors if the systolic blood pressure (SBP) is <90 mm Hg.[3] Mechanical circulatory support should be provided if there is no response to pharmacologic therapy. Diuretics and vasodilators should be considered if the SBP is >90 mm Hg.[3]

Indicators of good response to initial therapy that can be considered for discharge from ED observation unit include:[1,17]

- Patient-reported subjective improvement
- Resting heart rate <100 beats/min, respiratory rate <20 breaths/min
- Lack of orthostatic hypotension
- Adequate diuresis (urinary spot sodium ≥50–70 mEq/L after 2 hours or urine output ≥100–150 mL/hour after 6 hours)
- SpO_2> 95% in room air
- Decrease in body weight
- No significant alterations in renal function and electrolytes

TABLE 1: Predictors of risk in patients with ADHF in the ED.[3,15,16]

Risk category	Clinical and laboratory findings	Management
Immediate risk	Hypoxia, shock/hypoperfusion, respiratory distress, anuria, acute and worsening conditions (stroke, sepsis, ACS, and arrhythmia)	Needs immediate medical attention with admission to ICU
Intermediate risk	New-onset HF, low BP without shock or hypoperfusion, tachycardia, renal dysfunction, hyponatremia, hepatic dysfunction, elevated cardiac troponin (without ACS), and degree of BNP elevation	Needs immediate medical attention with admission to ICU/ward
Lower risk	Normal BP and HR, brisk response to initial IV diuretic, rapid resolution of symptoms in the ED, normal renal and liver function, normal cardiac biomarkers (BNP and cardiac troponin)	Observation in ED

(ACS: acute coronary syndrome; ADHF: Acute decompensated heart failure; BNP: Brain natriuretic peptide; BP: blood pressure; ED: emergency department; HF: heart failure; HR: heart rate; IV: intravenous)

- Absence of acute triggers (e.g., sepsis, acute coronary syndrome, and arrhythmias)

In recent years, numerous risk scores have been developed to successfully triage ADHF patients presenting in ED. Few commonly used are enumerated here.

- *Heart failure triage scale (HFTS)*:[18] It has four decision points—basic criteria, high-risk criteria, ECG criteria, and low-risk criteria to triage ADHF patients into levels 1, 2, 3, and 4, respectively.[18] Level 1 refers to immediate (life threatening, critical), level 2 is emergency (could become life threatening), level 3 is urgent (not life threatening), and level 4 is nonurgent (not life threatening). The HFTS is described in **Flowchart 3**.
- *HEARTRISK6 Scale*:[19] Has six variables, with scores ranging from 0 to 12, which helps triaging ADHF patients into 3 categories (low: score 0–1, medium: 2–5, and high: 6 to ≥10).[19] It predicts short-term serious outcomes.
  - History of valvular heart disease (moderate or severe from prior cardiology or imaging notes): Score 1
  - *Heart rate*: ≥100 to <120 beats/min—score 2 ≥120 beats/min—score 3
  - Treated with noninvasive ventilation (treated with BiPAP within 1 hour of initial assessment): score 2
  - *Creatinine*: ≥150 to <300 μmol/L—score 2 ≥300 μmol/L—score 3
  - *Troponin*: ≥3× or 4× upper reference level—score 1 ≥5× upper reference level—score 2
  - *Failed reassessment after ED treatment*: Resting vital signs abnormal (SaO_2 <90% on room air or usual O_2, or heart rate ≥110 beats/min, or respiratory rate ≥28 breaths/min) *or* unable to start or complete 3-minute walk test—score 1

The high-risk patients should be immediately admitted while the more low-risk patients can be safely discharged.[19]

Congestion at rest
No
Yes
Evidence of low perfusion at rest
No
Yes
Warm and dry
Warm and wet
Cold and dry
Cold and wet

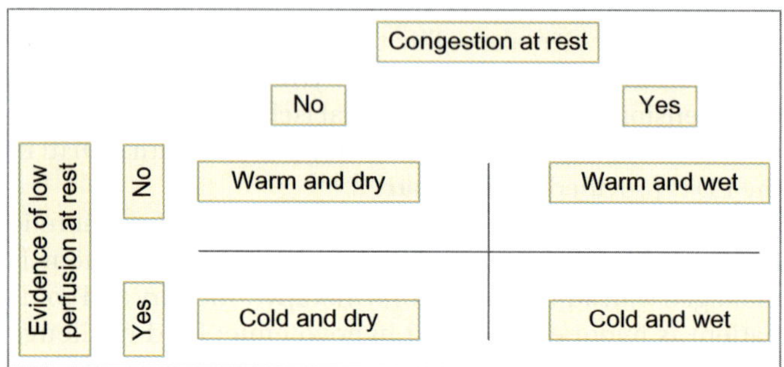

FLOWCHART 1: Assessment of hemodynamic profile of ADHF patients.

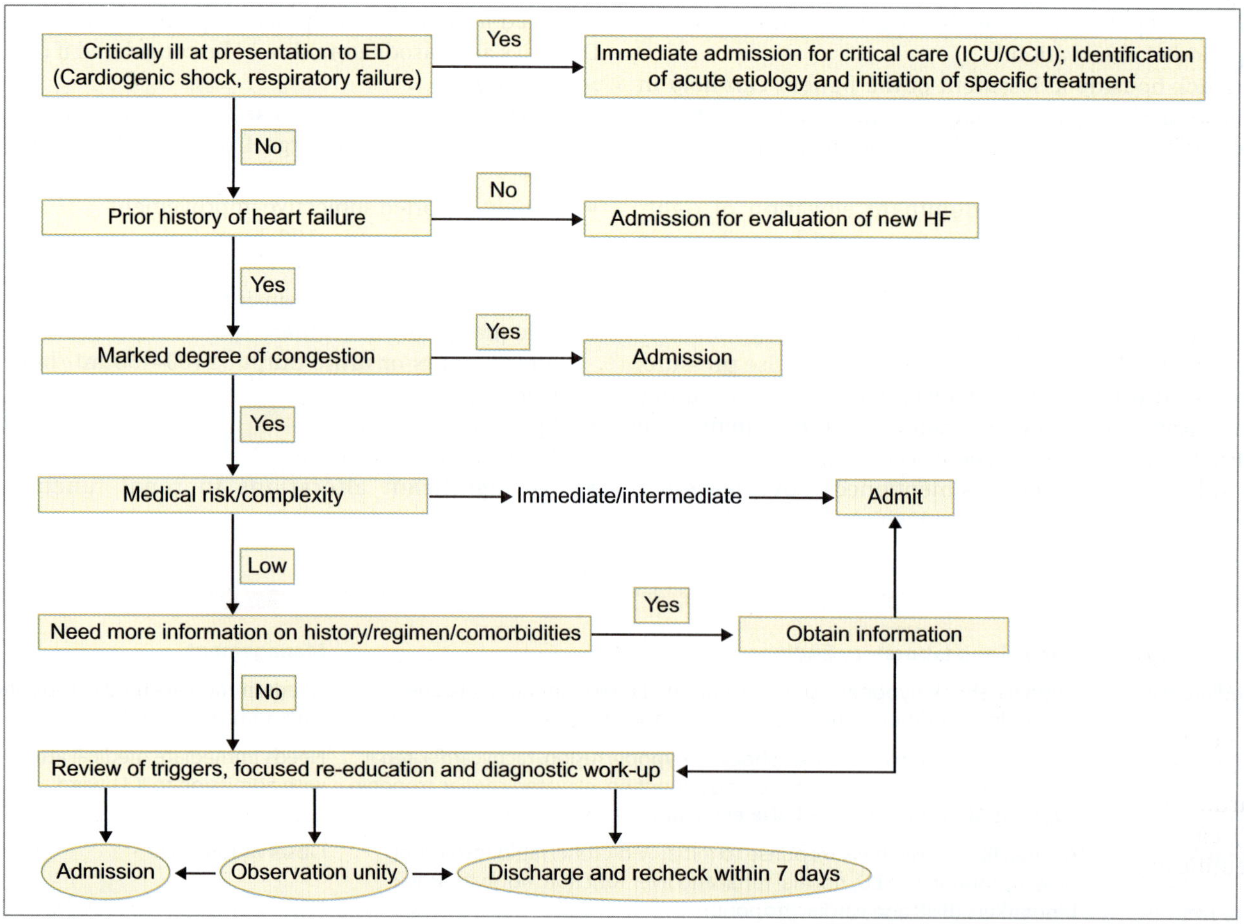

Critically ill at presentation to ED (Cardiogenic shock, respiratory failure)
Yes
Immediate admission for critical care (ICU/CCU); Identification of acute etiology and initiation of specific treatment
No
Prior history of heart failure
No
Admission for evaluation of new HF
Yes
Marked degree of congestion
Yes
Admission
Yes
Medical risk/complexity
Immediate/intermediate
Admit
Low
Need more information on history/regimen/comorbidities
Yes
Obtain information
No
Review of triggers, focused re-education and diagnostic work-up
Admission
Observation unity
Discharge and recheck within 7 days

FLOWCHART 2: Risk stratification algorithm for ADHF patients.

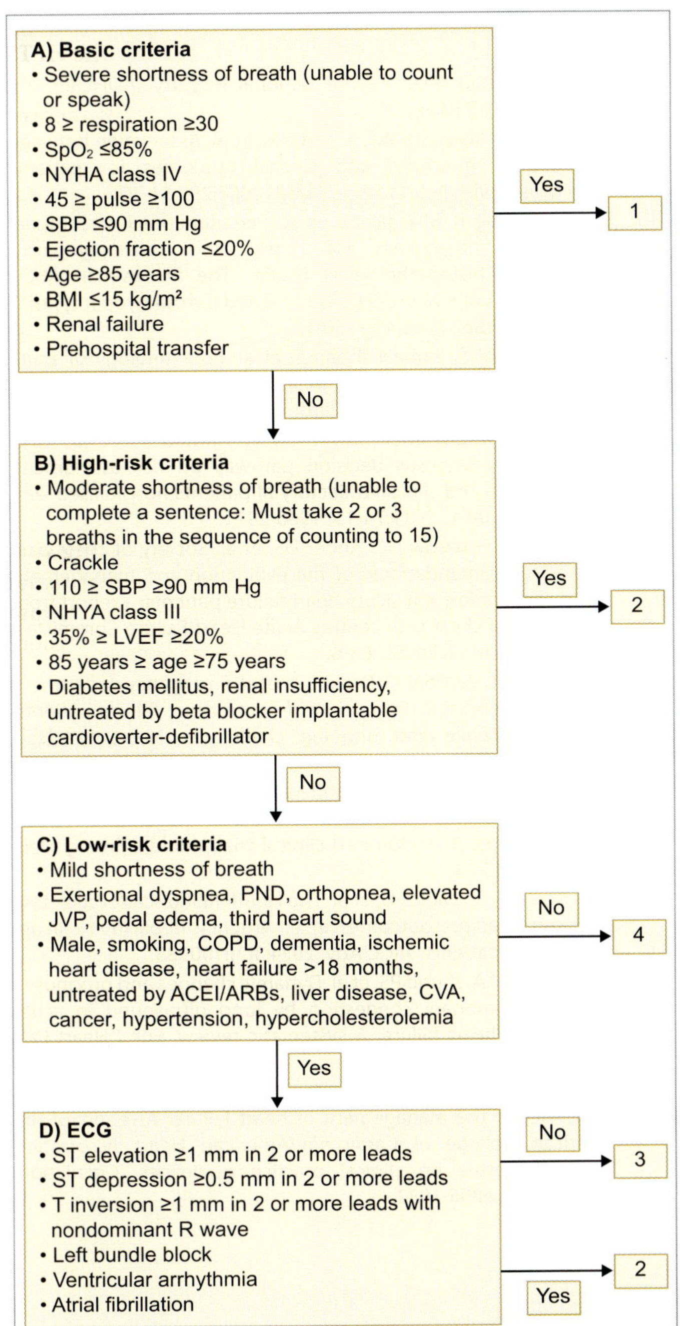

FLOWCHART 3: The heart failure triage scale.

In addition to the triaging scores mentioned above, the Emergency Heart Failure Mortality Risk Grade (EHMRG), EHMRG30-ST, Ottawa Heart Failure Risk Scale (OHFRS), Multiple Estimation of risk based on the Emergency department Spanish Score in patients with AHF (MEESSI-AHF) can also be used to stratify patients with ADHF presenting in the ED.[17]

Role of imaging in triaging ADHF patients: Echocardiography and lung ultrasound (LUS) may be useful for initial evaluation of ADHF patients and also for monitoring treatment.[17] Immediate echocardiography is recommended in the initial evaluation of ADHF patients, which are hemodynamically unstable.[17] In a systematic review of studies, LUS was used to detect the dynamic changes of pulmonary congestion (expressed as the number of B-lines) and correlate it with heart failure prognosis.[20] In ADHF patients, the detection of >15 B-lines on a 28-zone LUS was found to be associated with an increased risk of adverse outcomes, including HF readmission or death.[20] Hence, LUS is a potential tool to stratify these patients as well as monitor response to therapy. However, few other studies carried out in the ED on ADHF patients have failed to demonstrate any usefulness of LUS in risk stratification.[17] ED-based large trials are warranted to determine the usefulness of LUS.

CONSIDERATIONS FOR DISCHARGE OF PATIENTS HOSPITALIZED FOR ADHF

The following factors should be considered for discharging hospitalized ADHF patients[3]:

- All triggering factors addressed
- Optimal volume status achieved
- Successful transition from intravenous to oral diuretic therapy
- No intravenous vasodilator or inotropic therapy for 24 hours
- Optimal GDMT achieved; regimen stable for 24 hours prior to discharge
- Cessation of smoking initiated
- Adequate ambulation achieved

What do the guidelines say? ACC/AHA/HFSA and the European Guidelines on acute and chronic heart failure offer excellent guidance on the diagnosis and management of patients with acute and chronic heart failure, but very little on the methods of triaging and disposition of patients with ADHF in the ED.[4,21] Guidelines for early and efficient triaging of these patients are of utmost importance to prevent unnecessary admissions to the ICU/ward and safely discharge the low-risk patients.

CONCLUSION

Acute decompensated heart failure is one of the most common causes of hospitalization in individuals >65 years of age. It contributes to significant morbidity and mortality including hospital readmissions among patients with heart failure. Although advances have been made in understanding the pathophysiology and making a diagnosis of heart failure, there are no clear-cut guidelines in triaging patients with ADHF who come to the ED. Various algorithms and risk scores are available which do help in the risk stratification of these patients, but the development of a universal algorithm to efficiently triage and dispose patients with ADHF is the need of the hour.

REFERENCES

1. Mauro C, Chianese S, Cocchia R, et al. Acute Heart Failure: Diagnostic-Therapeutic Pathways and Preventive Strategies—A Real-World Clinician's Guide. J Clin Med. 2023;12:846.
2. Bozkurt B, Coats AJS, Tsutsui H, et al. Universal definition and classification of heart failure: A report of the Heart Failure Society of America, Heart Failure Association of the European Society of Cardiology, Japanese Heart Failure Society and Writing Committee of the Universal definition of Heart Failure: Endorsed by the Canadian Heart Failure Failure Society, Heart Failure association of India, Cardiac Society of Australia and New Zealand, and Chinese Heart Failure Association. Eur J Heart Fail. 2021;23:352-80.
3. Felker GM, Teerlink JR. Diagnosis and management of acute heart failure. In: Zipes DP, Libby P, Bonow R, et al (Eds). Braunwald's Heart Disease a textbook of Cardiovascular Medicine, 12th edition. Philadelphia, PA: Elsevier; 2021. pp. 946-74.
4. McDonagh TA, Metra M, Adamo M, et al. 2021 ESC guidelines for the diagnosis and treatment of acute and chronic heart failure. Eur Heart J. 2021;42:3599-726.
5. Chaturvedi V, Parakh N, Seth S, et al. Heart failure in India: the INDUS study. J Pract Cardiovasc Sci. 2016;2:28-35.
6. Kaul U, Das MK, Agarwal R, et al. Consensus and development of document or management of stabilised acute decompensated heart failure with reduced ejection fraction in India. Indian Heart J. 2020;72:477-81.
7. Sharma A, Gopichandran L, Seth S. A randomised control to assess the effectiveness of structured discharge counselling on heart failure outcomes. J Pract Cardiovasc Sci. 2018;4(2):102-4.
8. Seth S, Ramakrishnan S, Parekh N, et al. Heart failure guidelines for India: update 2017. J Pract Cardiovasc Sci. 2017;3:133-8.
9. Gheorghiade M, Zannad F, Sopko G, et al. Acute heart failure syndromes: Current state and framework for future research. Circulation. 2005;112:3958-68.
10. Fonarow GC, Abraham WT, Albert NM, et al. Influence of a performance-improvement initiative on quality of care for patients hospitalized with heart failure: Results of the Organized Program to Initiate Lifesaving Treatment in Hospitalized Patients With Heart Failure (OPTIMIZE-HF). Arch Intern Med. 2007;167:1493-502.
11. Fonarow GC, Heywood JT, Heidenreich PA, et al.; ADHERE Scientific Advisory Committee and Investigators. Temporal trends in clinical characteristics, treatments, and outcomes for heart failure hospitalizations, 2002 to 2004: Findings from Acute Decompensated Heart Failure National Registry (ADHERE). Am Heart J. 2007;153:1021-8.
12. Fonarow GC, Abraham WT, Albert NM, et al. Association between performance measures and clinical outcomes for patients hospitalized with heart failure. JAMA. 2007;297:61-70.
13. Seth S, Narang R, Bhargava B, et al. Percutaneous intracoronary cellular cardiomyoplasty for nonischemic cardiomyopathy: Clinical and histopathological results: The first-in-man ABCD (Autologous Bone Marrow Cells in Dilated Cardiomyopathy) trial. J Am Coll Cardiol. 2006;48:2350-1.
14. Seth S, Khanal S, Ramakrishnan S, et al. Epidemiology of acute decompensated heart failure in India: The AFAR study (Acute failure registry study). J Pract Cardiovasc Sci. 2015;1:35-8.
15. Hollenberg SM, Warner Stevenson L, Ahmad T, et al. 2019 ACC Expert consensus decision pathway on risk assessment, management, and clinical trajectory of patients hospitalised with heart failure. JACC. 2019;74(15):1966-2011.
16. Peacock WF, Fonarow GC, Ander DS, et al. Society of chest pain centres recommendations for the evaluation and management of the observation stay acute heart failure patients: a report from the Society of chest pain centres Acute Heart Failure Committee. Crit Pathw Cardiol. 2008;7:83-6.
17. Fountoulaki K, Ventoulis I, Drokou A, et al. Emergency department risk assessment and disposition of acute heart failure patients: existing evidence and ongoing challenges. Heart Fail Rev. 2023;28(4):781-93.
18. Pouyamehr A, Mirhaghi A, Sharifi MD, et al. Comparison between Emergency Severity Index and Heart Failure Triage Scale in heart failure patients: A randomised clinical trial. World J Emerg Med. 2019;10(4):215-21.
19. Stiell IG, Perry JJ, Eagles D, et al. The HEARTRISK6 scale: Predicting short-term serious outcomes in emergency department acute heart failure patients. JACC Adv. 2024;3(7):100988.
20. Platz E, Merz AA, Jhund PS, et al. Dynamic changes and prognostic value of pulmonary congestion by lung ultrasound in acute and chronic heart failure: A systematic review. Eur J Heart Fail. 2017;19(9):1154-63.
21. Heidenreich PA, Bozkurt B, Aguilar D, et al. 2022 ACC/AHA/HFSA Guideline for the management of heart failure: A report of the American College of Cardiology/American Heart Association Joint committee on clinical practice guidelines. Circulation. 2022;145(18):e895-1032.

CHAPTER 35

Gut Hypothesis of Heart Failure: Role of Gut Microbiota–Derived Metabolites

Puneet Rastogi

ABSTRACT

The gut–heart axis links intestinal microbiota alterations with heart failure pathogenesis. Dysbiosis, barrier dysfunction, and metabolites such as TMAO, SCFAs, and uremic toxins influence inflammation, metabolism, and neurohormonal activity. Emerging studies highlight their prognostic significance and therapeutic potential through dietary modulation, probiotics, and metabolite-targeting strategies, offering novel mechanistic and clinical perspectives in heart failure management.

Keywords: Gut–heart axis, microbiota, heart failure, TMAO, SCFAs, dysbiosis, intestinal barrier, inflammation, probiotics, metabolic modulation.

INTRODUCTION

Heart failure (HF) remains a major cause of morbidity and mortality worldwide. Despite advances in pharmacologic and device therapies, prognosis remains poor, and novel mechanisms are increasingly investigated to explain residual risk. One emerging paradigm is the *gut–heart axis*, which refers to the bidirectional communication between gut microbiota and cardiovascular function.[1-3]

Alterations in gut microbial composition (dysbiosis), intestinal barrier dysfunction, and shifts in microbial metabolites such as *trimethylamine N-oxide (TMAO)*, *short-chain fatty acids (SCFAs)*, and *uremic toxins* have been implicated in HF pathophysiology.[1,4-6] These mechanisms influence systemic inflammation, neurohormonal activation, oxidative stress, and endothelial function.[3,7,8]

This chapter synthesizes mechanistic evidence, clinical studies, therapeutic trials, biomarker data, and safety considerations.

GUT MICROBIOTA IN HEART FAILURE

Microbial Dysbiosis in Heart Failure

Patients with HF demonstrate consistent changes in gut microbial ecology. Studies show reduced microbial diversity, depletion of beneficial *SCFA-producing taxa* such as *Faecalibacterium prausnitzii*, and enrichment of proinflammatory or pathogenic bacteria.[4,9,10] Pasini et al.[4] reported that HF patients harbored greater proportions of gram-negative species and reduced commensals compared with healthy controls, indicating a shift toward a proinflammatory gut environment.

Drivers of dysbiosis in HF are multifactorial. *Intestinal hypoperfusion* due to reduced cardiac output, *venous congestion* causing bowel wall edema, and *polypharmacy* (including antibiotics, proton pump inhibitors, and diuretics) all disrupt microbial communities.[5,9] Furthermore, *dietary patterns* low in fiber and high in processed foods reduce SCFA production.[6] Comorbidities such as *chronic kidney disease (CKD)* and *type 2 diabetes* exacerbate dysbiosis and contribute to metabolic dysfunction.[5,11]

Pathophysiologic Consequences of Dysbiosis

Dysbiosis contributes to HF progression through several mechanisms:

- *Metabolic dysregulation:* A shift toward bacteria capable of metabolizing dietary choline and carnitine leads to increased trimethylamine (TMA) production, which is converted to TMAO in the liver. Elevated TMAO has been shown to worsen cardiovascular outcomes.[1,2,7] Meanwhile, reduced SCFA-producing bacteria deprive the host of beneficial metabolites essential for barrier integrity, immune regulation, and energy metabolism.[6,8]

- *Barrier dysfunction:* Gut wall edema and ischemia disrupt epithelial integrity, allowing bacterial products such as lipopolysaccharides (LPS) to enter the systemic circulation.[9] Biomarkers including *intestinal fatty acid-binding protein (I-FABP)* and *zonulin* correlate with disease severity and congestion in HF patients.[9,11]
- *Immune activation:* Bacterial translocation activates innate immune signaling pathways such as toll-like receptors (TLRs), promoting cytokine release and systemic low-grade inflammation.[3,12] Chronic inflammation contributes to myocardial remodeling, fibrosis, and reduced contractility.
- *Neurohormonal interplay:* Microbial metabolites such as TMAO interact with neurohormonal systems including the renin–angiotensin–aldosterone system (RAAS) and sympathetic nervous system, further driving sodium retention, vasoconstriction, and hypertrophy.[7,13]

Together, these mechanisms highlight the central role of the gut–heart axis in HF pathophysiology.

MICROBIAL METABOLITES AND THEIR RELEVANCE

Trimethylamine N-oxide

Trimethylamine N-oxide is produced by hepatic flavin monooxygenase-3 (FMO3) from microbially generated TMA, itself derived from dietary choline, carnitine, and phosphatidylcholine.[1,2] Tang et al.[1] demonstrated that higher plasma TMAO levels independently predicted long-term mortality in HF patients, even after adjustment for renal function and natriuretic peptides. A meta-analysis by Li et al.[2] confirmed that elevated TMAO levels are strongly associated with mortality and rehospitalization in HF, with hazard ratios ~1.8 across pooled cohorts. Mechanistically, TMAO enhances platelet hyperreactivity, promotes vascular inflammation, and accelerates myocardial fibrosis.[7]

Short-chain Fatty Acids

Short-chain fatty acids (acetate, propionate, and butyrate) are produced by microbial fermentation of dietary fibers. They maintain gut barrier integrity, modulate immune responses through G-protein coupled receptors (e.g., GPR41 and GPR43), and provide an energy source for colonocytes.[6,8] In HF, reduced SCFA levels correlate with dysbiosis and worsened outcomes.[4,6] Palm et al.[6] showed that SCFA supplementation improves metabolic efficiency and reduces systemic inflammation in experimental models.

Bile Acid Metabolites

Gut microbiotas convert primary bile acids into secondary bile acids, which signal via receptors such as *FXR* and *TGR5*. Altered bile acid pools in HF affect lipid and glucose metabolism, vascular tone, and inflammatory status[3] Dysregulation of this signaling pathway contributes to the metabolic abnormalities commonly observed in HF patients.[12]

Uremic Toxins

Indoxyl sulfate and p-cresyl sulfate are microbial metabolites of tryptophan and tyrosine, respectively. They accumulate particularly in patients with combined HF and CKD.[5] These toxins promote oxidative stress, endothelial dysfunction, and myocardial fibrosis, worsening HF progression. Rohrmann et al.[5] reported that higher circulating levels of these toxins were associated with increased hospitalization and mortality.

CLINICAL EVIDENCE: ASSOCIATIONS AND PROGNOSTIC SIGNIFICANCE

Observational and Cohort Studies

Numerous studies since 2015 have examined gut-derived metabolites and markers in HF prognosis. Tang et al.[1] first demonstrated that elevated TMAO predicted 5-year mortality independent of natriuretic peptides. Suzuki et al.[14] extended these findings to acute HF, showing that high TMAO levels predicted rehospitalization and all-cause mortality. A meta-analysis of over 5,000 patients by Li et al.[2] confirmed the robust association between high TMAO and adverse outcomes across different HF populations.

Markers of gut barrier dysfunction also hold prognostic value. Mayerhofer et al.[9] reported that *I-FABP* and *zonulin* were elevated in HF patients, correlating with NYHA functional class and NT-proBNP levels. Kitai et al.[11] further demonstrated that circulating I-FABP predicted adverse outcomes in HFpEF patients, suggesting that gut barrier disruption plays a role across HF phenotypes.

Microbiome profiling studies highlight consistent alterations. Pasini et al. [4] documented reduced diversity and depletion of SCFA-producing taxa in HF compared with controls. Huang et al.[10] provided similar evidence in HFpEF, noting reduced abundance of *Faecalibacterium prausnitzii* and altered bile acid metabolism.

Translational and Mechanistic Studies

Animal studies lend mechanistic support. Germ-free mice receiving fecal microbiota transplantation (FMT) from HF patients develop impaired ventricular function and heightened systemic inflammation.[3] Conversely, SCFA supplementation improves cardiac remodeling in preclinical models.[6,8]

Summary of Evidence

Taken together, these findings suggest that both microbial metabolites (e.g., TMAO, SCFAs, and uremic toxins) and barrier dysfunction markers (e.g., I-FABP and zonulin) have diagnostic and prognostic value. Microbiome compositional changes are consistent across HF phenotypes, underscoring the central role of gut dysbiosis in disease progression.[2-4,9,10]

THERAPEUTIC APPROACHES

Dietary Modulation

Diet is one of the strongest modulators of the gut microbiota. High-fiber, plant-based diets promote SCFA-producing bacteria, improve barrier function, and reduce systemic inflammation.[6,8] Marques et al.[15] and subsequent reviews highlighted that increased dietary fiber can beneficially shift the gut microbiome, with potential impact on cardiovascular health. Clinical studies show that dietary interventions improve surrogate biomarkers such as NT-proBNP and inflammatory markers.[15]

Probiotics and Synbiotics

Several small randomized and pilot trials suggest that probiotics and synbiotics may improve outcomes in HF. Marques et al.[15] reported reduced NT-proBNP and CRP following 12 weeks of synbiotic therapy in HFrEF patients. Pasini et al.[4,16] observed increased SCFA levels and reduced inflammation with combined dietary fiber and probiotic supplementation. Cui et al.[17] conducted an RCT in HFpEF, demonstrating improved exercise tolerance and lower NT-proBNP after 8 weeks of synbiotic therapy. A Brazilian trial.[18] using inulin plus probiotics in HFrEF also reduced NT-proBNP and showed a trend toward improved LVEF. A meta-analysis by Kazemi et al.[19] confirmed modest reductions in inflammatory biomarkers with probiotic/synbiotic use.

Antibiotics and Microbial Enzyme Inhibitors

While broad-spectrum antibiotics are not a sustainable solution, targeted antibiotics such as rifaximin have been explored for reducing endotoxemia in HF.[3] Novel small-molecule inhibitors of microbial TMA lyases have also been developed, showing efficacy in reducing TMAO levels and improving vascular function in preclinical models.[7,20]

Fecal Microbiota Transplantation

Fecal microbiota transplantation has been trialed in metabolic syndrome and insulin resistance but remains experimental in HF.[12] Concerns include safety, donor screening, and long-term ecological consequences. Nonetheless, mechanistic animal studies demonstrate that FMT from healthy donors can improve cardiac remodeling and reduce systemic inflammation.[3,8]

Engineered Microbiota and Next-generation Therapies

Synthetic biology approaches allow the engineering of commensal bacteria to secrete therapeutic molecules such as SCFAs or bile acid analogues.[12] These strategies remain preclinical but represent a precision approach to modulating the gut–heart axis.

Cardiometabolic Drugs and Indirect Modulation

Drugs such as *SGLT-2 inhibitors* and *GLP-1 receptor agonists*, now widely used in HF and diabetes, have been shown to alter gut microbial composition in animal and human studies.[12,13] These indirect effects may partly explain their anti-inflammatory and metabolic benefits.

BIOMARKERS, PATIENT SELECTION, SAFETY, AND REGULATION

Biomarkers

Among gut-derived biomarkers, *TMAO* is the most extensively studied. Multiple cohorts demonstrate that elevated TMAO predicts adverse outcomes in HF patients independent of natriuretic peptides.[1,2,7,14] A meta-analysis confirmed its reproducibility across >5,000 patients.[2]

Markers of intestinal barrier dysfunction, such as *I-FABP* and *zonulin*, also correlate with HF severity and congestion. Mayerhofer et al.[9] and Kitai et al.[11] showed associations with NYHA class, NT-proBNP, and outcomes in HF and HFpEF patients, respectively.

Emerging work is exploring *multimers signatures*. By integrating microbiome sequencing, metabolomics, and proteomics, researchers aim to refine risk stratification beyond single markers.[8,12] These approaches may identify HF phenotypes particularly susceptible to gut-driven inflammation and metabolic disruption **(Table 1)**.

Patient Selection

Not all HF patients are equally likely to benefit from microbiome-targeted therapies. High-yield populations may include:

- *Advanced HF with congestion:* Bowel wall edema exacerbates bacterial translocation and inflammation.[9,11]
- *HF with CKD:* Accumulation of uremic toxins worsens prognosis.[5,12]
- *HFpEF with metabolic syndrome/obesity:* Gut dysbiosis and altered bile acid metabolism are common in this subgroup.[10,12]
- *Patients with systemic inflammation despite optimal therapy:* Those with persistently elevated CRP or IL-6 may particularly benefit from anti-inflammatory microbiome interventions.[3,19]

Safety and Regulation

Probiotics and synbiotics are generally safe but rare cases of bacteremia have been reported in immunocompromised hosts.[16,19] FMT carries risks of pathogen transmission, requiring stringent donor screening and regulatory oversight.[12]

TABLE 1: Key clinical studies linking gut-derived biomarkers to HF prognosis.

Author/Year	Design and population	Marker(s)	Key findings	Reference
Pasini et al., 2016	Cross-sectional, 40 HF vs. 20 controls	Microbiota profiling	Reduced microbial diversity, loss of SCFA-producing taxa	[4]
Tang et al., 2016	Prospective cohort, $n \approx 720$ chronic HF	Plasma TMAO	Higher TMAO predicted 5-year mortality independent of BNP	[1]
Suzuki et al., 2016	Cohort, $n \approx 223$ acute HF	TMAO	Elevated TMAO predicted rehospitalization and mortality	[14]
Mayerhofer et al., 2017	Cohort, 155 HF patients	I-FABP, zonulin	Higher levels correlated with NYHA class, NT-proBNP	[9]
Rohrmann et al., 2019	HF + CKD population	Indoxyl sulfate, p-cresyl sulfate	Higher toxins linked to hospitalization and mortality	[5]
Kitai et al., 2020	190 HFpEF patients	I-FABP	Elevated levels predicted adverse outcomes	[11]
Li et al., 2022	Meta-analysis, >5,000 HF patients	TMAO	Higher TMAO associated with worse composite outcomes	[2]
Huang et al., 2022	HFpEF cohort	Gut microbiome sequencing	Lower diversity, reduced *Faecalibacterium prausnitzii*	[10]
Palm et al., 2022	Mechanistic models	SCFAs	SCFA supplementation improved remodeling, reduced inflammation	[6]

Engineered microbial therapies raise additional concerns, including horizontal gene transfer and long-term ecological impacts on the microbiome.[12,13] Regulatory agencies such as the FDA and EMA are developing frameworks to ensure safety while allowing innovation in microbiome therapeutics.

Future Directions

The gut–heart axis is a rapidly expanding field with multiple promising avenues:

- *Large-scale randomized controlled trials (RCTs):* Current probiotic and synbiotic trials are underpowered. Well-designed RCTs with hard clinical endpoints (mortality and HF hospitalization) are urgently needed.[17-19]
- *Mechanistic multiomics studies:* Integration of *metagenomics*, *metabolomics*, and *host transcriptomics* will enable a systems-level understanding of the gut–heart axis.[8,12]
- *Novel therapeutic strategies:* Future options may include *postbiotic supplementation* (direct delivery of SCFAs), *targeted TMA-lyase inhibitors*, and *engineered bacteria* capable of restoring metabolic balance.[7,12]
- *Precision medicine approaches:* Combining microbiome-derived biomarkers with clinical and imaging data could identify subgroups most likely to benefit from microbiome modulation, enabling *personalized therapy*.[2,8]
- *Regulatory and safety frameworks:* Long-term registries for probiotics, FMT, and engineered microbiota will be essential to establish safety profiles.[12,13]

Ultimately, gut microbiome modulation may complement existing HF therapies, bridging *metabolic*, *immune*, and *neurohormonal* pathways with cardiovascular outcomes.

Practical Recommendations for Clinicians (Evidence-informed)

While awaiting definitive outcome trials, clinicians can adopt several pragmatic, low-risk strategies informed by current knowledge:

- *Optimize congestion management:* Diuretics and other measures that reduce venous congestion help restore intestinal perfusion and reduce mucosal edema—an effective upstream intervention for gut barrier dysfunction.[9,11]
- *Encourage a fiber-rich, balanced diet:* Diets rich in nonrefined plant foods support SCFA-producing bacteria. Dietary counseling tailored to HF patients may help improve metabolic and inflammatory profiles.[6,15]
- *Be judicious with antibiotics and PPIs:* Unnecessary antibiotic use disrupts microbiota, while prolonged proton pump inhibitor (PPI) therapy alters gut ecology. Both should be reassessed periodically to minimize microbiome disruption.[3,12]
- *Consider synbiotic or probiotic adjuncts cautiously:* For motivated patients, probiotic or synbiotic supplementation may be considered as part of clinical trials or case-by-case. Evidence shows improvements in surrogate markers such as NT-proBNP and inflammation, but no definitive effect on hard outcomes yet.[15-19] Adverse events are rare but should be monitored, especially in immunocompromised patients.[16,19]
- *Stay informed about emerging biomarkers:* Biomarkers such as TMAO and I-FABP show strong associations with outcomes but should not yet guide routine therapy

outside research settings.[1,2,9] Clinicians should interpret results with caution and continue to prioritize established guideline-directed HF therapy.

CONCLUSION

The gut microbiota represents a biologically plausible and clinically relevant contributor to heart failure pathophysiology. Since 2015, a burgeoning literature has linked gut dysbiosis, intestinal barrier dysfunction, and microbial metabolites (notably TMAO and SCFAs) to HF severity and prognosis. Translational studies demonstrate mechanistic links, and a growing, but still preliminary, set of interventional human trials suggests that dietary, probiotic, and metabolite-targeting approaches can modulate biomarkers and may improve clinical status. However, large, randomized outcome trials demonstrate that microbiome-directed therapies reduce HF hospitalizations or mortality are lacking. For now, clinicians should prioritize evidence-based HF care, optimize congestion (thereby helping gut integrity), promote healthy fiber-rich diets, and consider microbiome interventions within clinical trials. The next 5 years will likely see decisive trials and the emergence of targeted microbial therapeutics—a development with the potential to materially change HF management.

REFERENCES

1. Tang WHW, Wang Z, Fan Y, et al. Gut microbiota-dependent trimethylamine N-oxide pathway contributes to both development of renal insufficiency and mortality risk in chronic heart failure. Eur J Heart Fail. 2016;18(7):857-64.
2. Li X, Su C, Jiang Z, et al. Trimethylamine N-Oxide in Heart Failure: A Meta-Analysis. Front Cardiovasc Med. 2022;9:930209.
3. Trøseid M, Andersen GØ, Broch K, et al. The gut microbiome in coronary artery disease and heart failure. EBioMedicine. 2020;52:102649.
4. Pasini E, Aquilani R, Testa C, et al. Pathogenic gut flora in patients with chronic heart failure. JACC Heart Fail. 2016;4(3):220-7.
5. Rohrmann S, Linseisen J, Allenspach M, et al. Uremic toxins and cardiovascular disease in heart failure with chronic kidney disease. Nephrol Dial Transplant. 2019;34(10):1720-29.
6. Palm CL, Schaub JA, Cresci GA, et al. Short-chain fatty acids in the metabolism of heart failure: mechanistic insights. Cardiovasc Res. 2022;118(6):1298-312.
7. Zhang Y, Wang Y, Guo R, et al. TMAO: how gut microbiota contributes to heart failure. Transl Res. 2021;232:1-14.
8. Lu Y, Fan C, Li P, et al. Microbiota-derived short-chain fatty acids and implications for cardiovascular disease. Front Cardiovasc Med. 2022;9:789012.
9. Mayerhofer CCK, Kummen M, Holm K, et al. Intestinal microbiota-dependent and -independent markers of gut barrier function in patients with heart failure. ESC Heart Fail. 2017;4(3):282-90.
10. Huang Z, Mei X, Jiang C, et al. Gut microbiota in heart failure with preserved ejection fraction. Front Cardiovasc Med. 2022;9:856123.
11. Kitai T, Kato M, Yahata T, et al. Circulating intestinal fatty acid-binding protein is associated with disease severity and outcome in heart failure with preserved ejection fraction. ESC Heart Fail. 2020;7(6):3363-73.
12. Lupu VV, Ignat A, Mitroi G, et al. The implication of the gut microbiome in heart failure: mechanistic insights and therapeutic perspectives. Int J Mol Sci. 2023;24(4):3456.
13. Trøseid M, Andersen GØ, Broch K, et al. Gut microbiota and cardiovascular disease: mechanisms and potential therapies. Lancet. 2020;396:1469-84.
14. Suzuki T, Heaney LM, Bhandari SS, et al. Trimethylamine N-oxide and prognosis in acute heart failure. Heart. 2016;102(11):841-8.
15. Marques FZ, Mackay CR, Kaye DM, et al. Gut microbiota and cardiovascular disease: role of gut-derived metabolites as biomarkers and therapeutic targets. Curr Opin Pharmacol. 2017;33:17-24.
16. Kitzinger J, Karall D, Mülleder U, et al. Probiotic yogurt in chronic heart failure: pilot clinical outcomes. Nutrients. 2019;11(9):1970.
17. Cui X, Ye L, Li J, et al. Effects of synbiotic supplementation on heart failure with preserved ejection fraction: a randomized controlled trial. Nutr Metab Cardiovasc Dis. 2020;30(10):1761-9.
18. Frontiers in Nutrition Trial Investigators, Silva B, Santos R, et al. Randomized trial of inulin + probiotic mix in HFrEF. Front Nutr. 2021;8:642223.
19. Kazemi A, Soltani S, Ghorabi S, et al. The effect of probiotic/synbiotic supplementation on inflammatory biomarkers: systematic review and meta-analysis. Clin Nutr. 2020;39(11):3249-59.
20. Jing L, Li Y, Xu S, et al. Role of Trimethylamine N-Oxide in Heart Failure: A Review. Cardiol Rev. 2024;32(2):89-99.

CHAPTER 36

Diuretic Potentiation Strategies in Acute Heart Failure

SK Dwivedi, Somil Verma

ABSTRACT

Acute heart failure (AHF) is a leading cause of morbidity, hospitalization, and mortality worldwide. It is characterized by rapid-onset or worsening of congestion, due to fluid retention and maladaptive neurohormonal activation. Loop diuretics are the cornerstone of AHF management; however, resistance to these agents is frequently encountered, resulting in inadequate decongestion and adverse clinical outcomes, and often requiring escalation of therapeutic strategies. In recent years, substantial clinical trial evidence has emerged supporting adjunctive diuretic strategies, namely, sequential nephron blockade with thiazides or carbonic anhydrase inhibitors and addition of sodium-glucose cotransporter 2 (SGLT2) inhibitors, vasopressin antagonists, and mineralocorticoid receptor antagonists (MRAs). While many strategies improve short-term congestion relief, their impact on long-term mortality remains uncertain. A stepwise, patient-focused strategy is emphasized, with the goal of maximizing symptom relief and minimizing complications. This chapter reviews the latest evidence and practical aspects of diuretic potentiation, underlying pathophysiology while incorporating global perspectives, updated clinical practices, diagnostic innovations, and limitations, with emphasis on resource-appropriate adaptation for Indian hospitals.

Keywords: Acute heart failure, diuretic resistance, loop diuretics, sequential nephron blockade, thiazides, acetazolamide, SGLT2 inhibitors, vasopressin antagonists.

INTRODUCTION

Heart failure (HF) poses a significant public health challenge worldwide. Acute heart failure (AHF), characterized by sudden or subacute deterioration in cardiac function, accounts for a substantial proportion of emergency hospital admissions and healthcare costs, especially in elderly. Despite advancements in chronic HF management, AHF hospitalizations remain associated with high in-hospital and postdischarge mortality. In India, 1-year mortality rates in AHF patients with reduced ejection fraction approaches 37%, with readmission rates as high as 30%.[1]

BURDEN OF HEART FAILURE IN INDIA AND WORLDWIDE

Heart failure affects an estimated 64 million individuals worldwide. In India, the prevalence is projected at approximately 1.3–22.7 million cases, with 0.5–1.8 million new cases diagnosed each year.[2] This rising burden is driven by an aging population, high rates of coronary artery disease, hypertension, rheumatic fever, and diabetes. Compared to Western population, Indian patients often present at a younger age, with more advanced disease, higher comorbidities, and limited access to specialized heart failure care.[3] Hospital-based registries in India such as the INTER-CHF and Trivandrum Heart Failure Registry highlight a younger age of presentation (mean age ~60 years), higher prevalence of ischemic etiology and rheumatic heart disease, and a greater proportion of patients presenting with acute decompensation on a background of chronic heart failure.

PATHOPHYSIOLOGY OF FLUID RETENTION

Acute heart failure arises from abrupt increase in cardiac filling pressures due to impaired contractility, elevated afterload, regurgitant lesions, or arrhythmias. The resultant congestion triggers a cascade:

- *Neurohormonal activation:* Renin–angiotensin–aldosterone system (RAAS) activation and sympathetic nervous system stimulation with vasopressin (antidiuretic hormone) secretion causes enhanced sodium and water retention.
- *Renal hemodynamics:* Low cardiac output causes decreased renal perfusion, which in turn causes decline in the glomerular filtration rate (GFR), further promoting sodium retention.
- *Tubular adaptation:* Acute loop diuretic use promotes sodium and water loss but with chronic use, there is compensatory increase in distal tubule sodium reabsorption (nephron remodeling), hence lowering diuretic efficacy.

TYPES OF DIURETICS

Diuretics encompass multiple pharmacological classes, of which loop and thiazide diuretics remain the mainstay in practice. Their mechanisms and corresponding sites of renal action are outlined in **Table 1** and illustrated in **Figure 1**.

DIURETIC RESISTANCE

Diuretic resistance is defined as a reduced natriuretic and diuretic effect despite appropriate dosing and persistent fluid overload, representing a frequent and clinically significant challenge in the management of AHF, where it is reported in roughly 20–30% of cases.[2] More quantitative definition is failure of high-dose oral furosemide (160 mg twice daily or equivalent) to raise sodium excretion by ≥90 mmol over 3 days. Alternatively, a spot urine sample obtained 1–2 hours after loop diuretic administration showing a sodium level <50 mmol predicts inadequate natriuresis and resistance.[4] Contributing comorbidities such as chronic kidney disease, hypoalbuminemia, and the use of nonsteroidal anti-inflammatory drugs further impair natriuresis. Diuretic resistance is associated with persistent congestion, longer hospital stays, higher readmission rates, and increased mortality.

Mechanisms of Diuretic Resistance

It arises from a combination of factors including:

- Reduced drug delivery due to gut edema (poor oral absorption) and hypoalbuminemia

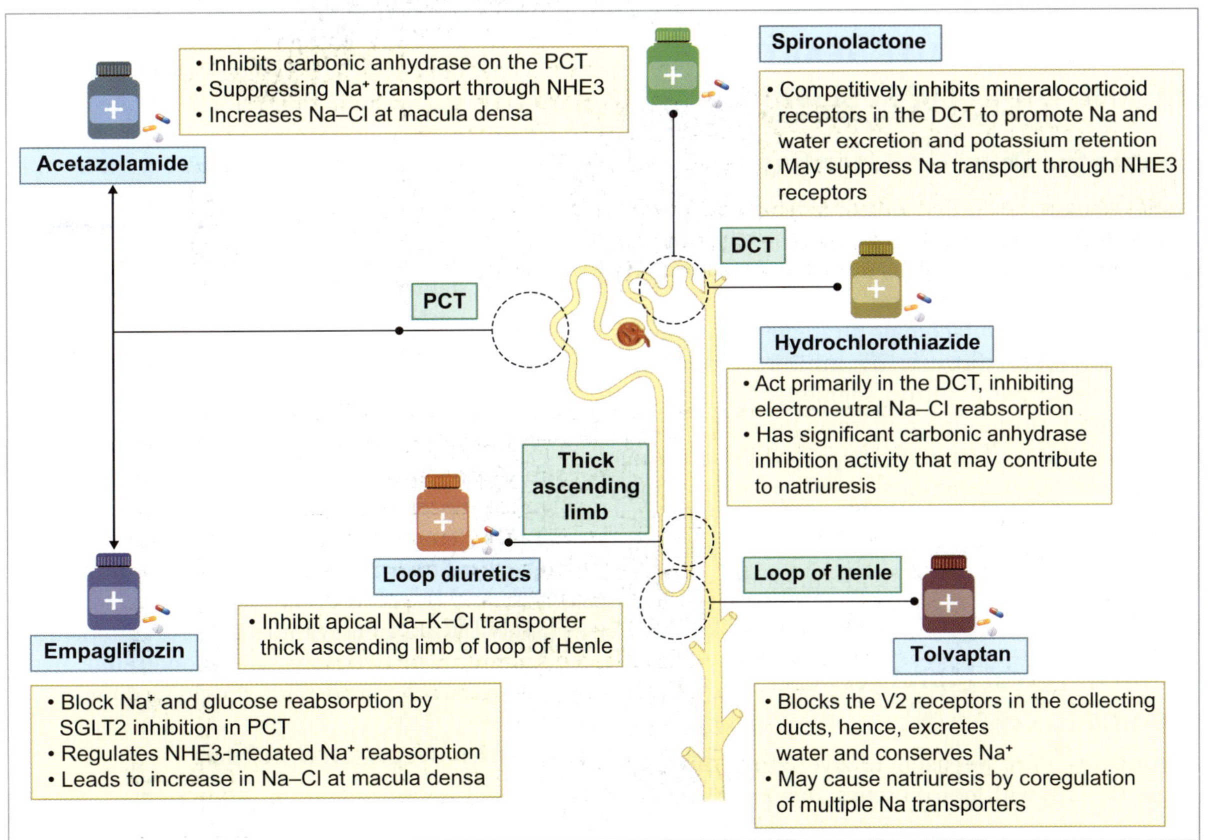

FIG. 1: Site of action and mechanism for different diuretics.

Source: Siddiqi et al. (2015).

(DCT: distal convoluted tubule; NHE3: sodium–hydrogen exchanger 3; PCT: proximal convoluted tubule; TAL: thick ascending limb; V2: vasopressin 2)

TABLE 1: Sites of action of diuretic classes in the nephron.

Drug class	Site of action	Mechanism
Loop diuretics	Thick ascending limb	Inhibit Na–K–2Cl cotransporter
Thiazides	Distal convoluted tubule	Inhibit Na–Cl symporter
Carbonic anhydrase inhibitors	Proximal tubule	Inhibit bicarbonate reabsorption and Na^+ exchange
SGLT2 inhibitors	Proximal tubule	Inhibit sodium-glucose cotransport
MRAs	Collecting duct/DCT	Block aldosterone-mediated sodium reabsorption
Vasopressin antagonists	Collecting duct	Block V2 receptors, induce aquaresis

- Enhanced proximal and distal sodium reabsorption
- RAAS and sympathetic activation
- Prolonged loop diuretic exposure causing "braking phenomenon" in which the nephron adapts by increasing sodium transport downstream of the loop of Henle
- Reduced renal perfusion resulting from acute reduction of cardiac output leading to cardiorenal syndrome
- *Pharmacokinetic issues:* Choice of therapy also results in variable natriuresis with loop diuretics being the choice. Among loop diuretics, furosemide has lower oral bioavailability (~50%), shorter half-life, and larger inter-individual variability compared to torsemide.

MANAGEMENT OF ACUTE HEART FAILURE AND DIURETIC RESISTANCE

Rationale for Diuretic Potentiation

Loop diuretics remain the cornerstone of AHF management, yet diuretic resistance, especially with chronic exposure is common and must be addressed, as unresolved congestion is linked to higher morbidity and mortality. Over the past decade, several pharmacologic strategies have been developed to augment diuresis by inhibiting sodium reabsorption at multiple nephron segments (sequential nephron blockade), promoting aquaresis, or modulating neurohormonal pathways. Sequential nephron blockade can be achieved by combining loop diuretics with agents acting on the PCT (e.g., acetazolamide and SGLT2 inhibitors), DCT (e.g., thiazides), or collecting duct (e.g., mineralocorticoid receptor antagonists and vasopressin antagonists), thus offering means to overcome this therapeutic challenge.[5]

Pharmacological Management Strategies

Various strategies may be used to overcome diuretic resistance, particularly with loop diuretics. They are discussed as follows:

Initiation and Intensification of Loop Diuretics

- *Mechanism:* Loop diuretics act by inhibiting the Na-K-2Cl transporter in the thick ascending limb, blocking approximately 25% of filtered sodium reabsorption, facilitating rapid natriuresis.
- *Dosing strategies and infusion approaches:* In AHF, intravenous administration is preferred over oral, for prompt absorption. Higher IV doses—typically about double the patient's usual oral dose—are advised at the time of admission.
- *Clinical evidence:*
    - *DOSE trial:* This trial compared high- versus low-dose and bolus versus continuous intravenous furosemide infusion in AHF. The results are as follows:
        - *High versus low dose:* High dose regimen (2.5 times the oral daily dose) aims to overcome reduced drug delivery to the nephron in AHF and was more beneficial as it yields greater urine output, more weight loss, and modest dyspnea improvement at 72 hours. Transient serum creatinine elevation is common but usually reversible with similar adverse event rates as with low-dose therapy.
        - *Bolus versus continuous infusion:* There was no superiority of continuous IV infusion over bolus delivery, but continuous infusion was associated with minimal pharmacodynamic peaks and troughs.[6]
- *Torsemide versus furosemide:* Meta-analyses and post-hoc analyses suggest torsemide may improve congestion with similar or better long-term morbidity compared to furosemide; however, the 2023 TRANSFORM-HF trial found no difference in all-cause mortality at 1 year.[7] **Table 2** compares pharmacokinetics of both the drugs.
- *Practical issues:* The efficacy of loop diuretic should be assessed by monitoring urine output, which should be >100–150 mL/hour within 6 hours of administration. Also, monitoring of hypokalemia, hyponatremia, hypotension, and renal function decline should be done.

Sequential Nephron Blockade

Use of add-on diuretic from different class may break the resistance and increase diuresis.

Thiazide/Thiazide-like Diuretics

Thiazides (hydrochlorothiazide, chlorothiazide, and metolazone) block the Na–Cl symporter in the distal tubule,

TABLE 2: Pharmacokinetics and clinical considerations: Furosemide versus Torsemide.

Parameter	Furosemide	Torsemide
Oral bioavailability	~50%	>85%
Half-life	1.5–2 h	3–6 h
Dosing intervals	Multiple/day	1–2/day
Mortality outcome	Similar in RCT	Similar in RCT[8]

preventing distal sodium reabsorption, thus countering the increased distal sodium delivery caused by loop diuretics.

Role in diuretic resistance:

- Thiazides are particularly effective for "braking phenomenon" when distal nephron adapts to loop diuretics inhibition.
- Metolazone is commonly used in practice, as it remains effective even in severe renal dysfunction.
- Chlorothiazide (IV) can provide a rapid effect but is expensive.

Clinical Evidence

- *CLOROTIC trial:* It found that adding a thiazide diuretic, such as oral hydrochlorothiazide (HCTZ) (50–100 mg/day), to a loop diuretic such as furosemide in patients hospitalized with AHF improved diuretic response and weight loss at 72 hour but did not improve dyspnea or hard outcomes. However, this combination was associated with a higher incidence of renal impairment, including more frequent hypokalemia and elevations in serum creatinine, though it did not affect short-term mortality or hospital readmission rates.[9]
- *Recent head-to-head cohort studies:* IV chlorothiazide may provide greater acute diuresis than metolazone without inducing additional electrolyte or creatinine derangements, but cost and accessibility limits widespread use **(Table 3)**.[10]

Acetazolamide

Acetazolamide acts by inhibiting carbonic anhydrase in the proximal tubule, increasing sodium delivery to loop diuretic sites, thus reducing sodium/bicarbonate reabsorption.

Acetazolamide has been shown to be particularly effective in metabolic alkalosis and in patients with profound diuretic resistance. It is inexpensive and widely available; but often underutilized.

Clinical Evidence

ADVOR trial (2022): This trial showed that adding intravenous acetazolamide (500 mg daily) to IV loop diuretics in AHF patients with volume overload achieved higher rates of successful decongestion by 72 hour without significant increase in serious adverse events, though rise in serum creatinine occurred more often.[11]

SGLT2 Inhibitors

Sodium-glucose cotransporter 2 inhibitors (empagliflozin and dapagliflozin) block sodium/glucose cotransport in the proximal tubule, producing natriuresis and glucosuria, and provide cardiovascular, renal, and mortality benefit.

Mechanisms in AHF:

- Reduced preload and afterload via osmotic diuresis
- Attenuation of neurohormonal activation
- Improved cardiac energetic status and reverse remodeling
- Renoprotection

Clinical Evidence

- *EMPULSE trial (2022):* Empagliflozin initiated in-hospital in AHF patients improved clinical outcomes at 90 days, including all-cause death, heart failure hospitalization, and KCCQ score improvements.[12]
- *Meta-analyses* confirm benefit across the ejection fraction spectrum, irrespective of diabetes.[13]

Practical Issues

Sodium-glucose cotransporter 2 inhibitors should be started once the patient is hemodynamically stable and not volume-depleted. Monitoring for genitourinary infections and rare cases of ketoacidosis is essential.

Vasopressin Receptor Antagonists (Vaptans)

Vaptans (e.g., tolvaptan) block V2 receptors in the collecting duct, promoting free water excretion ("aquaretic" effect).

They have been used in the treatment of severe hyponatremia and volume overload unresponsive to loop/thiazide therapy despite having a less robust effect on sodium excretion.

Clinical Evidence

EVEREST and SECRET of CHF trial: Tolvaptan produced greater weight loss and symptomatic improvement at 7 days, especially in hyponatremic patients, but did not reduce mortality or hospitalization at 10 months.[14,15]

Practical issues: Aquaretics can be life saving in euvolemic/hypervolemic hyponatremia but requires close sodium monitoring to avoid overly rapid correction.

TABLE 3: Efficacy and safety of thiazide as an add-on diuretic in AHF.

Drug	Route	24-hour urine output Δ (mL)	Key adverse effects
Metolazone	Oral	↑ ~1,100	Hypokalemia and hypomagnesemia
Chlorothiazide	IV	↑ ~2,100	Hypomagnesemia

Note: Thiazide selection should be individualized based on renal function, cost, and local formulary availability.

TABLE 4: Clinical trials summary (2019–2025).[2]

Trial (year)	Population	Intervention	Comparator	Key endpoints	Decongestion	Symptom benefit	Clinical outcome
DOSE (2011)	AHF, *n* = 308	High dose Infusion Loop	Low dose Bolus	Weight loss, dyspnea, and sCr	✓✓	✓✓	Similar at 60 days
CLOROTIC (2023)	AHF, resistant, *n* = 230	HCTZ + Loop	Loop alone	Weight loss and dyspnea	✓	×	No difference, more AKI
ADVOR (2022)	AHF with overload, *n* = 519	Acetazolamide + Loop	Loop alone	Decongestion at 72 hours	✓✓	✓	No mortality difference
EMPULSE (2022)	AHF, stabilized, *n* = 530	Empagliflozin	Placebo	Death, AHF event, and KCCQ	✓	✓✓	✓✓
EVEREST (2007)	AHF, *n* = 4133	Tolvaptan	Placebo	Death, HFH, and symptoms	✓	✓	×
ATHENA-HF (2017)	AHF, *n* = 360	Spironolactone	Placebo	Congestion and NT-proBNP	×	×	×

Note: ✓✓: robust; ✓: modest; ×: no effect.

(AHF: acute heart failure; AKI: acute kidney injury; HFH: heart failure hospitalization; HCTZ: hydrochlorthiazide; KCCQ: Kansas City Cardiomyopathy Questionnaire; sCr- serum creatinine)

Mineralocorticoid Receptor Antagonists

Mineralocorticoid receptor antagonists (spironolactone and eplerenone) blunt aldosterone-mediated distal sodium/water retention. Their chronic use in HFrEF is established.

Role in Acute Heart Failure

Selected patients with refractory edema and persistent hypokalemia may benefit from short-term, low-dose therapy.

Clinical Evidence

ATHENA-HF: High-dose spironolactone (100 mg/day) as adjunct to IV loop diuretics did not enhance net diuresis, clinical improvement, congestion scores or decrease natriuretic peptides peptides at 96 h compared with placebo, although they were generally safe **(Table 4)**.[16]

KEY FINDINGS FROM TRIALS OF DIURETIC STRATEGIES IN ACUTE HEART FAILURE

- *Symptom and weight reduction:* Significant bodyweight loss and dyspnea relief occurred only when loop diuretics were intensified or a vasopressin antagonist was added. Adding either a thiazide diuretic or a vasopressin antagonist reduced bodyweight by the end of treatment.
- *Limited early biomarker response:* Most potentiation approaches did not consistently lessen clinical signs of fluid retention or lower natriuretic peptide levels within the first 3–7 days.
- *Enhanced diuresis with specific agents:* Sodium-glucose cotransporter-2 inhibitors (SGLT2i), acetazolamide, and higher-dose loop diuretics produced notable increase in urine output during the initial treatment.
- *Renal effects:* All intensified diuretic regimens were associated with transient rise in serum creatinine.
- *Clinical outcomes:* Short-term diuretic augmentation has not translated into improved long-term cardiovascular outcomes.

MONITORING OF DIURETIC THERAPY

Monitoring of diuretic therapy includes the following:

- *Symptom relief:* Symptomatic relief from congestion is the most commonly targeted end point in AHF. But assessment of congestion has varied across trials with some relying on patient symptoms and others on physical signs. Trials like EMPULSE assessed symptoms at 90 days while ADVOR evaluated physical signs at

36 hours. Among trials reporting dyspnea response, DICTATE-AHF, SECRET of CHF, EVEREST, and DOSE indicate tolvaptan and high-dose loop diuretics reduced dyspnea. Thus, dyspnea showed the most consistent early improvement with the use of intensified loop diuretic therapy and vasopressin antagonists.

- *Weight loss:* Body-weight change is commonly measured in AHF trials but is subject to variability and confounding. Several studies (CLOROTIC, SECRET of CHF, EVEREST, ADVOR, and DOSE) showed short-term weight loss linked to decongestion, yet this reduction did not improve postdischarge outcomes such as mortality or rehospitalization. Only the intensification of loop diuretic agents or the addition of a thiazide diuretic or a vasopressin antagonist was consistently accompanied by a decrease in body weight.
- *Volume loss/urine output:* The efficacy of loop diuretic should be assessed by monitoring urine output, which should be >100–150 mL/hour within 6 hours of administration. Short term increase in urine output was observed with intensified loop therapy, acetazolamide, and SGLT2 inhibitors, with the greatest effects seen with empagliflozin and high-dose loop diuretics. In contrast, hydrochlorothiazide, high-dose spironolactone, and dapagliflozin produced minimal change.
- *Biomarkers:* Across multiple AHF trials, diuretic potentiation strategies produced no significant early reductions in NT-proBNP. Small decreases were noted only with empagliflozin in EMPAG-HF and EMPULSE. Overall, natriuretic peptide levels remained largely unchanged during the first week of therapy.
- *Natriuresis-guided therapy*: Urinary sodium (spot or 6-hour collection) after loop diuretic administration predicts clinical response; values <50–70 mmol suggest resistance and the need to escalate therapy. Recent trials favor urinary biomarker guidance for timely adjustment.[17]

PRACTICAL MANAGEMENT ALGORITHM

Practical management algorithm is as follows **(Flowchart 1)**:

- *Initial assessment:*
  - Confirm clinical signs of congestion (dyspnea, edema, elevated JVP, and rales).
  - Assess baseline renal function, electrolytes, hemodynamics.
  - Evaluate patients home diuretic dose.
- *Initiation:*
  - Administer loop diuretic as first-line treatment.

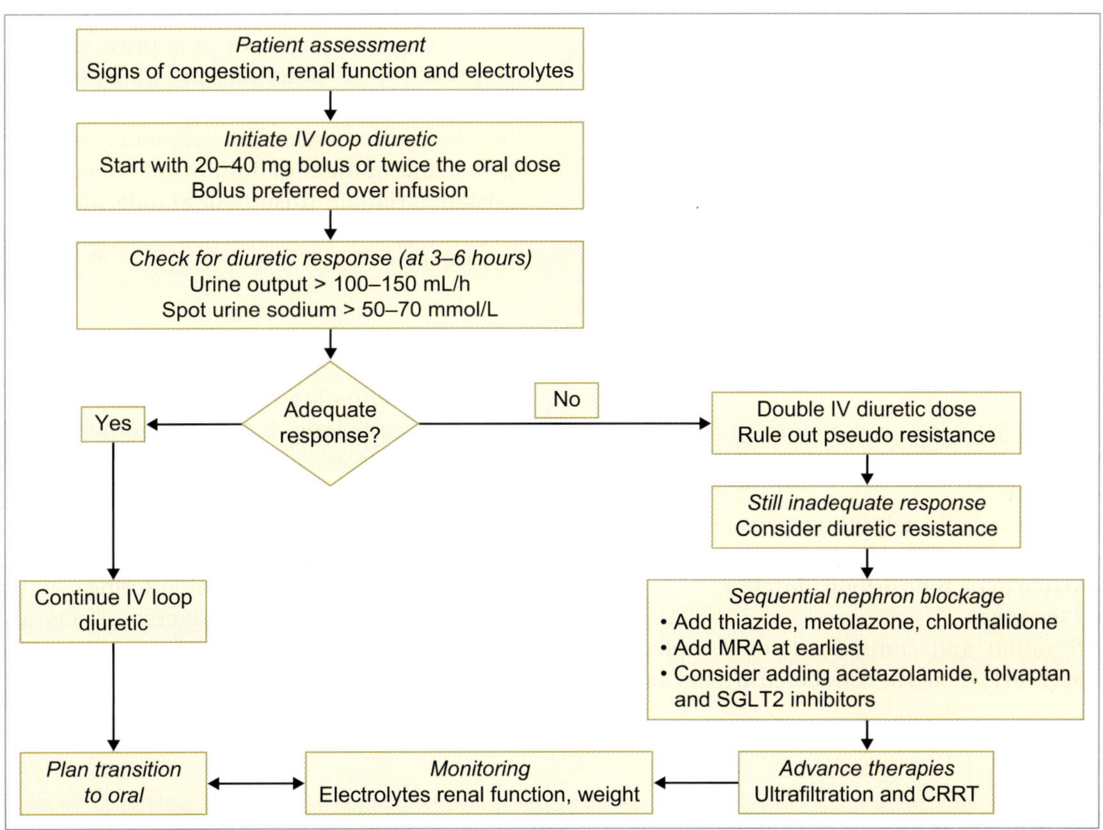

FLOWCHART 1: Diuretic potentiation strategies.

- *Dose:* At least 2 times the patient's home oral dose or 20–40 mg IV if diuretic naïve.
- *Route:* IV preferred for prompt effect
- Bolus preferred over continuous infusion
- Monitor urine output hourly.

- *Early response assessment at 6 hours:*
  - *Check urine output:* Target >100–150 mL/hour.
  - *Measure spot urine sodium (if available):* Target ≥50–70 mmol/L.
  - Urine output <100–150 mL/hour or spot urine sodium <50 mmol/L signals diuretic resistance.
  - Rule out pseudo-resistance (inadequate dosing, poor IV access, excessive intake).
  - *If adequate response (urine output and urine sodium targets met)*
    - Continue current loop diuretic dosing.
    - Monitor clinical status, electrolytes, and renal function.
    - Transition to oral loop diuretics once stable and euvolemic.
  - *If inadequate response (urine output <100–150 mL/hour or urine sodium <50 mmol/L)*
    - Double the loop diuretic dose.
    - Ensure correct administration and no pseudoresistance causes (e.g., poor IV access and excessive oral intake).
- *Persistent resistance despite escalated loop diuretic dose:* Add sequential nephron blockade agents based on clinical profile for diuretic potentiation:
  - Add thiazide/metolazone/chlorothiazide if persistent congestion:
    - Target distal convoluted tubule sodium reabsorption.
    - Especially useful for "braking phenomenon"
    - Use IV chlorothiazide for rapid effect if available.
  - Consider acetazolamide early, especially with metabolic alkalosis or severe overload.
  - Initiate SGLT2 inhibitor once patient is hemodynamically stable and euvolemic.
  - Tolvaptan for refractory hyponatremia or severe fluid overload.
- *Mineralocorticoid receptor antagonists (spironolactone)*:
  - Add early after hemodynamic and renal function stabilization.
  - They are especially helpful for persistent edema or refractory cases, while also preventing hypokalemia caused due to high-dose loop diuretics.
- *Advanced therapies*:
  - Ultrafiltration and continuous renal replacement therapy (CRRT) should be considered in refractory cases.
- *Monitoring and adjustment*:
  - Monitor weight, urine output, electrolytes (K^+, Na^+, Mg^{2+}), and renal function daily.
  - Mild rise in creatinine (≤0.5 mg/dL) during decongestion is acceptable and may not require stopping diuretics.
  - Replace electrolytes as needed.
  - Adjust diuretic regimen based on clinical and biochemical response.
  - Avoid overt diuresis causing hypotension or kidney injury.
- *Transition to oral and plan follow-up*: Early outpatient review, education regarding diet, adherence, and symptom monitoring.

Special Clinical Scenarios

- *Hyponatremia:* Tolvaptan is preferred if available; hypertonic saline is rarely used due to monitoring needs.
- *Cardiorenal syndrome:* Combination strategies with close creatinine monitoring are essential; ultrafiltration is limited to tertiary centers.
- *Right heart failure:* Diuretic responsiveness may be blunted; combination with thiazides often needed.

LIMITATIONS AND AREAS FOR FUTURE RESEARCH

Despite short-term efficacy in improving decongestion and symptoms, most potentiation strategies (except SGLT2i) have not improved mortality or rehospitalization in RCTs.[2] The ideal patient selection, sequence and combination of agents, and optimal definitions of congestion and diuretic resistance remain unsettled. Standardizing assessment of congestion and more robust head-to-head comparative trials are needed.

CONCLUSION

Diuretic potentiation in AHF is indispensable for patients unresponsive to loop diuretic monotherapy. Well-designed clinical trials in recent years provide a roadmap for rational use of thiazide diuretics, acetazolamide, SGLT2 inhibitors, and vaptans. Implementing a tailored, stepwise approach emphasizing early recognition of resistance, individualized drug selection, and dynamic monitoring can optimize short-term outcomes. Limiting adverse effects and obtaining sustained long-term benefits remain critical clinical priorities for the next decade.

REFERENCES

1. Philip A, Shastry CS, Utagi B, et al. Unveiling the impact of an Indian-specific heart failure checklist on heart failure with reduced ejection fraction management in the South Indian population. Clin Epidemiol Glob Health. 2024;27:101556.
2. Siddiqi TJ, Packer M, Ezekowitz JA, et al. Diuretic potentiation strategies in acute heart failure. JACC Heart Fail. 2025;13(1):14-27.
3. Kole A, Agarwal A, Seth B, et al. Epidemiology of heart failure in rural Chhattisgarh, India. Natl Med J India. 2024;36(3):163-6.
4. Wilcox CS, Testani JM, Pitt B. Pathophysiology of diuretic resistance and its implications for the management of chronic heart failure. Hypertension. 2020;76(4):1045-54.
5. Frăţilă GV, Obrişcă B, Ismail G. A practical approach to sequential nephron blockade in acute decompensated heart failure. Rom J Cardiol. 2023;33(3):83-92.
6. Felker GM, Lee KL, Bull DA, et al. Diuretic strategies in patients with acute decompensated heart failure. N Eng J Med. 2011;364(9):797-805.
7. Mentz RJ, Anstrom KJ, Eisenstein EL, et al. Effect of torsemide vs furosemide after discharge on all-cause mortality in patients hospitalized with heart failure. JAMA. 2023;329(3):214-23.
8. Mentz RJ, Hasselblad V, DeVore AD, et al. Torsemide versus furosemide in patients with acute heart failure (from the ASCEND-HF Trial). Am J Cardiol. 2016;117(3):404-11.
9. Trullàs JC, Morales-Rull JL, Casado J, et al. Combining loop with thiazide diuretics for decompensated heart failure: the CLOROTIC trial. Eur Heart J. 2023;44(5):411-21.
10. Gibson CM, Beard MM, Escano AK, et al. Metolazone versus chlorothiazide in acute heart failure patients with diuretic resistance and renal dysfunction: A retrospective cohort study. J Cardiovasc Pharmacol. 2024;84(4):451-6.
11. Mullens W, Dauw J, Martens P, et al. Acetazolamide in acute decompensated heart failure with volume overload. N Eng J Med. 2022;387(13):1185-95.
12. Biegus J, Voors AA, Collins SP, et al. Impact of empagliflozin on decongestion in acute heart failure: The EMPULSE trial. Eur Heart J. 2023;44(1):41-50.
13. Rahil AI, Bhavsar T, Fatima R, et al. Efficacy and safety of SGLT2 inhibitors in acute heart failure: A systematic review and meta-analysis of randomized controlled trials. Front Cardiovasc Med. 2025;12:1543153.
14. Konstam MA, Gheorghiade M, Burnett JC Jr, et al. Effects of oral tolvaptan in patients hospitalized for worsening heart failure: The EVEREST Outcome Trial. JAMA. 2007;297(12):1319.
15. Konstam MA, Kiernan M, Chandler A, et al. Short-term effects of tolvaptan in patients with acute heart failure and volume overload. J Am Coll Cardiol. 2017;69(11):1409-19.
16. Butler J, Anstrom KJ, Felker GM, et al. Efficacy and safety of spironolactone in acute heart failure. JAMA Cardiol. 2017; 2(9):950.
17. Natriuresis-guided diuretic therapy in acute heart failure: a pragmatic randomized trial. Nat Med. 2023;29(10):2625–2632.

CHAPTER 37

Approaches in Heart Failure with Mildly Reduced and Preserved Ejection Fraction

Vidyut Jain, Avani Jain

ABSTRACT

Heart failure (HF) remains a major global health challenge, associated with frequent hospitalizations and high mortality. Echocardiography is an essential and widely accepted tool for assessing left ventricular (LV) function. By calculating the ejection fraction, it allows classification of LV dysfunction into three categories: Heart failure with preserved ejection fraction (HFpEF), heart failure with reduced ejection fraction (HFrEF), and heart failure with mildly reduced ejection fraction (HFmrEF). The management of HFmrEF is particularly challenging, as patients in this group often share clinical characteristics with both HFrEF and HFpEF. Evidence suggests that patients with HFmrEF may derive some benefit from therapies proven effective in HFrEF, though the degree of benefit is limited.[1] Currently, therapeutic options for patients with HFpEF and HFmrEF remain limited compared to those for HFrEF. A more individualized approach—incorporating clinical features, echocardiographic parameters, phenotyping, and biomarker profiling—may help guide therapy and improve outcomes in these patients. Long-term studies are needed to better define the impact of different therapeutic strategies and their prognostic implications in HFpEF and HFmrEF populations.

Keywords: Heart failure with preserved ejection fraction (HFpEF), heart failure with mildly reduced ejection fraction (HFmrEF), heart failure (HF).

INTRODUCTION

Chronic heart failure (HF), associated with increased cardiovascular (CV) morbidity and mortality worldwide, is now recognized as a multisystem disorder. The prevalence of HF has risen steadily over the past two decades, with epidemiological studies estimating that 10–25% of patients fall into the heart failure with mildly reduced ejection fraction (HFmrEF) category.[2]

According to a study cited by Tout, the annual incidence of HFmrEF was 6.7 per 10,000 persons, which was lower but still clinically significant compared with heart failure with preserved ejection fraction (HFpEF) (26.9) and heart failure with reduced ejection fraction (HFrEF) (34.9).[3] Recognition of this subgroup was formalized in the 2021 ESC guidelines, which defined HFmrEF as a left ventricular ejection fraction (LVEF) of 41–49%. Patients with HFpEF and HFmrEF often demonstrate overlapping manifestations, adding to the complexity of diagnosis and management.[4]

Although research exploring the risk factors and mechanisms underlying these entities remains limited, existing evidence is informative. For example, Tromp and colleagues reported that individuals with diabetes and microvascular dysfunction were at higher risk of developing HFpEF. This observation has encouraged further exploration into the etiology, clinical course, and long-term outcomes of this group.[5]

Heart failure with preserved ejection fraction, in particular, is typically driven by chronic systemic stressors in combination with long-standing CV and metabolic disease. Because its clinical signs and symptoms often mimic those of other conditions, establishing a reliable diagnosis of HFpEF remains a significant challenge.[2]

DIAGNOSTIC AIDS AND VALUE OF BIOMARKERS

Biomarkers and cardiac imaging play a pivotal role in the early diagnosis and severity assessment of HF, and are widely accepted as essential tools in screening suspected cases. Clinical guidelines provide specific diagnostic standards for HFpEF, with NT-proBNP > 125 pg/mL frequently employed as a threshold. In HFmrEF, the average NT-proBNP level has been reported as 1,540 pg/mL, and higher values are associated with a two-fold increase in all-cause mortality and heart failure hospitalizations (HFHs) (HR 1.48; 95% CI 1.36–1.61).[6] In HFpEF, enhanced activation of inflammatory markers is well documented. The BIOSTAT-HF study demonstrated that HFmrEF patients show a biomarker injury profile resembling HFrEF, while also sharing certain HFpEF traits, such as extracellular matrix remodeling and β-catenin pathway activation.[7]

Biomarkers in HFpEF and HFmrEF are now widely recognized as being sensitive for both early diagnosis and prognostication.[8] Regardless of ejection fraction category, elevated levels of NT-proBNP, growth differentiation factor-15 (GDF-15), and high-sensitivity troponin T (hs-TnT) are consistently linked with worse HF outcomes. Emerging research highlights the potential role of microRNAs (miRNAs)—small, circulating noncoding RNAs capable of distinguishing between HF phenotypes. Their diagnostic and prognostic utility may represent the next frontier in precision medicine for HF.[9]

IMAGING

Multimodality imaging is essential for the early detection of HF, identification of its underlying etiology, and evaluation of the response to therapy.[10] Echocardiographic global longitudinal strain (GLS) provides greater sensitivity than conventional LVEF in predicting outcomes. GLS is a simple, reproducible bedside tool with particular value in patients with preserved EF (LVEF > 45%). Other echocardiographic parameters, such as left atrial (LA) compliance (measured as the ratio of LA reservoir strain to E/é) during exercise versus rest, and the exercise E/é ratio, are commonly used noninvasive tools for assessing diastolic dysfunction and diagnosing HFpEF.[11]

Importantly, more than half of HF patients present with symptomatic disease despite preserved or mildly reduced ejection fraction. These patients frequently have multiple noncardiac comorbidities, making guideline-directed therapy difficult to apply, and their long-term outcomes remain uncertain.[12]

COMORBIDITIES

The presence of comorbidities exerts a substantial negative impact on the prognosis of HF. Many patients are elderly, frail, and on polypharmacy, increasing the risk of adverse outcomes. Data from the PINNACLE registry (n = 697,542) reported that 46.5% of patients had HFpEF and 8.1% had HFmrEF. Among these, hypertension, diabetes mellitus, atrial fibrillation, chronic kidney disease (CKD), COPD, and obesity were common in the HFpEF group, whereas systemic hypertension, coronary artery disease (CAD), and peripheral artery disease (PAD) were more frequent in HFmrEF.[13]

Additional studies highlight geographic and population-based variations. A Japanese prospective study reported high rates of hypertension, dyslipidemia, CKD, anemia, and sleep apnea among HFpEF patients.[14] Similarly, analysis of the Swedish registry (2000–2018) compared comorbidity patterns between primary care and secondary care cohorts. The prevalence of ischemic heart disease (54.3% vs. 56.7%), kidney disease (44.3% vs. 61.7%), hypertension (62.2% vs. 76.6%), and anemia (33% vs. 40.8%) differed between the two, with HFpEF patients generally demonstrating a slightly higher burden of comorbidities than HFmrEF patients.[15]

Obesity and diabetes play a central role in the pathophysiology of both HFpEF and HFmrEF. Obesity, in particular, is an independent risk factor for HFpEF. Excess adipose tissue contributes to adverse remodeling through several mechanisms: (1) Reduced natriuretic peptide levels due to aldosterone production from adipocytes; (2) myocardial stiffness and vascular dysfunction driven by extracellular matrix remodeling; and (3) systemic proinflammatory state mediated by dysfunctional adipocytes. Recent studies, such as PROMISE-HFpEF, demonstrated that increased epicardial adipose tissue (EAT) exerts inflammatory damage via adipokines. Elevated EAT has been associated with venous and vascular endothelial dysfunction, increased LV end-diastolic pressure, impaired coronary flow reserve, and adverse prognosis.[16]

TREATMENT

Heart failure is a chronic condition that often coexists with multiple comorbidities. Numerous randomized controlled trials (RCTs) have evaluated pharmacological interventions, focusing primarily on the composite outcome of CV death and HFH. However, these studies had several limitations, including heterogeneity in inclusion criteria and endpoints. Consequently, the full application of guideline-directed therapies to the highly diverse HFmrEF/HFpEF populations remains challenging. Many patients in these groups are currently treated with combined regimens—targeting both HF and associated comorbidities.

A key distinction lies in the strength of evidence. Unlike HFrEF, where therapies such as ACE inhibitors/angiotensin receptor–neprilysin inhibitor (ARNI), beta-blockers, mineralocorticoid receptor antagonists (MRAs), and sodium-glucose cotransporter-2 (SGLT-2) inhibitors have robust Class IA recommendations, the evidence for HFmrEF/HFpEF is considerably weaker. This population is typically older, frailer, and burdened by multiple comorbidities, increasing their vulnerability to polypharmacy, drug interactions, and side effects.

It is also observed that the HFmrEF/HFpEF is more prevalent among older individuals and those who carry greater frailty and comorbid disease burden, leading to increased CV and noncardiovascular morbidity. The patients in HFmrEF/HFpEF often require polypharmacy and are potentially vulnerable to drug interactions and side effects. The effects of combination pharmacotherapy, working through various routes in individuals with HFmrEF or HFpEF, were evaluated in a meta-analysis of over 30,000 patients with a median follow-up of 33 months. Treatment with ACE/ARNI, selective beta-blocker, MRA, and SGLT2 inhibitor reduced the HFH, composite of CV death (HR 0.47; 95% CI 0.31–0.70), and CV death (HR 0.55; 95% CI 0.70).[17] SGLT-2 inhibitor, Dapagliflozin regardless of baseline NYHA class, dapagliflozin consistently decreased the risk of the primary endpoint when compared with a placebo in a prespecified analysis of the DELIVER study. Additionally, patients with NYHA III–IV showed a greater improvement in quality of life.[18] Across a broad spectrum of renal functioning, empagliflozin's effectiveness on the primary outcome of HFH or CV death remained constant.

■ Pharmacological Therapy

These patients usually require combination therapy along with treatment for noncardiac comorbidities. A large meta-analysis of >30,000 patients with a median follow-up of 33 months evaluated combination therapy with ACE inhibitors/ARNI, beta-blockers, MRAs, and SGLT2 inhibitors. This regimen reduced the risk of HFH, CV death, and the composite endpoint (HR 0.47; 95% CI 0.31–0.70 for composite outcome; HR 0.55; 95% CI 0.70 for CV death).[17]

Sodium-glucose Cotransporter-2 Inhibitor

Sodium-glucose cotransporter-2 inhibitors have emerged as the most consistent therapy in this group. In the DELIVER trial, dapagliflozin significantly reduced the risk of the primary endpoint compared with placebo, regardless of baseline NYHA class. Patients with NYHA III–IV also demonstrated greater improvement in quality of life (QoL).[18]

Empagliflozin maintained its efficacy across a broad spectrum of renal function in reducing the composite of HFH or CV death. A pooled analysis by Bhatt et al. combining DAPA-HF and DELIVER (n = 11,007) demonstrated that dapagliflozin improved Kansas City Cardiomyopathy Questionnaire (KCCQ) scores across all LVEF ranges as early as 3 months, with benefits sustained at 8 months.[19]

A larger meta-analysis of 14 RCTs (n = 21,737) confirmed that SGLT-2 inhibitors improved QoL across the spectrum of LVEF, with particularly strong effects in patients with recent HF worsening.[20]

The landmark outcome trials: DELIVER (dapagliflozin) and EMPEROR-Preserved (empagliflozin) demonstrated significant reductions in the composite endpoint of CV death or HFH compared with placebo.[21] In EMPEROR-Preserved trial, patients with LVEF >40% treated with empagliflozin showed a significantly lower risk of CV death or worsening HF events (HFH or urgent ER visit requiring escalation of diuretics).[22]

Mineralocorticoid Receptor Antagonists

Mineralocorticoid receptor antagonists act by blocking mineralocorticoid receptors (MRs), thereby preventing aldosterone or 11-deoxycorticosterone from inducing receptor activation. This blockade reduces inflammation and adverse cardiac remodeling, ultimately helping to preserve or improve HF symptoms and outcomes. The STRUCTURE study demonstrated that spironolactone improved exercise capacity and E/é, particularly in HFpEF patients with normal LV filling pressures at rest but increased filling pressures during activity.[23]

A patient-level meta-analysis of 984 HFpEF patients from HOMAGE, Aldo-DHF, and TOPCAT trials showed that spironolactone was associated with improved systolic and diastolic function, along with reductions in LA volume, LV mass, and wall thickness.[24]

In the TOPCAT trial, spironolactone reduced the risk of the composite outcome (CV death, aborted cardiac arrest, or HFH) in specific subgroups. Patients without a prior HFH in the preceding year experienced greater benefit. Importantly, significant regional variations were observed: Benefit was noted in North and South America, but not in Russia and Georgia, where paradoxical harm was suggested.[25]

The FINEARTS-HF trial evaluated finerenone, a novel nonsteroidal MRA, in patients with HFmrEF/HFpEF. Over a median follow-up of 32 months, finerenone significantly reduced the primary outcome of total worsening HF events or CV death compared with placebo (rate ratio: 0.84; 95% CI 0.74–0.95; p = 0.007). Total worsening HF events were also lower in the finerenone group (rate ratio 0.82; 95% CI 0.71–0.94; p = 0.006). Mortality benefit was less pronounced (HR 0.93; 95% CI 0.78–1.11).[26] These results suggest finerenone may be a valuable therapeutic option in selected patients with HFmrEF/HFpEF.

Angiotensin Receptor–Neprilysin Inhibitors

Angiotensin receptor–neprilysin inhibitors therapy, well established in HFrEF, is increasingly studied in HFmrEF and HFpEF. By blocking RAAS activation and enhancing natriuretic peptide pathways, ARNIs provide dual neurohumoral modulation. In the PARAGON-HF trial, sacubitril/valsartan narrowly missed statistical significance for the primary endpoint in HFpEF overall but demonstrated subgroup benefits, particularly in women and in patients with LVEF between 45 and 57%, where the risk of CV death or HFH was reduced compared with valsartan.[27] In HFmrEF, initiation of sacubitril/valsartan has also been linked to a reduced need for new loop diuretic therapy during follow-up, reflecting improved volume management.

Semaglutide

Semaglutide, a glucagon-like peptide 1 (GLP-1) agonist, a hypoglycemic drug with anti-inflammatory properties, was given once weekly at a dose of 2.4 mg for a year in the STEP-HFpEF trial. It significantly reduced body weight in obese HFpEF patients (13.3% loss compared to 2.6% in the placebo group) and improved their KCCQ clinical summary score, 6-minute walk distance. It also improved NYHA Class II–IV, natriuretic peptide levels. Most of the enrolled patients (84%) had LVEF ≥ 50%, and semaglutide reduced NT-proBNP levels by around 15% more than a placebo.[28]

Examining the potential benefits of cardiac contractility modulation (CCM) in 47 patients with HFpEF was the aim of the single-arm, multicenter pilot study CCM-HFpEF. KCCQ, the main outcome, rose 18.0 (±16.6) points ($p < 0.001$). In the study, the event-free rate was 93.6%, and the safety profile was fairly good.[29]

SUBGROUP ANALYSIS BY LEFT VENTRICULAR EJECTION FRACTION

Evidence suggests that the therapeutic benefit of ARNI, MRA, and SGLT-2 inhibitors differs according to LVEF range: A meta-analysis showed that triple therapy (ARNI + MRA + SGLT-2 inhibitor) reduced the primary outcome substantially in HFmrEF (HR 0.28; 95% CI 0.15–0.54). In HFpEF, the effect was more modest (HR 0.62; 95% CI 0.42–0.93), with SGLT-2 inhibitors driving most of the benefit. In patients with LVEF 50–60%, triple therapy yielded a clear reduction in HFHs (HR 0.62; 95% CI 0.45–0.85). In patients with LVEF > 60%, the benefit was attenuated (HR 0.72; 95% CI 0.52–0.99) and limited mainly to HFHs rather than CV death.[17]

REAL-WORLD EFFECTIVENESS

Real-world data on pharmacologic therapy in HFmrEF and HFpEF remain heterogeneous due to differences in trial inclusion criteria, comorbidity burden, endpoints, and variable drug dosing driven by hemodynamic status.

DISCUSSION

Evidence from pooled analyses suggests that a combination of SGLT-2 inhibitors, ARNI, MRAs, and β-blockers can be highly effective in patients with HFmrEF, particularly in reducing the composite of CV death, HFH, and cardiac death. Interestingly, even in the absence of β-blockers, outcomes were favorable, highlighting the incremental role of SGLT-2 inhibitors. These agents consistently reduced HFH, although their effect on all-cause mortality was not significant, even when used in combination with RAAS inhibitors. Future trials may clarify the benefits of new drug combinations.[30]

Therapy in HFmrEF/HFpEF must take into account the heterogeneity of these populations. Efforts at phenotyping—through clinical, imaging, and biomarker-guided approaches—will be critical for guiding individualized treatment. Importantly, not all drugs should be initiated simultaneously, since risks and responses differ between HF categories.[31]

The FINEARTS-HF trial demonstrated that the novel nonsteroidal MRA finerenone reduced the composite of CV death and total HF events in patients with LVEF > 40%, with additional improvements in quality of life.[26]

The role of β-blockers in HFmrEF and HFpEF remains less clear. No large RCT has shown a significant benefit in patients with LVEF > 40%.[30] About 70% of this population is already prescribed β-blockers, often for comorbidities such as CAD, atrial fibrillation, or hypertension.[31-33] However, evidence suggests no added benefit of β-blockers over triple therapy with SGLT-2 inhibitor, ARNI, and MRA in these patients.[34] A lower resting heart rate in HFpEF is paradoxically linked to poor outcomes, and β-blockers may be considered selectively, particularly in cases of excess sympathetic activity. Digoxin is generally discouraged in elderly HFpEF patients due to safety concerns.[35]

The STRONG trial, which included HF patients across all EF categories, suggested improved outcomes with early initiation and rapid titration of β-blockers in combination therapy.[36] Importantly, the addition of SGLT-2 Inhibitors have shown the most robust and consistent benefits in terms of safety and efficacy across the full LVEF spectrum. Patients who improve from HFrEF into the HFmrEF or HFimpEF (improved EF) spectrum benefit from continuation of HFrEF guideline-directed therapy, as rapid sequencing of neurohormonal antagonists accelerates recovery. Across all EF categories, SGLT-2 inhibitors have the strongest and most consistent evidence, and they should be considered cornerstone therapy alongside management of comorbidities and etiologies.[22]

CONCLUSION

Heart failure with mildly reduced ejection fraction and HFpEF impose a growing burden on global healthcare due to their high morbidity and mortality. Since its formal recognition in the 2021 ESC guidelines, HFmrEF has been a challenging category because of its overlapping features with both HFrEF and HFpEF. Advanced imaging modalities—such as 2D speckle-tracking echocardiography (2D-STE), 3D-STE, T1 mapping, and cardiac magnetic resonance feature tracking (CMR-FT)—along with emerging biomarkers, can help identify high-risk patients and improve phenotyping. Treatment for HFmrEF should generally follow HFrEF guidelines, as most of the benefit is derived from neurohormonal antagonism. For HFpEF, optimal management requires a multidisciplinary approach, given its complex pathophysiology, elderly patient population, and frequent comorbidities.

REFERENCES

1. McDonagh TA, Metra M, Adamo M, et al. 2021 ESC Guidelines for the diagnosis and treatment of acute and chronic heart failure: Developed by the Task Force for the diagnosis and treatment of acute and chronic heart failure of the European Society of Cardiology (ESC) With the special contribution of the Heart Failure Association (HFA) of the ESC. Eur Heart J. 2021;42(36):3599-726.
2. Ponikowski P, Voors AA, Anker SD, et al. 2016 ESC Guidelines for the diagnosis and treatment of acute and chronic heart failure: The Task Force for the diagnosis and treatment of acute and chronic heart failure of the European Society of Cardiology (ESC) Developed with the special contribution of the Heart Failure Association (HFA) of the ESC. European Heart J. 2016;37:2129-200.

3. Groenewegen A, Rutten FH, Mosterd A, et al. Epidemiology of heart failure. Eur J Heart Fail. 2020;22:1342-56.
4. Lam CSP, Voors AA, Piotr P, et al. Time to rename the middle child of heart failure: Heart failure with mildly reduced ejection fraction. Eur Heart J. 2020;41:2353-5.
5. Tromp J, Lim SL, Tay WT, et al. Microvascular disease in patients with diabetes with heart failure and reduced ejection versus preserved ejection fraction. Diabetes Care. 2019;42(9):1792-9.
6. McMurray JJV, Adamopoulos S, Anker SD, et al. ESC Guidelines for the diagnosis and treatment of acute and chronic heart failure 2012: The Task Force for the Diagnosis and Treatment of Acute and Chronic Heart Failure 2012 of the European Society of Cardiology. Developed in collaboration with the Heart. Eur J Heart Fail. 2012;14:803-69.
7. Voors AA, Anker SD, Cleland JG, et al. A systems BIOlogy Study to TAilored Treatment in Chronic Heart Failure: rationale, design, and baseline characteristics of BIOSTAT-CHF. Eur J Heart Fail. 2016;18(6):716-26.
8. Bayes-Genis A, Rosano G. Unlocking the potential of natriuretic peptide testing in primary care: A roadmap for early heart failure diagnosis. Eur J Heart Fail. 2023;25:1181-4.
9. Parvan R, Hosseinpour M, Moradi Y, et al. Diagnostic performance of microRNAs in the detection of heart failure with reduced or preserved ejection fraction: A systematic review and meta-analysis. Eur J Heart Fail. 2022;24:2212-25.
10. Moura B, Aimo A, Al-Mohammad A, et al. Diagnosis and management of patients with left ventricular hypertrophy: Role of multimodality cardiac imaging. A scientific statement of the Heart Failure Association of the European Society of Cardiology. Eur J Heart Fail. 2023;25:1493-506.
11. Harada T, Kagami K, Shina T, et al. Diagnostic value of reduced left atrial compliance during ergometry exercise in heart failure with preserved ejection fraction. Eur J Heart Fail. 2023;25:1293-303.
12. Lakhani I, Leung KSK, Tse G, et al. Novel mechanisms in heart failure with preserved, midrange, and reduced ejection fraction. Front Physiol. 2019;10:874.
13. Ibrahim NE, Song Y, Cannon CP, et al. Heart failure with mid-range ejection fraction: characterization of patients from the PINNACLE Registry®. ESC Heart Fail. 2019;6(4):784-92.
14. Yoshihisa A, Sato Y, Kanno Y, et al. Prognostic impacts of changes in left ventricular ejection fraction in heart failure patients with preserved left ventricular ejection fraction. Open Heart. 2020;7(1):e001112.
15. Lindberg F, Lund LH, Benson L, et al. Patient profile and outcomes associated with follow-up in specialty vs. primary care in heart failure. ESC Heart Fail. 2022;9(2):822-33.
16. Rodrigues MM, Falcão LM. Pathophysiology of heart failure with preserved ejection fraction in overweight and obesity - Clinical and treatment implications. Int J Cardiol. 2025;430:133182.
17. Zafeiropoulos S, Farmakis IT, Milioglou I, et al. Pharmacological Treatments in Heart Failure With Mildly Reduced and Preserved Ejection Fraction: Systematic Review and Network Meta-Analysis. JACC Heart Fail. 2024;12(4):616-27.
18. Yang M, Butt JH, Kondo T, et al. Dapagliflozin in patients with heart failure with mildly reduced and preserved ejection fraction treated with a mineralocorticoid receptor antagonist or sacubitril/valsartan. Eur J Heart Fail. 2022;24:2307-19.
19. Bhatt AS, Kosiborod MN, Vaduganathan M, et al. Effect of dapagliflozin on health status and quality of life across the spectrum of ejection fraction: Participant-level pooled analysis from the DAPA-HF and DELIVER trials. Eur J Heart Fail. 2023;25:981-8.
20. Zheng SL, Chan FT, Nabeebaccus AA, et al. Drug treatment effects on outcomes in heart failure with preserved ejection fraction: a systematic review and meta-analysis. Heart. 2018;104(5):407-15.
21. Solomon SD, McMurray JJV, Claggett B, et al. Dapagliflozin in heart failure with mildly reduced or preserved ejection fraction. N Engl J Med. 2022;387(12):1089-98.
22. Anker SD, Butler J, Filippatos G, et al.; the EMPEROR-Preserved Trial Investigators. Empagliflozin in Heart Failure with a Preserved Ejection Fraction. N Engl J Med. 2021;385(16):1451-61.
23. Kosmala W, Rojek A, Przewlocka Kosmala M, et al. Effect of aldosterone antagonism on exercise tolerance in heart failure with preserved ejection fraction. J Am Coll Cardiol. 2016;68:1823-34.
24. Ferreira JP, Cleland JG, Girerd N, et al. Spironolactone effect on cardiac structure and function of patients with heart failure and preserved ejection fraction: A pooled analysis of three randomized trials. Eur J Heart Fail. 2023;25:108-13.
25. Pitt B, Pfeffer MA, Assmann SF, et al. Spironolactone for heart failure with preserved ejection fraction. N Engl J Med. 2014;370(15):1383-92.
26. Solomon SD, McMurray JJV; FINEARTS-HF Committees and Investigators. Finerenone in Heart Failure with Mildly Reduced or Preserved Ejection Fraction. N Engl J Med. 2024;391(16):1475-85.
27. Chatur S, Claggett BL, Vardeny O, et al. Sacubitril/valsartan and loop diuretic requirement in heart failure with preserved ejection fraction in the PARAGON-HF trial. Eur J Heart Fail. 2023;25: 87-94.
28. Kosiborod MN, Abildstrøm SZ, Borlaug BA, et al. Semaglutide in patients with heart failure with preserved ejection fraction and obesity. New Engl J Med. 2023;389:1069-84.
29. Linde C, Grabowski M, Ponikowski P, et al. Cardiac contractility modulation therapy improves health status in patients with heart failure with preserved ejection fraction: A pilot study (CCM-HFpEF). Eur J Heart Fail. 2022;24:2275-84.
30. Xiang B, Zhang R, Wu X, et al. Optimal pharmacologic treatment of heart failure with preserved and mildly reduced ejection fraction: a meta-analysis. JAMA Netw Open. 2022;5(9).
31. Anker SD, Usman MS, Anker MS, et al. Patient phenotype profiling in heart failure with preserved ejection fraction to guide therapeutic decision making. A scientific statement of the Heart Failure Association, the European Heart Rhythm Association of the European Society of Cardiology, and the European Society of Hypertension. Eur J Heart Fail. 2023;25(7):936-55.
32. Cleland JGF, Bunting KV, Flather MD, et al. Beta-blockers for heart failure with reduced, mid-range, and preserved ejection fraction: an individual patient-level analysis of double-blind randomized trials. Eur Heart J. 2018;39(1):26-35.
33. Palau P, Seller J, Domínguez E, et al. Effect of b-blocker withdrawal on functional capacity in heart failure and preserved ejection fraction. J Am Coll Cardiol. 2021;78(21):2042-56.
34. Silverman DN, Plante TB, Infeld M, et al. Association of β-blocker use with heart failure hospitalizations and cardiovascular disease mortality among patients with heart failure with a preserved ejection fraction: a secondary analysis of the TOPCAT trial. JAMA Netw Open. 2019;2(12).
35. Llàcer P, Núñez J, Bayés-Genís A, et al. Digoxin and prognosis of heart failure in older patients with preserved ejection fraction: importance of heart rate. Results from an observational and multicenter study. Eur J Intern Med. 2019;60:18-23.
36. Mebazaa A, Davison B, Chioncel O, et al. Safety, tolerability and efficacy of up-titration of guideline-directed medical therapies for acute heart failure (STRONG-HF): a multinational, open label, randomised, trial. Lancet. 2022;400(10367):1938-52.

CHAPTER

38

Characteristics and Outcomes of Patients with Valvular Cardiogenic Shock

Sumanyu Suresh, Harikrishnan Sivadasanpillai

ABSTRACT

Valvular cardiogenic shock (VCS) is an under-recognized etiology of cardiogenic shock that accounts for about 16% of cases and is caused by acute severe native or prosthetic valve dysfunction. Unlike myocardial pump failure, VCS is caused by sudden hemodynamic collapse brought on by mechanical obstruction or regurgitation, with 30-day and 1-year mortality rates are 28% and 44%, respectively, and are both considerably higher than those of nonvalvular shock. Early recognition of the VCS and underlying valvular pathology is important for timely intervention and better outcomes. Conventional management was restricted by the high surgical risk in these patients, but recent advances, such as transcatheter aortic valve replacement, edge-to-edge mitral repair, and mechanical circulatory support, have expanded treatment options, leading to improved short- and mid-term outcomes.

Keywords: Valvular cardiogenic shock, acute valvular dysfunction, acute on chronic valvular dysfunction, high mortality, emergent transcatheter aortic valve implantation, transcatheter valve therapy, mechanical circulatory support.

INTRODUCTION

Cardiogenic shock (CS) is the most severe form of acute heart failure, characterized by inadequate tissue perfusion caused by primary cardiac dysfunction, leading to multiorgan hypoperfusion and high mortality rates.[1] Although the most common cause of CS is still acute myocardial infarction, valvular heart disease, especially acute severe lesions, is a clinically significant but frequently under-recognized etiology.[2] There are a few noteworthy distinctions between ischemic and nonischemic myocardial causes of shock and VCS. In VCS, hemodynamic compromise is often sudden and caused by mechanical obstruction or regurgitation, rather than being a result of primary myocardial pump failure. Second, a dramatic hemodynamic recovery can occur after addressing the underlying valvular pathology, which can usually be done surgically or through transcatheter means. This emphasizes the significance of prompt diagnosis and timely intervention.

The epidemiological burden of VCS is not negligible. Primary valvular pathology accounted for 16% of all CS admissions in a recent Cleveland Clinic cohort, with approximately 70% VCS having native valve dysfunction and the rest due to prosthetic valve dysfunction.[3] The short-term mortality rate for these patients was noticeably higher than that of patients with nonvalvular CS.[3] Historically, management of VCS was limited by elevated operative mortality in unstable patients. Treatment options have increased thanks to the advent of minimally invasive valve therapies, better perioperative care, and mechanical circulatory support (MCS) devices. The need for ongoing advancements in early recognition, hemodynamic optimization, and procedural timing is underscored by the fact that in-hospital mortality remains as high 17% even after definitive intervention.[4]

This chapter provides a comprehensive synopsis of current knowledge on VCS, highlights emerging data from registries and clinical trials, and outlines future research priorities.

DEFINITION AND CLASSIFICATION

Valvular cardiogenic shock (VCS) is defined as a clinical syndrome of inadequate tissue perfusion and end-organ hypoperfusion caused by primary acute severe valvular dysfunction or acute-on-chronic worsening of primary valvular disease, in the absence of hypovolemia and with evidence of poor cardiac output (CO).[1,2] A combination of clinical, hemodynamic, and biochemical criteria supports the diagnosis.

The *hemodynamic profile* of CS, as per the Society for Cardiovascular Angiography and Interventions (SCAI) and European Society of Cardiology (ESC), typically includes:

- *Systolic blood pressure (SBP)*: <90 mm Hg or need for vasopressor support to maintain SBP ≥ 90 mm Hg
- *Cardiac index (CI)*: <2.2 L/min/m²
- *Pulmonary capillary wedge pressure (PCWP)*: >15 mm Hg (in left-sided failure)
- *Evidence of end-organ hypoperfusion*: For example, oliguria, altered mental status, and elevated lactate.

While these thresholds help in diagnosis, CS is increasingly recognized as a continuum rather than a binary state, leading to the adoption of the SCAI shock staging system (A–E), which captures progression from "at risk" (Stage A) to "extremis" as mentioned in **Table 1**.[5]

The hemodynamic and clinical characteristics of VCS are depicted in **Table 2**.[1,4,6,7]

DEMOGRAPHIC CHARACTERISTICS

Patients with VCS tend to be *older* (median age 70 years vs. 64 years in non-VCS cohorts) with slight *female* dominance (40% vs. ~32% in non-VCS), and have a *higher comorbidity burden*, e.g., chronic kidney disease, atrial fibrillation, and prior valve interventions.[3,4,6]

PATHOPHYSIOLOGY

Valvular cardiogenic shock is a complex hemodynamic syndrome characterized by tissue hypoperfusion and low CO caused by severe mechanical valve dysfunction and the heart's inability to generate sufficient forward flow. The hemodynamic derangements are best understood using pressure–volume loop (P–V loop) analysis.

Valve-specific Hemodynamic Patterns

Critical aortic stenosis (AS): It leads to severe pressure overload with markedly elevated left ventricular (LV) systolic pressures (>200 mm Hg), reduced stroke volume (SV) despite preserved ejection fraction (EF), and elevated PCWP (>18 mm Hg) due to diastolic dysfunction. The P–V loop shows a rightward shift with a narrow, tall configuration as shown in **Figure 1A**. In the presence of a decompensating event like arrhythmia, ischemia, infection, or progressive valve obstruction, CO falls suddenly. The ventricle can no longer augment SV, and CO falls rapidly, in compensation, afterload increases. These patients have a poor prognosis and need early intervention.[8-10]

Acute severe aortic regurgitation (AR): Immediate and severe LV volume overload due to the diastolic regurgitant blood

TABLE 1: The SCAI shock staging system.

SCAI stage	Description	Clinical features	Mortality (%)
A: At risk	Patient not having CS but at risk (e.g., severe valvular disease)	No hypotension or hypoperfusion	<5
B: Beginning shock	Patient has relative hypotension, but no hypoperfusion	SBP < 90 mm Hg or MAP drop >30 mm Hg without hypoperfusion	10–20
C: Classic shock	Hypoperfusion that needs intervention beyond volume resuscitation	Evidence of hypoperfusion requiring inotropes/pressors or MCS	20–30
D: Deteriorating	Similar to stage C but worsening despite initial interventions	Failure to respond to interventions after 30 minutes	40–60
E: Extremis	Circulatory collapse with ongoing CPR or multiple acute interventions	Cardiovascular collapse, refractory arrest, and ECPR	70–90

(CPR: cardiopulmonary resuscitation; ECPR: extracorporeal cardiopulmonary resuscitation; MAP: mean arterial pressure; MCS: mechanical circulatory support)

TABLE 2: Hemodynamic and clinical characteristics of VCS.

Parameter	Normal	Cardiogenic shock	Valvular shock specifics
Systolic BP (mm Hg)	>90	<90 or requiring support	May be maintained in acute MR
Cardiac index (L/min/m²)	>2.5	<2.2	Often severely reduced
PCWP (mm Hg)	<12	>15–18	Markedly elevated in MR/MS
CVP (mm Hg)	<8	Variable	Elevated in AS with RV dysfunction
SVR (dynes-s/cm^{-5})	800–1,200	>1,200	Variable based on valve lesion
Lactate (mmol/L)	<2.0	>2.0	Often markedly elevated
Mixed venous O_2 sat (%)	>65	<60	Severely reduced

(AS: aortic stenosis; CVP: central venous pressure; MR: mitral regurgitation; MS: mitral stenosis; PCWP: pulmonary capillary wedge pressure; RV: right ventricular; SVR: systemic vascular resistance)

from the aorta. In contrast to chronic AR, in acute AR, the left ventricle has limited compliance, which leads to combined pressure and volume overload with rapid ventricular dilation, markedly increased left ventricular end diastolic pressure (LVEDP) (>25 mm Hg), reduced diastolic blood pressure (<40 mm Hg), and compensatory tachycardia. As shown in **Figure 1B**, in chronic AR, there is a minimal change in LVEDP despite the large volume overload as seen by the shift in the diastolic pressure–volume curve to the right (green loop). Low systemic diastolic pressures result in a brief isovolumetric phase and early complete ejection. The isovolumetric relaxation phase is not seen, because the incompetent valve permits filling of the left ventricle from the aorta during diastole, even before opening of the mitral valve. In contrast, when acute severe AR (blue loop) occurs, a characteristic triangular P–V loop is observed. The LV compliance is preserved, and a rapid *increase in LVEDP* from regurgitated blood rapidly led to *increased left atrial pressure (LAP)* and pulmonary congestion.[8,10-12]

Chronic mitral regurgitation (MR): In chronic MR, the shape of the pressure–volume loop as shown in **Figure 1C**, is shifted to the right; the loop has an increased area, a highly increased end-diastolic volume, a marginally increased LVEDP, an absence of isovolumic contraction phase, because of the left ventricle starts ejecting into left atrium (LA) with the beginning of LV contraction, a sustained ejection phase as the left ventricle continues to eject in a highly compliant LA, a very short isovolumic relaxation phase as the mitral valve opens early because of increased left atrial volume and pressure.[8,10,13,14] This rightward shift of the P–V loop is compensated by the preserved LV function initially, but when LV dysfunction sets in as a part of myocardial remodeling, fibrosis, contractile dysfunction, or any other precipitating event, there is a decline in forward CO, resulting in CS.[13]

Acute severe MR: Most classically happens after papillary muscle rupture following a myocardial infarction. It leads to acute volume overload of a noncompliant LA and left ventricle, resulting in significantly elevated PCWP (>25 mm Hg) with giant v-waves, reduced forward CI (<2.0 L/min/m^2), normal systemic vascular resistance (SVR), pulmonary venous congestion, and flash pulmonary edema. Forward

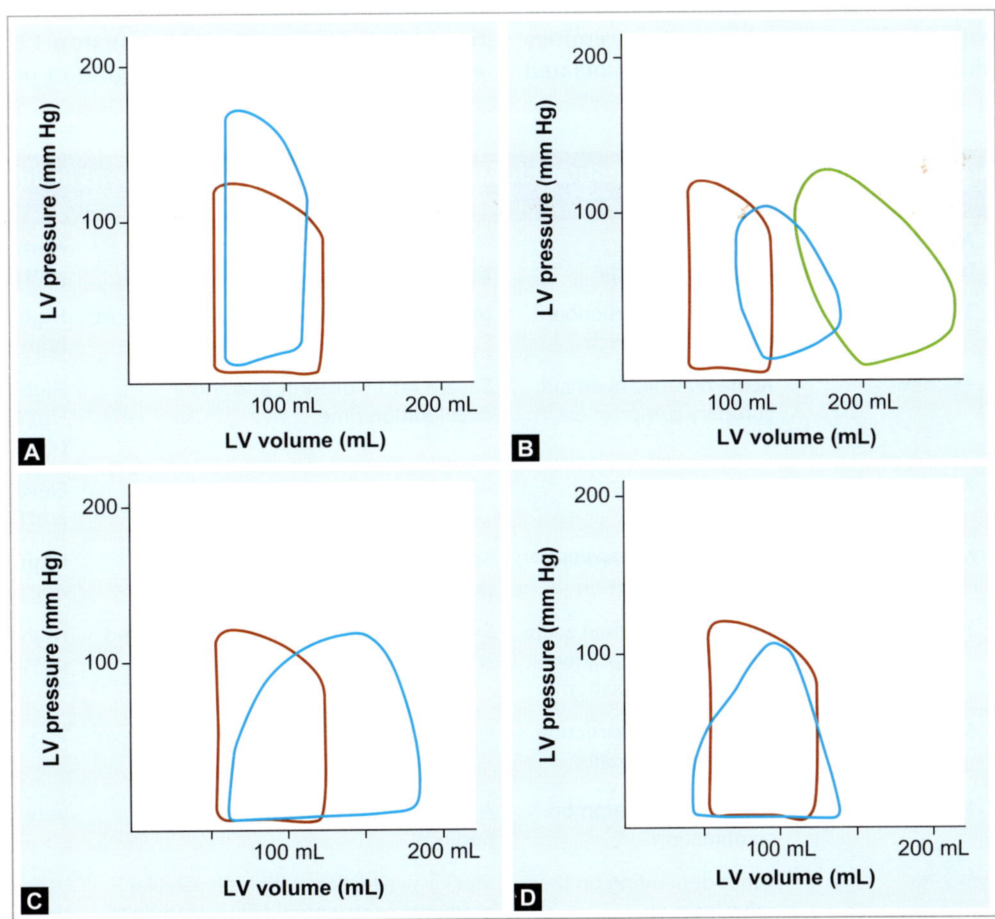

FIGS. 1A TO D: Pressure–Volume loops in (A) Red loop is normal, and blue loop is suggestive of severe aortic stenosis; (B) Red loop is normal, blue loop suggests acute aortic regurgitation, and red loop suggests chronic severe aortic regurgitation; (C) The red loop is normal, and the blue loop suggests chronic mitral regurgitation; (D) The red loop is normal; the blue loop suggests acute severe mitral regurgitation.

effective SV is less, as a large portion of each SV is lost retrograde. The P–V loop is shown in **Figure 1D**, a minimal increase in LV end-diastolic volume and a variable increase in LVEDP, depending on the severity of MR, a short isovolumic contraction phase as the left ventricle empties blood into the LA early during systole, prolonged ejection phase as the left ventricle continues to eject into the LA until the LV pressure equals the LAP during systole, a reduced end-systolic LV volume, and a short isovolumic relaxation phase as the mitral valve opens early because of a relatively high LAP followed by rapid LV filling.[8,10,13,14]

The valvular lesion, its pathophysiology, and hemodynamic pattern are summarized in **Table 3**.[3,4,6,9,12,15-22]

LABORATORY AND IMAGING FINDINGS

On assessment, there will be classic signs of low CO: Cool extremities, oliguria (less than 0.5 mL/kg/h), sustained hypotension (SBP < 90 mm Hg or the need for vasopressors), altered mental status, pulmonary edema, elevated jugular venous pulse (JVP), depending on the dysfunctional valve and clinical clues to the valvular pathology (such as a holosystolic murmur in MR or a harsh mid systolic murmur in AS).[1,5,7] Pulse volume discrepancy between extremities should raise suspicion of aortic dissection and associated AR. Laboratory results show rising blood urea nitrogen and creatinine levels, suggesting end-organ dysfunction, markedly elevated natriuretic peptides (BNP/NT-proBNP often >5,000 pg/mL) linked to wall stress, raised lactate levels (>2.0 mmol/L) reflecting tissue hypoperfusion, and elevated troponin indicative of myocardial injury or supply–demand mismatch. Even though markedly elevated troponin suggests acute myocardial infarction with papillary muscle rupture leading to acute MR, troponin levels were a better prognostic marker than NT-proBNP in predicting 30-day mortality in non-ACS CS patients.[23] Transthoracic echocardiogram (TTE) plays a major role in the rapid diagnosis of valvular pathology, and a transesophageal echocardiogram (TEE) is useful in establishing the etiology of valve dysfunction and in the evaluation of prosthetic valve dysfunction.[19-21]

MANAGEMENT

Intensive care

2025 concise clinical guidance by ACC on the evaluation and management of CS emphasizes the early diagnosis of CS by prompt recognition of symptoms and signs, monitoring urine output, peripheral perfusion,12-lead ECG, and echocardiogram and early recognition of the etiology and

TABLE 3: Summary of pathophysiology, echocardiographic findings, and hemodynamic patterns in different valvular lesions with CS.

Valve lesion	Approximate frequency in VCS	Pathophysiology	Key echo findings	Hemodynamic pattern
Critical AS	35–45%	LV outflow obstruction, afterload mismatch	Mean gradient >40 mm Hg, AVA < 1.0 cm^2	High PCWP, low CI, high SVR
Acute severe AR	15–20%	Acute diastolic overload, coronary compromise	Severe AR, LV dilation, and short deceleration time	High LVEDP (>25 mm Hg), low diastolic BP (<40 mm Hg)
MR (as a whole)	25–35%	–	–	Elevated LA pressure and PCWP
Acute severe MR	6.9–10%	Acute volume overload, no LA/LV adaptation	Severe MR, normal LA/LV size, pulmonary edema	High PCWP, low CI, and normal SVR
Chronic severe MR	15–25%	More common than acute MR, chronic adaptation with decompensation	Severe MR, dilated LA/left ventricle, and reduced EF	High PCWP, low CI, and possible high SVR
Acute MS	5–10%	Mitral inflow obstruction, LA pressure elevation	Mean gradient >10 mm Hg, MVA <1.5 cm^2	Very high PCWP, low CI
Mixed valvular disease	10–20%	AS + MR most common combination	A combination of individual valve findings	Very high PCWP, low CI
Prosthetic valve dysfunction	5–29%	Varies depending on the valve location	Stuck valve leaflets with high valvular gradients or structural failure leading to severe regurgitation	Varies depending on the valve location, low CI

(AR: aortic regurgitation; AS: aortic stenosis; AVA: aortic valve area; CI: cardiac index; EF: ejection fraction; LA: left atrium; LV: left ventricular; LVEDP: left ventricular end diastolic pressure; MR: mitral regurgitation; MS: mitral stenosis; TR: tricuspid regurgitation; MVA: mitral valve area; PCWP: pulmonary capillary wedge pressure; RAP: right atrial pressure; RVSP: right ventricular systolic pressure; SVR: systemic vascular resistance)

transfer of the patient to a tertiary care facility for ICU care or to a cardiac catheterization laboratory for coronary angiogram (CAG), RHC, or temporary MCS within 90 minutes.[24] More than 30% of patients with severe valvular disease who need to be admitted to the ICU suffer from acute respiratory failure.[24] When using mechanical ventilation in VCS, clinician needs to be vigilant to contemplate regarding the effect of valve pathology and hemodynamics.[25] Positive pressure ventilation (PPV) has different effects: The benefits being that it lowers LV preload, afterload, and myocardial oxygen demand. Risks are that it reduces RV output by reducing venous return and increasing pulmonary vascular resistance. The overall impact depends on the severity of valve lesion, biventricular function, the preload, and afterload conditions. In severe AR, PPV can assist in reducing the pressure in the LV, whereas in severe mitral stenosis, PPV may lower the venous return, which could lower CO.[25] Volume optimization in VCS can be challenging and depends on the valvular pathology. In AS, it is dependent on preload; aggressive diuresis may lead to further hemodynamic deterioration. In acute MR, reducing the volume may help lower the regurgitant fraction. AR patients need gradual volume reduction while preserving forward flow.[25]

Pharmacological Management of Cardiogenic Shock

In CS, the primary objective of pharmacological therapy is to alleviate congestion, maximize CO, and improve perfusion to essential organs.[26,27] If a congestive phenotype exists, it should be managed with intravenous loop diuretics, thiazide diuretics for augmentation, and renal replacement therapy for ultrafiltration if the congestion is refractory to the medications. Intravenous vasoactive medications can be initiated to address hypoperfusion.[24] Inotropes enhance cardiac function by improving the myocardium's load-independent contractility. More precisely, cardiac calcitropes, such as phosphodiesterase 3 inhibitors and catecholamines, boost intracellular calcium levels to improve contractility. Interestingly, these compounds influence myocardial forces rather than having indirect effects on vascular tone and chronotropy, which is desirable in CS. When chronotropes increase CO mostly through an increase in heart rate, inodilators, such as milrinone or dobutamine, maximize CO, and decrease afterload via systemic vasodilation. Dopamine, norepinephrine, and epinephrine are inotropes that increase CO while increasing SVR.[26,27]

Forward CO can be enhanced by afterload reduction in suitable valve defects, mainly regurgitant lesions. It is noteworthy that angiotensin receptor blockers (ARBs) and angiotensin converting enzyme (ACE) inhibitors should not be used in hemodynamically unstable patients, and vascular dilators such as hydralazine or nitroglycerin have to be carefully used. Contraindications of afterload reduction include severe AS, which may precipitate hemodynamic deterioration.[25,27] In acute MR, avoid agents increasing afterload; milrinone and levosimendan are preferred for balanced inodilation. However, dobutamine is recommended in cases with severe AS, because excessive vasodilation must be avoided and preload must be maintained. Bradycardia is avoided in acute AR, and positive chronotropic medications are helpful.[24,25,27]

Advanced Therapy in Cardiogenic Shock

Mechanical circulatory support systems have been extensively studied in CS due to acute myocardial infarction, and the majority of studies show no significant benefit.[28,29] However, the effectiveness of MCS may differ in valvular CS; it needs to be supported by high-volume studies.

Intra-aortic Balloon Pump

Most commonly used MCS in CS, intra-aortic balloon pump (IABP) counter pulsation lowers afterload, enhances coronary perfusion, and modestly improves CO. Particularly helpful for acute MR, but not recommended for severe AR (may exacerbate regurgitant flow), and has a limited role in managing severe AS.[30-32]

Impella

Impella is a nonpulsatile, axial flow device, designed to pump blood from the left ventricle into the aorta.[32] The devices offer direct flow support and LV unloading, which is useful in post-TAVR patients and for native valves with mitral disease, with caution. There have been reports of successful deployment as a bridge in acute valvular CS to intervention.[31-36]

Venoarterial-extracorporeal Membrane Oxygenation

Venoarterial-extracorporeal membrane oxygenation (VA-ECMO) stabilizes the patient physiologically and reduces the risk of ongoing iatrogenic injury. ECMO also regulates gas exchange, perfusion, and provides adequate time for diagnosis, treatment, and recuperation from primary heart injury or disease.[37] When used in severe refractory shock, VA-ECMO provides full cardiac and respiratory support, particularly in cases of respiratory failure or biventricular dysfunction. Unrepaired aortic dissection and severe AR (which worsens LV distension) are absolute contraindications.[31,37-39]

DEFINITE MANAGEMENT

Transcatheter Aortic Valve Implantation

Transcatheter aortic valve implantation (TAVI) has become a game-changing treatment option for patients with severe AS. Initially, TAVI was reserved for inoperable or high-risk patients, but now it has been demonstrated to have comparable or superior outcomes to SAVR in intermediate[40,41] and even low-risk populations[42,43] in multicenter randomized controlled trials. The clinical application of TAVI is being extended with the introduction of so-called "emergent TAVI". In patients who were considered traditionally high-risk or unfit for intervention, selective TAVI is a feasible and acceptable option with favorable short- and long-term outcomes than the nonintervention group, even though it had a slightly increased risk of acute kidney injury and 30-day mortality compared to the elective TAVI patients.[15,44,45] The STS/ACC TVT Registry, the German Aortic Valve Registry (GARY), and another European multicenter registry suggest that timely TAVI may help restore hemodynamic stability, lower the need for vasopressors or mechanical support, and increase survival in selected patients despite the elevated periprocedural complications and early mortality rates.[45-47] In a large retrospective analysis by Llah et al., including 11,000 hospitalizations of severe AS with CS, TAVI has shown better results in terms of in-hospital outcomes compared to BAV, but had increased risk of stroke and pacemaker implantation.[48]

Transcatheter Mitral Valve Edge-to-edge Repair

In more than 85% of CS cases, transcatheter mitral valve edge-to-edge repair (M-TEER) has been associated with device success, with a reduction of MR to ≤2 in 88% cases and a significant reduction in 1-year all-cause mortality with an adjusted hazard ratio of 0.49 (95% CI 0.41–0.59; $p < 0.001$).[49] TEER is a promising management option for functional or myxomatous severe MR with CS and elevated surgical risk, which improves short-term and intermediate-term mortality, but requires additional research.[50-53]

OUTCOMES OF VALVULAR CARDIOGENIC SHOCK

Mortality rates are much higher in patients with VCS compared to those without valvular pathology, and results vary greatly depending upon the type of valve lesion, timing of intervention, and comorbidities.[2,3] When compared to definitive valve replacement, medical management alone carries the highest mortality risk, with hazard ratios of 3.69 (95% CI 2.04–6.66).[15] According to recent data, the 30-day mortality rate for VCS is 28% and 20% in non-VCS, while the 1-year mortality rate is 44% and 37%, respectively ($p < 0.001$).[3] The 30-day mortality rate for emergent TAVI for AS-related CS is 19% (95% CI 17–20%) compared to 39% (95% CI 32–46%) for emergency balloon aortic valvuloplasty, while the in-hospital mortality rate is 11% for emergent TAVI and 40% for the latter.[48] Although the 1-year mortality rate after emergent TAVI is roughly 29% (95% CI 20–40%), patients who survive the first 30 days have comparable long-term outcomes to those who received elective treatment.[44,54] With a 2-year survival rate of roughly 54% and an in-hospital mortality rate of 26.3% for surgery compared to 27.1% for transcatheter interventions ($p = 1.000$), surgical procedures show similar results to transcatheter approaches.[55] Baseline CO < 3.0 L/min, acute kidney injury, mechanical ventilation, and delayed intervention >48 hours from symptom onset are the factors that are independently linked to mortality.[56] Overall, valvular CS is a less common subset of CS patients with poor prognosis and rapid deterioration without timely intervention.

CONCLUSION

Valvular cardiogenic shock represents a unique and high-risk subset of CS with rapid hemodynamic deterioration driven by acute or chronic valve dysfunction. VCS has a poor prognosis compared to non-VCS; early recognition, multidisciplinary coordination, and tailored intensive care are important in the management. The recent advances, such as emergent TAVI, TEER, and mechanical circulatory devices, when used timely in selected patients, yield safe and better short- and medium-term outcomes.

REFERENCES

1. Van Diepen S, Katz JN, Albert NM, et al. Contemporary Management of Cardiogenic Shock: A Scientific Statement from the American Heart Association. Circulation. 2017;136(16):e232-68.
2. Harjola VP, Lassus J, Sionis A, et al. Clinical picture and risk prediction of short-term mortality in cardiogenic shock. Eur J Heart Fail. 2015;17(5):501-9.
3. Nair RM, Chawla S, Alkhalaileh F, et al. Characteristics and Outcomes of Patients With Valvular Cardiogenic Shock. JACC Adv. 2024;3(11):101303.
4. Carnicelli AP, Miller PE, Berg DD, et al. Characteristics and Outcomes of Patients With Cardiogenic Shock and Clinically Significant Valvular Heart Disease: From the Critical Care Cardiology Trials Network. J Card Fail. 2025;0(0):1-10.
5. Baran DA, Grines CL, Bailey S, et al. SCAI clinical expert consensus statement on the classification of cardiogenic shock: This document was endorsed by the American College of Cardiology (ACC), the American Heart Association (AHA), the Society of Critical Care Medicine (SCCM), and the Society of Thoracic Surgeons (STS) in April 2019. Catheter Cardiovasc Interv. 2019;94(1):29-37.
6. Parlow S, Weng W, Di Santo P, et al. Significant Valvular Dysfunction and Outcomes in Cardiogenic Shock: Insights From the Randomized DOREMI Trial. Can J Cardiol. 2022;38(8):1211-9.
7. Jentzer JC, van Diepen S, Barsness GW, et al. Cardiogenic Shock Classification to Predict Mortality in the Cardiac Intensive Care Unit. J Am Coll Cardiol. 2019;74(17):2117-28.
8. Klabunde RE. (2013). Cardiovascular Physiology. Ventricular Pressure-Volume Loop Changes in Valve Disease. [online] Available from https://cvphysiology.com/heart-disease/hd009 [Last accessed November, 2025].
9. Miller PE, Senman BC, Gage A, et al. Acute Decompensated Valvular Disease in the Intensive Care Unit. JACC Adv. 2024;3(12).

10. Brener MI, Rosenblum HR, Burkhoff D. Pathophysiology and Advanced Hemodynamic Assessment of Cardiogenic Shock. Methodist Debakey Cardiovasc J. 2020;16(1):7.
11. Ivascu NS, Hartman GS, Skubas NJ. Valvular Heart Disease. Anesthesia Key. [online] Available from https://aneskey.com/valvular-heart-disease-11/ [Last accessed November, 2025].
12. de Assis LU, Mondellini GM, van den Dorpel MMP, et al. Incidence and Pathology of Aortic Regurgitation. Interv Cardiol. 2025;20:e07.
13. Neema PK, Panidapu N. The Mechanisms and Pathophysiology of Mitral Regurgitation: A Narrative Review. Ann Card Anaesth. 2025;28(2):109.
14. Kelly RV, Cohen MG, Stouffer GA. Mitral regurgitation. Thoracic Key. [online] Available from https://thoracickey.com/12-mitral-regurgitation/ [Last accessed November, 2025].
15. Nair RM, Chawla S, Abdelghaffar B, et al. Comparison of Contemporary Treatment Strategies in Patients With Cardiogenic Shock Due to Severe Aortic Stenosis. J Am Heart Assoc. 2024;13(10):33601.
16. Hochman JS, Buller CE, Sleeper LA, et al. Cardiogenic shock complicating acute myocardial infarction - Etiologies, management and outcome: A report from the SHOCK Trial Registry. J Am Coll Cardiol. 2000;36(3 SUPPL. A):1063-70.
17. Lurz P, Besler C. Mitral Regurgitation in Cardiogenic Shock: A Novel Target for Transcatheter Therapy? JACC Cardiovasc Interv. 2021;14(1):12-4.
18. Pillai AA, Balasubramonian VR, Munuswamy H, et al. Acute severe mitral regurgitation with cardiogenic shock following balloon mitral valvuloplasty: echocardiographic findings and outcomes following surgery. Cardiovasc Interv Ther. 2019;34(3):260-8.
19. Cáceres-Lóriga FM, Pérez-López H, Santos-Gracia J, et al. Prosthetic heart valve thrombosis: Pathogenesis, diagnosis and management. Int J Cardiol. 2006;110(1):1-6.
20. Zoghbi WA, Adams D, Bonow RO, et al. ASE GUIDELINES AND STANDARDS Recommendations for Noninvasive Evaluation of Native Valvular Regurgitation A Report from the American Society of Echocardiography Developed in Collaboration with the Society for Cardiovascular Magnetic Resonance. J Am Soc Echocardiogr. 2017;30:303-71.
21. Baumgartner H, Hung J, Bermejo J, et al. Echocardiographic Assessment of Valve Stenosis: EAE/ASE Recommendations for Clinical Practice. J Am Soc Echocardiogr. 2009;22(1):1-23; quiz 101-2.
22. Masson JB, Forcillo J. Mixed-Valve Disease: Management of Patients with Aortic Stenosis and Mitral Regurgitation: Thresholds for Surgery Versus Percutaneous Therapies. US Cardiol. 2021;15:e26.
23. Schupp T, Rusnak J, Forner J, et al. Cardiac Troponin I but Not N-Terminal Pro-B-Type Natriuretic Peptide Predicts Outcomes in Cardiogenic Shock. J Pers Med. 2023;13(9):1348.
24. Sinha SS, Morrow DA, Kapur NK, et al. 2025 Concise Clinical Guidance: An ACC Expert Consensus Statement on the Evaluation and Management of Cardiogenic Shock: A Report of the American College of Cardiology Solution Set Oversight Committee. J Am Coll Cardiol. 2025;85(16):1618-41.
25. Boldt J. Clinical review: Hemodynamic monitoring in the intensive care unit. Crit Care. 2002;6(1):52.
26. Blumer V, Marbach J, Veasey T, et al. Role of medical management of cardiogenic shock in the era of mechanical circulatory support. Curr Opin Cardiol. 2022;37(3):250-60.
27. Riccardi M, Pagnesi M, Chioncel O, et al. Medical therapy of cardiogenic shock: Contemporary use of inotropes and vasopressors. Eur J Heart Fail. 2024;26(2):411-31.
28. Thiele H, Zeymer U, Thelemann N, et al. Intraaortic Balloon Pump in Cardiogenic Shock Complicating Acute Myocardial Infarction: Long-Term 6-Year Outcome of the Randomized IABP-SHOCK II Trial. Circulation. 2019;139(3):395-403.
29. Thiele H, Zeymer U, Neumann FJ, et al. Intraaortic Balloon Support for Myocardial Infarction with Cardiogenic Shock. New Engl J Med. 2012;367(14):1287-96.
30. Dekker ALAJ, Reesink KD, van der Veen FH, et al. Intra-aortic balloon pumping in acute mitral regurgitation reduces aortic impedance and regurgitant fraction. Shock. 2003;19(4):334-8.
31. Nishimoto Y, Ohbe H, Matsui H, et al. Trends in mechanical circulatory support use and outcome of patients with cardiogenic shock in Japan, 2010–2020: a nationwide inpatients database study. Am J Cardiol. 2023;203:203-11.
32. Nakata J, Yamamoto T, Saku K, et al. Mechanical circulatory support in cardiogenic shock. J Intensive Care. 2023;11(1):1-14.
33. Tello CM, Jamil D, Tran HHV, et al. The Therapeutic Use of Impella Device in Cardiogenic Shock: A Systematic Review. Cureus. 2022;14(10):e30045.
34. Harada R, George TJ, Schaffer J, et al. Management Of Cardiogenic Shock With Impella In Patient With Transcatheter Aortic Valve. J Card Fail. 2023;29(4):581-2.
35. Bhardwaj A, Salas De Armas I, Al Rameni D, et al. Use of Impella 5.5 in patients with cardiogenic shock as a bridge to decision, recovery, or destination therapy. IHJ Cardiovasc Case Reports (CVCR). 2023;7(2):61-4.
36. Harada R, George TJ, Schaffer J, et al. Case report: management of refractory cardiogenic shock with Impella 5.5 in patients with transcatheter aortic valves. Eur Heart J Case Rep. 2023;7(8):ytad381.
37. Nambiar PM, Sharma J, Mehta Y, et al. Extracorporeal Membrane Oxygenation in Cardiogenic shock – A Review. J Cardiac Crit Care TSS. 2023;7(1):35-9.
38. Xie A, Phan K, Yi-Chin Tsai M, et al. Venoarterial extracorporeal membrane oxygenation for cardiogenic shock and cardiac arrest: A meta-analysis. J Cardiothorac Vasc Anesth. 2015;29(3):637-45.
39. Thiele H, Desch S, De Waha S. Mechanical circulatory support: The last resort in cardiogenic shock? EuroIntervention. 2018;13(18):e2099-101.
40. Leon MB, Smith CR, Mack MJ, et al. Transcatheter or Surgical Aortic-Valve Replacement in Intermediate-Risk Patients. New Engl J Medicine. 2016;374(17):1609-20.
41. Reardon MJ, Van Mieghem NM, Popma JJ, et al. Surgical or Transcatheter Aortic-Valve Replacement in Intermediate-Risk Patients. New Engl J Med. 2017;376(14):1321-31.
42. Mack MJ, Leon MB, Thourani VH, et al. Transcatheter Aortic-Valve Replacement with a Balloon-Expandable Valve in Low-Risk Patients. New Engl J Med. 2019;380(18):1695-705.
43. Popma JJ, Deeb GM, Yakubov SJ, et al. Transcatheter Aortic-Valve Replacement with a Self-Expanding Valve in Low-Risk Patients. New Engl J Med. 2019;380(18):1706-15.
44. Sattar Y, Hamza M, Yasmin F, et al. Cardiovascular outcomes of emergent vs elective transcatheter aortic valve replacement in severe aortic stenosis: regression matched meta-analysis. Am J Cardiovasc Dis. 2024;14(2):54.
45. Kolte D, Khera S, Vemulapalli S, et al. Outcomes Following Urgent/Emergent Transcatheter Aortic Valve Replacement: Insights From the STS/ACC TVT Registry. JACC Cardiovasc Interv. 2018;11(12):1175-85.
46. Piriou PG, Plessis J, Guerin P. Transcatheter aortic valve replacement in patients with cardiogenic shock: safe and effective, but the most critical patients require further investigations. Eur Heart J. 2024;45(11):966-7.
47. Fraccaro C, Campante Teles R, Tchétché D, et al. Transcatheter aortic valve implantation (TAVI) in cardiogenic shock: TAVI-shock registry results. Catheter Cardiovasc Interven. 2020;96(5):1128-35.

48. Llah ST, Sharif S, Ullah S, et al. TAVR vs balloon aortic valvotomy for severe aortic stenosis and cardiogenic shock: An insight from the National Inpatient Sample database. Cardiovasc Revascular Med. 2023;55:1-7.
49. Simard T, Vemulapalli S, Jung RG, et al. Transcatheter Edge-to-Edge Mitral Valve Repair in Patients With Severe Mitral Regurgitation and Cardiogenic Shock. J Am Coll Cardiol. 2022;80(22):2072-84.
50. Jung RG, Simard T, Di Santo P, et al. Transcatheter edge-to-edge repair in patients with mitral regurgitation and cardiogenic shock: A new therapeutic target. Curr Opin Crit Care. 2022;28(4):426-33.
51. Elkaryoni A, Stone GW. Mitral Valve Transcatheter Edge-to-Edge Repair in Patients With Cardiogenic Shock and Severe Mitral Regurgitation. J Am Coll Cardiol. 2023;81(15):e129.
52. Lurz P, Besler C. Transcatheter Treatment of Mitral Regurgitation in Cardiogenic Shock: Promises and Pitfalls. J Am Coll Cardiol. 2022;80(22):2085-8.
53. Jung RG, Simard T, Kovach C, et al. Transcatheter Mitral Valve Repair in Cardiogenic Shock and Mitral Regurgitation: A Patient-Level, Multicenter Analysis. JACC Cardiovasc Interv. 2021;14(1): 1-11.
54. Kühne SG, Patrignani A, Elvinger S, et al. Emergency interventions for cardiogenic shock due to decompensated aortic stenosis: a systematic review and meta-analysis. Open Heart. 2025;12(1):e003110.
55. Hohri Y, Faridmoayer E, Zhao Y, et al. Outcomes of following transcatheter and surgical interventions in patients with acute valvular dysfunction with cardiogenic shock. JTCVS Open. 2024;24:217.
56. Frerker C, Schewel J, Schlüter M, et al. Emergency transcatheter aortic valve replacement in patients with cardiogenic shock due to acutely decompensated aortic stenosis. EuroIntervention. 2016;11(13):1530-6.

CHAPTER 39

Hemodynamic Assessment by Right Heart Catheterization in Management of Heart Failure

Bijay Prakash Pandey, Rajat Kar

ABSTRACT

First introduced in 1945, right heart catheterization (RHC), nowadays being increasingly used to assess and monitor more complex patients of heart failure. It has now become the key for patient cantered approach before implantation of ventricular assist devices or cardiac transplant. It is an invasive procedure that directly measures pressure in right-sided chambers of heart, cardiac output and indirectly measures vascular resistance and left-sided pressures. Hemodynamic parameters obtained from RHC have very in-depth impact expanded over entire spectrum of heart failure management.

Keywords: Right heart catheterization, heart failure, ventricular assist devices, cardiac transplant, invasive procedure, right sided heart pressure, cardiac output, vascular resistance, hemodynamic parameters, heart failure management.

INTRODUCTION

Heart failure (HF) is a complex clinical syndrome characterized by the inability of the heart to pump blood adequately to meet the body's metabolic needs or to do so only at elevated filling pressures.[1]

It can be caused by systolic dysfunction [reduced ejection fraction, (HFrEF)], diastolic dysfunction [preserved ejection fraction, (HFpEF)], or both.

The clinical presentation varies widely—from asymptomatic ventricular dysfunction to advanced, refractory HF requiring specialized interventions.

Accurate assessment of hemodynamics is crucial for:

- Establishing diagnosis when noninvasive data are inconclusive.
- Guiding acute therapy in decompensated HF.
- Risk stratification and prognostication.
- Determining candidacy for advanced therapies such as cardiac transplantation or mechanical circulatory support.

While noninvasive tools such as echocardiography, Doppler, and biomarker measurements are essential, right heart catheterization (RHC) remains the gold standard for direct measurement of cardiac filling pressures, output, and pulmonary hemodynamics **(Fig. 1)**.

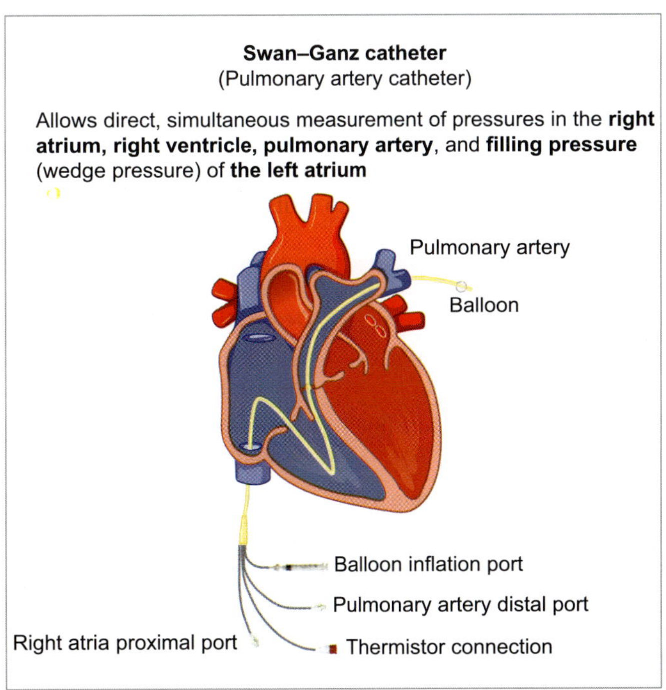

FIG. 1: Schematic diagram showing course of Swan–Ganz catheter during right heart catheterisation.[2]

BASICS OF RIGHT HEART CATHETERIZATION

Definition

Right heart catheterization is an invasive procedure in which a balloon-tipped, flow-directed catheter (Swan-Ganz catheter) is introduced via a central vein (internal jugular, subclavian, or femoral) into the right atrium (RA), right ventricle (RV), pulmonary artery (PA), and pulmonary capillary wedge position (PCWP).[3]

Key Hemodynamic Parameters Measured (Table 1)

Technical Considerations

Accurate data require correct zeroing of transducers at the mid-thoracic level, measurements at end-expiration, avoiding artifacts from damping or respiratory swings, and using directly measured VO_2 for Fick calculations, when possible, though thermodilution is often preferred.[6]

Advanced Calculated Metrics

- *Right ventricular stroke work index (RVSWI)*: The RVSWI is a measure of the work done by the right ventricle to pump blood. It is a hemodynamic parameter that reflects the systolic function of the right ventricle and is used to assess myocardial contractility.
  - The RVSWI is calculated using the following formula:

    – RVSWI = (mean pulmonary artery pressure – right atrial pressure) × stroke volume index × 0.0136

  - The factor 0.0136 is used to convert the units of pressure and volume to units of work ($g{\cdot}m/m^2$).[7-9]
- *Pulmonary artery pulsatility index (PAPi)*: Again an RV indices used to assess right ventricular function. It is particularly useful for predicting right ventricular failure in specific conditions, such as after an inferior myocardial infarction or following the implantation of a left ventricular assist device.
  - The PAPi is calculated using data obtained from a right heart catheterization and is a ratio of the pulmonary artery pulse pressure to the right atrial pressure.
  - *The formula is*:

    $$\text{PAPi} = \{\text{PASP} - \text{PADP}\}/\{\text{RAP}\}$$

    Where:
    PASP: Pulmonary artery systolic pressure; PADP: Pulmonary artery diastolic pressure; RAP: right atrial pressure.
  - A lower PAPi value is associated with an increased risk of right ventricular dysfunction, as well as higher rates of morbidity and mortality in various patient populations, including those with advanced heart failure and cardiogenic shock.[10-12]
- Right atrial pressure/PCWP ratio—helpful in advanced HF and RV failure prediction. The right atrial pressure to pulmonary capillary wedge pressure (RAP/PCWP) ratio is used to assess the synchronicity between the right and left heart.
  - An elevated RAP/PCWP ratio is an important prognostic indicator and is associated with right ventricular dysfunction.
  - The ratio is an independent predictor of in-hospital mortality, particularly in patients undergoing procedures like the implantation of a left ventricular assist device (LVAD). A high preoperative RAP/PCWP ratio can help identify patients at higher risk of postoperative right ventricular failure.

TABLE 1: Different parameters and their normal values measured during right heart catheterization.[4,5]

Parameters	Description	Normal range	Significance
Right atrial pressure (RAP/CVP)	Reflects systemic venous return and RV preload	2–8 mm Hg	Elevated in RV failure
Right ventricular pressure (RVP)	RV systolic function and pulmonary pressure	• Systolic 15–30 mm Hg • Diastolic 2–8 mm Hg	Elevated in PH and RV dysfunction
Pulmonary artery pressure (PAP)	Pressure beyond pulmonary valve	• Systolic 15–30 mm Hg • Diastolic 4–12 mm Hg	Pulmonary vascular status
Pulmonary capillary wedge pressure (PCWP)	Reflects LA pressure	6–12 mm Hg	Surrogate of LVEDP
Cardiac output (CO)	By thermodilution or Fick's method	4–8 L/min	Overall pump function and perfusion adequacy
Cardiac index (CI)		2.5–4 L/min/m^2	
Systematic vascular resistance (SVR)	For afterload assessment	900–1,400 dyn.s/cm^5	For pump failure and afterload mismatch
Pulmonary vascular resistance (PVR)	Differentiation between pre-capillary and postcapillary PH	20–130 dyn.s/cm^5	For vasodilator reversibility testing and choice for therapy in PH

- A RAP/PCWP ratio can also be used to differentiate between conditions. For example, a ratio >0.8 may suggest cardiac tamponade, while a ratio <0.8 may suggest constrictive pericarditis.[13-15]

INDICATIONS AND GUIDELINE RECOMMENDATIONS

Guideline-based Use[16,17]

International guidelines (ACC/AHA, ESC) advise RHC in:
- Heart failure with uncertain volume status, unresolvable via noninvasive tools.
- Decompensated HF is unresponsive to diuretics or standard therapy.
- Cardiogenic shock to determine shock phenotype, guide therapy, and escalate care.

Evidence from Evaluation Study of Congestive Heart Failure and Pulmonary Artery Catheterization Effectiveness Trial[18]

The ESCAPE (Evaluation Study of Congestive Heart Failure and Pulmonary Artery Catheterization Effectiveness) trial found no survival or hospitalization benefit from routine RHC in stable decompensated HF patients. This influenced guidelines to limit RHC use to complex or severe cases.

Cardiogenic Shock, Acute Heart Failure (Heart Failure with Reduced Ejection Fraction and Heart Failure with Preserved Ejection Fraction)[19]

In cardiogenic shock (CS), defined by hypoperfusion from inadequate CO absent hypovolemia, RHC is invaluable for diagnosis, staging (e.g., SCAI stages C–E), risk stratification, and guiding mechanical or pharmacologic escalation.

In acute decompensated HF (ADHF) without shock, RHC is not routine but useful in diagnostic dilemmas (e.g., restrictive vs constrictive physiology).

Heart failure with reduced ejection fraction shows elevated RAP, PCWP, and low CI. Decongestion is the cornerstone of treatment.

Heart failure with preserved ejection fraction shows PCWP rising disproportionately during exercise or volume challenge. Reducing LA pressure is the cornerstone of treatment.

Advanced Therapy Risk Assessment

- *Transplant evaluation*: Elevated PVR is a relative contraindication; vasodilator challenge via RHC can differentiate reversible from fixed pulmonary hypertension, guiding candidacy.
- *Left ventricular assist device candidates*: Preoperative RAP >15 mm Hg, elevated RAP/PCWP ratio, reduced RVSWI, or low PAPi predict postoperative RV failure. Hemodynamic ramp studies help optimize LVAD speed post-implant.

HEMODYNAMIC PROFILES AND MANAGEMENT IMPLICATIONS

Forrester-like Subsets in Modern Practice

Although originally derived in acute myocardial infarction, the "warm/dry, warm/wet, cold/dry, cold/wet" schema is adapted in HF (**Table 2**):[20]

Pulmonary Hypertension and Heart Failure

Postcapillary pulmonary hypertension (PH)—evidenced by mPAP ≥20 mm Hg and PCWP >15 mm Hg—is common in HF. PVR >2 wood units indicate a precapillary component, with implications for transplant eligibility and prognosis.[21]

Prognostic Hemodynamic Metrics

In advanced systolic HF, higher baseline RAP and PVR are significant predictors of adverse outcomes. Following inotropic challenge, elevated mPAP portends worse prognosis. A combined algorithm using these measures helps stratify risk.[22]

Right Ventricular Failure and Left Ventricular Assist Device[23,24]

Key indices for RV failure risk post-LVAD include:
- Preoperative RAP >15 mm Hg
- Elevated RAP/PCWP ratio
- Reduced RVSWI
- Low PAPi

Remote Hemodynamic Monitoring[25,26]

Technologies such as ReDS (remote dielectric system) offer noninvasive estimation of pulmonary congestion, correlating with PCWP and aiding outpatient risk stratification. Elevated ReDS (>34%) may warrant confirmatory RHC.

TABLE 2: Heart failure subtypes and possible treatment in each subtype.

	Dry	Wet
Warm	Adequate perfusion and volume—optimize baseline therapy	Congestion with preserved output—diuretics and vasodilation
Cold	Hypoperfusion without congestion—fluid challenge or inotropes	Both congestion and hypoperfusion—aggressive inotropic and diuretic therapy

EMERGING TRENDS AND INNOVATIONS

Noninvasive Surrogates and Artificial Intelligence[27]

Novel approaches such as artificial intelligence (AI)-enhanced echocardiography (e.g., the MePH model) significantly improve non-invasive estimation of mPAP and PVR, narrowing the gap with RHC accuracy and potentially reducing need for invasive procedures.

Advanced Hemodynamic Modeling[28]

Computational cardiovascular models, integrating RHC-derived data, enable "deep phenotyping" in transplant recipients, offering detailed tracking of recovery trajectories and predicting graft dysfunction through serial comparisons.

Exercise Right Heart Catheterization[19]

In HFpEF or unexplained dyspnea, exercise RHC helps unmask abnormal filling pressures and impaired CO reserve—not apparent at rest—and provides diagnostic and prognostic clarity.

Hemodynamic Ramps in Left Ventricular Assist Device Management[29]

Ramp studies combining hemodynamics and echocardiography guide LVAD speed adjustment to optimize filling pressures, improving outcomes, and potentially reducing readmissions.

Continuous Monitoring and Future Tools[30]

Implantable sensors (e.g., pulmonary artery pressure monitors) afford continuous hemodynamic surveillance, enabling proactive intervention before HF decompensation—though RHC remains indispensable when precise calibration is required **(Table 3)**.

TABLE 3: Different target hemodynamic parameters for optimum benefits from heart failure treatment.[19]

Cardiogenic shock management	• CVP 8–12 mm Hg • PCWP 15 mm Hg • Cardiac index >2.2 L/min/m^2
Heart transplant evaluation	• Cardiac index <1.8 L/min/m • PCWP >15 mm Hg • Systolic BP <90 mm Hg • Status 1–3 for transplant
	• PA systolic >50 mm Hg • Trans pulmonary gradient >15 mm Hg • PVR >3 WU • Indications for vasodilator challenge
Left ventricular assist device	• RV risk score • Hemodynamic ramp study

LIMITATIONS AND RISKS

Risks[31]

- *Invasive nature*: Vascular injury, bleeding, and infection
- Arrhythmias during catheter passage or manipulation
- Rarely pulmonary artery rupture and thrombosis
- Thromboembolic risks and procedural complications

Limitations[19]

- Spot measurements may not capture dynamic changes or diurnal/respiratory variability.
- Accuracy depends on technical execution—pressure transducer leveling, respiratory timing, patient factors (e.g., obesity, arrhythmias).
- ESCAPE trial demonstrated no benefit in stable inpatient HF, limiting routine use.
- Right heart catheterization use is specialized and depends on institutional expertise and clinical integration.

Noninvasive Alternatives[27]

While echocardiography, impedance cardiography, biomarkers, and physical examination are valuable, they lack the precision of RHC—though improving tools (e.g., AI models for echocardiography) may reduce reliance on catheterization in the future.

CONCLUSION

- Right heart catheterization remains the gold standard for detailed hemodynamic assessment in HF.
- It is indicated in advanced or refractory HF, cardiogenic shock, diagnostic ambiguity, and in assessment for transplant or LVAD.
- Hemodynamic data (e.g., RAP, PCWP, PVR, mPAP, RVSWI, and PAPi) guide targeted therapy, risk stratification, and advanced intervention planning.
- Noninvasive tools—especially AI-enhanced imaging and remote monitoring—are promising adjuncts but not replacements when precision is required.
- Procedure risks and resource demands necessitate judicious, guideline-aligned use.
- Future directions include integrated physiologic modeling, continuous monitoring, and noninvasive surrogate metrics to optimize patient outcomes.

REFERENCES

1. American Heart Association. (2025). TRIPLE Your Impact to Help Save Lives. [online] Available from www.heart.org. [Last accessed October 2025].
2. Swan HJ, Ganz W, Forrester J, et al. Catheterization of the heart in man with use of a flow-directed balloon-tipped catheter. N Engl J Med. 1970;283(9):447-51.
3. Krishnan A, Markham R, Savage M, et al. Right Heart Catheterisation: How To Do It. Heart Lung Circ. 2019;28(4):e71-8.
4. Sorajja P, Borlaug BA, Dimas VV, et al. SCAI/HFSA clinical expert consensus document on the use of invasive hemodynamics for the diagnosis and management of cardiovascular disease. Catheter Cardiovasc Interv. 2017;89(7):E233-47.
5. Saxena A, Garan AR, Kapur NK, et al. Value of Hemodynamic Monitoring in Patients With Cardiogenic Shock Undergoing Mechanical Circulatory Support. Circulation. 2020;141(14):1184-97.
6. Argueta EE, Paniagua D. Thermodilution Cardiac Output: A Concept Over 250 Years in the Making. Cardiol Rev. 2019;27(3):138-44.
7. Armstrong HF, Schulze PC, Kato TS, et al. Right ventricular stroke work index as a negative predictor of mortality and initial hospital stay after lung transplantation. J Heart Lung Transplant. 2013;32(6):603-8.
8. Jeong YH, Yang SM, Cho H, et al. The Prognostic Role of Right Ventricular Stroke Work Index during Liver Transplantation. J Clin Med. 2021;10(17):4022.
9. Kanjanahattakij N, Sirinvaravong N, Aguilar F, et al. High Right Ventricular Stroke Work Index is Associated with Worse Kidney Function in Patients With Heart Failure With Preserve Ejection Fraction. Cardiorenal Med. 2018;8(2):123-9.
10. Lim HS, Gustafsson F. Pulmonary artery pulsatility index: physiological basis and clinical application. Eur J Heart Fail. 2020;22(1):32-8.
11. Mazimba S, Welch TS, Mwansa H, et al. Haemodynamically Derived Pulmonary Artery Pulsatility Index Predicts Mortality in Pulmonary Arterial Hypertension. Heart Lung Circ. 2019;28(5):752-60.
12. Wei J, Kee A, Dukes R, et al. The Association of the Pulmonary Artery Pulsatility Index and Right Ventricular Function after Cardiac Surgery. Crit Care Res Pract. 2024;2024:5408008.
13. Grodin JL, Drazner MH, Dupont M, et al. A disproportionate elevation in right ventricular filling pressure, in relation to left ventricular filling pressure, is associated with renal impairment and increased mortality in advanced decompensated heart failure. Am Heart J. 2015;169(6):806-12.
14. Mostertz WC, Chang PP. Chronic heart failure, Cardiovascular Hemodynamics for the Clinician. Wiley Online Lib. 2025;225-41.
15. Kraus MJ, Veshapeli A, Reich C, et al. Risk prediction in heart failure using invasive hemodynamics. Clin Res Cardiol. 2025;114(10):1388-99.
16. Behnoush AH, Khalaji A, Naderi N, et al. ACC/AHA/HFSA 2022 and ESC 2021 guidelines on heart failure comparison. ESC Heart Fail. 2023;10(3):1531-44.
17. Zeder K, Mak S, Galie N, et al Right heart catheterization in heart failure: indications, interpretation, and pitfalls. Eur Heart J. 2025;46(34):3354-72.
18. Binanay C, Califf RM, Hasselblad V, et al. ESCAPE Investigators and ESCAPE Study Coordinators. Evaluation study of congestive heart failure and pulmonary artery catheterization effectiveness: the ESCAPE trial. JAMA. 2005;294(13):1625-33.
19. Rajagopalan N, Borlaug BA, Bailey AL, et al. Practical Guidance for Hemodynamic Assessment by Right Heart Catheterization in Management of Heart Failure. JACC Heart Fail. 2024;12(7):1141-56.
20. Abbas, Amr E. From Killip to Forrester to Echocardiography: Beyond Myocardial Infarction. J Am Soc Echocardiogr. 2022;35(4):443-44.
21. Humbert M, Kovacs G, Hoeper MM, et al. 2022 ESC/ERS Guidelines for the diagnosis and treatment of pulmonary hypertension. Eur Heart J. 2022;43(38):3618-731.
22. Ruopp NF, Cockrill BA. Diagnosis and treatment of pulmonary arterial hypertension. JAMA. 2022;327(14):1379-91.
23. Rajapreyar I, Soliman O, Brailovsky Y, et al. Late Right Heart Failure After Left Ventricular Assist Device Implantation: Contemporary Insights and Future Perspectives. JACC Heart Fail. 2023;11(8 Pt 1):865-78.
24. Cameli M, Loiacono F, Sparla S, et al. Systematic Left Ventricular Assist Device Implant Eligibility with Non-Invasive Assessment: The SIENA Protocol. J Cardiovasc Ultrasound. 2017;25(2):39-46.
25. Scheeren TWL, Ramsay MAE. New Developments in Hemodynamic Monitoring. J Cardiothorac Vasc Anesth. 2019;33 Suppl 1:S67-S72.
26. Clephas PRD, de Boer RA, Brugts JJ. Benefits of remote hemodynamic monitoring in heart failure. Trends Cardiovasc Med. 2024;34(7):468-76.
27. Yang J, Huang T, Ding S, et.al. AI-Enabled Accurate Non-Invasive Assessment of Pulmonary Hypertension Progression via Multi-Modal Echocardiography. Cornell University. 2025.
28. Colunga AL, Kim KG, Woodall NP, et al. Deep phenotyping of cardiac function in heart transplant patients using cardiovascular systems models. J Physiol. 2020;598(15):3203-22.
29. Imamura T, Narang N. Advances in Hemodynamic Monitoring in Heart Failure Patients. Intern Med. 2021;60(2):167-71.
30. Radhoe S, Brugts J. CardioMEMS™: A Tool for Remote Hemodynamic Monitoring of Chronic Heart Failure Patients. Future Cardiol. 2022;18(3):173-83.
31. Raco J, Peterson B, Muallem S. Assessment of Volume Status in Hospitalized Patients with Chronic Heart Failure. Cardiol Res. 2023;14(1):2-11.

SECTION

6

Cardiomyopathy

Section Outline

40. Sudden Cardiac Death in Hypertrophic Cardiomyopathy
R Alagesan, C Narasimhan, Muthiah Subramanian

41. Polygenic Inheritance in Hypertrophic Cardiomyopathy
Ajay Bahl

42. Dual (Ischemic and Nonischemic) Cardiomyopathy: A Wolf in Sheep's Clothing
Chandra Bhan Meena, Himanshu Mahla, Mayank Nausran

43. Vasovagal Syncope: What Treatment Can We Offer in 2025?
Nishad Chitnis, Hygriv B Rao

44. Role of Clonal Hematopoiesis in the Pathogenesis of Dilated Cardiomyopathy
Ganesan Manohar, Karthikaa Saminathan

45. Dilated Cardiomyopathy in Systemic Immune-mediated Diseases
Ganesh Seth, Mahima Saran, Himanshu Gupta

46. Arrhythmia-induced Cardiomyopathy
Arindam Mitra, Aditi Rastogi, Jayanta Saha

47. Alcoholic Cardiomyopathy
Shishu Shankar Mishra, Biswaranjan Mishra, Asharam Panda

CHAPTER 40

Sudden Cardiac Death in Hypertrophic Cardiomyopathy

R Alagesan, C Narasimhan, Muthiah Subramanian

ABSTRACT

Sudden cardiac death (SCD) in hypertrophic cardiomyopathy (HCM) arises from complex structural and electrical remodeling that predisposes to malignant ventricular arrhythmias. Key predictors include the traditional risk factors of family history of SCD, severe left ventricular (LV) hypertrophy, nonsustained ventricular tachycardia, and unexplained syncope. The newer risk enhancers are late gadolinium enhancement in cardiac MRI, LV apical aneurysm, and LV reduced EF <50%. The electrocardiogram (ECG), genetic markers, and LV global longitudinal strain are also useful to further refine risk assessment. Periodic evaluation and individualized medical, surgical, and intracardiac defibrillator therapy have significantly improved clinical outcomes in patients with HCM.

Keywords: Hypertrophic cardiomyopathy, sudden cardiac death, risk predictors, ventricular arrhythmia, late gadolinium enhancement, ejection fraction.

"There are known knowns, known unknowns and unknown unknowns".

INTRODUCTION

The above quote made in relation to the Iraq war (Donald Henry Rumsfeld, United States Secretary of Defense, 2002) can be applied to the problem of sudden cardiac death (SCD) due to various cardiac causes. Our understanding of etiology, mechanisms, prevention, and treatment is continuously evolving, and there are important gaps in our knowledge. Hypertrophic cardiomyopathy (HCM) is one of the common inherited cardiomyopathies with significant SCD events. In this chapter, we summarize the major risk markers, additional risk enhancers, and lesser understood markers for SCD. We look at the emerging role of left ventricular (LV) global longitudinal strain (GLS) and left atrial (LA) strain in predicting SCD events.

SUDDEN CARDIAC DEATH

Sudden cardiac death is defined as unexpected natural death due to cardiac causes, occurring within 1 hour of symptom onset (witnessed) or within 24 hours of having been seen alive and asymptomatic (unwitnessed).[1]

Hemodynamically, it is due to sudden decrease or stoppage of systemic circulation resulting in syncope and death. The cardiac output decreases due to loss of effective contraction resulting from Ventricular tachycardia/Ventricular fibrillation (VT/VF) or severe bradyarrhythmia/asystole.[2]

HYPERTROPHIC CARDIOMYOPATHY—INCIDENCE, NATURAL HISTORY, CAUSES OF DEATH, AND CONTEMPORARY OUTCOME

Incidence

Echocardiography-defined (phenotypic) HCM occurs in approximately 1 in 500 adults (~0.2%).[3] Genotype-based studies show sarcomere mutations in up to 1 in 200–250 individuals, although many genotype-positive patients never develop overt phenotype or may manifest only later/mildly due to variable penetrance and expressivity.[4]

Clinical Course and Overall Mortality

The clinical course is benign in ~80% of patients, while ~20% develop more symptomatic disease with increased morbidity and mortality.[5] All-cause mortality in HCM is approximately 1–2% per year, compared with ~0.4% per year in the general population.[6] With multidisciplinary care in specialized

HCM centers [individualized drug therapy, septal reduction, implantable cardioverter-defibrillators (ICDs) for high-risk patients, AF/HF management], overall survival has improved and approaches that of the general population.[7]

Causes of Death in Hypertrophic Cardiomyopathy

Broad distributions from historical autopsy/athlete registries and referral cohorts versus modern clinic cohorts show that sudden cardiac arrest continues to be the major cause of death:

- *SCD*: ~40–60% of HCM-related deaths[5,6]
- *Progressive (end-stage) heart failure (HF)*: ~20–40%
- *Stroke from atrial fibrillation (AF)*: ~5–15%

Older cohorts reported a split of SCD ≈ 51%, HF ≈ 36%, and AF/stroke ≈ 13%, but these vary with population studied. In older autopsy and athlete registries, 30–50% of SCDs occurred in previously undiagnosed individuals, underscoring the silent or minimally symptomatic phenotype and missed screening.[8] In modern, specialized HCM clinics, most SCDs occur in known patients, but the absolute event rate is much lower due to ICD implantation, better risk stratification, and lifestyle guidance.[7]

Timing of events—SCD tends to occur earlier in life (<40 years); heart-failure deaths and AF-related complications are more frequent in older patients.[6] A minority of deaths are therapy/procedure-related (ICD, myectomy, and transplant).

PATHOPHYSIOLOGY AND MECHANISMS OF SUDDEN CARDIAC DEATH IN HYPERTROPHIC CARDIOMYOPATHY

Sudden cardiac death in HCM typically results from malignant ventricular arrhythmias, most notably sustained VT or VF, occurring in structurally abnormal myocardium.[9] The pathogenesis is multifactorial, rooted in the profound architectural and cellular remodeling that characterizes HCM. The myocardial substrate comprises myocyte hypertrophy, disarray, interstitial and replacement fibrosis, and small-vessel disease.[10]

Histological studies consistently demonstrate chaotic alignment of cardiomyocytes forming a disorganized meshwork that disrupts normal electrical propagation and creates zones of slow conduction and reentry.[11] Interstitial fibrosis, detected noninvasively through cardiac magnetic resonance (CMR) with late gadolinium enhancement (LGE), further contributes to arrhythmogenesis by forming barriers to uniform impulse transmission.[12] Microvascular ischemia, caused by narrowed intramural coronary arterioles, exacerbates the substrate by inducing local injury and fibrosis.[13]

The arrhythmogenic substrate in HCM is dynamic. Over time, increasing hypertrophy, progressive fibrosis, and alterations in autonomic tone enhance arrhythmia vulnerability. Adrenergic stimulation, particularly during intense physical activity, is a recognized trigger for ventricular arrhythmias.[14,15] This is especially concerning in adolescents and young adults, in whom the SCD incidence is disproportionately higher.

While VT/VF is the predominant mechanism in most cases, other arrhythmias such as AF with rapid ventricular response can precipitate hemodynamic collapse in severe left ventricular outflow tract obstruction (LVOTO) or restrictive physiology. In rare instances, bradyarrhythmias or conduction system disease contribute to SCD, particularly in advanced disease or apical aneurysms.[16]

Modern imaging and electrophysiologic tools have expanded understanding of these mechanisms. High-resolution electroanatomic mapping in selected patients undergoing VT ablation demonstrates fractionated and delayed electrograms in areas of dense scar, often matching LGE on CMR.[17]

SUDDEN CARDIAC DEATH RISK ASSESSMENT IN HYPERTROPHIC CARDIOMYOPATHY

Sudden cardiac death risk assessment is critical and should be done at the first diagnosis and repeated every 1–2 years. Major risk markers and additional risk enhancers are listed in **Table 1**.

Family History of Sudden Cardiac Death

Sudden, unexpected death in a first-degree relative at a young age—parent, sibling, or child—or sudden death at any age is treated as a positive family history[18] **(Figs. 1A and B)**. This binary risk factor derives from large cohort analyses by Maron et al., establishing familial clustering of SCD and its prognostic importance.[19-21]

Nonsustained Ventricular Tachycardia

Nonsustained ventricular tachycardia (NSVT) ≥ 3 consecutive ventricular beats at >120–150 bpm lasting <30 seconds. Risk

TABLE 1: Traditional risk factors and risk enhancers for SCD in HCM.

Traditional major risk factors	Additional/Emerging risk enhancers
Family history of SCD	Late gadolinium enhancement (LGE) on CMR
Nonsustained ventricular tachycardia (NSVT)	LV apical aneurysm
Maximum LV wall thickness	LV systolic dysfunction ("end-stage" HCM)
Unexplained syncope	Abnormal BP response (<40 years)

(CMR: cardiac magnetic resonance; HCM: hypertrophic cardiomyopathy; LV: left ventricular; SCD: sudden cardiac death)

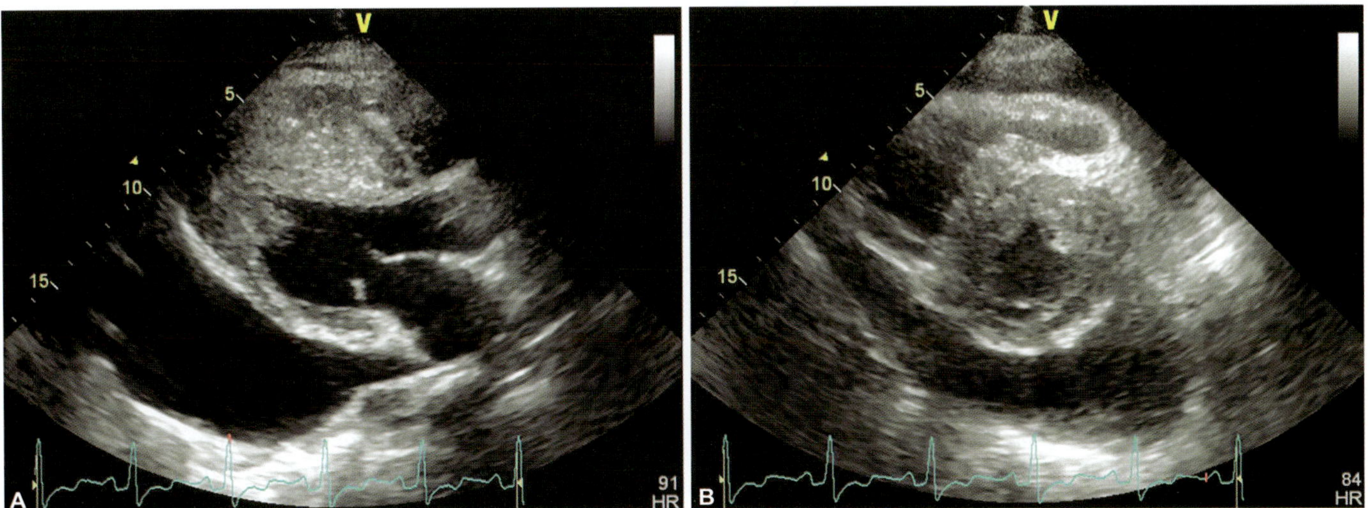

FIGS. 1A AND B: A 45-year-old male with HCM recurrent pericardial effusion asymptomatic sister with known HCM suffered SCD. He underwent pericardiectomy and ICD implantation.
(HCM: hypertrophic cardiomyopathy; ICD: implantable cardioverter-defibrillator; SCD: sudden cardiac death)

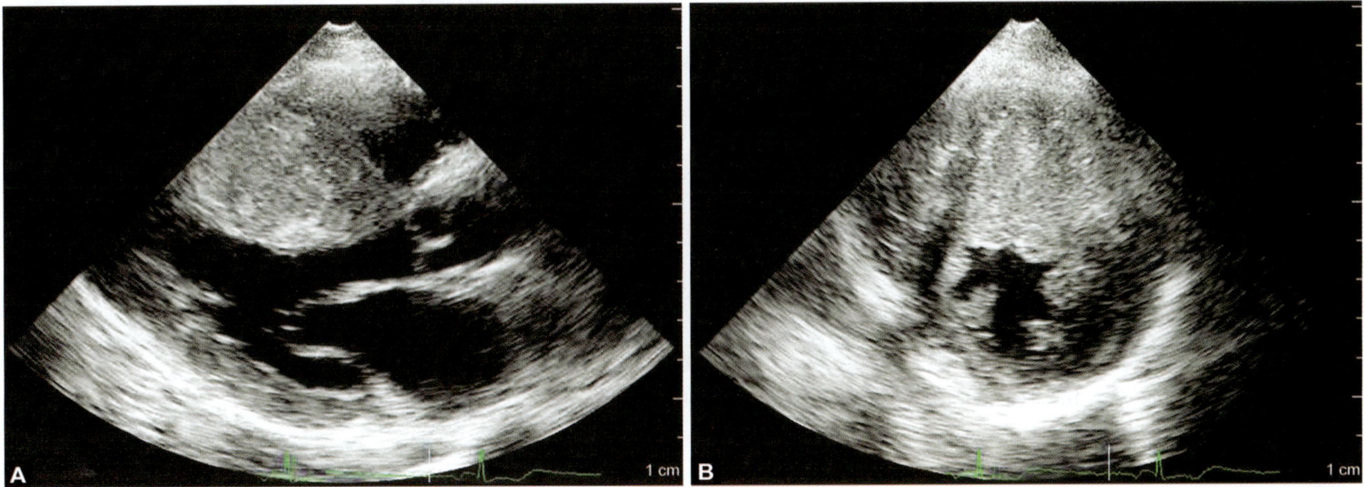

FIGS. 2A AND B: A 25-year-old male HCM with IVS, LV anterior wall thickness of 37 mm.
(HCM: hypertrophic cardiomyopathy; LV: left ventricular)

is higher when runs are frequent, long (>10–15 beats), very fast (>200 bpm), or occur in patients < 30 years.[22,23] NSVT is identified by ambulatory Holter monitoring, telemetry, or exercise testing. Isolated short runs in older patients are less predictive.

Maximum Left Ventricular Wall Thickness

Hypertrophic cardiomyopathy was first described pathologically by Donald Tearein 1958.[24] Subsequent clinicopathologic and imaging series demonstrated that greater maximal LV wall thickness ("massive" hypertrophy) is associated with worse prognosis and higher SCD incidence.[25] The European Society of Cardiology (ESC) HCM risk-SCD model treats wall thickness as a continuous variable,[6] whereas the American Heart Association/American College of Cardiology (AHA/ACC) guidelines consider extreme wall thickness > 30 mm a major risk factor **(Figs. 2A and B)**.[26,27] For pediatric HCM, a *Z*-score > 10–20 represents marked hypertrophy.

Transthoracic echocardiography (TTE) is first line for measurement; CMR is preferred if image quality is suboptimal. Extreme hypertrophy is associated with myocyte disarray, microvascular ischemia, and fibrosis. Imaging studies show that greater wall thickness correlates with more LGE, but not perfectly; combining both parameters refines risk assessment.[12,28]

Unexplained Syncope

Unexplained syncope is a transient loss of consciousness not clearly vasovagal or orthostatic, occurring within 6 months—especially during exertion or at rest without prodrome—and may reflect ventricular tachyarrhythmia. This is considered a marker of possible ventricular tachyarrhythmia, especially in the absence of severe LVOTO.

Late Gadolinium Enhancement on Cardiac Magnetic Resonance

There are two relevant types of fibrosis in HCM:

1. *Replacement fibrosis*: Patchy LGE on contrast CMR, often at RV insertion points, septum, and hypertrophied segments. LGE presence and extent are associated with increased SCD risk in a continuous fashion. Multiple studies and meta-analyses show incremental SCD risk with increasing LGE burden. An LGE extent > 15% of LV mass is associated with substantially higher SCD risk and is incorporated as a risk enhancer in the 2020 AHA/ACC guideline[12,28] **(Figs. 3A and B)**.
2. *Diffuse interstitial fibrosis*: It is detected with T1 mapping and extracellular volume (ECV) quantification. It correlates with diastolic dysfunction and possible propensity to arrhythmias. However, evidence is less robust than for LGE, and this parameter is not yet a risk marker.

Left Ventricular Apical Aneurysm

Left ventricular apical aneurysm in HCM (classically associated with midventricular obstruction) is an independent risk factor for SCD, HF, and thromboembolic stroke. Reported event rates for ventricular arrhythmia/SCD are substantially higher (several percent per year in cohorts), often due to monomorphic VT from reentrant scar circuits.[29,30] Risk is not simply related to aneurysm size and can occur even with preserved LV ejection fraction (EF). Thrombus formation and embolic stroke are more common with larger aneurysms **(Figs. 4A and B)**.

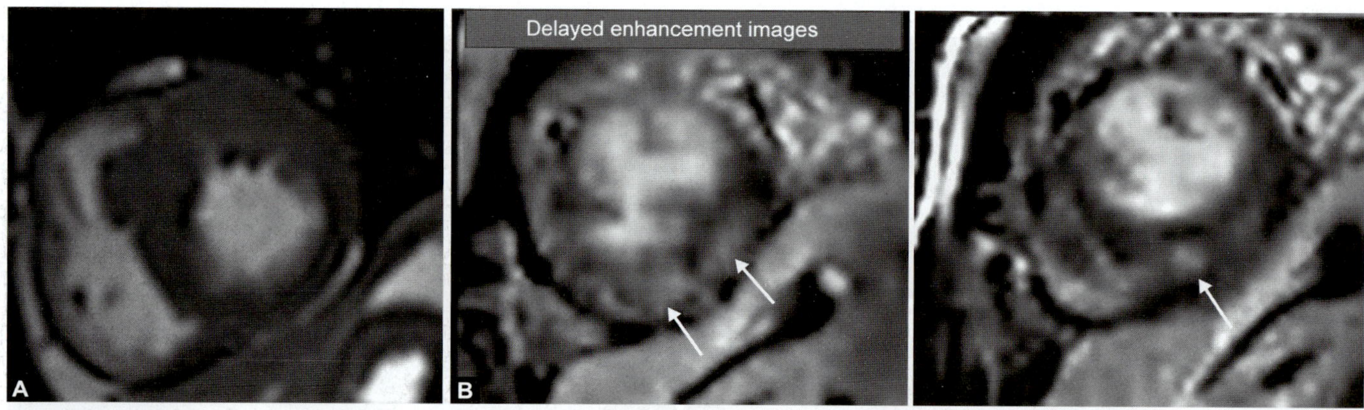

FIGS. 3A AND B: HCM with 10% LGE in interventricular septum and RV insertion points (white arrow).
(HCM: hypertrophic cardiomyopathy; LGE: late gadolinium enhancement)

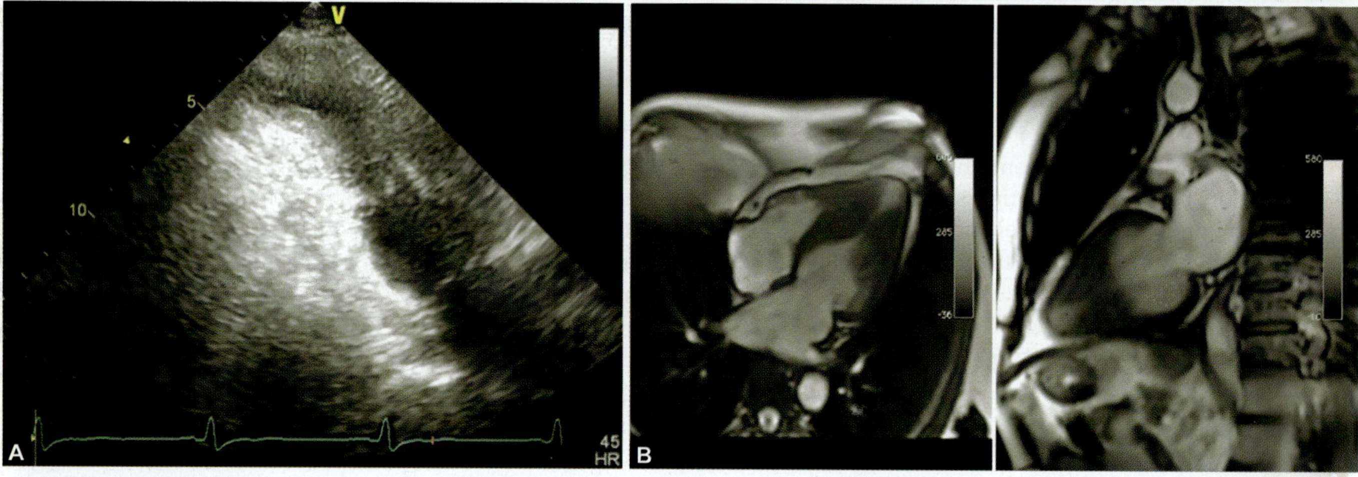

FIGS. 4A AND B: A 60-year-old male with HCM developed mid-LV obstruction, LV apical aneurysm around 68 years, now 80 years, on mild diuretics, anticoagulation, and doing well without ICD.
(HCM: hypertrophic cardiomyopathy; ICD: implantable cardioverter-defibrillator; LV: left ventricular)

Left Ventricular Systolic Dysfunction and "End-stage" Hypertrophic Cardiomyopathy

Most patients with HCM have normal or hyperdynamic systolic function. However, ~5–10% progress to LV systolic dysfunction (EF < 50%) with wall thinning and adverse remodeling—the "end-stage" HCM phenotype. These patients have higher risks of SCD and HF mortality and may require HFrEF therapy, ICD therapy, or transplantation **(Figs. 5A and B)**.[16,31] HF can also occur with preserved EF due to myocardial fibrosis producing diastolic dysfunction **(Figs. 6A to D)**.

CONTEMPORARY RISK STRATIFICATION MODELS

To improve the precision of SCD prediction in HCM, modern risk stratification tools have been developed that extend beyond the conventional "major risk factors" approach. Two primary paradigms dominate current clinical practice: The quantitative model endorsed by the ESC and the "qualitative framework proposed by the AHA/American College of Cardiology Foundation (ACCF)."[6,26,27]

European Society of Cardiology Risk-SCD Model

The ESC HCM risk-SCD calculator, introduced in 2014, is a multivariable risk prediction tool derived from a large European registry of over 3,000 patients. It uses the following seven variables to estimate a patient's individualized 5-year SCD risk **(Fig. 7A)**:

1. Age (years)
2. Maximal LV wall thickness (mm)
3. LA diameter (mm)
4. LVOT gradient (rest or provoked)
5. Family history of SCD
6. Unexplained syncope
7. NSVT on Holter monitoring

These inputs are processed using a logistic regression formula to yield a percentage estimate of 5-year SCD risk, with guideline-recommended ICD thresholds as follows:[32]

- *Low risk (<4%)*: No ICD is recommended.
- *Intermediate risk (4–6%)*: ICD may be considered on a case-by-case basis.
- *High risk (>6%)*: ICD is recommended.

This tool has gained popularity in Europe due to its objectivity and reproducibility, and its use is endorsed by ESC guidelines. However, critics note several limitations: It may underestimate risk in younger individuals, those with extreme hypertrophy, and patients with high-risk genetic variants. Moreover, this model does not incorporate findings from CMR, such as LGE, or novel markers, such as GLS or electrocardiogram (ECG) findings.[33]

American Heart Association/American College of Cardiology Foundation Risk-based Framework

In contrast, the AHA/ACCF guidelines (2011, reaffirmed in 2020)[26,27] do not rely on a scoring system. Instead, they utilize a binary, risk marker-based framework built upon five major clinical criteria:

1. Family history of SCD
2. Unexplained syncope
3. Maximal LV wall thickness ≥ 30 mm
4. NSVT on ambulatory monitoring
5. Abnormal blood pressure response to exercise (in patients <40 years old)[34]

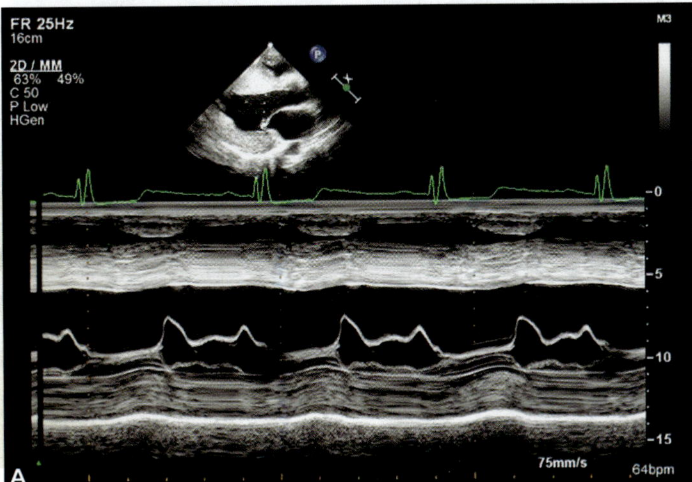

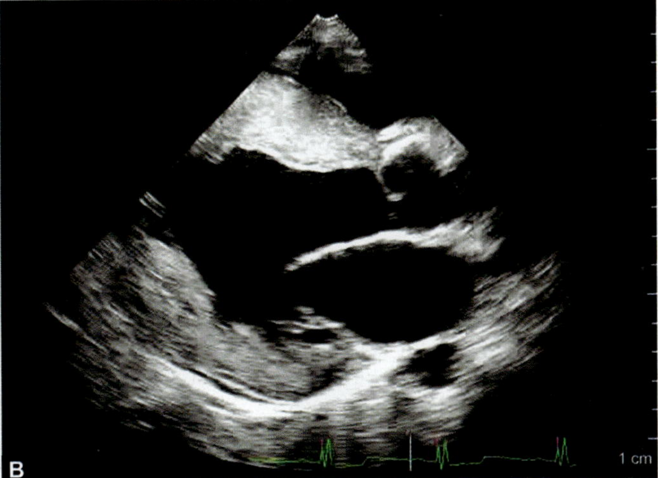

FIGS. 5A AND B: HCM in a 62-year-old male with heart failure reduced ejection fraction.
(HCM: hypertrophic cardiomyopathy)

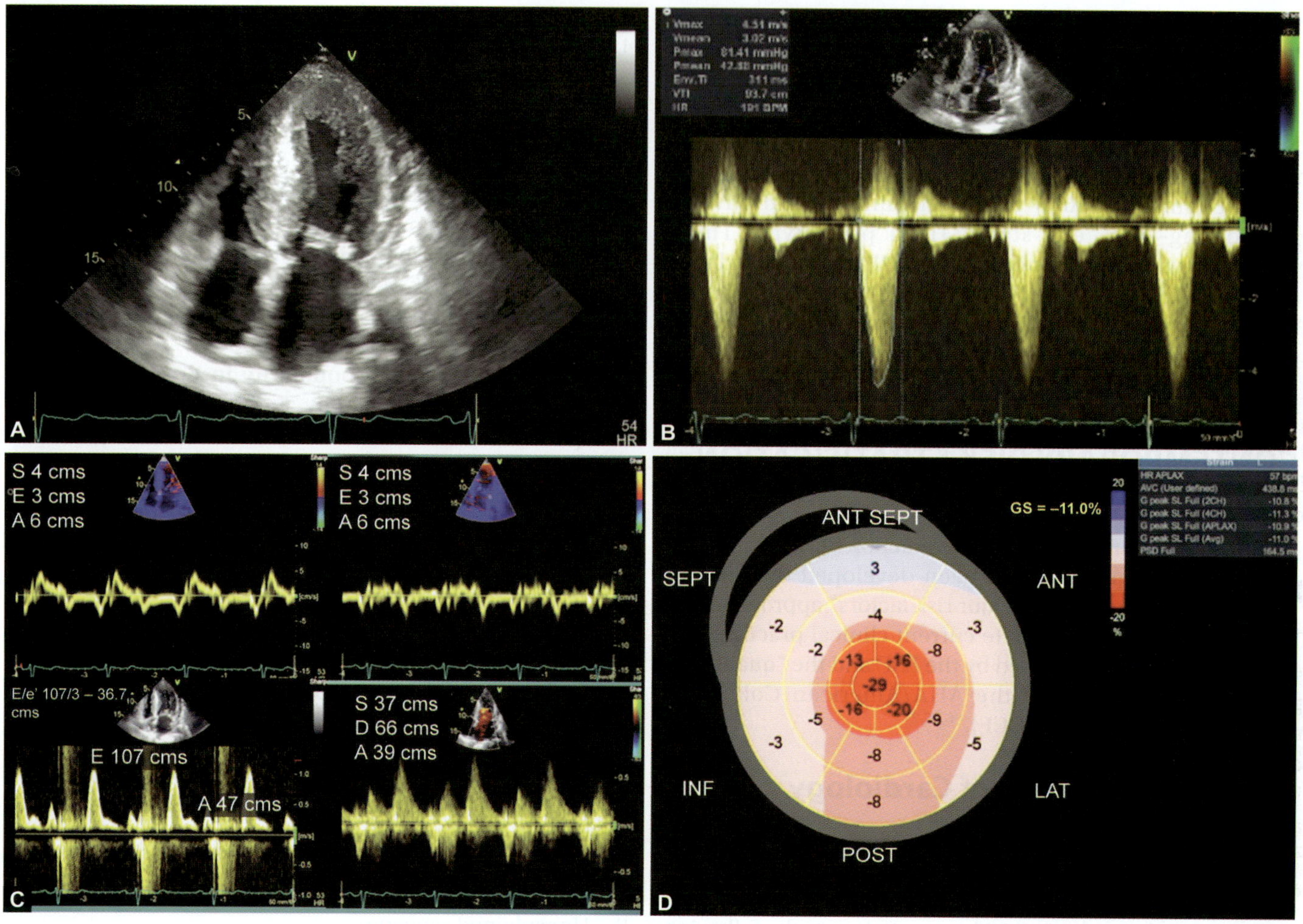

FIGS. 6A TO D: Heart failure with preserved EF in a 43-year-old male HOCM with severe LVOTO, restrictive pattern, PHT, markedly decreased LV GLS.

(GLS: global longitudinal strain; LV: left ventricular; LVOTO: left ventricular outflow tract obstruction)

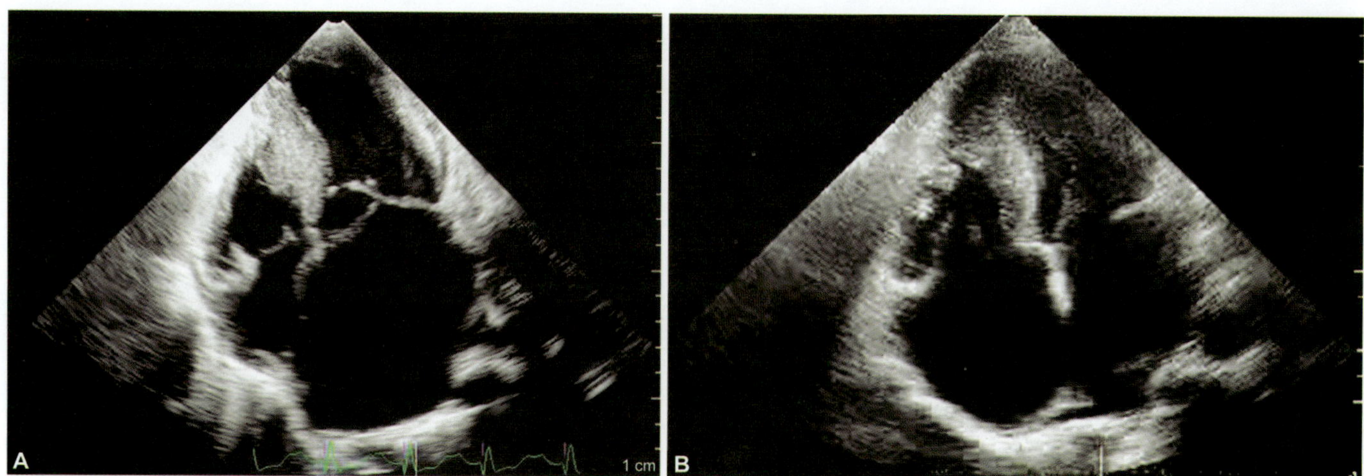

FIGS. 7A AND B: (A) A 15-year-old female with HOCM, marked LVH, severe LVOTO, severe MR, and markedly dilated LA; (B) HCM involving LV and RV with dilated LA, RA due to AF.

(HCM: hypertrophic cardiomyopathy; LV: left ventricular; LVOTO: left ventricular outflow tract obstruction)

The AHA model emphasizes the presence or absence of these individual risk markers and supports ICD implantation in patients with ≥1 major risk factor, particularly when the risk is felt to be significant and consistent with shared decision-making. Notably, the AHA guidelines do not specify a numerical SCD risk threshold but instead rely on clinical judgment, often supplemented by expert interpretation of imaging, family history, and genotype–phenotype correlations.

One advantage of the AHA approach is that it allows for clinical nuance, such as weighing the significance of borderline findings or integrating additional risk factors not captured in the ESC calculator (e.g., apical aneurysm, extensive LGE, or sarcomeric mutations). This flexibility, however, comes at the cost of interobserver variability, and its more qualitative nature may limit reproducibility between centers.

ELECTROCARDIOGRAPHIC PREDICTORS

The 12-lead ECG, while often considered a routine screening tool, holds substantial prognostic value in HCM. Virtually all patients with overt HCM demonstrate ECG abnormalities, reflecting the underlying structural and electrical myocardial derangements.[35] Although ECG findings are not formally included in most current guideline-based SCD risk models, accumulating evidence supports their role in refining risk stratification—particularly when integrated with imaging and clinical data.

Several specific ECG features have been associated with an increased risk of ventricular arrhythmias and SCD in HCM **(Table 2)**.

Q Waves and Pseudoinfarction Patterns

Pathological Q waves, particularly in the inferolateral leads, are present in approximately 25–30% of patients and often reflect severe septal hypertrophy and delayed septal depolarization.[36] Although not specific for arrhythmic risk, their presence signifies significant structural remodeling and regional electrical inhomogeneity **(Figs. 8A and B)**.

Giant Negative T Waves

Deep, symmetric T-wave inversions in precordial leads (especially V_{4-6}) are most often associated with apical HCM and correlate with apical hypertrophy and fibrotic burden.[37] In some reports, giant negative T waves have been associated with increased incidence of NSVT and syncope.

ST-T Abnormalities

Diffuse ST depression and T-wave abnormalities reflect repolarization heterogeneity, a potential arrhythmic substrate. These changes may also result from ischemia due to microvascular dysfunction.[38]

Fragmented QRS Complexes

Fragmented QRS (fQRS), defined as the presence of notching or additional R′ waves in two contiguous leads, correlates

TABLE 2: Electrocardiographic abnormalities associated with sudden cardiac death in HCM.

ECG feature	Mechanism/Pathophysiologic basis	Prognostic implication	Key references
Q waves and pseudoinfarction patterns	Reflect localized depolarization delay due to marked septal hypertrophy and regional electrical remodeling	Indicates significant structural remodeling; not specific for arrhythmic risk but correlates with disease severity	Yoshida et al.[36]
Giant negative T waves	Represent repolarization abnormalities caused by apical hypertrophy and underlying fibrosis	Associated with apical HCM phenotype; linked with NSVT and syncope; may reflect higher fibrotic burden	Yamaguchi et al.[37]
ST-T abnormalities	Result from repolarization heterogeneity and microvascular ischemia related to coronary flow impairment	Serve as markers of diffuse myocardial stress and ischemia; potential arrhythmic substrate	Cecchi et al.[38]
Fragmented QRS (fQRS) complexes	Caused by delayed conduction through fibrotic myocardium; correlates with CMR-detected late gadolinium enhancement	Surface marker of myocardial fibrosis; associated with higher NSVT incidence and arrhythmic events	Ono et al.[39]
Increased QT dispersion	Reflects spatial heterogeneity of ventricular repolarization and instability of action-potential recovery	Associated with polymorphic ventricular arrhythmias and adverse events, though independent predictive value remains debated	Haghjoo et al.[40]
Left atrial enlargement and P-wave abnormalities	Indicate left-atrial remodeling, elevated filling pressures, and conduction delay across the atria	Predict atrial fibrillation and diastolic dysfunction; indirectly worsen hemodynamics and clinical outcomes	Afonso et al.[41]

Note: Major electrocardiographic features linked with arrhythmic or hemodynamic risk in hypertrophic cardiomyopathy.

(CMR: cardiac magnetic resonance; ECG: electrocardiogram; HCM: hypertrophic cardiomyopathy; NSVT: nonsustained ventricular tachycardia)

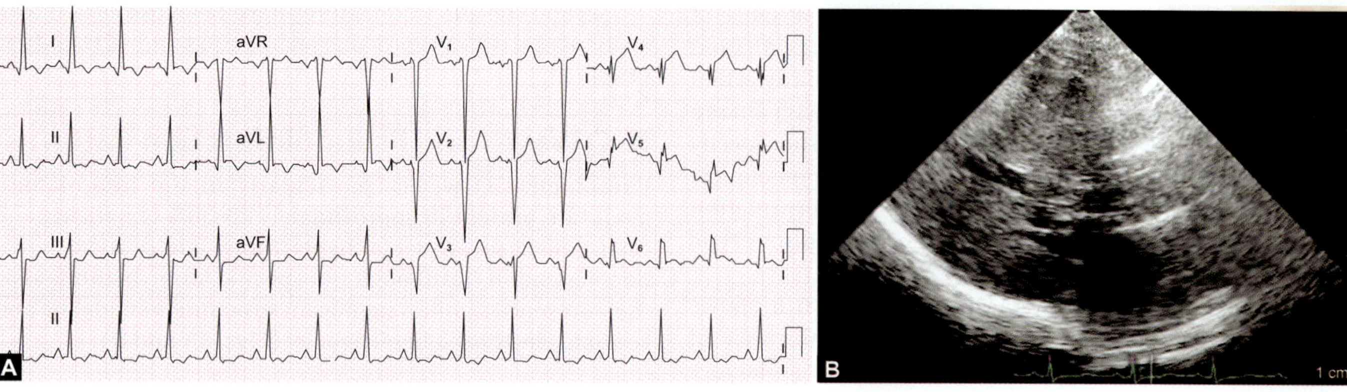

FIGS. 8A AND B: A 56-year-old male with HOCM, pseudoinfarct pattern, and Q waves in anterior leads.

with myocardial fibrosis identified on CMR. fQRS has been associated with increased prevalence of NSVT and higher arrhythmic burden in HCM.[39]

Increased QT Dispersion

Prolonged and dispersed QT intervals reflect repolarization instability and predispose to polymorphic ventricular arrhythmias. Some studies have shown that increased QT dispersion is more common in patients with adverse events, although its independent predictive value remains controversial.[40]

Left Atrial Enlargement and P-wave Abnormalities

Prolonged P-wave duration and interatrial block may reflect structural remodeling and elevated LA pressure. While not directly predictive of SCD, they correlate with an increased risk of atrial arrhythmias, which may indirectly affect hemodynamic status in patients with restrictive physiology.[41]

CARDIAC IMAGING

Cardiac imaging is central to the diagnosis, phenotyping, and risk stratification of HCM. While TTE remains the first-line modality, CMR has become indispensable, particularly for evaluating arrhythmogenic substrates such as myocardial fibrosis and apical aneurysms.

ECHOCARDIOGRAPHY

Echocardiography is widely available and provides high-resolution, real-time assessment of cardiac morphology, hemodynamics, and function.

Key echocardiographic features that correlate with increased SCD risk are summarized in **Table 3**.

Maximal Wall Thickness

The extent of LV hypertrophy is a well-established predictor of arrhythmic events. A maximal wall thickness (MWT) ≥ 30 mm is recognized as a major SCD risk factor in both AHA and ESC guidelines.[42] However, even lesser degrees of hypertrophy—especially when diffuse or involving midventricular or apical segments—may contribute to electrical instability and arrhythmogenesis **(Figs. 1, 2, 7, and 9)**.

Left Ventricular Outflow Tract Obstruction

Dynamic LVOTO, defined as a peak gradient ≥ 30 mm Hg at rest or with provocation, is associated with exertional syncope, ischemia, and increased wall stress.[43] Severe gradients may augment afterload, raise intracavitary pressures, and promote ventricular arrhythmias through mechanical–electrical interaction **(Figs. 6 and 9)**.

Left Atrial Enlargement

An increased left atrial volume index (LAVI > 34 mL/m^2) serves as a marker of chronically elevated LV filling pressures.[44] LA enlargement correlates with AF risk, heart-failure progression, and adverse outcomes. Although not a direct SCD marker, atrial arrhythmias can precipitate hemodynamic compromise and occasionally obscure malignant ventricular rhythms **(Figs. 7A and B)**.

Left Atrial Strain

The value of LA strain measured using speckle tracking needs to be mentioned. The reservoir strain has been found to be reduced <20% in HCM patients. This helps to assess the diastolic function. Impaired LA reservoir strain is common in HCM, even when LA size is normal.[45-47] This helps to differentiate HCM from physiologic LVH (athlete's heart) and hypertensive LVH. Impaired LA strain reflects elevated LV filling pressures and diastolic dysfunction. LA strain is more sensitive than LA volume in detecting LA remodeling and is a strong predictor of new-onset AF.[28] Impaired LA strain is associated with exercise limitation, HF symptoms, and hospitalization and has been an independent predictor of all-cause mortality.[47] It is not reported to indicate ventricular arrhythmias and is not a risk marker for SCD in HCM **(Figs. 9 and 10)**.[47]

TABLE 3: Echocardiographic abnormalities associated with SCD in HCM.

Echocardiographic parameter	Mechanism/pathophysiologic basis	Prognostic implication	Key references
Maximal wall thickness (MWT)	Reflects the extent of myocyte hypertrophy and disarray; extreme thickness increases wall stress and ischemia	MWT ≥30 mm is an established major SCD risk factor; lesser degrees, when diffuse or mid/apical, may still increase arrhythmic vulnerability	O'Mahony et al.[42]
Left ventricular outflow tract (LVOT) obstruction	Dynamic obstruction leads to elevated intracavitary pressures, ischemia, and mechanical–electrical interaction	Associated with exertional syncope, ischemia, and possibly higher ventricular arrhythmic risk; indicates advanced disease	Maron et al.[43]
Left atrial enlargement	Results from chronically elevated LV filling pressures and diastolic dysfunction	Predicts atrial fibrillation, HF progression, and adverse outcomes; not a direct SCD marker but worsens hemodynamic status	Nistri et al.[44]
Left atrial (LA) strain	Reflects LA compliance and reservoir function; reduction indicates elevated LV filling pressures and diastolic burden	Strong predictor of new-onset AF, HF symptoms, and mortality; helps differentiate HCM from physiologic LVH; not a marker for SCD	Sun et al., Debonnaire et al., and Hiemstra et al.[45-47]
Global longitudinal strain (GLS)	Measures global LV systolic deformation; reduced values correspond to myocardial fibrosis and subclinical dysfunction	Correlates with LGE on CMR and increased arrhythmic events; useful for early identification of high-risk patients	Reant et al.[48]
Apical aneurysm	Localized akinetic or dyskinetic apical segment with fibrotic scar formation	Strong predictor of sustained VT, thromboembolism, and SCD; represents a high-risk morphological feature	Maron et al.[49]

Note: Major echocardiographic findings associated with arrhythmic and hemodynamic risk in HCM.

(AF: atrial fibrillation; CMR: cardiac magnetic resonance; HCM: hypertrophic cardiomyopathy; HF: heart failure; LGE: late gadolinium enhancement; LV: left ventricle; SCD: sudden cardiac death)

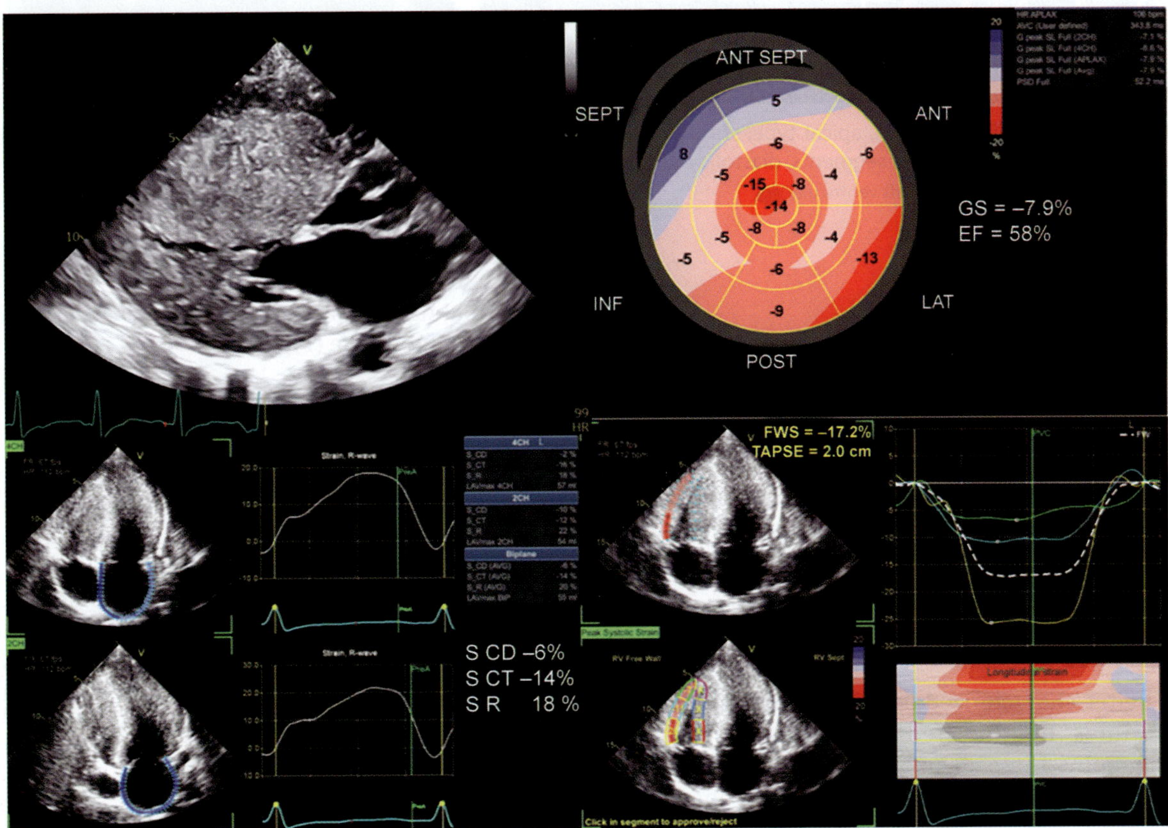

FIG. 9: A 16-year-old male with IVS thickness of 40 mm and LVOT and RVOT obstruction. LV GLS is markedly decreased (−7.9%). RV free wall strain is mildly decreased (−17.2%) and LA reservoir strain is markedly decreased (18%).

(LV: left ventricular; LVOT: left ventricular outflow tract)

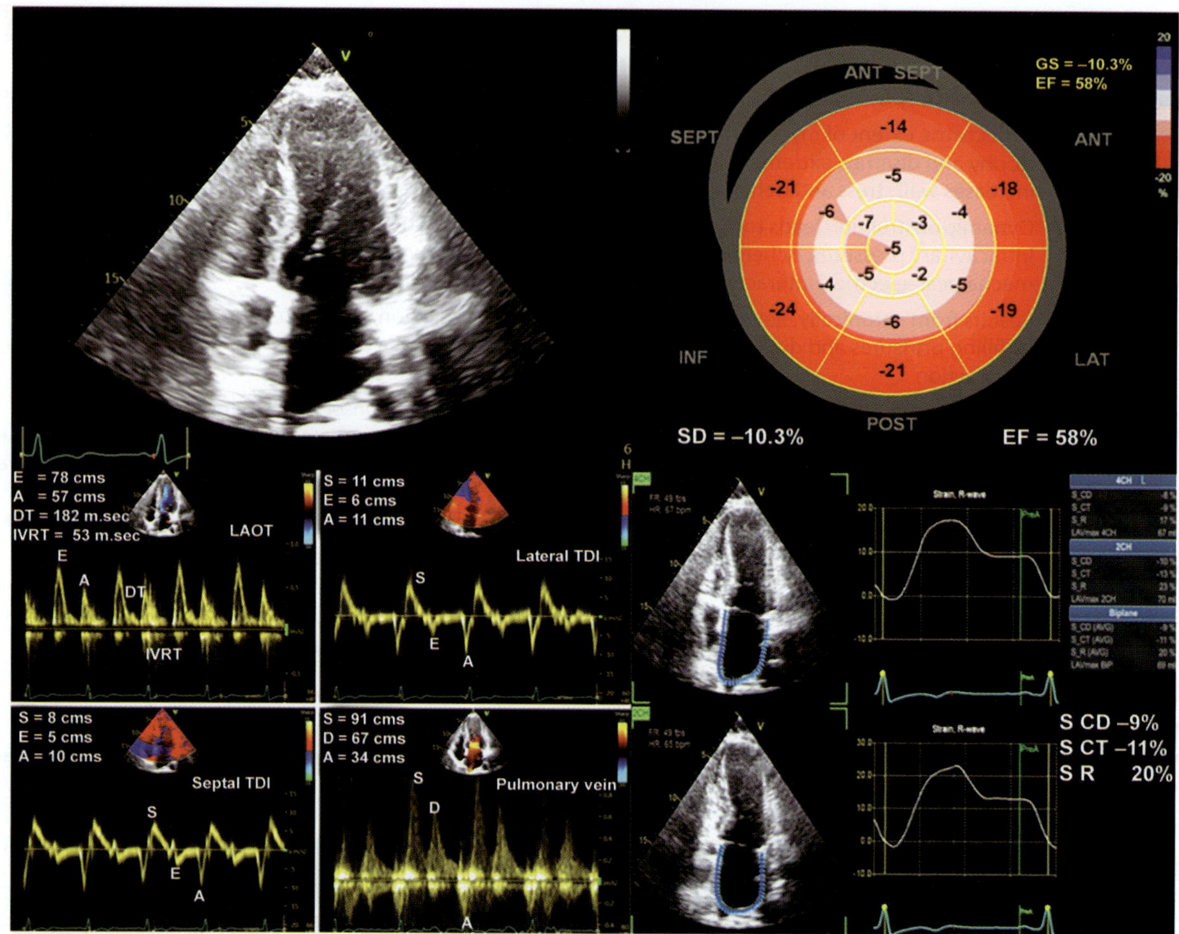

FIG. 10: A 56-year-old male with HCM, apical type, showing LV GLS of –10.3%, marked decrease in strain in the apical midventricular segment and preserved strain in basal segments, diastolic dysfunction grade 1 and decreased LA reservoir strain.
(HCM: hypertrophic cardiomyopathy; LV: left ventricular)

Left Ventricular Global Longitudinal Strain

Advanced echocardiographic techniques such as speckle-tracking strain imaging have demonstrated that impaired LV GLS—particularly in the presence of preserved EF—can indicate subclinical myocardial dysfunction and fibrosis. Reduced GLS correlates with LGE on CMR and arrhythmic risk.[48] This may be a useful marker to identify patients for further evaluation **(Figs. 9 and 10)**.

Apical Aneurysms

Although better characterized on CMR, apical aneurysms can sometimes be detected on contrast-enhanced echocardiography. These aneurysms are a high-risk feature for sustained monomorphic VT, thromboembolism, and SCD.[49]

Despite its many advantages, echocardiography has limitations in visualizing the apex and assessing myocardial tissue characteristics. This is where CMR offers complementary value **(Fig. 4)**.

CARDIAC MAGNETIC RESONANCE

Cardiac magnetic resonance offers superior spatial resolution and unparalleled myocardial tissue characterization, making it the gold standard for defining hypertrophy patterns and identifying myocardial fibrosis in HCM. It is particularly valuable in patients with suboptimal echocardiographic windows or equivocal findings, and it refines both phenotypic classification and arrhythmic risk assessment. Key CMR abnormalities associated with SCD are summarized in **(Table 4)**.

Late Gadolinium Enhancement

The most robust CMR predictor of SCD in HCM is the extent of LGE, which reflects areas of replacement fibrosis. Multiple studies have shown that LGE > 15% of LV mass confers a

TABLE 4: Cardiac magnetic resonance (CMR) abnormalities associated with sudden cardiac death (SCD) in hypertrophic cardiomyopathy (HCM)

CMR parameter	Mechanism/Pathophysiologic basis	Prognostic implication	Key References
Late gadolinium enhancement (LGE)	Focal replacement fibrosis in hypertrophic and insertion regions leads to conduction delay and re-entry	LGE >15% LV mass strongly associated with increased SCD risk; used as risk enhancer in guidelines	Chan et al.[12]
Apical/midventricular aneurysm	Localized scarring and wall thinning leads to electrical heterogeneity and re-entrant VT circuits	Independent predictor of sustained VT, SCD, and thromboembolism; risk independent of EF	Maron et al.[49] Rowin et al.[50]
Diffuse fibrosis (T1 mapping/ECV)	Tracks interstitial matrix expansion; identifies diffuse myocardial fibrosis not captured by LGE	Correlates with diastolic dysfunction and arrhythmias; *not yet a validated independent SCD risk marker*	Ommen et al.[27] Olivotto et al.[31]

TABLE 5: Genetic mutations associated with increased risk of SCD in HCM.

Genetic variant/category	Mechanistic basis/phenotype	SCD risk association	References
TNNT2 (cardiac troponin T) mutations	Altered calcium sensitivity and impaired relaxation despite mild hypertrophy	Disproportionately high SCD risk even with modest wall thickness	Watkins et al.[51]
MYBPC3 truncating mutations	Haploinsufficiency → progressive fibrosis, contractile instability	Associated with arrhythmic events and heart-failure progression	Ho et al.[52]
Compound/Multiple pathogenic variants ("double-hit" genotypes)	Additive or synergistic sarcomeric dysfunction	Higher penetrance and earlier, more severe phenotype with greater SCD risk	Lopes et al.[53]

(HCM: hypertrophic cardiomyopathy; SCD: sudden cardiac death)

two- to fourfold increase in SCD risk.[54] Even smaller extents (5–15%) may carry incremental risk, particularly among younger patients or those with coexisting risk factors. LGE typically localizes to the interventricular septum and right-ventricular insertion points, regions prone to myocyte disarray and fibrotic scarring. Current guideline models increasingly recognize quantitative LGE as an adjunct in ICD decision-making for borderline-risk individuals **(Fig. 3)**.

Apical and Midventricular Aneurysms

Cardiac magnetic resonance enables precise detection of apical or midventricular aneurysms, which may be missed on standard echocardiography due to limited apical visualization. These aneurysms represent zones of thinned myocardium, fibrosis, and electrical heterogeneity, predisposing to scar-related monomorphic VT.[50] Their presence indicates a distinct high-risk substrate, associated with SCD, thromboembolic events, and HF progression—even in patients without traditional risk factors **(Fig. 4)**.

Diffuse Fibrosis by T1 Mapping and Extracellular Volume

Beyond focal LGE, quantitative CMR techniques such as native T1 mapping and ECV estimation provide insight into diffuse interstitial fibrosis. Increased T1 values and elevated ECV fractions correlate with higher arrhythmic burden, progressive diastolic dysfunction, and adverse clinical outcomes, even when overt LGE is absent.[55] These markers offer a sensitive means of detecting early myocardial remodeling and may help identify patients at risk for arrhythmias before overt scar formation develops.

Summary

Cardiac magnetic resonance complements echocardiography by offering quantitative assessment of myocardial fibrosis, precise evaluation of aneurysmal morphology, and comprehensive mapping of hypertrophy patterns. Integrating CMR-derived indices—particularly extent of LGE and presence of apical aneurysm—into multimodal risk-assessment frameworks substantially enhances prediction of adverse events and guides ICD decision-making in HCM.

GENETIC RISK MARKERS

Genetic testing in HCM has long been used for diagnosis and family screening, but its role in SCD prediction is now increasingly recognized.[56] Approximately 50–60% of clinically diagnosed HCM cases harbor pathogenic or likely pathogenic variants in sarcomeric genes, most commonly *MYH7* (β-myosin heavy chain) and *MYBPC3* (myosin-binding protein C).[51,52] Certain variants are linked to more malignant arrhythmic phenotypes, independent of conventional structural risk factors **(Table 5)**.

Mutations in *TNNT2* (cardiac troponin T) are consistently associated with a disproportionately high risk of SCD despite relatively mild hypertrophy.[51] Similarly, compound heterozygosity or truncating MYBPC3 variants may confer increased arrhythmic potential and earlier disease expression.[52,53]

Emerging genotype–phenotype correlation algorithms integrate these variants with imaging markers—such as extent of fibrosis (LGE) or presence of apical aneurysm—to refine risk stratification.[57]

In parallel, polygenic risk score (PRS) approaches are under investigation. PRS models aggregate the minor additive effects of multiple common variants to estimate arrhythmic or penetrance risk in genetically ambiguous or sarcomere-negative patients.[58]

Genetic data are therefore evolving from a purely diagnostic to a prognostic and risk-refining tool, complementing clinical, electrocardiographic, and imaging markers in modern SCD prediction frameworks.

CONCLUSION

Sudden cardiac death remains one of the most feared complications of HCM, particularly in younger individuals. While traditional risk factors such as massive left-ventricular hypertrophy, family history of SCD, and NSVT continue to play a central role in risk assessment, these parameters alone are insufficient to capture the full complexity and heterogeneity of arrhythmic risk in HCM.

Contemporary approaches to SCD prediction have evolved beyond single-marker assessment to include multivariable risk models, such as the ESC HCM risk-SCD calculator and the more qualitative AHA framework. In parallel, the use of advanced cardiac imaging—especially CMR with LGE—and recognition of electrocardiographic markers of arrhythmogenicity have provided clinicians with more refined tools for identifying high-risk patients.

Genetic testing is now increasingly recognized not only for family screening but also for its prognostic implications, particularly in the presence of high-risk sarcomeric mutations or adverse genotype–phenotype correlations. Emerging modalities—including machine-learning-based ECG analysis, serum fibrosis biomarkers, and polygenic risk scoring—may soon enable more individualized and dynamic risk prediction.

Current models may both over- and underestimate risk, especially in patients at the extremes of age, those with atypical phenotypes, or in settings with limited access to advanced imaging or genetic diagnostics. Thus, clinical judgment and shared decision-making remain paramount when considering primary-prevention ICD therapy.

In the absence of randomized trials, observational and registry data continue to guide current management. Ongoing efforts to integrate imaging, genetic, biomarker, and electrophysiological parameters into unified predictive frameworks will be essential to advance precision medicine and further reduce the burden of sudden death in HCM.

REFERENCES

1. Myerburg RJ, Castellanos A. Cardiac arrest and sudden cardiac death. N Engl J Med. 2005;352:1749-60.
2. Zipes DP, Wellens HJ. Sudden cardiac death. Circulation. 1998; 98:2334-51.
3. Maron BJ, Gardin JM, Flack JM, et al. Prevalence of hypertrophic cardiomyopathy in a general population of young adults. Circulation. 1995;92:785-9.
4. Semsarian C, Ingles J, Maron MS, et al. New perspectives on the prevalence of hypertrophic cardiomyopathy. J Am Coll Cardiol. 2015;65:1249-54.
5. Maron BJ, Spirito P, Olivotto I, et al. Epidemiology of hypertrophic cardiomyopathy–related death: revisited in the contemporary era. Circulation. 2000;102:858-64.
6. O'Mahony C, Jichi F, Pavlou M, et al. A novel clinical risk prediction model for sudden cardiac death in hypertrophic cardiomyopathy (HCM risk-SCD). Eur Heart J. 2014;35:2010-20.
7. Rowin EJ, Maron MS, Olivotto I, et al. Contemporary natural history and management of non-obstructive hypertrophic cardiomyopathy. J Am Coll Cardiol. 2017;69:830-41.
8. Maron BJ, Doerer JJ, Haas TS, et al. Sudden deaths in young competitive athletes: analysis of 1866 deaths in the United States, 1980–2006. Circulation. 2009;119:1085-92.
9. Spirito P, Maron BJ. Pathophysiology of hypertrophic cardiomyopathy. Prog Cardiovasc Dis. 1989;32:23-57.
10. Maron MS, Olivotto I, Zenovich AG, et al. Hypertrophic cardiomyopathy is predominantly a disease of left ventricular outflow tract obstruction. Circulation. 2003;108:450-7.
11. Varnava AM, Elliott PM, Mahon N, et al. Relation between myocyte disarray and outcome in hypertrophic cardiomyopathy. Am J Cardiol. 2001;88:275-9.
12. Chan RH, Maron BJ, Olivotto I, et al. Prognostic value of late gadolinium enhancement by cardiac magnetic resonance in hypertrophic cardiomyopathy. Circulation. 2014;130: 484-495.
13. Cecchi F, Olivotto I, Gistri R, et al. Coronary microvascular dysfunction and prognosis in hypertrophic cardiomyopathy. N Engl J Med. 2003;349:1027-35.
14. Maron BJ, Thompson PD, Puffer JC, et al. Cardiovascular pre-participation screening of competitive athletes. Circulation. 1996;94:850-6.
15. Corrado D, Basso C, Schiavon M, et al. Screening for hypertrophic cardiomyopathy in athletes. N Engl J Med. 1998;339:364-9.
16. O'Mahony C, Akhtar MM, Anastasiou Z, et al. Clinical spectrum of end-stage hypertrophic cardiomyopathy. Heart. 2012;98: 1207-11.
17. Roberts JD, Veinot JP, Rutberg J, et al. Electroanatomic mapping of ventricular arrhythmias in hypertrophic cardiomyopathy. Heart Rhythm. 2015;12:1899-1908.

18. Bagnall RD, Weintraub RG, Ingles J, et al. A population-based study of sudden cardiac death in the young. N Engl J Med. 2016;374:2441-52.
19. Maron BJ, Casey SA, Poliac LC, et al. Clinical course of hypertrophic cardiomyopathy in a regional United States cohort. JAMA. 1999;281:650-5.
20. Maron BJ, Spirito P, Shen WK, et al. Implantable cardioverter-defibrillators and prevention of sudden death in hypertrophic cardiomyopathy. N Engl J Med. 2000;342:365-73.
21. Maron BJ, Maron MS. Hypertrophic cardiomyopathy. Lancet. 2013;381:242-55.
22. Spirito P, Bellone P, Harris KM, et al. Magnitude of nonsustained ventricular tachycardia and risk in hypertrophic cardiomyopathy. J Am Coll Cardiol. 2009;54:220-7.
23. Monserrat L, Elliott PM, Gimeno JR, et al. Non-sustained ventricular tachycardia in hypertrophic cardiomyopathy: relation to sudden death. Eur Heart J. 2003;24:1586-94.
24. Teare D. Asymmetrical hypertrophy of the heart in young adults. Br Heart J. 1958;20:1-8.
25. Spirito P, Maron BJ, Bonow RO, et al. Clinical course and outcomes in hypertrophic cardiomyopathy with massive left ventricular hypertrophy. N Engl J Med. 2000;342:1778-85.
26. Gersh BJ, Maron BJ, Bonow RO, et al. 2011 ACCF/AHA guideline for the diagnosis and treatment of hypertrophic cardiomyopathy: a report of the American College of Cardiology Foundation/American Heart Association Task Force on Practice Guidelines. Developed in collaboration with the American Association for Thoracic Surgery, American Society of Echocardiography, American Society of Nuclear Cardiology, Heart Failure Society of America, Heart Rhythm Society, Society for Cardiovascular Angiography and Interventions, and Society of Thoracic Surgeons. J Am Coll Cardiol. 2011;58:e212-60.
27. Ommen SR, Mital S, Burke MA, et al. 2020 AHA/ACC guideline for the diagnosis and treatment of hypertrophic cardiomyopathy: a report of the American College of Cardiology/American Heart Association Joint Committee on Clinical Practice Guidelines. Circulation. 2020;142:e558-631.
28. Elliott PM, Anastasakis A, Borger MA, et al. 2014 ESC guidelines on diagnosis and management of hypertrophic cardiomyopathy: the task force for the diagnosis and management of hypertrophic cardiomyopathy of the European Society of Cardiology (ESC). Eur Heart J. 2014;35:2733-79.
29. Olivotto I, Maron BJ, Autore C, et al. Assessment and significance of left ventricular outflow obstruction in hypertrophic cardiomyopathy. Eur Heart J. 2004;25:2058-66.
30. Maron MS, Olivotto I, Betocchi S, et al. Effect of left ventricular outflow tract obstruction on clinical outcome in hypertrophic cardiomyopathy. N Engl J Med. 2003;348:295-303.
31. Olivotto I, Maron BJ, Adabag AS, et al. Myocardial fibrosis and risk of sudden death in hypertrophic cardiomyopathy. J Am Coll Cardiol. 2008;52:1796-1804.
32. Lakdawala NK, Weinberger HD, Sagner G, et al. Hypertrophic cardiomyopathy in children: clinical features and outcomes. Circulation. 2017;136:1897-1907.
33. O'Mahony C, Jichi F, Pavlou M, et al. A novel clinical risk prediction model for SCD in HCM (ESC Risk-SCD). Eur Heart J. 2014;35:2010-2020.
34. Maron BJ, Maron MS. Clinical impact of contemporary management strategies for hypertrophic cardiomyopathy. Prog Cardiovasc Dis. 2012;54:502-12.
35. Maron BJ, Spirito P, Shen WK, et al. Implantable cardioverter-defibrillators and prevention of sudden cardiac death in hypertrophic cardiomyopathy. N Engl J Med. 2000;342[6]:365-73.
36. Yoshida N, Ikeda U, Shimada K, et al. Electrocardiographic Q-wave abnormalities and regional left ventricular hypertrophy in hypertrophic cardiomyopathy. J Am Coll Cardiol. 1988;12[1]:146-53.
37. Yamaguchi H, Nishiyama S, Nakanishi S, et al. Apical hypertrophic cardiomyopathy: clinical and electrocardiographic features, long-term outcome, and comparison with other forms of HCM. J Am Coll Cardiol. 2003;41[6]:987-93.
38. Cecchi F, Olivotto I, Gistri R, et al. Coronary microvascular dysfunction and prognosis in hypertrophic cardiomyopathy. N Engl J Med. 2003;349[11]:1027-35.
39. Ono N, Hayashi T, Kawamura S, et al. Fragmented QRS complexes are associated with myocardial fibrosis and ventricular arrhythmias in hypertrophic cardiomyopathy. Heart Rhythm. 2015;12[3]:551-8.
40. Haghjoo M, Arya A, Sadr-Ameli MA, et al. QT dispersion and risk of arrhythmic events in hypertrophic cardiomyopathy. Europace. 2009;11[5]:643-9.
41. Afonso LC, Bernal J, Bax JJ, et al. Electrocardiographic predictors of atrial fibrillation in hypertrophic cardiomyopathy: the role of P-wave indices. J Electrocardiol. 2016;49[3]:355-62.
42. O'Mahony C, Jichi F, Pavlou M, et al. A novel clinical risk prediction model for sudden cardiac death in hypertrophic cardiomyopathy (HCM Risk-SCD). Eur Heart J. 2014;35[30]:2010-20.
43. Maron MS, Olivotto I, Zenovich AG, et al. Hypertrophic cardiomyopathy is predominantly a disease of left ventricular outflow tract obstruction. Circulation. 2003;108[4]:450-7.
44. Nistri S, Olivotto I, Betocchi S, et al. Prognostic significance of left atrial size in patients with hypertrophic cardiomyopathy (Italian Registry Study). Eur Heart J. 2006;27[22]:2513-8.
45. Sun BJ, Park JH, Lee JH, et al. Left atrial strain as a predictor of atrial fibrillation in hypertrophic cardiomyopathy. J Am Soc Echocardiogr. 2020;33[9]:1189-99.
46. Debonnaire P, Joyce E, Hiemstra Y, et al. Left atrial size and function in hypertrophic cardiomyopathy and its relation to left ventricular diastolic function and fibrosis. Heart. 2017;103[9]:672-9.
47. Hiemstra YL, Debonnaire P, Bootsma M, et al. Clinical utility of left atrial strain for predicting outcome in hypertrophic cardiomyopathy. Eur Heart J Cardiovasc Imaging. 2021;22[1]:94-103.
48. Reant P, Reynaud A, Pillois X, et al. Global longitudinal strain is associated with fibrosis and ventricular arrhythmias in hypertrophic cardiomyopathy. J Am Soc Echocardiogr. 2016;29[12]:1069-78.
49. Maron MS, Finley JJ, Bos JM, et al. Prevalence, clinical significance, and natural history of left ventricular apical aneurysms in hypertrophic cardiomyopathy. J Am Coll Cardiol. 2008;51[25]:2346-52.
50. Rowin EJ, Maron MS, Haas TS, et al. Hypertrophic cardiomyopathy with left ventricular apical aneurysm: implications for risk stratification and management. J Am Coll Cardiol. 2017;69[7]:761-73.
51. Watkins H, Ashrafian H, Redwood C. Inherited cardiomyopathies. N Engl J Med. 2011;364:1643-56.
52. Ho CY, Day SM, Ashley EA, et al. Genotype and lifetime burden of disease in hypertrophic cardiomyopathy: insights from the Sarcomeric Human Cardiomyopathy Registry (SHaRe). Circulation. 2018;138:1387-98.

53. Lopes LR, Rahman MS, Elliott PM. A systematic review of genotype–phenotype associations in hypertrophic cardiomyopathy. Heart. 2013;99:1800-11.
54. Chan RH, Maron BJ, Olivotto I, et al. Prognostic value of quantitative late gadolinium enhancement in hypertrophic cardiomyopathy. Circulation. 2014;130[6]:484-95.
55. Puntmann VO, Peker E, Chandrashekhar Y, Nagel E. T1 mapping in characterizing myocardial disease: a comprehensive review. Circ Res. 2016;119[2]:277-99.
56. Ingles J, Semsarian C. The role of genetic testing in hypertrophic cardiomyopathy: when and how to test. Heart. 2014;100:355-61.
57. Ingles J, Burns C, Bagnall RD, Semsarian C. Genetics of hypertrophic cardiomyopathy: insights and implications for clinical management. Clin Genet. 2015;88:437-46.
58. Tadros R, Francis C, Xu X, et al. Shared genetic pathways contribute to risk of hypertrophic and dilated cardiomyopathies with clinical implications for polygenic risk prediction. Nat Genet. 2021;53:1476-84.

CHAPTER

41

Polygenic Inheritance in Hypertrophic Cardiomyopathy

Ajay Bahl

ABSTRACT

Hypertrophic cardiomyopathy (HCM) is typically considered to be an autosomal dominant disorder due to mutations in genes encoding sarcomeric proteins. However, HCM is much more complex. The single-gene model does not explain the disease phenotype in a large number of patients, and more complex models need to be considered. The four models are: (1) Single-mutation model, (2) multiple-mutation model, (3) polygenic model, and (4) multifactorial model. Each of these models may predominate in a given patient, with overlaps between them. Identification of specific factors in a given patient may result in a personalized approach to the management of HCM in future.

Keywords: Hypertrophic cardiomyopathy, polygenic, sequence variation.

INTRODUCTION

Hypertrophic cardiomyopathy (HCM) is traditionally considered to be an autosomal dominant disorder caused by mutations in genes encoding sarcomeric proteins. This single-gene model is simple, with genetic counseling being easy and straightforward. However, HCM is much more complex, and the single-gene model does not explain the disease in a large number of patients. More complex models need to be considered in many patients. The four models are: (1) *Single-mutation model,* (2) *multiple-mutation model,* (3) *polygenic model,* and (4) *multifactorial model* **(Flowchart 1)**. Each of these models may predominate in a given patient with overlaps between them. Thus, the disease may be best explained by a single-gene model in some patients while in others a different model example polygenic model may apply.

FLOWCHART 1: Potential models for disease phenotype in hypertrophic cardiomyopathy.

SINGLE-MUTATION MODEL

In this model, a single mutation is responsible for the disease. This implies that if a relative carries the causative mutation found in the family, he/she is at risk of developing HCM. In case a relative does not carry the mutation, he/she would not develop the disease in the future, and no further follow-up is needed. This model best applies when the family tree clearly shows an autosomal dominant inheritance pattern with a similar disease pattern in affected relatives.

There are several limitations of this model. Firstly, mutations in sarcomeric genes are identified only in 40–50% patients. Some of these could be due to as yet unidentified mutations. However, this model does not explain the cause of HCM in a majority of patients in whom more complex models need to be considered. Secondly, disease heterogeneity due to similar mutations and variability within the same family is also not explained. A given mutation should give rise to a similar phenotype in all affected patients if other factors are not involved. An example of variable expression are the mutations in the troponin I gene (*TNNI3*), which may manifest with different phenotypes including asymmetrical septal hypertrophy, apical hypertrophy, end-stage disease, restrictive cardiomyopathy as well as several other.[1] This variability suggests that factors other than a single mutation contribute to the disease phenotype.

MULTIPLE-MUTATION MODEL

One of the factors contributing to variation in disease morphology and severity could be the presence of more than one mutation in HCM causing genes with each mutation having an intermediate or large effect on the disease phenotype. Of HCM patients, two mutations are detected in 3–7.8% while 0.8% carry three mutations.[2-6] Individuals with more than one mutation are more likely to have a more severe phenotype and end-stage disease.[5] This model in which each variant makes a significant contribution to the phenotype is primarily responsible for disease only in a small number of patients (around 5%).

POLYGENIC MODEL

This model looks beyond mutations in sarcomeric genes and toward genetic variations that are common in the general population. Unlike Mendelian disorders, where a single mutation is responsible for the disease, each variant in the polygenic model has only a minor effect on the disease phenotype and large numbers of these variants may be present in each patient. Identifying these variants is thus challenging. These variants are identified by genome-wide association studies. These are usually present in non-HCM causing genes. Common examples of polygenic diseases include coronary artery disease and diabetes mellitus.

A large number of variants that affect the cardiac phenotype, including hypertrophy and contractility, have been identified. Examples include angiotensin-converting enzyme (*ACE*) gene insertion/deletion (I/D), angiotensin receptor type 1 gene (*AGTR1*), cardiac troponin I-interacting kinase gene (*TNNI3K*), *OBSCN*, nebulette gene (*NEBL*), and calmodulin gene (*CALM3*) polymorphisms.[7-9] A combination of all these variants may modulate the disease in mutation carriers. Some of these may have conflicting effects on disease phenotype. In addition to modulating the disease phenotype, multiple such variants may cause HCM even in the absence of a mutation.

Identifying and targeting these pathways in each patient is a potential for the future. This may result in a personalized approach to the management of HCM.

MULTIFACTORIAL MODEL

In addition to genetic factors, nongenetic conditions also contribute to the disease phenotype. These include hypertension, exercise, especially resistance training, and obesity. Males have higher left ventricular mass compared to females. Left ventricular hypertrophy due to long-standing poorly controlled hypertension may be difficult to distinguish from HCM.

INDIAN DATA

Each sequence variation first occurs *de novo* in an individual who is called the founder. This individual may then pass on the mutation to his/her children, who in turn pass it on to their descendants. Like all populations, Indians have their own founders. Thus, Indians have differences in sequence variations in cardiomyopathy causing/modulating genes compared to other populations. Though a large number of sequence variations are similar, over a third have been reported to be novel in Indians. Regional differences within the country are also present. Considerable data supports the polygenic model for HCM in Indians with several nonsarcomeric genetic variants, contributing to the HCM phenotype.

The most common variant that modulates the cardiomyopathy phenotype is a 25 bp deletion in intron 32 in the gene encoding cardiac myosin binding protein C (*MYBPC3*).[10] Since the founder lived thousands of years back, he/she would have a large number of descendants over many generations. This deletion is now found in around 4% of Indians and increases the risk of cardiomyopathies and heart failure. Another variant *MyBPC3* p.Asp389Val that occurs only in persons carrying the 25 basepair deletion is associated with hyperdynamic left ventricular contractility and unfavorable energetic state.[11]

Angiotensin-converting enzyme insertion/deletion (I/D) polymorphism is another important variant.[7,8] Individuals with HCM who carry the D genotype have higher septal thickness compared to those with the I phenotype. Variations in other genes, including angiotensin receptor type 1 (*AGTR1*), cardiac troponin I-interacting kinase (*TNNI3K*), and calmodulin (*CALM3*) have also been shown to modulate the HCM phenotype in Indians.[9]

IMPLICATIONS

Approaching HCM as a polygenic, multifactorial disorder would imply identifying different factors that contribute to the disease phenotype in each individual patient. This may identify new pathways that can potentially be targeted in each individual patient. This would result in a personalized approach to the management of HCM.

Family screening may also be more complex. Genetic counseling is straightforward in autosomal dominant disorders. In these, if a relative does not carry the mutation causing disease in the family, he/she can be reassured that there is no risk of disease in future. In case of multiple mutations, polygenic or multifactorial disorders, family screening and counseling has to consider multiple factors and can be far more complex.

CONCLUSION

Recent data indicates that the etiopathogenesis of HCM is complex. In a significant number of patients, the disease phenotype is largely due to a single mutation (single-mutation model) transmitted in an autosomal dominant pattern. In around 5%, the disease is caused by more than one mutation (multiple-mutation model). The role of multiple common variants, each with only a minor effect modulating the disease phenotype (polygenic model), is increasingly being recognized. The contribution of nongenetic factors such as hypertension (multifactorial model) is also important in some patients. In a given patient, any of these models may predominate with some overlap between them. Recognizing these complex pathways may result in a personalized medicine approach to the management of HCM.

REFERENCES

1. Mogensen J, Murphy RT, Kubo T, et al. Bahl A, Frequency and clinical expression of cardiac troponin I mutations in 748 consecutive families with hypertrophic cardiomyopathy. J Am Coll Cardiol. 2004;44:2315-25.
2. Viswanathan SK, Sanders HK, McNamara JW, et al. Hypertrophic cardiomyopathy clinical phenotype is independent of gene mutation and mutation dosage. PLoS One. 2017;12:e0187948.
3. Girolami F, Ho CY, Semsarian C, et al. Clinical features and outcome of hypertrophic cardiomyopathy associated with triple sarcomere protein gene mutations. J Am Coll Cardiol. 2010;55:1444-53.
4. Ingles J, Doolan A, Chiu C, et al. Compound and double mutations in patients with hypertrophic cardiomyopathy: implications for genetic testing and counselling. J Med Genet. 2005;42:e59.
5. Hiruma T, Inoue S, Dai Z, et al. Association of Multiple Nonhypertrophic Cardiomyopathy-related Genetic Variants and Outcomes in Patients with Hypertrophic Cardiomyopathy. JACC Heart Fail. 2024;12:2041-52.
6. Richard P, Charron P, Carrier L, et al.; EUROGENE Heart Failure Project. Hypertrophic cardiomyopathy: distribution of disease genes, spectrum of mutations, and implications for a molecular diagnosis strategy. Circulation. 2003;107:2227-32.
7. Rai TS, Dhandapany PS, Ahluwalia TS, et al. ACE I/D polymorphism in Indian patients with hypertrophic cardiomyopathy and dilated cardiomyopathy. Mol Cell Biochem. 2008;311:67-72.
8. Rani B, Kumar A, Bahl A, et al. Renin-angiotensin system gene polymorphisms as potential modifiers of hypertrophic and dilated cardiomyopathy phenotypes. Mol Cell Biochem. 2017;427:1-11.
9. Kumar A, Rani B, Sharma R, et al. ACE2, CALM3 and TNNI3K polymorphisms as potential disease modifiers in hypertrophic and dilated cardiomyopathies. Mol Cell Biochem. 2018;438:167-74.
10. Dhandapany PS, Sadayappan S, Xue Y, et al. A common MYBPC3 (cardiac myosin binding protein C) variant associated with cardiomyopathies in South Asia. Nat Genet. 2009;41:187-91.
11. Viswanathan SK, Puckelwartz MJ, Mehta A, et al. Association of Cardiomyopathy With MYBPC3 D389V and MYBPC3Δ25bp Intronic Deletion in South Asian Descendants. JAMA Cardiol. 2018;3:481-8.

CHAPTER 42

Dual (Ischemic and Nonischemic) Cardiomyopathy: A Wolf in Sheep's Clothing

Chandra Bhan Meena, Himanshu Mahla, Mayank Nausran

ABSTRACT

Dual cardiomyopathy is defined as the coexistence of both ischemic and nonischemic myocardial pathology in the same patient. It is underdiagnosed in our hospital settings and is often missed due to lack of awareness. Advances in imaging and histopathology have revealed that many patients previously classified under a single cardiomyopathy subtype actually have overlapping findings such as ischemic scar superimposed on dilated or infiltrative cardiomyopathy findings.

This coexistence leads to ventricular remodeling and myocardial fibrosis, thereby worsening systolic and diastolic dysfunction, increasing arrhythmic burden and worsening overall prognosis. The diagnostic challenge lies in differentiating the ischemic component from already existing nonischemic disease, as management strategies must be curated to address both entities simultaneously.

Coronary revascularization may not fully reverse dysfunction if an underlying nonischemic pathology persists, while device therapy and pharmacological interventions often require adjustment to the combined pathology. Recognition of dual cardiomyopathy is essential for symptomatic improvement and improved long-term outcomes.

This chapter highlights the epidemiology, pathophysiological mechanisms, diagnostic modalities, and management of dual cardiomyopathy.

Keywords: Dual cardiomyopathy, ischemic cardiomyopathy, nonischemic cardiomyopathy, dilated cardiomyopathy, myocardial fibrosis, heart failure, arrhythmia, sudden cardiac death, cardiac imaging, catheter ablation, implantable cardioverter-defibrillator (ICD).

INTRODUCTION

Dual cardiomyopathy refers to the existence of two distinct forms of heart muscle disease in the same patient, commonly ischemic and nonischemic cardiomyopathies. This condition is often underrecognized and can present subtly, truly acting as a wolf in sheep's clothing.[1]

Patients who are known cases of coronary artery disease (CAD) and referred for cardiovascular magnetic resonance (CMR) imaging, 1 of every 6 patients had nonischemic cardiomyopathy (NICM) or dual (both ischemic and nonischemic) cardiomyopathy.[2]

Patients with both, CAD and NICM, or dual cardiomyopathy, suffer worse long-term prognosis in form of recurrent heart failure hospitalizations and mortality in comparison to those with ischemic cardiomyopathy (ICM) undergoing coronary revascularisation.[2]

Several studies and trials done have not shown any benefit of revascularization in terms of prognosis and survival in CAD patients. This may be possibly due to coexistence of NICM in these patients.[1] It has been seen that around 17% of CAD patients, assessed via cardiac MRI, had features of NICM or dual cardiomyopathy.[1]

DEFINITION

Cardiomyopathy is defined as a myocardial disorder in which heart muscle is structurally and functionally abnormal, in absence of CAD, hypertension (HTN), valvular disease, and congenital heart disease sufficient to cause observed myocardial abnormality.[3]

Cardiomyopathy was defined as the presence of one or more of the following:

- Reduced left ventricular ejection fraction (LVEF; <50%)

- Late gadolinium enhancement (LGE) on cardiac MRI
- Morphological abnormalities of NICM [moderate or severe left ventricular hypertrophy (LV), moderate or severe LV dilatation, and regional wall motion abnormalities due to stress cardiomyopathy].[2]

In most of the studies, CAD was taken as at least 70% stenosis in proximal part of epicardial coronary artery or 50% stenosis in left main coronary artery.[2]

Nonischemic cardiomyopathy is defined as a reduction in left ventricular systolic function in the absence of obstructive CAD. Causes include entities such as valvular heart disease, inflammatory cardiomyopathies, arrhythmogenic cardiomyopathy, and genetic dilated cardiomyopathy.[4]

HISTORICAL PERSPECTIVES

The historical perspective of ischemic ICM dates back to recognition of CAD as a major cause of heart failure and left ventricular dysfunction. Early diagnosis relied heavily on clinical history of CAD or prior myocardial infarction and physical findings including signs of heart failure. Over time, diagnostic modalities evolved from chest X-rays and electrocardiograms to echocardiography, cardiac stress tests, and eventually invasive coronary angiography. These tools aimed to identify myocardial ischemia, viability, and extent of coronary artery involvement.

In more recent years, advanced imaging such as CMR with tissue characterization has enhanced understanding, especially for complex overlapping phenotypes such as dual ICM (ischemic plus nonischemic features). The historical progression highlights improved precision in diagnosis and tailored management of ischemic cardiomyopathy with guideline-directed therapies, coronary revascularization, device therapies (ICD, cardiac resynchronization), and heart transplantation for end-stage disease.[2]

PATHOPHYSIOLOGY

Dual cardiomyopathy arises from the coexistence of two distinct pathological processes affecting the myocardium, typically ischemic and nonischemic mechanisms, which may interact and overlap in complex ways.

Ischemic cardiomyopathy generally results from CAD leading to myocardial ischemia, infarction, and subsequent remodeling. Repeated or chronic ischemic insults cause myocyte loss, fibrosis, and ventricular dilation impairing contractility.

- Nonischemic cardiomyopathy includes a heterogenous group of conditions including genetic, inflammatory, infiltrative, and toxic myocardial diseases. NICM leads to myocardial dysfunction through diverse mechanisms such as myocyte hypertrophy, disarray, fibrosis, and impaired energetics.
- The coexistence may reflect coincidence—the patient having independent ischemic and nonischemic myocardial diseases—or interaction, where chronic ischemia predisposes to or exacerbates nonischemic damage through remodeling and fibrosis.
- Chronic ischemia-induced myocardial remodeling may facilitate susceptibility to secondary nonischemic pathology, including fibrosis or infiltration, blurring clinicopathological boundaries.
- This complex interplay often leads to heterogeneous myocardial tissue characteristics that challenge diagnosis and influence prognosis.[1,2]

Morphological traits used to describe cardiomyopathy phenotypes:

- Ventricular hypertrophy—left and or right
- Ventricular dilatation—left and or right
- Nonischemic ventricular scar and other myocardial tissue characterization features on cardiac magnetic resonance (CMR).

Functional traits:

- Ventricular systolic dysfunction (global regional)
- Ventricular diastolic dysfunction (rest physiology; **Fig. 1**).[5]

Patients typically present with symptoms of heart failure such as dyspnea, fatigue, palpitations, and exercise intolerance, which are nonspecific and common in both ischemic and nonischemic cardiomyopathies.

- Clinical examination may reveal signs of volume overload, arrhythmias, or conduction abnormalities.
- The overlap of dual pathology leads to variable clinical courses—some patients may have stable symptoms, while others exhibit progressive deterioration.
- The dual pathology often complicates treatment response, with some patients showing suboptimal improvement postrevascularization due to concurrent nonischemic damage.
- Diagnostic suspicion should be raised in patients with known CAD who are not improving clinically after revascularization.
- Multimodality imaging and tissue characterization may reveal mixed patterns of scarring, fibrosis, or hypertrophy, prompting further evaluation.
- Awareness of dual cardiomyopathy in clinical practice is essential for timely diagnosis and tailored management strategies.[5]

ETIOLOGY

- *Coronary artery disease (70%):* The largest segment, indicating that most patients with cardiomyopathy have an ischemic origin due to CAD
- *Nonischemic cardiomyopathy (NICM, 20%):* Represents a significant portion of cases where cardiomyopathy results from causes unrelated to CAD, such as genetic, inflammatory, or infiltrative processes
- *Other (8%):* Includes uncommon or miscellaneous etiologies that do not fall under ischemic, inherited, or nonischemic mechanisms

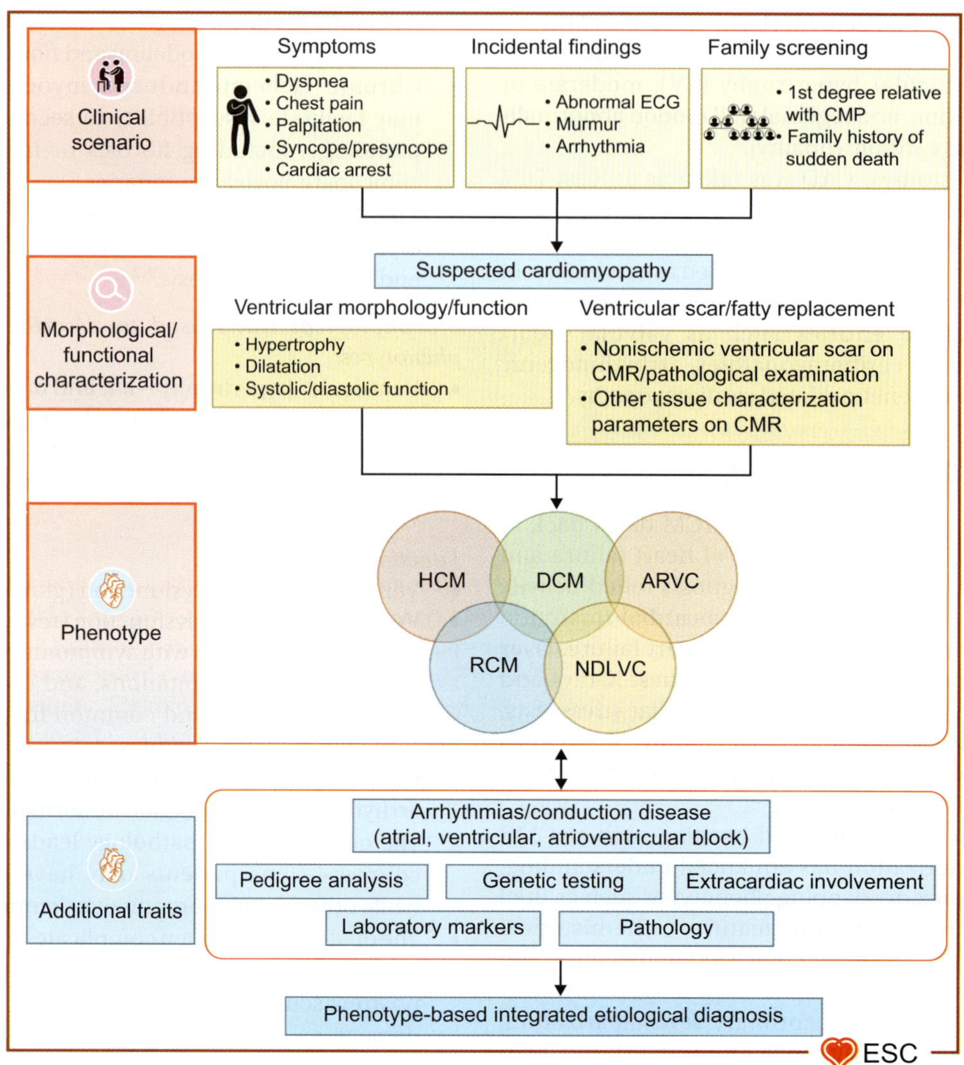

FIG. 1: Clinical diagnostic workflow of cardiomyopathy.[5]

(ARVC: arrhythmogenic right ventricular cardiomyopathy; CMP: cardiomyopathy; CMR: cardiac magnetic resonance; DCM: dilated cardiomyopathy; ECG: electrocardiogram; HCM: hypertrophic cardiomyopathy; NDLVC: non-dilated left ventricular cardiomyopathy)

Source: Adapted from Arbelo E, Protonotarios A, Gimeno JR. 2023 ESC Guidelines for the management of cardiomyopathies. Eur Heart J. 2025;44(37):3503-626.

- *Inherited cardiomyopathies (2%):* A smaller proportion of cases are due to direct genetic mutations leading to inherited cardiomyopathy forms.[6]

Figure 2 summarizes the causes, risk factors, triggers, and myocardial substrate characteristics of NICM. Each donut chart highlights different aspects associated with NICM, providing a visual overview of its complex biology.

Causes of NICM: Nonischemic cardiomyopathy can arise from various underlying problems such as idiopathic dilated cardiomyopathy, substance abuse, chemotherapy, connective tissue diseases, HIV, infiltrative diseases, peripartum cardiomyopathy, myocarditis, and hypertrophic cardiomyopathy (HCM). These causes are mostly noncoronary and unrelated to reduced blood supply to the heart.

Risk factors of NICM: The main risk factors include age, genetics, chronic kidney disease (CKD), diabetes, and male gender. These are patient attributes or comorbidities that increase the likelihood of developing NICM.

Triggers of NICM: Common triggers that can worsen NICM or precipitate symptoms are ischemia (oxygen shortage), inflammation, autonomic dysfunction, and heart failure. These events can make underlying NICM more symptomatic or severe.

Myocardial substrate in NICM: The structural changes in the heart muscle due to NICM include replacement fibrosis, interstitial fibrosis, impaired myocardial cell coupling, and dispersion of repolarization. These changes are important

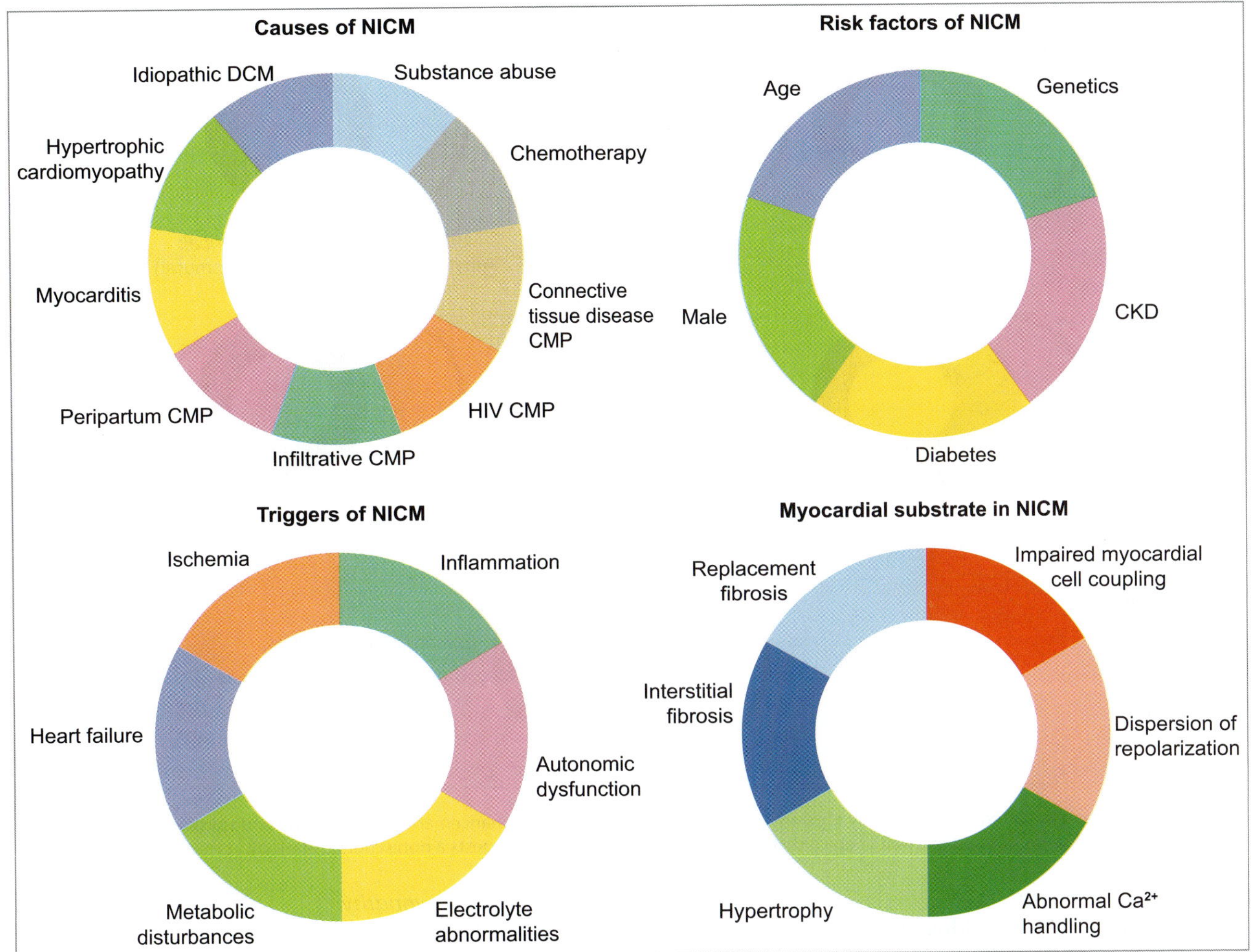

FIG. 2: Nonischemic cardiomyopathy (NICM): Causes, risk factors, triggers, and myocardial substrate.[6]

because they contribute to arrhythmias and deterioration of cardiac function.

This structured outline helps in understanding the wide range of etiologies, contributing factors, acute triggers, and pathological changes that together define NICM.[6]

IMAGING

Routine use of cardiac MRI and other advanced imaging techniques is suggested to delineate cause of heart failure in such patients so that timely decisions can be taken regarding choosing the course of treatment.[2]

Figure 3 illustrates the typical cardiac MRI LGE patterns seen in different heart diseases, helping distinguish ischemic from nonischemic etiologies.

Subendocardial and transmural enhancement:

- *Subendocardial:* Infarct shows gadolinium uptake along the inner (subendocardial) layer of the left ventricle, which is classic for ischemic myocardial infarction.
- *Transmural:* Infarct presents with enhancement extending through the entire wall thickness (from endocardium to epicardium), indicating a full-thickness (transmural) infarct, also typical of ischemic injury.

Subendocardial circumferential enhancement:

Subendocardial circumferential: Amyloidosis involves enhancement around the entire circumference of the sub endocardium and may also be transmural, commonly seen in cardiac amyloidosis.

Midmyocardial enhancement:

- *Midmyocardial:* HCM and midwall—myocarditis/idiopathic dilated CM patterns show mid-layer (midmyocardial) enhancement, a hallmark of nonischemic cardiomyopathies.
- *Midmyocardial enhancement:* Myocarditis and sarcoidosis demonstrates a similar midmyocardial enhancement pattern, seen in inflammatory conditions such as myocarditis or infiltrative diseases such as sarcoidosis.

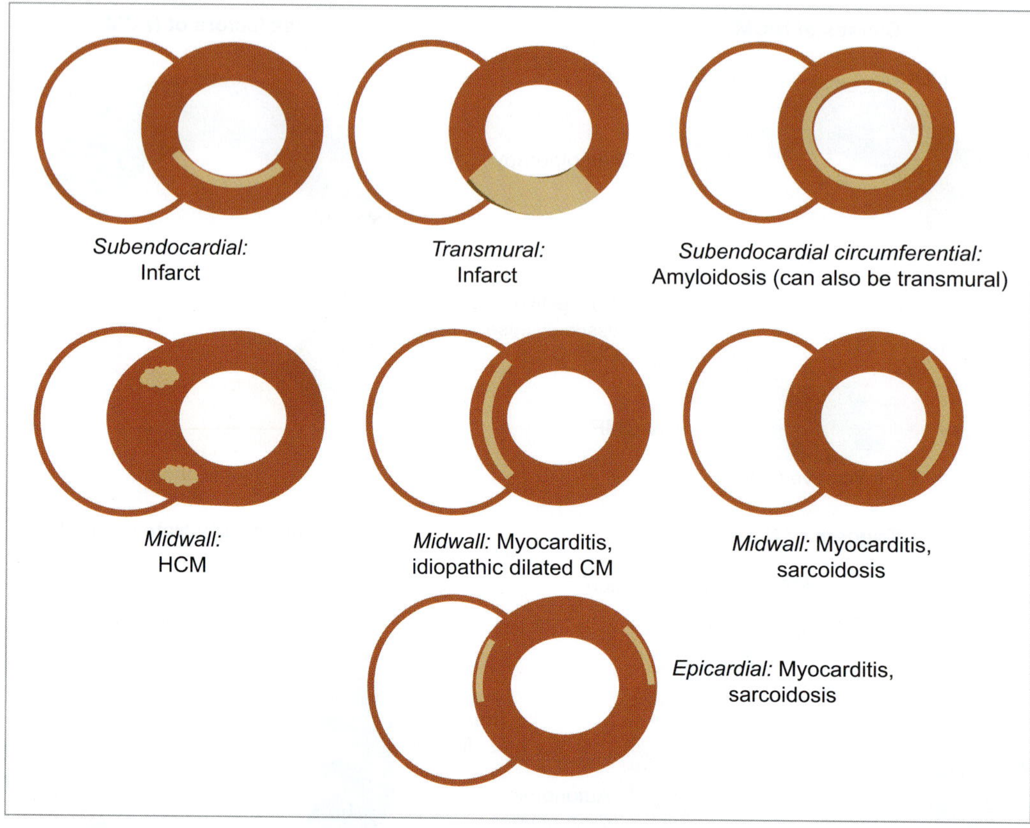

FIG. 3: Hyperenhancement patterns that one may encounter in clinical practice. If hyperenhancement is present, the endocardium should be involved in patients with ischemic disease. Isolated midwall or epicardial hyperenhancement strongly suggests a nonischemic etiology.[7]

Epicardial enhancement:
Epicardial: Myocarditis, sarcoidosis features enhancement in the outer layer (epicardium), which is typical for myocarditis and sarcoidosis.

Diagnostic steps:
Assess EF (CINE):
- *Step 1:* Measure ejection fraction (EF) using cine imaging.
- Normal EF typically means normal heart function, while EF < 50% suggests dysfunction.

Evaluate LGE pattern:
- *Step 2:* Check for LGE on cardiac MRI.
- LGE helps identify scar or fibrosis within the myocardium and can suggest the underlying pathology.

Check CAD status:
- *Step 3:* Assess for CAD.
- Having CAD or not changes the diagnosis between ischemic and nonischemic causes.
- Flow outcomes.

Normal myocardium:
- Normal EF + No LGE + No CAD
- Indicates a normal heart muscle.

Dilated cardiomyopathy (DCM):
- EF < 50% + No LGE + No CAD
- Points to DCM, a NICM.

Ischemic cardiomyopathy:
- MI-type LGE + CAD
- Suggests ICM, with myocardial infarction-type scarring and coronary disease.

Nonischemic cardiomyopathy:
- Non-MI LGE + No CAD
- Indicates NICM, etiologies include myocarditis, sarcoid, and genetic causes.

Dual cardiomyopathy:
- Mixed LGE + CAD
- Indicates both ischemic and nonischemic patterns, termed "Dual CM" (ICM + NICM).[2]

Positron emission tomography (PET) scan depicted myocardial fibroblast activation in NICM, which correlated with impaired ventricular contractile function. PET scan has the potential to depict fibrogenic pathogenesis and disease severity.[8]

MANAGEMENT CONSIDERATIONS (FIG. 4)

Solely targeting CAD via revascularization in CAD with NICM patients do not extend expected benefits of revascularization, and hence, results in poor prognosis of such patients.[2] It has been seen that patients with obstructive CAD with NICM have higher rates of hospitalization than patients with NICM

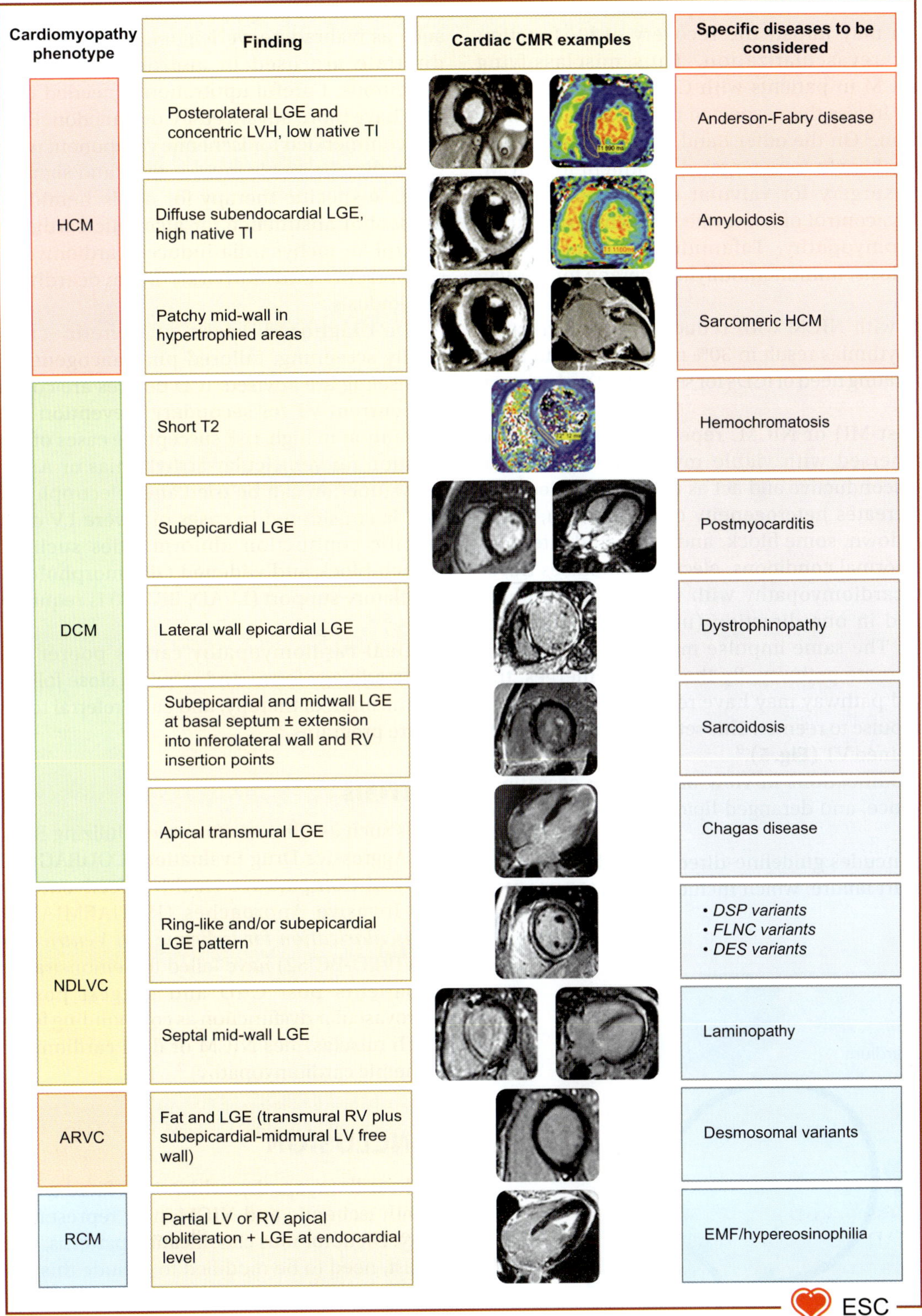

FIG. 4: Management of cardiomyopathies.[5]

(ARVC: arrhythmogenic right ventricular cardiomyopathy; CMR, cardiac magnetic resonance; DCM, dilated cardiomyopathy; GDMT, guideline-directed medical therapy; HCM, hypertrophic cardiomyopathy; HF, heart failure ICD, implantable cardioverter defibrillator; LVOTO, left ventricular outflow tract obstruction; MCS, mechanical circulatory support; NDLVC, non-dilated left ventricular cardiomyopathy; PVR, pulmonary vascular resistance; RCM, restrictive cardiomyopathy; SCD, sudden cardiac death)

Source: Adapted from Arbelo E, Protonotarios A, Gimeno JR. 2023 ESC Guidelines for the management of cardiomyopathies. Eur Heart J. 2023;44(37):3503-626.

or ICM alone.[2] NICM or dual CM in patients with CAD and LV dysfunction may impair the recovery of LV function after coronary revascularization. Thus misclassifying NICM or dual CM in patients with CAD, or labeling it as ICM may result in less than expected results after coronary revascularization.[2] On the other hand, patients with NICM or dual CM may benefit from targeted treatment for NICM, such as valve surgery for valvular dysfunction-related cardiomyopathy, control of heart rate for tachyarrhythmia-induced cardiomyopathy, Tafamidis for transthyretin cardiac amyloidosis, immunomodifying therapy for cardiac sarcoidosis.[2]

In patients with NICM with reduced ejection fraction (EF< 35%), arrhythmias result in 30% mortality due to SCD, thereby necessitating need of ICDs for secondary and primary prevention.[9]

In ICM (post-MI) or NICM, repeated injury leads to fibrosis interspersed with viable myocardium. Fibrotic patches are nonconductive and act as anatomical/electrical barriers. This creates heterogeneity of conduction, some impulses slow down, some block, and some find alternate routes. Under normal conditions, electrical impulses travel uniformly. In cardiomyopathy with fibrosis, an impulse may be blocked in one direction (unidirectional block) due to fibrosis. The same impulse may propagate slowly through an alternate pathway. By the time it emerges, the initially blocked pathway may have recovered excitability, allowing the impulse to reenter. This sets up a reentry circuit, producing sustained VT **(Fig. 5)**.[9]

Lifestyle modifications in view of smoking cessation, alcohol abstinence, and deranged lipids are recommended in specific cases.

Treatment incudes guideline-directed medical therapy (GDMT) for heart failure, which includes ACEI/ARB/ARNI, β-blockers, MRA, diuretics, and SGLT2 inhibitors. Drugs such as ivabradine, vericiguat, and hydralazine-isosorbide dinitrate are used in appropriate patients in specific conditions. Careful uptitration is needed because patients may have more advanced LV dysfunction. Revascularization is recommended for ischemic component with PCI or CABG when there is viable myocardium and significant ischemia. Disease-specific therapy for nonischemic etiologies such as alcohol abstinence for alcoholic cardiomyopathy, rate control for tachycardia-induced cardiomyopathy, immune suppresants and antivirals in myocarditis, Tafamids in amyloidosis.

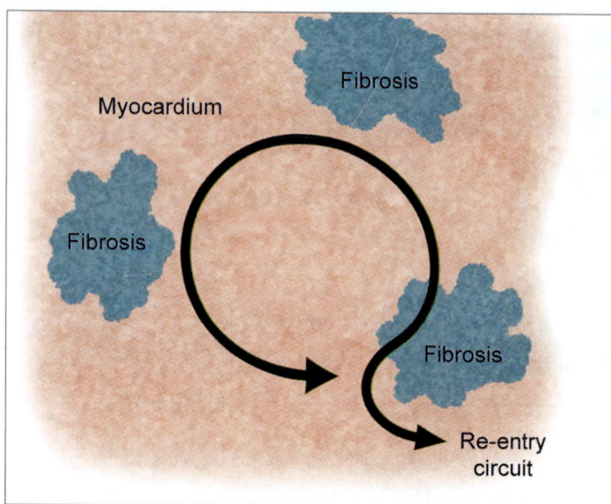

FIG. 5: Re-entry circuit in arrhythmia due to fibrosis.[9]

In diagnosed cases of genetic cardiomyopathy family screening, tailored pharmacogenetic therapy and counseling are advised. ICD devices are considered in case of recurrent VT for secondary prevention and for primary prevention in high-risk susceptible cases of NICM. Catheter ablation for ventricular arrhythmias or AF if contributing to dysfunction can be tried after electrophysiology studies. CRT is considered in cases of severe LV dysfunction with specific conduction abnormalities such as left bundle branch block and widened QRS morphology. Mechanical circulatory support (LVAD, BiVAD) is required in refractory cases.[5]

Dual cardiomyopathy carries poorer outcomes than single-etiology forms and requires close follow-up, frequent optimization of therapy, and early referral to advanced heart failure programs.[5]

Trials

Trials such as Clinical Outcomes Utilizing Revascularization and Aggressive Drug Evaluation (COURAGE), International Study of Comparative Health Effectiveness with Medical and Invasive Approaches (ISCHAEMIA), *Percutaneous Revascularization for Ischemic Left Ventricular Dysfunction* (REVIVED-BCIS2) have failed to demonstrate improvement in patients post CAD and suggest possible coronary microvascular dysfunction as confounding factor responsible which misclassifies NICM or dual cardiomyopathy as ICM (ischemic cardiomyopathy).[2]

CONCLUSION

Dual cardiomyopathy, which is defined as the coexistence of both ischemic and NICM, now represents as a separate entity. Dichotomous classification patterns, which were used in past, need to be modified to include this newly identified pattern. Cardiac MRI and advanced echocardiographic algorithms are need of an hour to identify this entity at earliest in outdoor. Future research must include artificial intelligence and advanced curated algorithms to identify patients having dual pathology at earliest so that targeted treatment can be done at earliest presentations.

REFERENCES

1. Juncà G, Delgado V. Dual (Ischemic and Nonischemic) Cardiomyopathy: A Wolf in Sheep's Clothing. Circulation. 2024;149(11):822-4.
2. Bawaskar P, Thomas N, Ismail K, et al. Nonischemic or Dual Cardiomyopathy in Patients with Coronary Artery Disease. Circulation. 2024;149(11):807-21.
3. Elliott P, Andersson B, Arbustini E, et al. Classification of the cardiomyopathies: a position statement from the european society of cardiology working group on myocardial and pericardial diseases. Eur Heart J. 2008;29(2):270-6.
4. Bozkurt B, Colvin M, Cook J, et al. Current Diagnostic and Treatment Strategies for Specific Dilated Cardiomyopathies: A Scientific Statement from the American Heart Association. Circulation. 2016;134(23):e579-646.
5. Arbelo E, Protonotarios A, Gimeno JR. 2023 ESC Guidelines for the management of cardiomyopathies. Eur Heart J. 2023;44(37):3503-626.
6. Chrispin J, Merchant FM, Lakdawala NK, et al. Risk of Arrhythmic Death in Patients with Nonischemic Cardiomyopathy: JACC Review Topic of the Week. J Am Coll Cardiol. 2023;82(8):735-47.
7. Senthilkumar A, Majmudar MD, Shenoy C, et al. Identifying the etiology: a systematic approach using delayed-enhancement cardiovascular magnetic resonance. Heart Fail Clin. 2009;5(3):349-67.
8. Marques-Alves P, Gonçalves L, Ferreira MJ. PET-CT Imaging in Hypertrophic Cardiomyopathy: A Narrative Review on Risk Stratification and Prognosis. Diagnostics. 2025;15(2):133.
9. Heidenreich PA, Bozkurt B, Aguilar D, et al. 2022 AHA/ACC/HFSA Guideline for the Management of Heart Failure: A Report of the American College of Cardiology/American Heart Association Joint Committee on Clinical Practice Guidelines. Circulation. 2022;145(18):E895-1032.

CHAPTER

43

Vasovagal Syncope: What Treatment Can We Offer in 2025?

Nishad Chitnis, Hygriv B Rao

ABSTRACT

Reflex vasovagal syncope (VVS), or neurocardiogenic syncope, is the most common cause of transient loss of consciousness, affecting up to 30–40% of the population during their lifetime. VVS is often triggered by upright posture, emotional stress, pain, or medical settings and is characterized by prodromal symptoms such as diaphoresis, pallor, nausea, and vasodepressor hypotension or bradycardia. Diagnosis relies primarily on a detailed history, eyewitness accounts, and head-up tilt table test (HUTT), which also facilitates classification according to the Vasovagal Syncope International Study (VASIS) system. Management involves a structured, stepwise approach combining nonpharmacological measures—including patient education, hydration, physical counterpressure maneuvers, tilt training, and yoga-based interventions such as *Tadasana*—with pharmacologic therapy reserved for refractory cases. Pacemaker implantation is limited to patients with predominantly cardioinhibitory syncope with documented asystole, while cardioneuroablation has emerged as a novel option for selected refractory cases. Systematic protocols such as the HySyn VVS protocol have demonstrated long-term efficacy in preventing syncope and improving quality of life, emphasizing the importance of a holistic, patient-centered approach to management.

Keywords: Reflex vasovagal syncope, neurocardiogenic syncope, transient loss of consciousness, head-up tilt table test, VASIS classification, nonpharmacological therapy, *Tadasana*, tilt training, pacemaker therapy, cardioneuroablation.

INTRODUCTION

Reflex vasovagal syncope (VVS) or neurocardiogenic syncope is the most important cause of transient loss of consciousness (TLOC) and occurs in 30–40% of humanity during their lifetime.[1]

As per the 2017 ACC/AHA guidelines on syncope, VVS: (1) May occur with upright posture (standing or seated or with exposure to emotional stress, pain, or medical settings); (2) typically is characterized by diaphoresis, warmth, nausea, and pallor; (3) is associated with vasodepressor hypotension and/or inappropriate bradycardia; and (4) is often followed by fatigue. Typical features may be absent in older patients. VVS is often preceded by identifiable triggers and/or by a characteristic prodrome. The diagnosis is made primarily on the basis of a thorough history, physical examination, and eyewitness observation, if available.[2]

DIAGNOSIS

History

A detailed history is pivotal to the diagnosis of VVS. No diagnostic test can give an unequivocal diagnosis of VVS. Detailed narrative from a witness is vital for making a diagnosis by a trained expert.

Head-up Tilt Table Test

The head-up tilt table test (HUTT) is an important objective tool to diagnose VVS. The test entails strapping down the patient on the tilt-table and incrementally increasing the angle of tilt of the table. Heart rate and blood pressure are monitored throughout. The aim is to document changes in heart rate and blood pressure during upright tilt and to confirm whether the said changes correlate with reproduction of the patient's symptoms during the test.[3]

TABLE 1: VASIS classification.

Type 1	*Mixed*: Heart rate falls during syncope but does not fall to <40 beats/min or falls to <40 beats/min for <10 seconds. Blood pressure falls before the heart rate falls
Type 2A	*Cardioinhibition without asystole*: Heart rate falls to <40 beats/min for >10 seconds but asystole of >3 seconds does not occur. Blood pressure falls before the heart rate falls
Type 2B	*Cardioinhibition with asystole*: Asystole occurs for >3 seconds. Blood pressure fall coincides with or occurs before the heart rate fall
Type 3	*Vasodepressor*: Heart rate does not fall >10% from its peak at the time of syncope
Exception 1	*Chronotropic incompetence*: No heart rate rise during tilt testing (i.e., <10% from the pre-tilt rate)
Exception 2	*Excessive heart rate rise*: An excessive rise in heart rate both at the onset of the upright position and throughout its duration before syncope (i.e., >130 beats/min)

New Vasovagal Syncope International Study Classification

A positive HUTT result is used to classify syncope as per the Vasovagal Syncope International Study (VASIS) classification based on predominance of hypotensive or bradycardic response and sequence of events. The classification is given in **Table 1**.[4]

The VASIS classification has practical implications. The cardioinhibitory form (type 2) differs from the vasodepressor form (type 3), while the mixed form (type 1) shows both cardioinhibition and vasdepression. The fundamental principles of management are generally the same for the three groups and are based on tilt training exercises.[4] Pacemakers may be useful in the cardioinhibitory forms, especially in those with asystole, and when carotid sinus hypersensitivity may be associated. In the latter case, cardiac pacing is of proven efficacy. The role of pacing in severe cardioinhibitory forms will most likely be limited to very rare, selected cases.

MANAGEMENT OF VASOVAGAL SYNCOPE

Despite being a ubiquitous medical problem, no universally accepted protocols exist. Patients present to physicians of different specialties, resulting in nonuniform management. Patients with frequent syncope episodes may suffer from social anxiety, lack of confidence, and depression. A holistic approach to management is required for best results. In the recent times, our group has worked on evolving a systematic protocol—Hysyn to treat VVS.[5] This protocol is easy to teach and learn, time and cost-effective for patients, and most importantly proven to be effective in the long term in preventing syncopal episodes.

HySyn Vasovagal Syncope Protocol[5]

We demonstrated consistent benefits with a protocol involving patient education, diet counseling, *Tadasana*, and other measures in a structured stepwise manner. The protocol recommends two steps of care. The first step involves education, hydration, syncope avoidance methods, physiotherapy, and *Tadasana*. The second step, used in patients who remain symptomatic, involves increasing salt intake, elastic stockings, and pharmacotherapy. The protocol is elaborated in **Table 2**. The protocol has demonstrated impressive success with near complete elimination of syncope and presyncope events over a period of 3 years **(Fig. 1)**.

TABLE 2: The HySyn protocol for management of vasovagal syncope.

Step 1	Education and counseling
	Hydration
	Syncope avoidance
	Physiotherapy (conditioning program, tilt training, and physical countermeasures)
Step 2	Reinforcement of step 1
	Increase salt intake
	Elastic stockings
	Pharmacotherapy

The components of the protocol are described in detail here.

General Measures[6]

The most important component of the management of VVS is patient reassurance and education. Patient and his family should be counseled that this is benign and a common condition. It is not a life-threatening condition and does not affect the longevity of life. Though not a serious condition, the injuries associated with syncopal episodes can be life threatening. Hence, syncope avoidance maneuvers should be taught to the patient. This includes switch to a supine position when they feel a prodrome of syncope. Simple measures can improve quality of life in most patients. They should avoid triggers such as prolonged standing or suddenly standing up from sitting or lying positions.

Counter-maneuvers can be attempted during the prodrome to abort the syncope. Each of these measures has individually shown to be effective in a subset of patients. Hysyn protocol encompasses most of these in a single algorithm which is easy to practice.

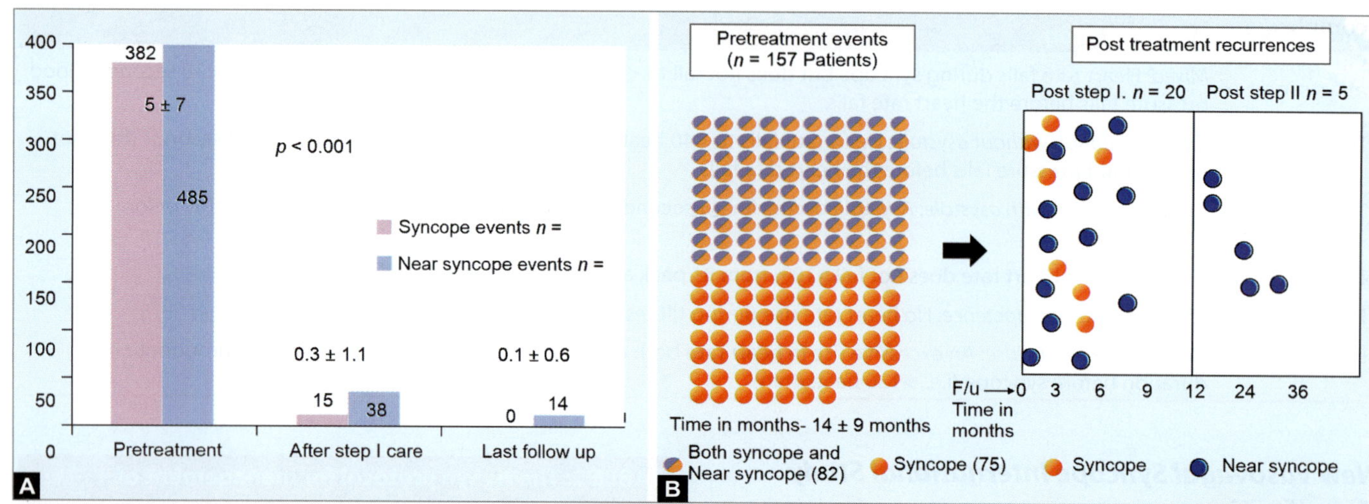

FIGS. 1A AND B: (A) Comparison of clinical outcomes (syncope and near syncope) before treatment, after step I and at final follow-up. It shows freedom from syncope at last follow-up and a marked reduction in near syncope events. (B) Illustration depicting number of patients with clinical events before and after treatment with the protocol. In a cohort of 157 patients, after 1st step, 20 had recurrences and at the end of follow-up, only 5 had near syncope events.

Source: Reproduced with permission from Rao BH, et al. (2024)[5]

Nonpharmacological Therapy

- *Fluid and salt intake:* Fluid and salt intake should be liberalized to increase blood volume and consequently venous return (ESC 2018 Class 1, AHA 2017 Class IIb). Around three liters of fluid should be consumed per day, mainly in the form of water. Salt intake should be around 8–10 g/day, preferably through food, alternatively via salt tablets. In patients with heart failure, these goals may not be achievable.[2,7,8]
- *Medication review and withdrawal:* Patients' medication should be reviewed, and possible offending medications should be withdrawn or reduced (ESC 2018 Class IIa, AHA 2017 Class IIb). Diuretics and vasodilators such as nitrates and alpha-adrenergic blockers are especially prone to precipitate reflex syncope. Regardless, all antihypertensives and several neurological and neuropsychiatric drugs can precipitate VVS and OH. Dosage reduction or switch over to alternative agents may be required.[2,7,9]
- *Compression garments:* Compression garments reduce venous pooling and increase venous return. A pressure of 20–30 mm Hg can be beneficial in reducing frequency of syncope (ESC 2018, AHA 2017 Class 1). Since abdominal venous pooling plays a major role in the pathophysiology of VVS, waist-high, pantyhose style garments are recommended. These are uncomfortable and often not tolerated. In such cases, athletic compression wear can be advised.[2,6,7]
- *Physical counterpressure maneuvers:* Physical counter-pressure maneuvers are useful in patients with prodrome to abort a syncopal episode (ESC 2018, AHA 2017 Class IIA). Following two maneuvers are commonly used. In case syncope still comes on, the patient should take a supine position (get down and stay down).[2,7]
    - *Leg crossing and lower body muscle testing* is done in standing position. The legs are crossed, and the muscles of the legs, buttocks, and abdomen are tensed.[10]
    - *Arm tensing* is done by linking one's hands in front of the body and pulling them apart.[11]
- *Tilt training:* Tilt training (ESC 2018, AHA 2017 Class IIb) is used in highly motivated patients. Patients are subjected to progressively longer duration of upright posture in order to develop advantageous physiologic regulatory mechanisms. An example is 30 minutes vertical wall stand for 6 days a week for at least 4 weeks. A simple home tilt training method is head-up sleeping.[2,7,12]

Yoga

Yoga is a mind-body therapy which encompasses a combination of *asanas* (postures), synchronous breathing (*pranayama*) and meditation. *Tadasana* involves asana and *pranayam*. It is important to consider *yogasana* as a movement-based contemplative practice or a psychospiritual practice. When one holds a posture for a certain period associated with synchronized breathing and mindful awareness, it gradually results in voluntary control of protective reflexes. These gradually correct the orthostatic imbalance by gaining control of protective neuromuscular reflexes, thus addressing the core of pathophysiology of VVS. *Asana* is not just holding a posture but holding the posture comfortably with the mind in an expansive state, focusing on infinity in a relaxed state. VVS is associated with complex neurohumoral alterations, including for instance catecholamines, adrenomedullin and vasopressin surges, alterations. Yoga is also known to beneficially reduce many of these neurohumoral effects, which may partially account for its effectiveness in VVS.

Recent studies have demonstrated the benefits of yoga for the therapy of syncope. Several studies have demonstrated the benefits of yoga on autonomic modulation by achieving a balance between the sympathetic and parasympathetic tone.[13] Gunda et al. were the first to demonstrate the benefits of yoga in reducing the incidence and severity of syncope and improving quality of life in 2015.[14] Two randomized studies from India demonstrated an impressive reduction in VVS frequency and improvement on quality of life using comprehensive yoga protocols.[13,15]

However, these studies used guided yoga sessions consisting of several *yogasanas* done daily with a daily session of 30–60 minutes. Though these may be very effective, in real-world long-term compliance is unlikely. We demonstrated in a systematic study the benefit of a single yogasana—Tadasana—in reducing VVS frequency.[16] Eight to twelve cycles of *Tadasana* were advised twice a day. Effective compliance was achieved over a period of over 2 years. The method of *Tadasana* is shown in **Figure 2**.

Pharmacological Therapy

The role of drug therapy in the treatment of VVS is limited. None of the drugs proposed have been consistent in preventing syncope. Consequently, there is no drug which has a class 1 recommendation. Drugs are only recommended in patients who are symptomatic despite nonpharmacological measures, with the caveat that they may not benefit from drugs either. The drugs used in the treatment of reflex syncope are given in **Table 3**.

Pacemaker Implantation

Implantation of dual-chamber pacemaker has been used for treatment of syncope. Pacemakers have shown benefit only in patients with predominantly cardioinhibitory syncope with asystole (VASIS classification type 2B) on HUTT. Patients with predominantly vasodepressor or a mixed response do not benefit from pacemaker implantation.

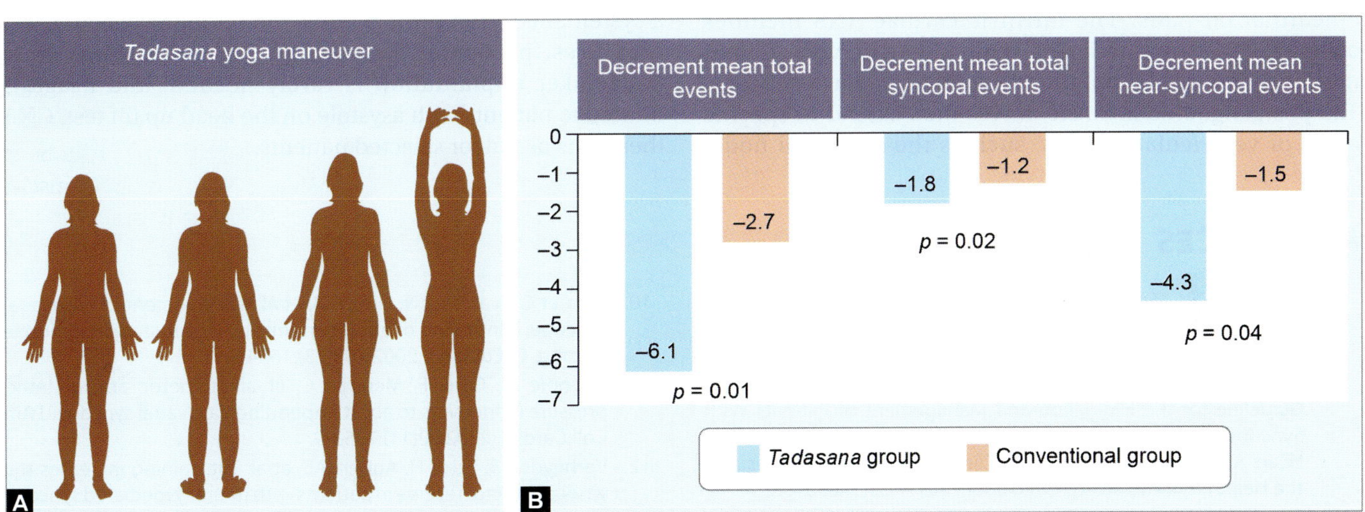

FIGS. 2A AND B: (Left) Tadasana steps. (1) Stand straight with feet together and arms by the side against wall with support. (2 and 3) Alternate dorsi flexion and plantar flexion of the ankle and foot. (4) Isometric contraction of quadriceps: Stand on toes keeping shoulders relaxed and straight; extend arms upward to keep them facing and parallel to each other. Breathe normally for 10 seconds. (Right) Comparison of decrement of total events, syncopal events, and near-syncopal events in the Tadasana and conventional groups in relation to pretreatment event burden. The Tadasana group demonstrated greater reduction in all three event categories.

Source: Reproduced with permission from Rao BH, et al. (2022)[16]

TABLE 3: Drugs used for treatment of syncope.

Drug	Class of recommendation	Indications
Midodrine	IIA	This alpha agonist is recommended in recurrent VVS with no hypertension, HF, or urinary retention
Fludrocortisone	IIB	This mineralocorticoid is used in recurrent VVS with inadequate response to salt and water. Hypokalemia can occur
Beta-blockers	IIB	Patients of 42 years or older with recurrent VVS
Selective serotonin reuptake inhibitors (SSRIs)	IIB	Fluoxetine and paroxetine have shown some benefit in small RCTs. They may be considered in recurrent VVS

The ACC/AHA/HRS 2017 guidelines recommend dual-chamber pacing as a Class IIB indication for patients with significantly symptomatic neurocardiogenic syncope associated with bradycardia documented spontaneously or at the time of tilt-table testing. However, the ESC 2018 guideline lists pacing as a Class IIA recommendation for patients over 40 years of age with spontaneous symptomatic pause >3 seconds, asymptomatic pause >6 seconds due to sinus arrest, atrioventricular block, or a combination.[17]

Cardioneuroablation Therapy

Parasympathetic hyperactivity has a central role in the mechanism of most forms of VVS. Hence, inhibition of parasympathetic activity has been proposed as a method of therapy for refractory VVS. Cardioneuroablation (CNA) is being evaluated as therapy for refractory syncope. CNA entails radiofrequency cardiac ablation of postganglionic parasympathetic neurons in the ganglionated plexi (GP) located in the epicardial fat pads and atrial walls.[18]

The cardiac ANS can be divided into the extrinsic and intrinsic components. Most of the neurons of the intrinsic cardiac ANS converge at several GP within the epicardial fat pads. The intrinsic cardiac ANS includes efferent parasympathetic and sympathetic nerves, afferent neurons, and local circuit neurons/intermediate neurons. The postganglionic intrinsic nerves then extend to specific atrial or ventricular regions, such as the sinoatrial node, atrioventricular (AV) node, and the roots of pulmonary veins. GP integrates preganglionic and postganglionic nerve fibers to affect heart rate and cardiac function. By targeting the GP with catheter ablation, CNA has emerged as a novel and effective therapy for VVS by ablating the endocardial neuromyocardial interface and GP. Since the atrial wall is around 3 mm thick, radiofrequency ablation energy can be transmitted to the epicardial fat pad by intra-atrial ablation catheter.[19]Cardioneuroablation was first proposed by Pachon et al. They used bi-atrial ablation and demonstrated significant relief from symptoms.[20] Scanacava et al. used high-frequency stimulation to locate target GP and succeeded in simplifying the procedure.[21] However, the results with this therapy have not been uniformly encouraging.[22-24]

CONCLUSION

Vasovagal syncope is a very common clinical problem faced by physicians. History from a witness is crucial to arriving at this diagnosis. It is important to avoid unnecessary investigations. VVS can be effectively managed by following a systematic Hysyn protocol involving nonpharmacological measures, particularly a specific *yogasana—Tadasana*. Pacemaker implantation is rarely needed, and usage is limited to patients with asystole on the head up tilt test. CNA therapy is useful for selected patients.

REFERENCES

1. Hamrefors V, Spahic JM, Nilsson D, et al. Syndromes of orthostatic intolerance and syncope in young adults. Open Heart. 2017;4(1):e000585.
2. Shen WK, Sheldon RS, Benditt DG, et al. 2017 ACC/AHA/HRS Guideline for the Evaluation and Management of Patients With Syncope: A Report of the American College of Cardiology/American Heart Association Task Force on Clinical Practice Guidelines and the Heart Rhythm Society. Circulation. 2017;136(5):e60-122.
3. Aponte-Becerra L, Novak P. Tilt Test: A Review. J Clin Neurophysiol. 2021;38(4):279-86.
4. Brignole M, Menozzi C, Del Rosso A, et al. New classification of haemodynamics of vasovagal syncope: beyond the VASIS classification. Analysis of the pre-syncopal phase of the tilt test without and with nitroglycerin challenge. Vasovagal Syncope International Study. Europace. 2000;2(1):66-76.
5. Rao BH, Gowlikar V, Vooturi S, et al. Management of patients with Reflex Vasovagal syncope with a protocol involving a yoga maneuver Tadasana. Int J Cardiol. 2024;412:132302.
6. Ballantyne BA, Letourneau-Shesaf S, Raj SR. Management of vasovagal syncope. Auton Neurosci. 2021;236:102904.
7. Brignole M, Moya A, de Lange FJ, et al. 2018 ESC Guidelines for the diagnosis and management of syncope. Eur Heart J. 2018;39(21):1883-948.
8. Lu CC, Diedrich A, Tung CS, et al. Water ingestion as prophylaxis against syncope. Circulation. 2003;108(21):2660-5.
9. Alsop K, Mac Mahon M. Withdrawing cardiovascular medications at a syncope clinic. Postgrad Med J. 2001;77(908):403-5.
10. Krediet CT, van Dijk N, Linzer M, et al. Management of vasovagal syncope: controlling or aborting faints by leg crossing and muscle tensing. Circulation. 2002;106(13):1684-9.
11. Brignole M, Croci F, Menozzi C, et al. Isometric arm counter-pressure maneuvers to abort impending vasovagal syncope. J Am Coll Cardiol. 2002;40(11):2053-9.
12. Verheyden B, Ector H, Aubert AE, et al. Tilt training increases the vasoconstrictor reserve in patients with neurally mediated syncope evoked by head-up tilt testing. Eur Heart J. 2008;29(12):1523-30.
13. Sharma G, Ramakumar V, Sharique M, et al. Effect of Yoga on Clinical Outcomes and Quality of Life in Patients With Vasovagal Syncope (LIVE-Yoga). JACC Clin Electrophysiol. 2022;8(2):141-9.
14. Gunda S, Kanmanthareddy A, Atkins D, et al. Role of yoga as an adjunctive therapy in patients with neurocardiogenic syncope: a pilot study. J Interv Card Electrophysiol. 2015;43(2):105-10.
15. Shenthar J, Prabhu MA, Banavalikar B, et al. Etiology and Outcomes of Syncope in Patients With Structural Heart Disease and Negative Electrophysiology Study. JACC Clin Electrophysiol. 2019;5(5):608-17.
16. Rao BH, Gowlikar V, Vooturi S, et al. "Tadasana" Yoga Maneuver for Preventing Vasovagal Syncope Recurrences: A Pilot Study. JACC Clin Electrophysiol. 2022;8(2):253-4.
17. Akella K, Olshansky B, Lakkireddy D, et al. Pacing Therapies for Vasovagal Syncope. J Atr Fibrillation. 2020;13(1):2406.
18. Garcia A, Marquez MF, Fierro EF, et al. Cardioinhibitory syncope: from pathophysiology to treatment-should we think on cardio-neuroablation? J Interv Card Electrophysiol. 2020;59(2):441-61.

19. Li L, Po S, Yao Y. Cardioneuroablation for Treating Vasovagal Syncope: Current Status and Future Directions. Arrhythm Electrophysiol Rev. 2023;12:e18.
20. Pachon JC, Pachon EI, Lobo TJ, et al. "Cardioneuroablation"--new treatment for neurocardiogenic syncope, functional AV block and sinus dysfunction using catheter RF-ablation. Europace. 2005;7(1):1-13.
21. Scanavacca M, Hachul D, Pisani C, et al. Selective vagal denervation of the sinus and atrioventricular nodes, guided by vagal reflexes induced by high frequency stimulation, to treat refractory neurally mediated syncope. J Cardiovasc Electrophysiol. 2009;20(5):558-63.
22. Aksu T, Padmanabhan D, Shenthar J, et al. The benefit of cardioneuroablation to reduce syncope recurrence in vasovagal syncope patients: a case-control study. J Interv Card Electrophysiol. 2022;63(1):77-86.
23. Piotrowski R, Baran J, Sikorska A, et al. Cardioneuroablation for Reflex Syncope: Efficacy and Effects on Autonomic Cardiac Regulation-A Prospective Randomized Trial. JACC Clin Electrophysiol. 2023;9(1):85-95.
24. Sud S, Massel D, Klein GJ, et al. The expectation effect and cardiac pacing for refractory vasovagal syncope. Am J Med. 2007;120(1):54-62.

CHAPTER

44

Role of Clonal Hematopoiesis in the Pathogenesis of Dilated Cardiomyopathy

Ganesan Manohar, Karthikaa Saminathan

ABSTRACT

The global burden of cardiovascular disease is projected to rise from 598 million (2025) to 1.14 billion (2050), including ischemic heart disease, cardiomyopathies, myocarditis, endocarditis, hypertensive heart disease, nonrheumatic valvular disorders, and peripheral arterial disease. Emerging genetic contributors such as clonal hematopoiesis of indeterminate potential (CHIP)—commonly involving DNMT3A, ASXL1, and JAK2 mutations—drive expansion of mutant myeloid cells (monocytes/macrophages) that secrete proinflammatory cytokines (IL-1β, IL-6, and TNF-α) and activate the NLRP3 inflammasome, producing chronic myocardial inflammation. Persistent immune activation promotes fibrosis and structural remodeling via TGF-β-mediated collagen deposition, leading to left ventricular dilation and dysfunction and eventual dilated cardiomyopathy (DCM). These changes increase susceptibility to arrhythmias and sudden cardiac death. Detection of clonal hematopoiesis in DCM is feasible with next-generation sequencing (NGS) and variant allele fraction (VAF) analysis to quantify clonal burden. Although causal pathways suggest therapeutic opportunities, translation remains exploratory: Candidate approaches include anti-inflammatory agents (e.g., colchicine, canakinumab), and advanced cellular or gene-editing strategies (CAR-T, BiTEs, and CRISPR–Cas9) as precision interventions. Integrating molecular detection with imaging and clinical phenotyping could refine risk stratification and guide personalized therapy **(Flowchart 1)**.

Keywords: Clonal hematopoiesis, dilated cardiomyopathy, clonal hematopoiesis of indeterminate potential, variant allele frequency, clonal hematopoiesis driver mutations, NLR family pyrin domain containing 3.

Increasing prevalence of cardiovascular disease burden from 2025 to 2050 (598 million in 2025 to 1.14 billion in 2050) (Including IHD, cardiomyopathies and myocarditis, endocarditis, HHD, nonrheumatic VHD, peripheral arterial disease)

↓

Need to explore all possible risk factors including genetic factors (Including clonal hematopoiesis)
Role of clonal hematopoiesis in DCM

↓

Clonal hematopoiesis of indeterminate potential (CHIP) (DNMT3A, ASXL1, and JAK2 mutations)

↓

Expansion of mutant myeloid cells (Monocytes, and macrophages)

↓

Proinflammatory cytokines, IL-1β, IL-6, TNF-α, NLRP3 activation

↓

Myocardial inflammation persistent immune activation | Fibrosis and remodeling (TGF-β, collagen deposition)

↓

Left ventricular dilation and dysfunction dilated cardiomyopathy

↓

Arrhythmias and sudden cardiac death

↓

- Detection of CH in DCM
- Next-generation sequencing
- VAF detection

- Potential therapies
- *Anti-inflammatory:* Colchicine, canakinumab
- *Cellular:* CAR-T, BiTEs, CRISPR-Cas9
- Precision medicine strategies

Future research directions:
- Clonal expansion dynamics
- Mutation-specific risks
- CH as biomarker for risk stratification

FLOWCHART 1: Central illustration showing the role of clonal hematopoiesis in the pathogenesis of DCM.

INTRODUCTION

The global crude prevalence of cardiovascular disease (CVD) is projected to increase from 598 million in 2025 to 1.14 billion in 2050, representing a 3.6% annual rise.[1] The Southeast Asia, East Asia, and Oceania super-region are forecasted to have the largest number of CVD cases, estimated to reach 407 million by 2050.[1] The multifactorial and heterogeneous nature of CVDs—shaped by cultural, genetic, socioeconomic, and other region-specific determinants—poses significant challenges to implementing universal strategies for managing the global burden of CVDs. Hence, it has become the need of the hour to explore all possible risk factors including the genetic determinants and develop targeted therapies for better outcomes.

OVERVIEW OF CLONAL HEMATOPOIESIS AND SOMATIC MUTATIONS

Cells throughout the body accumulate mutations over time as an organism ages, resulting in somatic mosaicism.[2] Clonal hematopoiesis (CH) is the clonal expansion of blood cells originating from hematopoietic stem or progenitor cells that have undergone somatic mutation in some driver genes. The mutations are responsible for a selective growth advantage that leads to a large proportion of blood cells carrying the same genetic alterations. CH is usually seen in the aging population and is linked with a higher risk of hematological malignancies and other chronic illness, such as CVD and heart failure. The condition when identified without overt hematological malignancy is referred to as clonal hematopoiesis of indeterminate potential (CHIP).

POPULATION GENETICS AND CLONAL HEMATOPOIESIS IN DILATED CARDIOMYOPATHY COHORTS

Dilated cardiomyopathy (DCM) is a primary myocardial disorder that may result from various genetic or acquired causes. Population-based studies indicate that CH is prevalent in DCM cohorts, especially in the older population. Importantly, the occurrence of CH driver mutations predicts worse clinical outcomes independently from traditional risk factors or the germline genetic background of DCM patients. Increased prevalence of CH in population studies confirms the magnitude of risk modification CH plays in cohorts with differing risk profiles.

Myocardial inflammation from CH may be a key trigger for DCM development in susceptible hearts (e.g., in presence of genetic variants, environmental triggers, and comorbidities).[3] Broad immunosuppressive therapy may have effects in DCM patients with increased myocardial inflammation, although there are currently limited targeted immunomodulation strategies. Due to the association between CH and inflammation, CH could serve as both a marker and a potential target for immunomodulatory treatment in individuals with DCM. Thus, we shall explore the role of CH in the pathogenesis of DCM.

VARIANT ALLELE FREQUENCY AND CLONAL BURDEN AS GENETIC RISK MODIFIERS

Variant allele frequency (VAF) quantifies the percentage of blood cells that contain a somatic mutation and is a surrogate measure of clonal burden. Higher levels of VAF (≥2%) can be associated with increased risk of adverse cardiovascular outcomes, including increased mortality.[20] VAF serves as a modifier of genetic risk, with low-grade CH possible, especially in old age or if found along with a higher clonal burden of a somatic mutation, and thereby increasing the risk of progressive cardiac dysfunction.

CLONAL HEMATOPOIESIS OF INDETERMINATE POTENTIAL AND CARDIOVASCULAR DISEASE

Clonal hematopoiesis of indeterminate potential refers to clonal hematopoiesis driver mutations (CHDMs) in at least 4% of circulating unnucleated blood cells. The size of the clone can be measured by the VAF (VAF in blood of ≥2% is considered significant).[4,5] Risk factors of CHDMs are aging, smoking, and chemotherapy.

The accumulation of CHIP-associated somatic mutations increases with age and has been linked to a higher risk of coronary heart disease.[22] CHDMs mainly occur in genes for epigenetic enzymes (e.g., DNMT3A, TET2, and ASXL1); spliceosome components (e.g., SRSF2 and SF3B1); signaling proteins (e.g., JAK2), or members of the DNA damage response (DDR) (e.g., PPM1D and TP53).[5] By the age of 70 years, 20–50% of persons harbor a CH clone, frequently found by sequencing blood DNA.[15]

GENETIC MECHANISMS LINKING CLONAL HEMATOPOIESIS TO INFLAMMATION AND DILATED CARDIOMYOPATHY

Although it is still uncertain whether inflammation is the cause or a result of the disease, certain immunosuppressive therapies have shown benefits for selected patients with chronic DCM.[12,13] Furthermore, there is cumulative evidence that CH driver mutations induce inflammation.

The build-up of somatic mutations in CH driver genes may lead to a proinflammatory environment, increased levels of cytokines (e.g., IL-1β and IL-6), and NLRP3 inflammasome activation in immune cells, which together promote myocardial injury and remodeling in individuals with DCM. The presence of dysfunctional macrophages and state of chronic inflammation leads to cardiac systolic dysfunction, fibrosis, and eventual adverse outcomes in individuals with DCM in a mutation-specific manner (with specific ASXL1 mutations). ASXL1 mutations were specifically reported to impact the severity of cardiac dysfunction (e.g., greater degree of ventricular dilation, lower EF) in DCM models, acting as a unique exacerbate to cardiac dysfunction in DCM.

Patients with DNMT3A-mediated CH showed an increased TH17/Treg ratio. Individuals with TET-2-mediated CH demonstrated elevated levels of circulating monocytes and increased serum concentrations of IL-1β and IL-6 (TOPMed cohort).[17] TET-2 deficient immune cells were associated with aggravated heart failure phenotypes through elevated IL-1β signaling. As a result, inhibitors targeting IL-1β and IL-6 signaling pathways may potentially lower cardiovascular risk in patients with DNMT3A or TET-2-mediated CH.

INTERACTION BETWEEN CLONAL HEMATOPOIESIS SOMATIC MUTATIONS AND GERMLINE DILATED CARDIOMYOPATHY MUTATIONS

In recent studies, myocyte CH mutations were shown to combine with germline mutations in cardiomyopathy-associated genes, affecting both prognosis and the severity of the disease. The negative effect of ASXL1-driven CH can be even more pronounced in patients with germline truncating TTN mutations, leading to greater myocardial fibrosis and functional impairment.

Thus, CH promotes cardiovascular inflammation, influencing the progression of atherosclerosis and ischemic heart failure. Notably, it has been demonstrated to have prognostic significance in nonischemic DCM, regardless of clone size. CHIP is linked to a twofold increase in the risk of cardiac mortality among patients with nonischemic DCM over a 10-year follow-up period.[11]

Cardiac fibrosis is a recognized risk factor for malignant ventricular arrhythmias and sudden cardiac death in individuals with DCM. Intracardiac inflammation can diminish cardiac function and promote fibrosis, even in the absence of overt atherosclerotic disease.

Recent research has shown that monocytes from heart failure patients with DNMT3A mutations can stimulate the release of heparin-binding epidermal growth factor-like growth factor, leading to activation of cardiac fibroblasts and subsequent cardiac fibrosis. Furthermore, in a murine HFpEF model, Tet2-mediated CH was linked to increased cardiac fibrosis.[10] The presence of large CH clones in patients correlated with increased myocardial fibrosis as detected by cardiac magnetic resonance imaging.[19] These findings suggest that CH may contribute to cardiac fibrosis independently of its association with inflammation. However, there are currently no studies specifically examining the relationship between CH and cardiac fibrosis in DCM patients.

SECOND HIT HYPOTHESIS IN DILATED CARDIOMYOPATHY[3]

The precise role of CH in DCM pathogenesis is unclear, with current studies showing only associative correlation. The presence of large clones at a younger age in DCM patients may indicate a direct role for CH, though DCM triggers such as chemotherapy and inflammation could also drive CH mutations. While these links are indirect, they help shape future research directions.

ASSOCIATION BETWEEN CLONAL HEMATOPOIESIS AND HEART FAILURE

CHIP increases heart failure risk by 25% and doubles the likelihood of worse clinical outcomes in carriers compared to noncarriers.[6,7] These results indicate that CHIP mutations are adversely related to cardiomyopathy progression.

The largest and longest follow-up study found that CH is significantly linked to incident HF, primarily because of ASXL1, TET2, and JAK2 mutations, regardless of age.[6] Two population studies found TET2 mutations linked to new cases of HFpEF, but not HFrEF.[8,9] Overall, CH is primarily associated with HFpEF incidence due to TET2 mutations, and this effect may be modified by age.

The study by Dorsheimer et al.[16] showed that chronic heart failure patients with TET2- or DNMT3A-mediated CH exhibit a worse prognosis.

A study examined whether CH could serve as a predictor of mortality in patients with cardiogenic shock, involving 686 participants, 65% of whom had nonischemic cardiomyopathy. The prevalence of CH mutations was higher among patients with cardiogenic shock compared to ambulatory heart failure patients, and this correlated with reduced survival too.[14]

ARRHYTHMIAS AND CLONAL HEMATOPOIESIS

Clonal hematopoiesis is independently associated with supraventricular arrhythmias, bradyarrhythmias, and ventricular arrhythmias, irrespective of heart failure or coronary artery disease status. In a study by Schuermans et al., the elevated risk was predominantly observed among individuals harboring TET2, ASXL1, PPM1D, or TP53 mutations.[19] Arrhythmias, including atrial fibrillation (AF), are frequently observed in patients with DCM, and may also contribute to its pathogenesis, as seen in cases such as tachycardiomyopathy.

Recent studies indicate that CHIP may be involved in the development and progression of AF.[19] Mechanistic research has shown that mutations in genes such as TET2 and DNMT3A result in increased production of proinflammatory cytokines, including interleukin-1 (IL-1) and IL-6. These cytokines are linked to atrial remodeling and fibrosis, altered calcium signaling, and contribute to the formation of a substrate that can promote arrhythmias. CHIP is also associated with oxidative stress and endothelial dysfunction, which appear to increase the vulnerability of atrial tissue to arrhythmogenesis. Additionally, CHIP has been connected to hypercoagulability, potentially raising the risk of thromboembolic events in AF, such as ischemic stroke and systemic embolism. CH driver mutations have been correlated with a more progressive form of AF, marked by longer duration of AF episodes, increased atrial volume, higher E/E′ values, and unfavorable clinical outcomes, including heart failure, ischemic stroke, and mortality.[21] Collectively, CH appears to influence the trajectory of arrhythmias and may contribute to the development of heart failure. The relationship among arrhythmias, DCM, and CH in disease progression presents an intriguing area for further research, which has yet to be explored.

THERAPY-RELATED CLONAL HEMATOPOIESIS AND CARDIOMYOPATHY

Therapy-related clonal hematopoiesis (t-CH) represents an aggressive subtype of CH that arises in individuals who have received oncological therapies.[23] t-CH is commonly linked with genes involved in the DDR, such as TP53 and PPM1D, which are associated with cellular resistance to genotoxic stress. Research suggests that TP53 and PPM1D mutant HSPCs pre-exist initially as small clones and may undergo rapid clonal expansion following cytotoxic therapy, likely due to a survival advantage under genotoxic stress provided by these mutations upon the stem cells. Such cytotoxic therapies (including anthracyclines) can give rise to cardiomyopathy.

While cytotoxic agents can directly damage the heart by acting on cells of the myocardium, it has been proposed that the cardiac toxicity associated with long latency periods could be due in part to the effects of t-CH that develops in this patient population.

Recent studies have shown that Trp53 and Ppm1d driver genes can contribute to HF and/or atherosclerotic CVD. The study by Sano et al. provides evidence to suggest that t-CH may be associated with cardiac toxicity in cancer patients treated with anthracyclines, potentially through increased infiltration and activation of neutrophils. While these experimental findings indicate a potential role for t-CH in the development of DCM among cancer survivors, there is currently a lack of robust clinical evidence to confirm this association. Addressing this gap may be possible by investigating the links between CH and cardiovascular outcomes in populations of cancer survivors. If future studies validate these observations, it would suggest that t-CH could serve as a predictive biomarker for DCM in this group, and that these patients might experience greater therapeutic benefits from anti-inflammatory treatments.

GENOMIC TECHNOLOGIES FOR DETECTING CLONAL HEMATOPOIESIS MUTATIONS IN DILATED CARDIOMYOPATHY PATIENTS

Identifying CH driver mutations in DCM patients uses next-generation sequencing methods, i.e., whole exome sequencing or deep-targeted sequencing to identify somatic variants at lower VAFs (<2%). Reverse calling methods and trinucleotide profiling help with identifying mutations that arise from the spontaneous process of normal hematopoietic stem cell (HSC) divisions. Sensitive sequencing is important for identifying CHIP and quantifying clonal burden.

POTENTIAL IMMUNOMODULATORY TREATMENT TARGETS IN FUTURE

Given the pivotal role of inflammation in the progression of CHIP-driven heart failure, immunomodulatory therapies represent a promising targeted management strategy.

Targeting the NLRP3 inflammasome, an essential element in the inflammatory pathway is particularly relevant, as it is activated in CHIP-associated heart failure.

Colchicine, a medication primarily prescribed for gout, exerts inhibitory effects on the inflammasome and has demonstrated efficacy in reducing cardiovascular events among patients with atherosclerosis; this suggests potential benefits for individuals with CHIP-driven heart failure as well.

An ongoing phase II study is currently evaluating the effects of colchicine in patients with CH and ischemic heart failure with reduced ejection fraction (HFrEF) (2021-001508-13, European Union Clinical Trials Register). Colchicine is a broad-spectrum anti-inflammatory agent that inhibits microtubule polymerization and partially inhibits the NLRP3-inflammasome, which may be dose-dependent. The primary endpoint of this study is endothelial function measured by flow-mediated dilation after 60 days of treatment; however, this outcome is not specifically relevant for patients with DCM. At present, there are no studies or trials examining CH-guided immunomodulatory therapy for individuals with DCM.

Targeting Cytokines

Canakinumab, an IL-1β neutralizing antibody, has demonstrated efficacy in decreasing cardiovascular events and heart failure-related hospitalizations among patients with a history of myocardial infarction and elevated C-reactive protein levels, particularly in individuals exhibiting TET2 CH of indeterminate potential (CHIP).[18]

CAR T-cell Therapy

Selective elimination of mutated blood cells represents an additional therapeutic strategy. Accurate identification of cell surface antigens unique to CH cells is essential for this approach. One promising method is chimeric antigen receptor T-cell therapy, which involves engineering a patient's T-cells to target and eradicate CH cells that display specific antigens.

Another method involves bispecific T-cell engagers, which are engineered proteins capable of binding both a T-cell and a target cell at the same time. These T-cell engagers facilitate the proximity of T-cells and CH cells, resulting in the subsequent elimination of CH cells.

A more invasive option in severe cases is gene editing using CRISPR–Cas9 to address mutations in HSCs responsible for CH. This process entails collecting HSCs from the patient, performing mutation correction ex vivo, and then reinfusing the modified cells into the patient. This technique presents significant challenges but may offer therapeutic benefits for patients with HF.

Precision Medicine Strategies

Genetic testing for a patient's CHIP status can help tailor effective and personalized anti-inflammatory treatments and predict drug responses. Genetically informed therapies may one day be individualized toward mutation-specific risk, and a strategy targeting germline and somatic pathogenic variants may improve heart failure outcomes for DCM patients.

PROMISING AVENUES FOR RESEARCH IN CLONAL HEMATOPOIESIS

Understanding the Dynamics of Clonal Hematopoiesis

Advanced DNA sequencing techniques indicate that nearly all middle-aged individuals possess blood cells with CH-related mutations at very low frequencies. Determining the factors that influence whether a mutant HSC remains quiescent and indolent or progresses to form a significant clonal population holds considerable clinical relevance. Applying whole genome sequencing method to a large sequencing dataset led to the identification of inherited genetic variance in the *TCL1A* gene as an important modulator of the fitness advantage of several commonly mutated driver genes in CH. The data available to date lead to two major conclusions. Firstly, the expansion rates of mutant hematopoietic clones differ significantly, depending on the specific driver gene involved. Although further investigation is warranted, current evidence indicates that mutations in epigenetic regulatory genes tend to expand at a slower pace compared to those affecting splicing regulators or genes associated with the DDR pathway. Secondly, even when examining identical mutated genes or hotspot mutations, considerable variability in clone expansion rates exists among individuals. This observation suggests that the dynamics of CH are strongly influenced by nonmutational factors, which remain to be elucidated.

CONCLUSION

Clonal hematopoiesis may arise as a result of various etiologies of DCM, such as chemotherapy, but may also initiate mechanisms that contribute to the onset and progression of DCM, including inflammation and AF. The tissue inflammation associated with CH represents a potential therapeutic target. Future research should systematically assess the role of CH in DCM, clearly delineate the DNA sequencing methodologies employed, ensure rigorous phenotyping of study cohorts, and apply robust statistical analyses. Such measures are essential for facilitating effective comparisons across studies and for developing clinical trials investigating CH-based treatment stratification **(Table 1)**.

TABLE 1: Key studies linking *CHIP* genes and dilated cardiomyopathy.

Study (Year)	Sikking et al., JACC: Heart Failure (2024)	Inoue et al., JACC: Basic to Translational Science (2024)	Wu et al., ESC Heart Failure (2022)
Country/Center	Netherlands (Maastricht University Medical Center)	Japan (Multicenter University Hospitals)	Germany (University Hospital Jena)
Design	Prospective observational cohort	Observational cohort with genomic profiling	Prospective cohort (DCM and ICM analyzed separately)
Population	Dilated cardiomyopathy (DCM)	Nonischemic DCM on guideline-directed therapy	DCM ($n = 52$) and ischemic cardiomyopathy (ICM, $n = 48$)
N (participants)	520	198	100
CHIP prevalence (n, %)	109 (21%) overall; 45 (9%) with VAF ≥ 2%	22 (11%) with CHIP driver mutations	DCM: 10/52 (19%); ICM: 6/48 (13%)
Sequencing method	Ultradeep smMIP-based targeted sequencing of CHIP driver genes (high sensitivity, ~0.01% VAF detection)	Whole exome + deep targeted sequencing (germline cardiomyopathy genes and CHIP drivers)	NGS panel of 54 CHIP-associated genes

Continued

Continued

Study (Year)	Sikking et al., JACC: Heart Failure (2024)	Inoue et al., JACC: Basic to Translational Science (2024)	Wu et al., ESC Heart Failure (2022)
VAF thresholds used	Data-driven: 0.36% (cardiac death), 0.06% (all-cause mortality)	Not specified in abstract; deep sequencing and standard CHIP calling applied	Standard CHIP definition applied; study reports clone sizes, not single-fixed threshold in abstract
Dominant *CHIP* genes	DNMT3A, TET2 (others possible; panel of CH drivers)	DNMT3A most frequent (others present)	DNMT3A, followed by TET2 and CUX1
Primary endpoint(s)	Cardiac death; all-cause mortality	Left ventricular reverse remodeling (LVRR) over ~1 year	Composite of all-cause death or all-cause hospitalization
Primary endpoint(s)	Cardiac death HR 2.33 (95% CI 1.24–4.40); all-cause mortality HR 1.72 (95% CI: 1.10–2.69)	LVRR less frequent in CHIP carriers vs. noncarriers (22.7% vs. 47.2%; $p = 0.023$). CHIP independently predicted lower odds of LVRR in multivariable models	Trend toward worse outcome in DCM carriers of DNMT3A/TET2, but not statistically significant over median 3.1 years
Follow-up duration	Median 6.5 years (IQR 4.7–9.7)	≈1 year for remodeling assessment	Median 3.1 years
Key adjustments	Adjusted for age and established DCM prognostic factors (per study)	Adjusted for known prognostic variables and germline cardiomyopathy variants	Cox proportional hazards models; details in full text
Notes	Risk elevated independent of age and clone size; very low VAFs still prognostic with data-driven cutoffs	Also included mouse experiments showing CHIP worsens systolic dysfunction/fibrosis under DCM stressors	Suggested age-independent occurrence of CHIP in DCM (mutations even <45 years); recommended larger cohorts
Citation (PMID/DOI)	PMID: 37747588; DOI:10.1016/j.jchf.2023.06.037	PMID: 39297129; DOI:10.1016/j.jacbts.2024.04.010	PMID: 35979940; PMCID: PMC9773636; DOI:10.1002/ehf2.14115

REFERENCES

1. Chong B, Jayabaskaran J, Jauhari SM, et al. Global burden of cardiovascular diseases: projections from 2025 to 2050. Eur J Prev Cardiol. 2024:zwae281.
2. Verdonschot JAJ, Fuster JJ, Walsh K, et al. The emerging role of clonal haematopoiesis in the pathogenesis of dilated cardiomyopathy. Eur Heart J. 2024;45(45):4797-807.
3. Sikking MA, Verdonschot JAJ. How Clonal Hematopoiesis Can Predict Treatment Response in Patients with Dilated Cardiomyopathy. JACC Basic Transl Sci. 2024;9(8):968-70.
4. Sikking MA, Stroeks SLVM, Henkens MTHM, et al. Clonal Hematopoiesis has Prognostic Value in Dilated Cardiomyopathy Independent of Age and Clone Size. JACC Heart Fail. 2024;12(5):905-14.
5. Schuermans A, Honigberg MC, Raffield LM, et al. Clonal hematopoiesis and incident heart failure with preserved ejection fraction. JAMA Netw Open. 2024;7:e2353244.
6. Reiner AP, Roberts MB, Honigberg MC, et al. Association of Clonal Hematopoiesis of Indeterminate Potential with Incident Heart Failure with Preserved Ejection Fraction. medRxiv [Preprint]. 2023.
7. Chimenti C, Russo MA, Frustaci A. Immunosuppressive therapy in virus-negative inflammatory cardiomyopathy: 20-year follow-up of the TIMIC trial. Eur Heart. J 2022;43:3463-73.
8. Scolari FL, Brahmbhatt DH, Abelson S, et al. Clonal hematopoiesis confers an increased mortality risk in orthotopic heart transplant recipients. Am J Transplant. 2022;22:3078-86.
9. Yura Y, Cochran JD, Walsh K. Therapy-related clonal hematopoiesis: a new link between cancer and cardiovascular disease. Heart Fail Clin. 2022;18:349-59.
10. Shumliakivska M, Luxán G, Hemmerling I, et al. DNMT3A clonal hematopoiesis-driver mutations induce cardiac fibrosis by paracrine activation of fibroblasts. Nat Commun. 2024; 15:606.
11. Wu JMF, Bekfani T, Hinze A, et al. Clonal haematopoiesis of indeterminate potential-related mutations and outcome in dilated and ischaemic cardiomyopathy. ESC Heart Fail. 2022;9: 3954-60.
12. Ahn HJ, An HY, Ryu G, et al. Clonal Haematopoiesis of Indeterminate Potential and Atrial Fibrillation: An East Asian Cohort Study. Eur Heart J. 2024;45:778-90.
13. Lin AE, Bapat AC, Xiao L, et al. Clonal Hematopoiesis of Indeterminate Potential with Loss of Tet2 Enhances Risk for Atrial Fibrillation Through Nlrp3 Inflammasome Activation. Circulation. 2024;149:1419-34.
14. Guillotin F, Mercier É, Fortier M, et al. Clonal Haematopoiesis of Indeterminate Potential in Patients with Venous Thromboembolism. J Thromb Thrombolysis. 2023;56:351-4.
15. Zon RL, Sekar A, Clapham K, et al. JAK2-Mutant Clonal Hematopoiesis Is Associated with Venous Thromboembolism. Blood. 2024;144:2149-54.

16. Liu Q, Smedby KE, Xue H, et al. Clonal Hematopoiesis of Indeterminate Potential and the Risk of Pulmonary Embolism: An Observational Study. EClinicalMedicine. 2024;74:102753.
17. Deftereos SG, Beerkens FJ, Shah B, et al. Colchicine in cardiovascular disease. In-depth review. Circulation. 2022;145:61-78.
18. Svensson EC, Madar A, Campbell CD, et al. TET2-driven clonal hematopoiesis and response to canakinumab: an exploratory analysis of the CANTOS randomized clinical trial. JAMA Cardiol. 2022;7:521-8.
19. Weinstock JS, Gopakumar J, Burugula BB, et al. Aberrant activation of TCL1A promotes stem cell expansion in clonal haematopoiesis. Nature. 2023;616:755-63.
20. Robertson NA, Latorre-Crespo E, Terradas-Terradas M, et al. Longitudinal dynamics of clonal hematopoiesis identifies gene-specific fitness effects. Nat Med. 2022;28:1439-46.
21. Fabre MA, de Almeida JG, Fiorillo E, et al. The longitudinal dynamics and natural history of clonal haematopoiesis. Nature. 2022;606:335-42.
22. van Zeventer IA, de Graaf AO, Salzbrunn JB, et al. Evolutionary landscape of clonal hematopoiesis in 3,359 individuals from the general population. Cancer Cell. 2023;41:1017-31.e4.
23. Uslu U, June CH. CAR T-cell therapy meets clonal hematopoiesis. Blood Cancer Discov. 2022;3:382-4.

CHAPTER

45

Dilated Cardiomyopathy in Systemic Immune-mediated Diseases

Ganesh Seth, Mahima Saran, Himanshu Gupta

ABSTRACT

Systemic immune-mediated diseases (SIDs), including autoimmune and autoinflammatory disorders, frequently affect the cardiovascular system, particularly the myocardium. Manifestations range from subclinical dysfunction to myocarditis, dilated cardiomyopathy, arrhythmias, and sudden cardiac death. Commonly implicated conditions include systemic lupus erythematosus, systemic sclerosis, rheumatoid arthritis, sarcoidosis, and granulomatosis with polyangiitis. Diagnosis relies on multimodal tools such as electrocardiography, echocardiography, biomarkers, cardiac MRI, PET, and, in select cases, endomyocardial biopsy. Management integrates immunosuppressive therapy for the underlying disease with guideline-directed therapy for cardiomyopathy. Early recognition and individualized strategies are critical, as myocardial involvement significantly worsens prognosis in SIDs.

Keywords: Systemic immune-mediated diseases, myocardial involvement, dilated cardiomyopathy, myocarditis, cardiac MRI.

INTRODUCTION

Systemic immune-mediated diseases (SIDs) are a group of disorders that include both autoimmune and autoinflammatory diseases that affect at least two organ systems.[1]

Autoinflammatory diseases are a group of conditions characterized by unprovoked inflammation caused by a primary innate immune system dysfunction. Autoimmune diseases are characterized by immune cell responses against self-antigens in genetically susceptible individuals. However, both may coexist in same individual, so it should be considered as a continuum. The relationship between SIDs and cardiovascular system has been established since long. It can involve all components of cardiovascular system including vessels (large, medium, and small) as well as heart.

Cardiac involvement in SIDs are not uncommon and are associated with poor outcomes.[2] Even in heart, SIDs can involve pericardium, myocardium as well as endocardium. At present, the diagnosis of cardiac involvement in SIDs is made very less often because of the absence of any standardized workup protocol that is probably due to variable degree of cardiac involvement in specific SID, late presentation, and also availability of scientific knowledge. Although SIDs can involve all component of heart structure, but this chapter will focus mainly on the involvement of myocardium. Myocardial involvement can present as (1) myocarditis which mainly presents as dilated cardiomyopathy and (2) endomyocarditis.

Common SIDs that can present with cardiac involvement are systemic lupus erythematosus (SLE), systemic sclerosis (SSc), rheumatoid arthritis (RA), polymyositis, dermatomyositis, eosinophilic granulomatosis (formerly Churg–Strauss syndrome), sarcoidosis, Sjögren's syndrome, spondyloarthropathies, and many others.

Dilated cardiomyopathy is the common cardiac phenotype, which is commonly observed in patients with SIDs, which is characterized by left ventricular or biventricular systolic dysfunction even in asymptomatic patients.[3] Even among patients with the same SID, the degree of cardiac involvement can vary significantly. Therefore, a disease-specific approach, rather than an involvement-specific one, is recommended for cardiac assessment.

CLINICAL FEATURE INDICATING MYOCARDIAL INVOLVEMENT

Sign and symptoms of myocardial involvement ranges from asymptomatic to life-threatening arrhythmias, sudden cardiac death, and cardiogenic shock. High-risk features can be unexplained breathlessness, chest pain with troponin rise, rhythm abnormalities, syncope, heart failure, aborted SCD, and shock.[4] Increased incidence of coronary artery diseases is also present in systemic inflammatory diseases and should be ruled out before making the diagnosis of myocarditis and LV dysfunction.[5,6]

DIAGNOSTIC TOOLS FOR ASSESSMENT OF CARDIAC INVOLVEMENT

Multiple diagnostic tests can be helpful in assessing degree and severity of myocardial involvement starting from noninvasive electrocardiogram to invasive endomyocardial biopsy (EMB).

- *ECG:* ECG abnormalities can be nonspecific including mild ST-T changes. It can also detect arrhythmias. Sometimes Holter can be helpful in patients presenting with sudden onset palpitation and/or syncope.
- *2D echocardiography*: It plays a crucial role in diagnosing dilated cardiomyopathy suggested by left atrial enlargement, left ventricular dilation, and sometimes right ventricular involvement.[7-9] Sometimes strain imaging can also be helpful in early stages. Doppler analysis can also detect valvular involvement in the form of regurgitation. Pericardial effusion can also be seen in many SIDs, especially in acute phase.
- *Biomarkers*: Rise in troponins as well as NT-ProBNP can be observed in many patients of SIDs. Biomarker levels also correlates with the severity of myocardial involvement; however, coronary artery disease should be ruled out in case of raised troponin.
- *Other disease specific biomarkers*: Many disease-specific biomarkers are available for underlying SIDs,[10,11] but it is unclear whether they can be considered as biomarker for myocardial involvement or not.
- *Cardiac MRI (CMR)*: It can be helpful in diagnosing cardiac involvement in many SIDs. It can also be helpful in tissue characterization and accessing the degree of involvement, valvular abnormalities as well as assessment of pericardial involvement. CMR can detect all three main pathophysiologic components of myocarditis, i.e., myocardial edema by T2-weighted imaging, regional hyperemia, and capillary leak by early gadolinium enhancement ratio, and myocardial necrosis or fibrosis by LGE imaging.[12] Several studies have suggested LGE pattern to be a strong prognostic marker,[13] and monitoring of LGE changes may identify a higher risk cohort than captured by serum troponins or inflammatory biomarkers.[14] The characteristic pattern of LGE in CMR (subepicardial or mid-myocardial or subendocardial) also helps in diagnosing particular SID;[15] at the same time, it also helps in ruling out coronary artery disease and has been shown to correlate with disease activity in RA, and in SSc.
- *Cardiac CT*: Especially useful in evaluating vascular involvement like large vessels as well as coronary artery disease. CT can also be useful in pericardial disease assessment.
- *Positron emission tomography (PET)*: It is very useful, especially in acute phase to detect inflammation such as in sarcoidosis.[16]
- *Endomyocardial biopsy*: It is the gold standard for suspected myocarditis with or without associated SID. It can detect inflammatory infiltrate of the myocardium with necrosis and/or degeneration of adjacent myocytes not typical of the ischemic damage associated with coronary artery disease.[17] With the application of immunological and histochemical staining techniques specific SIDs can also be identified **(Figs. 1A to D)**.[18-20]

SYSTEMIC LUPUS ERYTHEMATOSUS

Systemic lupus erythematosus is a systemic autoimmune disease that predominantly affects females with a ratio of 9:1 and affects all racial groups but more commonly those of Afro-Caribbean, Asian, and Chinese population. Cardiac involvement in SLE is common (more than 50% of the patients and may affect any heart structure.[21] Cardiac manifestations of SLE include pericarditis, myocarditis, endocarditis, aortitis, and coronary arteritis. Myocarditis can be present in up to 8–10% of SLE and most commonly is subclinical. SLE myocarditis may be associated with mutations in the gene encoding the 3’-5’ DNA exonuclease TREX1.[22] Symptoms of SLE myocarditis can be low-grade fever, unexplained dyspnea, and palpitation to severe heart failure. Increased levels of ESR, CRP, anti-ds DNA antibodies, troponin, and NT proBNP can occur and correlates with severity of involvement. Dilated cardiomyopathy is the most serious form of organ involvement in SLE carrying very high mortality.

The ECG typically shows nonspecific findings such as sinus tachycardia, ST or T-wave changes. Supraventricular or ventricular tachycardias may also occur. Echocardiography aids in assessment. Functional abnormalities may include segmental, regional, or global wall motion abnormalities; chamber dilation; and a reduced ejection fraction. CMR can be helpful in early diagnosis of myocardial involvement suggested by inflammation and fibrosis at the same time. It can also detect coronary artery disease.

Treatment of SLE myocarditis includes high-dose IV methylprednisolone followed by oral steroid along with other immunosuppressive drugs such as azathioprine, cyclophosphamide, or intravenous immunoglobulin (IVIg).[23]

SYSTEMIC SCLEROSIS

Cardiac abnormalities in SSc are mostly secondary to involvement of other organ systems like pulmonary (vascular or interstitial) disease[24] or kidney disease but sometimes primary cardiac involvement can occur and mostly in patients who have skeletal muscle myositis. Left ventricular systolic dysfunction is typical finding in SSc.[25] Left ventricular diastolic abnormality is also common. Right ventricular can also be involved along with left ventricle. Pulmonary

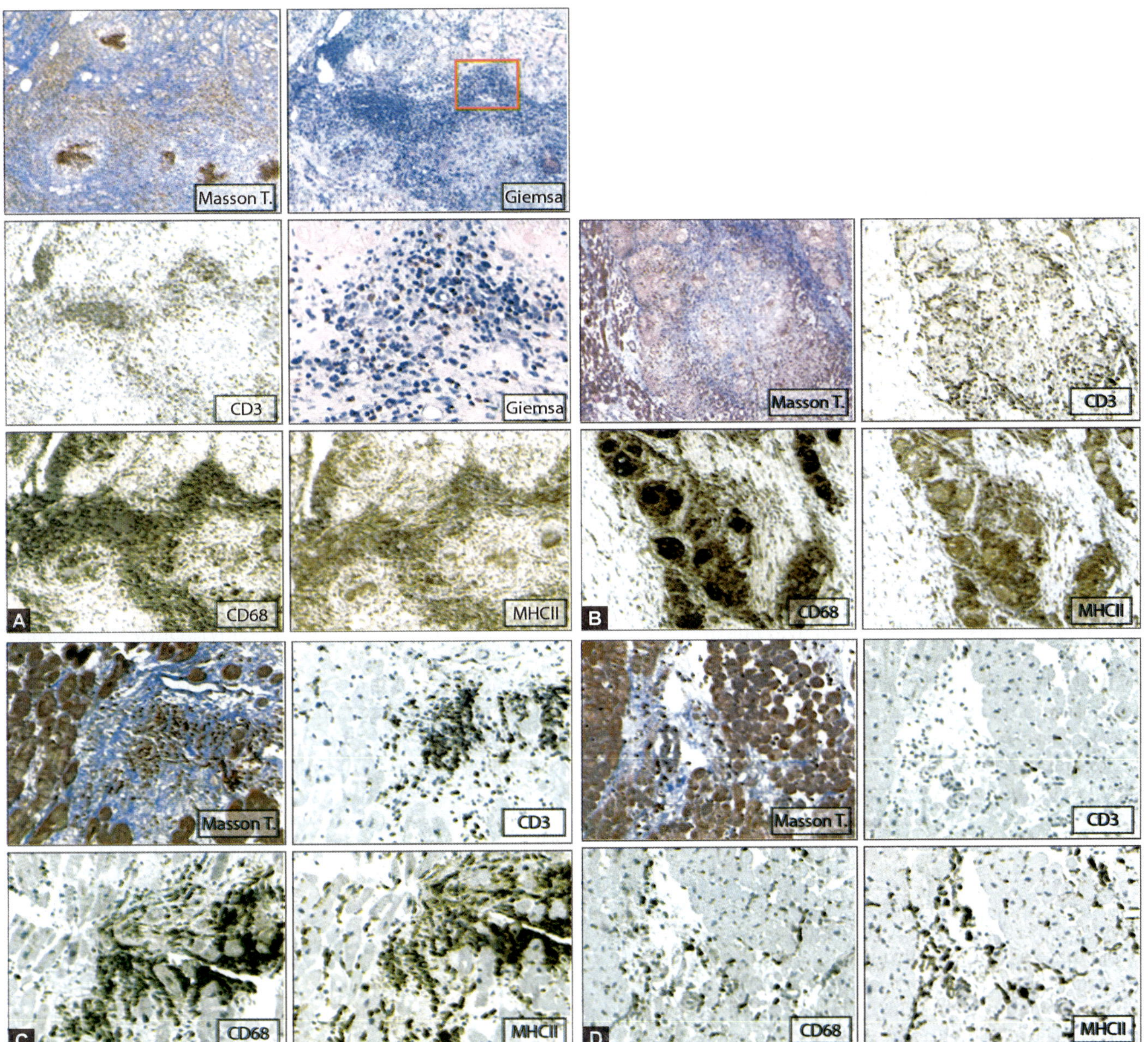

FIGS. 1A TO D: Endomyocardial biopsy examples of myocarditis in systemic immune-mediated diseases (SIDs). (A) Eosinophilic granulomatosis with polyangiitis, (B) Sarcoidosis, (C) Rheumatoid arthritis, and (D) Systemic sclerosis.

hypertension should be carefully evaluated. ECG abnormality can be present in up to 50% patients, and most common abnormality is the presence of left bundle branch block (LBBB).[26] SSc myocarditis can present as supraventricular and/or ventricular arrhythmias and can be a cause of sudden death in 5% of SSc patients.[27] Treatment of SSc myocarditis involves immunosuppressive drugs followed by standard treatment of heart failure.

SARCOIDOSIS

Sarcoidosis is a non-necrotizing granulomatous disease of multisystem disorder that frequently involves lymph node, lung, and skin lesions. The diagnosis is based upon clinical and noninvasive findings, along with diagnostic histological evidence of non-necrotizing granuloma.[28] Cardiac involvement can be seen in up to 10% of patients with sarcoidosis. Myocardial involvement in sarcoidosis presentation depends on location of granulomas in heart. Usual presentation is the presence of multiple types of arrhythmias long with variable degree of heart failure.

Sarcoidosis can present as variable degree of AV blocks along with ventricular tachycardias and can be a reason of sudden cardiac death in patients with sarcoidosis. Dilated cardiomyopathy is a common presentation of left ventricular involvement in this disorder. CMR and PET are especially helpful in making the diagnosis in these patients. EMB can also detect non-necrotizing granulomas in heart but because of patchy involvement it can be missed. Corticosteroids are the standard treatment of sarcoidosis along with heart failure therapy. Cardiac transplantation sometimes requires in end-stage diseases.

RHEUMATOID ARTHRITIS

Rheumatoid arthritis is the most common SID, affecting around 1% individuals. Although RA is primarily an inflammatory joint disease, it can affect other organs as well. Cardiac involvement in RA is common but usually asymptomatic and usually present as heart failure and associated with increased mortality.[29] Cardiac involvement can present as increased risk of CAD, pericarditis, myocarditis, and arrhythmias. Myocarditis occurs because of presence of diffuse necrotizing or granulomatous lesions in cardiac muscle, and sometimes these can involve conduction system and present with heart failure and arrhythmias, respectively.[30] Echocardiography and CMR can be useful in assessing the degree of LV dysfunction and myocardial involvement.

GRANULOMATOSIS WITH POLYANGIITIS (FORMERLY WEGENER'S GRANULOMATOSIS)

Granulomatosis with polyangiitis (GPA) is an uncommon necrotizing granulomatous SID, which mainly affect small to medium vessels. GPA which usually involves the upper and lower respiratory tract, but any other organ can be affected. Cardiac involvement in GPA usually presents as pericarditis, cardiomyopathy, coronary artery disease, and valve abnormalities.

Presence of congestive heart failure in patient with GPA carries poor prognosis and associated with 25% mortality in 1 year of diagnosis. Treatment includes immunosuppression with steroid and biologic agents along with standard treatment of cardiac involvement.

OTHERS SYSTEMIC IMMUNE-MEDIATED DISEASE

There are many other SIDs that can present with myocardial involvement characterized by dilated cardiomyopathy like dermatomyositis/polymyositis, Sjögren syndrome, adult still's disease, amyloidosis, and many others. Symptomatic cardiomyopathy is uncommon but poor prognostic feature. Dilated cardiomyopathy is a common phenotype, which is most of SIDs. EMB with immunohistochemical analysis can differentiate between different types of cardiomyopathies but rarely needed.

MANAGEMENT OF SYSTEMIC IMMUNE-MEDIATED DISEASE CARDIOMYOPATHY (FLOWCHART 1)

Systemic immune-mediated diseases and its cardiomyopathy treatment involve two components.

1. *Treatment of specific disease*: Immunosuppressive drugs are the mainstay of therapy of disease, especially in acute phases. It may involve IV corticosteroids followed by oral steroids. Biologic agents may be required in acute phases. Attempt should be made to avoid opportunistic infections and should be treated if occurs. Since corticosteroid use is also associated with adverse cardiovascular outcomes, so steroid-sparing therapy should be preferred if possible.
2. *Treatment of dilated cardiomyopathy*: Standard treatment of cardiomyopathy should be given in patient presenting with symptoms of heart failure. IV diuretics may be required in acute phase. All heart failure drugs (RAAS inhibitor, beta blocker, MRA, and SGLT-2 inhibitor) should be initiated as early as possible. There is high risk of incidence of hyperkalemia if there is simultaneous

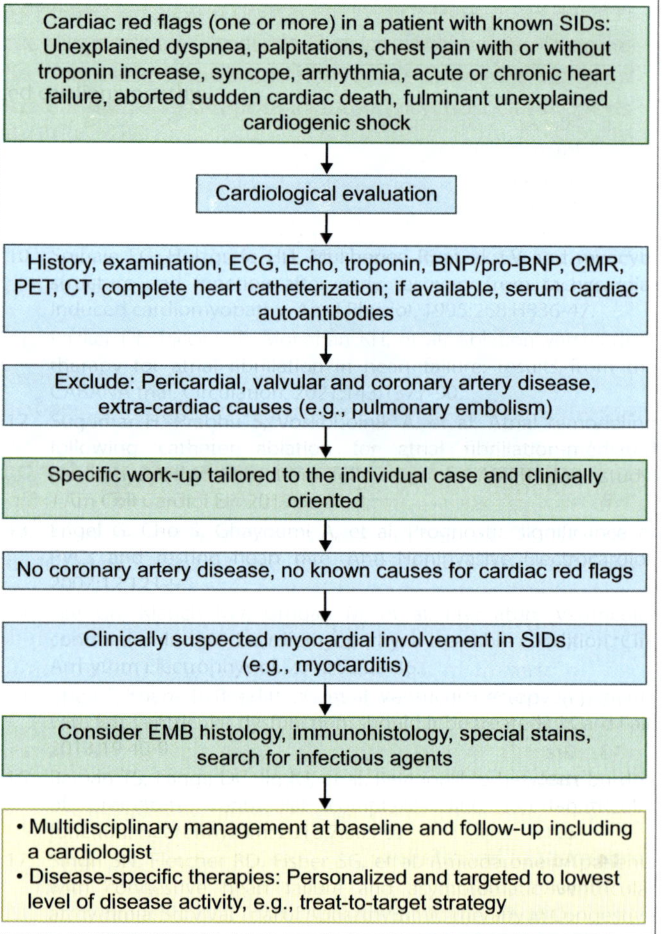

FLOWCHART 1: Myocardial involvement in SIDs: Diagnostic work-up and management.

renal involvement also. Benefit of ICD should be given in aborted SCD or fatal arrhythmia.

CONCLUSION

Cardiovascular system involvement in systemic inflammatory diseases is common, but usually asymptomatic. The pathogenesis of SIDs can include abnormalities in any structure of the heart, with significant heterogeneity in their presentation and severity. Dilated cardiomyopathy is a frequent manifestation of myocardial involvement and is associated with an unfavorable prognosis. Management includes treatment of specific disease along with heart failure therapy as per current guidelines.

REFERENCES

1. McGonagle D, McDermott MF. A proposed classification of the immunological diseases. PLoSMed. 2006;3:e297.
2. Comarmond C, Pagnoux C, Khellaf M, et al. Eosinophilic granulomatosis with polyangiitis (Churg-Strauss): clinical characteristics and long-term follow-up of the 383 patients enrolled in the French Vasculitis Study Group cohort. Arthritis Rheum. 2013;65:270-81.
3. Japp AG, Gulati A, Cook SA, et al. The diagnosis and evaluation of dilated cardiomyopathy. J Am Coll Cardiol. 2016;67:2996-3010.
4. Caforio AL, Pankuweit S, Arbustini E, et al.; European Society of Cardiology Working Group on Myocardial and Pericardial Diseases. Current state of knowledge on aetiology, diagnosis, management, and therapy of myocarditis: a position statement of the European Society of Cardiology Working Group on Myocardial and Pericardial Diseases. Eur Heart J. 2013;34:2636-48.
5. Faccini A, Kaski JC, Camici PG. Coronary microvascular dysfunction in chronic inflammatory rheumatoid diseases. Eur Heart J. 2016;37:1799-806.
6. Agewall S, Beltrame JF, Reynolds HR, et al. WG on Cardiovascular Pharmacotherapy. ESC working group position paper on myocardial infarction with non-obstructive coronary arteries. Eur Heart J. 2017;38:143-53.
7. Chow PC1, Ho MH, Lee TL, et al. Relation of arterial stiffness of left ventricular structure and function in adolescents and young adults with pediatric-onset systemic lupus erythematosus. J Rheumatol. 2007;34:1345-52.
8. Corrao S, Argano C, Pistone G, et al. Rheumatoid arthritis affects left ventricular mass: systematic review and meta-analysis. Eur J intern Med. 2015;26:259-67.
9. Sasson Z, Rasooly Y, Chow CW, et al. Impairment of left ventricular diastolic function in systemic lupus erythematosus. Am J Cardiol. 1992;69:1629-34.
10. Wahren-Herlenius M, Dörner T. Immunopathogenic mechanisms of systemic autoimmune disease. Lancet. 2013;382:819-31.
11. Suurmond J, Diamond B. Autoantibodies in systemic autoimmune diseases: specificity and pathogenicity. J Clin Invest. 2015;125:2194-202.
12. Kotanidis CP, Bazmpani MA, Haidich AB, et al. Diagnostic accuracy of cardiovascular magnetic resonance in acute myocarditis: a systematic review and meta-analysis. JACC Cardiovasc Imaging. 2018;11:1583-90.
13. Grani C, Eichhorn C, Biere L, et al. Prognostic value of cardiac magnetic resonance tissue characterization in risk stratifying patients with suspected myocarditis. J Am Coll Cardiol. 2017;70:1964-76.
14. Aquaro GD, Ghebru Habtemicael Y, Camastra G, et al. Prognostic value of repeating cardiac magnetic resonance in patients with acute myocarditis. J Am Coll Cardiol. 2019;74:2439-48.
15. Mavrogeni S, Karabela G, Stavropoulos E, et al. Imaging patterns of heart failure in rheumatoid arthritis evaluated by cardiovascular magnetic resonance. Int J Cardiol. 2013;168:4333-5.
16. Kusano KF, Satomi K. Diagnosis and treatment of cardiac sarcoidosis. Heart. 2016;102:184-90.
17. Leone O, Veinot JP, Angelini A, et al. 2011 consensus statement on endomyocardial biopsy from the association for European Cardiovascular Pathology and the Society for Cardiovascular Pathology. Cardiovasc Pathol. 2012;21:245-74.
18. Ardehali H, Howard DL, Hariri A, et al. A positive endomyocardial biopsy result for sarcoid is associated with poor prognosis in patients with initially unexplained cardiomyopathy. Am Heart J. 2005;150:459-63.
19. Austin BA, Duffy B, Tan C, et al. Comparison of functional status, electrocardiographic, and echocardiographic parameters to mortality in endomyocardial-biopsy proven cardiac amyloidosis. Am J Cardiol. 2009;103:1429-33.
20. Baccouche H, Mahrholdt H, Meinhardt G, et al. Diagnostic synergy of non-invasive cardiovascular magnetic resonance and invasive endomyocardial biopsy in troponin-positive patients without coronary artery disease. Eur Heart J. 2009;30:2869-79.
21. D'Cruz D, Khamashta M, Hughes GRV. Cardiovascular manifestations of systemic lupus erythematosus. In: Wallace DJ, Hahn BH (Eds). Dubois' Lupus Erythematosus. Philadelphia: Lippincott William and Wilkins; 2002. p. 645.
22. Lee-Kirsch MA, Gong M, Chowdhury D, et al. Mutations in the gene encoding the 3'-5' DNA exonuclease TREX1 are associated with systemic lupus erythematosus. Nat Genet. 2007;39:1065-7.
23. Tincani A, Rebaioli CB, Taglietti M, et al. Heart involvement in systemic lupus erythematosus, anti-phospholipid syndrome and neonatal lupus. Rheumatology. 2006;45:iv8-i13.
24. van den Hoogen F, Khanna D, Fransen J. 2013 classification criteria for systemic sclerosis: an American College of Rheumatology/ European League against Rheumatism collaborative initiative. Arthritis Rheum. 2013;65:2737-47.
25. Allanore Y, Meune C, Vonk MC; EUSTAR co-authors. Prevalence and factors associated with left ventricular dysfunction in the EULAR Scleroderma Trial and Research group (EUSTAR) database of patients with systemic sclerosis. Ann Rheum Dis. 2010;69:218-21.
26. Morelli S, Sgreccia A, Ferrante L, et al. Relationship between electrocardiographic and echocardiographic findings in systemic sclerosis (scleroderma). Int J Cardiol 1996;57:151-60.
27. Follansbee WP, Zerbe TR, Medsger TA. Cardiac and skeletal muscle disease in systemic sclerosis (scleroderma): a high risk association. Am Heart J. 1993;125:194-203.
28. Rudan I, Sidhu S, Papana A, et al. Prevalence of rheumatoid arthritis in low- and middle-income countries: A systematic review and analysis. J Glob Health. 2015;5(1):010409.
29. Wright K, Crowson CS, Gabriel SE. Cardiovascular comorbidity in rheumatic diseases: a focus on heart failure. Heart Fail Clin. 2014;10:339-52.
30. Lebowitz WB. The heart in rheumatoid arthritis (rheumatoid disease):a clinical and pathological study of sixty-two cases. Ann Intern Med. 1963;58:102-23.

CHAPTER

46 Arrhythmia-induced Cardiomyopathy

Arindam Mitra, Aditi Rastogi, Jayanta Saha

ABSTRACT

Arrhythmias coexist in patients with heart failure (HF) and left ventricular (LV) dysfunction. Tachycardias, atrial fibrillation, and premature ventricular contractions are known to trigger a reversible dilated cardiomyopathy referred as arrhythmia-induced cardiomyopathy (AiCM). AiCM should be suspected in patients with mean heart rate >100 beats/min, atrial fibrillation, and/or premature ventricular contractions burden ≥10%. Reversal of CM by elimination of arrhythmia not only confirms the diagnosis but may significantly improve outcomes. Ambulatory ECG monitoring and CMR are key to establishing the diagnosis of AiCM. Therapeutic choice depends on the culprit arrhythmia, patient preferences, and associated comorbidities. Following recovery of LV function, patients require continued follow-up for arrhythmia recurrence if an abnormal myocardial substrate is present.

Keywords: Arrhythmia, cardiomyopathy, heart failure, supraventricular tachycardia, atrial fibrillation, premature ventricular contractions.

INTRODUCTION

Arrhythmias are a common occurrence in patients of cardiomyopathies and frequently result in worsening of heart failure. Arrhythmia-induced cardiomyopathy (AiCM) is defined as atrial and/or ventricular dysfunction secondary to rapid and/or asynchronous/irregular myocardial contraction, partially or completely reversible after treatment of the causative arrhythmia.[1]

Arrhythmia-induced cardiomyopathy encompasses tachycardia-induced CM (T-CM), atrial fibrillation–induced CM (AF-CM), and premature ventricular contraction (PVC)-induced CM (PVC-CM) **(Fig. 1)**. This term does not include the more recently recognized forms of CM resulting from abnormalities in the conduction system, such as chronic right ventricular (RV) pacing, left bundle branch block, and cardiac pre-excitation **(Fig. 2)**.[2]

TACHYCARDIA-INDUCED CARDIOMYOPATHY

Tachycardia-induced cardiomyopathy (T-CM) is reversible LV dysfunction caused by increased ventricular rate irrespective of origin of tachycardia. A study by Medi C et al. in 345 patients showed that TCM occurred in 10% patients

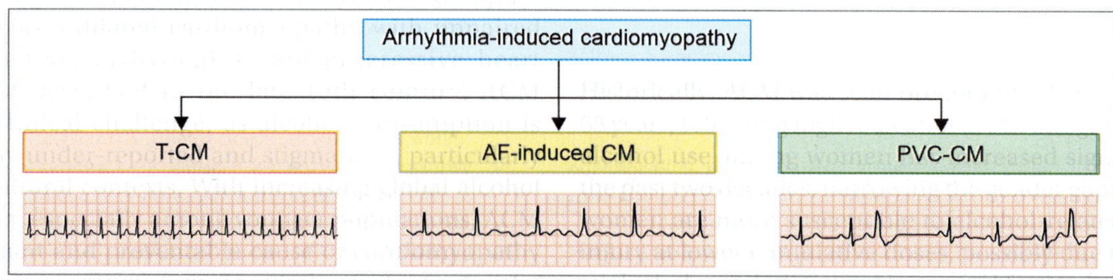

FIG. 1: Classification of AiCM.

	Tachycardia	Atrial fibrillation	Frequent PVCs
Triggers	Increased HR	• HR irregularity • Autonomic dysfunction • Loss of atrial contraction	• LV dyssynchrony • AV dissociation • HR irregularity • Intermittent tachycardia • Sympathetic dysregulation • Post-extrasystolic potentiation
Mediators	• Ca^{2+} Overload • Ca^{2+} Mishandling	Ca^{2+} Mishandling	• Ca^{2+} Mishandling • Ca^{2+} Overload
Effect	• Fibrosis • Myocyte and electrical remodeling • Contractile dysfunction • Neurohormonal activation	Contractile dysfunction	• Myocyte and electrical remodeling • Contractile dysfunction • ?? Fibrosis
Arrhythmia suppression	Ablation	Arrhythmia drug	
Recovery	• Normalized LVEF • Ventricular dilatation • Diastolic dysfunction • Reactive hypertrophy • Persistent fibrosis	Normalized LVEF	Normalized LVEF and dimensions

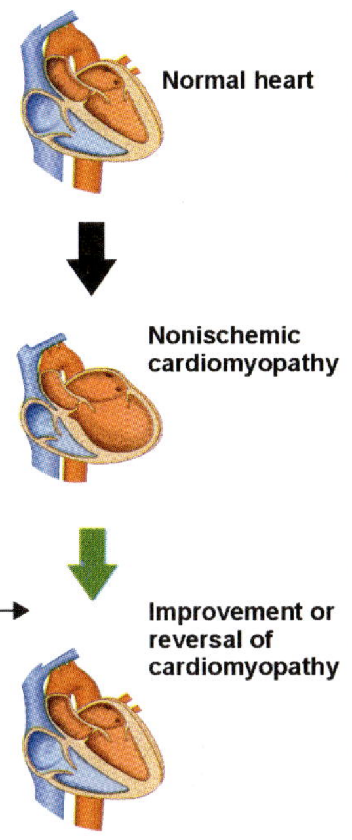

Normal heart

Nonischemic cardiomyopathy

Improvement or reversal of cardiomyopathy

FIG. 2: Arrhythmia induced cardiomyopathies: Possible triggers, mediators, effect, and recovery.

Courtesy: Huizar JF, Ellenbogen KA, Tan AY, et al. Arrhythmia-induced cardiomyopathy: JACC state-of-the-art review. J Am Coll Cardiol. 2019;73:2328-44.

with focal AT.[3] In another study by Jeremy P MOORE et al. on pediatric TCM showed that the most common arrhythmias were ectopic atrial tachycardia (59%), permanent junctional reciprocating tachycardia (23%), and ventricular tachycardia (7%).[4]

Etiology

Various arrhythmias implicated in causing TCM include atrial flutter and AF with rapid ventricular response (most common), atrial tachycardia, atrioventricular (AV) reciprocating tachycardia, AV nodal re-entrant tachycardia, sustained sinus tachycardia, various ventricular tachycardia (idiopathic, bundle branch, and fascicular), and pacemaker-mediated tachycardia can also lead to T-CM.

Pathophysiology and Mechanism

The pathophysiology of tachycardia-induced cardiomyopathy (T-CM) involves several key mechanisms, primarily driven by sustained increased ventricular rates regardless of tachycardia origin. The development of T-CM in clinical studies occurred between 3 and 120 days from the onset of tachycardia.

- *Structural and functional myocardial changes:* Persistent tachycardia leads to HF symptoms, LV systolic dysfunction and dilatation, decrease in LV dP/dt max (contractile function) and myocardial blood flow, and increase in LV wall stress and end-diastolic pressure and volume. Typically, biventricular dilation occurs without hypertrophy or change in overall heart mass, but with mild ventricular wall thinning.[5]
- *Cellular and molecular alterations:* Impaired calcium handling dynamics including reduced calcium transients (Ca^{2+}), L-type calcium current, and basal adenosine triphosphatase activity are correlated with the decrease in LV ejection fraction (LVEF).[6] There is impaired excitation-contraction coupling and diastolic dysfunction.
- *Hemodynamic and neurohormonal changes:* Systemic blood pressure decreases while LV and pulmonary artery pressures increase during tachycardia. Neurohormonal activation is indicated by elevated biomarkers such as B-type natriuretic peptide.

Cessation of tachycardia leads to the normalization of right atrial and arterial pressure, significant improvement of LVEF, and cardiac output within 48 hours, with full normalization occurring after 1–2 weeks.[5] Despite functional recovery, some histological and structural abnormalities may persist.

Clinical Presentation and Diagnosis

Patients of TCM present with palpitations (29%), HF class III and IV symptoms (47%), presyncope/syncope (12%), while the remaining may have no symptoms. Sudden cardiac death remains a risk in ≤8% to 12% of cases.[7]

Tachycardia-induced CM should be suspected in patients with LV dysfunction and a prior or persistent or frequent paroxysmal tachycardia without obvious etiology **(Table 1)**. A superimposed T-CM should be considered despite underlying secondary CM (ischemic, infiltrative, or toxic/drug-related) if the tachycardia is present. Thus, using an ambulatory ECG monitor for ≥2 weeks is essential to establish the T-CM diagnosis. Echocardiogram or cardiac magnetic resonance can assist in excluding other etiologies.[8] Neurohormonal markers such as B-type natriuretic peptide (BNP) and pro-BNP are commonly elevated and may precede LV dysfunction. The definitive diagnosis of T-CM can only be established after recovery or improvement of LV systolic function within the first 6 months after eliminating the culprit tachycardia.

Treatment

The primary treatment involves suppressing the primary arrhythmia using antiarrhythmic drugs (AADs) or ablation. Initiating or optimizing heart failure (HF) medications [beta-blockers, angiotensin receptor/neprilysin inhibitor (ARNi), angiotensin-converting enzyme inhibitors (ACEi) or angiotensin receptor blockers (ARB), diuretics, and aldosterone blockers/sodium-glucose cotransporter 2 inhibitors] is essential to promote reverse remodeling.

By resolving tachyarrhythmia, LV function typically improves within 4–12 weeks, and HF symptoms often improve by ≥1 NYHA functional class in most patients.[9] Full recovery of T-CM is not always achieved, and specific histopathologic abnormalities, diastolic dysfunction, and ventricular dilatation with hypertrophy may persist despite normalizing LV systolic function.[10]

Tachycardia recurrence can cause HF symptoms to reappear sooner than the initial event with at least the same severity compared with the initial presentation, hence permanent treatment of the tachycardia such as the ablation therapy becomes important especially for the tachycardias with high success rate **(Table 2)**.

TABLE 1: Reversible and irreversible causes of cardiomyopathy.

Reversible	Irreversible
Transient ischemia/after cardiac arrest	Extensive/multiple myocardial infarctions
Subacute valvular heart disease	Hypertrophic cardiomyopathy
Uncontrolled hypertension	Cardiac sarcoidosis
Abnormal conduction induced cardiomyopathy (i.e., LBBB-, pacing-, pre-excitation-induced cardiomyopathy)	End-stage valvular heart disease
Drug or alcohol abuse	Infectious (e.g., Chagas disease)
Endocrine (severe hypothyroidism)	
Arrhythmia induced cardiomyopathy (i.e., PVC-, AF-, and tachycardia-induced cardiomyopathy)	
Stress-induced cardiomyopathy	
Peripartum cardiomyopathy	
Inflammatory/infectious (e.g., myocarditis, sepsis)	

TABLE 2: Treatment options of tachycardia-induced cardiomyopathy based on tachyarrhythmia.

Arrhythmia	Treatment
Sinus tachycardia/thyrotoxicosis	BB + treatment of underlying disease
Atrial fibrillation with VR	Rhythm (PVI with or without AADs) vs. rate control vs. AVJ
Atrial flutter with RVR	Radiofrequency ablation
Atrial tachycardia	Radiofrequency ablation vs. AADs
AVRT/AVNRT	Radiofrequency ablation
Rapid atrial/ventricular pacing (pacemaker mediated tachycardia)	Reprogram pacemaker
Sustained ventricular tachycardia	Radiofrequency ablation with or without AADs

(AADs: antiarrhythmic drugs; AVJ: atrioventricular nodal ablation; AVNRT: atrioventricular nodal re-entry tachycardia; AVRT: atrioventricular re-entrant tachycardia; BB: beta-blockers; PVI: pulmonary vein isolation)

ATRIAL FIBRILLATION-INDUCED CARDIOMYOPATHY

Atrial fibrillation-induced cardiomyopathy (AF-CM) is defined as LV systolic dysfunction in patients with paroxysmal or persistent AF despite appropriate rate control.[9] The basic pathology involved is abnormal calcium dynamics due to irregular heart rate and loss of atrial contractility triggering sympathetic activation and subsequently increased filling pressures, functional mitral regurgitation, and diastolic dysfunction. Rate control is the key to distinguish between AF-CM from T-CM.

Clinical Presentation and Diagnosis

Patients usually present with HF symptoms. It is difficult to differentiate AF-induced cardiomyopathy from other cardiomyopathies with superimposed AF.[9] AF-induced CM should be suspected in nonischemic CM patients where no other secondary cause is found and with persistent AF where there is no improvement despite GDMT for HF and adequate rate control. A conclusive diagnosis of AF-CM can only be confirmed if LV systolic function improves or returns to normal after AF elimination.

Treatment

The clinical management of AF-CM includes guideline-directed medical therapy and rhythm control. The current evidence suggests that ventricular rate control alone during AF may not reliably predict CM reversibility. Various trials comparing rate control versus rhythm control via ablation have demonstrated superiority of rhythm control strategy. CABANA trial demonstrated that catheter ablation therapy resulted in survival benefit, improved QOL and freedom from AF recurrence compared to drug therapy.[11] CAMERA-MRI trial demonstrated reduced atrial myocardial fibrosis with improved remodeling in patients who underwent ablation.[12] Rhythm control strategy via ablation should be the first-line therapy in patients of AF-induced CM along with the GDMT for HF.

PREMATURE VENTRICULAR CONTRACTION CARDIOMYOPATHY

Premature ventricular contraction cardiomyopathy (PVC-CM) is defined as the development of LV dysfunction caused solely by frequent PVCs. Superimposed PVC-CM can be defined as worsening LVEF by at least 10% due to frequent PVCs in a previously known CM. Frequent PVCs are commonly referred to as PVC burden >5% and PVC burden ≥10% is considered high and significant enough to trigger PVC-CM.

Epidemiology of Premature Ventricular Contractions and Premature Ventricular Contraction Cardiomyopathy

The PVC prevalence is higher with age, especially in those ≥75 years (~70% prevalence), while rarely occurring in children <11 years old.[13,14] PVCs are often linked to postmyocardial infarction, coronary heart disease, dilated CM, and HF with reported prevalence above 90%.[13] Nearly one-half of NYHA functional class II and III patients display frequent PVCs (>1,000 PVCs/day).[15] PVCs are an independent predictor of all-cause and cardiovascular mortality.[13] There is a robust correlation between high PVC burden and LV dysfunction[16] **(Figs. 3A and B)**. PVC-CM was found in 9–30% of patients referred for PVC ablation.[16] A secondary analysis of the CHF-STAT (Survival Trial of Antiarrhythmic Therapy in Congestive

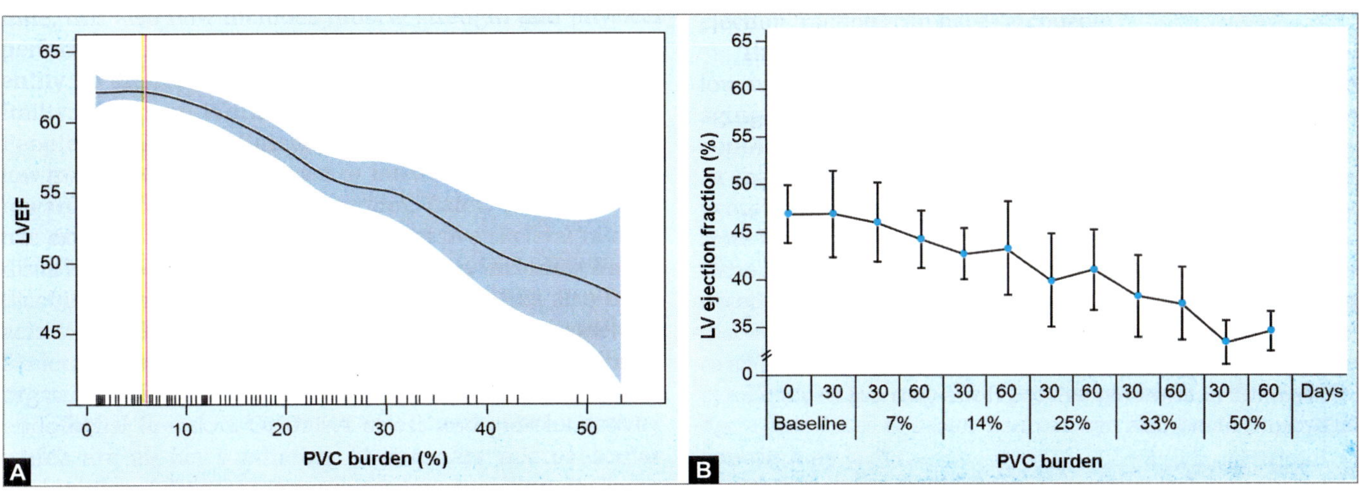

FIGS. 3A AND B: Linear decrease of LV ejection fraction with sequential increase in PVC burden in (A) clinical setting and (B) translational animal model.

Courtesy: Shoureshi P, Tan A, Koneru J, et al. Arrhythmia-induced Cardiomyopathy: JACC State-of-the-Art Review. JACC. 2024;83(22):2214-32.

Heart Failure) study[17] involving patients with both a PVC rate of >10 per hour and an LVEF of <40%, revealed an overall PVC-CM prevalence of 29% and ≤41% in patients with nonischemic CM alone.[18]

Potential Mechanism(S) of Premature Ventricular Contraction-induced Cardiomyopathy

The mechanism remains poorly understood. An animal study comparing the effects of atrial and ventricular bigeminy over a 12-week period observed that only PVCs led to significant changes in LV function when compared with a control and atrial bigeminy group. This suggests that neither increased heart rate nor irregularity alone can account for PVC-CM.[19] However, the proposed mechanisms are:

- *Disrupted calcium handling*: The primary cause of contractile dysfunction is related to disruptions in the Ca^{2+}-induced Ca^{2+} release mechanism within cardiac myocytes.
- *Electrophysiological remodeling and fibrosis*: Premature ventricular contraction-induced cardiomyopathy is associated with electrical remodeling, including changes in ion currents and prolonged action potential duration and there is myocardial fibrosis in the LV tissue, contributing to altered structural integrity and function.
- *Autonomic nervous system imbalance*: Premature ventricular contractions disrupt cardiac autonomic balance leading to chronic imbalanced sympathetic overload. PVCs with variable coupling intervals appear to disrupt cardiac autonomic balance most potently.[20]
- *Left ventricular dyssynchrony and post-extrasystolic potentiation (PESP)*: Left ventricular (LV) dyssynchrony caused by uncoordinated segment contractions related to PVCs leads to inefficient contractile function. PESP, a phenomenon related to the varying contractility following a PVC, also plays a role in worsening LV function.[21]
- *Hemodynamic impairment*: Atrioventricular (AV) dissociation during PVCs causes atrial contraction against a closed AV valve, raising left atrial pressure and impairing LV filling.

These interacting processes, cellular calcium mishandling, structural remodeling with fibrosis, autonomic imbalance, mechanical dyssynchrony, and impaired hemodynamics—collectively lead to the development and progression of PVC-CM.

Predictors of Premature Ventricular Contraction-induced Cardiomyopathy

- Premature ventricular contraction burden of ≥10%[16,21]
- Epicardial origin[22]
- Interpolated PVCs 50
- Premature ventricular contraction-QRS duration (>157 ms)[23]
- In RVOT PVCs, higher peak deflection index (time from QRS onset to peak of tallest R in inferior leads divided by total QRS duration)[24]
- Varying coupling interval[25]
- Male gender
- Genetic predisposition (R222Q missense variant of the Nav1.5 subunit of sodium channel).[26]
- A preclinical study suggests PVCs with variable coupling intervals cause higher cardiac neuronal disturbance than PVCs with short or long intervals, thereby contributing to the severity of PVC-CM.[27]
- The ABC-VT score (maximum 12 points) **(Fig. 4)** is used in frequent PVCs >5% burden. It is a risk stratification tool to predict development of LV remodeling and MACE: *Low risk*: 0–4 points; *intermediate risk*: 5–8 points; or *high risk*: 9–12 points.
- *Axis (superior)*: 1 point
- *Burden:*
  - *>10–20%*: 2 points
  - *>20%*: 3 points
- *Coupling interval (>500 ms)*: 4 points
- *Ventricular tachycardia*: 4 points

Clinical Presentation, Diagnosis, and Prognosis

Premature ventricular contraction-induced cardiomyopathy is a diagnosis of exclusion. PVC-CM should be suspected in patients with frequent PVCs (>10%), especially in nonischemic CM. PVC-CM can manifest with no symptoms of HF or syncope. Physical examination is frequently normal apart from irregular heart sounds and mild signs of HF.

Although the ECG is valuable, an extended ambulatory ECG monitor of minimum of 6 days is ideal to detect an individual's maximum PVC burden.[28]

"The riddle of the chicken and the egg still unanswered?" It is often challenging to determine whether PVCs caused the

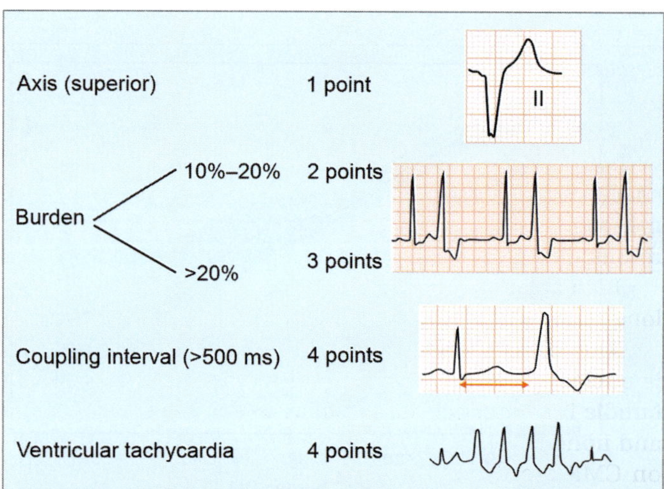

FIG. 4: ABC-VT risk score (maximum 12). Risk stratification tool to predict the development of LV remodeling and subsequent cardiac adverse events (minimum 24-hour burden over the 14-day monitoring period). *Low risk*: 0–4 points; *intermediate risk*: 5–8 points; or *high risk*: 9–12 points.

TABLE 3: Clinical and PVC features to identify PVC-CM.

CM resulting in PVCs		PVCs causing CM
Patient characteristics	Older with known heart disease	Otherwise healthy
Comorbidities	CAD, myocarditis, RV dysplasia	No prior cardiac history
Echocardiogram	Segmental hypokinesia, LVEF <25%	Global hypokinesia, LVEF 37±10%
Cardiac magnetic resonance imaging (late-gadolinium enhancement)	Significant scar	Absence or minimal scar burden (≤9 g)
PVC frequency	<5,000/24 hours (<5%)	≥10,000/24 h (≥10%)
PVC pattern	Multifocal	Monomorphic
QRS morphology	Nonspecific	RVOT/LVOT/epicardial
Response to PVC suppression	No change in LV function	Improvement of LV function

Source: Shoureshi P, Tan A, Koneru J, et al. Arrhythmia-induced Cardiomyopathy: JACC State-of-the-Art Review. JACC. 2024;83(22):2214-32.

cardiomyopathy or if the cardiomyopathy led to the PVCs. **Table 3** shows the clinical and PVC Features to Identify PVC Cardiomyopathy.

Premature ventricular contraction-induced cardiomyopathy is characterized by mild to moderate LV dysfunction, LV enlargement, mild mitral regurgitation, and left atrial enlargement, which typically resolves within 2–12 weeks after eliminating PVCs.

The ABC-VT scoring system predicts adverse LV remodeling and future clinical outcomes in patients with frequent PVCs, incorporating factors such as superiorly directed PVC axis, PVC burden, PVC coupling interval >500 ms, and nonsustained VT.

Recently, myocarditis has emerged as a possible trigger of frequent PVCs and CM.[29]

Treatment

Guidelines recommend PVC suppression in patients with CM and PVC burden of >15%.[30]

Patients with frequent PVCs (≥10% burden) without LV dysfunction, should be regularly monitored at least every 6–12 months.

Managing frequent PVCs (≥10% burden) in individuals without LV dysfunction (LVEF ≥50%) or symptoms is challenging. They need regular monitoring at least every 6–12 months. A study[31] highlighted high rates of spontaneous PVC resolution without ablation or AADs therapy.

Both ablation and AAD therapies have exhibited similar long-term PVC suppression rates ranging from 70 to 80%.[18]

The optimal PVC burden threshold for intervention is unclear. Patients with frequent PVCs and baseline left bundle branch block, nonsustained ventricular tachycardia and nonoutflow PVCs, and late gadolinium enhancement on CMR are usually treated.[32] Achieving successful PVC suppression is defined as a burden reduction of >80% compared with baseline.[33]

No randomized, prospective studies have directly compared ablation and AAD therapy outcomes. Ablation has complication rates range from 5 to 8%, and AADs have an approximately 10% discontinuation rate owing to short- and long-term side effects. A retrospective study has shown that only ablation has shown a statistically significant reduction in PVCs in patients with a <10% burden.[34]

Besides improving LVEF, PVC suppression in PVCCM should also improve LV dilatation, RV function, mitral regurgitation, and BNP levels. LVEF can improve by 10–15% after ablation.[34] Successful ablation can even restore RV function in patients with PVC-CM affecting the RV. However, it is unclear whether PVC suppression in the presence of abnormal CMR improves outcomes. CMR-assessed scar burden can predict responders and nonresponders to PVC suppression, especially when there is a substantial reduction (>20%) in PVC burden **(Flowchart 1)**.[35]

CONCLUSION

Arrhythmia-induced cardiomyopathy (AiCM) encompasses a spectrum of reversible cardiomyopathies caused by tachycardia, atrial fibrillation, and premature ventricular contractions. It is a *reversible form of cardiomyopathy* that can manifest with a significant variety of presentations, ranging from being asymptomatic to causing severe heart failure (HF) symptoms. Clinicians should have a *high index of suspicion* of superimposed AiCM even in patients with an obvious etiology. As such we must: (1) suspect T-CM in patients with paroxysmal or persistent SVTs, primarily AF/atrial flutter, atrial tachycardia, and persistent junctional reciprocating tachycardia with heart rates above 100 beats/min. (2) consider AF-CM in patients with nonischemic CM and paroxysmal, persistent, or permanent AF, even with appropriate rate control, whereas PVC-CM should be considered in patients with nonischemic CM and PVC burden ≥10%. The primary treatment for AICM involves suppressing the arrhythmia, often through antiarrhythmic drugs or ablation. Research is still needed to better understand the pathophysiological mechanisms and predictors of AICM in order to develop effective long-term preventive strategies.

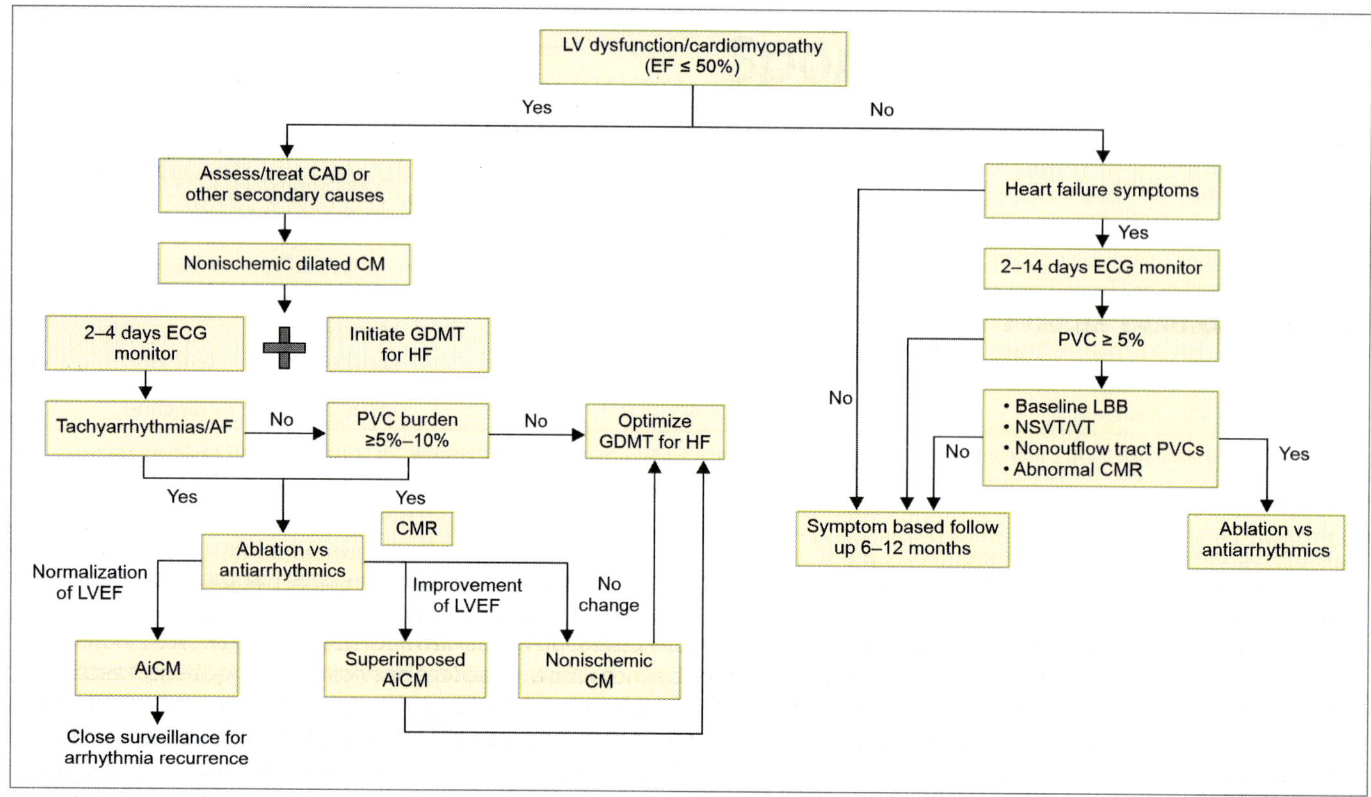

FLOWCHART 1: Proposed management algorithm for arrhythmia-induced cardiomyopathy.

REFERENCES

1. Gallagher JJ. Tachycardia and cardiomyopathy: the chicken-egg dilemma revisited. J Am Coll Cardiol. 1985;6:1172-3.
2. Shoureshi P, Tan A, Koneru J, et al. Arrhythmia-Induced Cardiomyopathy: JACC State-of-the-Art Review. JACC. 2024;83(22):2214-32.
3. Medi C, Kalman JM, Haqqani H, et al. Tachycardia-mediated cardiomyopathy secondary to focal atrial tachycardia: long-term outcome after catheter ablation. J Am Coll Cardiol. 2009;53:1791-7.
4. Moore JP, Patel PA, Shannon KM, et al. Predictors of myocardial recovery in pediatric tachycardia-induced cardiomyopathy. Heart Rhythm. 2014;11:1163-9.
5. Shinbane JS, Wood MA, Jensen DN, et al. Tachycardia-induced cardiomyopathy: a review of animal models and clinical studies. J Am Coll Cardiol. 1997;29:709-15.
6. O'Brien PJ, Moe GW, Nowack LM, et al. Sarcoplasmic reticulum Ca-release channel and ATP-synthesis activities are early myocardial markers of heart failure produced by rapid ventricular pacing in dogs. Can J Physiol Pharmacol. 1994;72:999-1006.
7. Nerheim P, Birger-Botkin S, Piracha L, et al. Heart failure and sudden death in patients with tachycardia-induced cardiomyopathy and recurrent tachycardia. Circulation. 2004;110:247-52.
8. Huizar JF, Ellenbogen KA, Tan AY, et al. Arrhythmia-induced cardiomyopathy: JACC state-of-the-art review. J Am Coll Cardiol. 2019;73:2328-44.
9. Watanabe H, Okamura K, Chinushi M, et al. Clinical characteristics, treatment, and outcome of tachycardia induced cardiomyopathy. Int Heart J. 2008;49:39-47.
10. Spinale FG, Holzgrefe HH, Mukherjee R, et al. LV and myocyte structure and function after early recovery from tachycardia-induced cardiomyopathy. Am J Physiol. 1995;268:H836-47.
11. Packer DL, Piccini JP, Monahan KH, et al. Ablation versus drug therapy for atrial fibrillation in heart failure: results from the CABANA trial. Circulation. 2021;143:1377-90.
12. Sugumar H, Prabhu S, Voskoboinik A, et al. Atrial remodeling following catheter ablation for atrial fibrillation-mediated cardiomyopathy: long term follow-up of CAMERA-MRI study. J Am Coll Cardiol EP. 2019;5:681-8.
13. Engel G, Cho S, Ghayoumi A, et al. Prognostic significance of PVCs and resting heart rate. Ann Noninvasive Electrocardiol. 2007;12:121-9.
14. Lee GK, Klarich KW, Grogan M, et al. Premature ventricular contraction-induced cardiomyopathy: a treatable condition. Circ Arrhythm Electrophysiol. 2012;5:229-36.
15. Chen T, Koene R, Benditt DG, et al. Ventricular ectopy in patients with left ventricular dysfunction: should it be treated? J Card Fail. 2013;19:40-9.
16. Baman TS, Lange DC, Ilg KJ, et al. Relationship between burden of premature ventricular complexes and left ventricular function. Heart Rhythm. 2010;7:865-9.
17. Singh SN, Fletcher RD, Fisher SG, et al. Amiodarone in patients with congestive heart failure and asymptomatic ventricular arrhythmia. Survival Trial of Antiarrhythmic Therapy in Congestive Heart Failure. N Engl J Med. 1995;333:77-82.

18. Huizar JF, Fisher SG, Kaszala K, et al. Amiodarone is an effective treatment of PVC-cardiomyopathy in the veteran population. Circulation. 2017;136:A14667.
19. Kowgli N, Jovin D, O'Quinn M, et al. Neither irregularity nor tachycardia are triggers of PVC-cardiomyopathy: comparing persistent atrial and ventricular ectopy in an animal model. Heart Rhythm. 2018;15:S594.
20. Tan AY, Elharrif K, Cardona-Guarache R, et al. Persistent proarrhythmic neural remodeling despite recovery from premature ventricular contraction-induced cardiomyopathy. J Am Coll Cardiol. 2020;75:1-13.
21. Shoureshi P, Kabadi R, James N, et al. Left ventricular remodeling in premature ventricular contraction-induced cardiomyopathy: effect of coupling intervals and atrioventricular dissociation. Heart Rhythm. O_2. 2023;4:556-64.
22. Bogun F, Crawford T, Reich S, et al. Radiofrequency ablation of frequent, idiopathic premature ventricular complexes: comparison with a control group without intervention. Heart Rhythm. 2007;4:863-7.
23. Park KM, Im SI, Lee SH, et al. Left ventricular dysfunction in outpatients with frequent ventricular premature complexes. Tex Heart Inst J. 2022;49.
24. Yamada S, Chung FP, Lin YJ, et al. Electrocardiographic characteristics for predicting idiopathic right ventricular outflow tract premature ventricular complex-induced cardiomyopathy. J Interv Card Electrophysiol. 2018;53:175-85.
25. Lee CH, Park KH, Nam JH, et al. Increased variability of the coupling interval of premature ventricular contractions as a predictor of cardiac mortality in patients with left ventricular dysfunction. Circ J. 2015;79:2360-6.
26. Mann SA, Castro ML, Ohanian M, et al. R222Q SCN5A mutation is associated with reversible ventricular ectopy and dilated cardiomyopathy. J Am Coll Cardiol. 2012;60:1566.
27. Hamon D, Rajendran PS, Chui RW, et al. Premature ventricular contraction coupling interval variability destabilizes cardiac neuronal and electrophysiological control: insights from simultaneous cardioneural mapping. Circ Arrhythm Electrophysiol. 2017;10(4):e004937.
28. Loring Z, Hanna P, Pellegrini CN. Longer ambulatory ECG monitoring increases identification of clinically significant ectopy. Pacing Clin Electrophysiol. 2016;39:592-7.
29. Tung R, Bauer B, Schelbert H, et al. Incidence of abnormal positron emission tomography in patients with unexplained cardiomyopathy and ventricular arrhythmias: the potential role of occult inflammation in arrhythmogenesis. Heart Rhythm. 2015;12:2488-98.
30. Cronin EM, Bogun FM, Maury P, et al. 2019 HRS/EHRA/APHRS/LAHRS expert consensus statement on catheter ablation of ventricular arrhythmias. Heart Rhythm. 2020;17:e2-e154.
31. Lee AKY, Andrade J, Hawkins NM, et al. Outcomes of untreated frequent premature ventricular complexes with normal left ventricular function. Heart. 2019;105:1408-13.
32. Hosseini F, Thibert MJ, Gulsin GS, et al. Cardiac magnetic resonance in the evaluation of patients with frequent premature ventricular complexes. J Am Coll Cardiol. 2022;8:1122-32.
33. Anastasiou-Nana MI, Menlove RL, Nanas JN, et al. Changes in spontaneous variability of ventricular ectopic activity as a function of time in patients with chronic arrhythmias. Circulation. 1988;78:286-95.
34. Zhong L, Lee YH, Huang XM, et al. Relative efficacy of catheter ablation vs antiarrhythmic drugs in treating premature ventricular contractions: a single-center retrospective study. Heart Rhythm. 2014;11:187-93.
35. Penela D, Martinez M, Fernandez-Armenta J, et al. Influence of myocardial scar on the response to frequent premature ventricular complex ablation. Heart. 2019;105:378-83.

CHAPTER 47

Alcoholic Cardiomyopathy

Shishu Shankar Mishra, Biswaranjan Mishra, Asharam Panda

ABSTRACT

Alcoholic cardiomyopathy (ACM) is a subtype of nonischemic dilated cardiomyopathy caused by chronic heavy alcohol consumption, typically sustained over a period of years. It is characterized by left ventricular dilatation, reduced systolic function, and the clinical syndrome of heart failure. The pathophysiology is multifactorial, involving direct myocardial toxicity, toxicity mediated by its metabolite acetaldehyde, oxidative stress, neurohormonal activation, nutritional deficiencies, and genetic susceptibility. Despite its prevalence, ACM is underdiagnosed, largely because of underreporting of alcohol intake and overlap with idiopathic dilated cardiomyopathy. Emerging evidence demonstrates that abstinence from alcohol can lead to significant improvement in ventricular function and prognosis. Drugs such as disulfiram, naltrexone, and acamprosate have demonstrated to achieve and sustain abstinence. Heart failure directed therapy includes the standard treatment for heart failure with reduced ejection fraction (HFrEF) along with nutritional support.

Keywords: Alcoholic cardiomyopathy, dilated cardiomyopathy, left ventricular dysfunction, heart failure with reduced ejection fraction.

INTRODUCTION

The cardiovascular effects of alcohol consumption have been described for centuries, with both harmful and purported protective associations. Moderate consumption has historically been linked with reduced risk of coronary artery disease, the so-called "French Paradox." However, recent studies have refuted such beneficial action of moderate drinking and alcohol is no more considered to have any beneficial effect.[1] Chronic and heavy alcohol use has unequivocally deleterious effects, particularly on the myocardium.[2]

Alcoholic cardiomyopathy (ACM) represents an advanced stage of alcohol-induced myocardial injury. It manifests as a dilated cardiomyopathy with impaired systolic function, arrhythmias, and progressive heart failure. First described in the late 19th century, ACM remains a clinical challenge, as alcohol consumption is often socially under-reported and stigmatized, particularly in certain cultural contexts. With increasing global alcohol consumption, especially among younger populations, ACM is an important and preventable cause of cardiomyopathy that physicians must remain vigilant. Importantly, timely recognition and intervention can alter its natural history, making it distinct from many other forms of cardiomyopathy.[3]

EPIDEMIOLOGY

The prevalence of ACM varies widely depending on definitions of "heavy drinking," geographic region, and cultural patterns of alcohol use. In Western countries, chronic alcohol abuse accounts for approximately 20–40% of all cases of dilated cardiomyopathy. In autopsy studies of alcoholics, myocardial changes consistent with ACM have been reported in up to 30% of subjects.[4]

Demographics

Historically, ACM was seen predominantly in men aged 35–65 years, reflecting higher alcohol use in this group. However, alcohol use among women has increased significantly over the past two decades, narrowing the gender gap. Importantly, women are more susceptible to alcohol-related myocardial injury at lower cumulative doses, possibly due to differences in alcohol metabolism and hormonal factors.[5]

Global Burden

In Europe and America, alcohol contributes substantially to cardiomyopathy-related heart failure hospitalizations. In low- and middle-income countries, including India, true prevalence is likely underestimated due to poor reporting and limited diagnostic facilities. With rising per capita alcohol consumption in India, the incidence of ACM is expected to increase.[6]

Threshold of Risk

Although risk correlates with dose and duration, not all chronic drinkers develop ACM, suggesting a role for genetic and environmental modifiers. Roughly 80–125 g/day for >5 years is commonly cited as the threshold for ACM development, though lower intakes may be harmful in susceptible individuals.[7]

PATHOPHYSIOLOGY

The pathogenesis of ACM is complex and multifactorial **(Fig. 1)**. Several interrelated mechanisms contribute to myocardial injury.[8]

Direct Myocyte Toxicity

Ethanol and its metabolite, acetaldehyde, directly impair myocardial protein synthesis, disrupt sarcomeric organization, and interfere with excitation-contraction coupling. Chronic exposure alters calcium handling, leading to impaired contractility and arrhythmogenesis.[9]

Mitochondrial Dysfunction

Alcohol induces mitochondrial structural abnormalities, including swelling and loss of cristae. Impaired oxidative phosphorylation reduces ATP production, while excess reactive oxygen species (ROS) generation promotes cellular apoptosis.[10]

Oxidative Stress

Increased production of free radicals overwhelms antioxidant defenses, leading to lipid peroxidation, DNA damage, and protein modification.[11]

Neurohormonal Activation

Alcohol enhances sympathetic activity and renin angiotensin aldosterone system (RAAS activation, further promoting myocardial remodeling, hypertrophy, and fibrosis).[12]

Metabolic Derangement

Alcohol impairs myocardial glucose utilization and promotes fatty acid oxidation, leading to intracellular lipid accumulation and liptoxicity.[13]

Inflammatory Pathways

Chronic alcohol use upregulates cytokines such as TNF-α and interleukins, perpetuating myocardial inflammation and fibrosis.

Nutritional Deficiencies

Chronic alcoholism is commonly associated with thiamine deficiency (leading to beriberi cardiomyopathy) as well as deficiencies in folate, magnesium, and selenium, which exacerbate myocardial dysfunction.[14]

Genetic Susceptibility

Certain genetic variants, such as polymorphisms in alcohol dehydrogenase and ALDH2 enzymes, influence metabolism of ethanol and may predispose individuals to ACM.

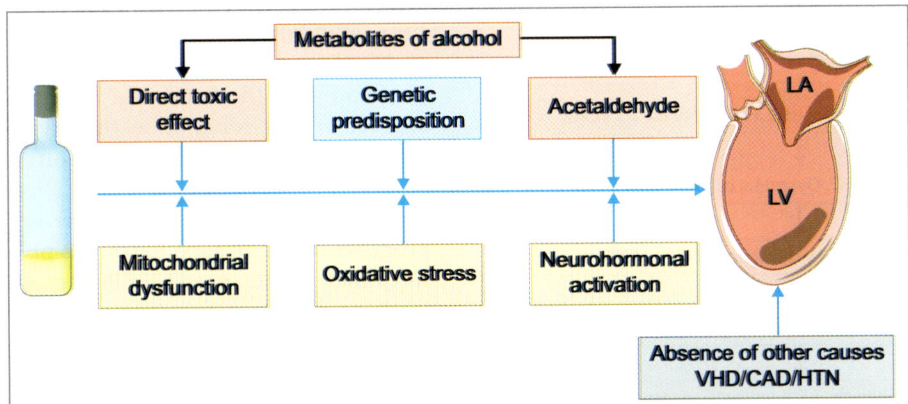

FIG. 1: Pathophysiology of alcoholic cardiomyopathy. Direct toxic effect of alcohol, effect of its metabolite acetaldehyde, and genetic predisposition lead to mitochondrial dysfunction, oxidative stress, and neurohormonal activation leading to alcoholic cardiomyopathy (ACM). Diagnosis of ACM is made in the absence of other diseases causing myocardial dysfunction.

(CAD: coronary artery disease; HTN: hypertensive heart disease; VHD: valvular heart disease)

The interplay of these mechanisms results in ventricular dilatation, wall thinning, myocardial fibrosis, and progressive systolic dysfunction.[15]

DIAGNOSTIC CRITERIA

There are no universally standardized diagnostic criteria, but most clinicians rely on the following triad.[16]

History of Chronic Heavy Alcohol Consumption

More than 80 g/day for at least 5 years, although lower thresholds may apply in women and genetically predisposed individuals.[17]

Dilated Cardiomyopathy Phenotype

Left ventricular (LV) dilatation >2 standard deviations from the normal value, with reduced ejection fraction (EF) <50% is taken as ACM where clinically suspected.[18]

Exclusion of Other Causes of Cardiomyopathy

Alcoholic cardiomyopathy diagnosis is made after excluding ischemic, valvular, genetic, or infiltrative etiologies of reduced systolic function. Given the overlap with idiopathic dilated cardiomyopathy, ACM is often a diagnosis of exclusion.[19] Diagnostic algorithm from clinical to investigations for comprehensive assessment of ACM is described in **Flowchart 1**.

CLINICAL FEATURES

Besides the history of alcoholism, there are no characteristic symptoms or signs of ACM which is different from dilated cardiomyopathy. Symptoms and signs are that of heart failure of any other etiology, though stigmata of chronic alcoholism such as hepatosplenomegaly, spider angiomas, palmar erythema, and tremors are seen in some cases.

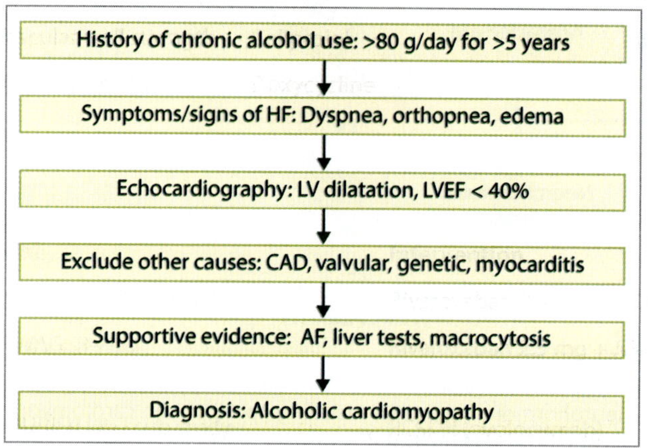

FLOWCHART 1: Diagnostic algorithm and steps in the comprehensive assessment of alcoholic cardiomyopathy.

Progressive exertional dyspnea, orthopnea, paroxysmal nocturnal dyspnea, fatigue, reduced exercise tolerance, lower limb swelling, and epigastric pain are characteristic symptoms. Palpitations, presyncope, or syncope related to atrial or ventricular arrhythmias may also occur including sudden cardiac death (SCD). Atrial fibrillation (AF) is particularly common and may precede overt ventricular dysfunction.[20]

Typical signs of congestive heart failure such as elevated JVP, displaced apical impulse, S3 gallop, pulmonary rales, hepatomegaly, ascites, and peripheral edema are seen in advance cases.

Alcohol withdrawal symptoms, macrocytic anemia, and deranged liver function tests often coexist, providing indirect evidence of chronic alcohol use.[21]

INVESTIGATIONS

Electrocardiography

Sinus tachycardia, left atrial enlargement, and left ventricular hypertrophy are common. Conduction delays such as left or right bundle branch block (LBBB or RBBB), fragmented QRS complexes may be seen **(Fig. 2)**. AF is a common association in ACM occurring in up to 38% of patients.[22] Various grades of AV block, ST and T-wave changes, and prolonged QRS are seen due to myocardial dysfunction. Electrolyte imbalances may also contribute to ECG changes. Low QRS voltages are seen in advanced cases. Paroxysmal AF may be linked to episodes of binge drinking known as holiday heart syndrome.[23]

Echocardiography

Transthoracic echocardiography (TTE) is the most common mode for diagnosis of ACM **(Figs. 3A to D)**. Dilated left ventricle >2 standard deviations from normal, global hypokinesia, and reduced LVEF to <50% as measured by biplane Simpson's method are the hallmark of ACM.[21] Various degrees of functional or secondary mitral regurgitation are present due to annular dilatation. Left atrium is usually enlarged, the volume of which should be measured as a prognostic marker and in follow-up echoes to determine progression of disease. Group 2 pulmonary hypertension secondary to increased LV filling pressure is often present in the form of high velocity tricuspid regurgitant (TR) jet. Right atrial enlargement and right ventricular dysfunction are also seen and are markers of advanced disease. Increased LV diastolic volume, increased LV mass, increased E/e' ratio are all described to be associated with ACM. Markedly decreased global longitudinal strain (GLS) is seen in ACM; GLS determined by speckle tracking can also be determined early in the course of disease before the EF is actually decreased. Other strain parameters such as twist, rotation,

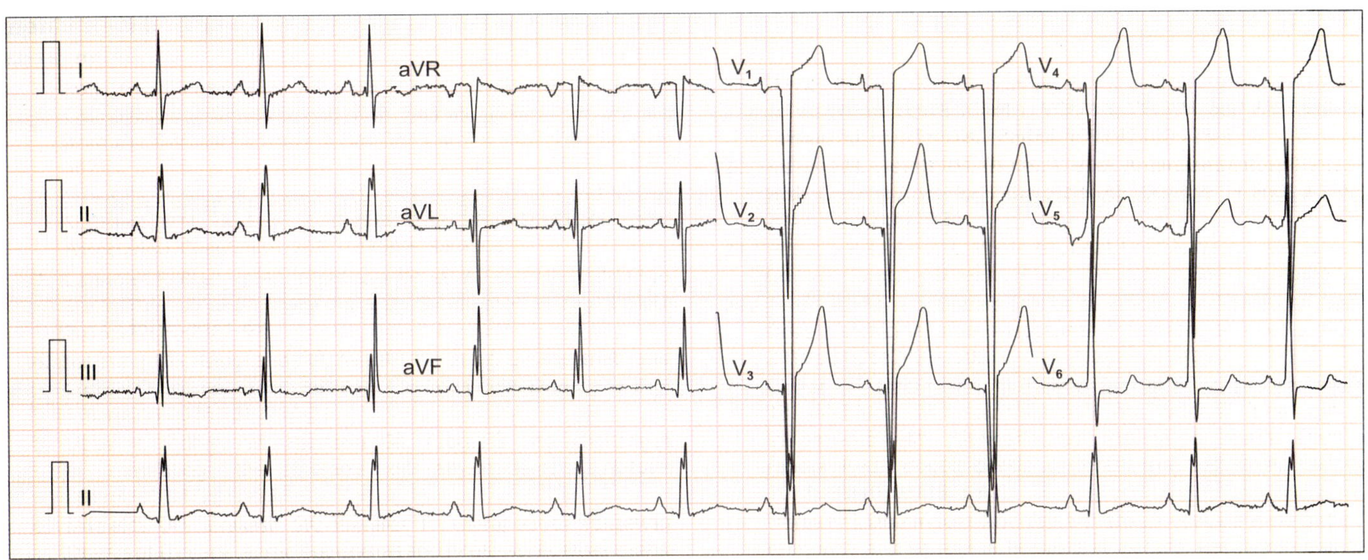

FIG. 2: ECG in a case of alcoholic cardiomyopathy showing left atrial enlargement, left ventricular hypertrophy, fragmented QRS complexes, and ST/T changes.

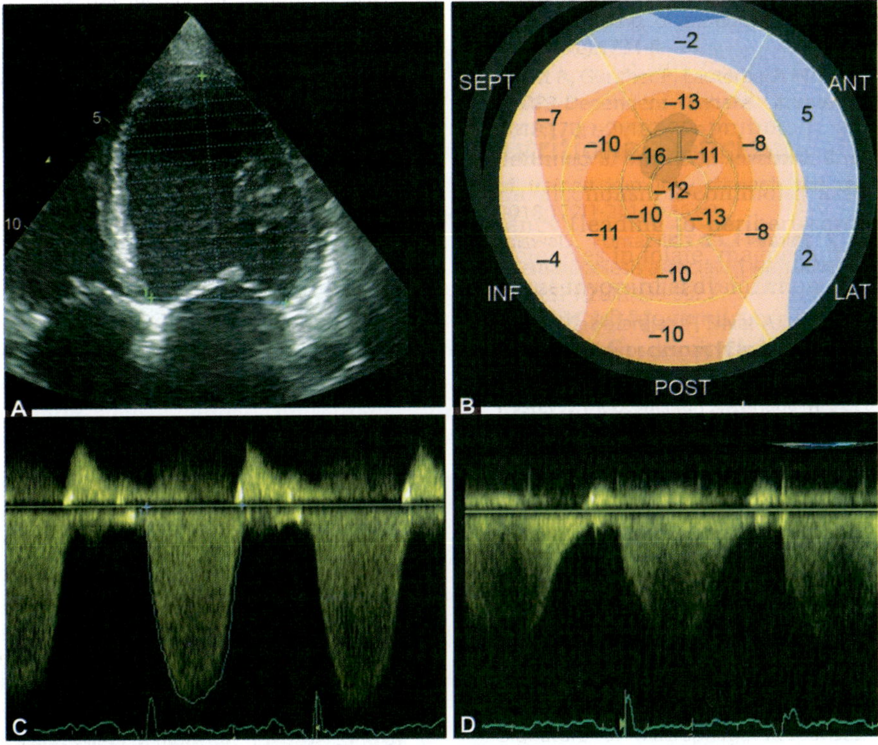

FIGS. 3A TO D: Echocardiography in a case of alcoholic cardiomyopathy. (A) 2D echo in apical 4-chamber view shows dilated left atrium and left ventricle. (B) Severely decreased global longitudinal strain is seen in the same patient. (C) Significant secondary mitral regurgitation is seen. (D) High velocity tricuspid regurgitation jet secondary to group 2 pulmonary hypertension is seen.

and circumferential strain are also studied and linked to prediction of ACM before EF reduction.[24] Early recognition of tissue Doppler and strain imaging findings should be done routinely in alcohol abusers to warn regarding progression to ACM. People with alcoholic habits can be checked with tissue Doppler and strain imaging for unexplained dyspnea and fatigue.

Cardiac Magnetic Resonance Imaging

Cardiac magnetic resonance imaging (MRI) is particularly useful for myocardial tissue characterization. Late gadolinium enhancement (LGE) in ACM is of nonischemic pattern, often patchy, mid-wall, or diffuse. MRI helps distinguish ACM from ischemic cardiomyopathy.[25]

Biomarkers

Natriuretic peptides such as BNP and NT-proBNP are used for heart failure (HF) assessment. Biomarkers of chronic alcohol intake such as gamma-glutamyl transferase (GGT) and carbohydrate-deficient transferrin (CDT), mean corpuscular volume (MCV) may be used to assess chronic alcohol consumption. Thiamine, magnesium, and folate levels should be assessed when deficiency of these nutrients is suspected.[26]

Coronary Angiography

Coronary angiography (CAG) is necessary to exclude ischemic cardiomyopathy in high-risk populations and when other evidence of coronary artery disease such as history of myocardial infarction, ECG, or echo evidence of old infarction is present.[27] CT CAG and coronary calcium scoring can be done in relevant cases.

Endomyocardial Biopsy

Endomyocardial biopsy (EMB) is not indicated to make a diagnosis of ACM. It may be performed if EF does not improve after alcohol abstinence and HF directed drugs after excluding ischemic and genetic causes. Biopsy shows nonspecific findings including myocyte hypertrophy, vacuolization, interstitial fibrosis, and lipid accumulation.[28]

DIFFERENTIAL DIAGNOSIS

Differential diagnosis includes idiopathic dilated cardiomyopathy, ischemic cardiomyopathy, tachycardia-induced cardiomyopathy, nutritional cardiomyopathies (thiamine deficiency), viral myocarditis, genetic/familial cardiomyopathies, peripartum cardiomyopathy, and infiltrative cardiomyopathy (amyloidosis and sarcoidosis). In clinical context, laboratory parameters can differentiate each of these conditions.[29]

MANAGEMENT

Alcohol Abstinence

Complete abstinence is the single most important intervention. Abstinence leads to stabilization or recovery of LV function in many patients, often within 6–12 months **(Figs. 4A and B)**. It requires structured interventions, including counseling, pharmacotherapy, and support groups. Pharmacotherapy for alcohol abstinence includes the following options.[30]

Disulfiram

Disulfiram is an aldehyde dehydrogenase (ALDH) inhibitor that causes unpleasant reactions when alcohol is consumed, deterring drinking. It is effective but should be used cautiously in mild cases of ACM without overt heart failure, as it can cause palpitations, tachycardia, chest pain, or hypotension.

Naltrexone

Naltrexone is an opioid antagonist that reduces the rewarding effects of alcohol. It is effective in reducing alcohol-related hospitalizations and does not have cardiac-related contraindications.

Acamprosate

Acamprosate is a noncompetitive N-methyl-D-aspartate (NMDA) receptor blocker that helps maintain abstinence by reducing cravings. It is also safe for use in patients with ACM.

Studies suggest that disulfiram is more effective in increasing abstinence days, but naltrexone and acamprosate

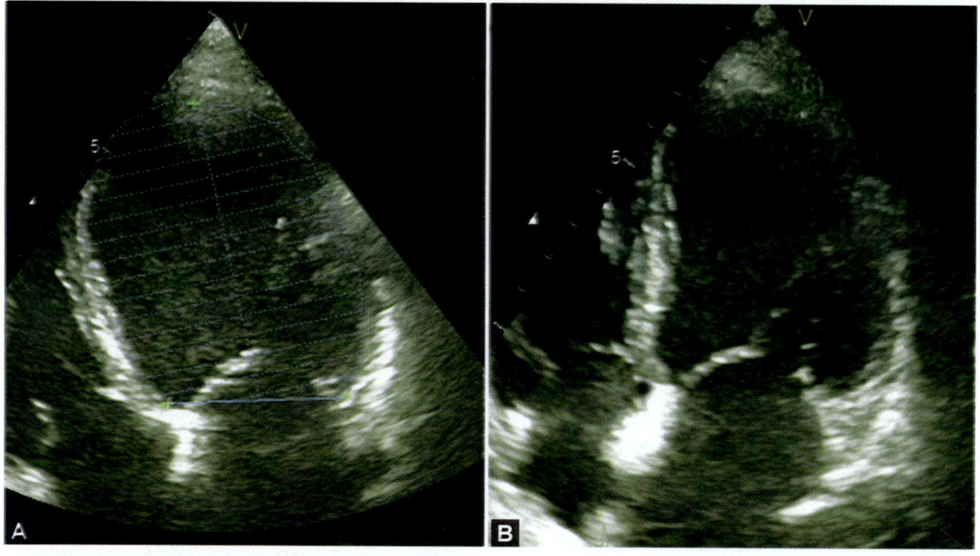

FIGS. 4A AND B: Significant improvement in left ventricular (LV) echo parameters is seen with complete abstinence. (A) Markedly dilated left ventricle is seen. (B) After 6 months of complete abstinence, the LV volume shows reduction in its volume.

are safer options for patients with cardiac conditions. Combination therapy with naltrexone and acamprosate has also shown effectiveness.[31]

Guideline-directed Medical Therapy

Guideline-directed medical therapy (GDMT) for heart failure with reduced ejection fraction (HFrEF) with ACE inhibitors/ARBs/ARNIs, beta-blockers (carvedilol, bisoprolol, and metoprolol succinate), mineralocorticoid receptor antagonists (MRAs), SGLT-2 inhibitors (dapagliflozin and empagliflozin) and diuretics for symptom relief in congestion are all indicated as in HFrEF of any other etiology.[32]

Arrhythmia Management and Device Therapy

Atrial fibrillations when present are managed by rate/rhythm control, anticoagulation based on CHA_2DS_2-VASc score. Ventricular arrhythmia treatment, implantable cardioverter defibrillator (ICD) for secondary prevention are done as indicated including cardiac resynchronization therapy (CRT) based on standard criteria. Advanced HF therapies including LV assist devices and transplantation are reserved for refractory cases. However, active alcohol use is a contraindication to heart transplant.[33] Before deciding on transplant, patients must demonstrate abstinence and psychosocial stability. Management algorithm is enumerated in **Flowchart 2**.

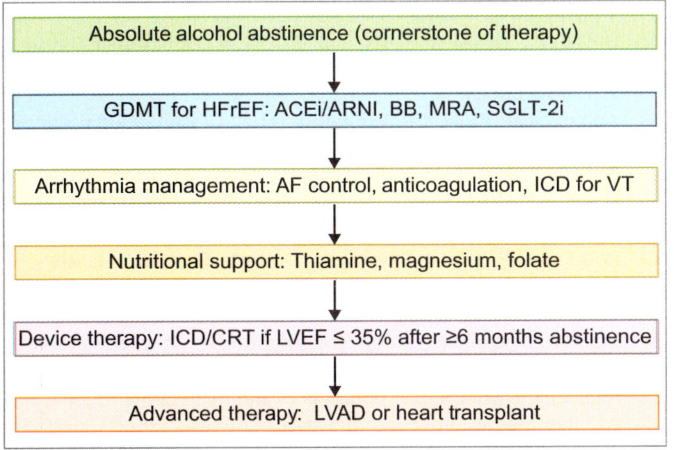

FLOWCHART 2: Management algorithm and different aspects of treatment in a case of alcoholic cardiomyopathy.

Nutritional and Lifestyle Measures

Correction of nutritional deficiency such as thiamine and multivitamin supplementation should always be done in ACM including correction of magnesium and electrolyte imbalances. Lifestyle changes such as regular exercise and low-salt, low-calorie, and high-fiber diets are part of medical management.

Prevention Strategies

Alcoholism is a familial, social, community, and economic problem with a huge economic burden. Screening for alcohol misuse and patient education are essential. Public education in educational institutions, in medias, and in general educational curriculum is essential to educate children in their formative age against the perils of alcohol abuse, so that they do not initiate alcohol consumption.[34]

PROGNOSIS

Prognosis is strongly determined by alcohol abstinence. Patients who achieve sustained abstinence have 5-year survival rates comparable to those with idiopathic DCM. Continued alcohol use is associated with progressive HF, recurrent arrhythmias, and higher mortality. Predictors of poor prognosis are persistent alcohol use, advanced LV dysfunction at diagnosis, coexistent liver disease, and recurrent arrhythmias **(Table 1)**. Women are more vulnerable at lower doses of alcohol and do worse if ACM develops. Coexistent cirrhosis complicates prognosis and management. Genetic screening and counseling are required for families with alcohol exposure.[35]

CONCLUSION

Alcoholic cardiomyopathy is a distinct, preventable, and potentially reversible cause of dilated cardiomyopathy. A high index of suspicion of alcoholism by physicians is essential to identify ACM in dilated cardiomyopathy. Early recognition and intervention centered around alcohol abstinence and guideline-directed heart failure therapy can dramatically improve outcomes. As alcohol use continue to increase among younger generation and women, ACM will remain a key focus in the management of nonischemic dilated cardiomyopathies and its prevention.

TABLE 1: Prognostic factors in alcoholic cardiomyopathy. Left-side column shows favorable factors and right-side column shows factors associated with poor prognosis.

Favorable prognostic factors	Poor prognostic factors
Sustained alcohol abstinence	Continued alcohol consumption
Early diagnosis and treatment	Advanced LV dysfunction at diagnosis
Good response to GDMT	Coexistent liver cirrhosis
Absence of major arrhythmias	Recurrent ventricular arrhythmias

REFERENCES

1. Mustroph J, Baier MJ, Unsin D, et al. Ethanol-induced atrial fibrillation results from late INa and can be prevented by ranolazine. Circulation. 2023;148:698-700.
2. Mustroph J, Drzymalski M, Baier M, et al. The Ca/calmodulin-dependent kinase II inhibitor RA608 improves contractile function and prevents arrhythmias in heart failure. ESC Heart Fail. 2020;7:2871-83.
3. Luczak ED, Wu Y, Granger JM, et al. Mitochondrial CaMKII causes adverse metabolic reprogramming and dilated cardiomyopathy. Nat Commun. 2020;11:4416.
4. Seferović PM, Tsutsui H, McNamara DM, et al. Heart Failure Association of the ESC, Heart Failure Society of America and Japanese Heart Failure Society position statement on endomyocardial biopsy. Eur J Heart Fail. 2021;23:854-71.
5. Tayal U, Gregson J, Buchan R, et al. Moderate excess alcohol consumption and adverse cardiac remodelling in dilated cardiomyopathy. Heart. 2022;108:619-25.
6. Artico J, Merlo M, Asher C, et al. The alcohol-induced cardiomyopathy: a cardiovascular magnetic resonance characterization. Int J Cardiol. 2021;331:131-7.
7. Lazarević AM, Nakatani S, Nešković AN, et al. Early changes in left ventricular function in chronic asymptomatic alcoholics: relation to the duration of heavy drinking. J Am Coll Cardiol. 2000;35: 1599-606.
8. McDonagh TA, Metra M, Adamo M, et al. 2021 ESC guidelines for the diagnosis and treatment of acute and chronic heart failure. Developed by the task force for the diagnosis and treatment of acute and chronic heart failure of the European Society of Cardiology (ESC) with the special contribution of the Heart Failure Association (HFA) of the ESC. Eur Heart J. 2021;42:3599-726.
9. Heidenreich PA, Bozkurt B, Aguilar D, et al. 2022 AHA/ACC/HFSA guideline for the management of heart failure: a report of the American College of Cardiology/American Heart Association joint committee on clinical practice guidelines. Circulation. 2022; 145:E895-1032.
10. SEC Working Group for the 2021 ESC guidelines for the diagnosis and treatment of acute and chronic heart failure and SEC Guidelines Committee. Comments to the 2021 ESC guidelines for the diagnosis and treatment of acute and chronic heart failure. Rev Esp Cardiol. 2022;75:458-65.
11. Zeppenfeld K, Tfelt-Hansen J, de Riva M, et al. 2022 ESC guidelines for the management of patients with ventricular arrhythmias and the prevention of sudden cardiac death. Eur Heart J. 2022;43: 3997-4126.
12. Soulaidopoulos S, Goulis I, Cholongitas E. Pulmonary manifestations of chronic liver disease: a comprehensive review. Ann Gastroenterol. 2020;33:237-49.
13. Liu H, Nguyen HH, Yoon KT, et al. Pathogenic mechanisms underlying cirrhotic cardiomyopathy. Front Netw Physiol. 2022;2:849253.
14. Park SK, Moon K, Ryoo JH, et al. The association between alcohol consumption and left ventricular diastolic function and geometry change in general Korean population. Eur Heart J Cardiovasc Imaging. 2018;19:271-8.
15. Andersson C, Schou M, Gustafsson F, et al. Alcohol intake in patients with cardiomyopathy and heart failure: consensus and controversy. Circ Heart Fail. 2022;15:e009459.
16. Biddinger KJ, Emdin CA, Haas ME, et al. Association of habitual alcohol intake with risk of cardiovascular disease. JAMA Netw Open. 2022;5:e223849.
17. Lota AS, Hazebroek MR, Theotokis P, et al. Genetic architecture of acute myocarditis and the overlap with inherited cardiomyopathy. Circulation. 2022;146:1123-34.
18. Tsai MK, Gao W, Wen CP. The relationship between alcohol consumption and health: J-shaped or less is more? BMC Med. 2023;21:228.
19. Negreira-Caamaño M, Abellán-Huerta J. La paradoja del consumo de alcohol: cautela ante una evidencia en desarrollo. Rev Esp Cardiol. 2022;75:190-1.
20. Manivannan A, Schou M, Monahan KM, et al. Prognostic importance of atrial fibrillation and anticoagulation in alcoholic versus dilated cardiomyopathy. Alcohol Alcohol. 2023;58:159-63.
21. Fernández-Solà J. The effects of ethanol on the heart: alcoholic cardiomyopathy. Nutrients. 2020;12:572.
22. Fauchier L, Babuty D, Poret P, et al. Comparison of long-term outcome of alcoholic and idiopathic dilated cardiomyopathy. Eur Heart J. 2000;21:306-14.
23. Gavazzi A, De Maria R, Parolini M, et al. Alcohol abuse and dilated cardiomyopathy in men. Am J Cardiol. 2000;85:1114-8.
24. Piano MR, Mazzuco A, Kang M, et al. Cardiovascular consequences of binge drinking: an integrative review with implications for advocacy, policy, and research. Alcohol Clin Exp Res. 2017;41:487-96.
25. Mustroph J, Wagemann O, Lebek S, et al. SR Ca^{2+}-leak and disordered excitation-contraction coupling as the basis for arrhythmogenic and negative inotropic effects of acute ethanol exposure. J Mol Cell Cardiol. 2018;116:81-90.
26. Garcia-Pavia P, Kim Y, Restrepo-Cordoba MA, et al. Genetic variants associated with cancer therapy-induced cardiomyopathy. Circulation. 2019;140:31-41.
27. Huizar JF, Ellenbogen KA, Tan AY, et al. Arrhythmia-induced cardiomyopathy: JACC state-of-the-art review. J Am Coll Cardiol. 2019;73:2328-44.
28. Aggarwal M, Bozkurt B, Panjrath G, et al. Lifestyle modifications for preventing and treating heart failure. J Am Coll Cardiol. 2018;72:2391-405.
29. Day E, Rudd JHF. Alcohol use disorders and the heart. Addiction. 2019;114:1670-8.
30. Rodrigues P, Santos-Ribeiro S, Teodoro T, et al. Association between alcohol intake and cardiac remodeling. J Am Coll Cardiol. 2018;72:1452-62.
31. Maisch B. Alcoholic cardiomyopathy: the result of dosage and individual predisposition. Herz. 2016;41:484-93.
32. Münzel T, Daiber A. The potential of aldehyde dehydrogenase 2 as a therapeutic target in cardiovascular disease. Expert Opin Ther Targets. 2018;22:217-31.
33. Mustroph J, Lebek S, Maier LS, et al. Mechanisms of cardiac ethanol toxicity and novel treatment options. Pharmacol Ther. 2019;197:1-10.
34. Kim Y, Hack LM, Ahn ES, et al. Practical outpatient pharmacotherapy for alcohol use disorder. Drugs Context. 2018;7:212308.
35. Li H, Liu FY, Li XL, et al. Clinical effects of carvedilol and trimetazidine for the treatment of alcoholic myocardiopathy. Exp Ther Med. 2016;12:979-82.

SECTION

7

Congenital Heart Disease

Section Outline

48. Expanding Future of Sinus Venosus Atrial Septal Defect Closure
Rishika Mehta, Amitabha Chattopadhyay

49. Clinical Risk Assessment and Prediction in Congenital Heart Disease Across the Lifespan
Anita Saxena

50. Early Intervention for Tetralogy of Fallot, but at What Cost?
Mahua Roy, Sucheta Barman

51. Novel Imaging Techniques for Congenital Heart Disease
D Seshagiri Rao, Ramya Pechetty

52. Evaluation and Management of Chronic Heart Failure in Children and Adolescents with Congenital Heart Disease
Jonaki Pal, Debasree Gangopadhyay

53. Advancing New Solutions for Adult Congenital Heart Diseases-related Heart Failure
Prafulla Kerkar, Ujjwala Tulluri

54. Care for Congenital Heart Disease in India: The Evolving Landscape
R Krishna Kumar

55. Echocardiography for Childhood Left Ventricular Noncompaction
Sura Kishore Mishra, Bitan Mohanty

56. Adults with Congenital Heart Disease: What Every Cardiologist Should Know About Their Care?
Arun Gopalakrishnan, Shyam S Kothari

57. Quest for a Lifelong Pulmonary Valve in Repaired Tetralogy of Fallot
Ronak Sheth, Snehal Kulkarni

CHAPTER 48

Expanding Future of Sinus Venosus Atrial Septal Defect Closure

Rishika Mehta, Amitabha Chattopadhyay

ABSTRACT

The gold standard of correction of sinus venosus atrial septal defect (SV-ASD) has been surgery since ages with redirection of the superior vena cava (SVC) flow to the right atrium and that of the partial anomalous right pulmonary vein to the left atrium. The last decade has revolutionized the treatment of SV-ASD in the cardiac catheterization laboratory by placing a covered stent in the SVC and flaring its lower end in the right atrium, which redirects flow of the anomalous vein back to the left atrium (LA), making transcatheter closure of the defect possible. This technique was first described by Abdullah et al. at the Congenital and Structural Interventions conference in Frankfurt in 2013, and the series from Evelina Children's hospital in London (Hansen).[1]

Keywords: SV-ASD, transcatheter, stenting, RUPV obstruction.

INTRODUCTION

Sinus venosus atrial septal defect (SV-ASD) is the most common interatrial communication outside the fossa ovalis. They make up 5% of ASDs, of which 90% are superior defects. Surgical repair of SVD is in totality excellent with a very low mortality of less than 1%, but like all other open-heart procedures, there is a morbidity of sternotomy and cardiopulmonary bypass. A single-patch, double-patch, or the Warden procedures are performed to close the defect. The double-patch technique uses one patch to close the ASD and another to enlarge the SVC at the cavoatrial junction. The right atrium (RA) incision extends onto the SVC, and so the sinus node may undergo iatrogenic dysfunction requiring pacemaker implantation.

Unlike patch procedures, the Warden procedure though avoids a cavoatrial incision and the risk of sinus node damage; however, SVC obstruction has been described. 2–8.6% sinus node dysfunction, 2.7–7.7% pulmonary vein, and SVC obstruction have been reported in a meta-analysis of over 900 patients. However, individual series report higher complication rates, as high as sinus node dysfunction in 35%, right upper pulmonary vein (RUPV) obstruction in 22.5%, SVC narrowing or obstruction in 20%, and postoperative atrial fibrillation in 14%. Warden operation uses an interposition graft, which can cause complications of thrombosis. Hence, in the last decade, transcatheter repair has become a feasible and encouraging option for SV-ASD repair.

Choosing the right patient, preprocedural screening, multimodality imaging for case planning and guidance, 3D modeling, balloon interrogation of the SVC, and procedural steps are the keys to a successful percutaneous intervention. The procedural concept depends upon understanding the anatomy of the defect. The RUPV ostium, the SVC orifice, the RA, and the left atrium (LA) form a crossroad above the level of the unroofed atrial septum **(Figs. 1A to D)**.

UNDERSTANDING THE ANATOMY OF THE SUPERIOR SINUS VENOSUS ATRIAL SEPTAL DEFECT

Embryologically SV-ASD results from deficient infolding of the atrial wall, which forms the SVC posterior wall and RUPV anterior wall. It lies inferior to the SVC–RA junction. The RUPV drains into the SVC mouth in the RA rather than the LA. It is almost always associated with anomalous connection of one or more of the right-sided pulmonary veins. Caudal the defect, more are the chances of PAPVC of the inferior right pulmonary vein **(Figs. 1A to D)**.

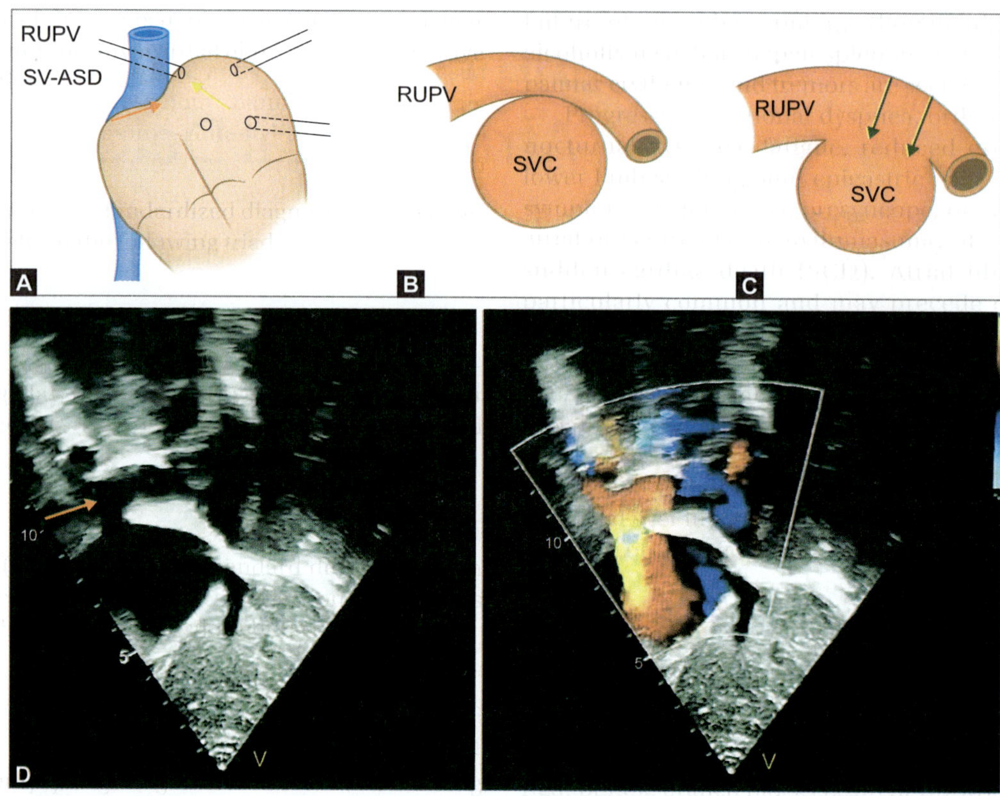

FIGS. 1A TO D: Pictorial diagram depicting the 2D gap in the IAS, just below the SVC–RA junction, marked with the red arrow—the sinus venosus defect (A). The RUPV and the SVC share a common wall, as depicted in (B). The yellow arrow points toward the RUPV orifice in the LA, which drains into the RA instead of the LA, because the common wall between the RUPV and the SVC is missing in these cases (green arrows) (C). The echocardiographic equivalent from the subcostal view is shown in **Figure B**, with a left to right flow (D).

CONCEPT OF THE TRANSCATHETER CLOSURE A

A long, covered stent is to be positioned in the SVC–RA junction to close the defect, so that the SVC flow is directed into the RA and the RUPV flow around the stent is redirected into the LA. The technique might seem simple but requires detailed multimodality preprocedural planning.[2] A proper transesophageal echocardiogram (TEE), balloon interrogation of the SVC echocardiographically as well as angiographically, computed tomography (CT) scan, sometimes patient-specific 3D printed models with simulation of stent implantation, and holographic augmented reality are needed for optimal planning. Proper measurements of SVC diameter at various levels and the length for correct choice of stent and balloon to achieve accurate placement of the stent are the keys to a successful procedure **(Figs. 2A to D)**.

PLANNING AND IMAGING

Transthoracic Echocardiography and Transesophageal Echocardiography

They are the primary imaging modalities used to assess the defect size and position, its dimensions, pulmonary venous drainage, single or bilateral SVC, tricuspid regurgitation, and RV and LV function.

Electrocardiography-gated Cardiac Computed Tomography

It first confirms the diagnosis and is used to assess the defect, its anatomy, and the surrounding structures. The exact delineation of the shape and the size of the defect, length and diameter of the SVC at the caudal and the cranial ends of the defect, the presence of single or bilateral SVCs, the pulmonary venous drainage, presence and the number of anomalously draining veins, their diameter, the location and relationship with the defect—whether it is too high or low which might not be amenable to percutaneous closure, and the presence of any accessory veins, are the points to be noted. However, a smaller accessory vein of low hemodynamic significance draining into the SVC away from the SVC–RA junction and higher than the main RUPV, especially if it is too far to be surgically addressed and the flow volume can be confirmed on cardiac MRI, is not a contraindication for percutaneous closure.

Patients with bilateral SVC with an absence of interconnecting vein are excellent candidates for percutaneous closure as right SVC is smaller than the normal size; there is

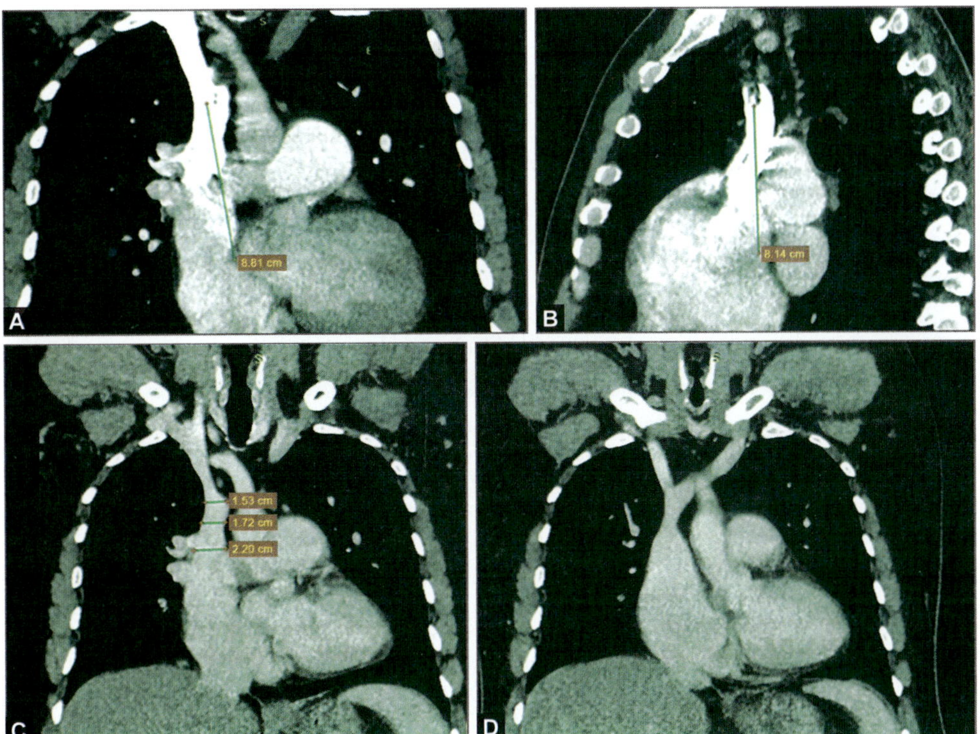

FIGS. 2A TO D: (A and B) Length of the covered stent estimated in coronal and sagittal sections of CT angiogram; (C) The diameter of the SVC is measured at multiple points in the coronal section; (D) The distance of the innominate vein from the SVC–RA junction is measured, to estimate the length available for anchoring of the stent.

a longer landing zone which helps in firm stent placement without the risk of innominate vein obstruction as higher stent placement is possible. Interruption of the inferior vena cava with azygos continuation should be ruled out in CT **(Figs. 3A to C)**.

Specific CT acquisition protocol should be implemented to achieve all the desired information. The box of acquisition should cover the entire thorax including the heart, the SVC, and the innominate vein with allowance for the delay of acquisitions for opacifications of both the systemic venous return and pulmonary venous return and performing submillimeter slicing to the spatial resolution.

Cardiac Magnetic Resonance Imaging

It is not usually required for planning the procedure. It can be used as a complimentary imaging technique for flow dynamic assessment of the shunt, and in some cases for confirming the flow from the anomalous accessory RUPV branches in few selected cases.

3D Printing

Even after a detailed echocardiogram and CT scan, virtual 3D model simulation and 3D printing seems suitable in selected cases to prevent procedural failure due to the variable and complex anatomical features of SV-ASD and their variable morphology. This helps to convert medical images obtained with the CT scan into a physical model, which replicates the anatomical study which can even be converted to simulation models, so that technique optimization, stent placement, and size selection in SVD closure can be done. If the software are integrated, the 3D CT scan data set can be merged with fluoroscopy for better procedural guidance.

Procedure

All procedures should be performed under general anesthesia with transesophageal echocardiographic and fluoroscopic guidance. Both right and left internal jugular veins, both right and left femoral veins, and the left femoral arterial accesses are to be taken. Intravenous heparin is given to keep the activated clotting time between 200 and 250 seconds. Atrial septal puncture is done using a Brockenbrough needle inside an 8F Mullins sheath through the left femoral vein access, and a 5F MPA II catheter is positioned in the RUPV throughout the procedure to monitor pressures and give injections for visualization and possible balloon protection. Innominate vein injection can be given through the LIJV access, if any or by passing a 5F RCA catheter through the RIJV access into the innominate vein, in the anteroposterior view. This injection helps us to assess the distance of the innominate vein from the SVC–RA junction, whereby the available landing zone for the stent may be estimated. If there are bilateral SVCs with no innominate vein, this same injection may be obtained by a dye flush through the RIJV access **(Fig. 4)**.

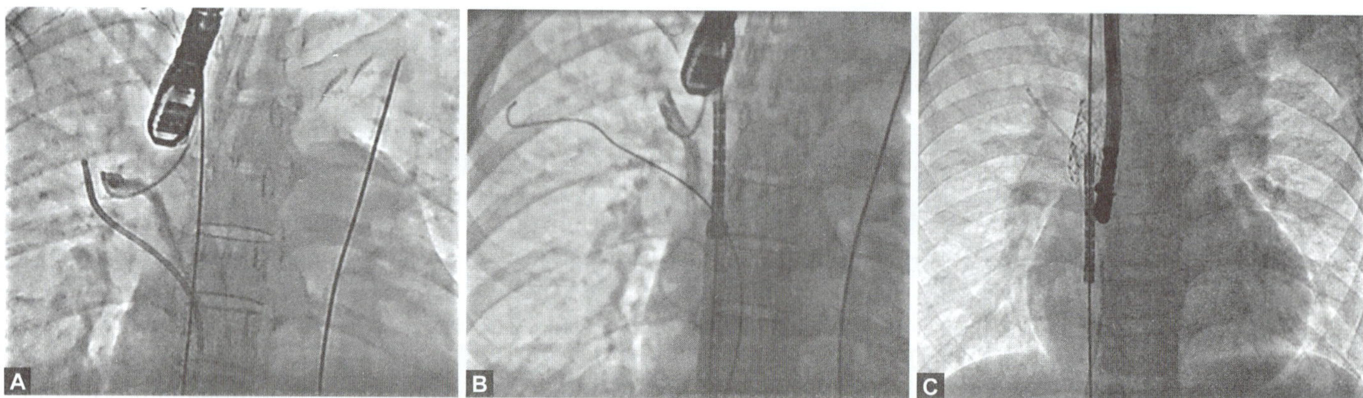

FIGS. 3A TO C: Angiographic views, depicting an additional pulmonary vein, above the RUPV (marked by 5F multipurpose catheter, through the septostomy) (A), while another additional right-sided pulmonary vein is seen to be draining into the SVC, opacified by the dye through the 5F RCA catheter from the internal jugular vein access (B). While closing the defect, special precautions were taken so as *not* to obstruct the upper vein, hence a separate anchoring stent was provided, thereafter the covered stent was placed below it, in a telescoping manner, so as not to cause any obstructions to any of the pulmonary veins (C).

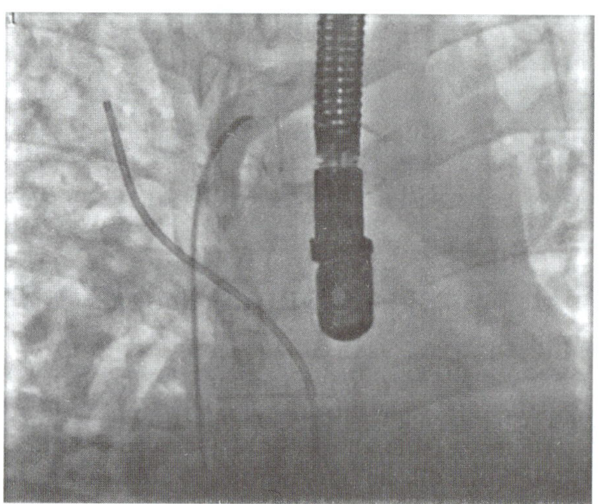

FIG. 4: Innominate vein injection through a MP catheter from the groin access, giving an estimation of the distance from the innominate to the SVC–RA junction.

BALLOON INTERROGATION OF THE SINUS VENOSUS ATRIAL SEPTAL DEFECT

A venovenous loop is formed from the right femoral vein to the RIJV and an 0.035-Lunderquist wire (Cook Medical) is exteriorized via the RIJV. An Amplatzer sizing balloon (Abbott) or a balloon 2–4 mm larger than the SVC diameter measured on CT imaging is chosen, if the sizing balloon is not available. A Z-Med (Nu Med) or Atlas (Andramed) of the desired diameter of 60 or 80 mm length is inflated in the anticipated stent landing zone until TEE confirms abolition of the shunt and the unobstructed flow in the RUPV. An increase in gradient of more than 4 mm on continuous Doppler across the RUPV–LA poses a high risk of obstruction of RUPV flow during stent implantation. The same findings are reconfirmed using angiograms; SVC flow occlusion is confirmed by an SVC angiogram through the RIJV, and RUPV patency is checked from the MPA-II catheter placed inside the RUPV. If any obstruction of the RUPV is seen, the "protective balloon technique" can be used by placing a noncompliant balloon—8–12 mm depending upon the size of the RUPV during stent implantation inside the SVC. It helps to prevent excessive bulging of the SVC stent into the pulmonary vein **(Figs. 5A and B)**.

COVERED STENT IMPLANTATION

This is the step where the complexity of the procedure begins as stent placement in the SVC is challenging due to the patulous and distensible nature of SVC at its cranial end. Also, there is absence of stenosis, which would provide a landing zone to anchor the stent at the cranial end. The caudal end of the stent is to be placed in a manner where the complete defect gets covered without obstructing the entry of RUPV into the LA, which might require the flaring of the caudal end up to three times the stent diameter causing an unpredictable degree of foreshortening.

The diameter of the balloon is chosen, which is 4 mm larger than the measured SVC diameter. A balloon expandable stent is crimped over the desired balloon (manually or with a commercially available crimper) and is advanced through a large sheath (16F Cook or 14-Fr Dry Seal based on the availability) from the right femoral vein over the Lunderquist wire. The stent is deployed by balloon inflation and the stability of the stent is assessed. Postdilation can be performed at the upper part to further stabilize the stent. Thereafter the unobstructed flow of the pulmonary vein to the left atrium and the presence of residual flow are assessed on the TEE and angiography, and postdilation of the lower part of the stent is to be performed with a larger balloon until

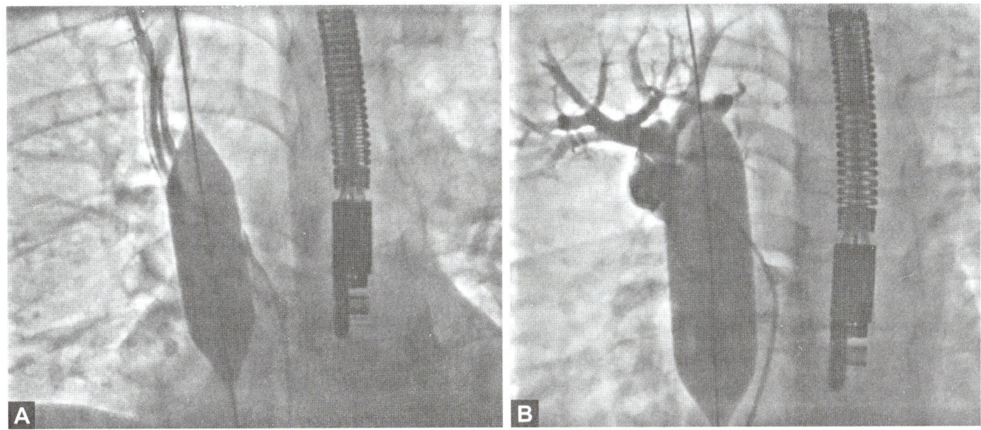

FIGS. 5A AND B: (A) SVC injection postballoon occlusion—demonstrating there are no residual flows while the SVC had been blocked totally by balloon inflation, without causing any flow impedance to the RUPV, which is draining into the LA without any obstruction (B).

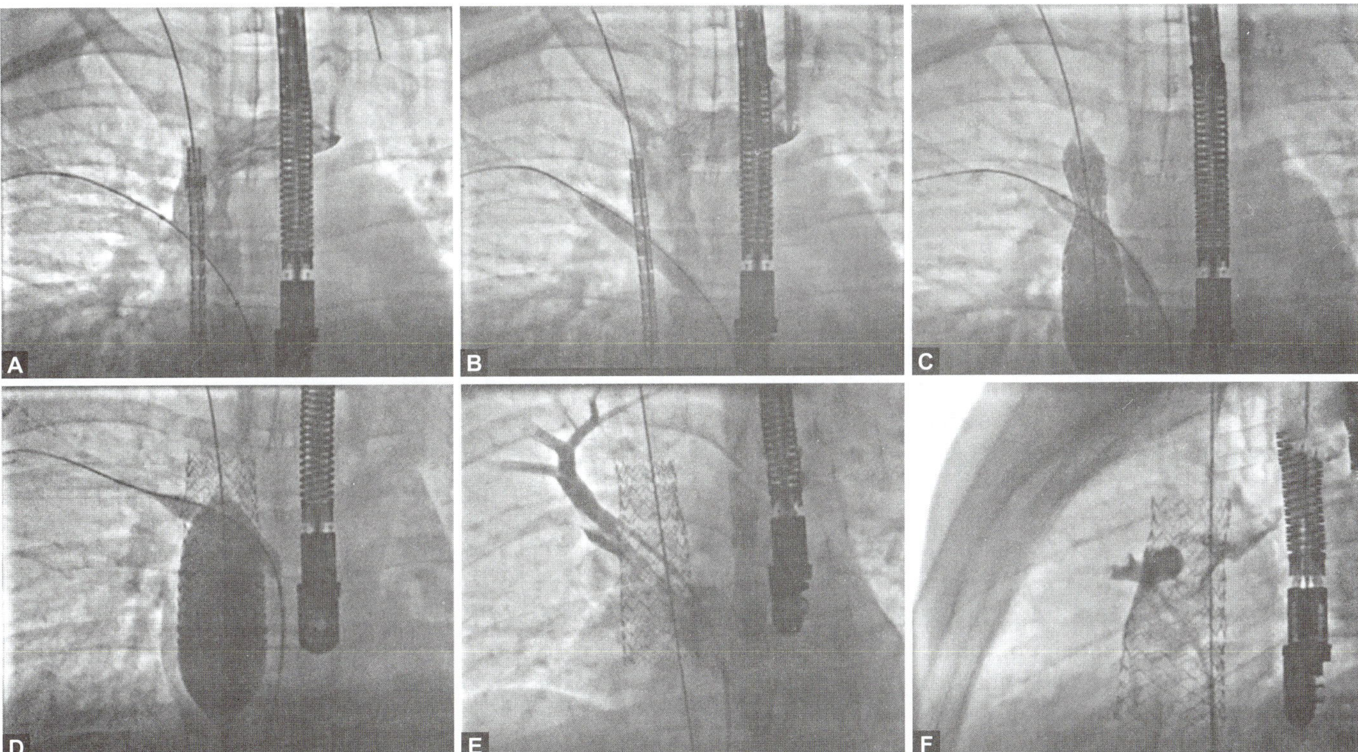

FIGS. 6A TO F: Delivery of the stent: (A) Passage of the stent crimped on the balloon over the Lunderquist wire, through the 16F delivery system; (B) Stent position being confirmed with innominate vein injection, with the RUPV balloon protection on; (C) The balloon stent assembly being inflated up to a predetermined diameter; (D) Lower end of the stent being flared, so as to appose the stent with the upper edge of the remaining part of the IAS; (E and F) Unobstructed pulmonary venous return after deployment of the stent, both from AP and lateral views.

any residual shunt is obliterated. Small residual flow may disappear over time when the enlarged RA shall remodel to a smaller size, which shall allow the caudal edge of the defect to oppose to the covered stent. Another stent can be used telescoping the previous one if the whole defect is not covered using the original stent. The jailing of the azygous vein is not given any significance. The innominate vein should be free to drain in the SVC **(Figs. 6A to F)**.

CHOICE OF STENTS AND BALLOONS

Since the early reports, procedures mainly used a 10-zig-covered CP stent, but the use of other covered balloon expandable stents—Zephyr (Sahajanand Laser Technology); Advanta V; Andra Stent (AndraMed GmbH); Optimus—CVS (AndraTec); BeGraft (Bentley InnoMed); long G-ARMOR (Numed Inc.), and self-expandable stents has been reported. The 10-zig-covered CP stent is available in lengths of 50, 55, and 60 mm. The stent was initially available in versions up to 110 mm length and up to 34-mm diameter. However, as the lengths above 60 mm did not receive CE mark, they are not very widely available. The Optimus XXL covered stent (15-zig design) has been used for pre stenting for percutaneous pulmonary valve implantation and aortic coarctation, and a covered 99-mm-long Optimus is specifically designed for SV-ASD correction. Balloons available for mounting purposes are BIB balloon, Gemini Balloon (AndraTec GmbH), which inflates like a BIB balloon and Z-Med (NuMed).

An open-cell "hybrid stent" consisting of a partially covered and partially uncovered stent—Zephyr (Sahajanand Laser Technology); Optimus Stent (AndraTec GmbH) have recently found use as the cranial bare portion gives a longer anchorage without obstructing additional veins or the innominate vein. However, what might still create a problem is positioning of the covered portion, and the bare end might still crush the additional PV orifice.

COMPLICATIONS AND TECHNICAL MODIFICATIONS

Stent Instability and Migration

Stent instability is caused due to a shorter segment apposed to the SVC, i.e., if the distance between the cranial end of the stent and the beginning of the flared segment is not long enough and the firm apposition of the stent is not achieved. Various technical modifications have evolved to provide stent stability and prevent stent migration.

Anchor Stent

When it is felt that the apposition is short and insufficient to provide secure anchoring, an additional overlapping bare-metal stent is deployed in the upper segment of the SVC below the innominate vein, so that it overlaps the cranial portion of the covered stent. If the initial stent is long enough, the need of the anchoring stent becomes minimal **(Figs. 3A to C)**.

Landing Zone Stent

A bare metal stent which is supposed to grip the SVC better forms a landing zone inside which the covered stent is deployed. However, it is noticed that the covered stent might migrate from landing zone stent while dilating the caudal end of the stent to achieve complete closure.

Sandwich Stent

A landing zone bare-metal stent was placed in the SVC followed by a covered CP stent, and the top end sandwiched with a third bare-metal stent. It locks the covered stent and prevents the later migration of the stent; however, it is expensive.

Jugular Suture Control Technique

Jugular suture-holding technique was first described by Hejazi et al., which allows precise placement of stent using a surgical suture, which is looped around the uncovered strut of the stent.[3] The stent-balloon assembly is then advanced from the RIJV into the RA by pushing on the stent and pulling the balloon from the RFV into the RIJV sheath. After that a small vascular balloon is inflated, and the stent is partially expanded in the SVC, and the stent position is readjusted. This balloon is then removed, and the desired balloon is put inside the stent for full dilatation with the suture being held. After the desired position and diameter are achieved, the suture is released.

Pulmonary Vein Stenosis or Occlusion

The RUPV obstruction is an uncommon entity as it is already confirmed during balloon interrogation of the defect. However, still few techniques are applied to prevent any vein stenosis **(Figs. 5A and B)**.

Pulmonary Vein Balloon Rescue Technique

A noncompliant vascular balloon is inflated during the time of SVC stent dilatation, so that it indents the SVC stent without causing the vein obstruction.[4]

Pulmonary Vein Stent Rescue Technique

A stent is overdilated into the pulmonary vein, it can mold the stent toward SVC and restore adequate flow.

Innominate Vein Obstruction

It can be prevented by using a hybrid stent (Zephyr or Optimus) where the cranial uncovered portion can prevent the occlusion innominate vein.

ABSOLUTE CONTRAINDICATIONS FOR SUPERIOR VENA CAVA STENTING IN SINUS VENOSUS ATRIAL SEPTAL DEFECT

Right pulmonary vein obstruction during balloon interrogation of the SVC in a patient in whom pulmonary vein balloon protection is expected to fail.

FOLLOW-UP

All patients undergoing SVC stenting for the defect receive aspirin for 6 months; some centers use concomitant clopidogrel for 2 months. A comprehensive clinical evaluation, a 12-lead electrocardiogram, and transthoracic echocardiography should be performed at 3, 6, and 12 months after the procedure. A CT scan should be performed at 2–3 months to evaluate the stent position and the pulmonary venous drainage.

FUTURE

Early- and medium-term results are promising; longer follow-up studies are required to see the role of this transcutaneous intervention and the need for follow-up, especially in children.

CONCLUSION

Transcatheter correction of SV-ASD using a covered stent is a safe and effective alternative to surgery in carefully selected patients. It achieves physiological redirection of venous flow while avoiding sternotomy and bypass-related morbidity. With advances in imaging, stent technology, and procedural planning, outcomes are promising. Long-term studies are warranted to confirm durability and assess results, especially in younger patients.

REFERENCES

1. Hansen JH, Duong P, Jivanji SGM, et al. Transcatheter Correction of Superior Sinus Venosus Atrial Septal Defects as an Alternative to Surgical Treatment. J Am Coll Cardiol. 2020;75(11):1266-78.
2. Baruteau AE, Hascoet S, Malekzadeh-Milani S, et al. Transcatheter Closure of Superior Sinus Venosus Defects. JACC Cardiovasc Interv. 2023;16(21):2587-99.
3. Hejazi Y, Hijazi ZM, Saloos HA, et al. Novel technique for transcatheter closure of sinus venosus atrial septal defect: The temporary suture-holding technique. Catheter Cardiovasc Interv. 2022;100(6):1068-77.
4. Rosenthal E, Jones MI. Covered Stent Correction of Sinus Venosus Atrial Septal Defects—Continued Technical Modifications Drive the Procedure Forward. J Soc Cardiovasc Angiogr Interv. 2025;4(2):102572.

CHAPTER

49

Clinical Risk Assessment and Prediction in Congenital Heart Disease Across the Lifespan

Anita Saxena

ABSTRACT

With timely management, over 90% of children born with congenital heart disease (CHD) survive to adulthood. However, for vast majority long-term surveillance is required due to various morbidities that may arise as they age. Risk assessment and prediction of adverse events aid the clinician in decision-making and management. Besides the complexity of CHD, a number of cofounders, such as residual defects, hemodynamic and electrophysiological abnormalities, presence of genetic syndrome, etc., affect long-term prognosis due to intervening events from time-to-time. Several prediction models are available for adults with acquired heart disease, but very few for CHDs. This is due to the relatively heterogenous population of CHDs, the complexity of disease, varying from simple lesions such as atrial septal defect, to very complex lesions like univentricular hearts. Most available risk scores are derived from retrospective studies and are not validated in large cohorts. As the population of adults with CHD is growing, we need better risk assessment tools and prediction models, not only to prognosticate but to guide appropriate therapy. In the era of big data, use of artificial intelligence should be the way forward for creating validated prediction models for CHD patients.

Keywords: Congenital heart disease, risk assessment, risk scores, lifespan.

INTRODUCTION

Advances in surgical and catheter-based procedures have resulted in long-term survival of patients with congenital heart disease (CHD). If treated in time, over 90% of children survive to adulthood as is evident in high income countries.[1] In these regions, adults exceed the number of children with CHD.[2] However, in low- and middle-income countries, significant proportions do not have access to timely management and continue to face adverse events. Mortality, in-hospital or 30-day after the procedure has been the main consideration in 1990s.[3] As the postintervention population is increasing, even in developing countries, greater emphasis is being placed on long-term morbidity, need for intervention, and mortality. Whenever a child with CHD is advised surgery or an intervention, the expected question from the parents is related to long-term prognosis and quality of life. Therefore, risk assessment through development of risk prediction models is an obvious need for such patients. Prediction models estimate the risk of a certain outcome in an individual patient across the lifespan. This information helps the clinician to inform patients and their parents about prognosis over a long period of time and aids the clinician in decision-making and management of the patient. These models are primarily derived from risk assessment of the disease and the hazard ratios.

RISK ASSESSMENT

As for any disease, risk is the probability of an adverse event or set of events over a given period. Lifetime risk should include both mortality and morbidity. This period in CHD, native or postintervention, relates to several decades of life. With improved survival over long period, many of the CHD patients also face the burden of acquired heart disease, further compounding the clinical risk assessment. Clinical risk assessment aims to identify patients for whom outcomes can be improved by providing information to the clinician so that he/she can choose the best option for management.

Overall, patients with CHD have a higher mortality risk, the standardized mortality ratio (SMR) ranging from 2.2 to 2.6.[4,5] The SMR further increases if older patients are included. At a mean age of 41.8 ± 15.3 years, overall average predicted 10-year mortality for the CHD cohort was 13.7 ± 15.8% and it increased to 29.8 ± 3.0% for those above 50 years of age.[6] Additional acquired comorbidities (cardiovascular and others) due to increasing age are contributory. Inactivity, obesity, low body mass index, diabetes mellitus, neoplasms, and other acquired cardiovascular disease are likely to be as prevalent, if not more, in patients with CHD as in an age-matched general population.

FACTORS INFLUENCING THE LIFETIME RISK OF CONGENITAL HEART DISEASE (FIG. 1)

Complexity of Congenital Heart Disease

Patients with CHD of great complexity have the highest predicted risk of morbidity and mortality. Several studies consider CHD as a whole, not specifically addressing the subgroup of patients with simple CHD, who are likely to do much better than those with higher complexity.

In a Danish registry of 17,157 patients with simple CHDs consisting of atrial septal defect (ASD), ventricular septal defect (VSD), patent ductus arteriosus (PDA), and pulmonary stenosis, the lifetime risks of all comorbidities were still higher for patients than for sex and birth year matched controls, except for neoplasm.[7] Males had higher risk for stroke, heart failure, and myocardial infarction, females had high risk for stroke, heart failure, and atrial fibrillation. The association of CHD with stroke was mainly driven by ASD, which is further increased by atrial fibrillation. Treated CHDs had lower risk of stroke, myocardial infarction, and heart failure than untreated.

As complexity of CHD increases, the risk also increases. In a study of 406 adult patients, median age of 41.8 ± 15.3 years, 10-year mortality risk was 17.6 ± 2.7% for simple CHDs, 25.5 ± 2.3% for moderately complex CHD and 53.0 ± 7.7% for more severe complex CHD.[6] The list of simple, moderate, and severe complex CHDs was as per an earlier article.[8]

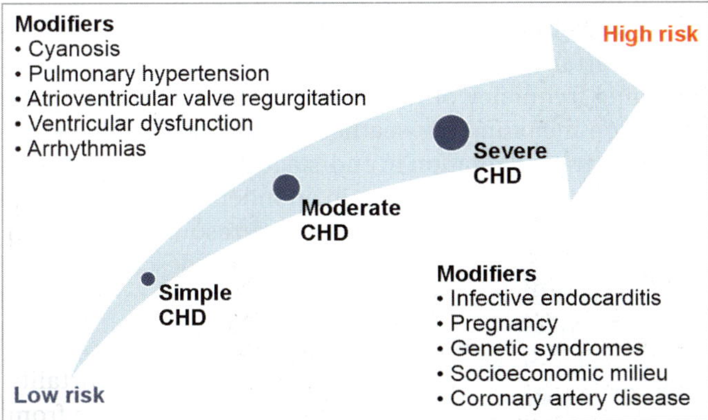

FIG. 1: Factors influencing the lifetime risk of congenital heart disease (CHD).

HEMODYNAMIC AND OTHER ANATOMICAL AND PHYSIOLOGICAL FACTORS

In addition to the anatomic complexity, other independent risk factors that have been found to increase mortality include presence of cyanosis, univentricular physiology, ventricular dysfunction, residual hemodynamic lesions such as pulmonary outflow tract obstruction, significant atrioventricular valve regurgitation, and severe pulmonary hypertension. Acquired late complications such as infective endocarditis, aortic aneurysm, and coronary artery disease also pose risk. These factors which are over and above the anatomical categorization can partly explain different mortality patterns for the same CHD.

The SMR was high at 5.22 (95% CI 4.5–6.0) and median age at death was 55.6 years (95% CI 50–61) if one of the above risk factors was present (996 patients), highest being for cyanosis and single ventricle physiology. In contrast, SMR was only 1.14 and median age at death was 83.7 years (95% CI 82–87) for those with no risk factor (2,315 patients), same as for the reference population.[5]

OTHER FACTORS

Association with genetic syndrome: About 15% of all CHDs are associated with genetic syndromes, the specific type is often associated with specific CHDs, e.g., atrioventricular septal defect with Down syndrome. Some of these genetic syndromes have risk of their own. For example, increased risk of sudden death during anesthesia induction in Williams syndrome.[9] Down syndrome has high risk of neoplasia and dementia in older patients.

Social determinants of health: These include education, income, geography etc., which influence healthcare access through the entire lifespan of CHD patients. Race and ethnicity are also likely to be important factor due to biological differences between the various ethnic groups.[10] Lack of insurance, psychological and mental health challenges, and employability are some of the other factors influencing the lifetime risk of premature mortality.

Pregnancy: In women, pregnancy is a very important determinant of risk. CARPREG II defined predictors of maternal risk during pregnancy.[11] These included prior cardiac events or arrhythmias, poor functional class or cyanosis, high-risk valve disease/left ventricular outflow tract obstruction, systemic ventricular dysfunction, no prior cardiac interventions, mechanical valves, high-risk aortopathies, pulmonary hypertension, coronary artery disease, and presenting late in pregnancy. Some of these factors are important for lifetime risk in these women.

Arrhythmia: Electrophysiological abnormalities are common cardiovascular complication of CHD and their prevalence increases with time. These include both brady- and tachyarrhythmias, risks are dependent on the underlying CHD, type of surgical intervention done and hemodynamically significant residual defects. Lifetime prevalence of arrhythmias has been estimated to be >50%, which is much higher than that seen in age-matched controls.[12,13]

COMPOSITE RISK ASSESSMENT

Risk of CHD across the lifespan is influenced by a number of factors described above; the contribution of each factor is likely to vary in an individual patient. There is no simple algorithm which can reliably predict morbidity and mortality in adults with CHD. Ombelet F, et al. published the predictive value of different disease severity and functional indices for 15-year all-cause and cardiac mortality in 629 patients with CHD (median age = 24 years; 60% men).[14] Five indices used were:

1. The Bethesda disease complexity classification categorizes patients into three groups: (i) simple, (ii) moderate, and (iii) severely complex CHDs based on the anatomical complexity.
2. The NYHA class which has four functional classes pertaining to the patient's day-to-day level of functioning and experienced symptoms.
3. The ability index scores patients on their capacity to work, capacity to be active, and ability to go through uncomplicated pregnancies (if applicable). It assigns patients to four classes:
   a. *Grade 1:* Normal life. Full time work or school. Can manage pregnancy.
   b. *Grade 2:* Able to do part time work. Life modified by symptoms.
   c. *Grade 3:* Unable to work. Noticeable limitation of activities.
   d. *Grade 4:* Extreme limitation. Dependent. Almost housebound.
4. The disease severity index compiles information on the patient's history of surgical and/or catheter-based interventions and whether they have persistent cyanosis, allocating patients to one of three categories:
   a. *Low severity:* ≤1 cardiovascular procedure
   b. *Moderate severity:* >1 cardiovascular procedure
   c. *High severity:* Persistent cyanosis or single ventricle physiology
5. *Congenital heart disease functional index (CHDFI):* It has five categories, comprising different elements of the patient's status: Surgical history, clinical status, functional capacity, and current frequency of follow-up based on disease complexity or on the physician's professional opinion:
   a. *Class 1:* No surgery, good clinical status, and medical follow-up not strictly necessary.
   b. *Class 2:* With or without surgery, functionally perfect, postoperative normalization of clinical condition, medical checkup every 3–5 years, and competitive sports permitted.
   c. *Class 3:* With or without surgery, functionally good, medical restrictions, medical checkup every 1–2 years, and recreational sports permitted.
   d. *Class 4:* With or without surgery, moderate functional status, functioning at own pace, and medical checkup every year.
   e. *Class 5:* With or without palliative surgery, bad functional status, cyanosis, and medical checkup every 6–12 months.

With the exception of disease severity index, all scales predicted all-cause and cardiac mortality. The CHDFI fared best to detect adults with CHD at high risk. This index is easy to use in clinical practice. Patients falling into class 4 and 5 require more exhaustive assessment to look for a cause such as pulmonary hypertension, ventricular dysfunction or an acquired heart disease. This data required further validation in a larger study.

RISK PREDICTION MODELS

Advancements in technology and computation have enabled big data analysis and advanced statistical modeling. This has been applied to medicine for the development of prediction models which estimate the risk of an individual affected with a particular disease and calculates outcomes based on set of risk factors. Several risk scores have been developed for acquired cardiovascular diseases and are widely used. There are prediction models for coronary artery disease,[15] heart failure,[16] risk of stroke in atrial fibrillation,[17,18] outcome after cardiac surgery, and many others. One needs lifetime risk predictions for CHD. Only few studies have reported prediction models in CHD over long period of time. Small sample size, limited data sources, heterogeneity of population in terms of anatomy and surgical approach, low event rates, and unmeasured confounding factors are the main reasons for the lack of such models for CHD.[19] Risk prediction models are important for guiding management of CHD patients including frequency of follow-up visits, need for treatment escalation including transcatheter or surgical interventions and heart transplantation in end-stage disease. These models must have external validation in an independent sample for further tuning, better outcomes, and resource allocation. Some of the examples of risk calculators are described below.

Geenen LW, et al. published a risk calculator in adults with CHD, based on data from two large prospective cohort studies including a total 1,351 moderately to severely complex adult CHD patients.[20] A prospective cohort of 602 patients in Netherlands was merged with Boston adult CHD Biobank study, a prospectively enrolled cohort of 749 patients who visited a referral center in Boston between 2012 and 2017, the later was used for external validation. In the final model, five predictors were included, namely NYHA class, use of cardiac medications, reintervention, BMI, and NT-proBNP. Hazard ratios of the model variables in the merged dataset were: NYHA class ≥ II = 1.91 (95% CI 1.50–2.43), cardiac medication use = 2.53 (95% CI 1.92–3.35), ≥1 reintervention = 1.55 (95% CI 1.20–2.00), BMI = 1.03 (95% CI 1.01–1.05) kg/m^2; and log2 NT-proBNP = 1.44 (95% CI 1.35–1.54) pmol/L. The risk calculator is available online https:// achdwebcalculator-updated.shinyapps.io/achdshinyweb/.

The observed risk for patients in the highest sextile of predicted risk was 37.7% versus 0.5%, for patients in the lowest sextile. Follow-up strategy can be based on this risk score, those in lowest sextile can have a less stringent follow-up as compared to those in higher sextiles. The validation of this score in a large, independent, prospective cohort study makes it a good model for moderate and severely complex CHDs. There are two caveats in this model, it cannot be used for simple CHDs and age was not included in the final model.

Another model is for prediction of heart failure hospitalizations in adult CHD patients. Heart failure is the leading cause of hospital admissions and death in adults with ACHD.[21] Several models exist for heart failure risk prediction, but ACHD patients are excluded in these. Cohen et al. have published a risk prediction model for heart failure-related hospitalizations in adults with CHD.[22] The cohort included 29,991 adults with CHD, aged 18–64 years who were followed for 648,457 person-years. The cumulative risk of heart failure-related hospitalization by age of 65 years was 12.58%. One-year predictors for heart failure-related hospitalization were age ≥ 50 years, male sex, severity of CHD, history of heart failure hospitalization in last 12 months, pulmonary arterial hypertension, chronic kidney disease, coronary artery disease, systemic arterial hypertension, and diabetes mellitus. The created risk score ranged from 0 to 19 as shown in **Table 1**. The risk scoring system demonstrated excellent prediction performance. For a score of 7, risk of heart failure hospitalization was only 1.63%, increasing to 75% for a score of 19.

TABLE 1: Risk factor scoring for heart failure hospitalization in adults with congenital heart disease (CHD).

Risk factor	Points
Heart failure in past 12 months	3
Pulmonary hypertension (lifetime)	3
Chronic kidney disease (lifetime)	3
Coronary artery disease (lifetime)	3
Systemic arterial hypertension (lifetime)	2
CHD lesion: Severe vs. shunt	2
CHD lesions: Valve vs. shunt	1
Diabetes mellitus (lifetime)	1
Sex: Male vs. female	1
Age: ≥50 vs. <50 years	1
Total score (possible points)	0–19

CLINICAL RISK ASSESSMENT AND PREDICTION ACROSS THE LIFESPAN IN SPECIFIC DISEASES

Post-Fontan Operation

Fontan operation or one of its modifications is performed in CHD with univentricular physiology where a biventricular repair is not possible, the classical examples are tricuspid atresia and, double inlet left ventricle (LV). Due to the unphysiological circulation, these patients are at risk for adverse events during their entire lifespan. The risk depends on a number of variables starting with their preoperative anatomy and hemodynamics. The year of surgery, the type of surgery, intraoperative, and early postoperative factors, all play a part in risk assessment. Their long-term outcome is affected by several complications, such as protein losing enteropathy, plastic bronchitis, liver fibrosis, etc., primarily related to high systemic venous pressure. Long-term outcome measures vary greatly between studies in Fontan patients making assessment of mortality hazard very challenging.

A systematic review of 28 studies including 6,707 post-Fontan patients was published in 2016 where authors evaluated risk factors for long-term mortality.[23] Authors identified 35 risk factors for late mortality which were classified into nine categories. The most relevant risk factors were combined into a simple risk score, based on pooled hazard ratios. The risk score ranged from 0 to 100. The final score included eight risk factors; weightage was given according to the hazard ratio **(Table 2)**.

These risk scores are easy to evaluate in outpatient settings, however, they need further validation. Large registry with multinational collaboration will help in further refining the prediction models. Some studies have shown the predictive value of brain natriuretic peptide (BNP), exercise testing, and cardiovascular magnetic imaging, which could also be included in future models.

REPAIRED TETRALOGY OF FALLOT

Tetralogy of Fallot (TOF) is the most common cyanotic CHD beyond infancy. After a successful repair, a 20-year survival has been reported to be >90%. Long-term complications include pulmonary regurgitation and arrhythmias. Sudden death has also been reported rarely. Risk factors such as enlarged right ventricle (RV), RV dysfunction, broad QRS duration, atrial arrhythmias, and LV dysfunction have been listed for adverse outcome in various published reports. An International Multicenter TOF Registry (INDICATOR),[24] identified RV mass-to-volume ratio ≥ 0.3 g/mL (HR

TABLE 2: Risk scores for late mortality in Fontan patients.

Risk factor	Hazard ratio range	Risk score
Anatomic risk factors (hypoplastic left heart or heterotaxy)	42.8–12.7	13
Elevated preoperative pulmonary artery pressure >15 or Fontan pressure >20 mm Hg postoperatively	1.14–3.5	6
Atriopulmonary Fontan	3.7–6.2	18
Heart failure symptoms or need for diuretic use	1.58–9.16	7
Arrhythmia	1.79–6	9
Moderate/severe ventricular dysfunction or moderate/severe AV valve regurgitation	4.02–7.17	25
Protein-losing enteropathy	1.97–8.5	9
End-organ disease including cirrhosis or renal insufficiency	2.49–19	13

5.04; 95% CI 2.3–11.0; $p < 0.001$), left ventricular ejection fraction (LVEF) z-score < –2.0 (HR 3.34; 95% CI 1.59–7.01; $p = 0.001$), and history of atrial tachyarrhythmia (HR: 3.65; 95% CI 1.75–7.62; $p = 0.001$) to be predictive of death and sustained ventricular tachycardia. LV dysfunction was equally important to RV dysfunction for adverse outcome. Using Kaplan–Meier analysis, 98% of patients had freedom from death or sustained VT at 5 and 10 years if none of the above predictors were present. Patients who had all three risk factors (RV mass-to-volume ratio ≥ 0.3 g/mL and LVEF z-score <–2.0 and history of atrial arrhythmias), the freedom from death and sustained VT was only 43%.

Significant late gadolinium enhancement of RV on cardiac MRI has also been found to be associated with adverse event (sustained ventricular tachycardia).[25]

ATRIAL ARRHYTHMIAS AFTER ATRIAL SEPTAL DEFECT CLOSURE

Atrial septal defect is a common CHD, the expected survival is excellent with >97% reaching adulthood. One of the major factors for morbidity is onset of atrial arrhythmias, though closure during childhood is relatively protective against arrhythmias as compared to closure during adult life. In a study by Van De Bruaene A, et al., data of 155 patients who had undergone ASD closure (surgical or device) during adult life was analyzed for atrial arrhythmias.[26] Nine (5.8%) had permanent atrial fibrillation, 7 (4.5%) had persistent atrial fibrillation, and 23 (14.8%) had paroxysmal atrial fibrillation. Multivariate analysis showed that male gender (HR 2.18; 95% CI 1.11–4.29; $p = 0.024$), pulmonary hypertension (HR 4.34; 95% CI 2.17–9.09; $p < 0.0001$), atrial arrhythmia before repair (HR 3.52; 95% CI 1.75–7.14; $p < 0.0001$), and atrial arrhythmia within 1 month after repair (HR 6.63; 95% CI 2.38–20.00; $p < 0.0001$) were independently associated with the occurrence of atrial arrhythmia >1 month after ASD repair. The risk score was calculated using these variables and risk was calculated for 1, 2, 3, 4, and 5 years **(Table 3)**. Likelihood of arrhythmia increased as follow-up period increases. Kaplan–Meier analysis revealed that a risk score of <4 was associated with no risk till 4 years follow-up and a very low risk of 0–10% at 5 years. On the other hand, a score of >20 predicted atrial arrhythmias in 80% of cases as early as, at 1 year. Use of this tool may allow for individualization and optimization of treatment strategies after ASD closure.

TABLE 3: Predictive model for atrial arrhythmia after ASD closure.

Risk factor	Score
Gender male	4
Gender female	0
Atrial arrhythmias before repair	6
Atrial arrhythmias ≤1 month after repair	10
Mean pulmonary artery pressure ≥ 25 mm Hg	8
Total maximum	28

CONCLUSION

Significant advances have been made in management of CHD and increasing number of patients are undergoing early surgical or transcatheter interventions. Many of these are at lifetime risk of morbidity and mortality which is higher than those of age-matched control population. Available risk scores for predicting adverse events are few and most are derived from retrospective studies. Many are not internally or externally validated. We need more adequately validated risk scores which not only be very useful in clinical practice, but will also be an important step toward personalized medicine. Since the population of CHD is very heterogenous, multicenter, national and international, collaboration with well-designed studies, and use of artificial intelligence will go a long way in creating good prediction models for CHD population. A recent study from Boston Children's Hospital assesses the utility of an artificial intelligence-enhanced ECG model for risk stratification in a large cohort of pediatric and adult patients with CHD.[27] Artificial intelligence-enhanced ECG model outperformed traditional clinical measures, including age, QRS duration, and LVEF. Patients classified as high risk by the model had an HR > 4 (based on the first or random ECG) and >7 when using the most recent ECG. Artificial intelligence is suitably poised to benefit CHD patients given their heterogeneity and growing numbers.

REFERENCES

1. Warnes CA. The adult with congenital heart disease. J Am Coll Cardiol. 2005;46:1-8.
2. Marelli AJ, Mackie AS, Ionescu-Ittu R, et al. Congenital heart disease in the general population: changing prevalence and age distribution. Circulation. 2007;115:163-72.
3. Price S, Jaggar S, Jordan S, et al. Adult congenital heart disease: intensive care management and outcome prediction. Intensive Care Med. 2007;33:652-9.
4. Diller GP, Kempny A, Alonso-Gonzalez R, et al. Survival prospects and circumstances of death in contemporary adult congenital heart disease Patients under follow-up at a large tertiary centre. Circulation. 2015;132:2118-25.
5. Oliver JM, Gallego P, Gonzalez Garcia AE, et al. Risk factors for excess mortality in adults with congenital heart diseases. Eur Heart J. 2017;0:1-10.
6. Fernandes SM, Lui GK, Long J, et al. Predicting 10-year mortality in adults with congenital heart disease. Int J Cardiol Congenit Heart Dis. 2021;2:100057.
7. El-Chouli M, Meddis A, Christensen DM, et al. Lifetime risk of comorbidity in patients with simple congenital heart disease: a Danish nationwide study. Eur Heart J. 2023;44:741-8.
8. Warnes CA, Williams RG, Bashore TM, et al. ACC/AHA 2008 guidelines for the management of adults with congenital heart disease: a report of the American college of cardiology/American heart association task force on practice guidelines. J Am Coll Cardiol. 2008;52:e143-263.
9. Brown ML, Nasr VG, Toohey R, et al. Williams syndrome and anesthesia for noncardiac surgery: high risk can be mitigated with appropriate planning. Pediatr Cardiol. 2018;39:1123-8.
10. Davey B, Sinha R, Lee JH, et al. Social determinants of health and outcomes for children and adults with congenital heart disease: a systematic review. Pediatr Res. 2021;89:275-94.
11. Silversides CK, Grewal J, Mason J, et al. Pregnancy outcomes in women with heart disease: The CARPREG II Study. J Am Coll Cardiol. 2018;71:2419-30.
12. Labombarda F, Hamilton R, Shohoudi A, et al. Increasing prevalence of atrial fibrillation and permanent atrial arrhythmias in congenital heart disease. J Am Coll Cardiol. 2017;70:857-65.
13. Bouchardy J, Therrien J, Pilote L, et al. Atrial arrhythmias in adults with congenital heart disease. Circulation. 2009;120:1679-86.
14. Ombelet F, Goossens E, Apers S, et al. Predicting 15-year mortality in adults with congenital heart disease using disease severity and functional indices. Can J Cardiol. 2019;35:907-13.
15. Wilson PW, D'Agostino RB, Levy D, et al. Prediction of coronary heart disease using risk factor categories. Circulation. 1998;97(18):1837-47.
16. Levy WC, Mozaffarian D, Linker DT, et al. The Seattle heart failure model: prediction of survival in heart failure. Circulation. 2006;113:1424-33.
17. Gage BF, van Walraven C, Pearce L, et al. Selecting patients with atrial fibrillation for anticoagulation: stroke risk stratification in patients taking aspirin. Circulation. 2004;110:2287-92.
18. Lip GY, Nieuwlaat R, Pisters R, et al. Refining clinical risk stratification for predicting stroke and thromboembolism in atrial fibrillation using a novel risk factor-based approach: THE Euro heart survey on atrial fibrillation. Chest. 2010;137:263-72.
19. Opotowsky AR, Khairy P, Diller G, et al. Clinical Risk Assessment and Prediction inCongenital Heart Disease Across the Lifespan: JACC Scientific Statement. J Am Coll Cardiol. 2024;83:2091-111.
20. Geenen LW, Opotowsky AR, Lachtrupp C, et al. Tuning and external validation of an adult congenital heart disease risk prediction model. Eur Heart J Qual Care Clin Outcomes. 2022;8:70-8.
21. Engelings CC, Helm PC, Abdul-Khaliq H, et al. Cause of death in adults with congenital heart disease - an analysis of the German National Register for Congenital Heart Defects. Int J Cardiol. 2016;211:31-6.
22. Cohen S, Liu A, Wang F, et al. Risk prediction models for heart failure admissions in adults with congenital heart disease. Int J Cardiol. 2021;322:149-57.
23. Alsaied T, Bokma JP, Engel ME, et al. Predicting long-term mortality after Fontan procedures: A risk score based on 6707 patients from 28 studies. Congenit Heart Dis. 2017;12(4):393-8.
24. Valente AM, Gauvreau K, Assenza GE, et al. Contemporary predictors of death and sustained ventricular tachycardia in patients with repaired tetralogy of Fallot enrolled in the INDICATOR cohort. Heart. 2014;100:247-53.
25. Kakarla J, Ishikita A, Suszko A, et al. Risk scores inconsistently predict sudden death and ventriculararrhythmias in repaired tetralogy of Fallot. Heart Rhythm. 2025.
26. Van De Bruaene A, Moons P, Belmans A, et al. Predictive model for late atrial arrhythmia after closure of an atrial septal defect. Int J Cardio. 2013;164:318-22.
27. Mayourian J, El-Bokl A, Lukyanenko P, et al. Electrocardiogram-based deep learning to predict mortality in paediatric and adult congenital heart disease. Eur Heart J. 2025;46:856-68.

CHAPTER 50

Early Intervention for Tetralogy of Fallot, but at What Cost?

Mahua Roy, Sucheta Barman

ABSTRACT

Infants with Tetralogy of Fallot (TOF) typically undergo operative correction in their first year of life. However, some neonates with unfavorable anatomy may present with symptomatic cyanosis and need early intervention. Controversy surrounds the optimal management strategy of symptomatic neonates with TOF (sTOF). Options are primary repair (PR) or staged repair (SR). Among SR, initial palliation (IP) by surgically putting aortopulmonary shunt (modified BT shunt) or transcatheter procedure such as ductal stenting and/or right ventricular outflow tract (RVOT) stenting or balloon pulmonary valvuloplasty (BPV) is followed by complete repair (CR). Early intervention with staged approach for TOF may improve outcomes, but it comes with potential costs, including financial burdens, potential complications, and needs of long-term monitoring.

Keywords: Tetralogy of Fallot, primary repair, staged repair, right ventricular outflow tract stenting, ductal stenting, balloon pulmonary valvuloplasty.

INTRODUCTION

Infants born with Tetralogy of Fallot (TOF) typically undergo surgical correction in their first year of life. Elective anatomic repair beyond early infancy is associated with a low risk of mortality. However, a subset with unfavorable anatomy presents with symptomatic cyanosis at neonatal period, prompting early intervention. There is still debate about the optimal management strategy for neonatal symptomatic TOF (sTOF). The treatment options include primary repair (PR) or staged repair (SR), in which an initial palliation (IP) is followed by complete repair (CR). Previously, aortopulmonary shunt was the only palliative option in these patients. Recent expansion in transcatheter options for palliation [balloon pulmonary valvuloplasty (BPV), right ventricular outflow tract (RVOT) stent, and/or ductal stent] has made the debate even more complicated.[1] Early intervention for TOF is generally recommended to improve outcomes, but it comes with potential costs, including financial burdens, potential complications, and long-term monitoring needs.

EARLY INTERVENTIONS IN BRIEF

- *Treatment options for cyanotic young infants with TOF:*
  - Primary repair
  - Staged repair—IP is followed by CR:
    - Surgical palliation—aortopulmonary shunt (modified BT shunt, central shunt, etc.)
    - *Transcatheter palliation:*
      - RVOT stent
      - Ductal stent
      - BPV

Although each procedure has its own advantages and limitations, costs associated with early intervention for TOF can be broadly categorized as follows:

- *Financial costs:* Including surgery, hospitalization, postprocedure care, long-term monitoring, and reintervention
- *Potential complications:* Immediate- and long-term complications, and rarely developmental impact
- *Other considerations:* Psychological impact and impact on quality of life
- **Primary repair**:[2]
  - *Potential advantages:*
    - Provides a definitive correction of the heart defect, potentially eliminating the need for further interventions
    - Single exposure to general anesthesia (GA) and cardiopulmonary bypass (CPB)
    - Reduces the duration of cyanosis

- Avoids the risks of a potentially unstable circulation in the period between IP and CR
- Can lead to normal pulmonary blood flow and oxygen saturation
- May improve long-term outcomes and quality of life

- *Limitations:*
  - Requires open-heart surgery under CPB, which carries inherent risks
  - May be associated with higher mortality and morbidity in infants with complex anatomy or prematurity
  - May require a *transannular patch,* which can lead to long-term complications
  - May require reintervention (e.g., patch angioplasty) to address pulmonary artery stenosis

- **Staged repair**:
  - *Whom to do:*
    - PGE1 dependent
    - Severely cyanosed and trickle of antegrade flow due to poor anatomy of RVOT
    - Poor anatomy of pulmonary artery tree (hypoplastic PAs, MAPCAs, Z score < −2)
    - Coexisting neonatal comorbidities—prematurity, LBW, infection, and neurological injury
    - Abnormal coronary artery distribution
  - *Potential advantages:*[2]
    - By delaying complete operative correction, SR reduces exposure to GA and CPB in the neonatal period, during which neurological development may be especially vulnerable.
    - Allowing for interval growth of the patient and their pulmonary arteries may also reduce the risks of perioperative adverse outcomes and postoperative reintervention(s).
- *Interventions as palliation:* The transcatheter options are technically feasible, well-tolerated and effective in improving systemic oxygen saturation and promoting pulmonary arterial growth, thus reducing the risk of surgical repair.[3] This approach promotes more symmetric growth of the pulmonary artery as compared to the modified BT shunt, presumably due to a more uniform pulmonary blood flow. Despite being less durable than surgical palliation, either RVOT stenting **(Fig. 1)** or ductal stenting **(Fig. 2)** show comparable clinical sequelae and early mortality rates, which are significantly better than those resulting from surgical palliation **(Table 1)**. Although, the choice of transcatheter options depends on institutional and cardiologist's preference, ductal stenting should be preferred in case of anticipated spontaneous improvement or the need for larger stents in future, and RVOT stenting should be selected in case of early CR or complex duct anatomy **(Table 2)**. Rarely, both options might be proposed in sequence over time, where it is mandatory to prolong the lifespan of the stented tracts.

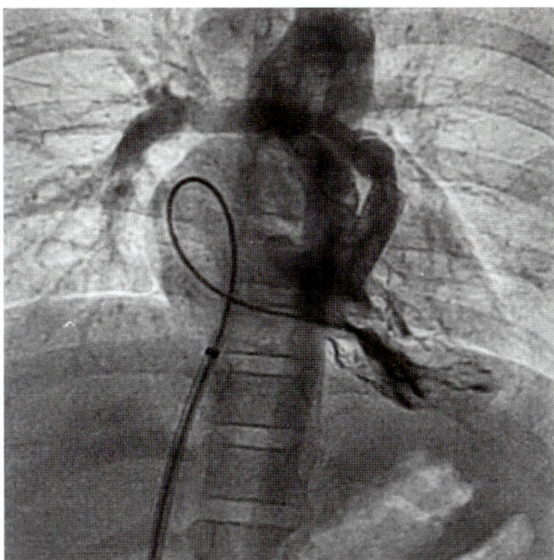

FIG. 1: Right ventriculogram showing right ventricular outflow tract (RVOT) stent in situ with opacification of lungs through branch pulmonary arteries.

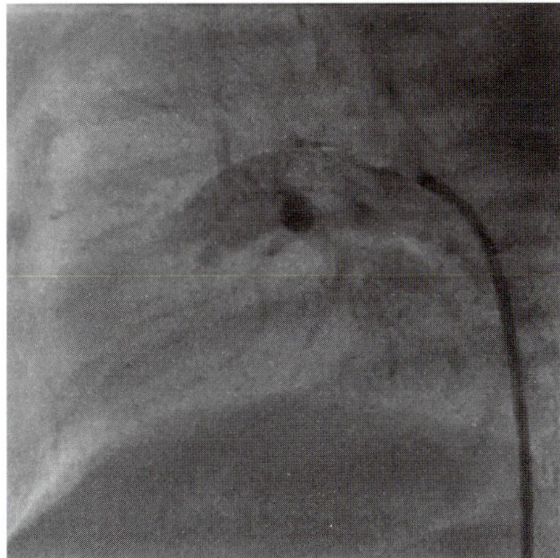

FIG. 2: Aortogram showing flow across the ductal stent and opacification of branch pulmonary arteries.

Either RVOT stenting or ductal stenting enables a balanced increase in systemic arterial saturation by mimicking the physiologic pattern of pulmonary blood flow. However, some differences should be reported in view of a patient-tailored approach.

- *RVOT stent:*[5]
  - Safer and effective management strategy
  - More recent
  - More physiologic than aortopulmonary shunt
  - *Indications:* No established indications
    - High risk for conventional surgical palliation
    - Low risk for conventional surgical palliation but with an anticipated need for short-term support to pulmonary circulation due to early surgical repair

TABLE 1: Differences between surgical and transcatheter initial palliation.[4]

	Surgical (aortopulmonary shunt)	Transcatheter (ductal stent)
Early bending or thrombosis of stent or conduit	More	Less
Reintervention	Less	More
PA growth	Asymmetric	Balanced, particularly in patients with hypoplastic MPAs
Redilatation	Not possible	Possible
Risk of pulmonary overcirculation and CHF	Higher	Significantly decreases
Longevity	Longer	Less durable
Morbidity and mortality	Higher	Lower
Cost-effective	Less	More
Safety and effectiveness	Less	More
Superiority in terms of complications, length of hospital stay, and mortality and costs	No	Yes
Contraindication		Previous branch PA stenosis

TABLE 2: Pathophysiologic differences in transcatheter palliation approaches.[3]

	RVOT stent	Ductal stent
Type of pulmonary blood flow	Only systolic	Continuous but not always balanced flow due to the origin and orientation of the duct
Stent size depends on	• Right ventricular outflow tract (RVOT) anatomy • Size of the pulmonary valve annulus	• Duct anatomy • PA anatomy
Complications	• Rhythmic contraction of the RV infundibulum often results in stent strut fractures → early recurrence of RVOT obstruction • PA rupture • Stent embolization to PA or aorta • Stent in-growth stenosis	• Potential flow streaming might worsen any potential original size discrepancy between the pulmonary arteries • PS at the site of duct implantation

- *Advantages:*
  - Decreases mortality compared to MBTS and PR
  - Overcomes the difficulties of CPB, especially ≤2 kg
  - Balanced pulmonary blood flow → more constant symmetrical growth of branch PAs
  - More physiologic
  - Improved oxygenation → relief of hypoxia
  - Less invasive → decreases immediate surgical risks (safer)
  - Faster recovery
  - Improve growth of patient and weight gain
- *Limitations:*
  - Technically difficult, especially in small infants
  - High burden of reintervention
  - Prevents valve-sparing anatomic repair → needs TAP or conduit
  - May complicate subsequent anatomic repair (90–95% case: Stents removed entirely)
  - Temporary solution
  - Stent-related complications
  - Growth-related issues
  - Radiation exposure—ALARA principle; marker of increased cancer risk

- *Ductal stent:[3]*
  - *Indications:*
    - High-risk profile for surgery, having an anatomically suitable ductus arteriosus and more than one source of pulmonary blood flow.
    - Low risk for surgical palliation but with an anticipated need for short-term support for pulmonary circulation due to early surgical repair or while waiting for the evolution of clinical scenarios.
  - *Advantages:*
    - Can be a lifesaving procedure for newborns with duct-dependent pulmonary blood flow, providing a source of pulmonary blood flow when the RVOT is severely obstructed or atretic.

- May lead to better pulmonary artery growth compared to surgical shunts due to more even distribution of blood flow.
- Can be used as a bridge to CR or as a temporary measure until the infant is older and can undergo surgery.

- *Limitations:*
  - High rate of PA stenosis
  - Requires careful monitoring to ensure the stent does not migrate or cause complications
  - May require reintervention if the ductus arteriosus starts to narrow or close
  - May not be suitable for all patients, especially those with complex heart defects or other medical conditions

- *BPV:*
  - Not gained widespread acceptance
  - Subvalvular muscular obstruction → unresponsive to BPV alone

RECENT DATA

Tetralogy of Fallot is one of the most common cyanotic CHDs but its incidence is very low (3–5 per 10,000 live births). Still, the public health impact is magnified by its cost. TOF is the 3rd most costly congenital cardiac diagnosis and 14th most costly overall pediatric diagnosis based on in-hospital spending each year.[2]

Small number of babies become symptomatic at birth, those are a more vulnerable group. They are at a higher risk of morbidity and mortality, and they use more health care resources and cost more to treat. To find out the optimal strategy for repair is important because it can lead to better long-term health and quality of life.

The recent multicenter retrospective cohort study from the Congenital Cardiac Research Collaborative (CCRC) included neonates with TOF undergoing intervention at ≤30 days of age between January 1, 2011 and December 31, 2017, evaluating for differences in clinical outcome between those undergoing PR and SR **(Table 3)**.[2]

TABLE 3: Comparative results of clinical outcomes between primary repair and staged repair from Congenital Cardiac Research Collaborative (CCRC) cohort study.

	Primary repair (n = 131)	Staged repair (n = 193)	p-value
Mortality:			
• Through 3 months	5 (6)	1 (1)	0.02
• Through 18 months	7 (9)	4 (7)	0.19
Procedural complications	47 (61)	37 (72)	0.10
Reintervention	11 (15)	17 (33)	0.20
ECMO	6 (8)	1 (1)	0.004
Ventilation, day	3 (1–8)	4 (2–8)	0.14
Hospital length of stay, day	21 (14–35)	32.5 (22–49)	<0.001
ICU length of stay, day	8 (5–18)	12 (8–19.5)	<0.001

Note: Values are %(n) or median (IQR).

It is challenging to apply the present data into clinical practice and achieve the best outcome for these vulnerable neonates. When traditional outcomes are similar, lower costs support pursuing a strategy, as it represents good value relative to the more costly alternative. Also, on average, sicker patients consume more medical care (laboratories, imaging, and medication along with longer duration of care) and, in so doing, incur more costs. Total medical costs can provide a composite measure of morbidity, combining the range of adverse events into a single metric that quantifies morbidity not captured in disparate traditional outcome measures.

They conclude that PR was associated with superior value and lower cost with similar mortality risk, through 18 months of age. Hence, PR should be considered as the primary strategy for management of neonates with sTOF where feasible and appropriate. Future data from a broader range of centers, greater experience with transcatheter palliation, and inclusion of longer-term clinical and functional health outcomes could influence these conclusions.

The hypothesis that delaying operative correction and sending a larger baby to the surgeon would reduce the risk of both mortality and morbidity sounds reasonable. However, a recent multicenter retrospective cohort study showed that the early survival benefit of SR goes down if cases are followed through their eventual CR. In that study, there was not much difference between management strategies regarding risks of hospital and procedural complications, and reintervention. If there is no significant difference in the likelihood of meaningful, measurable clinical outcomes, deciding on the optimal approach to sTOF is more complicated.

Transcatheter approach included BPV (48%), RVOT stent (14%), and PDA stent (38%). Of these transcatheter palliation patients, 13% underwent a subsequent surgical aorto-pulmonary shunt prior to CR (i.e., crossover from transcatheter to surgical palliation). Advanced facilities and increased experience may be associated with improved outcomes and reduced cost. But, the cost of necessary devices (e.g., drug-eluting coronary stents) and interstage reinterventions may offset potential savings. Transcatheter interventions carry higher device costs, whereas operative interventions incur longer length of stay and accompanying costs.

It is also noticed that neurodevelopment, cardiopulmonary exercise performance, and health-related quality of life are diminished in cohorts of repaired TOF patients. The impact of PR or SR on these important outcomes in this vulnerable cohort was not incorporated into this study. Incorporating these measures into ongoing research is critical to determining the optimal care of the next generation of neonates with sTOF.

CONCLUSION

Early intervention in case of symptomatic young infants with TOF is crucial to improve outcomes. We should meticulously select the treatment option on individual basis depending upon various factors. At the same point, it is important to carefully weigh the financial, medical, and psychological costs and benefits for each individual case.

REFERENCES

1. Ratnayaka K, Nageotte SJ, Moore JW, et al. Patent ductus arteriosus stenting for all ductal dependent cyanotic infants: waning use of Blalock-Taussig shunts. Circ Cardiovasc Interv. 2021;14:e009520.
2. O'Byrne ML, Glatz AC, Huang YV, et al. Comparative Costs of Management Strategies for Neonates with Symptomatic Tetralogy of Fallot. J Am Coll Cardiol. 2022;79(12):1170-80.
3. Scalera ST, Pizzuto A, Marchese P, et al. Personalized Approach in Transcatheter Palliation of Congenital Heart Disease with Duct-Dependent Pulmonary Circulation: Right Ventricular Outflow Tract Stenting vs. Arterial Duct Stenting. J Pers Med. 2024;14(3):302.
4. Rendón-Elías FG, Castro-Medina M, de la Cerda-Belmont GA, et al. Palliative Surgical Procedures vs Duct or Right Ventricular Outflow Stent in neonates with ductus dependent pulmonary blood flow. Cir Card Mex. 2021;6(2):40-53.
5. Pizzuto A, Cuman M, Assanta N, et al. Right Ventricular Outflow Tract Stenting as Palliation of Critical Tetralogy of Fallot: Techniques and Results. Hearts. 2021;2(2):278-87.

CHAPTER

51

Novel Imaging Techniques for Congenital Heart Disease

D Seshagiri Rao, Ramya Pechetty

ABSTRACT

Congenital heart diseases (CHD) are highly dependent on imaging for their accurate diagnosis and treatment. Apart from traditional imaging modalities such as echocardiography, cardiac CT (CCT), and cardiac MRI (CMR), recent times has seen the growth of various novel tools in the imaging of CHD such as 3D echocardiography, ultrafast ultrasound imaging, fusion imaging, etc. As these innovations continue to evolve, they hold the potential to transform the clinical approach to CHD, enabling earlier detection, minimally invasive interventions, and improved long-term outcomes.

Keywords: Congenital heart disease, cardiac computerized tomography, cardiac magnetic resonance, 3-dimensional echocardiography, virtual reality, artificial intelligence, machine learning, deep learning, left ventricle/right ventricle, ejection fraction, tetralogy of Fallot, atrial septal defect/ventricular septal defect.

INTRODUCTION

Congenital heart disease (CHD) presents with intricate anatomical variations that demand precise and detailed imaging for accurate diagnosis, effective treatment planning, and long-term management. While traditional modalities such as echocardiography, cardiac CT (CCT), and cardiac MRI (CMR) continue to play a central role, emerging technologies are increasingly complementing these tools. These innovations aim to enhance visualization, improve diagnostic accuracy, and optimize the overall continuum of care for patients with CHD.

Some of the new and emerging tools in the imaging of CHD are as follows[1] **(Fig. 1)**:

- *Advances in echocardiography*:
  - 3D echocardiography (3DE), rendering techniques, and blood speckle tracking
  - Ultrafast ultrasound imaging
- Advances in CCT
- Advances in CMR
- 3D rotational angiography
- *Advanced digital technologies*:
  - Fusion imaging
  - D printing and virtual reality
  - Virtual procedural planning (VPP)
- Artificial intelligence (AI) and machine learning (ML)

ADVANCES IN ECHOCARDIOGRAPHY

Two-dimensional echocardiography is the first-line investigation for any patient of suspected or diagnosed congenital heart disease. However, newer techniques have been developed in recent years which further improve the diagnosing capability of 2D echocardiography. These are 3D echocardiography (3DE) and ultrafast ultrasound imaging.

THREE-DIMENSIONAL ECHOCARDIOGRAPHY

Three-dimensional echocardiography is an important imaging tool for evaluating CHD. "The Three-dimensional Echocardiography in Congenital Heart Disease: An Expert Consensus Document" from EACVI and ASE emphasize the role of 3DE in the evaluation of various congenital heart diseases.[2]

Three-dimensional echocardiography can also be done in children using high-frequency (6–7 MHz) pediatric transthoracic transducers with a small footprint.[3] The 3D display modes for CHD include volume rendered, surface rendered, and multiplanar reformatted (MPR) image displays. Combining 3D and TEE has been found to enable better images.

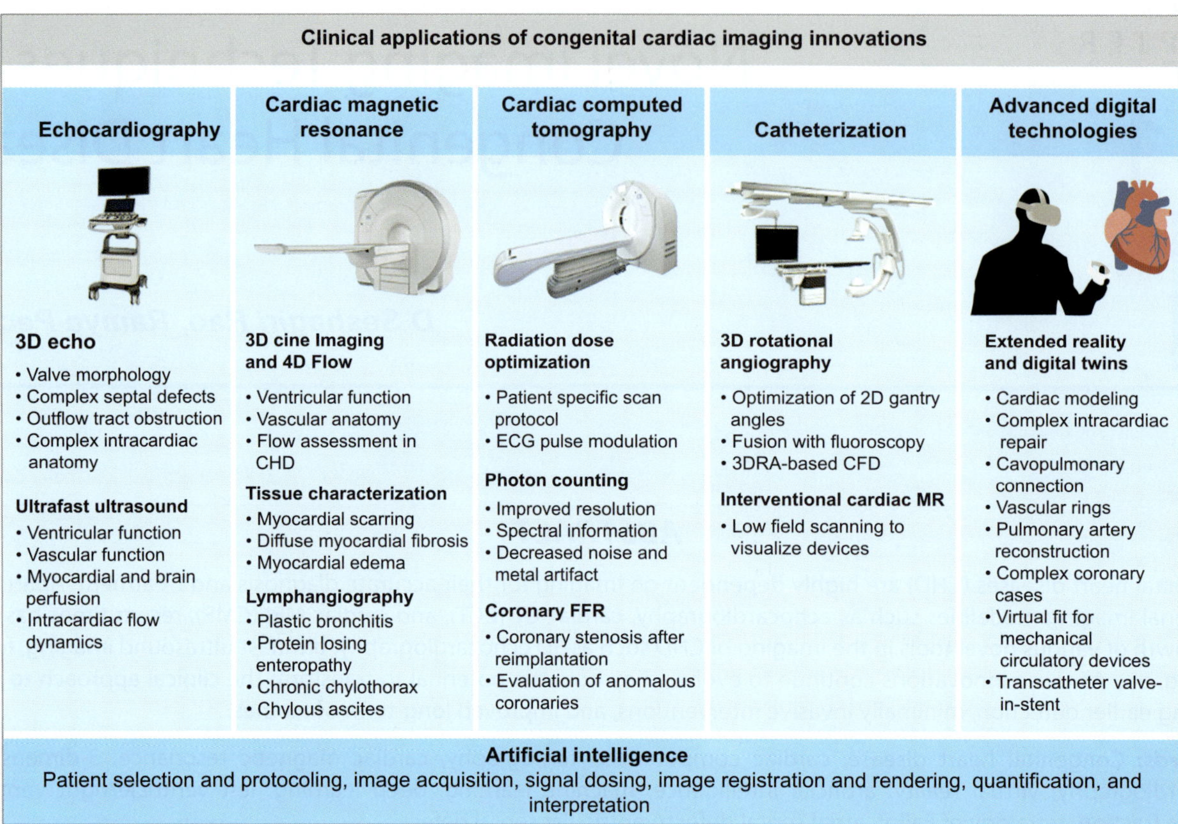

FIG. 1: Innovations in cardiac imaging.

Source: Adapted from Sachdeva R, Aimee K. Armstrong, Rima Arnaout, et al. Novel Techniques in Imaging Congenital Heart Disease: JACC Scientific Statement. JACC J. 2024;83(1):63-81.

Three-dimensional Echocardiography in Assessment of Congenital Heart Diseases

Three-dimensional echocardiography has been found to complement 2D echocardiography images and provide diagnostic as well as prognostic information. The role of 3DE in some common congenital heart defects has been summarized in **Table 1**.[4-8]

Three-dimensional Echocardiography to Guide Catheter Intervention

Three-dimensional echocardiography is recommended to assist interventional procedures such as device closure of selected ASDs and VSDs, particularly multiple, irregularly shaped, or residual defects. Pre-procedure assessment of site of defect, size of defects, surrounding structures, and important landmarks help in planning the procedure. Real-time 3D imaging assists in visualization of catheters, delivery systems, and devices during catheter intervention.[9,10]

Three-dimensional echocardiography guidance can also assist in catheter-based closure of Fontan fenestrations, prosthetic valve para-valvar leaks, ruptured sinus of Valsalva aneurysms, coronary artery fistulas, atrial switch baffle leaks, or obstruction and others.

Three-dimensional Echocardiography in Assessment of RV and LV Function

Assessment of RV size and function by TTE may be limited due to its anterior location, poor endocardial border delineation, complicated RV geometry and location of RV inflow and outflow tracts in different imaging planes. 3DE has potential advantages for assessment of RV volume and function, particularly in patients with repaired tetralogy of Fallot (TOF), surgeries utilizing RV to pulmonary artery conduit, where RV measurements help to determine the timing of pulmonary valve replacement[11,12] **(Fig. 4)**.

Assessment of LV volume and function is important in patients, especially in pediatric populations where assumption in LV shape may give erroneous findings. 3DE can accurately measure the LV volumes and calculate the EF due to its superior endocardial border definition. 3DE has been found to be comparable to MRI, however, 3DE has a systematic bias to produce lower volumes than MRI.[13,14] Segmental assessment of LV for dyssynchrony and calculation of LV mass is also possible. LV dyssynchrony has been found to impact outcomes in children with Kawasaki disease, those with dilated cardiomyopathy and tricuspid atresia patients after Fontan surgery.

TABLE 1: Application of 3D echocardiography in CHD.

Pathology	Role of 3D echocardiography	Comments
ASD	Size/number/shape/location of defects especially multiple defects, residual leaks, spiral defects[4-5] **(Figs. 2A to C)**	Less valuable in PFO
VSD	Size/number/shape/location of defects, multiple defects, unusually located defects[6-7]	
AV valve	Leaflet morphology, chordae, papillary muscle, delineation, and mechanism/severity of regurgitation[8] **(Figs. 3A and B)**	
Aortic valve/LVOT	Morphology of aortic valve leaflets, mechanism of aortic regurgitation, morphology of subaortic obstruction and aortic valve, imaging of aortic valve leaflets more difficult by 3D TTE, 3D TEE preferred **(Figs. 3A and B)**	
Pulmonary valve/RVOT	PV morphology and function, RVOT morphology, site of RVOT obstruction	Less useful than TTE
Anomalous systemic and pulmonary vein drainage	Pulmonary veins can be imaged	Less useful
AV septal defects	Size of atrial and ventricular defects, leaflet morphology and chordal support, delineation of regurgitant jets, measurement of valve size, ventricular function	
TOF	VSD size/location and RVOT anatomy, specific concerns, e.g., VSD position or RVOT anatomy, RV volume estimation postoperatively	
DORV	Relationship of AV valves, VSD size and location, relative position of great arteries, guiding appropriate type of repair	
DTGA/LTGA	Location and size of associated VSDs, right and LV outflow tract size and obstruction, MV and TV morphology and size, planning surgical procedures	

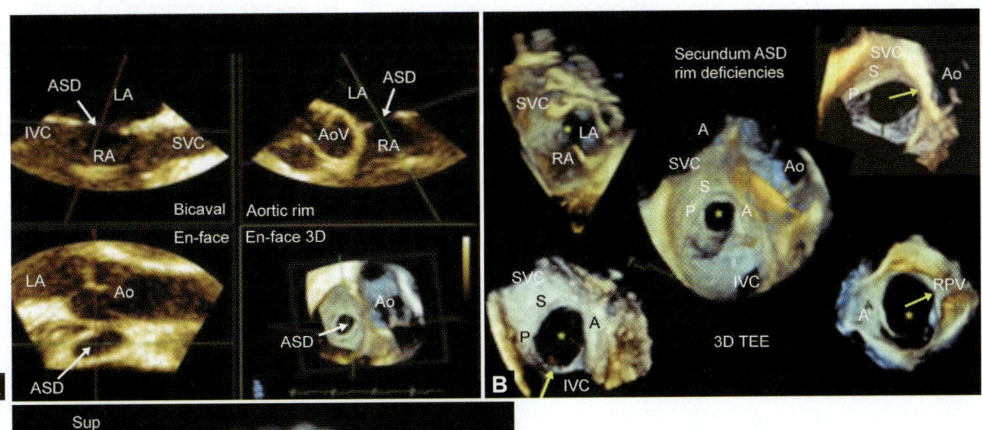

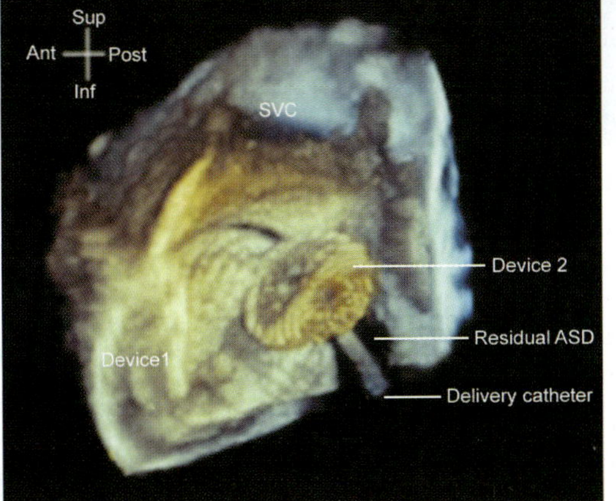

FIGS. 2A TO C: 3D TEE showing a secundum atrial septal defect. (A) Shows ostium secundum ASD in bicaval view, short axis view, long axis view and enface views showing adequate rims for device closure; (B) Shows ostium secundum ASD en-face views with deficient aortic, right pulmonary vein and superior vena caval rims, making it unsuitable for device closure; (C) Transesophageal real-time 3D image showing the deployment of a second septal occluder to close a residual atrial septal defect.

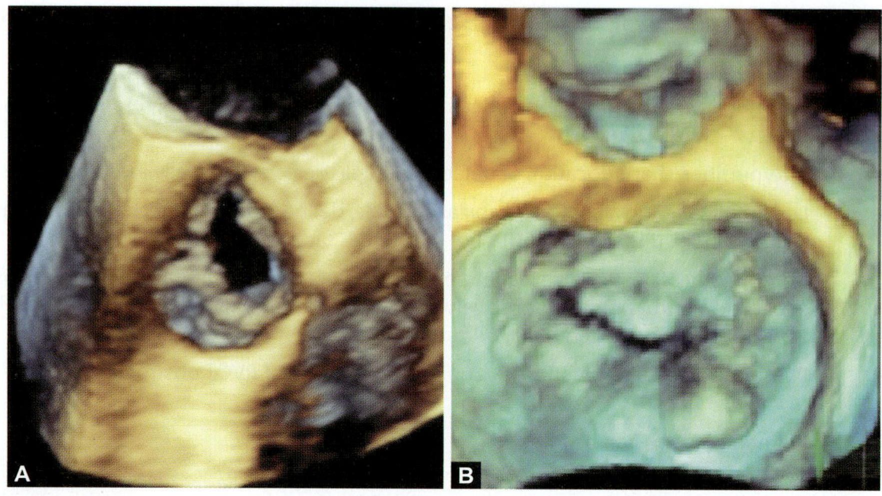

FIGS. 3A AND B: 3D TEE showing bicuspid aortic valve (A) and Mitral P3 prolapse (B).

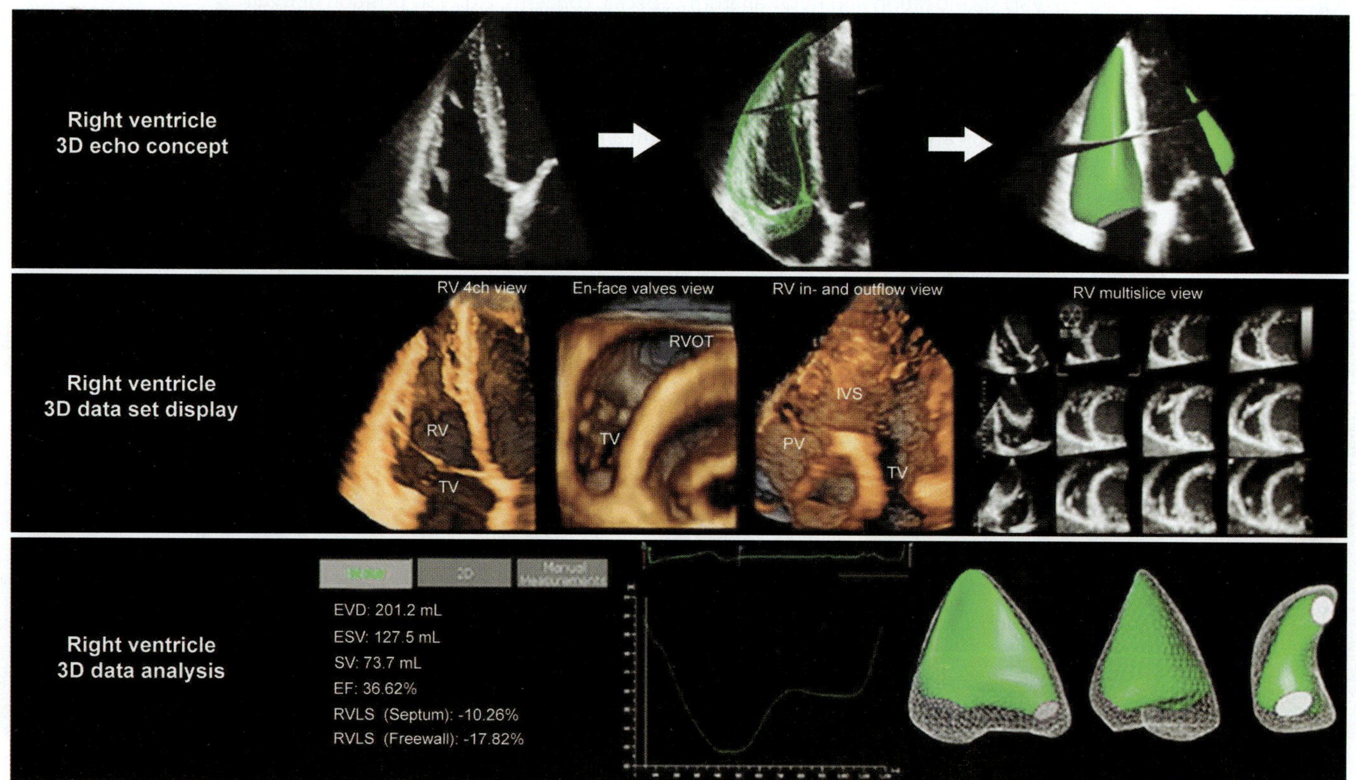

FIG. 4: 3D echocardiography showing assessment of right ventricular volumes and EF.

Novel Rendering Techniques in Three-dimensional Echocardiography

- *Transillumination rendering*: A tool that uses virtual light source in three dimensions to enhance depth perception and improve details, making it easier to delineate orifices, septal defects, assess valve areas, and thin structures like chordae. AI-generated refinements to render cardiac structures as if they are transparent, like glass can be added to light imaging[15,16] **(Figs. 5A to D and 6A to E)**.
- *Tissue-transparent display*: A tool that highlights the blood-pool tissue interface thereby improving the diagnosis and localizing chordal ruptures, leaflet clefts and assist in transcatheter edge-to-edge valve repairs.[17]
- *Fusion imaging*: 3DE datasets can be co-registered with other imaging modalities (fluoroscopy, CT angiography,

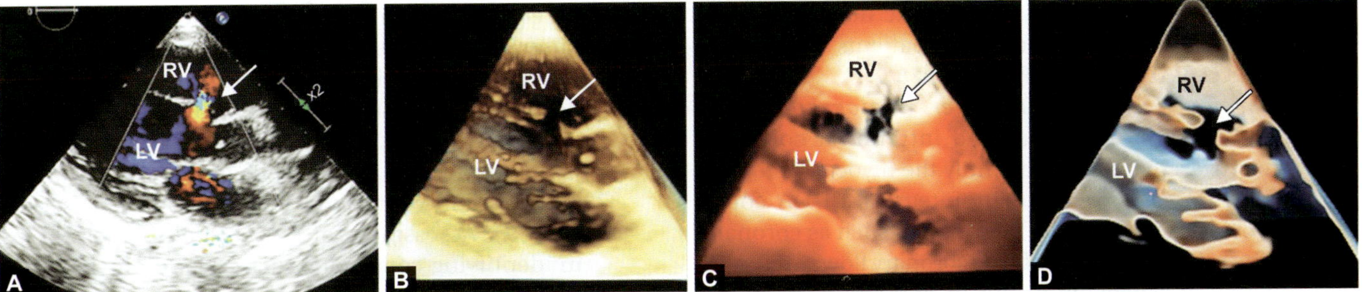

FIGS. 5A TO D: Transthoracic echocardiogram showing perimembranous ventricular septal defect; (A) 2D echocardiogram; (B) Traditional 3D; (C) Light rendered TEE/TrueVue light; (D) TrueVue glass images.

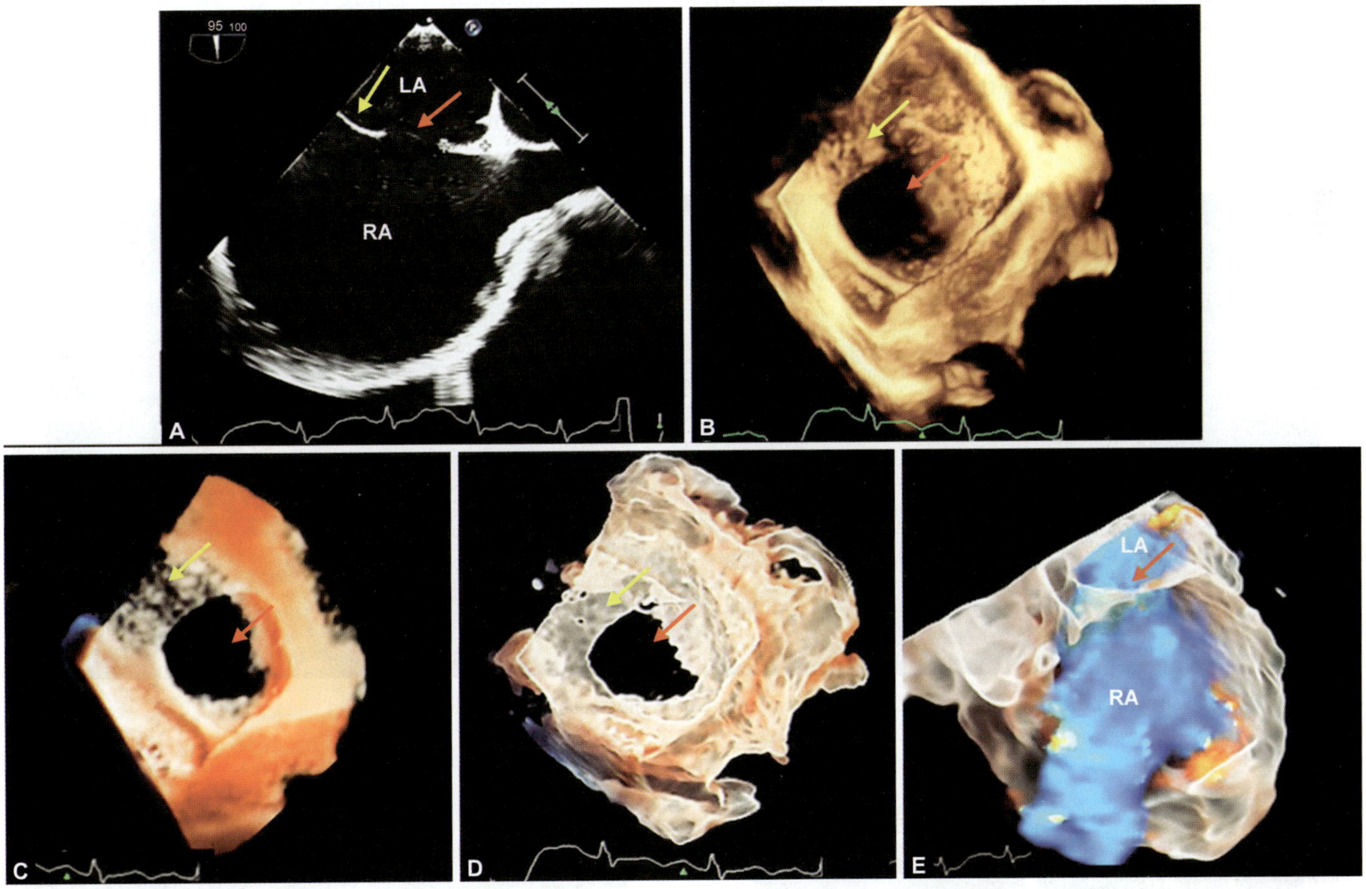

FIGS. 6A TO E: (A) The 2D; (B) Traditional 3D; (C) TrueVue Light; (D) TrueVue Glass; (E) TrueVue Glass showing left to right shunt in OS type of atrial septal defect.

and MRI), will allow for both automated anatomic orientation of 3DE.

ULTRAFAST ULTRASOUND IMAGING

Ultrafast ultrasound imaging uses high frame rates, which are 100 times greater than conventional methods to capture rapidly moving structures such as myocardium and complex blood flows. The spatial resolution of the image is improved by using multiple plane waves at different angles (called coherent plane wave compounding).[18] Ultrafast ultrasound can be used to assess the following:

- *Imaging of blood flow:* Ultrafast vector flow imaging (VFI), coronary ultrafast Doppler angiography (CUDA)
  - *Vector flow imaging/blood speckle flow imaging*: This is based on the use of ultrafast ultrasound in tracking of blood speckles, without the use of contrast agents. It enables visualization and estimation of the direction and velocities of blood flow indifferent directions from any angle. By using 3D and 4D VFI

one can measure the intracardiac flow velocities, vorticity, and energy losses in patients with septal defects, PAH, etc.[19,20] **(Figs. 7 and 8)**.
 - *Coronary ultrafast Doppler angiography* can evaluate the epicardial and intramural coronary microvasculature and quantify the myocardial blood flow. Using power-velocity integrals, CUDA could provide hemodynamic information such as coronary flow reserve and quantify the coronary flow variations, which is especially useful in patients undergoing complex cardiac surgeries.[21]
- *Myocardial stiffness:* Natural shear wave imaging, shear wave elastography, electromechanical wave imaging
  - *Natural shear wave imaging, shear wave elastography:* Ultrafast ultrasound imaging uses a higher frame rate which enables visualization of short-lived myocardial tissue motion that cannot be detected by conventional techniques. Natural shear wave imaging detects myocardial mechanical waves that occur naturally (at the time of valve closure or following electrical depolarization). Shear wave elastography detects acoustic signals by transmitting an external mechanical wave. By tracking the shear waves and measuring their velocity, degree of myocardial stiffness and ventricular function can be assessed **(Fig. 9)**. Assessment of myocardial stiffness helps in identifying conditions such as cardiomyopathies and extent of myocardial fibrosis in myocarditis.[22] Myocardial stiffness also helps in the understanding of systolic and diastolic dysfunction in children.[23]
  - *Electromechanical wave imaging (EWI)*: Electromechanical coupling is a very short-lived cardiac event between electrical and mechanical activation. EWI measures the motion induced by the electromechanical coupling, which can estimate the mechanical activation timing and map it. In a study

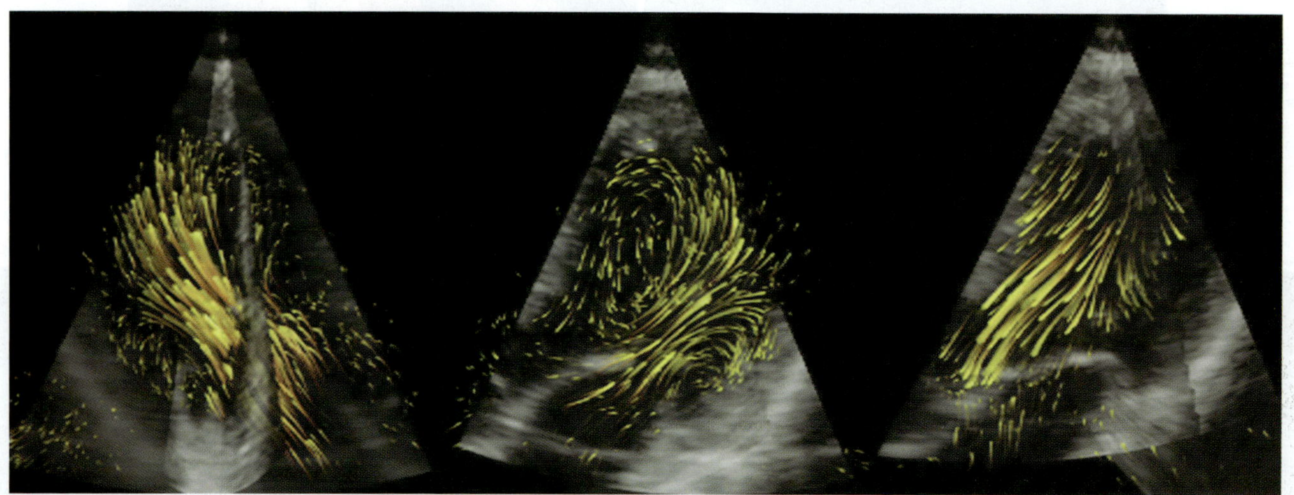

FIG. 7: 4D VFI showing the flow of blood during ventricular diastole, diastasis, and systole.

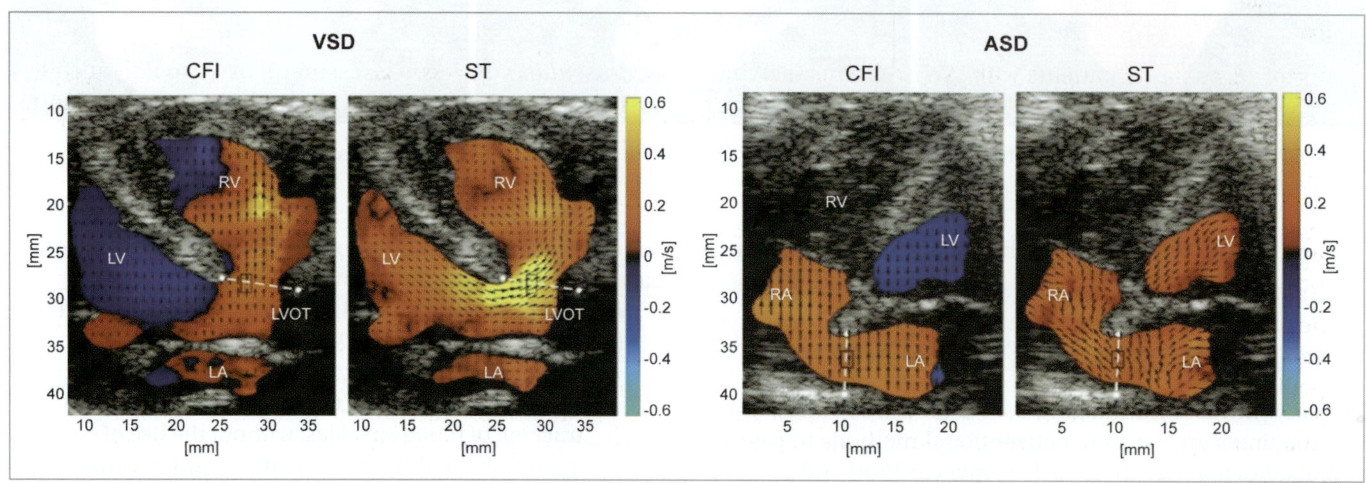

FIG. 8: Comparison between conventional color flow imaging and vector flow imaging by speckle tracking in ventricular septal defect shunt (VSD) and atrial septal defect shunt (ASD).

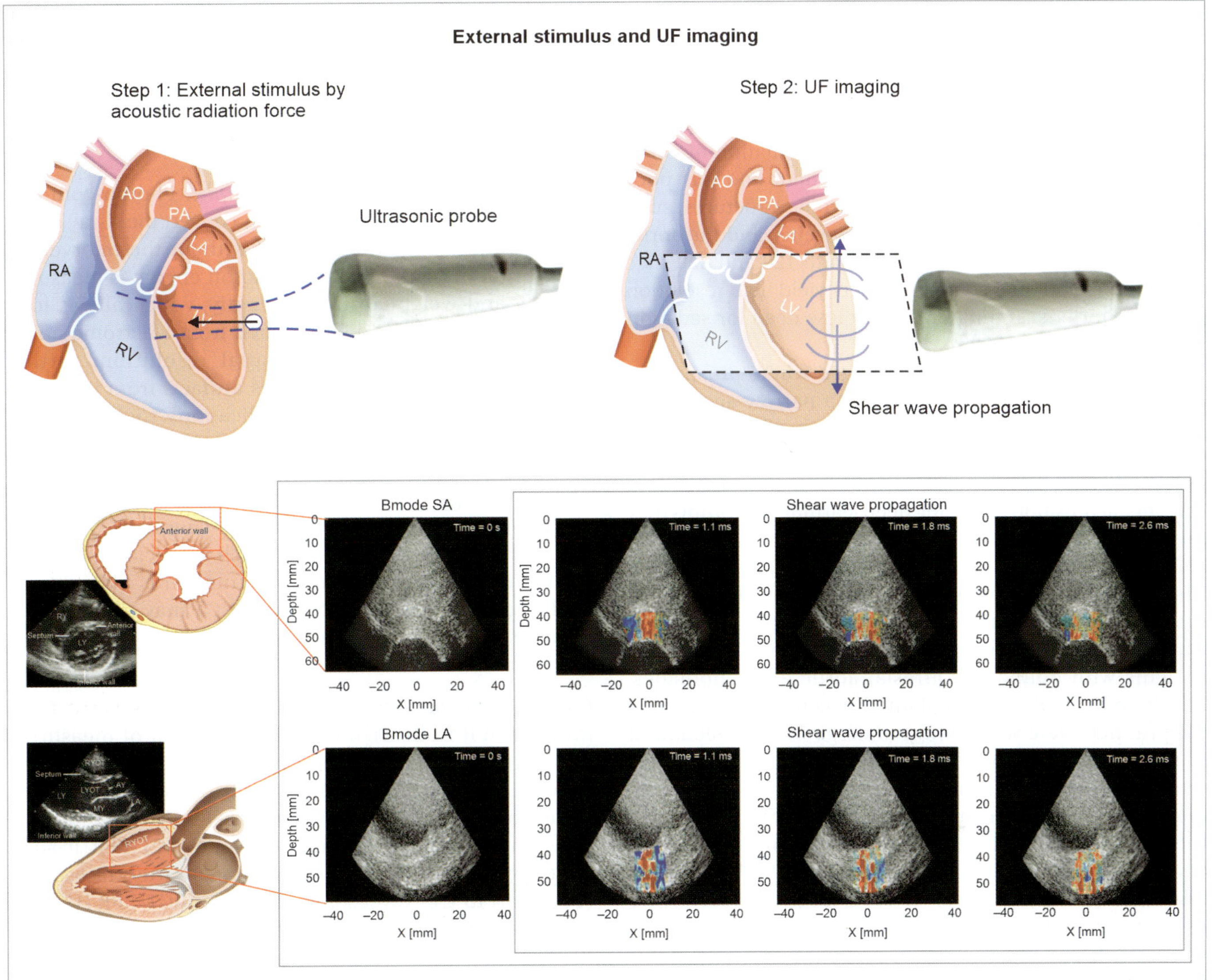

FIG. 9: Shear wave elastography measuring the propagation of the shear wave and deduced shear wave speed after an external stimulus.

of 15 pediatric patients with Wolff-Parkinson-White syndrome, EWI was capable of consistently localizing accessory pathways.[24]

- *Myocardial fiber array—Backscatter tensor imaging (BTI), elastic tensor imaging (ETI):* Ultrafast ultrasound can measure the degree of myocardial disarray. In patients with hypertrophic cardiomyopathy, ETI has shown that fractional disarray/anisotropy is more compared to healthy volunteers.[25] Myocardial fiber array assessment can assess the degree of ventricular remodeling in pediatric patients.[26]
- *Myocardial perfusion*: Ultrafast ultrasound can measure blood flow to the myocardium more accurately than contrast echocardiography.
- *Vascular stiffness:* Assessment of vascular stiffness helps in evaluation of patients with coarctation of aorta, carotid artery disease and in those undergoing prosthetic vascular implants.

By reducing the time needed to image rapidly moving structures, ultrafast ultrasound imaging may reduce the need for more invasive imaging tests like cardiac MRI or those requiring radiation like cardiac CT.[27] Better diagnosis and devising individualized treatment can improve care of patients with CHD. However, ultrafast imaging currently provides a segmented rather than a global myocardial analysis and is still an experimental imaging tool that needs more widespread clinical application especially in pediatric population.

ADVANCES IN CARDIAC COMPUTED TOMOGRAPHY

Cardiac computed tomography plays a vital role in evaluating congenital heart disease (CHD). While echocardiography is the primary technique used for the evaluation of CHD, it is limited by being operator dependent and has poor acoustic windows to evaluate extracardiac structures, such as the pulmonary arteries, pulmonary veins, and the aortic arch and great vessels.[28] 16-MDCT up to 128 and 320 slice CT scanners and dual source scanners yield high resolution images, shorter scanning time, with less need for sedation and less radiation exposure.

Low-dose CT imaging has emerged where prospective ECG gating, limits radiation dose to a narrow acquisition window with cine imaging. This allows reduction of radiation dose by 85–90%.[29] Use of increasingly sophisticated image processing tools that decrease noise in the reconstructed data sets after acquisition and using deep learning algorithms may further reduce radiation dose.

Cardiac computed tomography can be considered the first-line imaging technique for evaluation of suspected systemic or pulmonary vein anomalies, vascular ring or sling,[30] suspected aortopulmonary collateral arteries in patients with pulmonary atresia, aortic arch anomalies, and in individuals with implanted pacemakers and metal surgical hardware who cannot undergo MRI. Detection or exclusion of coronary anomalies and coronary fistulas is another important use of CCT. Multiplanar reformatted and 3D reconstructed images can be helpful in guiding the treatment in patients with coronary anomalies.[31] CCT is also useful in post operative follow up of CHD patients undergoing interventional or surgical procedures. CCT can assess the patency of shunts such as BT shunt, RV-PA conduits, Glenn shunt, Fontan pathways and also stents such as in coarctation of aorta. In patients with coarctation of aorta, CCT can assess the accurately depict the location, extent, and severity; presence of collateral vessels; plan the appropriate treatment and monitor for post-surgical or post-interventional complications such as residual or recurrent stenosis, aneurysm formation, or stent-related issues[32] **(Figs. 10A to C to 12)**.

Photon-counting computed tomography: Photon-counting detectors are a new technology that convert the X-ray signal directly into an electronic signal without the intervening conversion to light. Individual photon energy is measured directly and weighted independently, which allows low-energy photons to be differentiated from electronic noise. This technology improves spatial resolution, further reduces radiation, and minimizes artifacts from implants, with potential for advanced applications such as virtual non-contrast scans (calcium maps, iodine maps) and measurement of extracellular volume or coronary plaque quantity[33] **(Figs. 13A to C)**.

Some studies suggest that photon-counting CT (PCCT) can minimize motion artifacts, which is crucial in imaging infants and young children where motion is a significant challenge. Research indicates that PCCT may eliminate the need for ECG gating in some cases, simplifying the imaging process and further reducing radiation exposure.[34,35]

Computed tomography-derived fractional flow reserve: Non-invasive FFR from CT imaging is a method of measuring FFR with the use of computational fluid dynamics. Several randomized controlled trials have demonstrated good correlation between invasive FFR and computed tomography-derived fractional flow reserve (CT-FFR) in adult patients undergoing evaluation of coronary artery disease[36,37] **(Figs. 14A to C)**. Novel software such as uCT-FFR (United-Imaging Computed Tomography-Derived Fractional Flow Reserve) and machine learning-based approaches enable rapid on-site and real-time computation of FFR.[38]

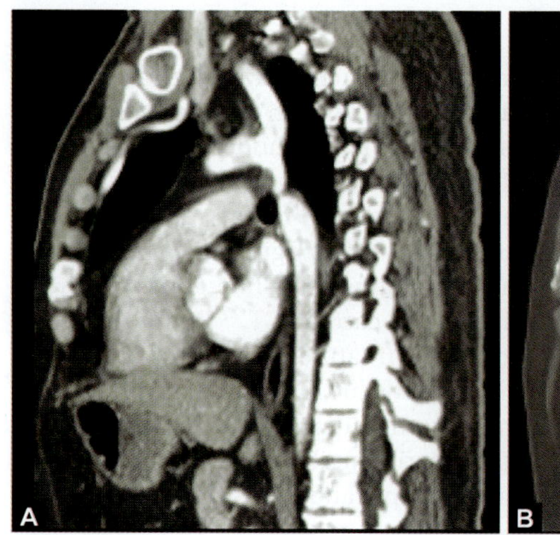

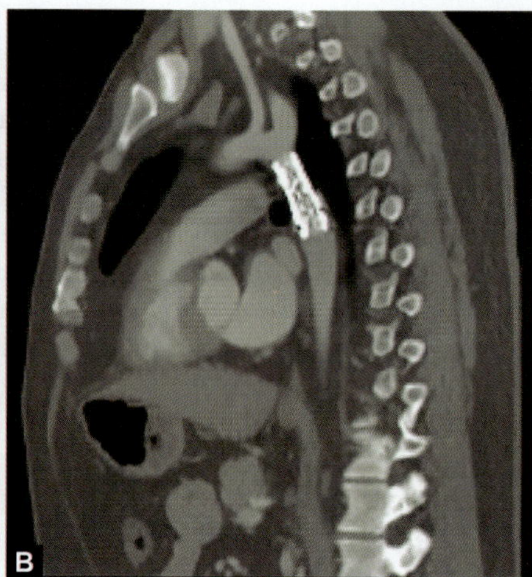

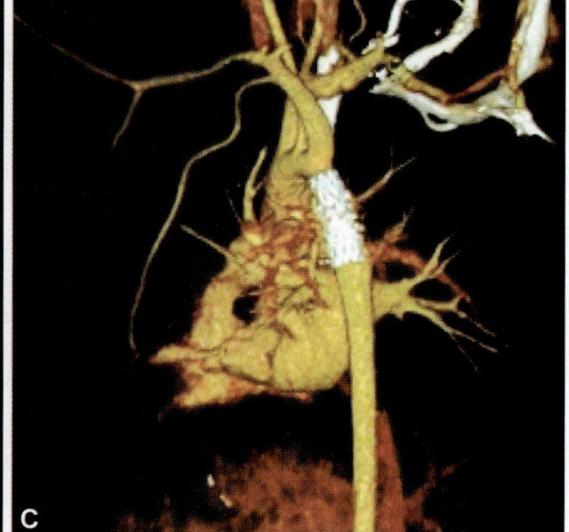

FIGS. 10A TO C: Computed tomography angiography of the aorta in the sagittal planes demonstrating (A) severity of the coarctation; (B) CoA after successful stenting; (C) Three-dimensional reconstruction displaying the luminal surface of the Cheatham-Platinum covered stent.

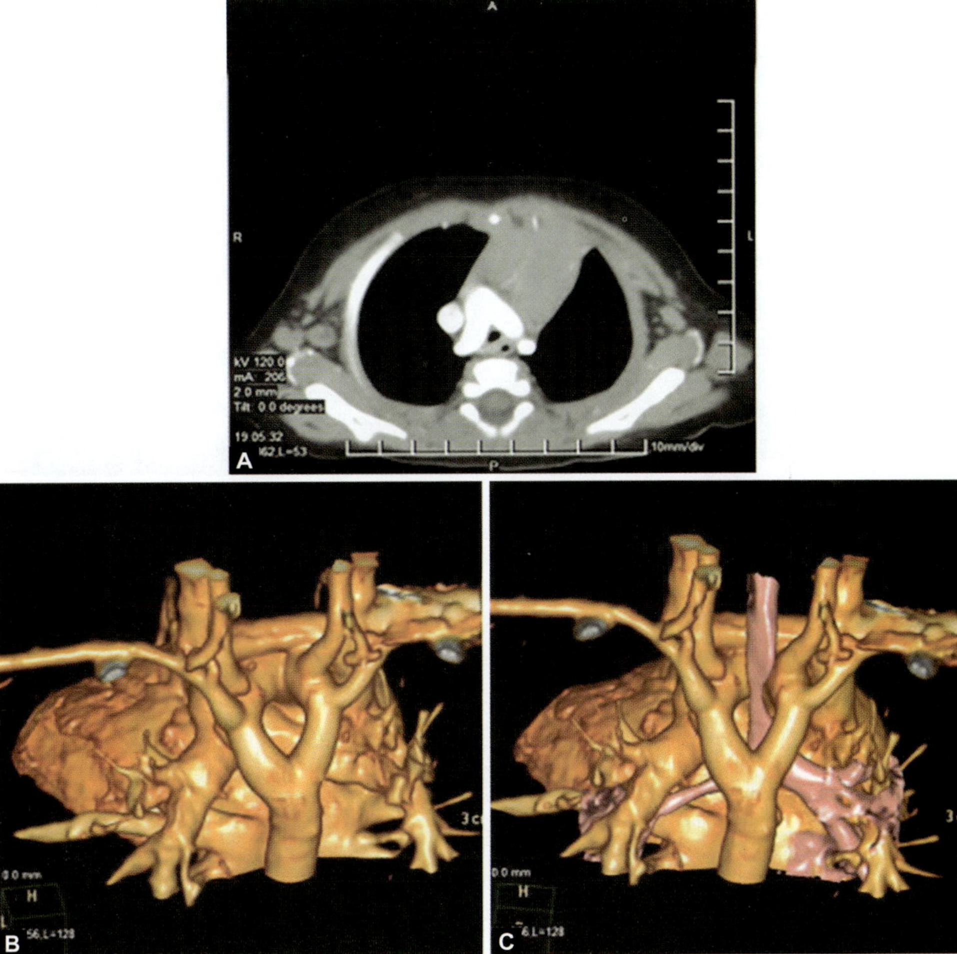

FIGS. 11A TO C: Codominant double aortic arch; (A) Axial contrast-enhanced CT showing the double aortic arch compressing the trachea; (B and C) Volume-rendered, posterior view shows the double aortic arch forming a complete ring encircling and compressing the trachea.

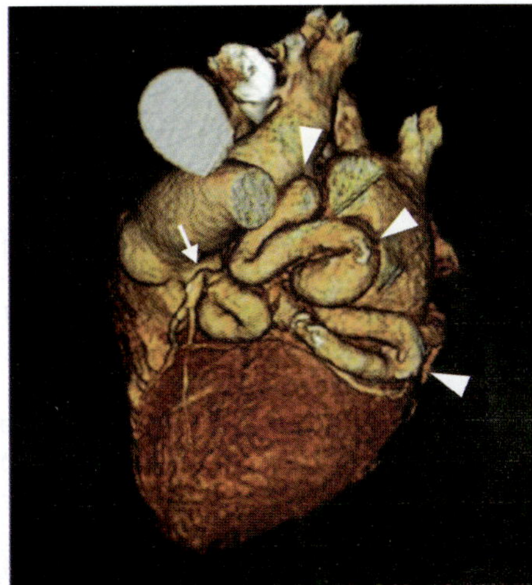

FIG. 12: Tortuous, dilated left circumflex artery and fistula in a 3-dimensional volume-rendered CT image.

Computed tomography-derived fractional flow reserve may have utility in patients with anomalous aortic origin of a coronary artery (AAOCA), coronary artery stenosis after reimplantation as part of CHD surgery and in patients with Kawasaki's disease.[39,40] However, further studies are needed to guide the clinical use of CT FFR in pediatric and CHD patients.

ADVANCES IN CARDIAC MAGNETIC RESONANCE IMAGING

Magnetic resonance imaging is a non-invasive tool in the imaging of CHD. MRI is superior to CT in delineation of soft tissue and to study the tissue characteristics.[41] Lack of ionizing radiation makes it especially useful in children and young adults. The Task Force of the European Society of

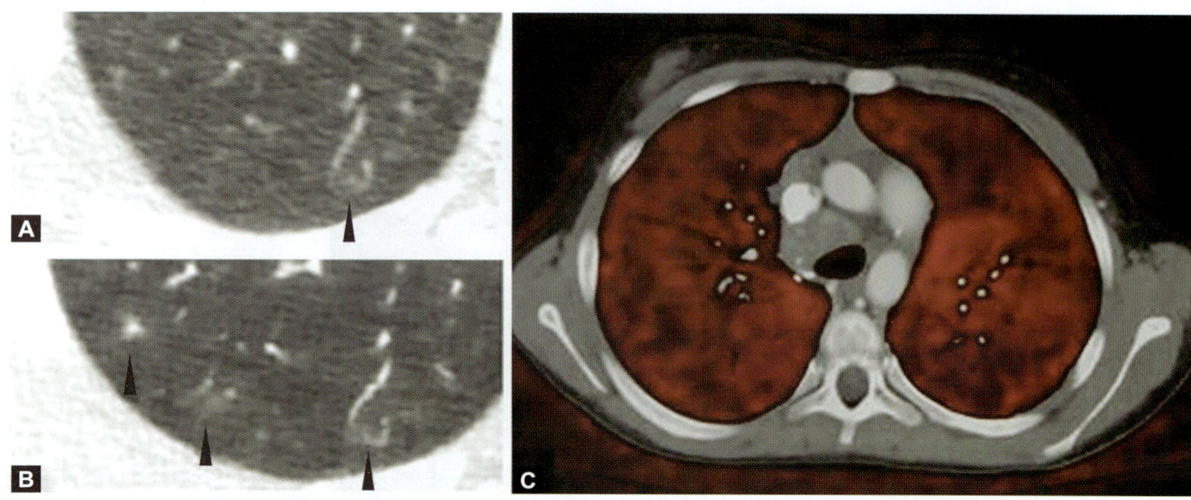

FIGS. 13A TO C: Photon counting CT in hereditary hemorrhagic telangiectasia. Shows better detection of peripheral arteriovenous malformations than conventional CT. PCCT of lung showing heterogeneous perfusion of the lung parenchyma.

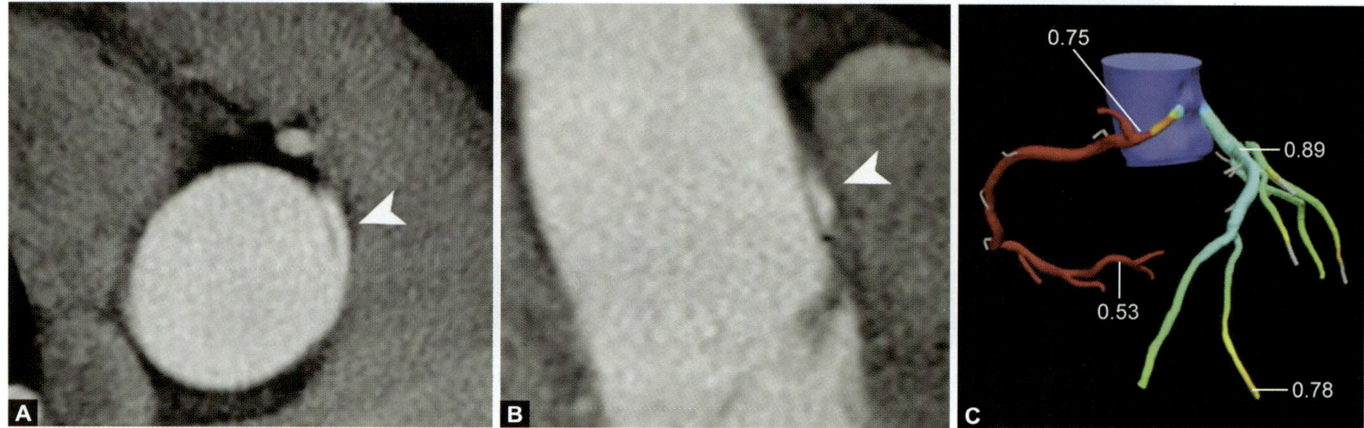

FIGS. 14A TO C: Coronary CTA and FFR-CT (CT guided fractional flow reserve) images of right coronary arteries with anomalous aortic origin and intramural path showing a take-off angle of <30° (A), elliptic coronary ostium with luminal narrowing of >50% (B) and FFR-CT value of 0.75 in proximal RCA \(C).

Cardiology[42] has established the role of MRI in patients with congenital heart disease as follows:

- Anatomical identification of cardiac structures
- Evaluation of thoracic aortic anomalies such as coarctation of aorta, right aortic arch, MAPCA, aberrant subclavian arteries
- Non-invasive detection of direction of flow and quantification of shunts, stenoses and regurgitations
- Evaluation of conotruncal malformations and complex anomalies
- Identification of pulmonary and systemic venous anomalies
- Postoperative-palliative shunts (BT shunt), RV-PA conduits, post-TOF surgery pulmonary artery size, RV function after Fontan repairs

However, cardiac MRI has major limitations with respect to longer acquisition time, need for anesthesia in children and need for contrast agents. To overcome these limitations novel techniques have emerged.[43]

Cardiac Magnetic Resonance Imaging Parametric Mapping

Cardiac magnetic resonance imaging parametric mapping consists of tissue characterization techniques, which rely on relative variations in image intensities to highlight abnormal tissues. They provide direct visualization of tissue properties such as T1, T2, T2* and ECV in absolute denominations (e.g., in milliseconds).[44]

Magnetic resonance imaging can provide tissue characterization by non-invasive assessments of myocardial fibrosis, edema, and iron deposition, which is increasingly being applied for risk stratification and to determine the timing of reintervention in repaired defects. Prolonged myocardial T1 times and expanded extracellular volume (ECV) are considered as markers of diffuse fibrosis and have been associated with decreased myocardial contractility in patients with TOF.[45] Prolonged T2-signal decay times can determine the presence of an inflammatory component due to edema such as in acute myocarditis.[46]

Magnetic Resonance Lymphangiography

Magnetic resonance (MR) can assess the anatomy and physiology of the lymphatic system[47] by using static MR lymphangiography and/or dynamic contrast-enhanced magnetic resonance lymphangiography (DCMRL). MR lymphangiography can help in the assessment of lymphatic disorders that complicate CHD such as after Fontan surgery patients developing protein-losing enteropathy, plastic bronchitis, and chylous effusions due to increase in lymphatic pressures. Greater lymphatic burden, assessed by T2-weighted imaging, in these patients are associated with adverse outcomes.[48]

Three-dimensional/Four-dimensional Magnetic Resonance Imaging, Four-dimensional Flow Magnetic Resonance Imaging

By adding a third spatial dimension, 3D or sometimes 4-dimensional (4D) cine and 4D phase contrast MR imaging enables rapid acquisition of the whole data set with offline processing. Comparable automatic volume assessments right and left ventricles and their functional analysis is possible.[49-50]

Four-dimensional flow CMR refers to phase-contrast CMR (ECG gated) with flow-encoding in all three spatial directions, in typical transverse, sagittal, and coronal planes with time as the 4th dimension along the cardiac cycle. The velocities are color coded and represented as flow patterns.[51]

Four-dimensional flow provides information on advanced hemodynamic measures, such as vorticity, helicity, intra cavitary blood flow kinetic energy, wall shear stress, atrioventricular valve inflow and regurgitation, pressure gradients, shunt flows and pulse-wave velocity.[52,53] Kinetic energy represents the amount of energy present in the blood flow due to movement, and its loss is a marker of ventricular insufficiency. In patients with TOF, abnormal kinetic energy was noted, indicating ventricular dysfunction much before abnormalities in EDVI, ESVI, and EF. Higher kinetic energy in RVOT suggest pulmonary regurgitation in TOF cases[54] **(Figs. 15A to D)**. 4D flow MRI can also accurately assess pulmonary valve or branch stenosis and quantify the PV regurgitant flow after TOF repair.

Four-dimensional MRI can assess ventricle function, valvular regurgitation, patency of the Fontan pathway, and presence of collateral flow after Fontan's surgery. Post surgical decrease in the pulmonary artery flow can also be assessed[55] **(Fig. 16)**.

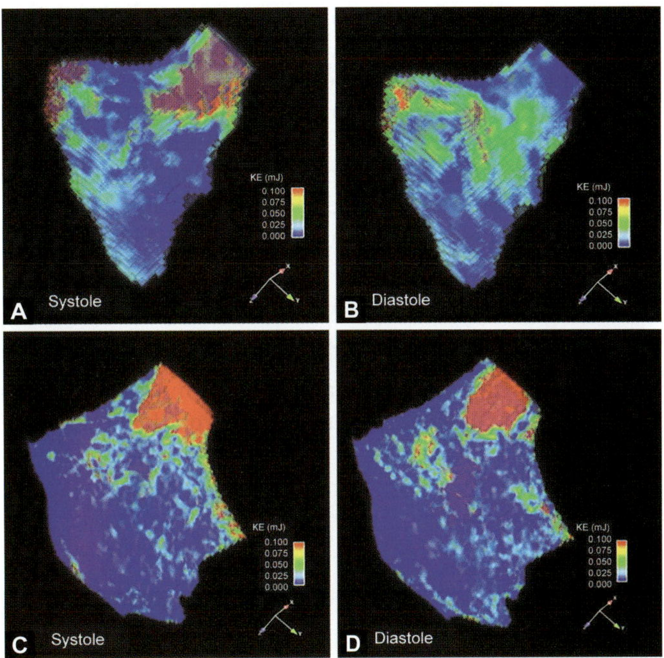

FIGS. 15A TO D: (A and B) Normal RV Kinetic energy maps in a long axis orientation; (C and D) Higher kinetic energies (redder) are seen along the RV outflow tract during systole and along the RV inner curvature during diastole due to the presence of pulmonic regurgitation on a TOF patient.[55]

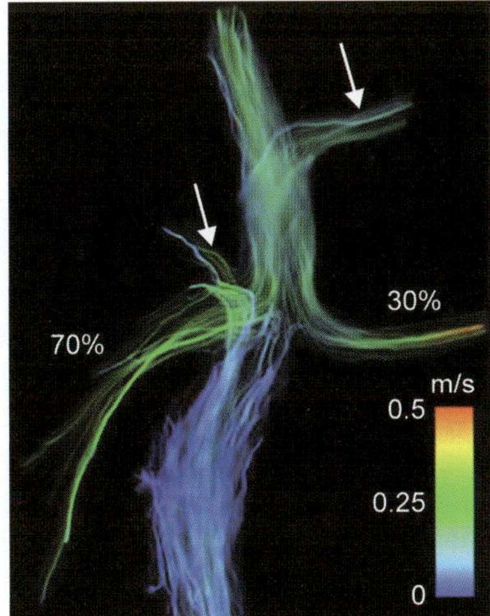

FIG. 16: 4D flow MRI in a total cavo-pulmonary connection with flow distribution 70% into the RPA and 30% in LPA.
(LPA: left pulmonary artery; RPA: right pulmonary artery)

Cardiac Magnetic Resonance Finger Printing

Magnetic resonance finger printing is a rapid, multi-parametric tissue property mapping that allows simultaneous efficient measurements of multiple tissue properties with one acquisition, thereby improving the efficiency of cardiac

MRI examination.[56] It involves a three-step process—data acquisition, pattern matching and tissue property visualization. T1 and T2 values obtained with MRF studies have shown good correlation with conventional T1 and T2 mapping methods. Information about tissue perfusion, ECV, fat deposition, T2* can provide similar information as MR imaging, without the need for contrast agent, thereby enabling widespread clinical applications[57,58] **(Fig. 17)**.

Invasive Cardiovascular Magnetic Resonance Imaging

Invasive cardiovascular magnetic resonance imaging (iCMR) of cardiac catheterization provides real-time anatomical visualization of the cardiovascular structures[59] and hemodynamic data, without radiation exposure, especially in children. Conditioned catheters and guidewires with gadolinium-filled balloon are used in CMR-guided cardiac catheterization to measure cardiac output and the QP/QS ratio by phase contrast imaging. Ventricular and atrial volumes, EF, and functional analysis with tissue characterization can also be done. Reddy et al. demonstrated the potential of iCMR in diagnostic right and left heart studies, CoA diagnosis, and in hemodynamic testing after Fontan fenestration occlusion.[60]

The balloon attached to the tip of the catheter is filled with diluted gadolinium and guided using a conditioned guide toward the structures to be evaluated hemodynamically

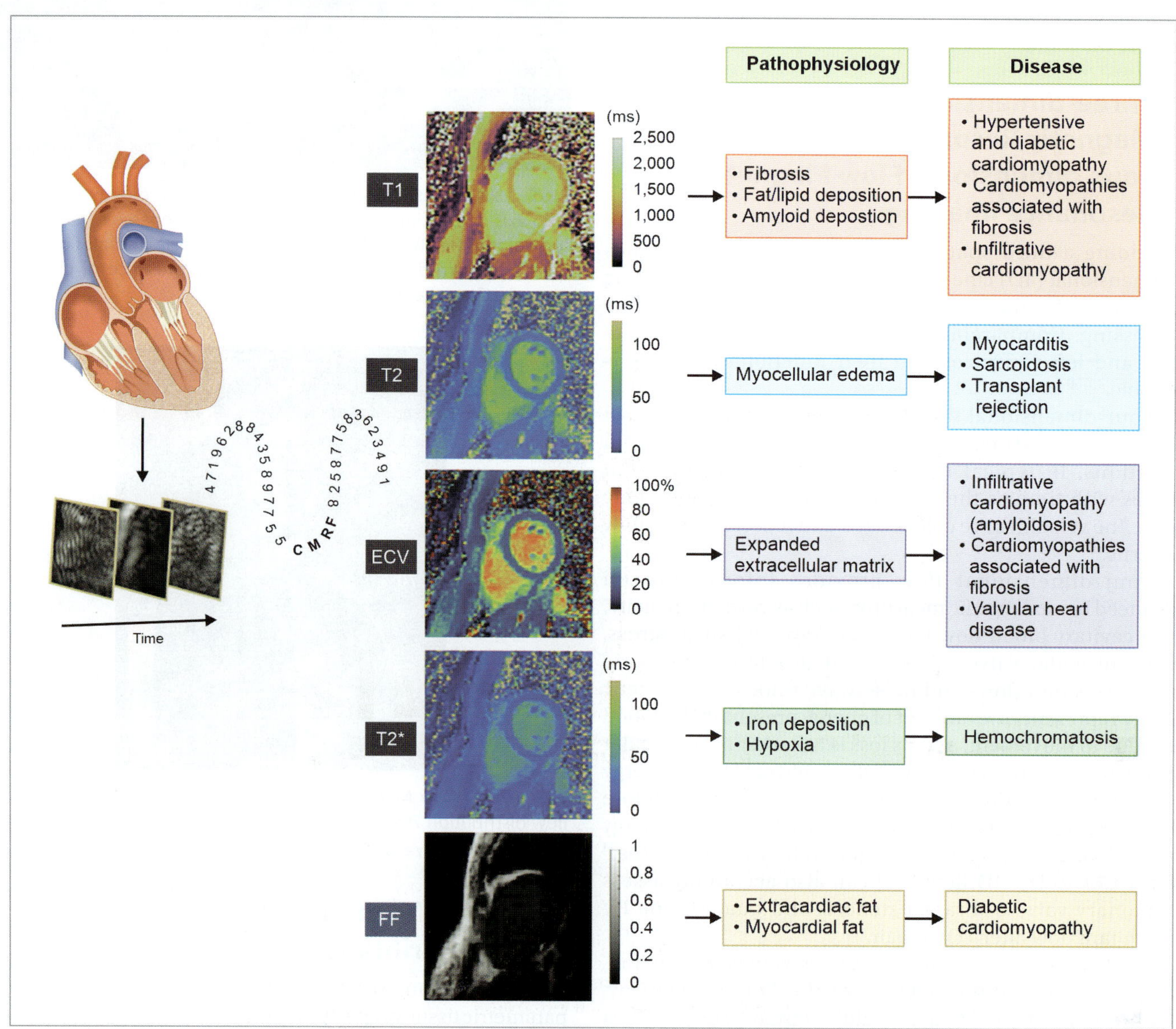

FIG. 17: Role of cardiac magnetic resonance fingerprinting (cMRF) in the assessment of an array of myocardial diseases.
(ECV: extracellular volume fraction; FF: fat fraction)
Source: Adapted from Liu Y, Hamilton J, Rajagopalan S, et al. Cardiac Magnetic Resonance Fingerprinting: Technical Overview and Initial Results. JACC Cardiovasc Imaging. 2018;11(12):1837-53.

(Figs. 18A to G). However, further studies and evaluation are needed for its widespread availability.

Three-dimensional Rotational Angiography

Three-dimensional rotational angiography (3DRA) consists of the single-plane C-arm flat panel detector rotating around the patient over 4–5 seconds during contrast injection. A real time 2D angiogram images with 200°–240° of viewing can be obtained, which allows 3D reconstruction and multiplanar reformatting. Advantage over CT is the better visualization of soft tissues and airway with spatial resolution enabling the understanding of the orientation of cardiac structures and vessels with the surrounding structures.[61] Optimal angle for imaging can be selected reducing the radiation and contrast dose.[62]

Most of the software can automatically register and overlay images onto live fluoroscopy images which can improve procedural efficiency.[63,64] Intraluminal fly-through and clipping-plane views allow an endovascular assessment of stents, aneurysms, vessel wall irregularities, and calcification.

By integrating data from 3D rotational angiography images with other imaging modalities, 3D printing and virtual procedural planning can be done.[65] Further advances in using 3DRA involves combining the hemodynamic data with computational fluid dynamics (CFD) assessment. This permits virtual stenting, and prediction of hemodynamic outcomes after intervention.[66]

FUSION IMAGING

In Fusion imaging, 3D reconstructions from echocardiography, CMR, CCT, and angiography are fused with fluoroscopy for real-time procedural guidance.[67] This technique enhances understanding of complex anatomy, facilitates navigation, and improves procedural guidance, potentially reducing radiation exposure and improving outcome. This technique has shown excellent safety and usability in children.[68]

Fusion imaging is being increasingly used for a variety of transcatheter procedures, such as closure of septal defects, balloon valvuloplasty, stenting of pulmonary veins, and pulmonary valve implantations[69-71] **(Figs. 19A to F)**.

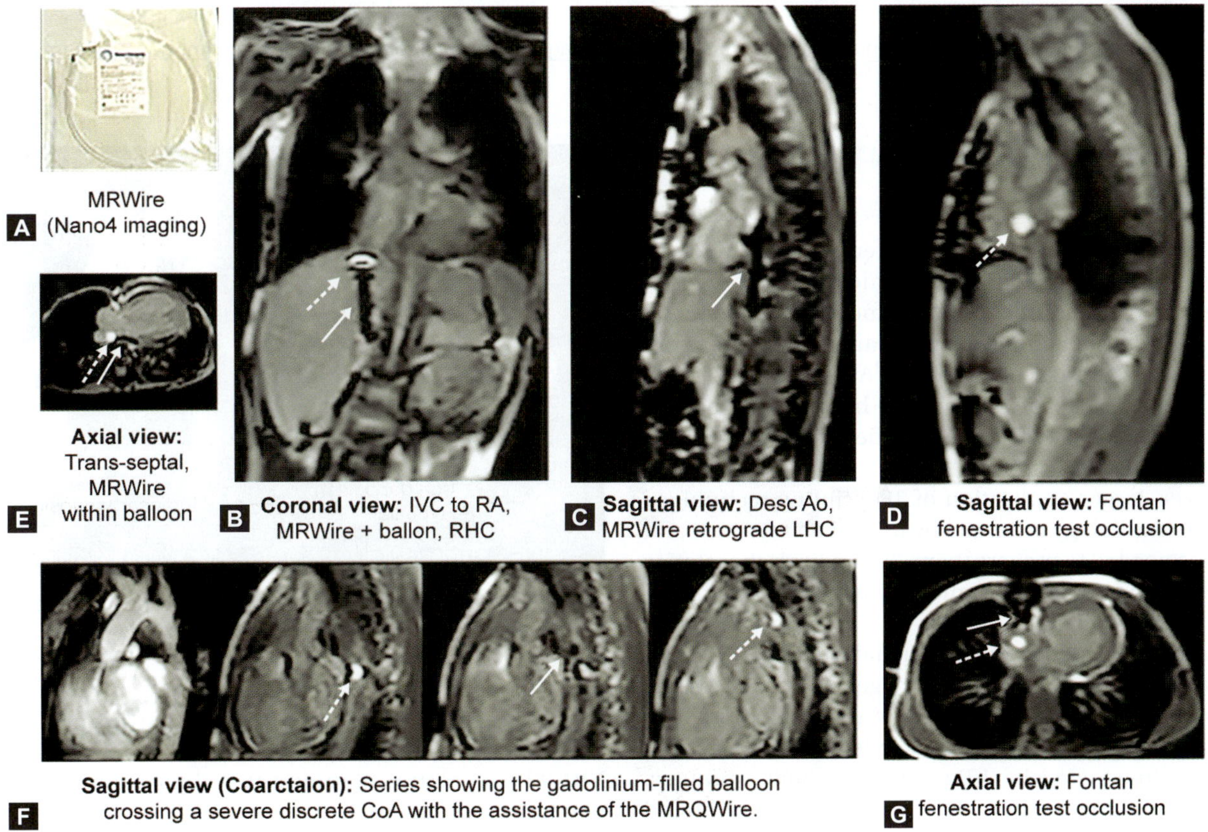

FIG 18 A TO G: Invasive Magnetic resonance imaging. (A) shows MR wire, (E) shows transeptal MR wire (white arrow) with gadolinium-filled balloon (dashed white arrow), (B) shows right heart catheterisation (RHC) being done, (C) shows Left heart catheterisation (LHC) being done, (D) shows Fontan fenestration test occlusion, (F) shows Gadolinium filled balloon crossing a severe coarctation of aorta, and (G) shows axial view of Fontan fenestration occlusion test.

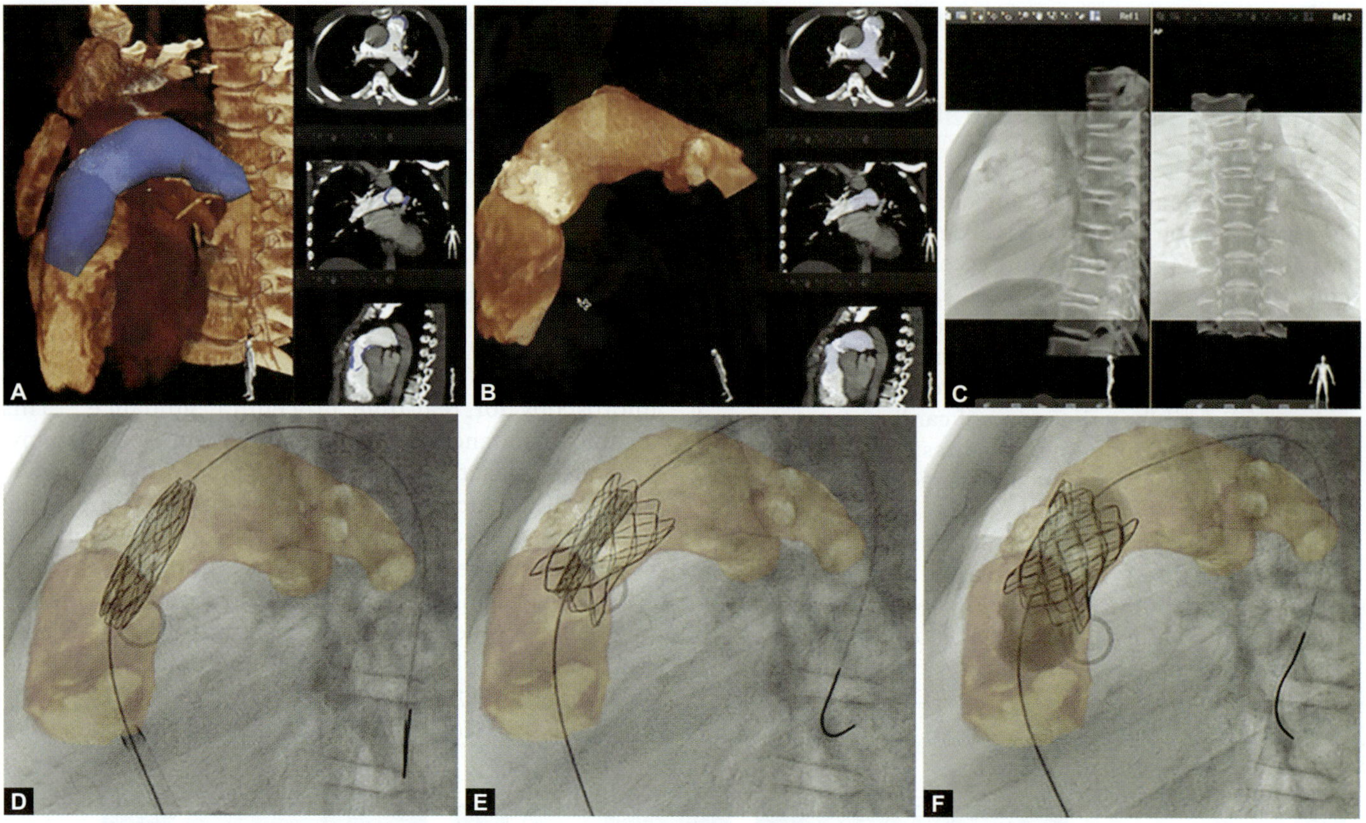

FIGS. 19A TO F: Automatic three-dimensional (3D) fusion images of CT images with live fluoroscopy during pulmonary valve implantation (Melody valve).[71]

THREE-DIMENSIONAL PRINTING AND VIRTUAL REALITY

Three-dimensional (3D) printing technology involves creating a patient-specific anatomical model, which enhances the perception of depth, dimensions and spatial configuration of the complex cardiac anomalies, therefore facilitating the surgical planning.[72,73]A multicenter study showed that the use of 3D-printed heart CHD models enabled surgical decisions to be modified in around 50% of cases[74] **(Fig. 20)**.

However, larger application of 3D printing technology in pediatric cardiology is limited by its availability, cost, and longer time needed to prepare them. 3D medical laboratories are working to create anatomic digital twins which can display 3D images digitally.

An alternate technique is virtual reality (VR). VR transforms standard 2D medical images (CT scans, MRIs, echocardiograms) into dynamic, interactive 3D models of the heart[75] **(Fig. 21)**. Raimondi and colleagues showed that the median time to develop VR models was only 5 minutes, which is much less than 3D (8 hours).[76] Enhanced visualization helps in pre-procedural planning. VR also enables remote consultations and enhanced knowledge sharing.

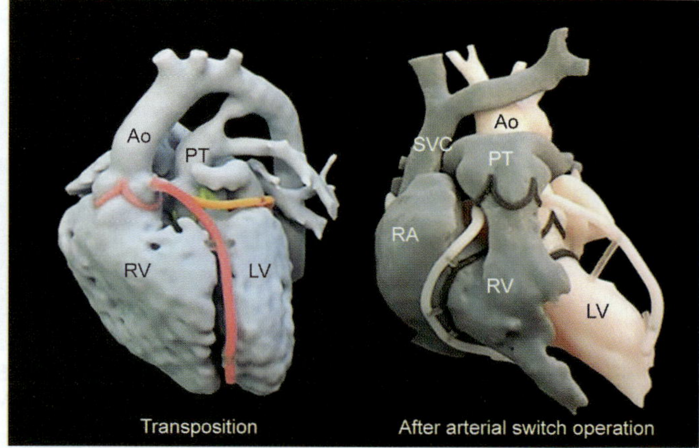

FIG. 20: D-printed models of transposition of the great arteries before and after arterial switch operation.

VIRTUAL PROCEDURAL PLANNING

Virtual procedural planning is a digital simulation of a planned procedure using patient-specific 3D anatomical data (from CT, MRI, or echocardiography). It allows clinicians to visualize complex anatomical structures, simulate surgeries or interventions virtually, assess the feasibility of

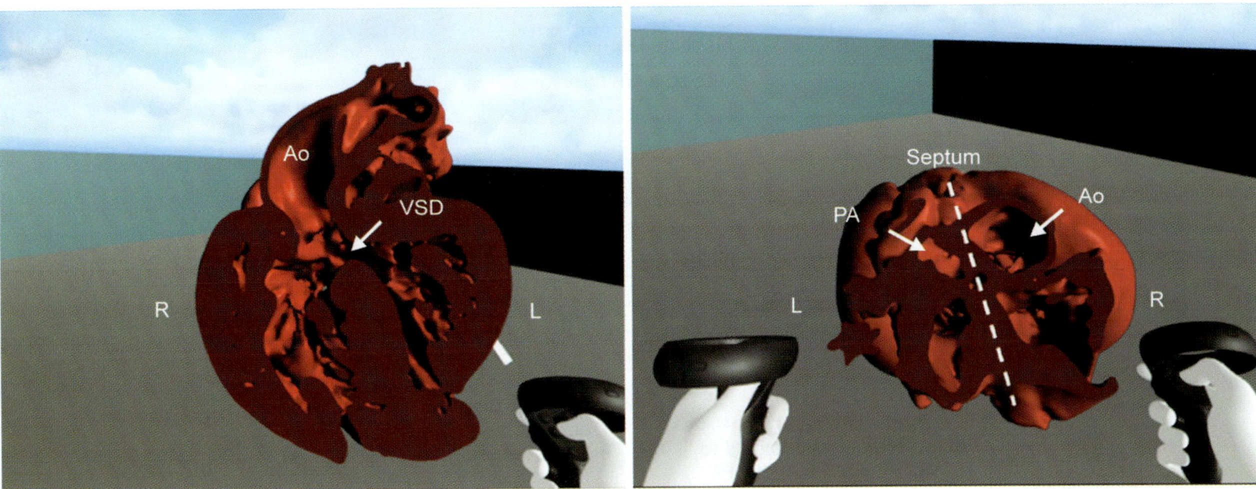

FIG. 21: Virtual reality (VR) images in a case of TOF showing aorta overriding and VSD.

procedures, plan strategies before the actual procedure and allows a multidisciplinary team collaboration by providing a shared visual reference.[77] By integrating imaging data with computational models and simulation, VPP is becoming an essential adjunct to conventional imaging, offering a more precise, personalized approach to CHD management.[78]

ARTIFICIAL INTELLIGENCE AND MACHINE LEARNING

Artificial intelligence (AI) is an upcoming and promising tool that is likely to have a wider spread application in the management of congenital heart diseases in future **(Fig. 22)**. Echocardiography-specific ML (machine learning) and deep learning (DL) algorithms can identify different echocardiographic views and improve the inferences from the images. By using AI, accurate and rapid assessment of LV structure and function is possible.[79-81] Similar applications of DL echocardiography can detect hypertrophic cardiomyopathy, pulmonary arterial anomalies, atrial septal defects, ventricular septal defects, and coarctation of the aorta.[82-83] Measurement of transvalvular gradients and diastolic dysfunction can be done with adequate reliability and precision .[84-85]

Artificial intelligence has the potential to rapidly analyze the entire data set of cardiac CT and MRI images and perform image segmentation of different regions of the heart. This can significantly reduce the time needed for post processing of images, and improve image interpretation.[86,87] Tandon et al. demonstrated that AI can be adapted for use in repaired tetralogy of Fallot cases, with a relatively small new training dataset.[88] Zhang et al. have developed a system for myocardial scar delineation using non-contrast cine and T1 images.[89] This is of particular importance in children where safety of gadolinium deposition is unclear.

Artificial intelligence also allows segmentation and analysis of coronary CT angiography images. Coenen et al.[90] developed a DL-based algorithm for non-invasive FFR measurement which can identify functionally significant obstructive coronary artery disease with 78% accuracy compared with visual assessment (58% accuracy).

Future advancements can involve development of CHD-specific AI algorithms which can reduce the image acquisition time, improve image processing, and yield better diagnostic accuracy. Development of completely automatic operator-independent AI-assisted imaging tools may be possible.[91] Other potential roles of AI in CHD imaging include:

- *Risk assessment and treatment planning*: ML models can predict the likelihood of complications, and guide personalized treatment plans including surgical approaches.
- *Research and drug development*: AI can analyze vast amounts of genomic and clinical data to understand the underlying genetic factors of CHD and develop new targets in drug development.
- *Telemedicine*: AI-based platforms can enable remote monitoring and consultations, improving the access to specialist care.
- *Patient education*: AI can provide patients and families with tailored educational information to improve their understanding of different heart diseases.

Limitations of Artificial Intelligence in Congenital Heart Diseases Imaging

- Most of the current AI algorithms are based on data from general cardiac patients, and not specific for CHD patients. Global collaboration is needed to improve the data set of congenital heart diseases.
- Limited availability of data in pediatric imaging and high rate of variability among them, makes AI application challenging.
- There are no published clinical trials comparing with MRI or CT images, making it difficult to establish the effectiveness of AI.

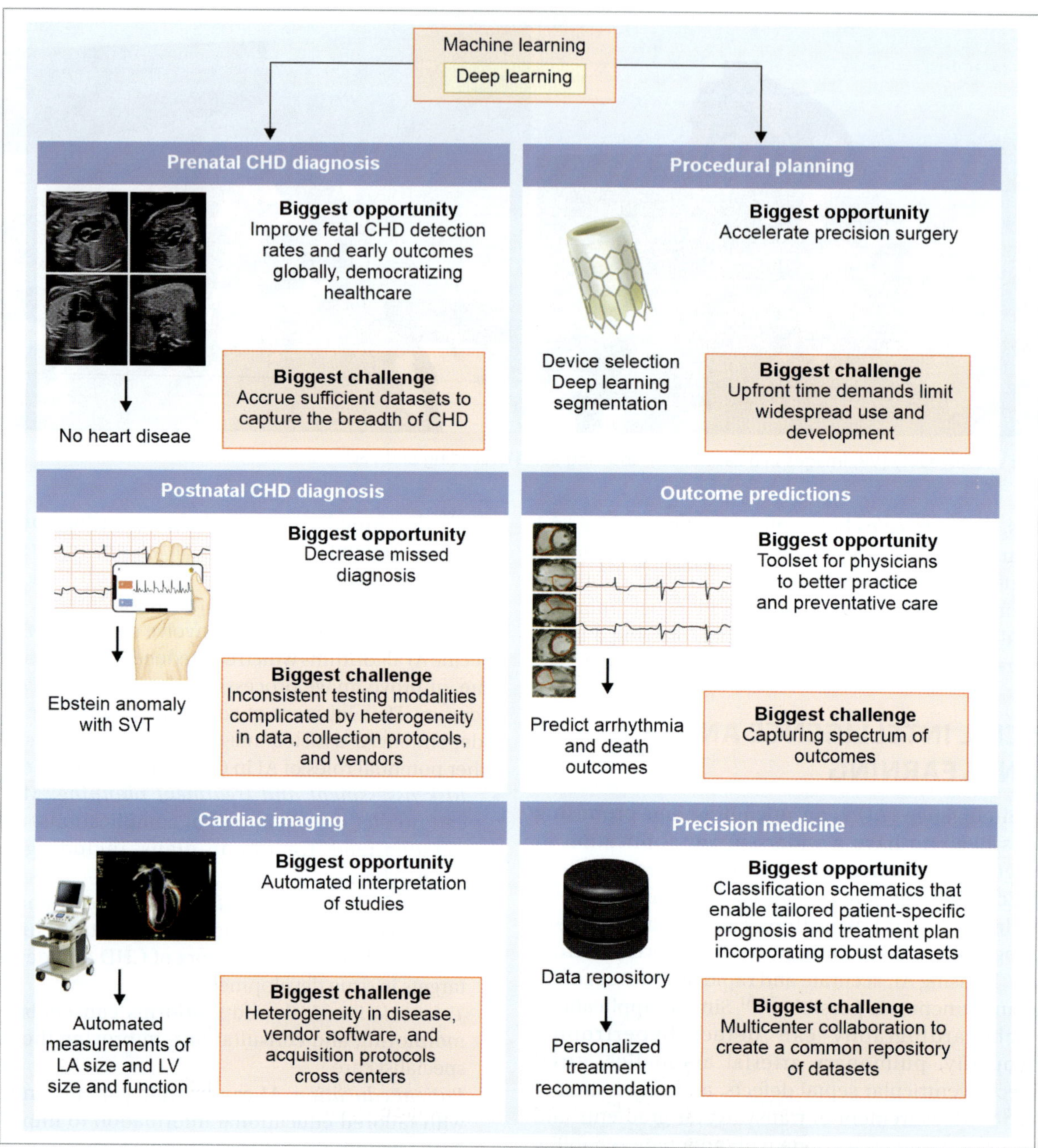

FIG. 22: Summary of the applications of AI in imaging of CHD.

Source: Adapted from Jone PN, Gearhart A, Lei H, et al. Artificial Intelligence in Congenital Heart Disease: Current State and Prospects. JACC Adv. 2022;1(5):100153.

- Inherent inertia to adopt and embrace AI technology limits its more widespread use.

CONCLUSION

Emerging imaging technologies are transforming the diagnosis and management of congenital heart disease. Techniques such as 3D echocardiography, 4D flow MRI, low-dose CT, and fusion imaging offer greater anatomical and functional detail, improving accuracy and guiding treatment **(Table 2)**. The growing role of AI further enhances efficiency and personalization. As these innovations continue to evolve, they hold the potential to transform the clinical approach to CHD, enabling earlier detection, minimally invasive interventions, and improved long-term outcomes. However, ongoing research, standardized protocols, and multidisciplinary collaboration remain essential to fully harness the benefits of these technologies in routine clinical practice.

TABLE 2: Novel tools in the imaging of CHD.

Name of the technique		Indications	Limitations
3D echocardiography	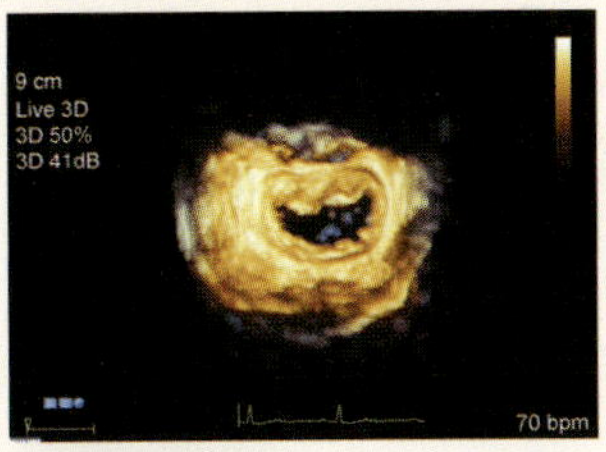	Septal defects, valve abnormalities, and complex congenital defects	Pulmonary valve/RVOT anomalies, anomalous systemic and pulmonary vein anomalies
Ultrafast ultrasound	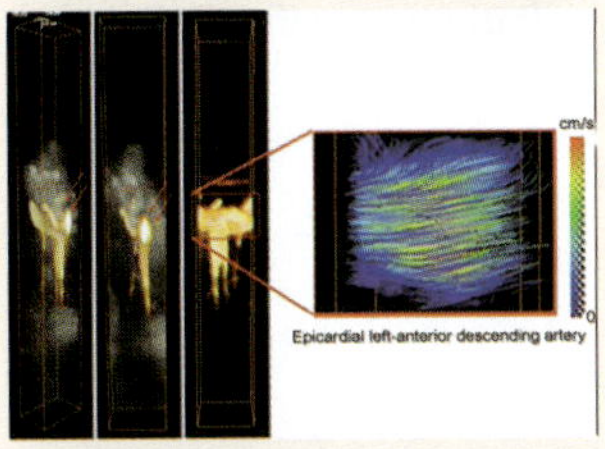	Blood flow velocity, myocardial function, and stiffness, coronary blood flow	Experimental, not widely available
Cardiac CT	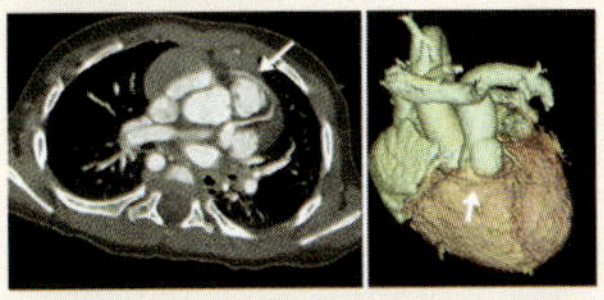	Complex cardiac defects, extra cardiac structures, such as pulmonary arteries, aorta, branch vessels, systemic and pulmonary veins	Radiation exposure, limited information on tissue characteristics
Cardiac MR	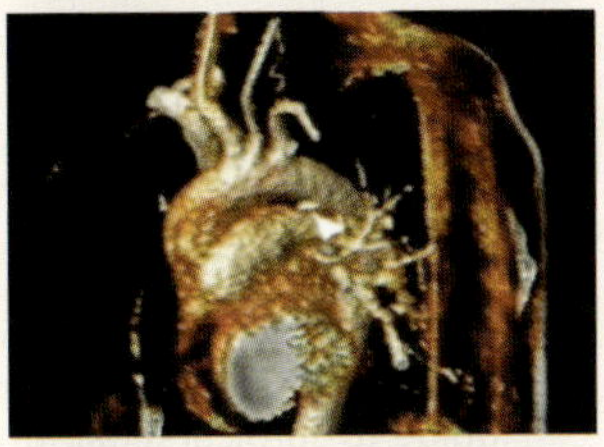	Complex cardiac anomalies, tissues characteristics, 4D flow, thoracic aorta anomalies	Longer acquisition time, need anesthesia in children
3D rotational angiography	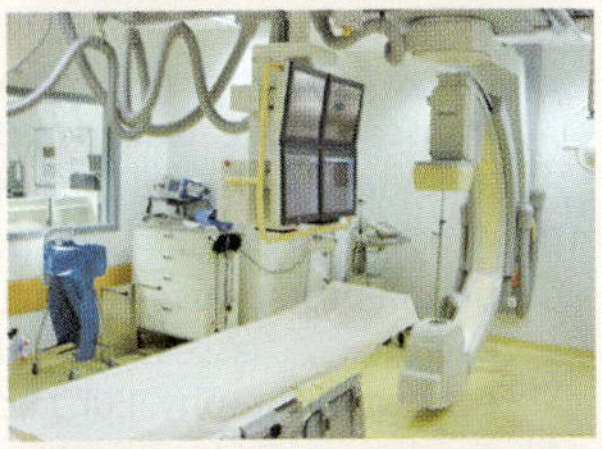	Real time views with analysis of relation to surrounding structures	Radiation exposure, limited information on tissue characteristics
Fusion imaging	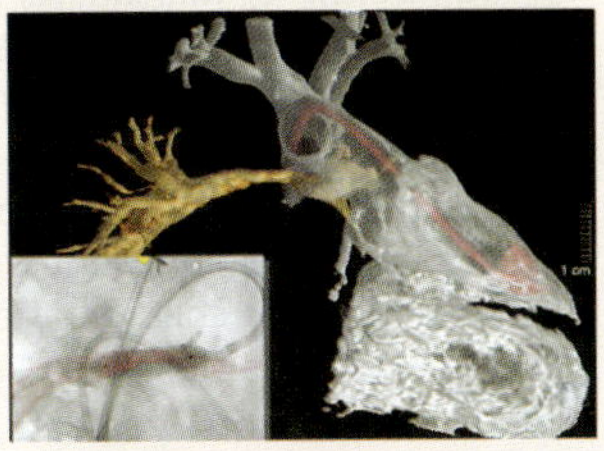	Understand complex anatomies, real time procedure guidance	Limited to certain procedures until now
3D printing	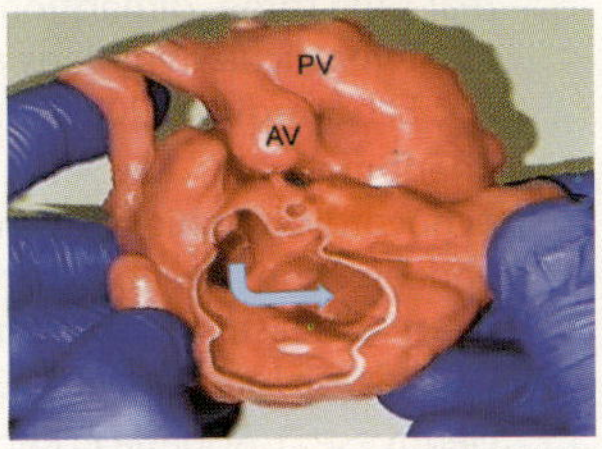	Understand anatomies and spatial configuration, facilitate procedures	Longer time to make, costly, limited availability

Continued

Continued

Name of the technique		Indications	Limitations
Virtual reality		Faster to develop. Facilitate procedure planning	Limited availability
Virtual procedure planning		Patient specific digital simulation	Limited availability
Artificial intelligence		Better diagnosis, interpretation of images, and precision planning	Developing field, and limited data in pediatric patients

REFERENCES

1. Sachdeva R, Aimee K. Armstrong, Rima Arnaout, et al. Novel Techniques in Imaging Congenital Heart Disease: JACC Scientific Statement. JACC J. 2024;83(1):63-81.
2. Simpson J, Lopez L, Acar P, et al. Three-dimensional echocardiography in congenital heart disease: an expert consensus document from the European Association of Cardiovascular Imaging and the American Society of Echocardiography. J Am Soc Echocardiogr. 2017;30(1):1-27.
3. Shah SS, A D, Madan N, et al. Initial experience with Pediatric 3D Transesophageal Echo Probe and Imaging System. Abstract presented at: 8th World Congress of Pediatric Cardiology and Cardiac Surgery; August 27–September 1, 2023; Washington, DC.
4. Pushparajah K, Miller OI, Simpson JM. 3D echocardiography of the atrial septum: anatomical features and landmarks for the echocardiographer. JACC Cardiovasc Imaging. 2010;3:981-4.
5. Roberson DA, Cui W, Patel D, et al. Three-dimensional transesophageal echocardiography of atrial septal defect: a qualitative and quantitative anatomic study. J Am Soc Echocardiogr. 2011;24:600-10.
6. Chen FL, Hsiung MC, Nanda N. Real time three-dimensional echocardiography in assessing ventricular septal defects: an echocardiographic-surgical correlative study. Echocardiography. 2006;23:562-8.
7. Charakida M, Qureshi S, Simpson JM. 3D echocardiography for planning and guidance of interventional closure of VSD. JACC Cardiovasc Imaging. 2013;6:120-3.
8. Rawlins DB, Austin C, Simpson JM. Live three-dimensional paediatric intraoperative epicardial echocardiography as a guide to surgical repair of atrioventricular valves. Cardiol Young. 2006;16:34-9.
9. Bhaya M, Mutluer FO, Mahan E. Live/real time three-dimensional transesophageal echocardiography in percutaneous closure of atrial septal defects Echocardiography. 2013;30:345-53.
10. Acar P, Abadir S, Aggoun Y. Transcatheter closure of perimembranous ventricular septal defects with Amplatzer occluder assessed by real-time three-dimensional echocardiography. Eur J Echocardiogr. 2007;8:110-5.
11. Tamborini G, Marsan N., Gripari P. Reference values for right ventricular volumes and ejection fraction with real-time three-dimensional echocardiography: evaluation in a large series of normal subjects, J Am Soc Echocardiogr. 2010;23:109-5.
12. Dragulescu A, Grosse-Wortmann L, Fackoury C. Echocardiographic assessment of right ventricular volumes: a comparison of different techniques in children after surgical repair of tetralogy of Fallot. Eur Heart J Cardiovasc Imaging. 2012;13:596-604.
13. Lu X, Nadvoretskiy V, Bu L, et al. Accuracy and reproducibility of real-time three- dimensional echocardiography for assessment of right ventricular volumes and ejection fraction in children. J Am Soc Echocardiogr. 2008;21:84-9.
14. Friedberg MK, Su X, Tworetzky W. Validation of 3D echocardiographic assessment of left ventricular volumes, mass, and ejection fraction in neonates and infants with congenital heart disease: a comparison study with cardiac MRI. Circ Cardiovasc Imaging. 2010;3:735-42.
15. Genovese D, Addetia K, Kebed K, et al. First clinical experience with 3-dimensional echocardiographic transillumination rendering. J Am Coll Cardiol Imaging. 2019;12(9):1868-71.

16. Sun F, Sun A, Chen Y, et al. Novel TrueVue series of 3D echocardiography: revealing the pathological morphology of congenital heart disease. Front Physiol. 2022;13:1000007.
17. Karagodin I, Addetia K, Singh A, et al. Improved delineation of cardiac pathology using a novel three-dimensional echocardiographic tissue transparency tool. J Am Soc Echocardiogr. 2020;33(11):1316-23.
18. Villemain O, Baranger J, Friedberg MK, et al. Ultrafast ultrasound imaging in pediatric and adult cardiology: techniques, applications, and perspectives. J Am Coll Cardiol Imaging. 2020;13(8):1771-91.
19. Nyrnes SA, Fadnes S, Wigen MS, et al. Blood speckle-tracking based on high-frame rate ultrasound imaging in pediatric cardiology. J Am Soc Echocardiogr. 2020;33(4):493-503.e495.
20. Marchese P, Cantinotti M, Van den Eynde J, et al. Left ventricular vortex analysis by high-frame rate blood speckle tracking echocardiography in healthy children and in congenital heart disease. Int J Cardiol Heart Vasc. 2021;37:100897.
21. Maresca D, Correia M, Villemain O, et al. Noninvasive imaging of the coronary vasculature using ultrafast ultrasound. J Am Coll Cardiol Imaging. 2018;11:798-808.
22. Villemain O, Correia M, Khraiche D, et al. Myocardial stiffness assessment using shear wave imaging in pediatric hypertrophic cardiomyopathy. J Am Coll Cardiol Imaging. 2018;11(5):779-81.
23. Sorensen K, Fadnes S, Mertens L, et al. Assessment of early diastolic intraventricular pressure difference in children by blood speckle-tracking echocardiography. J Am Soc Echocardiogr. 2023;36(5):523-32.e3.
24. Melki L, Grubb CS, Weber R, et al. Localization of accessory pathways in pediatric patients with Wolff-Parkinson-White syndrome using 3D-rendered electromechanical wave imaging. J Am Coll Cardiol. 2019;5:427-37.
25. Papadacci C, Finel V, Provost J, et al. Imaging the dynamics of cardiac fiber orientation in vivo using 3D ultrasound backscatter tensor imaging. Sci Rep. 2017;7(1):830.
26. Wigen MS, Fadnes S, Rodriguez-Molares A, et al. 4-D intracardiac ultrasound vector flow imaging–feasibility and comparison to phase-contrast MRI IEEE. Trans Med Imaging. 2018;37:2619-29.
27. Fadnes S, Nyrnes SA, Torp H, et al. Shunt flow evaluation in congenital heart disease based on two-dimensional speckle tracking Ultrasound Med Biol. 2014;40:2379-91.
28. Dillman JR, Hernandez RJ. Role of CT in the Evaluation of Congenital Cardiovascular Disease in Children. AJR. 2009;192(5): 1219-31.
29. Ali F, Rizvi A, Ahmad H, et al. Quality initiative to reduce cardiac CT angiography radiation exposure in patients with congenital heart disease. Pediatr Qual Saf. 2019;4(3):e168.
30. Hernanz-Schulman M. Vascular rings: a practical approach to imaging diagnosis. Pediatr Radiol. 2005;35:961-79.
31. Schmitt R, Froehner S, Brunn J, et al. Congenital anomalies of the coronary arteries: imaging with contrast-enhanced, multidetector computed tomography. Eur Radiol. 2005;15(6):1110-21.
32. Shih MC, Tholpady A, Kramer CM. Surgical and endovascular repair of aortic coarctation: normal findings and appearance of complications on CT angiography and MR angiography. AJR Am J Roentgenol. 2006;187(3):W302-12.
33. Kim NY, Im DJ, Youn JC, et al. Synthetic extracellular volume fraction derived using virtual unenhanced attenuation of blood on contrast-enhanced cardiac dual-energy CT in nonischemic cardiomyopathy. AJR Am J Roentgenol. 2022;218(3):454-61.
34. Tsiflikas I, Thater G, Ayx I, et al. Low dose pediatric chest computed tomography on a photon counting detector system—initial clinical experience. Pediatr Radiol. 2023;53(6):1057-62.
35. Perera Molligoda Arachchige AS, Verma Y. Role of photon-counting computed tomography in pediatric cardiovascular imaging. World J Clin Pediatr. 2025;14(1):99288.
36. Sand NPR, Veien KT, Nielsen SS, et al. Prospective Comparison of FFR Derived from Coronary CT Angiography with SPECT Perfusion Imaging in Stable Coronary Artery Disease: The ReASSESS Study. JACC Cardiovasc Imaging. 2018;11(11):1640-50.
37. Patel MR, Norgaard BL. 1-Year Impact on Medical Practice and Clinical Outcomes of FFRCT: The ADVANCE Registry. JACC. 2020;13(1):97-105.
38. Tang CX, Liu CY, Lu MJ. CT FFR for Ischemia-Specific CAD With a New Computational Fluid Dynamics Algorithm: A Chinese Multicenter Study. JACC Cardiovasc Imaging. 2020;13(4):980-90.
39. Adjedj J, Hyafil F, Halna du Fretay X, et al. Physiological evaluation of anomalous aortic origin of a coronary artery using computed tomography-derived fractional flow reserve. J Am Heart Assoc. 2021;10:7:e018593.
40. Molossi S, Doan T, Sachdeva S. Anomalous coronary arteries: a state-of-the-art approach. Cardiol Clin. 2023;41:1:51-69.
41. Di Salvo G, Miller O, Babu Narayan S, et al. Imaging the adult with congenital heart disease: A multimodality imaging approach—Position paper from the EACVI. Eur Heart J Cardiovasc Imaging. 2018;19:1077-98.
42. Task Force of the European Society of Cardiology, in collaboration with the Association of European Pediatric Cardiologist. The clinical role of magnetic resonance in cardiovascular disease. Eur Heart J. 1998;19:19-39.
43. Friedrich M. The future of cardiovascular magnetic resonance imaging. Eur Heart J. 2017;38:1698-701.
44. Ferreira VM, Piechnik SK. CMR Parametric Mapping as a Tool for Myocardial Tissue Characterization. Korean Circ J. 2020;50(8):658-76.
45. de Alba CG, Khan A, Woods P, et al. Left ventricular strain and fibrosis in adults with repaired tetralogy of Fallot: a case-control study. Int J Cardiol. 2021;323:34-3.
46. Cornicelli MD, Rigsby CK, Rychlik K, et al. Diagnostic performance of cardiovascular magnetic resonance native T1 and T2 mapping in pediatric patients with acute myocarditis. J Cardiovasc Magn Reson. 2019;21:1:40.
47. Chavhan GB, Lam CZ, Greer MC, et al. Magnetic resonance lymphangiography. Radiol Clin North Am. 2020;58(4):693-706.
48. Ghosh RM, Griffis HM, Glatz AC, et al. Prevalence and cause of early fontan complications: does the lymphatic circulation play a role? J Am Heart Assoc. 2020;9(7):e015318.
49. Moghari MH, van der Geest RJ, Brighenti M, et al. Cardiac magnetic resonance using fused 3D cine and 4D flow sequences: validation of ventricular and blood flow measurements. Magn Reson Imaging. 2020;74:203-12.
50. Van der Ven JPG, van Genuchten W, Sadighy Z, et al. Multivendor evaluation of automated MRI postprocessing of biventricular size and function for children with and without congenital heart defects. J Magn Reson Imaging. 2023;58:3:794-804.
51. Zhong L, Schrauben EM, Garcia J, et al. Intracardiac 4D flow MRI in congenital heart disease: Recommendations on behalf of the ISMRM flow & motion study group. J Magn Reson Imaging. 2019;50(3):677-81.
52. Kaur H, Assadi H, Alabed S, et al. Left ventricular blood flow kinetic energy assessment by 4D flow cardiovascular magnetic resonance: a systematic review of the clinical relevance. J Cardiovasc Dev Dis. 2020;7:3:37.
53. Gorecka M, Bissell MM, Higgins DM, et al. Rationale and clinical applications of 4D flow cardiovascular magnetic resonance in assessment of valvular heart disease: a comprehensive review. J Cardiovasc Magn Reson. 2022;24:1:49.

54. Jeong D, Anagnostopoulos PV, Roldan Alzate A, et al. Ventricular kinetic energy may provide a novel noninvasive way to assess ventricular performance in patients with repaired tetralogy of Fallot. J Thorac Cardiovasc Surg. 2015;149:1339-47.
55. Puricelli F, Voges I, Gatehouse P, et al. Performance of cardiac MRI in pediatric and adult patients with Fontan circulation. Radiol Cardiothorac Imaging. 2022;4(3):e210235.
56. Schuenke P, Redshaw Kranich C, Lutz M, et al. Open-source cardiac magnetic resonance fingerprinting. MAGMA. 2025;38(4):665-77.
57. Eck BL, Yim M, Hamilton JI, et al. Cardiac Magnetic Resonance Fingerprinting: Potential Clinical Applications. Curr Cardiol Rep. 2023;25(3):119-31.
58. Liu Y, Hamilton J, Rajagopalan S, et al. Cardiac Magnetic Resonance Fingerprinting: Technical Overview and Initial Results. JACC Cardiovasc Imaging. 2018;11(12).
59. Razavi R, Hill DL, Keevil SF, et al. Cardiac catheterisation guided by MRI in children and adults with congenital heart disease. Lancet. 2003;362:1877-82.
60. Surendranath R, Reddy V. Invasive cardiovascular magnetic resonance (iCMR) for diagnostic right and left heart catheterization using an MR-conditional guidewire and passive visualization in congenital heart disease. J Cardiovasc Magnet Reson. 2020;22:20.
61. Kang SL, Armstrong A, Krings G, et al. Three-dimensional rotational angiography in congenital heart disease: present status and evolving future. Congenit Heart Dis. 2019;14(6):1046-57.
62. Minderhoud SCS, Van der Stelt F, Molenschot MMC, et al. Dramatic dose reduction in three-dimensional rotational angiography after implementation of a simple dose reduction protocol. Pediatr Cardiol. 2018;39(8):1635-41.
63. Stenger A, Dittrich S, Glockler M. Three-dimensional rotational angiography in the pediatric cath lab: optimizing aortic interventions. Pediatr Cardiol. 2016;37(3):528-36.
64. Haddad L, Waller BR, Johnson J, et al. Radiation protocol for three-dimensional rotational angiography to limit procedural radiation exposure in the pediatric cardiac catheterization lab. Congenit Heart Dis. 2016;11(6):637-46.
65. Seckeler MD, Boe BA, Barber BJ, et al. Use of rotational angiography in congenital cardiac catheterisations to generate three-dimensional-printed models. Cardiol Young. 2021;31(9):1407-11.
66. Armstrong AK, Zampi JD, Itu LM, et al. Use of 3D rotational angiography to perform computational fluid dynamics and virtual interventions in aortic coarctation. Catheter Cardiovasc Interv. 2020;95(2):294-9.
67. Jone PN, Gearhart A, Lei H, et al. Artificial Intelligence in Congenital Heart Disease: Current State and Prospects. JACC Adv. 2022;1(5):100153.
68. Ehret N, Alkassar M, Dittrich S, et al. A new approach of three-dimensional guidance in paediatric cath lab: segmented and tessellated heart models for cardiovascular interventions in CHD. Cardiol Young. 2018;28:5:661-7.
69. Narayan SA, Qureshi S. Multimodality Medical Image Fusion: Applications in Congenital Cardiology. Future Cardiol. 2017;4.
70. Nobre C, Oliveira-Santos M, Paiva L, et al. Fusion imaging in interventional cardiology. Rev Port Cardiol (Engl Ed). 2020;39.
71. Goreczny S, Moszura T, Dryzek P. Three-dimensional image fusion guidance of percutaneous pulmonary valve implantation to reduce radiation exposure and contrast dose: A comparison with traditional two-dimensional and three-dimensional rotational angiographic guidance. Neth Heart J. 2017;25(2):91-9.
72. Lau I, Sun Z. Three-dimensional printing in congenital heart disease: A systematic review. J Med Radiat Sci. 2018;65:226-36.
73. Biglino G, Milano EG, Capelli C, et al. Three-dimensional printing in congenital heart disease: Considerations on training and clinical implementation from a teaching session. Intern J Art Organs. 2019;42:595-9.
74. Valverde I, Gomez-Ciriza G, Hussain T, et al. Three-dimensional printed models for surgical planning of complex congenital heart defects: An international multicentre study. Eur J Cardio-Thorac Surg. 2017;52:1139-48.
75. Ong CS, Krishnan A, Huang CY, et al. Role of virtual reality in congenital heart disease Congenit Heart Dis. 2018;13(3):357-61.
76. Raimondi F, Vida V, Godard C, et al. Fast-track virtual reality for cardiac imaging in congenital heart disease. J Cardiac Surg. 2021;36:2598-602.
77. Stephenson N, Pushparajah K, Wheeler G, et al. Simpson. Extended reality for procedural planning and guidance in structural heart disease—a review of the state-of-the-art Int J Cardiovasc Imaging. 2023;39(7):1405-19.
78. Sai TYT, Onuma Y, Zlahoda-Huzior A, et al. Merging virtual and physical experiences: extended realities in cardiovascular medicine. Eur Heart J. 2023;44(35):3311-22.
79. Zhang J, Gajjala S, Agrawal P, et al. Fully automated echocardiogram interpretation in clinical practice. Circulation. 2018;138(16):1623-35.
80. Ghorbani A, Ouyang D, Abid A, et al. Deep learning interpretation of echocardiograms. NPJ Digit Med. 2020;3:10.
81. Madani A, Arnaout R, Mofrad M, et al. Fast and accurate view classification of echocardiograms using deep learning. NPJ Digit Med. 2018;1:6.
82. Pereira F, Bueno A, Rodriguez A, et al. Automated detection of coarctation of aorta in neonates from two-dimensional echocardiograms. J Med Imaging (Bellingham). 2017;4(1):014502.
83. Wang J, Liu X, Wang F, et al. Automated interpretation of congenital heart disease from multi-view echocardiograms. Med Image Anal. 2021;69:101942.
84. Tromp J, Seekings PJ, Hung C-L, et al. Automated interpretation of systolic and diastolic function on the echocardiogram: a multicohort study. Lancet Digit Health. 2022;4(1):e46-e54.
85. Tromp J, Bauer D, Claggett BL, et al. A formal validation of a deep learning-based automated workflow for the interpretation of the echocardiogram. Nat Commun. 2022;13(1):6776.
86. Zhu Y, Fahmy AS, Duan C, et al. Automated myocardial T2 and extracellular volume quantification in cardiac MRI using transfer learning-based myocardium segmentation. Radiol Artif Intell. 2020;2(1):e190034.
87. Bai W, Sinclai M, Tarroni G, et al. Automated cardiovascular magnetic resonance image analysis with fully convolutional networks. J Cardiovasc Magn Reson. 2018;20(1):65.
88. Tandon A, Mohan N, Jensen C, et al. Retraining convolutional neural networks for specialized cardiovascular imaging tasks: lessons from tetralogy of Fallot. Pediatr Cardiol. 2021;42(3):578-89.
89. Zhang Q, Burrage MK, Shanmuganathan M, et al. Artificial intelligence for contrast free MRI: scar assessment in myocardial infarction using deep learning–based virtual native enhancement. Circulation. 2022;146(20):1492-503.
90. Coenen A, KimY-H, Kruk M, et al. Diagnostic accuracy of a machine-learning approach to coronary computed tomographic angiography–based fractional flow reserve: Result from the MACHINE Consortium. Circ Cardiovasc Imaging. 2018;11(6):e007217.
91. Douglas PS, De Bruyne B, Pontone G, et al. 1-year outcomes of FFRCT-guided care in patients with suspected coronary disease: The PLATFORM Study. J Am Coll Cardiol. 2016;68(5):435-45.

CHAPTER 52

Evaluation and Management of Chronic Heart Failure in Children and Adolescents with Congenital Heart Disease

Jonaki Pal, Debasree Gangopadhyay

ABSTRACT

Heart failure (HF) in children with congenital heart disease (CHD) is a complex syndrome. Chronic HF is the product of persistently increased volume/pressure loading conditions or myocardial injury secondary to hypoxia. Management requires a multidisciplinary approach and adaptation to the varying needs of different phases of childhood and adolescence. Treatment includes nutritional support, medications, and surgical interventions. Despite this, morbidity and mortality are high. A thorough follow-up and continued assessment are necessary to increase survival and ensure a good quality of life.

Keywords: Heart failure, congenital heart disease, NT-proBNP.

INTRODUCTION

Heart failure (HF) is a clinical syndrome characterized by symptomatic underperfusion and venous congestion resulting from impaired ventricular filling or ejection.[1] It is a common cause of morbidity and mortality in children and adolescents with congenital heart disease (CHD). Understanding the causes of HF, along with the complexities of diagnosis and management, is crucial for improving outcomes and ensuring optimal care for this growing population.

EPIDEMIOLOGY

Congenital heart disease accounts for 28% of all congenital birth defects, with a global incidence of 8–12/1000 live births. India represents a microcosm of the global situation.[2] As the population of children with unrepaired, palliated, or repaired CHD ages, chronic HF becomes a significant contributor to their ongoing morbidity. 40% of patients with CHD developed HF after surgery according to the Finnish National registry.[3] In lower- and middle-income countries, this is exacerbated by anemia or malnutrition. In India, the prevalence of HF is 40.8% amongst malnourished children with CHD.[4] CHDs are responsible for most pediatric HF-related emergency visits and hospitalizations. The requirement of advanced HF therapies such as extracorporeal membrane oxygenation (ECMO), ventricular assist device (VAD), and heart transplantation (HT) is significantly higher for children compared to adults.

DEFINITION OF CHRONIC HEART FAILURE IN PEDIATRIC CONGENITAL HEART DISEASE

Heart failure is defined as "a complex clinical syndrome with symptoms and signs that result from any structural or functional impairment of ventricular filling or ejection of blood."[5] Defined for adults with structurally normal hearts; this definition is pertinent to the pediatric population despite the hemodynamic, structural, and functional heterogeneity.[6] It can primarily be classified as two major types: Heart failure with reduced ejection fraction (HFrEF) and heart failure with preserved ejection fraction (HFpEF).

Heart Failure with Reduced Ejection Fraction (Systolic Dysfunction)

In clinical practice, HF is assessed based on the degree of left ventricular (LV) systolic dysfunction or ejection fraction (EF). This forms the basis of guideline-directed medical therapy (GDMT) in adults. However, it differs in CHDs with single ventricle (SV) physiology or discordant ventricular connections as in congenitally corrected transposition of great arteries (CCTGA), where LV is no longer the systemic ventricle. Estimating ventricular dysfunction in such situations has been subjective over the years, based on visual gradation. Although there are no set guidelines in the pediatric population, dysfunction of the systemic ventricle of LV morphology, as used in clinical practice, is summarized in

TABLE 1: Echocardiographic cut-off values and severity grading of heart failure with reduced ejection fraction (HFrEF) in the systemic ventricle of left ventricular morphology.

Type of heart failure, according to LVEF	Criteria
Normal function	• EF > 51% • FS between 26 and 45%
Mild dysfunction	• EF 41–51% • FS 20–25%
Moderate dysfunction	• EF of 30–40% • FS 15–19%
Severe dysfunction	• EF < 30% • FS ≤ 14%

(EF: ejection fraction; FS: fractional shortening)

Table 1. Use of surrogate markers such as tissue Doppler index (TDI) and its peak annular systolic velocity (S' wave) may be considered as a qualitative measure of global LV systolic function as well. A value of ≥10 cm/s in adults is considered normal. Functional assessment is more challenging in systemic ventricles of right or indeterminate morphology and is best done by cardiac magnetic resonance imaging (cMRI). Fractional area change (FAC) is an echocardiographic surrogate for right ventricular (RV) systolic function and is seen to correlate well with cMRI-derived RV-EF. RV FAC < 35% is considered abnormal in children with biventricular physiology [such as tetralogy of Fallot (TOF)]. Alternatively, RV tricuspid annular plane systolic excursion (TAPSE) assesses the RV longitudinal function, a value < 10 mm in children being an indicator of RV systolic dysfunction.

Despite these, visual gradation remains the most important method for functional assessment in neonatal and pediatric intensive care units. The trajectory of EF is the best prognostic indicator.

Heart Failure with Preserved Ejection Fraction (Diastolic Dysfunction)

Diastolic dysfunction (DD) in CHD is often related to chronic exposure to increased preload (atrioventricular or semilunar valve insufficiency) or afterload (aortic stenosis, coarctation of the aorta) or secondary to the effects of hemodynamic stressors like residual obstructions or myocardial fibrosis. It is assessed by the ratio of transmitral E and A velocities, which reflects the ratio of early and late diastolic filling. The early stages of DD are characterized by impaired relaxation with normal ventricular compliance, causing a reduction in the E/A ratio to <1. As the DD progresses, ventricular compliance decreases and diastolic pressure increases. An increased end-diastolic pressure (EDP) decreases the end-diastolic atrioventricular pressure gradient, causing A to decrease, and the E/A ratio returns to >1. Further decrease in ventricular compliance results in a restrictive physiology, causing significantly increased EDP, and the E/A ratio increases to >2 (as seen in TOF). Diastolic function can also be assessed using TDI, wherein early mitral annular E' velocity < 8 cm/s indicates DD. The E/E' ratio (Doppler early mitral inflow velocity/TDI early diastolic mitral annular velocity) is seen to correlate well with the pulmonary capillary wedge pressure and is a good predictor of elevated EDP. DD is a significant contributor to morbidity in post-Fontan patients.

PATHOPHYSIOLOGY

Congenital heart disease with outflow tract obstruction (pressure overload) or left-to-right shunt lesions (volume overload) typically present with HF secondary to reduced/fixed cardiac output (CO) and pulmonary overperfusion, respectively. They make a good recovery post-intervention when done at an appropriate age. However, SV physiology is more complicated, wherein the ventricular volume overload is as much as three times the normal CO. This results in ventricular dilatation and hypertrophy, leading to a further distorted geometry and atrioventricular valve regurgitation (AVVR). It is not until the stage II palliation (bidirectional Glenn) that volume unloading happens, but once set in, the AVVR does not resolve. AVVR in Fontan patients is associated with a two-fold increased risk of developing Fontan circulation failure compared to patients without AVVR. Additionally, formation of aortopulmonary collaterals places a significant hemodynamic burden due to left-to-right shunting, causing high-output cardiac failure.

The increased energy demand of the heart, achieved by increased consumption of metabolites, requires more oxygen/unit weight than any other organ in the body. This is exacerbated in children with cyanotic CHD, where the myocardium is at risk for subendocardial ischemia due to systemic hypoxemia. At rest, the myocardium is protected by increased oxygen extraction (60–75%), and a compensatory increase in hemoglobin maintains the oxygen-carrying capacity. However, during periods of increased myocardial demand, the oxygen content in an already cyanotic child becomes limiting, resulting in myocardial ischemia. Although the immediate impact is not detectable, it contributes to maladaptive remodeling over the years.

Moreover, hearts with SV physiology often have mismatched coronary perfusion. The typical coronary supply is inadequate for an enlarged, hypertrophied ventricle, resulting in the formation of ventricular-coronary fistulas (as in pulmonary atresia with intact ventricular septum and hypoplastic left heart syndrome with mitral stenosis and aortic atresia), which eventually leads to coronary steal and myocardial dysfunction. Furthermore, in staged palliations such as the Blalock–Taussig (BT) shunt, the diastolic runoff leads to coronary steal. Multistaged palliative pathways or prolonged cardiopulmonary bypass times also contribute to significant myocardial damage in the long run.

ASSESSING HEART FAILURE SEVERITY IN CONGENITAL HEART DISEASE

The clinical picture of HF in children and adolescents depends on age. While infants and toddlers commonly present with respiratory symptoms such as dyspnea, tachypnea, and diaphoresis, exacerbated by physical activity or feeding, older children exhibit fatigue, shortness of breath, and exercise intolerance. Oliguria, pedal oedema (pitting), hepatomegaly, and pleural effusion may develop later. Growth retardation and failure to thrive are common due to increased metabolic demands. Obstructive lesions often present with syncope and palpitations due to decreased CO and arrhythmias. These children eventually manifest with signs of cerebral hypoperfusion, such as convulsions.

HEART FAILURE STAGES

The grading of HF severity is based on the child or the parent reporting signs and symptoms. The Ross classification and the New York Heart Association (NYHA) classification recognize four functional classes with increasing severity, from I to IV, and are commonly used in clinical practice **(Table 2)**. While the Ross classification assesses severity in infants and toddlers (up to 5 years of age), the NYHA classification has been validated in adults and is used to assess HF symptoms in children > 5 years of age. A modified Ross classification, proposed in 2012, has been hard to acclimate in clinical practice.

A summary of the framework proposed by the AHA Scientific Committee **(Table 3)** may be used as a comprehensive approach to characterize HF severity in children.[6]

- *Exercise stress tests*: Cardiopulmonary exercise testing (CPET) is a valuable tool for monitoring children with CHD and chronic congestive HF. Serial myocardial oxygen consumption (MVO_2) on metabolic exercise stress tests is used to characterize HF severity. However, young children (≤8 years of age) are often not able to perform optimally or up to completion, making assessment difficult. Furthermore, MVO_2 varies by age, which makes using this parameter cumbersome. Although a treadmill test (Bruce protocol) is the ideal method, a cycle ergometer is sometimes preferred in children. A decline in peak VO_2, heart rate (HR), and exercise oscillatory ventilation has been observed to be a

TABLE 2: Heart failure severity classifications.

Class	NYHA	Ross
I	No limitation of physical activity. Ordinary physical activity does not cause undue fatigue, palpitation, shortness of breath, or chest pain	No limitations or symptoms
II	Slight limitation of physical activity. Comfortable at rest. Ordinary physical activity results in fatigue, palpitation, shortness of breath, or chest pain	Mild tachypnea or diaphoresis with feeding in infants. Dyspnea on exertion in older children. No growth failure
III	Marked limitation of physical activity. Comfortable at rest. Less than ordinary activity causes fatigue, palpitation, shortness of breath, or chest pain	Marked tachypnea or diaphoresis with feeding, or exertion, and prolonged feeding times with growth failure
IV	Symptoms of heart failure at rest. Any physical activity causes further discomfort	Symptomatic at rest with tachypnea, retractions, grunting, or diaphoresis

TABLE 3: Severity grading of chronic heart failure in children and adolescents with congenital heart disease.

Heart failure severity	Normal	Mild	Moderate	Severe
• NYHA (≥ 5 years) • Ross (<5 years)	1	2	3	4
Growth percentile (weight for length)	–2z < Z-score < 2z	–3z < Z-score < -2z	–3z < Z-score < –4z	Z-score < –4z
NT-proBNP	Normal	2 times	>2–4 times	>4 times
MVO_2 on exercise stress test	>75% predicted	50–74% predicted	25–49% predicted	<25% predicted
Cardiac catheterization measurements:				
• Cardiac index	>2.5L/min/m^2	1.5–2.4 L/min/m^2	<1.5L/min/m^2	<1.5L/min/m^2
• LVEDP	<15 mm Hg	15–17 mm Hg	18–20 mm Hg	>20 mm Hg
Hospitalizations for heart failure	0	1	2	≥2

(NYHA: New York Heart Association Classification System; NT-proBNP: N-terminal pro-B-type natriuretic peptide; MVO_2: myocardial oxygen consumption; LVEDP: left ventricular end-diastolic pressure)

Source: Amdani S, Conway J, George K, et al. Evaluation and management of chronic heart failure in children and adolescents with congenital heart disease: A scientific statement from the American Heart Association. Circulation. 2024;150(2):e33-50.

predictor of transplantation and mortality among Fontan patients. Serial exercise testing may also be an adjunct for cardiac rehabilitation in these children.

- *Role of biomarkers*: N-terminal pro-B-type natriuretic peptide (NT-proBNP) is a widely studied cardiac biomarker in pediatric HF. A significant rise from the baseline level helps in differentiating patients with respiratory distress secondary to cardiac disease from pulmonary causes and healthy children. Serial levels during follow-up help in prognostication. The current NICE guidelines and ISHLT guidelines advise measuring NT-proBNP as a preliminary investigation in suspected HF because of its high diagnostic accuracy (Class I indication according to NICE guidelines).[7,8] It is the most sensitive and specific biomarker of cardiac dysfunction in children. In healthy children, NT-proBNP levels are highest in the first year of life, which decreases steadily throughout childhood to reach adult levels as the child approaches puberty.[9] NT-proBNP levels in females have higher baseline values than in males. Damaged cardiomyocytes release troponin into the bloodstream after hypoxic injury, and although prognostically inferior, hs-cardiac troponin (cTn) has also been used in pediatric HF. The LIFE Child study provides age-dependent reference values for hs-cTn-T and NT-proBNP **(Tables 4 and 5)**.[9]

SPECIAL CONSIDERATIONS IN SINGLE VENTRICLES AND ROLE OF ADVANCED IMAGING

Single ventricle hearts have an underlying physiological form of chronic HF due to low CO. Ventricular function is initially preserved but declines over time. Symptomatic HF in such conditions is a strong predictor of worse outcomes. Although cMRI is the standard for serial assessment of ventricular performance, 2-D echocardiography may be used for monitoring on a more frequent basis. DD is more difficult to assess noninvasively. Advanced technologies such as real-time 3-D echocardiography, strain and strain rate derived from speckle tracking imaging, pressure-strain loops, and velocity-vector imaging help in global and regional myocardial functional assessment even in subclinical forms of cardiac dysfunction. Abnormalities in biomarkers or exercise performance may also be used to gauge ventricular performance. NT-proBNP > 100 pg/mL is a marker of significant ventricular dilation or dysfunction in SV. Baseline

TABLE 4: Age-dependent and sex-adjusted reference values (5th, 50th, 75th, 95th, and 97.5th percentiles) for NT-proBNP (values in ng/L) (Adapted from the LIFE Child Study).[9]

	5th		50th		75th		95th		97.5th	
Age (years)	**Male**	**Female**	**Male**	**Female**	**Male**	**Female**	**Male**	**Female**	**Male**	**Female**
0.25	54.3	46.7	157.8	139.7	230.8	204.1	388.5	345.2	458.8	409.9
0.5	50.6	44.1	147.2	133.0	215.6	194.7	363.5	330.3	429.4	392.4
1	44.1	39.8	129.4	121.5	190.0	178.6	321.2	304.6	379.7	362.6
2	35.5	33.5	105.5	105.3	155.5	156.2	264.4	269.2	313.1	321.5
3	30.8	29.2	93.0	94.6	137.7	141.5	235.4	246.7	279.3	295.6
4	28.6	26.0	87.5	87.0	130.2	131.3	223.8	231.4	265.9	278.3
5	27.4	24.0	85.2	82.9	127.3	126.3	220.1	225.3	262.0	271.8
6	26.5	22.9	83.5	81.6	125.4	125.4	218.1	226.2	260.1	273.9
7	25.4	21.2	81.3	78.3	122.6	121.5	214.5	221.9	256.2	269.6
8	23.9	18.7	77.8	71.6	117.8	112.2	207.4	207.3	248.1	252.8
9	22.2	16.1	73.1	63.8	111.3	101.0	197.0	189.0	236.2	231.3
10	19.9	14.1	66.8	57.9	102.1	92.7	181.9	175.6	218.4	215.7
11	17.6	12.8	59.8	54.8	91.9	88.5	164.7	169.8	198.1	209.4
12	15.4	11.5	53.3	50.9	82.3	83.1	148.4	161.6	178.9	200.1
13	13.6	9.5	48.0	43.8	74.6	72.3	135.2	142.4	163.3	177.0
14	12.3	7.2	44.1	34.8	68.9	58.1	125.7	115.9	152.0	144.6
15	11.3	5.3	41.2	26.7	64.6	45.1	118.6	91.3	143.7	114.4
16	10.5	4.0	39.0	20.8	61.4	35.6	113.5	73.0	137.8	91.8
17	10.1	3.1	37.9	16.8	60.1	29.0	111.7	60.3	135.9	76.2

exercise performance is markedly impaired, with a mean maximal peak oxygen consumption of 60% predicted in post-Fontan patients.

- *Invasive assessment*: Despite ongoing advancements, invasive hemodynamic assessment by cardiac catheterization remains the gold standard in the assessment of systemic ventricular EDP, pulmonary vascular resistance (PVR), and anatomic contributors of ventricular dysfunction.

GENETIC TESTING

Syndromic associations account for 20–30% of all CHDs and typically have a known genetic cause, such as aneuploidies, copy number variants, or single-gene mutations. Clinical phenotype usually guides genetic testing. Prenatal genetic tests may be undertaken when either parent has a cardiovascular trait or an identified variant. A knowledge of gene-disease relationships is required for a targeted approach. Cytogenetic testing (e.g., microarrays) or a gene panel should be used when syndromic CHD is suspected. Common syndromes to consider include Down syndrome, Noonan syndrome, CHARGE (*C*oloboma, *H*eart defects, *A*tresia choanae, *R*etardation of growth, *G*enital and urinary abnormalities, and *E*ar abnormalities and deafness), Williams-Beuren, and Marfan syndrome.

MEDICAL MANAGEMENT

Treatment of HF in children is dependent on age and the underlying cause. The principle of management includes supportive measures, decongestive therapy, treating underlying causes and morbidities, and promoting psychosocial health.

Supportive Management

General supportive measures and nutritional support are of paramount importance. For infants and toddlers, adequate calories should be provided to permit weight gain. They require significantly higher calories than their healthy counterparts, due to increased metabolic demands, decreased intake, and malabsorption. In infants, a caloric intake of about 150 kcal/kg/day is required with preferably small and frequent meals that are better tolerated. Mother's milk or hypercaloric feeds (e.g., concentrated formula feeds) should be given to meet the child's demands. Enteral nutrition with

TABLE 5: Age-dependent and sex-adjusted reference values (5th, 50th, 75th, 95th, and 97.5th percentiles) for hs-cardiac troponin T (values in ng/L) (adapted from the LIFE Child study).[9]

	5th		50th		75th		95th		97.5th	
Age (years)	Male	Female	Male	Female	Male	Female	Male	Female	Male	Female
0.25	8.35	6.11	17.71	16.22	22.25	20.47	32.38	28.26	37.72	31.66
0.5	5.14	3.92	10.81	10.12	13.51	12.71	19.67	17.49	23.04	19.61
1	2.56	2.05	5.32	5.04	6.58	6.26	9.63	8.58	11.43	9.64
2	1.73	1.50	3.59	3.45	4.37	4.21	6.52	5.75	8.02	6.50
3	1.39	1.44	2.90	3.15	3.49	3.80	5.33	5.19	6.83	5.93
4	1.39	1.37	2.91	2.93	3.47	3.50	5.41	4.81	7.18	5.56
5	1.36	1.42	2.81	2.99	3.31	3.55	5.20	4.94	7.05	5.80
6	1.28	1.48	2.58	3.12	3.02	3.69	4.70	5.21	6.36	6.24
7	1.36	1.40	2.64	2.96	3.08	3.49	4.67	5.04	6.20	6.16
8	1.51	1.28	2.81	2.75	3.25	3.24	4.79	4.78	6.18	5.98
9	1.53	1.28	2.74	2.81	3.16	3.33	4.52	5.02	5.65	6.41
10	1.62	1.22	2.80	2.74	3.22	3.26	4.49	5.04	5.47	6.54
11	1.66	1.30	2.81	3.01	3.23	3.60	4.42	5.66	5.27	7.45
12	1.66	1.25	2.77	3.00	3.19	3.61	4.31	5.78	5.07	7.67
13	1.62	1.25	2.71	3.12	3.13	3.80	4.21	6.16	4.91	8.18
14	1.71	1.23	2.88	3.25	3.34	4.01	4.51	6.55	5.26	8.66
15	1.72	1.30	2.97	3.67	3.47	4.59	4.75	7.54	5.57	9.88
16	1.61	1.38	2.93	4.22	3.45	5.38	4.83	8.87	5.77	11.48
17	1.45	1.37	2.84	4.64	3.39	6.04	4.97	10.00	6.14	12.77
18	1.18	1.56	2.63	5.98	3.18	8.00	5.07	13.31	6.71	16.76

a nasogastric tube or parenteral nutrition may be considered if the child is unable to feed. Deficiency of micronutrients, iron, vitamin D, and carnitine, and, in those with Fontan circulation, protein-losing enteropathy must be addressed. Anemia and iron deficiency are associated with worse outcomes, and intravenous therapy should be considered at hemoglobin levels < 10 g/dL. Additionally, blood pressure control and promotion of physical activity are mandatory.

Pharmacotherapy

Pharmacotherapy for HF is primarily guided by the neurohormonal paradigm. HF activates compensatory mechanisms such as the adrenergic nervous system, the renin–angiotensin–aldosterone system (RAAS), and the pro-inflammatory cytokine system. The therapeutic goal is to inhibit these pathways to prevent HF decompensation, thereby reducing hospitalization and mortality. While adult guidelines provide a comprehensive framework for GDMT, a contemporary, standardized recommendation for the pediatric population is lacking. Nonetheless, the empirical application of GDMT in children with CHD has shown favorable outcomes. Medications should be initiated at the lowest feasible doses and gradually uptitrated to the highest tolerated doses in accordance with the established guidelines **(Table 6)**.

- *Diuretic agents*: Loop diuretics are the first-line therapy for pediatric HF. They play a key role in symptomatic management by reducing volume overload. Furosemide, bumetanide, and torsemide act on the loop of Henle and inhibit sodium and chloride reabsorption. Thiazides (hydrochlorothiazide or metolazone) are added in those who do not respond adequately to loop diuretics. These agents act at the distal convoluted tubule. Together, these diuretics help in relieving congestive symptoms by optimizing fluid balance and improving the quality of life.
- *RAAS inhibitors*: This group includes angiotensin-converting enzyme inhibitors (ACEIs), angiotensin receptor blockers (ARBs), and angiotensin receptor-neprilysin inhibitors (ARNis). They act by downregulation of the RAAS, reducing afterload, decreasing wall stress, and preventing adverse remodeling secondary to myocardial fibrosis and Drug Administration approved sacubitril/valsartan (Entresto) for the treatment of symptomatic pediatric HF with systemic LV systolic dysfunction in patients aged ≥ 1 year.[10] For systemic RV dysfunction, it is considered on a case-by-case basis.
- *β-blockers*: Beta-blockers provide the greatest mortality benefit in adults and are recommended as part of GDMT in children with HFrEF. Carvedilol is the preferred first-line agent in pediatric patients; however, alternatives such as metoprolol, propranolol, or bisoprolol may be considered in cases with coexisting arrhythmias, hypertension, or intolerance to carvedilol. Children on beta-blockers should be closely monitored for hypotension, bradycardia, and hypoglycemia (especially infants). SV or systemic RV dysfunction treated with beta-blockers has shown worse outcomes, and such groups entail caution before use.
- *Mineralocorticoid receptor antagonists (MRA)*: MRAs such as spironolactone and eplerenone promote reverse myocardial remodeling due to their antifibrotic effects. However, in patients at risk of renal dysfunction or hyperkalemia, close monitoring is essential. Initiation of MRAs is contraindicated in individuals with an estimated glomerular filtration rate (eGFR) ≤ 30 mL/min/1.73 m^2 or serum potassium ≥ 5.0 mmol/L.[5] Among MRAs, eplerenone demonstrates greater selectivity and a more favorable side-effect profile compared to spironolactone. However, this group may not be effective in children with SV physiology or underlying RV morphology, as fibrosis is not a primary contributor to HF in them.[6]
- *Digoxin*: Digoxin, an oral inotropic drug, has been used empirically in children with both biventricular and SV CHD with no history of arrhythmia, and is associated with significantly reduced interstage mortality. Although traditionally a mainstay treatment for pediatric HF, its use is challenged due to its mechanism of action (improved CO at the cost of increased myocardial oxygen consumption) and the chance of hemodynamic collapse in a failing myocardium.
- *Sodium-glucose cotransporter-2 (SGLT-2i) inhibitors*: SGLT-2i (dapagliflozin) have demonstrated benefits in adult patients with symptomatic chronic HFrEF. Its experience in children is currently limited, but it is being increasingly used as a part of established GDMT. Side effects include glycosuria. Patients should be monitored for volume depletion, hypotension, hypoglycemia, and urinary tract infections. Studies suggest it to be safe and efficacious, even in those with systemic RV.[11]
- *Ivabradine*: Ivabradine, a sinoatrial node modulator that selectively inhibits the *I*(f) current, acts by reducing the HR. It has shown favorable outcomes in HF in children with dilated cardiomyopathy, but studies in CHD are lacking.
- *Soluble guanylyl cyclase (sGC) stimulators*: Novel drugs such as Vericiguat directly bind and stimulate sGC and increase cyclic guanosine monophosphate (cGMP) production. cGMP has potential beneficial effects in HF, including vasodilation, improvement in endothelial function, as well as reduced fibrosis and reverse remodeling of the heart. An RCT including children > 28 days is underway to evaluate the efficacy of vericiguat in pediatric patients with HF due to LV systolic dysfunction.[12]

THERAPIES FOR CONGENITAL HEART DISEASE WITH ADVANCED HEART FAILURE

Mechanical circulatory support (MCS) therapies for patients with CHD are intricate and complex, and include patient-specific risk factors (size, anatomy, prior surgery, etc.). ECMO has been the most used MCS for postcardiotomy support,

TABLE 6: Commonly used doses in pediatrics for heart failure medications.

Drug	Dosage			Maximum daily dose
Diuretics	*Starting dose*		*Interval*	
Furosemide	0.5–2 mg/kg/dose PO/IV		Twice to four times /day	600 mg
Bumetanide	0.015–0.1 mg/kg/dose PO/IV		Once to twice /day	10 mg
Torsemide	0.1–1 mg/kg/day PO		Once/day	50 mg
Chlorothiazide	10–20 mg/kg/dose PO		Twice/day	2,000 mg
Hydrochlorothiazide	1–2 mg/kg/dose PO		Twice/day	200 mg
Metolazone	0.2–0.4 mg/kg/day PO		Once to twice /day	20 mg
ACEi	*Starting dose*		*Interval*	
Enalapril	0.1–0.5 mg/kg/day PO		Twice/day	20 mg
Captopril	0.1–2 mg/kg/dose PO		Thrice/day	6 mg/kg/day
Ramipril	0.05–0.2 mg/kg/day PO		Once/day	10 mg
ARNI				
Sacubitril + Valsartan	*Titration Step Dose (twice daily) every 2 weeks*			
	Starting	*Second*	*Final*	
Patients < 40 kg	1.6 mg/kg	2.3 mg/kg	3.1 mg/kg	
Patients at least 40 kg, <50 kg	24/26 mg	49/51 mg	72/78 mg	
Patients at least 50 kg	49/51 mg	72/78 mg	97/103 mg	
β-blockers	*Starting dose*		*Interval*	
Carvedilol	0.05–0.8 mg/kg/dose PO		Twice/day	25 mg
Metoprolol	1–2 mg/kg/dose PO		Twice/day	100 mg
Bisoprolol	0.2–0.4 mg/kg/day PO		Twice/day	20 mg
Propranolol	0.5–2 mg/kg/dose/day PO		Twice to four times/day	80 mg
MRA	*Starting dose*		*Interval*	
Spironolactone	1–4 mg/kg/day PO		Twice/day	75 mg
Eplerenone	0.5–1 mg/kg/dose PO		Once to twice/day	50 mg
Digoxin				
	Digitalizing dose		*Maintenance dose*	
Premature infants	20 µg/kg		5 µg/kg/day	
Newborn infants	30 µg/kg		8 µg/kg/day	
<2 years	40–50 µg/kg		10–12 µg/kg/day	
>2 years	30–40 µg/kg		8–10 µg/kg/day	
SGLT-2i inhibitors	*Starting dose*		*Interval*	
Dapagliflozin	5–10 mg/kg/day		Once/day	10 mg
Ivabradine	0.02–0.05 mg/kg/day		Twice/day	15 mg

(ACEi: angiotensin-converting enzyme inhibitor; ARNI: angiotensin receptor-neprilysin inhibitor; MRA: mineralocorticoid receptor antagonists; SGLT-2i: sodium-glucose cotransporter-2 inhibitor)

even though the mortality has been high.[1] There is also growing experience for the use of VAD, particularly in Failing Fontan patients. VAD support is maximal when systolic ventricular dysfunction is the primary cause of Fontan failure. Poorer results are reported when it is used in prior stages of palliation. This has brought into practice the completion of Fontan circulation at the time of VAD implantation and has demonstrated superior survival.[13] Common options for support in infants and small children include a pulsatile device (EXCOR; Berlin Heart Inc., Berlin, Germany) or a continuous-flow device (PediMag and CentriMag, Abbott, Chicago, IL; or Rotaflow, Getinge, Gothenburg, Sweden).[14]

HEART TRANSPLANTATION

Heart-lung transplantation remains the gold standard and definitive treatment for advanced HF, provided there are no contraindications. However, its use is significantly limited by donor organ shortages and by the complex anatomical and pathophysiological characteristics commonly seen in CHD. These include vascular anomalies, extensive collateral vessels, prior surgical interventions, intrathoracic scars and adhesions, and altered immunologic status due to previous blood transfusions. Transplantation may be considered not only in patients who are inotrope dependent or receive durable MCS but also in those with worsening exercise intolerance, diminished quality of life, presence of extracardiac organ dysfunction, or lymphatic dysfunction. Despite improvements in patient selection and perioperative management, morbidity and mortality remain high.

COMORBIDITIES AND OUTCOMES

Patients with CHD have increased lifetime risks of various comorbidities. Atrial tachycardia is common in patients with CCTGA, Ebstein anomaly, post-operative atrial switch (i.e., Mustard/Senning procedures), or Fontan completion. Ventricular dysfunction, maladaptive pulmonary vascular remodeling secondary to increased PVR, is detrimental in the long run. Obstructions in the Fontan pathways may lead to a failing Fontan if not addressed timely. These patients present with symptoms of HF or result in specific complications such as plastic bronchitis and protein-losing enteropathy secondary to lymphatic dysfunction, which ultimately entails the patient as a candidate for HT. Polycythemia in patients with cyanotic CHD predisposes them to thrombosis affecting coronary blood flow, leading to ventricular dysfunction.

CONCLUSION

Heart failure in children with CHD is complex due to the inherent hemodynamics, with fluctuating clinical courses over time. Current treatment strategies rely on expert consensus guidelines derived from evidence-based adult studies. Despite advances in therapy, morbidity and mortality are high. As the management and care of these children continue to improve, they will live longer; thus, potentially increasing the overall burden of pediatric HF. Competent multidisciplinary teams with suitable funding agencies will be required in the future to optimize the care of this growing population.

REFERENCES

1. In: Shady RE, Penny DJ, Feltes TF, et al. Moss and Adams' heart disease in infants, children, and adolescents: including the fetus and young adult, 10th edition. Philadelphia: Wolters Kluwer; 2022.
2. Nair SM, Zheleva B, Dobrzycka A, et al. A Population Health Approach to Address the Burden of Congenital Heart Disease in Kerala, India. Glob Heart. 2021;16(1):71.
3. Raissadati A, Haukka J, Pätilä T, et al. Chronic Disease Burden After Congenital Heart Surgery: A 47-Year Population-Based Study With 99% Follow-Up. J Am Heart Assoc. 2020;9(9):e015354.
4. Shaddy RE, George AT, Jaecklin T, et al. Systematic Literature Review on the Incidence and Prevalence of Heart Failure in Children and Adolescents. Pediatr Cardiol. 2018;39(3):415-36.
5. Heidenreich PA, Bozkurt B, Aguilar D, et al. 2022 AHA/ACC/HFSA Guideline for the Management of Heart Failure: A Report of the American College of Cardiology/American Heart Association Joint Committee on Clinical Practice Guidelines. Circulation. 2022;145(18):e895-1032.
6. Amdani S, Conway J, George K, et al. Evaluation and Management of Chronic Heart Failure in Children and Adolescents With Congenital Heart Disease: A Scientific Statement From the American Heart Association. Circulation. 2024;150(2):e33-50.
7. National Institute for Health and Care Excellence. (2025). Chronic heart failure in adults: diagnosis and management. [Online]. Available from https://www.nice.org.uk/guidance/ng106 [Last accessed October, 2025].
8. Lorts A, Conway J, Schweiger M, et al. ISHLT consensus statement for the selection and management of pediatric and congenital heart disease patients on ventricular assist devices Endorsed by the American Heart Association. J Heart Lung Transplant Off Publ Int Soc Heart Transplant. 2021;40(8):709-32.
9. Kiess A, Green J, Willenberg A, et al. Age-Dependent Reference Values for hs-Troponin T and NT-proBNP and Determining Factors in a Cohort of Healthy Children (The LIFE Child Study). Pediatr Cardiol. 2022;43(5):1071-83.
10. Shaddy R, Burch M, Kantor PF, et al. Sacubitril/Valsartan in Pediatric Heart Failure (PANORAMA-HF): A Randomized, Multicenter, Double-Blind Trial. Circulation. 2024;150(22):1756-66.
11. Konduri A, West C, Lowery R, et al. Experience with SGLT2 Inhibitors in Patients with Single Ventricle Congenital Heart Disease and Fontan Circulatory Failure. Pediatr Cardiol. 2025;46(1):81-8.
12. Sharp M, Dohme LLC. Efficacy, Safety, and Pharmacokinetics of Vericiguat in Pediatric Participants With Heart Failure Due to Left Ventricular Systolic Dysfunction (MK-1242-036). [Online] Available from https://clinicaltrials.gov/study/NCT05714085 [Last accessed October, 2025].
13. Maeda K, Nasirov T, Yarlagadda V, et al. Single Ventricular Assist Device Support for the Failing Bidirectional Glenn Patient. Ann Thorac Surg. 2020;110(5):1659-66.
14. Joong A, Maeda K, Peng DM, ACTION Learning Network Investigators. Ventricular Assist Device Outcomes in Infants and Children With Stage 1 Single Ventricle Palliation. ASAIO J Am Soc Artif Intern Organs 1992. 2022;68(11):e188-95.

CHAPTER 53

Advancing New Solutions for Adult Congenital Heart Diseases-related Heart Failure

Prafulla Kerkar, Ujjwala Tulluri

ABSTRACT

Heart failure (HF) among adults with congenital heart disease (ACHD) is increasingly recognized, largely due to improved survival rates following comprehensive surgical and medical interventions. Nonetheless, there remains a significant deficit in data and clinical guidelines pertaining to contemporary treatment options for this demographic, particularly for operated distinct anatomical conditions such as tetralogy of Fallot (TOF), single ventricle physiology, and transposition of the great arteries (TGA). Despite these challenges, numerous large-scale and smaller studies conducted across various regions have laid a foundational framework for developing management strategies that encompass both pharmacological and interventional techniques for the treatment of heart failure, as well as bridging therapies for candidates awaiting transplantation. This chapter delineates the available treatment modalities across the divergent anatomical presentations within the ACHD cohort.

Keywords: Adult congenital heart disease, recent advances, tetralogy of Fallot (TOF), congenitally corrected transposition of great arteries (ccTGA), dextro-transposition of the great arteries (dTGA), Fontan circulation, transcatheter valve replacement, mechanical circulatory support (MCS), cardiac resynchronization therapy (CRT), extracorporeal membrane oxygenation (ECMO).

INTRODUCTION

Adult congenital heart disease (ACHD) encompasses a variety of structural heart defects that are present at birth and can persist in adulthood, potentially leading to complications later in life. In recent years, significant advancements have been made in the management of heart failure, both with preserved and reduced ejection fraction, mainly due to large-scale trials that advocate for guideline-directed medical therapy. Additionally, new invasive methods for monitoring a patient's hemodynamic status have been developed.

However, the management of heart failure related to ACHD has not received the requisite attention. With the rapid advancements in surgical and medical therapies for congenital heart diseases identified in children, many patients are now entering adulthood, and a considerable number of them are developing heart failure. Currently, heart failure is the leading cause of death in this population.[1] Unlike heart failure from ischemic or hypertensive etiologies, ACHD-related heart failure arises from complex mechanisms, including congenital hemodynamic disturbances, surgical sequelae, and acquired factors such as arrhythmias or pulmonary vascular disease. Patients with high-risk lesions, including those with a systemic right ventricle, Fontan circulation, or persistent cyanosis may exhibit atypical features that complicate diagnosis and treatment.[2]

ETIOLOGY AND MECHANISM OF HEART FAILURE IN ADULT CONGENITAL HEART DISEASE

Patients with congenital heart disease (CHD) may develop heart failure due to a combination of genetic factors. Additionally, those who underwent cardiac surgery as children might experience residual health issues such as residual lesions, valvular disease, intracardiac shunting, neurohormonal activation, endothelial dysfunction, and ischemia. Arrhythmia can also be a significant contributing factor. Recent studies indicate that individuals with CHD may have a genetic predisposition to accelerated aging, as well as an increased vulnerability to chronic inflammation, which can further exacerbate their condition.[3]

Heart failure in ACHD patients depends on their underlying anatomy and physiology. Failure may be related to the systemic LV, the systemic RV, the subpulmonic RV, or worsening Fontan physiology. Dysfunction of the systemic LV is due to the resulting fibrosis, altering systolic and diastolic function. This occurs due to its susceptibility to abnormal pressure and/or volume overload, ventricular hypertrophy as a maladaptive remodeling response, myocardial ischemia, and effects of cyanosis, prior cardiopulmonary bypass, and/or ventriculotomy.[4]

Understanding RV function requires a good insight into its architecture, as it differs from that of the left, with the myocardial fibers transitioning from outward horizontal to deep longitudinal, and some fibers are shared with LV at the anterior interventricular sulcus, leading to a longitudinal contraction. LV further pulls the free RV wall in the direction of the septum, which protrudes into the RV as well, and permits volume change without significant energy expenditure. This enables RV to respond well to volume changes in the low-pressure, highly compliant pulmonary system. However, when placed in the systemic position, this architecture requires changes to support circulation, which may be maladaptive–the systemic RV requires dilatation, increased wall thickness, and muscle contractility, and this geometry makes contraction circumferential, resembling the systemic LV. Shifting of the septum leftward and contraction toward the center of the RV reverses the normal contractile pattern. Consequently, it may result in diminished myocardial work and reduced global function.[4]

The subpulmonic RV is affected by several factors, such as RV diastolic afterload, diastolic pressure gradient between the RV and the main pulmonary artery, intrinsic RV compliance, and capacitance of pulmonary arteries. Its susceptibility to failure may result from a prior history of repair of defects such as double outlet RV, truncus arteriosus, tetralogy of Fallot, pulmonary atresia, pulmonary stenosis, pretricuspid valve shunt, or intrinsic congenital heart disease-related pulmonary arterial hypertension.[4]

Eisenmenger syndrome is highly sensitive to any changes in hemodynamic homeostasis. The phenotype is associated with suprasystemic pulmonary artery pressures in ACHD patients with shunt lesions, leading to worsening pulmonary vascular disease and ultimately causing shunt reversal and central cyanosis. Moreover, associated comorbidities such as iron deficiency, arrhythmias, and thrombotic diathesis can play a part in the progression of heart failure symptoms.[4]

Other mechanisms include Fontan failure, extracardiac shunts, and collaterals that cause additional volume and/or pressure loading conditions. Occasionally, the tissue surrounding surgical scars or operative patches may act as a nidus for arrhythmias that worsen.[4]

CLINICAL PRESENTATION AND DIAGNOSIS

It is particularly challenging to diagnose heart failure in adults with congenital heart disease as they are habituated to decreased exercise tolerance and shortness of breath[3]. Hence, the patients do not view their limitations as abnormal. Symptoms to help identify heart failure in an individual with congenital heart disease were arbitrarily classified by Budts W et al. in 2016 in a position paper of the Working Group of Grown-Up Congenital Heart Disease and the Heart Failure Association of the European Society of Cardiology.[5] These included symptoms of systemic ventricular failure (fatigues, breathlessness, dry cough especially lying flat, reduced exercise tolerance, orthopnea, paroxysmal nocturnal dyspnea, and wheezing), symptoms of subpulmonary ventricular failure (fatigue, bloating, weight gain of >2 kg/week, loss of appetite, reduced exercise tolerance, and increased abdominal girth) and symptoms of congestive (biventricular) failure.[5] However, this classification does not include single ventricular or Fontan physiology. Clinical factors may be more reliable to identify heart failure in adults with CHD. These include cardiopulmonary exercise testing to assess changes in exercise capacity rather than absolute exercise capacity, functional classification, rate of hospitalization, presence of atrial arrhythmias, ventricular arrhythmias, monitoring of natriuretic peptides, hsCRP, liver function, renal function, and red cell distribution. Hemodynamic evaluation is particularly important in adults with CHD undergoing assessment for heart transplantation.[3]

MANAGEMENT AND TREATMENT STRATEGIES

The heart failure staging proposed by the 2022 American Heart Association (AHA)/American College of Cardiology (ACC)/Heart Failure Society (HFA) classification system can be applied to this cohort of adults with CHD. However, patients with CHD would start in stage B and progress to stage C and stage D when symptoms interfere with daily living and lead to recurrent hospitalizations despite optimal medical therapy.[3]

When patients enter stage C, initiation of diuretics may be attempted. However, its use in Fontan population has been studied to correlate with a 17-fold increase in risk of death or transplantation.[6]

Furthermore, the Guideline-directed medical therapy (GDMT) that has been standardized for the treatment of a general adult cardiology patient does not have similar evidence advocating it for its use in an adult with CHD. For a patient with biventricular circulation such as in tetralogy of Fallot, or with a systemic LV these guidelines are fairly extrapolated. GDMT which includes the four pillars—β-blockers, angiotensin receptor-neprilysin inhibitor [or angiotensin-converting enzyme inhibitor (ACEI) or angiotensin receptor blocker (ARB) as tolerated, mineralocorticoid receptor antagonist, sodium-glucose cotransporter-2 inhibitor (SGLT-2i), and other agents such as hydralazine and nitrate, is focused on neurohormonal pathways.[3] For the patients with systemic RV or those with

Fontan circulation (even if LV is the systemic ventricle), GDMT is used with abundant caution. This pertains to concerns about bradycardia with β-blockers and intolerance to ACEI/ARB/ARNI due to hypotension in patients with sRV [with dextro-transposition of the great arteries (dTGA) or with congenitally corrected transposition of the great arteries (ccTGA)]. In a single-ventricle patient with Fontan physiology, use of β-blockers is concerning due to sinus node dysfunction.[3] β-blockers such as carvedilol, metoprolol, and bisoprolol have been linked to improved systemic RV size and systolic function.[4,7] A few small-scale trials have shown no proven benefit of ACEIs with regard to exercise capacity, hemodynamics, ventricular size, or EF.[4,8,9]

Medication for patients with failure of the subpulmonic RV has been limited to those with repaired tetralogy of Fallot. Two studies—The ACE inhibitors for Potential PRevention Of the deleterious effects of Pulmonary Regurgitation In Adults with repaired TEtralogy of Fallot study (APPROPRIATE) trial[10] and Right vEntricular Dysfunction in tEtralogy of Fallot: INhibition of the rEnin–angiotensin–aldosterone system (REDEFINE) trial[11] did not show any statistically significant benefit in terms of improvement in RV EF with use of ramipril and losartan respectively, in adult patients with TOF. It has been hypothesized that pulmonary vasodilators may be potential strategy to overcome the so called "bottleneck" in patients with Fontan circulation relying on passive pulmonary blood flow, to improve filling of the heart[3,12] The increase in peak VO_2 has been a measure for primary endpoint in many trials assessing the efficacy of sildenafil, udenafil, bosentan, ambrisentan, and macitentan.[13-16] Although these drugs have not shown a significant improvement in peak VO_2, the TEMPO trial had demonstrated an improvement in peak VO_2 with bosentan and most others had shown improvement in submaximal exercise and ventilatory efficiency.[14]

The latest addition to the range of heart failure medications is SGLT-2i, which have been extensively studied for their benefits in patients with both reduced and preserved ejection fraction. Neijunhuis et al. conducted a recent study on the use of SGLT-2i in the ACHD patients, highlighting a significant increase in the prescription of these drugs over the past few years.[17] This international, retrospective, multicenter cohort study included 174 adults with congenital heart disease, of whom 162 were prescribed SGLT-2i for heart failure. This study is considered the largest trial to date with SGLT-2i in this specific population, revealed a threefold reduction in hospitalizations due to heart failure at follow-up compared to before treatment.[17] This significant outcome underscores the need for future prospective trials to further explore the potential of SGLT2i in patients with ACHD. Interestingly, a few case series have demonstrated positive results with weight loss, reduced BNP, increased oxygen saturation levels, glomerular filtration rate, and albumin with the use of SGLT-2i in adults with Fontan circulation and sRVs.[3,18,19] This further encourages future studies to assess their benefit with regard to Fontan cardiorenal syndrome and Fontan-associated liver disease.

Role of Cardiac Resynchronization Therapy

According to the 2014 guidelines from the Pediatric and Congenital Electrophysiology Society and the Heart Rhythm Society, cardiac resynchronization therapy (CRT) is recommended for patients with systemic LV with severely reduced ventricular function of 35% or less, with left bundle branch block, New York Heart Association (NYHA) class II–IV symptoms, sRV dilation, and a QRS duration exceeding 150 ms (class I level B) or 120–149 ms (class IIa level B). For those with systemic RV, it is recommended (class IIa, level C) in the presence of right ventricular dilatation, NYHA class II-IV, RBBB, and QRS duration ≥150 ms. Additionally, CRT is also recommended (class IIa, level C) for individuals with a single ventricle who exhibit ventricular dilation, NYHA class II–IV symptoms, and a QRS duration >150 ms.[20]

A recent multicenter study, the largest to date on the use of CRT in patients with ACHD, showed significant improvements in functional class and reductions in QRS duration for patients who underwent ventricular pacing prior to CRT. However, those who had de novo CRT implantation did not experience similar beneficial changes.[21]

Role of Implantable Hemodynamic Monitoring

In recent years, there has been increasing support for the use of implantable hemodynamic monitoring devices in adults with heart failure, particularly in noncongenital heart disease (non-CHD) populations. However, very little evidence exists regarding their utilization in ACHD patients. Following an initial study by Bradley EA, et al. in 2016 on the implantation of hemodynamic monitoring devices in patients with single ventricle Fontan anatomy,[22] a recent study by Salavitabar A, et al. explored the feasibility and technical aspects of implantation in selected complex ACHD patients.[23] This study shed some much needed light onto the practical aspects of CardioMEMS implantation in ACHD patients (single ventricle, Fontan, d-transposition of the great arteries and those with atrial switch) regarding implantation technique and sites with few patients receiving the device in right branch pulmonary artery due to left pulmonary artery stent, some with the device implanted distal to an LPA stent, and some requiring a long sheath due to a tortuous course of the atrial switch anatomy. Complications such as device shift and device migration were also studied. Nevertheless, future studies with larger cohorts and longer follow-up durations may shed more light on hemodynamic monitoring in ACHD patients and prevent recurrent hospitalization.

Role of Mechanical Circulatory Devices

Mechanical circulatory support (MCS) modalities, including extracorporeal membrane oxygenation (ECMO), intra-aortic balloon pump (IABP), Impella device, and ventricular assist devices (VADs), have been systematically evaluated in patients with congenital heart disease (CHD) as potential strategies for bridging to myocardial recovery or heart transplantation.[3,24] Although ECMO has been extensively researched as a method for facilitating recovery or providing durable hemodynamic support, it presents significant challenges associated with cannulation due to the complex venous anatomies and arterial shunts frequently present in this patient population. Additionally, a higher incidence of complications such as limb ischemia, hemolysis, acute kidney injury, stroke, and bleeding has been observed in ACHD who undergo ECMO.[3,25]

The use of IABP has shown promise as a bridge to transplantation within the pediatric demographic, as well as among patients with Fontan physiology.[3] Recent investigations involving IABP in adults with acute myocardial infarction complicated by cardiogenic shock indicate that it is associated with fewer vascular and hematological complications compared to the Impella device.[26]

The recent 2023 International Society of Heart and Lung Transplantation guidelines on durable MCS underscore the need for careful consideration of ACHD patients experiencing heart failure refractory to medical management, advocating for the evaluation of these individuals for durable MCS implantation prior to the progression of end-organ dysfunction.[27] These guidelines stipulate that ACHD patients supported by durable VADs exhibit survival rates comparable to those without congenital heart disease, highlighting the necessity of meticulous assessment and management of all comorbidities such as liver dysfunction, pulmonary hypertension, kidney dysfunction, and collateral circulation before the deployment of a durable VAD.[3,27]

In patients with a systemic left ventricle within a biventricular circulation, the application of VADs mirrors that seen in general adult cardiology patients diagnosed with stage D heart failure. Conversely, patients with single ventricular anatomy, particularly those with an sRV, encounter unique morphological challenges that complicate device implantation, particularly the optimal positioning of the inflow cannula.[3] Recent innovations, including the utilization of three-dimensional (3D) printing for the generation of structural models, have been proposed to enhance presurgical planning for cannula and device placement in ACHD populations.[28] In patients with systemic RV failure due to congenitally corrected TGA, VADs can effectively decompress the ventricle and support the systemic circulation in patients with systemic RV failure, such as due to ccTGA.[28] In cases involving Fontan circulation, understanding the etiology of Fontan failure is crucial, as patients with either reduced or preserved ejection fraction may derive substantial benefits from VAD support to either replace the failing ventricle or alleviate end-diastolic pressures, respectively. In contrast, patients exhibiting normal hemodynamics may benefit little from VAD implementation.[3] Notably, a multicenter study by Roche SL et al. reported a survival to hospital discharge rate of nearly 93% in patients with sRVs, despite numerous technical challenges.[29]

In the realm of transcatheter valve replacement, advancements in technology and procedural techniques present significant opportunities for managing heart failure in ACHD patients, particularly in addressing reversible conditions such as valvular disease that can exacerbate heart failure. A comprehensive study conducted by Bokma JP et al. established that pulmonary valve replacement considerably diminishes the occurrence of major adverse cardiac events, including mortality and arrhythmic episodes such as ventricular tachycardia, in adults with repaired tetralogy of Fallot (rTOF). This investigation represents the largest observational cohort study to date, encompassing 1,143 patients with rTOF.[30] While transcatheter aortic valve replacement (TAVR) is transforming adult cardiology practice, its application in the ACHD cohort remains less common, primarily attributed to factors such as the younger age of patients, the typically insufficient calcium for anchoring, and a predominance of regurgitant over stenotic lesions.[3]

Moreover, as technical innovations and enhanced understanding of procedural approaches continue to evolve, valve-in-valve procedures may gain increased integration into clinical practice, offering potential improvements such as shorter hospitalization periods and expedited recovery times.[3] The MitraClip and MitraClip XT R systems have undergone preliminary investigation in ACHD patients diagnosed with ccTGAs by several researchers, albeit with limited study numbers. Nonetheless, the initial results are promising, particularly concerning tricuspid regurgitation, left atrial pressures, and pulmonary vascular resistance.[31-33] Recently, the application of the PASCAL system in patients with ccTGA has demonstrated a significant reduction in tricuspid regurgitation and left atrial v-wave pressures.[34]

Future Perspectives

Although supportive evidence exists for the aforementioned strategies, a comprehensive multidisciplinary approach, inclusive of larger-scale clinical trials tailored to specific anatomical variations within the congenital heart disease population, is imperative. Such research endeavors are necessary to inform clinical practices and optimize management strategies for heart failure in this population. Additionally, a notable disparity exists in the availability of evidence from the Indian demographic, highlighting the urgent need for advanced percutaneous interventions and expanded collaborative networks to mitigate morbidity and mortality rates further in this patient population.

CONCLUSION

ACHD related heart failure represents an increasingly recognized clinical entity, though it remains under-studied. With advances in mechanical circulatory support, CRT, transcatheter valve interventions and the appropriate application of GDMT in this population, management strategies are evolving. Nevertheless further studies are warranted to optimize care pathways and understand their role as a bridge to transplant.

REFERENCES

1. Arnaert S, De Meester P, Troost E, et al. Heart failure related to adult congenital heart disease: prevalence, outcome and risk factors. ESC Heart Fail. 2021;8(4):2940-50.
2. Menachem JN, Schlendorf KH, Mazurek JA, et al. Advanced heart failure in adults with congenital heart disease. Heart Fail. 2020;8(2):87-99.
3. Vaikunth S, Sundaravel S, Saef J, et al. Novel therapeutic strategies in heart failure in adult congenital heart disease: of medicines and devices. Curr Heart Fail Rep. 2023;20(5):401-16.
4. Carazo M. Medical Therapy for Heart Failure in Adult Congenital Heart Disease Patients. Struct Heart. 2024;8(4):100297.
5. Budts W, Roos-Hesselink J, Rädle-Hurst T, et al. Treatment of heart failure in adult congenital heart disease: a position paper of the Working Group of Grown-Up Congenital Heart Disease and the Heart Failure Association of the European Society of Cardiology. Eur Heart J. 2016;37(18):1419-27.
6. Andrade L, Ortega-Legaspi JM, Awh K, et al. Diuretic use in the adult Fontan. Int J Cardiol Congenit Heart Dis. 2022;8:100387.
7. Josephson CB, Howlett JG, Jackson SD, et al. A case series of systemic right ventricular dysfunction post atrial switch for simple D-transposition of the great arteries: the impact of beta-blockade. Can J Cardiol. 2006;22(9):769-72.
8. van der Bom T, Winter MM, Bouma BJ, et al. Effect of valsartan on systemic right ventricular function: a double-blind, randomized, placebo-controlled pilot trial. Circulation. 2013;127(3):322-30.
9. Tutarel O, Meyer GP, Bertram H, et al. Safety and efficiency of chronic ACE inhibition in symptomatic heart failure patients with a systemic right ventricle. Int J Cardiol. 2012;154(1):14-6.
10. Babu-Narayan SV, Uebing A, Davlouros PA, et al. Randomised trial of ramipril in repaired tetralogy of Fallot and pulmonary regurgitation: the APPROPRIATE study (Ace inhibitors for Potential PRevention Of the deleterious effects of Pulmonary Regurgitation In Adults with repaired TEtralogy of Fallot). Int J Cardiol. 2012;154(3):299-305.
11. Bokma JP, Winter MM, Kornaat EM, et al. Right vEntricular Dysfunction in tEtralogy of Fallot: INhibition of the rEnin-angiotensin-aldosterone system (REDEFINE) trial: Rationale and design of a randomized, double-blind, placebo-controlled clinical trial. Am Heart J. 2017;186:83-90.
12. Gewillig M, Brown SC. The Fontan circulation after 45 years: update in physiology. Heart. 2016;102(14):1081-6.
13. Goldberg DJ, Zak V, Goldstein BH, et al. Results of the FUEL trial. Circulation. 2020;141(8):641-51.
14. Hebert A, Mikkelsen UR, Thilen U, et al. Bosentan improves exercise capacity in adolescents and adults after Fontan operation: the TEMPO (treatment with endothelin receptor antagonist in fontan patients, a randomized, placebo-controlled, double-blind study measuring peak oxygen consumption) study. Circulation. 2014;130(23):2021-30.
15. Cedars AM, Saef J, Peterson LR, et al. Effect of ambrisentan on exercise capacity in adult patients after the Fontan procedure. Am J Cardiol. 2016;117(9):1524-32.
16. Clift P, Berger F, Sondergaard L, et al. The efficacy and safety of macitentan in Fontan-palliated patients: results of the 52-week randomised, placebo-controlled RUBATO trial. Eur Heart J. 2022;43(Supplement_2):ehac544-1560.
17. Neijenhuis RM, Macdonald ST, Zemrak F, et al. Effect of sodium-glucose cotransporter 2 inhibitors in adults with congenital heart disease. J Am Coll Cardiol. 2024;83(15):1403-14.
18. Muneuchi J, Sugitani Y, Kobayashi M, et al. Feasibility and Safety of Sodium Glucose Cotransporter-2 Inhibitors in Adults with Heart Failure after the Fontan Procedure. Case Rep Cardiol. 2022;2022(1):5243594.
19. Saef J, Sundaravel S, Ortega-Legaspi J, et al. Safety and treatment experience with sodium/glucose cotransporter-2 inhib- itors (SGLT2i) in adult patients with congenital heart disease. J Card Fail. 2023;S1071-9164(23):00104-5.
20. Khairy P, Van Hare GF, Balaji S, et al. PACES/HRS Expert consensus statement on the recognition and management of arrhythmias in adult congenital heart disease: Executive Summary. Heart Rhythm. 2014;11(10):e81-101.
21. Kharbanda RK, Moore JP, Lloyd MS, et al. Cardiac resynchronization therapy for adult patients with a failing systemic right ventricle: a multicenter study. J Am Heart Assoc. 2022;11(22):e025121.
22. Bradley EA, Jassal A, Moore-Clingenpeel M, et al. Ambulatory Fontan pressure monitoring: results from the implantable hemodynamic monitor Fontan feasibility cohort (IHM-FFC). Int J Cardiol. 2019;284:22-7.
23. Salavitabar A, Bradley EA, Chisolm JL, et al. Implantable pulmonary artery pressure monitoring device in patients with palliated congenital heart disease: technical considerations and procedural outcomes. Catheter Cardiovasc Interv. 2020;95(2):270-9.
24. Perry T, Brown T, Misfeldt A, et al. Extracorporeal membrane oxygenation in congenital heart disease. Children. 2022;9(3):380.
25. Kops SA, White SC, Klewer SE, et al. ECMO in adults with congenital heart disease-analysis of a national discharge database. Int J Cardiol Congenit Heart Dis. 2022;8:100366.
26. Moustafa A, Khan MS, Saad M, et al. Impella support versus intra-aortic balloon pump in acute myocardial infarction complicated by cardiogenic shock: a meta-analysis. Cardiovasc Revasc Med. 2022;34:25-31.
27. Saeed D, Feldman D, El Banayosy A, et al. The 2023 International Society for Heart and Lung Transplantation guidelines for mechanical circulatory support: a 10-year update. J Heart Lung Transplant. 2023;42(7):e1-222.
28. Givertz MM, DeFilippis EM, Landzberg MJ, et al. Advanced heart failure therapies for adults with congenital heart disease: JACC state-of-the-art review. J Am Coll Cardiol. 2019;74(18):2295-312.
29. Roche SL, Crossland DS, Adachi I, et al. Mechanical circulatory support for the failing sub-aortic right ventricle in adults. Semin Thorac Cardiovasc Surg Ann. 2021;24:2-9.
30. Bokma JP, Geva T, Sleeper LA, et al. Improved outcomes after pulmonary valve replacement in repaired tetralogy of Fallot. J Am Coll Cardiol. 2023;81(21):2075-85.
31. Franzen O, von Samson P, Dodge-Khatami A, et al. Percutaneous edge-to-edge repair of tricuspid regurgitation in congenitally corrected transposition of the great arteries. Congenit Heart Dis. 2011;6(1):57-9.
32. Van Melle JP, Schurer R, Willemsen M, et al. Percutaneous tricuspid valve repair using MitraClip® for the treatment of severe tricuspid valve regurgitation in a patient with congenitally corrected transposition of the great arteries. Netherlands Heart J. 2016;24(11):696-7.
33. Picard F, Tadros VX, Asgar AW. From tricuspid to double orifice Morphology: Percutaneous tricuspid regurgitation repair with the MitraClip device in congenitally corrected-transposition of great arteries. Catheter Cardiovasc Interv. 2017;90(3):432-6.
34. Luedike P, Riebisch M, Weymann A, et al. Feasibility of a novel transcatheter valve repair system to treat tricuspid regurgitation in ccTGA. Case Rep. 2021;3(6):893-6.

CHAPTER

54

Care for Congenital Heart Disease in India: The Evolving Landscape

R Krishna Kumar

ABSTRACT

India has the largest burden of cardiovascular disease in the world. In the past few decades, there has been considerable attention given to acquired heart diseases. However, India also has the world's largest burden of congenital heart diseases. This affects the entire age range from newborn infants to adults. While there has been a steady growth in the quality of care as well as access to services for patients with congenital heart diseases in India, there is still a very substantial burden of unaddressed CHD. In the past three decades, while considerable progress has been made across a number of institutions in India in the outlook for CHD, there is a strongly felt need to address fundamental challenges that come in the way of equitable access to CHD care. This review seeks to examine the current landscape, outline the specific challenges and suggest a way forward.

Keywords: Congenital heart disease, healthcare access, health disparities.

INTRODUCTION

Congenital heart disease (CHD) is the most common congenital anomaly. The overall incidence of CHD is approximately 8–10 per 1,000 live births; 5–6 per 1,000 require specialized interventions, and approximately 50% of these are patients during the neonatal or early infancy period of critical CHD.[1]

While CHD is unlikely to be perceived as a pediatric health priority in regions with relatively high infant mortality rates (IMR), it is increasingly important as IMR declines. A declining trend in IMR is now being witnessed in almost every part of the world except for regions that are affected by armed conflict. This decline is almost entirely attributable to reductions in mortality from communicable diseases. Congenital heart defects have begun to surface as a significant health problem among infants and newborns in several regions that are now witnessing rapid and substantial improvements in human development indices.[2]

The clinical spectrum of CHD varies from critical CHD that requires immediate attention to minor CHD that needs occasional follow-up. The broad categories of CHD along with the implications for survival and the appropriate treatment approaches are presented in **Table 1**.

In the above table, the first two categories of critical and major CHD typically require to be addressed during the neonatal period or in the first 1–2 years of life. In most cases this will require heart surgery and in selected instances, catheter interventions can be considered. Without these procedures, most children with critical and many with major heart defects are unlikely to survive beyond early childhood. The small proportion of infants and children that survive without any form of definitive treatment often grow up with significant disabilities and limitations that result from irreversible changes in the heart and pulmonary vasculature.

In the past 2–3 decades there have been impressive advancements in the overall capability of taking care of children and adults with CHD in many centers in India and the overall outlook of CHD has improved impressively. The improvements relate to range of services provided, surgical outcomes, and results of catheter procedures. However significant problems remain. Large parts of the country do not have access to comprehensive care for CHD. In particular, access to safe infant and neonatal surgery remains highly variable in terms of access and quality.

ESTIMATES OF CONGENITAL HEART DISEASE BURDEN IN INDIA

Two surveys at birth have provided the basis of estimating the burden of CHD in India.[3,4] Vaidyanathan and others

TABLE 1: Broad categories of congenital heart disease, classified according to natural history.

Broad category	Implications for survival and treatment	Examples[a]
Critical CHD	Incompatible with survival without specific intervention in newborn period or early infancy	Transposition of the great arteries, obstructed TAPVC, duct-dependent pulmonary or systemic circulation
Major CHD	Intervention is required, often in early infancy, for optimal long-term outcome	TOF, DORV, large VSD, and PDA, complete atrioventricular canal, truncus arteriosus, aorto-pulmonary window, single ventricle physiology, unobstructed TAPVC, ALCAPA, severe outflow tract obstructions
CHD that typically manifests at an older age	Diagnosis seldom made in early childhood; intervention required to prevent long-term sequelae in adulthood	Moderate or large ASD, some forms of coarctation, some patients with Ebstein's anomaly, relatively less severe forms of aortic and pulmonary valve stenosis, congenitally corrected transposition of the great arteries with intact ventricular septum
Minor CHD	Long-term, symptom-free survival can be expected without any specific intervention in most cases	Small left-to-right shunts (ASD, VSD, and PDA), bicommissural aortic valve

[a]These examples are not a comprehensive list of conditions; many conditions are not listed. Numerous combinations are possible.

(ALCAPA: anomalous coronary artery from pulmonary artery; ASD: atrial septal defect; CHD: congenital heart disease; DORV: double outlet right ventricle; PDA: patent ductus arteriosus; TAPVC: total anomalous pulmonary venous communication; TOF: tetralogy of Fallot; VSD: ventricular septal defect)

(2011) reported 425 babies (7.75%) with CHD of the 5,487 consecutive newborns screened through echocardiography at a community hospital in Kerala, India. Of these, 17 (0.31%) had major CHD that was likely to require correction through heart surgery or catheter procedure in the first year of life; the rest had minor lesions, most of which normalized without intervention by age 6 weeks.[3] In a more recent study by Saxena et al. that involved a much larger population, 19,009 newborns screened, and 70 had major CHDs at birth (44 serious, 26 critical; overall prevalence of 0.037%).[4,5] The strength of both these studies was that all newborns that were screened had echocardiograms.

Estimates of CHD among older patients require school surveys or community-based surveys. These surveys are likely to pick up patients with less severe forms of CHD that are unlikely to manifest in the first few years of life. A community-based survey from Himachal Pradesh estimated a prevalence of 6.3/1,000[6] and a school-based survey from Andhra Pradesh estimated a prevalence of 9.2/1,000.[7] These numbers translate into a massive national burden.

Using the generally accepted statistic for all forms of CHD of 8/1,000, it can be estimated that there are 200–250,000 children born with CHD in India every year. This number would include CHD that do not require intervention of any kind because they may eventually close (such as a restrictive VSD) and defects such as atrial septal defect that need to be addressed later in life. Using estimates of major CHD incidence at birth,[2] it can be estimated that approximately 100,000 babies are born each year with CHD requiring intervention in the first year of life. Of these, ~37,000 have critical CHD requiring intervention in the first month of life. It is very difficult to estimate the burden of uncorrected CHD in older children and in adults.

WHAT IS REQUIRED TO DELIVER COMPREHENSIVE CARE FOR CONGENITAL HEART DISEASE?

Care of children with heart disease requires a highly coordinated effort from a team of specially trained personnel. Pediatric cardiologists, pediatric cardiac surgeons, intensive care physicians, and intensive care nurses should ideally constitute this team. **Flowchart 1** demonstrates the elements that are required for comprehensive care for patients with CHD. Perhaps the most significant driver for the resources is the expectation of safe and effective infant and neonatal heart surgery. This necessitates a significant amount of human resources and infrastructural requirements.[8]

Human resources: Taking care of children requires high-level of skills in distinct disciplines that include pediatric cardiac surgery, pediatric cardiology, and pediatric cardiac anesthesiology/intensive care. There is also requirement for other skilled personnel that include nurses, perfusion, technologists, and respiratory therapists. The role of a pediatric cardiologist is in making an accurate diagnosis and planning the surgery. While some conditions can be managed through catheter interventions, it is essential to have surgical back up in the rare event that there is a complication.[9]

Cohesive teamwork: It is not enough just to have individuals with skills. These individuals have to work together cohesively. Cohesive teamwork is perhaps the most critical component of a successful pediatric heart program.[9]

Infrastructure and equipment: The infrastructure and equipment for delivery of comprehensive pediatric cardiac care relate to comprehensive imaging that include

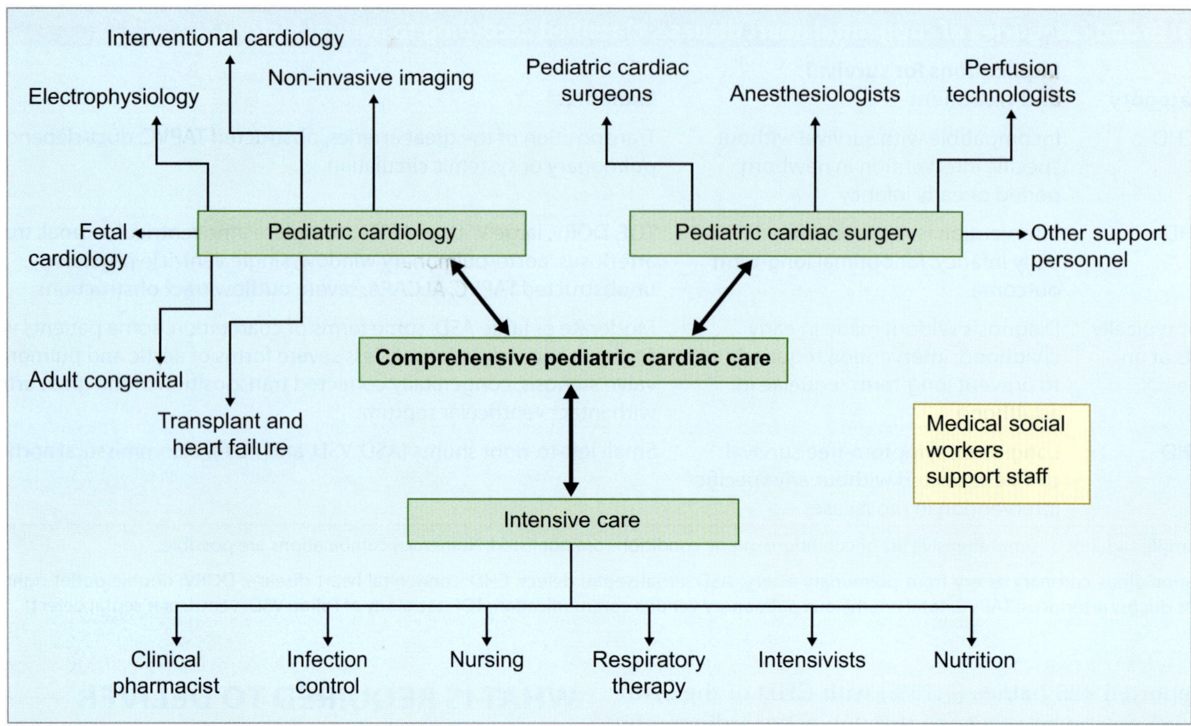

FLOWCHART 1: Components that constitute a comprehensive pediatric cardiac program that can adequately take care of patients with congenital heart disease across entire age range. As evident from this picture, the program needs to be constituted by a multidisciplinary team with caregivers from diverse training backgrounds who need to work cohesively together to enable the best outcomes for this very vulnerable group of patients.

echocardiography, CT and MRI, cardiac catheterization services, cardiac surgery and intensive care. Altogether, this is a substantial capital investment and contributes considerably to costs of care. While many hospitals advertise and display that they may have the most recent equipment and facilities such as robotic surgery, the truth is that the most advanced technology does not necessarily translate into consistent safe outcomes. To a substantial extent, individuals matter much more than machines and equipment.

Constant focus on quality improvement: Pediatric heart programs that have a conscious focus on quality improvement are likely to deliver the best results. Often such programs voluntarily share their results in multi-institutional collaborative networks. One example of such a program is the quality improvement collaboration for congenital heart disease (IQIC). Pediatric heart teams have a strong focus on quality improvement, also, invest a great deal in Infection control and quality of their nursing.[9]

EVOLUTION OF PEDIATRIC AND CONGENITAL HEART SERVICES IN INDIA

Figure 1 captures the distribution of pediatric heart programs in India in 1998 and 2025. Centers with capability of infant and neonatal heart surgery have been depicted here. Impressive progress has been made since 1998 when it was estimated that only 1.3–1.5% infants and neonates with congenital heart disease received timely attention in just 4 or 5 centers that had the capability of infant heart surgery. In the year 2025, there are over 60 centers with capability of infant and neonatal heart surgery. The collective numbers operated in them allow for ~20% of the national burden to be addressed. However, there are significant issues with geographic distribution of these centers. **Figure 2** is a pie chart that demonstrates the paucity of centers in North and East India as compared to South India that caters to a smaller population.

Outcomes: Over the last three decades there have been significant improvements in the surgical results for CHD in India. In a recent meta-analysis of 135 studies met the inclusion criteria and included 30,587 patients aged from 1 day to 65 years.[10] The pooled mortality rate of 43 Indian studies reporting multiple CHD surgical outcomes is 5.63% [95% confidence interval (CI) 4.26–7.16; I^2 = 93.9%], as against a pooled mortality rate of 2.65% for comparative western data. The estimated lesion-specific mortalities are also significantly higher than the Western data, except for the GUCH population and coarctation of the aorta. The higher mortality has been attributed to socioeconomic status, demographics, and health-care system accessibility.

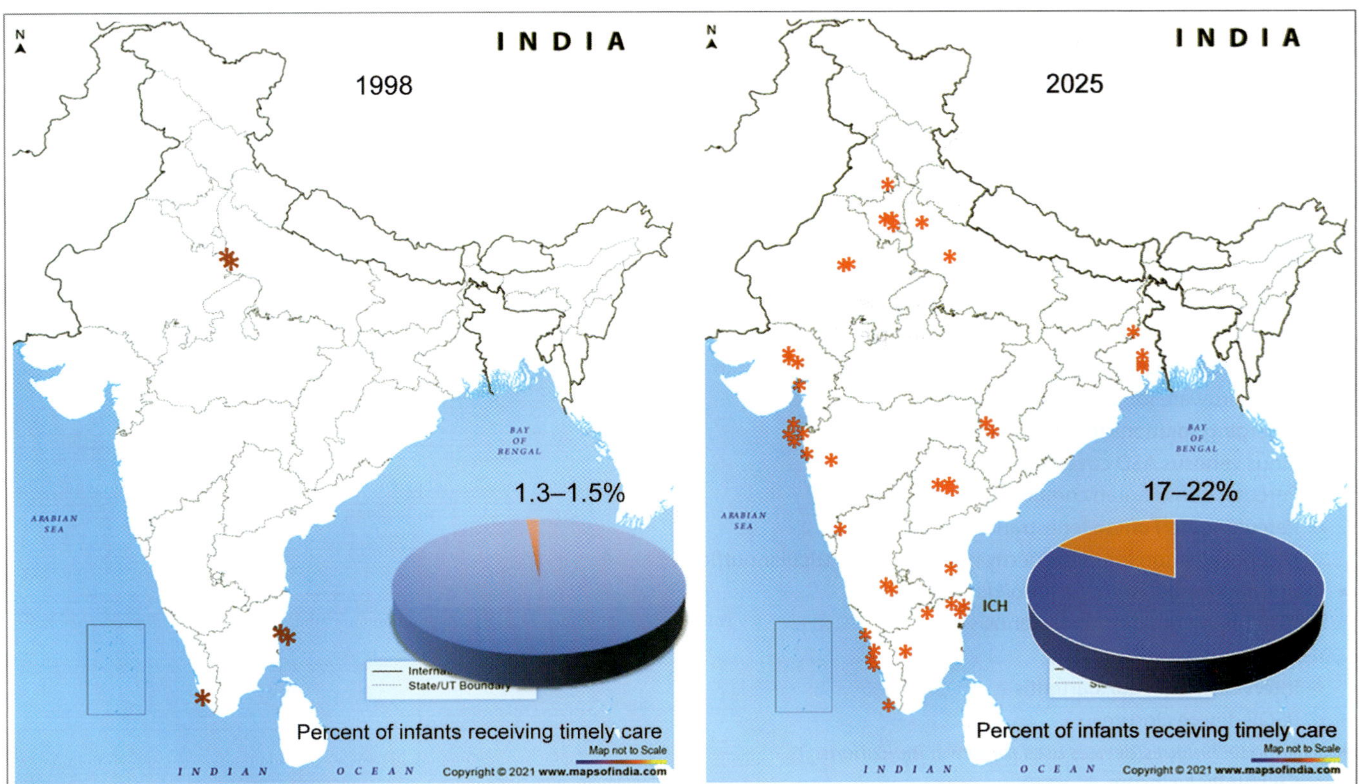

FIG. 1: Remarkable growth of pediatric and congenital cardiac services across the country in the last three decades. The pie charts indicate the progress that has been made in improving access to the average infant with CHD. Despite the substantial number increase in the number of centers, there is still nearly 80% of infants born in India that do not have access to timely care for congenital heart disease.

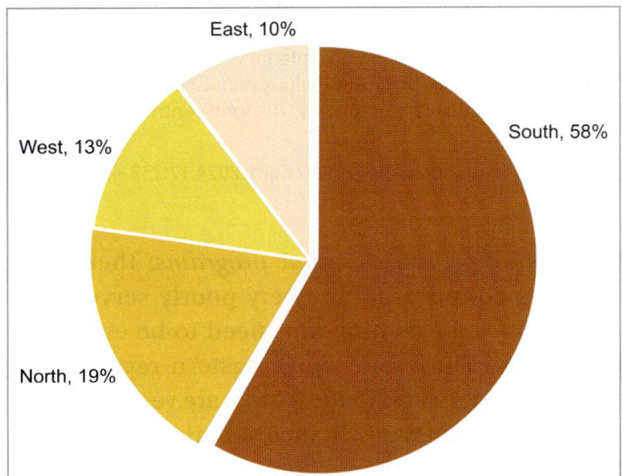

FIG. 2: Maldistribution of congenital heart centers in India that seem to be clustered in Southern India.

All these factors may contribute to a poor preoperative status. However, select Indian centers have managed to overcome these limitations and deliver outcomes compared to the west without significantly impacting costs of care.[11] This has required emphasis on systems that are essential to good outcomes. These cost very little and yield a high return on investment. These systems and programs include:

- Establishment of a robust infection control program,
- Implementation of a surgical safety checklist,
- Continued education and empowerment of nurses, and
- Creation of forums for communication amongst individual team members, enabling cohesion among members of the TEAM and proactively minimizing conflict.

INNOVATIONS FROM INDIA

A number of innovations from India have enabled the better conduct of catheter interventions at a relatively low cost. A recent review has summarized them **(Box 1)**.[12] These innovations have been accepted world-wide and have showcased the ingenuity that was necessitated by the shortage of resources.

Similarly, there have been important innovations in congenital heart surgery that include tissue-engineered patches, handmade conduits, and indigenous devices for surgical closure of multiple ventricular septal defects.[13] Several new surgical techniques have been described, and

Box 1: Selected list of innovative pediatric cardiac interventions from India.

- *New devices developed in India*:
  - Transcatheter pulmonary valve
  - The Konar MFO device for ventricular septal defects
  - Zephyr stent (bare and covered)
  - Python BZ sheath for delivery of transcatheter pulmonary valve
- *New techniques*:
  - Balloon-assisted ASD device deployment
  - Retroflection of the TEE probe for viewing the IVC rim
  - Various techniques for the closure of multiple ASDs
  - Ductal stents for retraining the left ventricle in TGA
  - CTO hardware for pulmonary atresia
  - Emerging solutions to purely surgical subsets
  - Sinus venosus ASD covered stent
  - Percutaneous Fontan completion
  - Percutaneous Fontan fenestration creation
  - Alcohol ablation for the hypertrophied right ventricular outflow
- *Interventions standardized/consolidated by India*:
  - PTMC in rheumatic mitral stenosis
  - Membranous VSD closure
  - Interventions in aortoarteritis
  - RSOV device closure
- *Existing techniques/devices used for newer indications*:
  - Coil for PDA closure
  - ADO II for VSD closure
  - AVP II and muscular VSD devices for difficult PDAs:
- *Innovative emergency bailouts*
  - RVOT stenting during a cyanotic spell
  - Manual autotransfusion for on-table spell
  - Balloon/stenting of obstructed TAPVC

(ADO: amplatzer duct occlude; ASD: atrial septal defect; AVP: amplatzer vascular plugs; CTO: chronic total occlusion; IVC: inferior vena cava; MFO: multifunction occlude; PDA: patent ductus arteriosus; PTMC: percutaneous transvenous mitral commissurotomy; TAPVC: total anomalous pulmonary venous connection; TEE: transesophageal echocardiography; TGA: transposition of great arteries; RSOV: ruptured sinus of Valsalva; RVOT: right ventricular outflow tract; VSD: ventricular septal defect)

Source: Modified from Mantoo MR, Ramakrishnan S. Pediatric cardiac interventions: Innovations from India. Ann Pediatr Card. 2024;17:233-42.

Indian surgeons have described some new anatomical entities. Innovations in imaging, including three-dimensional printing and virtual reality, are transforming preoperative planning and surgical education.

CURRENT NATIONAL CHALLENGES AND PRIORITIES

Overall magnitude versus resources: The total number of centers with capability of comprehensive pediatric cardiac team is completely inadequate to serve the needs of the population. Assuming an average capability of tackling 500 infant heart surgeries annually, India would need total of nearly 400 large pediatric cardiac programs. Therefore, there is a substantial absolute shortfall.

Distribution of pediatric cardiac programs: There are large areas of the country that are very poorly served **(Fig. 1)**. Newer pediatric heart programs need to be established in several states. The entire north-eastern region, much of north India, eastern and Central India are very poorly served. Most centers are clustered in metros and these centers often compete with each other. The number of pediatric heart programs that are exclusively funded by the government are a small minority in India. Due to budgetary constraints and lack of understanding of the specialized nature of this care, publicly funded hospitals find it challenging to recruit and retain the highly trained human resources and develop robust systems needed for pediatric cardiac care. Rigid hierarchies come in the way of empowering motivated leaders. Privately funded institutions, on the other hand, often do not see pediatric heart care as a profitable clinical field and are reluctant to invest in this area of care. In India they have stepped in in a very limited way. Another financial model involves charitable, not for profit institutions that have stepped in, but this is by no means enough to tackle the needs of the country.[14]

Fragile heath systems: We have recently described the concept of the pediatric care continuum to highlight the challenges in journey of a child with CHD **(Flowchart 2)**. The six stages of this continuum include initial recognition of disease, diagnosis and prioritization, referral, stabilization and tertiary treatment, and follow-up. It is necessary to address shortcomings at each stage of the care continuum for it to have a meaningful impact on the outcomes of patients with CHD. This is especially for the most vulnerable populations—neonates and infants.[15]

Capacity building for the future: While there has been some success with dedicated training programs for pediatric cardiology, there is a crisis of considerable magnitude when it comes to building the workforce in pediatric cardiovascular surgery.[16] The existing surgeons are perhaps so overburdened that very little efforts are made individually or collectively toward training future pediatric cardiac surgeons. There are a number of other unique challenges that make pediatric heart surgery a relatively unattractive career option for any young surgeon. Perhaps the most serious situation relates to the work force in pediatric cardiac intensive care. While provision of high quality pediatric cardiac intensive care is absolutely critical to outcomes after pediatric heart surgery, there is really no concerted effort whatsoever in building this component of the workforce. Both physician and nursing are short supply and training opportunities are extremely limited for ICUs. Additionally, opportunities for career development are limited by a serious shortfall of nurturing institutions.

Funding individual patients: Caring for children with heart disease is challenging and expensive because it requires sophisticated equipment and infrastructure together with a cohesive team of highly qualified health professionals that include pediatric heart surgeons, pediatric cardiologists, intensive care experts and specially trained nurses. The most vulnerable group, newborns and infants, require the maximum resources and expertise. It is not therefore, surprising that economic barriers come in the way of most Indian children receiving timely care for their heart conditions. The hardships faced by young parents that have just begun a family are enormous given their limited financial reserves. Furthermore, most medical insurance providers have specifically listed congenital heart defects as an exception to the list of conditions covered. Heart operations and catheter procedures in children are expensive because of the resources utilized (costs of consumables, intensive care etc.). As a result, the economic impact on families who pay from out of their pockets is often devastating.[17] Private insurance companies are quite reluctant to fund CHD operations and have often listed them as a specific exclusion.

THE WAY FORWARD

This section will describe a few specific initiatives that could serve as examples to build on nationally. The Rashtriya Bal Swasthya Karyakram (RBSK) is an innovative and ambitious program, focused on Child Health Screening and Early Intervention Services.[4] RBSK aims at the early detection and management of the "4Ds" prevalent in children—defects at birth, diseases in children, deficiencies, and developmental delays. This program includes CHD care, and the government has allocated substantial resources for its deployment.[17] With the addition of funds and commitment by the Government of Kerala, financial resources were made available for a dedicated program to address the CHD burden in the state. This program is named "Hridyam—for little hearts."[15] The program seeks to look at the entire life course of CHD from screening to identification to referral, surgery and follow-up rather than providing for the surgery alone **(Flowchart 2)**. This is in keeping with the vision of the RBSK. An innovative comprehensive web-based application has been developed to enable referral and track the progress through each

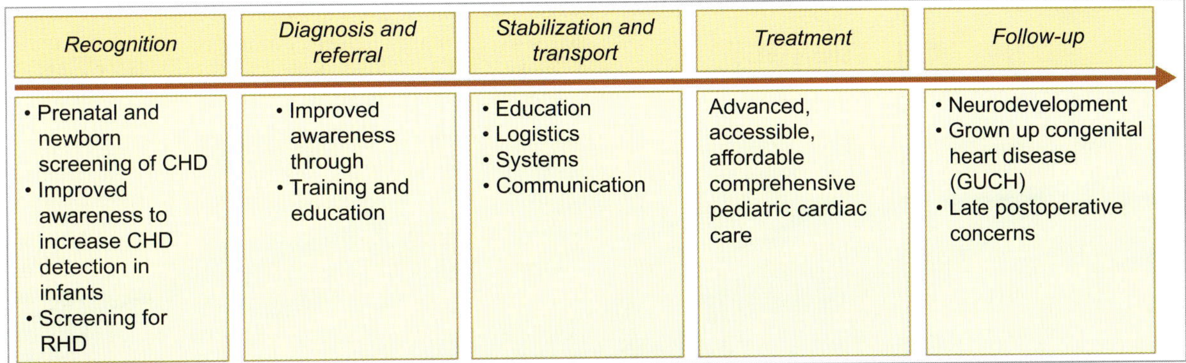

FLOWCHART 2: Care continuum for pediatric and congenital heart disease from screening to postprocedure follow-up.

stage. This program also functions as a registry for children 0–18 years with suspected CHD of all types. Comprehensive pediatric cardiac care that includes surgery and catheter procedures are delivered in two government and five private institutions across the state through a unique public-private partnership model. Hridyam has had a significant impact on CHD mortality in Kerala and perhaps enabled the achievement of a single digit infant mortality rate for the first time.

The Hridyam model needs to be sustained and scaled up nationally to make a meaningful impact. While this could be challenging, there are several tangible benefits of improving the outlook for CHD care nationally. The most important of which is the fact there is the massive potential for lives of children to be transformed by enabling them to become productive adults.

CONCLUSION

While impressive strides have been made for the care of CHD in India, particularly in the last three decades, there is much that needs to be done. The most significant challenge is in addressing the inequity that prevails in the care of children that is largely dictated by economic constraints and regional imbalances. There is also much to be done to develop an adequate workforce for care of patients, especially infants in newborn, with congenital heart disease.

REFERENCES

1. Wu W, He J, Shao X. Incidence and mortality trend of congenital heart disease at the global, regional, and national level, 1990–2017. Medicine (Baltimore). 2020;99(23):e20593.
2. Zimmerman MS, Smith AGC, Sable CA et al. Global, regional, and national burden of congenital heart disease, 1990–2017: a systematic analysis for the Global Burden of Disease Study 2017. Lancet Child Adolesc Health. 2020;4:185-200.
3. Vaidyanathan B, Sathish G, Mohanan ST, et al. Clinical screening for Congenital heart disease at birth: A prospective study in a community hospital in Kerala. Indian Pediatr. 2011;48:25-30.
4. Saxena A, Mehta A, Ramakrishnan S, et al. Pulse oximetry as a screening tool for detecting major congenital heart defects in Indian newborns. Arch Dis Child Fetal Neonatal Ed. 2015;100(5):F416-21.
5. Saxena A, Mehta A, Ramakrishnan S, et al. Birth prevalence of congenital heart disease: A cross-sectional observational study from North India. Ann Pediatr Cardiol. 2016;9(3):205-9.
6. Bhardwaj R, Kandoria A, Marwah R, et al. Prevalence of congenital heart disease in rural population of Himachal – A population-based study Indian Heart J. 2016; 68(1):48-51.
7. Kumari NR, Raju IB, Patnaik AN, et al. Prevalence of rheumatic and congenital heart disease in school children of Andhra Pradesh, South India. J Cardiovasc Dis Res. 2013;4(1):11-4.
8. Vervoort D, Jin H, Edwin F, et al. Global Access to Comprehensive Care for Paediatric and Congenital Heart Disease. CJC Pediatr Congenit Heart Dis. 2023;2(6Part B):453-63.
9. Mohsin S, Hasan B, Zheleva B, et al. Enhancing Quality of Congenital Heart Care Within Resource-Limited Settings. Pediatr Cardiol. 2025;46(1):27-38.
10. Kadiyani L, Kalaivani M, Iyer KS, et al. The outcome of surgery for congenital heart disease in India: A systematic review and metanalysis. Ann Pediatr Card. 2024;17:164-79.
11. McMahon CJ, Penny DJ, Kim M, et al. Achieving excellence in paediatric cardiac care in resource limited and resource plentiful settings and building successful care networks across different countries. Cardiol Young. 2024;34(11):2279-89.
12. Mantoo MR, Ramakrishnan S. Pediatric cardiac interventions: Innovations from India. Ann Pediatr Card. 2024;17:233-42.
13. Das D. Congenital cardiac surgery: Innovations from India. Ann Pediatr Card. 2024;17:389-400.
14. Murthy PR, Jandhyala S, Setty SP, et al. Free surgery for CHD through philanthropy-a sustainable model? Indian J Thorac Cardiovasc Surg. 2025;41(6):672-85.
15. Nair SM, Hesslein PS, Zheleva B, et al. A Population-Based Approach to Congenital Heart Disease in Kerala, India. Pediatrics. 2025;156(S1):e2025070739G.
16. Kumar RK. Training pediatric heart surgeons for the future: A global challenge. Ann Pediatr Cardiol. 2015;8(2):99-102.
17. Nair SM, Zheleva B, Dobrzycka A, et al. A Population Health Approach to Address the Burden of Congenital Heart Disease in Kerala, India. Glob Heart. 2021;16(1):71.

CHAPTER

55

Echocardiography for Childhood Left Ventricular Noncompaction

Sura Kishore Mishra, Bitan Mohanty

ABSTRACT

Left ventricular noncompaction (LVNC) is a rare cardiomyopathy characterized by a spongy myocardial structure due to excessive trabeculations and deep intertrabecular recesses. It is thought to result from incomplete myocardial compaction during embryogenesis, although genetic and acquired factors also contribute. In children, LVNC has a wide clinical spectrum, ranging from incidental detection to more severe presentations with heart failure, arrhythmias, or thromboembolic events.

Echocardiography remains the primary diagnostic tool for LVNC, yet the absence of universally accepted standards creates significant variability. Three major echocardiographic criteria are widely used. The *Chin method* evaluates the depth of trabecular recesses relative to myocardial thickness (X/Y ratio <0.5) and demonstrates high sensitivity and reproducibility, particularly at the apical level. The *Jenni method* assesses the noncompacted-to-compacted myocardium ratio (NC/C > 2), but pediatric studies show poor sensitivity and limited interobserver agreement. The *Stöllberger method* emphasizes trabeculation count and recess perfusion, offering greater specificity but depending heavily on operator expertise and image quality.

Comparative analyses suggest that the Chin criteria perform best overall, with Stöllberger adding diagnostic value in selected cases, while Jenni remains less reliable in children. Establishing standardized, multiparametric echocardiographic protocols may enhance diagnostic accuracy and improve early identification of LVNC in pediatric populations.

Keywords: Left ventricular noncompaction, echocardiography, pediatric cardiomyopathy, diagnostic criteria.

INTRODUCTION

Left ventricular noncompaction (LVNC) refers to an abnormality of myocardial architecture characterized by excessive trabeculations and deep intertrabecular recesses in the left ventricle. The myocardium appears to consist of two distinct layers: A thin compact outer layer and a thicker noncompacted (NC) inner layer. When this morphological abnormality is associated with functional impairment of the left ventricle, it is categorized as LVNC cardiomyopathy.[1]

The entity of isolated LVNC was first brought to clinical attention in 1984 when Engberding and Bender identified it by echocardiography as the persistence of primitive myocardial sinusoids.[1] Since then, LVNC has been recognized as a distinct, though heterogeneous, cardiomyopathy.

EMBRYOLOGY

The most widely accepted developmental explanation is that LVNC results from incomplete myocardial compaction during embryogenesis. In early cardiac development, cardiomyocytes derived from mesoderm form a primitive myocardial layer with trabecular projections into the ventricular cavity. These trabeculae enhance myocardial perfusion before the coronary circulation matures.[2]

Normally, compaction occurs between the 10th and 12th week of gestation and continues through the fourth month, with the trabecular myocardium progressively condensing into a compacted layer. Postnatally, the process is refined as systemic vascular resistance rises, eventually resulting in spiral fiber orientation that allows effective torsional contraction.[2,3]

In LVNC, interruption of this sequence leads to persistence of spongy myocardium and impaired contractile mechanics.

GENETICS

Left ventricular noncompaction is genetically heterogeneous. Approximately one-third of cases are familial, while the remainder occur sporadically.[5,6] Genetic investigations have identified mutations in sarcomeric, cytoskeletal, and mitochondrial genes. Importantly, no single genetic abnormality accounts for all cases.

Associations with Barth syndrome, mitochondrial cytopathies, and myotonic dystrophy suggest a shared pathway between metabolic derangements and abnormal trabecular remodeling.[7] Some patients with previously normal echocardiograms later developed LVNC morphology, indicating a possible acquired form and raising the possibility that LVNC may represent a morphological continuum with dilated or hypertrophic cardiomyopathy.[6]

Genes identified:

- Fbkp1a/Notch pathway
- *G4.5* gene/TAZ protein
- 14-3-3 deletion
- ZASP protein
- TNNT2 protein
- MYH7 protein
- TPM1 protein
- MYBPC3 protein
- ACTC1 protein

Genetic screening plays an important role in the evaluation of families affected by LVNC. Current guidelines, such as those from the Heart Rhythm Society, recommend offering genetic testing to relatives when a causative mutation has already been identified in the affected individual (Class I indication).[8] However, routine genetic testing for all patients with LVNC is not universally advised, as existing reviews of inherited cardiomyopathies suggest that the supporting evidence remains insufficient for blanket application in every case.

CLINICAL FEATURES

Left ventricular noncompaction in children presents with a wide range of clinical manifestations. Although the condition is congenital, the timing of symptom onset varies from the neonatal period to adolescence, and severity can range from incidental findings to life-threatening events.

Symptom Onset and Variability

- *Infants*: Feeding difficulties, poor weight gain, irritability, tachypnea, and failure to thrive are common early signs. These features reflect impaired cardiac output and early development of heart failure.[9]
- *Older children and adolescents*: Often present with exercise intolerance, easy fatigability, chest discomfort, palpitations, or dizziness; in some cases, syncope or presyncope may be the first manifestation.
- *Asymptomatic cases*: A subset of children are diagnosed incidentally during family screening or imaging for unrelated murmurs.

Heart Failure Features

Heart failure is the predominant clinical presentation in pediatrics:

- *Symptoms*: Dyspnea on exertion, orthopnea, and fatigue are common. Infants often display tachypnea and feeding difficulties rather than classic adult symptoms.
- *Signs*: Hepatomegaly, pulmonary rales, elevated jugular venous pressure, and peripheral edema may be observed.
- *Course*: Many children initially present with decompensated heart failure requiring hospitalization. In several pediatric series, more than half of affected patients showed impaired systolic function at the time of diagnosis.

Arrhythmias and Conduction Abnormalities

Electrophysiological abnormalities are frequent in pediatric LVNC:

- *Atrial arrhythmias*: Atrial fibrillation and supraventricular tachycardia can occur, producing palpitations or syncope.
- *Ventricular arrhythmias*: Ventricular tachycardia, though less frequent in children than adults, is a recognized complication and may lead to sudden cardiac arrest.
- *Conduction defects*: Atrioventricular block, intraventricular conduction delay, and bundle branch block have been described.[10,11]

Electrocardiographic changes such as T-wave inversion, ST-segment depression, and evidence of left ventricular hypertrophy are often documented.

Thromboembolic Phenomena

While systemic embolic events are well established in adult LVNC, their frequency in children appears lower. Nevertheless, embolic stroke and peripheral arterial occlusion have been reported. The pathophysiological basis is blood stasis within the intertrabecular recesses, especially when combined with systolic dysfunction or atrial arrhythmias.

Spectrum of Disease Severity

- *Severe course*: Infants and young children with marked systolic dysfunction often deteriorate rapidly, progressing to end-stage heart failure within months to years.

- *Milder course*: Some older children and adolescents maintain preserved ventricular function for long periods and remain minimally symptomatic.
- *Variable progression*: Even within families, the phenotype may range from asymptomatic to rapidly progressive disease, reflecting genetic and developmental heterogeneity.

Associated Clinical Clues

Certain extracardiac findings may accompany pediatric LVNC in some cohorts, including developmental delay or congenital anomalies. However, these associations are inconsistent and vary by population. Unlike adults, familial recurrence and features such as Wolff-Parkinson-White syndrome are not uniformly observed in children.

ECHO DIAGNOSIS

Echocardiography remains the most widely used imaging modality for identifying LVNC. However, lack of universally accepted diagnostic standards makes reproducibility challenging. Several diagnostic criteria sets have been proposed, each emphasizing different morphologic features.

- Chin et al.—measure the depths of intertrabecular recesses
- Jenni et al.—the ratio of NC to C myocardium
- Stöllberger et al.—the number of trabeculations

X/Y Ratio (Chin Criteria) (Fig. 1)[2]

The Chin method quantifies trabecular depth relative to myocardial thickness. It is performed as follows:

- *Measurements*:
  - X: Distance from the epicardial surface to the trough of the trabecular recess
  - Y: Distance from the epicardial surface to the peak of the trabeculation
  - X/Y ratio is then calculated
- *Diagnostic cutoff*: An X/Y ratio <0.5 in the apical regions (particularly apical anterior and apical lateral segments) is considered diagnostic of LVNC.

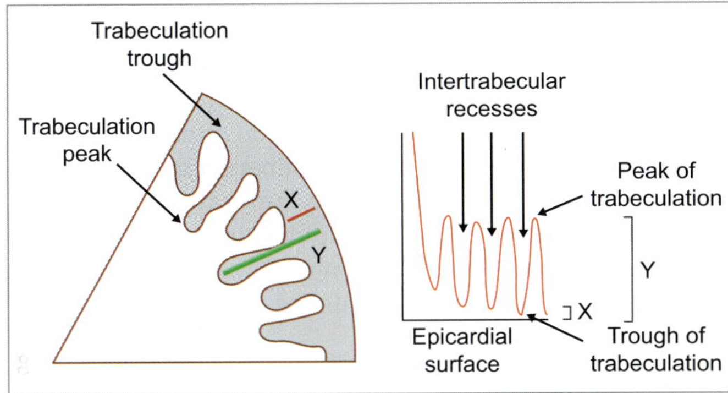

FIG. 1: Chin method.[2]

- *Preferred echocardiographic view*:
  - Parasternal short-axis view at the apical level
  - Ideally assessed during end-diastole, when trabecular recesses are most visible

Jenni Method (Fig. 2)[3]

The Jenni method highlights the two-layered myocardial structure that characterizes LVNC.

- *Measurements*:
  - The NC layer and the C layer are measured at the same site.
  - The NC/C ratio is calculated.
- *Diagnostic cutoff*: An NC/C ratio >2 is diagnostic.
- *Preferred echocardiographic views*:
  - Parasternal short-axis view (best for wall thickness assessment).
  - Apical 4-chamber and apical 2-chamber views can also demonstrate the layered myocardium.
  - Measurements are taken during end-systole, when the compacted layer is at its thickest and most distinct.
  - Trabeculations should show color Doppler evidence of blood flow into the recesses from the ventricular cavity, confirming that they are not artifact or false tendons.

Stöllberger Criteria (Fig. 3)[4]

The Stöllberger criteria rely on qualitative and functional evaluation of trabeculations.

- *Diagnostic requirements (all must be present)*:
  - More than three trabeculations seen along the LV endocardium in end-diastole.
  - Trabeculations must be clearly distinct from papillary muscles or false tendons.

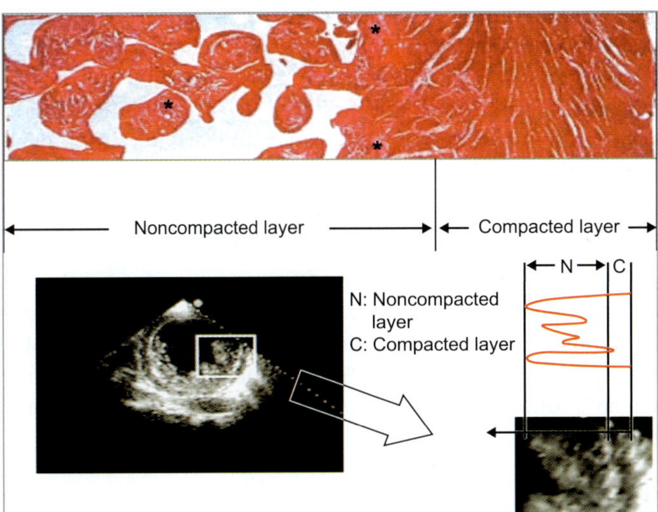

FIG. 2: Jenni method.[3]

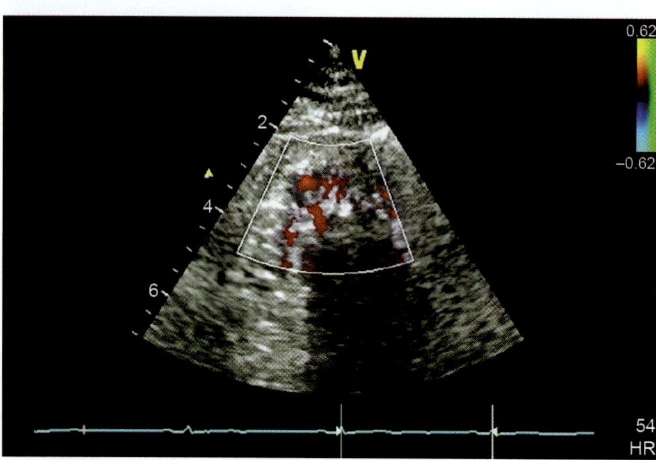

FIG. 3: Stöllberger method.[4]

- ○ Trabeculations must contract synchronously with the compacted myocardium.
- ○ Perfusion of the intertrabecular recesses should be demonstrated by color Doppler or contrast echocardiography, confirming their communication with the ventricular cavity.

Optimal view for assessing the number of trabeculations would be the parasternal short-axis view at the apical level, measured at end-diastole.

Apical trabeculations with perfusion of the intertrabecular spaces from the ventricular cavity are visualized by color Doppler echocardiography.

COMPARATIVE STATISTICAL ANALYSIS OF ECHOCARDIOGRAPHIC CRITERIA IN PEDIATRIC LEFT VENTRICULAR NONCOMPACTION

The diagnostic evaluation of LVNC in children remains challenging, and the reliability of echocardiographic criteria varies considerably. The three most frequently applied systems—Chin, Jenni, and Stöllberger—have been directly compared in pediatric cohorts, revealing striking differences in statistical validity.

Overall Diagnostic Accuracy

Among the three methods, the Chin criterion demonstrated the strongest diagnostic power. When applied to the apical anterolateral segment in short-axis view at end-diastole, the sensitivity reached 100%, with specificity ranging from 70–86%, depending on cutoff. Receiver operating characteristic (ROC) analysis yielded an AUC > 0.80, confirming robust discriminatory capacity. In contrast, the Jenni criterion produced AUC values close to 0.50, essentially no better than chance. The Stöllberger criterion showed intermediate validity, with AUC values between 0.75 and 0.85, depending on location and observer experience.[12]

Sensitivity and Specificity

- *Chin*: Highest sensitivity (approaching 100%), moderate-to-high specificity (70–86%); particularly reliable at apical levels, where trabeculation is most marked.
- *Jenni*: Sensitivity and specificity were both poor; many cases of LVNC were missed, while others were misclassified, leading to false negatives and false positives.
- *Stöllberger*: Sensitivity ~79–80% and specificity up to 93% at the apex, though performance declined at midventricular levels. Thus, statistically more specific than Chin but less sensitive.

Interobserver Reproducibility

- *Chin*: Showed the highest reproducibility, with kappa values reflecting good agreement across observers. Its numerical ratio minimized subjectivity.[13]
- *Stöllberger*: Moderate reproducibility; trabeculation counting depends on image quality and operator skill, making results variable between examiners.
- *Jenni*: The least reproducible; systolic measurement of NC/C ratio was highly inconsistent, especially in small pediatric hearts with rapid rates, leading to poor interrater reliability.

Summary of Statistical Comparison

- *Chin*: Best overall performer—maximal sensitivity, high AUC, strong reproducibility
- *Stöllberger*: Adds specificity, useful in obvious trabeculation, but more operator-dependent
- *Jenni*: Statistically weakest—poor sensitivity, specificity, AUC, and reproducibility

CONCLUSION

Echocardiographic assessment of LVNC continues to evolve. Current diagnostic methods differ in sensitivity and reproducibility, with the modified Chin criteria showing the greatest sensitivity and the Jenni method offering specificity at the cost of reproducibility. The Stöllberger criteria, though comprehensive, remain heavily operator-dependent. Future directions should include development of unified measurement protocols and possibly multiparametric echocardiographic scores to minimize diagnostic variability.

REFERENCES

1. Engberding R, Bender F. Identification of a rare congenital anomaly of the myocardium by two-dimensional echocardiography: persistence of isolated myocardial sinusoids. Am J Cardiol. 1984;53:1733-4.
2. Chin TK, Perloff JK, Williams RG, et al. Isolated noncompaction of left ventricular myocardium. A study of eight cases. Circulation. 1990;82:507-13.
3. Jenni R, Oechslin EN, van der Loo B. Isolated ventricular non-compaction of the myocardium in adults. Heart. 2007;93(1):11-5.
4. Stöllberger C, Finsterer J. Left ventricular hypertrabeculation/noncompaction. J Am Soc Echocardiogr. 2004;17(1):91-100.
5. Bhatia NL, Tajik AJ, Wilansky S, et al. Isolated noncompaction of the left ventricular myocardium in adults: a systematic overview. J Card Fail. 2011;17(9):771-8.
6. Oechslin E, Jenni R. Left ventricular non-compaction revisited: a distinct phenotype with genetic heterogeneity? Eur Heart J. 2011;32(12):1446-56.
7. Towbin JA. Left ventricular noncompaction: a new form of heart failure. Heart Fail Clin. 2010;6(4):453-69.
8. Bennett CE, Freudenberger R. The current approach to diagnosis and management of left ventricular noncompaction cardiomyopathy: review of the literature. Cardiol Res Pract. 2016;2016(1):5172308.
9. Hinton RB, Ware SM. Heart failure in pediatric patients with congenital heart disease. Circ Res. 2017;120(6):978-94.
10. Paszkowska A, Mirecka-Rola A, Piekutowska-Abramczuk D, et al. Spectrum of clinical features and genetic profile of left ventricular noncompaction cardiomyopathy in children. Cardiogenetics. 2021;11(4):191-203.
11. Vasichkina ES, Kovalchuk TS, Pervunina TM, et al. Spectrum of Cardiac Arrhythmias in children with left ventricular non-compaction. Eur Heart J. 2020 Nov;41(Supplement-2): ehaa946-0355.
12. Joong A, Hayes DA, Anderson BR, et al. Comparison of echocardiographic diagnostic criteria of left ventricular noncompaction in a pediatric population. Pediatr Cardiol. 2017;38(7):1493-504.
13. Kock TO, Børresen MF, Sillesen AS, et al. Left ventricular non-compaction in childhood: echocardiographic follow-up and prevalence in first-degree relatives. JACC Adv. 2024;3(3):100829.

CHAPTER 56

Adults with Congenital Heart Disease: What Every Cardiologist Should Know About Their Care?

Arun Gopalakrishnan, Shyam S Kothari

ABSTRACT

In India, there is a significant population with unoperated adults with congenital heart disease (ACHD), and a growing population with operated ACHD as well. With increasing lop sighted focus on interventional cardiology, an average cardiologist is not well prepared to treat patients with ACHD. We recount some essential core principles in the management of ACHD that should be known to every practicing cardiologist. Common disorders such as Eisenmenger syndrome (ES), Tetralogy of Fallot (TOF), atrial and ventricular septal defects (VSDs), and a few operated ACHD cases are included.

Keywords: Adult congenital heart disease, grown-up congenital heart disease, Eisenmenger syndrome, cyanotic congenital heart disease.

INTRODUCTION

The improvement in survival of children born with congenital heart diseases (CHD) due to early identification and definitive and/or palliative treatment has led to the advent of adult congenital heart disease (ACHD)/grown-up congenital heart disease (GUCH) as a new specialty in cardiology. The situation in India is peculiar, as a significant proportion of adult cardiologists prefer to be referred to as "consultant interventional cardiologists" with expertise limited to coronary interventions with no exposure and/or interest in the management of ACHD. In this chapter, we recount some of the important key areas that every cardiologist should be aware of.

UNOPERATED ADULT CONGENITAL HEART DISEASE

While over 90% of adults with CHD in developed countries have undergone one or more interventions for their disease in childhood, the vast majority of the ACHD population in India represents the natural survivors of unoperated CHD.[1] This section will outline most of the unoperated ACHD that a cardiologist in India is likely to encounter and some of the essential points in their management.

EISENMENGER SYNDROME

It is unfortunate to note that Eisenmenger syndrome (ES) is still not an uncommon diagnosis in the ACHD population in India. ES due to ventricular septal defect (VSD) or patent ductus arteriosus (PDA) is established very early in life (by 1–2 years or so), and it is unfortunate that some physicians still think ES is a disease that sets in by the second or third decade or beyond.

Patients with ES can present to the adult cardiologist with exertional dyspnea, fatigue, and occasionally syncope. Often, they report less symptoms as they are chronically adapted to lower levels of physical activity due to exercise-induced hypoxemia.[2] Chronic hypoxemia leads to multi-system involvement and adversely affects their quality of life.

Some salient points to note:

- ES in PDA is often missed in adult cardiology practice because these patients are often less symptomatic, and lower limb oxygen saturation is not routinely checked. Severe pulmonary arterial hypertension (PAH) in ES might be missed on transthoracic echocardiography, particularly in the absence of significant tricuspid regurgitation. When the ventricular septum is intact, a D-shaped septal configuration with an abnormal eccentricity index (>1.1) should be a clue to the diagnosis of pulmonary hypertension.[3] Midsystolic notching of the pulse doppler across the right ventricular outflow tract, and a pulmonary arterial acceleration time < 105 milliseconds are other features that reveal severe PAH.

- ES patients live longer than those with other forms of PAH. The reported 5-year, 10-year, and 15-year survival rates of ES are 86%, 79%, and 76% respectively.[4] This is in contrast to idiopathic pulmonary arterial hypertension (IPAH), which has an estimated median survival of 2.8 years from diagnosis, and 1-year, 3-year, and 5-year survival rates of 68%, 48%, and 34%, respectively.[5] Survival in all forms of PAH is improving with therapy in modern times compared to the past, though it is still very unsatisfactory. Survival in ES with complex CHD is comparatively significantly limited due to associated valvar regurgitation, ventricular dysfunction, and other additional issues.
- Anemia in ES patients is poorly tolerated, and the required hematocrit varies inversely with the degree of desaturation. A hemoglobin level of 14 g/dL may be anemia for a patient with oxygen saturation below 85%.[6] Iron studies are relevant to the management of ES, and iron supplementation should be considered in iron-deficient patients.
- Routine phlebotomies are contraindicated in ES as they can worsen iron deficiency and adversely affect oxygen delivery.[6] Only those with symptoms attributable to hyperviscosity syndrome should be considered for phlebotomy. Headache, dizziness, blurring of vision, amaurosis fugax, excessive fatigue, paresthesia, and presyncope may suggest hyperviscosity syndrome. Dehydration can precipitate hyperviscosity syndrome and end-organ dysfunction in ES.
- Care should be taken when patients with ES are considered for non-cardiac surgery (including hernia and other minor procedures), as ill-advised surgery or unplanned administration of an anesthetic agent may result in serious adverse events in ES. Systemic vasodilation that occurs during general anesthesia can aggravate right-to-left shunting in ES; the fixed vascular resistance in ES patients does not have the capacity for physiological adjustments, and a sudden change might trigger a vicious cycle that results in the death of the patient. In view of the greater risk of perioperative complications and mortality, noncardiac surgery in ES should be performed only at institutions with ACHD centers and anesthesiologists experienced in CHD care.
- Patients with ES should be counseled against pregnancy due to the increased risk of maternal mortality and worsening clinical status after delivery in survivors. Historically, pregnancy in ES has been associated with a 50% risk of maternal mortality. Although recent registries have reported maternal mortality of 20% in pregnancy,[7] morbidity outcomes remain grave in ES with a 55% incidence of heart failure during the second and third trimesters of pregnancy and early postpartum period.[8] There are increased chances of poor fetal outcomes with oxygen saturation below 85% in the mother. There are unique challenges that an adult cardiologist in India often encounters where the family is unwilling to terminate a pregnancy in ES. A midtrimester abortion in these patients is also risky. Hence, the decision should be made as early as possible in the early pregnancy. These patients should be managed by a dedicated heart team at the centers with expertise to ensure optimal fetal and maternal outcomes.[9] Successful deliveries in ES patients (with milder desaturation) have been reported with coordinated clinical care, but in general, it is best to avoid pregnancy.
- Routine anticoagulation is not indicated in ES and is associated with an increase in bleeding events. However, anticoagulation may be considered in ES patients who are otherwise candidates for the same due to atrial flutter or fibrillation, thromboembolic events, or who have mechanical prosthetic valves.
- Tricuspid regurgitation and heart failure are late events in ES secondary to post-tricuspid shunts (VSD and PDA), but patients with ES in atrial septal defects (ASDs) may present with heart failure. Similarly, cardiomegaly is common in ES associated with ASD, whereas ES with VSD or PDA has a normally sized heart till late in the course of the disease **(Figs. 1A to C)**. Why the ES heart functioning as a single unit against the systemic and pulmonary load in post-tricuspid shunts does not fail for so long is somewhat mysterious.
- ES is associated with an increased risk of sudden cardiac death. Age, atrial fibrillation, prolonged QRS duration, complete heart block, right atrial enlargement, right bundle branch block, increased right atrial pressure, impaired biventricular function, and the presence of a pacemaker were associated with increased risk of sudden cardiac death (SCD). Arrhythmias are common in ES and are a predictor of sudden cardiac death, and the risk may not be reduced by antiarrhythmic therapy alone.[10] Atrioventricular valve regurgitation is a risk factor for arrhythmia in ES. Disease-targeting therapy is considered a protective factor against all-cause mortality in ES.[10,11]
- Targeted PAH—directed therapies targeting multiple pathways can improve exercise capacity and hemodynamics in patients with ES and New York Heart Association class III symptoms. Bosentan has the most robust data till date in ES.[11] Phosphodiesterase inhibitors are considered a second-line therapy in ES.[12] The role of upfront combination PAH-therapies in ES is still unclear and needs to be addressed in further studies.
- In the past, there have been concerns regarding the safety of air travel in patients with ES. However, it has been found that shifts in the oxygen–hemoglobin dissociation curve tend to attenuate the effects of low oxygen tension during air travel, and most ES patients are able to fly safely without hassles.[13] However, patients should be advised to avoid dehydration and inactivity while embarking on

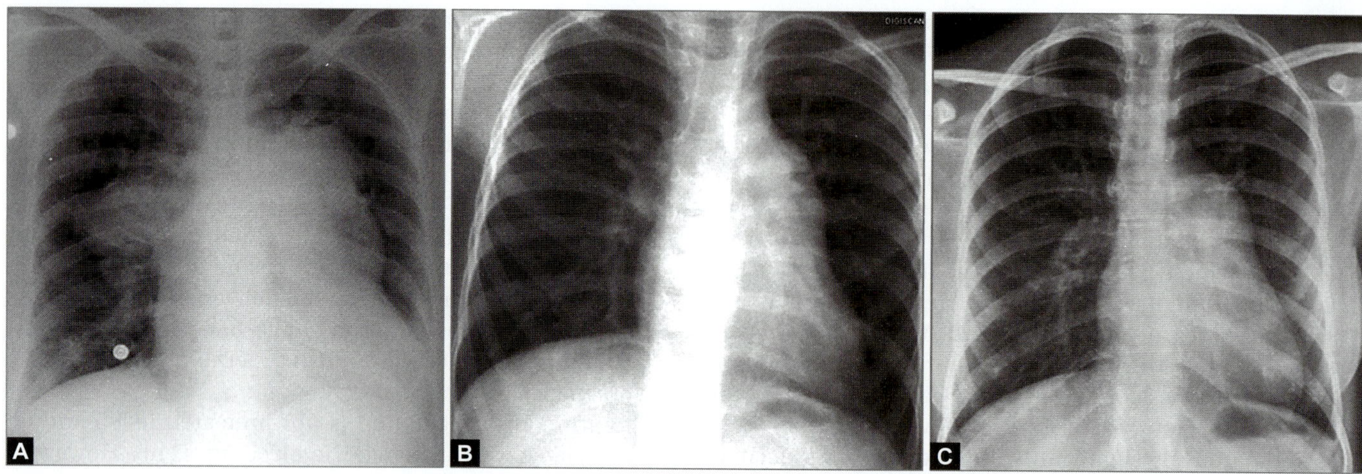

FIGS. 1A TO C: Chest X-ray of ASD ES, VSD ES, and PDA ES, respectively.
(ASD: atrial septal defect; ES: Eisenmenger syndrome; PDA: patent ductus arteriosus; VSD: ventricular septal defect)

air travel. Although there is no formal recommendation, supplemental oxygen may be used in selected patients with ES with oxygen saturation below 80%.[13]

- ES are not prone to infective endocarditis (IE) since there are no high velocity jets in the heart with ES. It is prudent to maintain good dental hygiene in CHD patients.
- ES patient with mild-moderate symptoms must NOT be referred for heart-lung transplant. Such a referral only reflects the ignorance of the referring physician regarding the natural history of ES and the understanding of the median survival of heart-lung transplant. The key indications for heart-lung transplant in ES include end-stage PAH refractory to maximal medical therapy with progressive symptoms and deteriorating right ventricular function with worsening hypoxemia. The median survival of ES after heart-lung transplant in the Nordic region is 12 years.[14] Based on personal communication, it is understood that survivors of heart-lung transplantation for ES in India to date are in single digits.
- Most ES can have a significant useful life span. It is a moral obligation on the treating physician to maintain a due cautious optimism in their care and not impose unnecessary restrictions in their lives.

ADULT TETRALOGY OF FALLOT

It is an unfortunate reality that patients with tetralogy of Fallot (TOF) are still newly diagnosed or discovered in adulthood in India. Adult patients constituted 14% of TOF repairs between 1991 and 2001 at AIIMS, New Delhi.[15] In India, one might rarely find an adult with TOF surviving on an aortopulmonary shunt done in infancy and never reported for a completion surgery or reassessment for the same thereafter. *Some salient points to note in adult TOF*:

- Every TOF patient should be operated on. Long survival in balanced VSD and PS (TOF) may sometimes be seen, but eventually right ventricular dysfunction and cyanosis-related complications curtail life.
- All forms of cyanotic heart diseases, including TOF, suffer from the complications of cerebrovascular accidents, brain abscess, IE, and polycythemia-related issues.
- It is a common misconception that a brain abscess will present with fever. Fever might be absent in 70%.[16] Thus, the onus of excluding brain abscess in TOF patients rests with the physician. More severe cyanotic patients might be more susceptible to brain abscess, but it might occur in patients with mild cyanosis. An unwary physician has diagnosed a brain tumor in a TOF patient that was an abscess!
- IE in TOF may present as pneumonia from embolism of the right-sided IE. The vegetations on the right ventricular outflow or in the pulmonary arteries might be missing.
- These patients are possibly more susceptible to tuberculosis than the general population, though systematic data on this aspect are scarce. Thus, a high index of suspicion for the above disorders in adult TOF patients should be maintained.
- The caution regarding anemia and venesection, as written for ES above, are equally important for TOF. In fact, venesection for TOF should only be needed in an inoperable pulmonary atresia patient with clear hyperviscosity syndrome. All others with TOF should be operated on.
- While TOF offers the best unoperated survival amongst the cyanotic CHDs, several factors adversely influence adult TOF patients. Chronic hypoxemia, long-standing right ventricular dysfunction, restrictive right ventricular physiology, aortopulmonary collaterals, left ventricular diastolic dysfunction, and aortopathy increase the operative mortality in adult TOF to 10%.[15,17] Adult TOF patients often benefit from detailed analysis with cardiac catheterization, angiography, and/or computed

tomography to delineate aortopulmonary collaterals, segmental pulmonary artery anatomy, and coronary artery anatomy.[18,19]
- Pregnancy in adult TOF is associated with high rates of fetal growth restriction, preterm births, and thromboembolic complications, although maternal mortality rates are not markedly elevated.[20] It is prudent to undertake pregnancy after corrective surgery for TOF.

TOTAL ANOMALOUS PULMONARY VENOUS CONNECTION

Total anomalous pulmonary venous connection (TAPVC) has a mortality rate of 90% in the first year of life without operation. However, several patients tend to present in adulthood in India.[21]

Salient points to note in adult TAPVC:
- Survival into adulthood in TAPVC is often associated with an unrestricted ASD, minimal obstruction to the pulmonary venous return, and the absence of advanced pulmonary vascular disease.[22]
- The clinical examination findings in adult TAPVC tend to mimic those of a large ASD, but with cyanosis. These include cardiomegaly, prominent right ventricular impulses, a wide fixed split of the second sound, and flow murmurs across the right ventricular outflow tract and tricuspid valve.
- Pulmonary hypertension is common in adult TAPVC. Cardiac catheterization should be offered to all adults with pulmonary hypertension before TAPVC repair.
- An arterial saturation of 85% or above generally indicates an operable lesion in TAPVC. Calculation of pulmonary vascular resistance index (PVRI) is problematic with all chambers showing nearly equal saturations. Theoretically, A fixed PVRI of >8 WU·m^2 with no demonstrable fall on administration of 100% oxygen or inhaled nitric oxide generally contraindicates surgical repair,[23] but a nuanced judgement is needed for this decision. It is interesting to note that in TAPVC repair, the cardiac anatomy is not altered (compared to a VSD ES repair), and whether different cutoff thresholds should apply is conjectural.

COMPLEX CONGENITAL HEART DISEASES

Some unoperated patients with complex CHDs survive well beyond adolescence and can present to the cardiologist in adulthood.

Patients with TOF and long-segment pulmonary atresia and pulmonary circulation perfused by adequate aortopulmonary collaterals often survive into adulthood. Those with the most balanced circulation tend to survive with the fewest symptoms. Segmental pulmonary hypertension is a peculiar concern in TOF with pulmonary atresia.[24] While aortopathy leading to significant aortic dilatation and aortic regurgitation is common, aortic dissection is extremely unusual. Those with advanced disease may present with pulmonary hemorrhage, ventricular dysfunction, heart failure, and arrhythmia.[25]

Patients with an unoperated single ventricle can occasionally survive well into adulthood with reasonable functional status. Most of these patients have ventricles of left ventricular morphology, and moderate to severe subpulmonary obstruction, ensuring a decent degree of pulmonary blood flow to maintain decent oxygen saturation with limited pulmonary overcirculation and heart failure. The median age at death of an unoperated cohort of unoperated single ventricle from Mayo Clinic was 56 years.[26]

ACYANOTIC CONGENITAL HEART DISEASES

Atrial Septal Defect

ASDs constitute the most common CHD diagnosed in adults. While most of them are asymptomatic and diagnosed incidentally, some may present with effort intolerance and dyspnea, and significant volume overload of the right heart chambers after a long asymptomatic period. While this could be related to long-standing shunt, the development of systemic hypertension, left ventricular diastolic dysfunction, and ventricular and vascular stiffening also contribute to increased shunt and worsening of the symptoms in these patients. Atrial fibrillation and flutter increasingly occur in ASD patients as they age and often add mitral and tricuspid regurgitation loads to the heart.

Some salient points to note in adult ASDs:
- ASD might be missed on echo or spuriously diagnosed. Sinus venosus ASD in adults should be investigated by transesophageal echo. Right ventricular dilatation with no apparent cause is often due to an unrecognized sinus venosus ASD or a partial anomalous pulmonary venous connection (PAPVC).
- Undiagnosed left ventricular diastolic dysfunction can result in pulmonary edema in adults after ASD closure. Patients with systemic hypertension and metabolic syndrome can have symptomatic worsening following an unplanned ASD closure. Some of these patients would need optimization of medications, followed by test ASD occlusion and assessment of LV end diastolic pressures and pulmonary capillary wedge pressures (PCWPs) before a decision on device closure. A rise in PCWP of >10 mm Hg from baseline or any value > 20 mm Hg is considered a high-risk subset. ASD closure with a fenestrated device/patch is a consideration in these patients.
- The decision to close an ASD in adults may be difficult. ASD may be inoperable with modest elevation of PA pressure since the intact ventricular septum does not mandate systemic systolic pressure (in contrast to VSD). Thus, it is not uncommon that a PA mean of 50 mm Hg in ASD might be associated with high PVRI and considered inoperable. But in general, age is not a contraindication

for closure. Even the elderly with Right ventricular volume load and tricuspid regurgitation benefit from the closure and have a better clinical course than without closure.[27] Closure before 25 years of age is associated with a reduction in arrhythmia later in life, and late closure might not change the incidence of atrial fibrillation, according to one study; however, closure is still indicated in appropriate patients.

- The PVRI cutoffs for closure in ASD have been drastically lowered more recently, but closing an ASD with PVRI 6 WU has been practiced for years and seems more appropriate. ASD ES is relatively rare, and only 20% of ASD patients would show raised PVRI.
- Some patients with ASD and inoperable PVRI have responded to pulmonary vasodilator therapy and have become operable. Please note that such a response has not been seen in VSD/PDA patients, and this strategy should not be adopted for post-tricuspid shunt patients.[28]
- Sinus venosus ASD closure with covered stents has been successfully done. The long-term results are not there yet. This strategy, as a routine, is not favored by the authors but might be utilized in selected patients.
- ASD patients might be cyanosed even without PAH because of several reasons. Lung diseases such as COPD may pose dilemmas for clinical management and require cardiac catheterization. Closure of ASD and reduction of shunt might be helpful in symptom amelioration in lung disease patients and should not be denied. Rarely, a left-to-right shunting ASD might be a cause of paradoxical embolism!

Ventricular Septal Defect

The common VSDs that are present in adulthood are the perimembranous (80%) and muscular (15–20%) types, while the inflow and outflow defects are less prevalent. Most of them present either with inconsequential shunts and cardiac murmurs or with severe pulmonary hypertension when they are inoperable.

Some salient points to note in adults with a small VSD:

- Patients with small VSD and no pulmonary hypertension do not require closure. There are a few reports of patients developing a cardiomyopathy-like picture from chronic volume overload; however, such an occurrence is a rarity, and most patients with small VSDs live well. The risks of IE were not an argument for surgical closure of VSD, and the same should apply to the device closure. However, adults with moderate VSD and a significant shunt (1.5:1) should have their VSD closed.
- The lifetime risks of IE in patients with VSD were estimated to be around 10–15%. Thus, advice to maintain oral hygiene and oral health should be seriously undertaken on every single visit. Patients with VSD and aortic regurgitation are at higher risk for IE.
- The risk of aortic regurgitation is higher with subpulmonary (subarterial/supracristal) VSDs followed by subaortic (perimembranous) defects.[29] The risk for aortic valve prolapses and regurgitation increases with age, but those who have not developed aortic regurgitation till 10 years of age do not develop it later. A small subpulmonary VSD < 5 mm in size without AR might be followed up medically alone. There is a lower threshold for operating for subpulmonary VSD than perimembranous VSD, as the former may be closed from the pulmonary artery and does not leave a cardiac scar.
- The patient should be followed up regularly, as sometimes they develop a double-chambered right ventricle or a subaortic membrane on follow-up. VSDs might also close during adult life also. An aneurysm of the membranous septum might serve as a nidus for thromboembolism or arrhythmia.

Patent Ductus Arteriosus

Adults who present with PDA often have moderate PDA with left heart volume overload and/or pulmonary hypertension. Those with large PDAs often have irreversible pulmonary vascular disease. The PDA with elevation of PVR *should not* have device closure done. There are several patients who would have lived well with their PDA who have developed severe PAH and right ventricular failure after ill-advised device closure. If the PA pressure falls significantly (<50% of systemic pressure) after temporary closure of PDA with a device or balloon, then it may be safer to do the device closure.[30] PDA with left ventricular volume overload and a persistent shunt should have their PDA closed at any age if the PVRI is within operable range. That range could be 6–8 WU, and not 3–4 WU as has been floated by some overly restrictive recent guidelines.

Infective endocarditis in patients with small PDA is often missed, and it may present as recurrent pneumonia from embolization of vegetations in the pulmonary artery.

Coarctation of the Aorta

Coarctation of the aorta (CoA) is an easily understood but often missed lesion that causes secondary hypertension, left ventricular hypertrophy, aortic dissection, intracranial bleed, and shorter life expectancy in adults.

Salient points to note in adult CoA:

- Hypertension in the upper limb with a systolic gradient of >20 mm Hg in the lower limb blood pressure is generally diagnostic of CoA, but may occur with aortic obstruction from other causes, such as Takayasu aortitis, coral reef aorta, aortic thrombus, and an obstructive dissection flap. Sometimes, hypertension might be absent or mild, and exercise hypertension may occur. A chest X-ray may reveal the diagnosis **(Fig. 2)**.
- Adults with CoA do not develop heart failure until late, in contrast to infants with CoA who present with severe heart failure. This bimodal distribution of heart failure has diagnostic utility, as patients with Takayasu aortitis often have heart failure in adults.

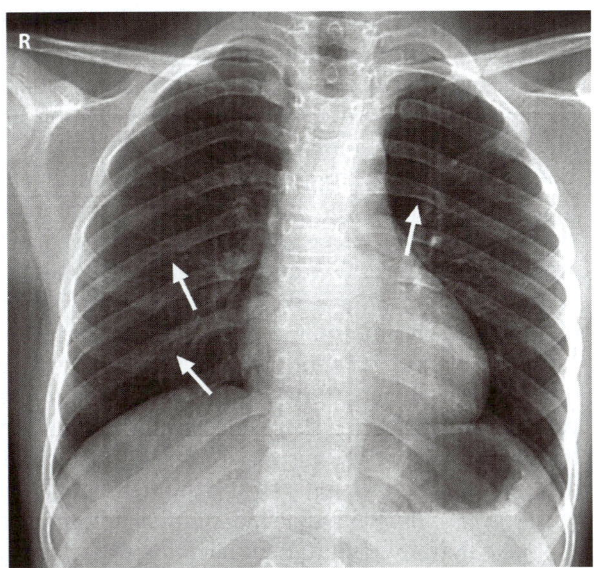

FIG. 2: Chest X-ray demonstrating rib notching in adult CoA. (Sometimes the aortic knob is inconspicuous instead of the typical 3 sign, though here it appears normal).

- Hypertensive emergencies are less common in patients with CoA for a similar degree of blood pressure elevation.
- Patients with CoA have a higher risk of developing aortic aneurysm (often in the post-CoA area) and aortic dissection. This is more common in patients with associated bicuspid valve (in 40–65% of patients), or associated with Turner syndrome, and during pregnancy.
- The absolute risks of complications of CoA during pregnancy are not high, and most patients might be able to undergo a successful pregnancy, though it is preferable to treat CoA before pregnancy.
- Hypertension might persist even after repair of CoA if done beyond early childhood, and patients with CoA have reduced life span and more susceptibility to atherosclerosis in some studies. Hence, risk factor management of these is important.
- An occasional patient of CoA with a ruptured Berry aneurysm might present with intracranial hemorrhage. Routine screening for evaluation of Berry aneurysm is not recommended (as it is seen in 2% of patients and management in unruptured aneurysm is controversial).
- IE in patients with CoA might be difficult to detect as it is endarteritis, but suspicion in a clinical context should be kept in mind. *Salmonella* species have a propensity to infect aneurysms, though most cases are not due to *Salmonella* IE in these patients.
- Percutaneous stenting is considered the treatment of choice for re-CoA and native coarctation with favorable anatomy, though balloon dilatation is effective in many patients.
- Surgery as a treatment for CoA in adults is generally reserved for complex CoA, aortic isthmic atresia, and long-segment CoA that needs an interposition graft. Risks of paraplegia after surgical correction are 2.6%.[31]
- Aortic tortuosity mimicking anatomic coarctation without gradient (pseudocoarctation) is sometimes seen and does not need treatment.

Pulmonary Stenosis

Valvar PS is more commonly a disease of childhood, but may occasionally present in adults. Mild PS with a gradient < 30 mm Hg in childhood does not progress, but more severe stenosis might worsen with the occurrence of severe secondary right ventricular hypertrophy and failure. In India, severe PS presenting with congestive heart failure in adults > 50 years old is occasionally seen. PS is commonly treated with balloon angioplasty with good results; however, sometimes it might be difficult to identify whether there is an organic obstruction from the muscles in the right ventricle that would need surgical relief. Commonly, secondary right ventricular hypertrophy regresses following balloon valvuloplasty. Dysplastic pulmonary valves are often associated with Noonan syndrome and often need repeated valvuloplasty with tougher balloons. Patients with gross congestive heart failure with severe PS might develop fatal pulmonary edema following balloon dilatation, and it is our practice to do staged dilatation in them. Isolated infundibular PS or double-chamber right ventricle should not be mistaken for valvar PS, and these lesions often require surgical correction.

Congenitally Corrected Transposition of the Great Arteries

Congenitally corrected transposition of the great arteries (CTGA) accounts for 1% of all CHD. This condition is characterized by double discordance (atrioventricular and ventriculoarterial) and therefore a normal physiology.

Salient points to note in CTGA:

- Patients with CTGA and no associated lesion can have excellent survival despite a systemic right ventricle that serves blood into the aorta.[32] This questions the common belief that the RV as a systemic chamber does not last a lifetime! However, most patients have associated lesions that influence natural history and survival.
- Patients with CTGA and VSD with PS (if balanced PS) can also have a long survival, and decisions in them about a high-risk surgery versus medical follow-up may be more nuanced, especially if they were to undergo Fontan palliation.
- Patients with mild to moderate PS or a moderate ASD should not be treated, as these conditions help maintain a favorable interventricular septal (IVS) profile that helps to reduce tricuspid regurgitation. The reasoning is like a palliative PA band offered to these patients during childhood. A palliative PA band leads to left ventricle overload (since PA arises from the left ventricle, which is well suited to the left ventricle's structure to generate pressure) and septal shift toward the right ventricle, which favorably influences tricuspid valve dynamics and reduces tricuspid regurgitation. TR can still occur if the

valve is morphologically abnormal, as often seen in CTGA patients. Such a band can keep LV prepared for a double switch surgery later in life and should be employed to train the ventricles during early childhood. Studies have shown that ventricles do not withstand a double switch surgery unless prepared before 4 years of age. Such preparations done later in life carry higher mortality and should be avoided.

- Complete heart block occurs in these patients at the rate of 2%/year, and conventional pacing often worsens the trajectory of the clinical course. Epicardial pacing might be a better option for them to preserve the systemic ventricular function.

  It is interesting to note that conduction problems are far less likely in patients who have CTGA in situs inversus. The reason for this is due to better alignment of the conduction axis in that developmental "ILL" loop configuration.
- Limited data suggest the utility of CRT in these patients if they develop systemic ventricular dysfunction, but it is technically challenging and should be done only at expert centers.
- Corrective surgery for CTGA patients (double switch surgery) is an appealing option in early childhood (before regression of the left ventricle in intact septum or development of raised PVRI in patients with VSD) but carries higher mortality and needs experienced congenital cardiac surgeons. Physiological repair alone leaves the right ventricle (RV) as a systemic chamber and is associated with heart failure in the long run in patients with VSD. In patients with no VSD and significant tricuspid regurgitation, tricuspid valve replacement often yields satisfactory results, provided the right ventricle has not developed dysfunction. A right ventricular end-diastolic dimension ≥ 60 mm and right ventricular ejection fraction < 40% are adverse outcomes after tricuspid valve replacement.[12,33] Assessment with magnetic resonance imaging (MRI) might be useful, but this judgement can be difficult in individual patients, and a heart transplant is indicated with severe right ventricular dysfunction.

■ Ebstein's Anomaly

Patients with Ebstein anomaly can present at any age, depending on the severity of the malformation. Patients with moderately severe disease are often present in adulthood with arrhythmia, or cyanosis, and heart failure. Echocardiogram is the diagnostic modality of choice, and MRI is increasingly utilized for morphoanatomical characterization before surgery. Displacement of septal leaflets > 20 or >8 mm/m^2 leading to "atrialization" of a portion of the right ventricle gives the diagnosis.[34]

Salient points to note in Ebstein's anomaly:

- Patients with mild Ebstein's anomaly might have a long, favorable clinical course with few symptoms, and some might only need treatment of arrhythmia by radiofrequency ablation. Multiple pathways (bypass tracts) are common, and they might need multiple procedures. Ventricular tachycardia and sudden death in Ebstein's anomaly are less well-recognized complications that should be remembered.
- The indications for surgery in Ebstein's anomaly include significant symptoms or deteriorating functional capacity, cyanosis (systemic oxygen saturation < 90%), paradoxical embolism, progressive cardiomegaly on chest X-ray (cardiothoracic ratio > 0.65), progressive right ventricular dilatation or dysfunction, and arrhythmia refractory to catheter ablation.[35] Tricuspid valve repair is the surgical treatment of choice. Cone repair is a form of tricuspid valve repair that involves delamination of the anterior tricuspid leaflet from the right ventricular endocardium, detaching and rotating it to bring the redundant leaflets to the level of the true tricuspid annulus to form a cone-shaped valve and longitudinal plication of the atrialized RV to restore RV geometry and function. A bidirectional Glenn shunt may be added in patients with relatively poor functional RV, thereby completing a one-and-a-half ventricle repair.

PALLIATED/CORRECTED CONGENITAL HEART DISEASES

An ACHD clinic in the west would cater primarily to treated CHD, unlike in India till date.[36,37] Simple heart diseases, such as treated VSD, ASD, and PDA, have a prognosis almost like the general population. Moderately complex and complex disorders need specific information and follow-up. General risk factor management and psychological support are required for all of them. Due to space constraints, only a few comments are included below. The management of adult CHD is well described in the recent guidelines.[12,38]

TETRALOGY OF FALLOT

While TOF repair in infancy and early childhood leads to excellent long-term survival into adulthood, all of them require long-term follow-up as they can present to the adult cardiologist with various issues.

Salient points to note in repaired TOF (rTOF):

- Severe pulmonary regurgitation leading to right ventricular dilatation, arrhythmia, and heart failure is one of the most common long-term complications of rTOF encountered in adult cardiology practice. Timely pulmonary valve replacement in rTOF is associated with survival benefit, freedom from ventricular arrhythmias, and improved quality of life.[39]
- The electrocardiogram provides a useful tool to follow up patients with progressive pulmonary regurgitation in rTOF. A markedly wide QRS (>180 ms) and QRS fragmentation are risk markers for ventricular arrhythmias and adverse clinical outcomes.[40]

- Dilated right ventricle as defined by increased end-diastolic indexed volume ≥ 160 mL/m^2, increased end-systolic indexed volume ≥ 80 mL/m^2, right ventricular systolic dysfunction, and progressive reduction in exercise tolerance are indications for pulmonary valve replacement.[38]
- Right ventricular outflow tract obstruction, residual VSDs, and aortopulmonary collaterals are other situations that may require intervention in adults with rTOF.
- Long-standing residual VSD, aortopulmonary collaterals, and branch pulmonary artery stenosis can lead to pulmonary hypertension in rTOF and can complicate the clinical course and natural history.[41]

TRANSPOSITION OF THE GREAT ARTERIES

Arterial switch operation in the neonatal period has revolutionized the long-term survival outcomes of transposition of the great arteries (TGA). In the past, atrial switch repair (Senning/Mustard repair) was the treatment of choice. It is not unusual for an adult cardiologist to encounter some of these patients in adulthood.

- Systemic right ventricular dysfunction is common in adults after Senning repair in childhood. While most patients are asymptomatic, some patients can present with exertional dyspnea, advanced right ventricular dysfunction, and secondary tricuspid regurgitation, and need heart failure management.
- Obstruction to the pulmonary and systemic venous baffles are reported in 15% of adults after Senning repair. Some of them need intervention for the same.
- Adults after Senning repair are at an increased risk of atrial arrhythmias and often need antiarrhythmics and electrophysiological studies for substrate modification.
- While arterial switch operation presents relatively better long-term clinical outcomes, some adults need reintervention for significant neoaortic valve regurgitation, neoaortic root dilatation, supravalvar pulmonary stenosis, supravalvar aortic stenosis, and coronary artery issues.

FONTAN CIRCULATION

Staged univentricular palliation culminating in total cavopulmonary communication, often referred to as the Fontan circulation, is being offered in several pediatric cardiac surgical centers across India, and there are increasing number of survivors into adulthood.

Salient points to note in Fontan circulation:

- The long-term survival of Fontan patients is excellent, 70–79% at 20 years, 76% at 25 years.[42,43] However, the Fontan circulation works only if the ventricle is functional, pulmonary resistance is low, and there is no obstruction along the pathway. The efficiency of the lungs and pulmonary vasculature are important determinant in their long-term clinical outcomes.
- Fontan patients require multidisciplinary surveillance with a holistic approach in adulthood. Dysfunction of the liver, kidney, lungs, and gut are not uncommon because of chronic systemic venous congestion in Fontan circulation.
- The adult cardiologist should be aware of the long-term complications of Fontan circulation including atrial and ventricular arrhythmias (30–70%), thrombosis (15–30%), need for surgical reintervention (12–20%), protein-losing enteropathy (3–15%), stroke (3–15%), Fontan-associated liver disease (5–25%), sudden cardiac death (9%).[44-47]
- Fontan patients cannot be cleared for high-intensity competitive sports as they have a relatively fixed cardiac output with limited ability to augment forward flow with increased requirements. In addition, chronotropic incompetence is also evident during activity, thereby limiting the exercise capacity of these patients. However, they should be encouraged to engage in low to moderate intensity aerobic activity.
- Pregnancy is associated with a high risk of adverse maternal and fetal outcomes in Fontan circulation and needs specialized care. The World Health Organization places a well-functioning Fontan in class III (high risk) and a Fontan with any complication in class IV (pregnancy not recommended). Well-functioning Fontan patients may be evaluated at dedicated Fontan clinics with a facility for dedicated high-risk pregnancy care for counseling and evaluation. Factors associated with a successful pregnancy outcome are younger age, normal body weight, absence of significant functional limitation, no Fontan-related complications, and well-functioning single ventricle physiology.[48]
- Patients with Fontan failure should be evaluated for heart transplantation at centers of expertise. Patients with ventricular dysfunction as the primary indication have excellent early survival after heart transplantation.[49] Worsening cyanosis, poor candidature for completion Fontan procedure due to severe atrioventricular valve regurgitation or pulmonary artery anatomy, protein-losing enteropathy, plastic bronchitis, and worsening systemic venous congestion are indications in those with normal ventricular function.

CONCLUSION

Every ACHD patient is a success story of survival of a birth defect into adulthood. Management of these patients requires an understanding of the natural and unnatural history of the disease and the given treatment. These patients require psychological support, vocational guidance, and specific cardiac advice, which requires not only a thorough understanding of the disease but also patient-specific issues. The care of an ACHD patient requires a team-based approach and a well-grounded cardiologist.

REFERENCES

1. Saxena A. Adult With Congenital Heart Disease in Developing Country: Scope, Challenges and Possible Solutions. Curr Treat Options Cardio Med. 2015;17(11):46.
2. Kempny A, Dimopoulos K, Uebing A, et al. Reference values for exercise limitations among adults with congenital heart disease. Relation to activities of daily life—single centre experience and review of published data. Eur Heart J. 2012;33(11):1386-96.
3. Mukherjee M, Rudski LG, Addetia K, et al. Guidelines for the Echocardiographic Assessment of the Right Heart in Adults and Special Considerations in Pulmonary Hypertension: Recommendations from the American Society of Echocardiography. J Am Soc Echocardiogr. 2025;38(3):141-86.
4. Saha A, Balakrishnan KG, Jaiswal PK, et al. Prognosis for patients with Eisenmenger syndrome of various aetiology. International J Cardiol. 1994;45(3):199-207.
5. McLaughlin VV, Presberg KW, Doyle RL, et al. Prognosis of Pulmonary Arterial Hypertension*: ACCP Evidence-Based Clinical Practice Guidelines. CHEST. 2004;126(1):78S-92S.
6. Arvanitaki A, Giannakoulas G, Baumgartner H, et al. Eisenmenger syndrome: diagnosis, prognosis, and clinical management. Heart. 2020;106(21):1638-45.
7. Keepanasseril A, Pillai A, Yavanasuriya J, et al. Outcome of pregnancies in women with pulmonary hypertension: a single-centre experience from South India. BJOG: Int J Obstet Gy. 2019;126(S4):43-9.
8. Arvanitaki A, Gatzoulis MA, Opotowsky AR, et al. Eisenmenger Syndrome. JACC. 2022;79(12):1183-98.
9. Justin Paul G, Anne Princy S, Anju S, et al. Pregnancy outcomes in women with heart disease: the Madras Medical College Pregnancy And Cardiac (M-PAC) Registry from India. Eur Heart J. 2023;44(17):1530-40.
10. Baskar S, Horne P, Fitzsimmons S, et al. Arrhythmia burden and related outcomes in Eisenmenger syndrome. Congenit Heart Dis. 2017;12(4):512-9.
11. Galiè N, Beghetti M, Gatzoulis MA, et al. Bosentan Therapy in Patients With Eisenmenger Syndrome. Circulation. 2006;114(1): 48-54.
12. Stout KK, Daniels CJ, Aboulhosn JA, et al. 2018 AHA/ACC Guideline for the Management of Adults With Congenital Heart Disease: A Report of the American College of Cardiology/American Heart Association Task Force on Clinical Practice Guidelines. J Am Coll Cardiol. 2019;73(12):e81-192.
13. Broberg CS, Uebing A, Cuomo L, et al. Adult patients with Eisenmenger syndrome report flying safely on commercial airlines. Heart. 2007;93(12):1599-603.
14. Hjortshøj CS, Gilljam T, Dellgren G, et al. Outcome after heart-lung or lung transplantation in patients with Eisenmenger syndrome. Heart. 2020;106(2):127-32.
15. Bisoi AK, Murala JSK, Airan B, et al. Tetralogy of Fallot in teenagers and adults: surgical experience and follow-up. Gen Thorac Cardiovasc Surg. 2007;55(3):105-12.
16. Udayakumaran S, Onyia CU, Kumar RK. Forgotten? Not Yet. Cardiogenic Brain Abscess in Children: A Case Series–Based Review. World Neurosurgery. 2017;107:124-9.
17. Abraham KA, Cherian G, Rao VD, et al. Tetralogy of Fallot in adults: A report on 147 patients. The American Journal of Medicine. 1979;66(5):811-6.
18. Rammohan M, Airan B, Bhan A, et al. Total correction of tetralogy of Fallot in adults-surgical experience. International Journal of Cardiology. 1998;63(2):121-8.
19. Bhushan R, Chugh V, Loona M, et al. Intracardiac Repair in Late Adolescent and Adult Tetralogy of Fallot — Early and Midterm Results from a Tertiary Care Centre. Braz J Cardiovasc Surg. 2022;37(4):511-6.
20. Keepanasseril A, Raj A, Plakkal N, et al. Maternal and perinatal outcomes of pregnant women with tetralogy of Fallot: a tertiary center experience from south-India. J Matern Fetal Neonatal Med. 2022;35(18):3483-8.
21. Bagaria V, Lahari B, Jagannath BR, et al. Total Anomalous Pulmonary Venous Connection in Adults: Should We Offer Surgery? World J Pediatr Congenit Heart Surg. 2024;15(3):319-24.
22. Rodriguez-Collado J, Attie F, Zabal C, et al. Total anomalous pulmonary venous connection in adults: Long-term follow-up. J Thorac Cardiovasc Surg. 1992;103(5):877-80.
23. Talwar S, Arora Y, Gupta SK, et al. Total Anomalous Pulmonary Venous Connection Beyond the First Decade of Life. World J Pediatr Congenit Heart Surg. 2019;10(2):185-91.
24. Dimopoulos K, Diller G, Opotowsky AR, et al. Definition and Management of Segmental Pulmonary Hypertension. J Am Heart Assoc. 2018;7(14):e008587.
25. Montanaro C, Merola A, Kempny A, et al. The outcome of adults born with pulmonary atresia: High morbidity and mortality irrespective of repair. International Journal of Cardiology. 2019; 280:61-6.
26. Poterucha JT, Anavekar NS, Egbe AC, et al. Survival and outcomes of patients with an unoperated single ventricle. Heart. 2016;102(3):216-22.
27. Humenberger M, Rosenhek R, Gabriel H, et al. Benefit of atrial septal defect closure in adults: impact of age. Eur Heart J. 2011;32(5):553-60.
28. Arvind B, Relan J, Kothari SS. "Treat and repair" strategy for shunt lesions: a critical review. Pulm Circ. 2020;10(2):2045894020917885.
29. Giridhara P, Poonia A, Sasikumar D, et al. Outflow Ventricular Septal Defect With Aortic Regurgitation: Optimal Timing of Surgery? Ann Thorac Surg. 2022;114(3):873-80.
30. Zhang DZ, Zhu XY, Lv B, et al. Trial occlusion to assess the risk of persistent pulmonary arterial hypertension after closure of a large patent ductus arteriosus in adolescents and adults with elevated pulmonary artery pressure. Circ Cardiovasc Interv. 2014;7(4): 473-81.
31. Wong CH, Watson B, Smith J, et al. The use of left heart bypass in adult and recurrent coarctation repair. Eur J Cardiothorac Surg. 2001;20(6):1199-201.
32. Beauchesne LM, Warnes CA, Connolly HM, et al. Outcome of the unoperated adult who presents with congenitallycorrected transposition of the great arteries. JACC. 2002;40(2):285-90.
33. Deng L, Xu J, Tang Y, et al. Long-Term Outcomes of Tricuspid Valve Surgery in Patients With Congenitally Corrected Transposition of the Great Arteries. J Am Heart Assoc. 2018;7(6):e008127.
34. Jaiswal PramodK, Balakrishnan KG, Saha A, et al. Clinical profile and natural history of Ebstein's anomaly of tricuspid valve. Int J Cardiol. 1994;46(2):113-9.
35. Saxena A, Relan J, Agarwal R, et al. Indian guidelines for indications and timing of intervention for common congenital heart diseases: Revised and updated consensus statement of the Working group on management of congenital heart diseases. Ann Pediatr Cardiol. 2019;12(3):254.
36. Willems R, Werbrouck A, Backer JD, et al. Real-world healthcare utilization in adult congenital heart disease: a systematic review of trends and ratios. Cardiol Young. 2019;29(5):553-63.

37. Saxena A. Congenital Heart Disease in India: A Status Report. Indian Pediatr. 2018;55(12):1075-82.
38. Baumgartner H, De Backer J, Babu-Narayan SV, et al. 2020 ESC Guidelines for the management of adult congenital heart disease: The Task Force for the management of adult congenital heart disease of the European Society of Cardiology (ESC). Endorsed by: Association for European Paediatric and Congenital Cardiology (AEPC), International Society for Adult Congenital Heart Disease (ISACHD). EurHeart J. 2021;42(6):563-645.
39. Bokma JP, Geva T, Sleeper LA, et al. Improved Outcomes After Pulmonary Valve Replacement in Repaired Tetralogy of Fallot. JACC. 2023;81(21):2075-85.
40. Bokma JP, Winter MM, Vehmeijer JT, et al. QRS fragmentation is superior to QRS duration in predicting mortality in adults with tetralogy of Fallot. Heart. 2017;103(9):666-71.
41. Venkatesh G, Kurup H, Raghuram K, et al. Pulmonary Arterial Hypertension After Repair of Classical Tetralogy of Fallot. Turk Kardiyol Dern Ars. 2025;53(5):358-61.
42. d'Udekem Y, Iyengar AJ, Galati JC, et al. Redefining expectations of long-term survival after the Fontan procedure: twenty-five years of follow-up from the entire population of Australia and New Zealand. Circulation. 2014;130(11 Suppl 1):S32-8.
43. Downing TE, Allen KY, Glatz AC, et al. Long-term survival after the Fontan operation: Twenty years of experience at a single center. J Thorac Cardiovasc Surg. 2017;154(1):243-53.e2.
44. Rao PS. Fontan Operation: Indications, Short and Long Term Outcomes. Indian J Pediatr. 2015;82(12):1147-56.
45. Pundi KN, Johnson JN, Dearani JA, et al. 40-Year Follow-Up After the Fontan Operation. JACC. 2015;66(15):1700-10.
46. Dennis M, Zannino D, du Plessis K, et al. Clinical Outcomes in Adolescents and Adults After the Fontan Procedure. JACC. 2018; 71(9):1009-17.
47. Gordon-Walker TT, Bove K, Veldtman G. Fontan-associated liver disease: A review. J Cardiol. 2019;74(3):223-32.
48. Montanaro C, Boyle S, Wander G, et al. Pregnancy in patients with the Fontan operation. Eur J Prev Cardiol. 2024;31(11):1336-44.
49. Krishnan GS, Gnanasekharan P, Sharma D, et al. Heart transplantation for patients with single ventricle physiology. Indian J Thorac Cardiovasc Surg. 2021;37(6):647-61.

CHAPTER 57

Quest for a Lifelong Pulmonary Valve in Repaired Tetralogy of Fallot

Ronak Sheth, Snehal Kulkarni

ABSTRACT

Tetralogy of Fallot (TOF) represents the most common cyanotic congenital heart defect, with right ventricular outflow tract (RVOT) dysfunction and pulmonary regurgitation (PR) as frequent sequelae after surgical repair. Chronic PR leads to progressive right and left ventricular dysfunction, arrhythmias, heart failure, and increased mortality. Pulmonary valve replacement (PVR), performed surgically or via transcatheter techniques, is key to restoring competence and preventing irreversible remodeling. Advances in imaging, valve technologies, and tissue-engineered heart valves (TEHVs) offer promising solutions, yet timing and durability remain challenges. Lifelong management of repaired tetralogy of Fallot (rTOF) requires careful risk stratification and individualized procedural planning.

Keywords: Tetralogy of Fallot, pulmonary regurgitation, right ventricular outflow tract, pulmonary valve replacement, transcatheter pulmonary valve.

INTRODUCTION

The incidence of congenital heart disease (CHD) is around 1%, approximately 20% of these affect the pulmonary valve or the right ventricular outflow tract (RVOT). Tetralogy of Fallot (TOF) is the fifth most common congenital heart defect and most common cyanotic congenital heart defect. Surgical repair of these pulmonary outflow lesions in early life (most commonly relief of obstruction or creation of a new outflow tract using a conduit) usually leave the outflow slightly stenotic or regurgitant. Over long-term follow-up, this may continue with progressive right ventricle (RV) outflow dysfunction. 40–85% of patients will have significant regurgitation at 5–10 years follow-up which in turn contributes to adverse RV remodeling.[1] Almost 50% of those who survive the primary repair will require a pulmonary valve replacement (PVR) in 30 years. Thus, pulmonary valve and RVOT reinterventions and resurgeries are one of the most common procedures required for these "grown-up congenital heart" (GUCH).

During reconstruction of RVOT, to relive RVOT obstruction, pulmonary valve integrity is lost which leads to immediate pulmonary regurgitation (PR) in most of the patients. This results in progressive RV dilatation and dysfunction of not only RV but also dysfunction of left ventricle as well due to interdependence of the ventricles. Some patients will need competent pulmonary valve placement either surgically or transcatheter techniques which depend upon anatomical characteristics of the RVOT. Patient selection and timing of the procedure are utmost important for this procedure. The competent pulmonary valve needs to be placed before significant RV dilatation and dysfunction sets in, so that recovery of RV is possible.

Many factors such as initial shunt placement, infundibular resection, transannular patch placement, reconstruction of branch pulmonary arteries, degree of residual stenosis, and regurgitation at the time of surgery need to be included in decision-making. Severity of PR is determined by regurgitant orifice area, RV compliance, diastolic pressure difference between main pulmonary artery and RV, capacitance and resistance of pulmonary arterial system, and duration of diastole. Although significant PR is common after TOF repair, the time course of PR progression, concomitant stenosis if present and their consequences differ considerably from patient to patient. A significant number of patients have tricuspid regurgitation due to dilatation of tricuspid valve, displacement of free wall papillary muscles, and distortion of septal attachment by VSD closure patch. In addition to PR, there is residual or recurrent RVOT obstruction. Left ventricular dysfunction is a key predictor of adverse outcomes. Volumetric criteria are useful when patients are asymptomatic or mildly symptomatic. Symptoms often are present when RV is significantly dilated and dysfunctional.

It is always debatable whether these patients can be benefited after having competent pulmonary valve.

NATURAL HISTORY OF REPAIRED TETRALOGY OF FALLOT

With newer diagnostic techniques and surgical expertise, results of TOF repair have significantly improved. This has resulted in improved survival and growing population of adults with repaired tetralogy of Fallot (rTOF). Residual RVOT obstruction and regurgitation are common sequelae after surgical repair which leads to electromechanical consequences and premature death. Though early survival during first year of repair is 98%, the morbidity and mortality start increasing during third decade of life due to sustained arrhythmias and heart failure.

Patients with rTOF often have PR of varying degrees. Although this pump inefficiency is well-tolerated for an extended time interval usually ranging from years to decades,[2] it ultimately leads to gradual process of adverse RV remodeling and complications. The brunt of these long-term sequelae is born by the RV with imminent long-term complications including arrhythmias, exercise intolerance, heart failure, and increased mortality risk **(Flowchart 1)**.

Globally we are now encountering an increasing population of adult congenital heart disease (ACHD), a large proportion of which is those with rTOF with dysfunctional RVOT **(Figs. 1 and 2)**.[3] There has been a 15-fold increase in the number of patients undergoing PVR annually over the last five decades[4] and there is a >50-fold increase in the number of rTOF patients living with a bioprosthetic pulmonary valve over the same period.

NATURAL HISTORY OF PULMONARY REGURGITATION

A large international cohort[5] trial showed that among propensity matched individuals with rTOF, those undergoing

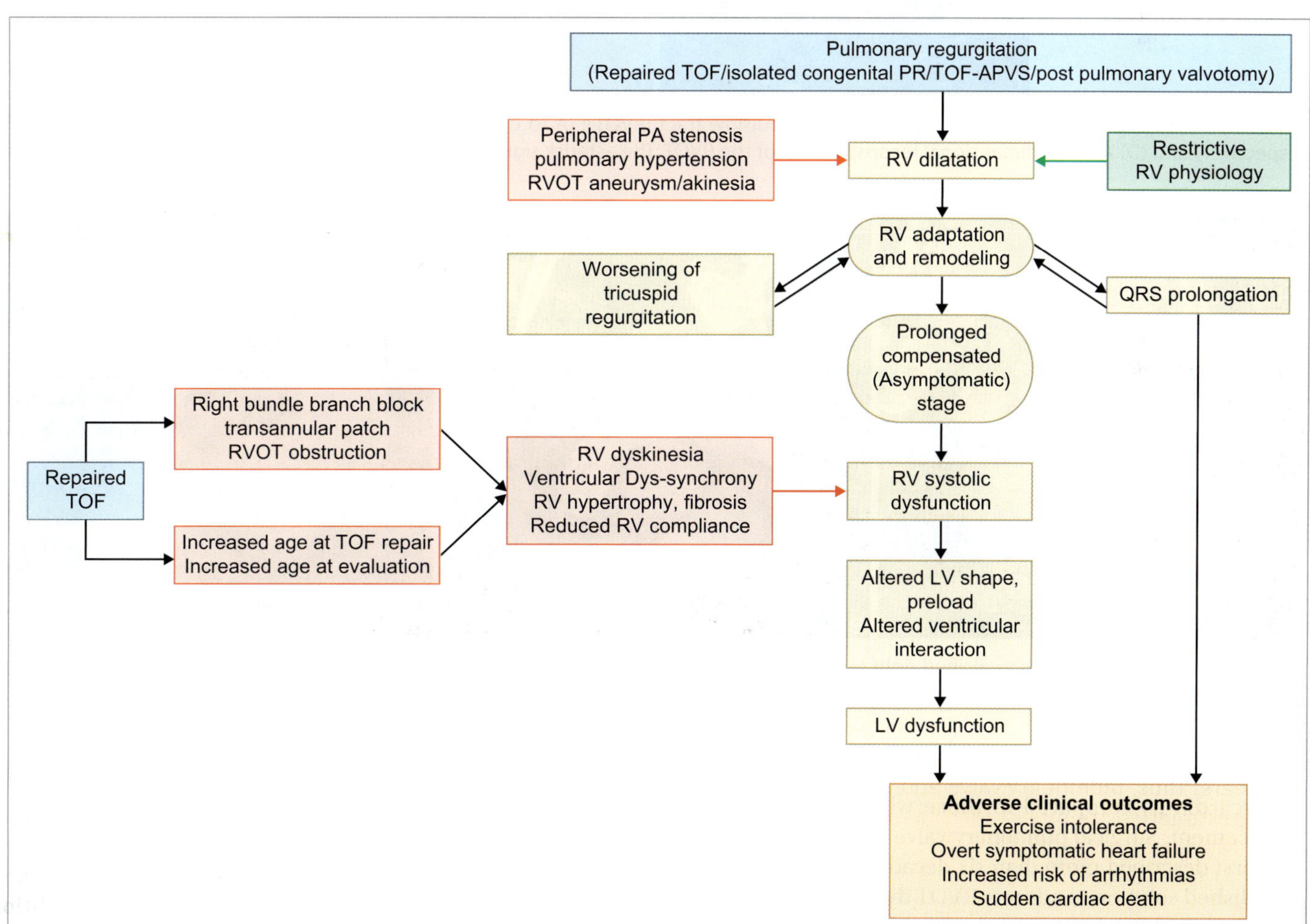

FLOWCHART 1: Pathophysiology of pulmonary regurgitation and repaired tetralogy of Fallot leading to adverse right ventricular (RV) remodeling and adverse long-term clinical outcomes. The boxes in red color are factors which aggravate the adverse effects on the RV whereas in green offers partial protection to it.

(PR: pulmonary regurgitation; RVOT: right ventricular outflow tract; TOF: tetralogy of Fallot)

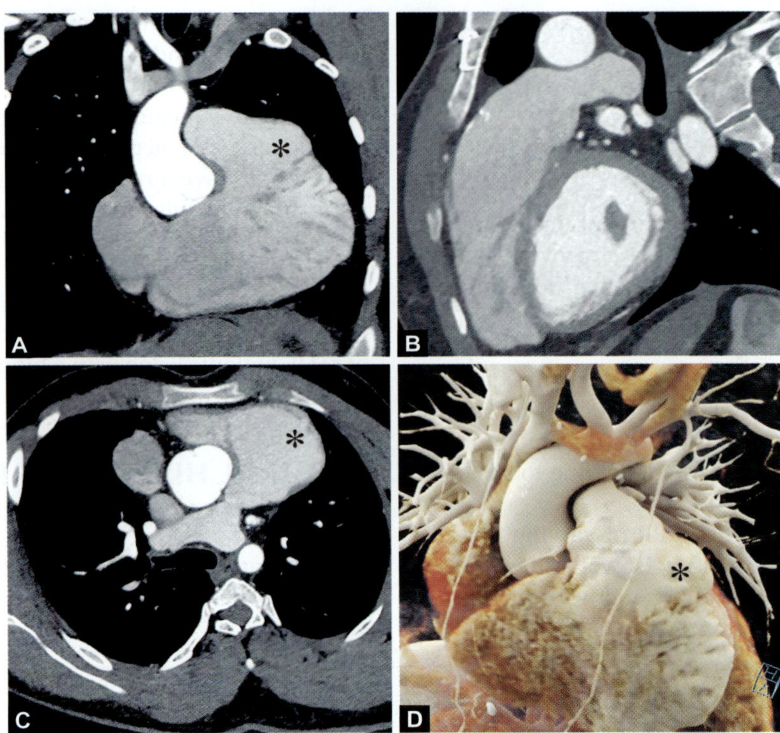

FIGS. 1A TO D: Dilated dysfunctional right ventricular outflow tract (RVOT): (A to C) Frontal, long-axis and short-axis views of the RVOT respectively and (D) A three-dimensional reconstruction of the RVOT. The asterisk sign depicts the aneurysmal RVOT.

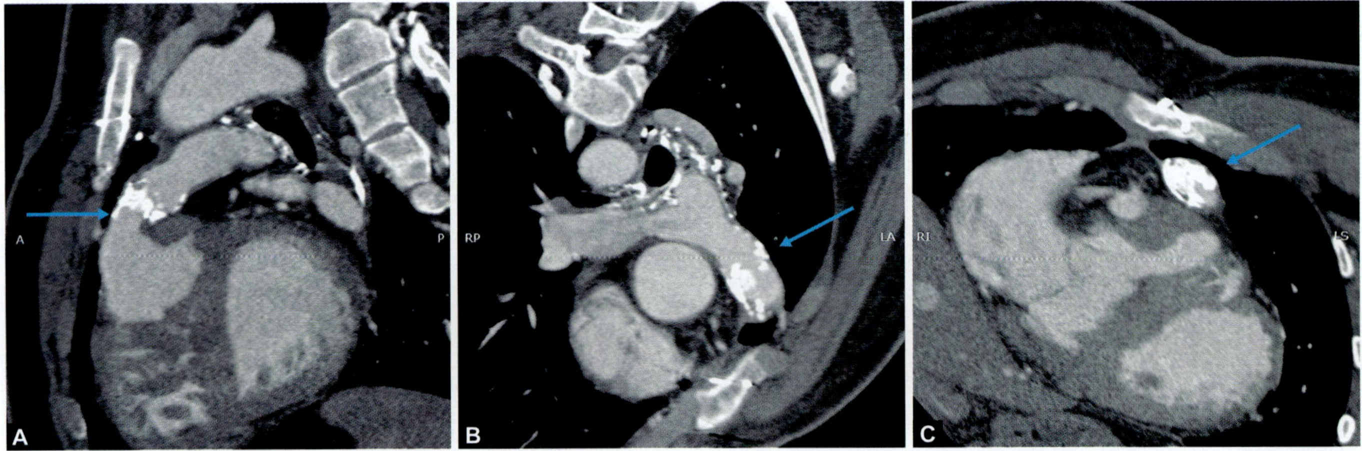

FIGS. 2A TO C: Stenotic heavily calcified right ventricular outflow tract (RVOT) typical of a calcified conduit: (A, B, and C) Long-axis, short-axis, and en face views of the RVOT. The blue arrow depicts the heavy circumferential calcification close to the proximal end of the conduit.

PVR are at a reduced risk of mortality or sustained ventricular tachycardia as compared to those who did not undergo replacement. Surgical pulmonary valve replacement (SPVR) was first described more than six decades ago and is a well-established solution to address RVOT dysfunction.[6]

The detrimental effects of chronic PR on RV function and exercise capacity; and the increased risk of arrhythmias and sudden cardiac death are well established.[1] Quantitation of PR through advanced imaging **(Fig. 3)** with regurgitant fraction and RV volume has facilitated stratifying these patients into risk categories and possibility of offering PVR before irreversible RV dysfunction sets in.

With advancing age, chronicity of PR, and adverse left heart dynamics including increased afterload and diastolic dysfunction, precipitates heart failure and exercise intolerance. The vast majority of patients with uncorrected PR in third and fourth decades of life are in NYHA functional Class II–IV and despite the chronicity of adverse RV remodeling, have a remarkable improvement in functional class following pulmonary valve implantation.[7]

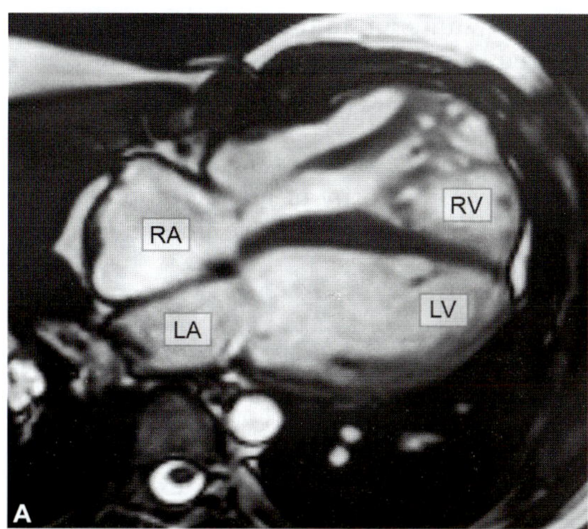

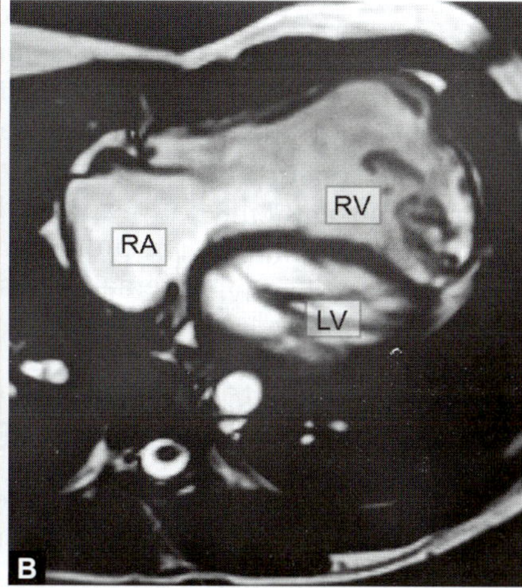

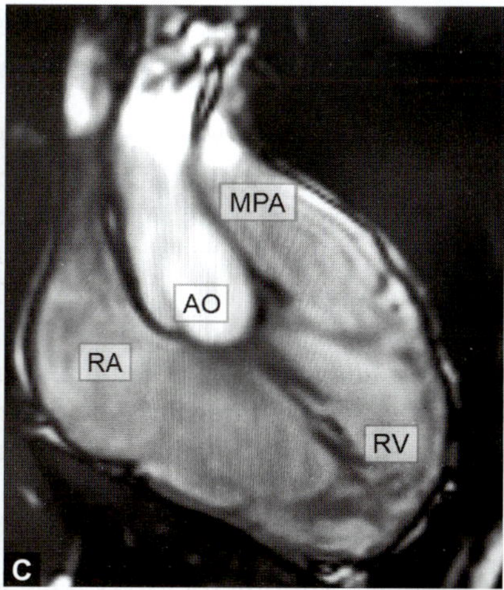

FIGS. 3A TO C: Cardiac magnetic resonance imaging (MRI) images depicting the significantly dilated right atrium and right ventricle (RV) in cine imaging. Still images depicted here (A) Four-chamber section; (B) RV focused apical section; and (C) RV inflow outflow section. This patient has mild biventricular systolic dysfunction. The cardiac MRI-derived estimated volumes are: RVEDVi = 231; RVESVi = 131, RVEF = 43%; LVEDVi = 107, LVESVi = 58, LVEF = 46%. The pulmonary regurgitant fraction is 50%.

TIMING AND INDICATIONS FOR PVR—BALANCING RISK STRATIFICATION AND LONG-TERM OUTCOMES

Although this debate remains and an answer to this question is still elusive, the predominant factors affecting the balance of decision-making are—preventing adverse outcomes by premeditating RV adverse remodeling before irreversible changes set in by using MRI volume criteria and thus deciding for PVR earlier versus the concern about valve longevity and durability and the cumulative risk of reinterventions and resurgeries that accrue over the lifetime of the patient. And the adult CHD specialist has to shoulder the responsibility of striking a fine balance considering all these factors with a sound judgment which takes into consideration the "lifetime" management of these patients.

A recent landmark study—INDICATOR trial—showed that there is a significant benefit of a proactive approach to PVR based on MRI RV volume criteria in asymptomatic patients.[5] On one hand, the interventionist's transcatheter heart valve (THV) portfolio has expanded multifold over the last few years, with advent of both balloon-expanding and self-expanding valve designs as well as sizes, which now include valves suitable for practically all sizes and morphologies of RVOTs; on the other hand, there have been limited advances in improving long-term durability of transcatheter pulmonary valves. Thus, despite many reinterventions now being amenable to transcatheter treatment with valve-in-valve implantations, the cumulative morbidity burden has not further reduced.

Certain patient clinical factors which contribute to a higher risk include:

- Transannular patch placement across RVOT
- Residual pulmonary stenosis/regurgitation after surgery
- Older age at the time of surgery
- Placement of RV-PA conduit—will need replacement
- Ventricular arrhythmias
- RV volumes quantification—pre-PVR RVEF< 40% is an independent predictor of adverse clinical outcome after PVR

Patients with higher end-diastolic volume index (EDVi) and end-systolic volume index (ESVi) values are at a higher risk of major cardiovascular adverse events (including heart failure hospitalization, life-threatening arrhythmia, transplant, stroke or death). Combination of RVESVi > 95 mL/m^2 and TAPSE/RV systolic pressure ratio < 0.4 are predictive of high risk of major cardiovascular adverse events.[8]

Follow-up after Pulmonary Valve Replacement and duration of QRS Complex

Right ventricular depolarization and repolarization characteristics improve after PVR partly in response to reduction in RV volume—especially QRS duration—which is strongly associated with RV function. Repaired patients with TOF having QRS duration of >180 ms are at risk of adverse events. There is no documented clinical relevance of change of QRS complex after pulmonary valve placement. Patients who lack improvement in QRS duration have poorer RV function and thus have higher risk of adverse cardiac events as compared with patients who improve in QRS duration after PVR.

Pulmonary valve replacement may not normalize the right and left ventricular dilatation and dysfunction in all patients. Some patients still persist to have RV dilatation and wide QRS complex and have high incidence of ventricular arrhythmias even with competent pulmonary valve. Many may need implantable cardioverter and defibrillator (ICD) on long-term follow-up.

COMPETENT PULMONARY VALVE—SURGICAL OPTIONS

During a surgical PVR, additional RVOT mechanics also need to be paid close attention, not only for ensuring valve longevity but also for facilitating future transcatheter therapies—these include the angulation of the pulmonary valve placement in relation to the RVOT, aneurysmorrhaphy, addressing hypertrophied RVOT muscle bundles and stenosis, correction of additional branch pulmonary artery distortion, discrete stenosis, aneurysmal dilatation; favorable valve positioning in relation to coronary arteries.[9]

Mechanical Pulmonary Valve

Mechanical pulmonary valves have a theoretical advantage of long durability; however, it comes at a real cost of lifelong anticoagulation; and high incidence of thromboembolic and hemorrhagic complications. Due to the inordinate risks involved, they are rarely used in the pulmonary position.[4,10]

Stented and stentless bioprosthetic valves: Though they are good options for RVOT obstruction and/or regurgitation and no need for anticoagulation, the durability and sizes are a big concern in children.

Biological Conduits

Homograft of Bovine jugular vein valved conduits (Contegra). Homografts get calcified on long-term follow-up and Contegra conduits need rereplacements often.

Handmade Pericardial Valves/conduits

Limited durability is the biggest disadvantage.

A large study of long-term follow-up of surgical pulmonary valve prosthesis showed a significantly higher incidence of prosthetic valve dysfunction in the bovine bioprosthesis group as compared to porcine.[11] Another large study also showed bovine bioprosthesis at a significantly higher risk of structural valve deterioration (SVD) at 5 years as compared to porcine valves.[12] Multiple theories have been proposed to explain the relative inferiority of bovine bioprosthesis in pulmonary position; but a conclusive inference as yet remains elusive **(Table 1)**.

TRANSCATHETER PULMONARY VALVE LONG-TERM OUTCOMES

Transcatheter PVR was first made possible by the pioneering work of Bonhoeffer et al.[13] The field has exponentially grown with a wide portfolio of transcatheter pulmonary valve therapies now available for clinical use in a wide variety of patient subsets.[14,15] Despite the global experience of transcatheter pulmonary valve implantation now ranging to more than two and half decades, there is limited understanding of long-term durability of transcatheter PVR. The major concerns with transcatheter PVR include procedural risks and long-term concerns of durability and risk of long-term device/valve in vivo including infective endocarditis (IE).

The longest follow-up of any prospective THV study—Melody Valve—Investigational Device Exemption (IDE) trial affirms the benefits with sustained symptomatic and hemodynamic improvement in majority of patients; with 10 years freedom from reintervention of 60% and freedom from valve dysfunction of 53%; and a TPV-related endocarditis annualized risk of 2% per year.[16] The Melody valve was more frequently replaced for indication of IE as compared to other Bioprosthetic valves.[4]

Multiple factors affect the longevity of transcatheter pulmonary valves including:[17]

TABLE 1: Currently available transcatheter pulmonary valve implants.

Valve models	Valve material	Frame/stent	Sizes available
Balloon-expanding valve models			
Melody: Medtronic Inc., Minneapolis, MN	Bovine jugular vein	Platinum Iridium	18, 20, and 22 mm
Sapien: Edwards Lifesciences, Irvine, CA	Bovine pericardium	Cobalt Chromium	20, 23, 26, and 29 mm
Myval: Meril Lifesciences, India	Bovine pericardium	Cobalt alloy	20–33.5 in 1.5 mm increments
Self-expanding valve models			
Harmony: Medtronic Inc., Minneapolis, MN	Porcine pericardium	Nitinol	22 and 25 mm
Venus-P: Venus Medtech, Shanghai, China	Porcine pericardium	Nitinol	18–36 in 2 mm increments
Pulsta: TaeWoong Medical Co, South Korea	Porcine pericardium	Nitinol	18–28 in 2 mm increments
MedZenith PT: China	Porcine pericardium	Nitinol	20, 23, and 26 mm
Self-expanding pre-stents (to be combined with suitable valve)			
Alterra: Edwards Lifesciences, Irvine, CA	–	Nitinol	Accommodates 29 mm Sapien 3 valve

- Pre-transcatheter pulmonary valve replacement (pre-TPVR) RVOT obstruction
- Post-TPVR peak velocity across pulmonary outflow
- Valve diameter < 22
- Age < 25 years at TPVR
- Occurrence of IE

Infective endocarditis is a major concern for transcatheter pulmonary valves affecting its long-term durability and long-term morbidity and reintervention rates. A recent study found a higher incidence of IE as well as requirement for secondary PVR among Melody THV as compared to SAPIEN valve; Incidence of IE and SecPVR of 5.5 and 7.6 per 100 patient years in Melody Group compared to 0.2 and 1.3 in Sapien valve group.[17]

The higher additional risk of IE in Melody valves adds a substantial incremental risk of TPVI graft failure.[17] Younger age at PVR and smaller valve diameters are independently associated with reduced valve longevity.[4]

Although the median redo PVR duration is 17 years, the curve is exponential even longest durability in current era is unlikely to be much higher than two decades. Considering the advancing life expectancy of these GUCH patients, and concurrent advances in management of other cardiac morbidities, thus most patients will require at least three valves over their lifetime.

Valve-associated Thrombosis

Studies are now forthcoming with the value of advanced imaging surveillance of TPVR using computed tomography (CT) to assess leaflet morphology and motion on follow-up. Beyond echocardiographic assessment of valve leaflet motion and doppler gradients, CT now provides additional data—the two most commonly being studies are hypoattenuating leaflet thrombosis (HALT) and hypoattenuation affecting motion (HAM). At 8 months median follow-up, the prevalence of HALT and HAM was 17 and 6%; they are associated with valve deterioration and increasing transvalvular gradients; it is not seen in patients on anticoagulation. HALT and HAM are proposed to reflect subclinical leaflet thrombosis and are potentially associated with poor valve longevity and although long-term studies are awaited, such early identification by CT helps in guiding treatment with anticoagulation.[18,19]

TRANSCATHETER PULMONARY VALVE REPLACEMENT VERSUS SURGICAL PULMONARY VALVE REPLACEMENT

Right heart remodeling and functional outcomes are better after TPVR; however, the benefits may be offset by a relatively higher incidence of prosthetic valve dysfunction predominantly due to higher incidence of endocarditis.[20] TPVR has a greater improvement in RA reservoir strain and RV global longitudinal strain at 1- and 3-year follow-up as compared to SPVR group. However, the TPVR group also had a higher incidence of prosthetic valve endocarditis and valve dysfunction as compared to the SPVR group; both groups had similar gradients and similar reintervention rates on follow-up.

IDEAL PULMONARY VALVE

Properties of the ideal valve:[21]

- Rapid and complete closure of leaflets
- High ratio of orifice area in open position to total valve area
- Mechanical stability with repetitive deformation and movements
- Nonthrombogenic—endothelial surface
- Resistant to structural deterioration, degradation, and calcification
- Resistant to infection
- Capable of self-repair of injuries
- Remodeling ability in response to local mechanical forces
- Growth potential
- Permanent viability
- Ease of implantation technique
- Cost-efficient

TISSUE-ENGINEERED HEART VALVES

Tissue engineering attempts to solve this problem to improve the longevity of RVOT rehabilitation and thus reduce morbidity and risks for patients with repaired RVOTs.[22] Tissue-engineered heart valves (TEHVs) are tissue-engineered valves designed to function as bioinstructive scaffolds which will guide in situ autologous valve leaflet generation capable of growth repair and remodeling thus behaving similar to natural valves and promising a normal like longevity. TEHVs offer the possibility for overcoming the limitations of current mechanical and bioprosthetic valves; acting as lifelong valve substitutes.[23]

The most pressing need for advancing this new innovative TEHVs is in pediatric and Grown congenital heart population as the results of heart valve replacement are inferior in this subset as compared to adults and also the prospect of growth regeneration and healing promises a long durability with reduced burden of reintervention.[21]

Need for Tissue-engineered Heart Valve

The indications for TPVR are expanding including lower risk patients and younger population.[14,24] However, this is offset by limitations of current TPVR therapies which involve use of glutaraldehyde fixed xenogenic tissues which make them prone to calcification and structural deterioration thus limiting their longevity raising concerns for use in younger patients for the sheer number of reinterventions that are potentially required over the patient's lifetime.

Next-generation TEHVs have repair, remodeling, regenerative, and growth capacities. These "native-equivalent" valves will help to address the Achilles heel of current generation of heart valve prosthesis and be an especially promising therapy for the pediatric and CHD population.[25] TEHV advantages include nonthrombogenicity, infection resistance, cellular viability, growth, regeneration, and healing.[21]

Initial results with a novel "biorestorative" valved conduit "Xeltis pulmonary valve" have shown promising results. It is a novel technology which allows for a "living and regenerating" heart valve. It is a novel synthetic porous bioabsorbable polymer. The implanted graft material attracts the patient's own cells and proteins thus triggering a cascade leading to tissue restoration; the native tissue invading the graft and leaflets, gradually organizing into natural valve tissue and structure while the implanted polymer scaffold gets bioabsorbed.[26]

The CorMatrix Cor Tricuspid valve is a tissue-engineered valve designed specifically for tricuspid position with the concept of "whole valve replacement"—it is designed to reconstitute the entire valve including the subvalvar apparatus, with remodeling and tissue ingrowth of native cells from annulus to papillary muscles within 3 months, thus remodeling RV geometry and function. Initial feasibility studies and first-in-man trials are now ongoing; and early results in human use are promising.[27]

Multiple TEHV models are nearing clinical translation and early clinical "in-human" feasibility studies.[28] TEHVs based on decellularized in vitro grown tissue-engineered matrices have shown feasibility in early studies and are on the verge of clinical application.[29] Broad-based clinical translation of TEHV technology depends on overcoming multiple challenges relating to immunohemocompatibility, good manufacturing, and laboratory practices, regulatory approvals, and standardization requirements.[25]

CONCLUSION

The lifelong management of repaired tetralogy of Fallot hinges on timely pulmonary adverse valve replacement to prevent irreversible right ventricular remodeling and dysfunction. While surgical and transcatheter approaches have advanced, valve durability and infective endocarditis remain major concerns. Emerging TEHVs hold promise for growth, regeneration, and long-term viability, potentially offering a lifelong solution for this complex congenital condition.

REFERENCES

1. Bouzas B, Kilner PJ, Gatzoulis MA. Pulmonary regurgitation: not a benign lesion. Eur Heart J. 2005;26(5):433-9.
2. Cuypers JA, Menting ME, Konings EE, et al. Unnatural history of tetralogy of Fallot: prospective follow-up of 40 years after surgical correction. Circulation. 2014;130(22):1944-53.
3. Van der Bom T, Zomer AC, Zwinderman AH, et al. The changing epidemiology of congenital heart disease. Nat Rev Cardiol. 2011;8(1):50-60.
4. Gröning M, Smerup MH, Munk K, et al. Pulmonary valve replacement in tetralogy of Fallot: procedural volume and durability of bioprosthetic pulmonary valves. J Am Coll Cardiol Intv.2024;17(2):217-27.
5. Bokma JP, Geva T, Sleeper LA, et al. Improved outcomes after pulmonary valve replacement in repaired tetralogy of Fallot. J Am Coll Cardiol. 2023;81(21):2075-85.
6. Lillehei CW, Levy MJ, Adams P, et al. Corrective surgery for tetralogy of Fallot. Long-term follow-up by postoperative recatheterization in 69 cases and certain surgical considerations. J Thorac Cardiovasc Surg. 1964;48:556-76.
7. Aldoss O, Carr K, Shahanavaz S, et al. Acute and mid-term outcomes of transcatheter pulmonary valve implantation in patients older than 40 years. Int J Cardiol Congenit Heart Dis. 2021;3:100084.
8. Egbe AC, Miranda WR, Said SM, et al. Risk stratification and clinical outcomes after surgical pulmonary valve replacement. Am Heart J. 2018;206:105-12.
9. Lee CH. Beyond the Valve: Lifelong Management of Right Ventricular Outflow Tract Lesion in Adult Congenital Heart Disease. Korean Circ J. 2022;52(8):632-4.
10. Hascoet S, Gatzoulis MA, Fraisse A. Quest for a Lifelong Pulmonary Valve in Repaired Tetralogy of Fallot: Valve Bioengineering Is Needed. JACC Cardiovasc Interv. 2024;17(2):228-30.
11. Kwak JG, Bang JH, Cho S, et al. Long-term durability of bioprosthetic valves in pulmonary position: pericardial versus porcine valves. J Thorac Cardiovasc Surg. 2020;160:476-84.
12. Ramchandani B, Sánchez R, Rey J, et al. A bicentric propensity matched analysis of 158 patients comparing porcine versus bovine stented bioprosthetic valves in pulmonary position. Korean Circ J. 2022;52:623-31.
13. Bonhoeffer P, Boudjemline Y, Saliba Z, et al. Percutaneous replacement of pulmonary valve in a right-ventricle to pulmonary-artery prosthetic conduit with valve dysfunction. Lancet. 2000;356(9239):1403-5.
14. Constantine A, Dimopoulos K, Heng EL, et al. Transcatheter pulmonary valve implantation: An option for the few becoming an option for the many. Int J Cardiol. 2023;373:44-6.
15. Patel ND, Levi DS, Cheatham JP, et al. Transcatheter Pulmonary Valve Replacement: A Review of Current Valve Technologies. J Soc Cardiovasc Angiogr Interv. 2022;1(6):100452.
16. Jones TK, McElhinney DB, Vincent JA, et al. Long-Term Outcomes After Melody Transcatheter Pulmonary Valve Replacement in the US Investigational Device Exemption Trial. Circ Cardiovasc Interv. 2022;15(1):e010852.
17. Houeijeh A, Batteux C, Karsenty C, et al. Long-term outcomes of transcatheter pulmonary valve implantation with melody and SAPIEN valves. Int J Cardiol. 2023;370:156-66.
18. Spagnolo P, Bevilacqua F, Perillo N, et al. Hypoattenuating Leaflet Thickening After Transcatheter Pulmonary Valve Implantation: An Urgent Call to Action. JACC Case Rep. 2025;30(17):103889.
19. Sefton C, Firth A, Curran K, et al. Outcomes of Hypoattenuating Leaflet Thickening Post-Transcatheter Pulmonary Valve Replacement. JACC Adv. 2025;4(3):101599.

20. Egbe AC, Salama AA, Miranda WR, et al. Right Heart Reverse Remodeling and Prosthetic Valve Function After Transcatheter vs Surgical Pulmonary Valve Replacement. JACC Cardiovasc Interv. 2024;17(2):248-58.
21. Mendelson K, Schoen FJ. Heart valve tissue engineering: concepts, approaches, progress, and challenges. Ann Biomed Eng. 2006;34(12):1799-819.
22. Almeida-Pinto R, Leite-Moreira AF, Brás-Silva C, et al. Pulmonary Valve Replacement: A New Paradigm with Tissue Engineering. Curr Probl Cardiol. 2023;48(8):101212.
23. Cordoves EM, Vunjak-Novakovic G, Kalfa DM. Designing biocompatible tissue engineered heart valves in situ. J Am Coll Cardiol. 2023;81(10):994-1003.
24. McCarthy E, Georgiev S, Zhang Y, et al. Long-term durability of Melody Valves implanted in small (<30kg) patients. J Soc Cardiovasc Angiogr Interv. 2025;4(5):102667.
25. Fioretta ES, Motta SE, Lintas V, et al. Next-generation tissue-engineered heart valves with repair, remodelling and regeneration capacity. Nat Rev Cardiol. 2021;18(2):92-116.
26. Morales DL, Herrington C, Bacha EA, et al. A novel restorative pulmonary valve conduit: early outcomes of two clinical trials. Front Cardiovasc Med. 2020;7:583360.
27. Gerdisch M, Stelly T, Slaughter M, et al. Early Results from the FDA Extracellular Matrix (ECM) Cylinder Valve Clinical Feasibility Trial. Struct Heart. 2020;4(S1):102.
28. Mirani B, Parvin Nejad S, Simmons CA. Recent Progress Toward Clinical Translation of Tissue-Engineered Heart Valves. Can J Cardiol. 2021;37(7):1064-77.
29. Motta SE, Lintas V, Fioretta ES, et al. Human cell-derived tissue-engineered heart valve with integrated Valsalva sinuses: towards native-like transcatheter pulmonary valve replacements. NPJ Regen Med. 2019;4:14.

SECTION

8

Valvular Heart Disease

Section Outline

58. Multiparametric Approach to Asymptomatic Aortic Stenosis
Ajay Kumar Pandey, Nikhil Gupta, Prashant Kumar Pandey

59. Secondary Mitral Regurgitation: Phenotypes, Proportionality, and Evolving Management
Arijit Ghosh, Arup Dasbiswas, Subhasis Roy Chowdhury, Mainak Mukhopadhyay

60. Mitral Annular Disjunction in Mitral Valve Prolapse
Biswaranjan Mishra

61. An Update on High-gradient Moderate Aortic Stenosis
Debika Chatterjee

62. Comprehensive Risk Phenotyping in Aortic Stenosis
Dipankar Ghosh Dastidar

63. When to Treat Young and Low-risk Patients with Aortic Stenosis
Gopala Krishna Koduru, Raghuram Palaparti, Venkata RS Subrahmanya Sarma

64. Acute Rheumatic Fever and Rheumatic Heart Disease: A Continuum (Recent Advances)
Mohit D Gupta, Girish MP, Gaurav Sharma, Mayank Shami

65. Comprehensive Approach to Aortic Valve Pathophysiology by Fibro-Calcific Imaging
Johann Christopher, Raja Ramesh Nukavarapu

66. Reimagining Valvular Heart Disease Management: Insights from the 2025 ESC/EACTS Guidelines
Mrinal Kanti Das

67. Rheumatic Heart Disease in India: An Imperative Tale to Tell
Sanjeev Asotra, Vinay Bhardwaj, Preetam Thakur

CHAPTER

58

Multiparametric Approach to Asymptomatic Aortic Stenosis

Ajay Kumar Pandey, Nikhil Gupta, Prashant Kumar Pandey

ABSTRACT

Aortic stenosis (AS) is the most prevalent valvular heart disease in elderly populations and poses significant clinical challenges, particularly during its asymptomatic phase. Historically, management focused on symptom-driven aortic valve replacement (AVR); however, recent data clearly indicate that adverse myocardial remodeling and subclinical dysfunction often precede symptom onset. Modern multiparametric risk stratification—integrating advanced echocardiographic deformation imaging, multimodality cardiac magnetic resonance (CMR) imaging and computed tomography (CT), circulating biomarkers [e.g., B-type natriuretic peptide (BNP), and high-sensitivity troponin], and objective exercise testing—enables improved identification of patients at imminent risk. This chapter synthesizes contemporary evidence and guideline recommendations to guide personalized management of asymptomatic severe AS, aimed at preventing irreversible myocardial damage and improving clinical outcomes.

Keywords: Aortic stenosis, asymptomatic, multiparametric risk stratification, echocardiography, cardiac magnetic resonance imaging, biomarkers, valve replacement.

INTRODUCTION

Aortic stenosis (AS) is the leading valvular heart disease affecting older adults globally. Epidemiological studies estimate that 3–5% of individuals aged over 75 have AS, with recent data suggesting up to 12% prevalence when including mild/moderate disease, and 3–4% having severe AS.[1,2] As global populations age and longevity improves, burdened by multimorbidity, the number of patients living with asymptomatic moderate-to-severe AS is expanding.

Management historically pivots around symptom-driven intervention, supported by trials showing survival benefit after aortic valve replacement (AVR) in symptomatic patients.[3] However, subclinical myocardial injury (interstitial and replacement fibrosis) and impaired ventricular mechanics frequently predate symptom onset, elevating risk for sudden cardiac death, heart failure hospitalizations, and irreversible left ventricular (LV) damage.[4,5] Many patients classified clinically as "asymptomatic" show advanced subclinical pathology on modern imaging and biomarker assays—challenging traditional paradigms that dictate intervention only upon symptom emergence.

Multiparametric risk stratification employing advanced echocardiographic deformation imaging [e.g., global longitudinal strain (GLS)], multimodal imaging including cardiac magnetic resonance (CMR) with late gadolinium enhancement (LGE), computed tomography (CT) valve calcium quantification, dynamic circulating biomarkers (BNP, high-sensitivity troponin), and objective exercise stress testing (EST) facilitates early identification of patients at greatest risk. This integrated approach enables tailored clinical decision-making, targeting timely AVR to improve outcomes.

This chapter systematically reviews current evidence and guideline recommendations on multiparametric evaluation of asymptomatic AS, with emphasis on pragmatic clinical application and future directions.

PATHOPHYSIOLOGY AND NATURAL HISTORY OF AORTIC STENOSIS

Aortic stenosis arises largely from progressive fibrocalcific degeneration of the aortic valve. The predominant etiology in adults over 65 years is degenerative calcific AS, responsible for 80–90% of cases, while congenital bicuspid aortic valve (BAV) significantly contributes to younger patients.[6]

Molecular and Cellular Mechanisms

The progression to stenosis involves active inflammation and osteogenic transformation. Mechanical endothelial injury, compounded by systemic risk factors such as hypertension, diabetes, and dyslipidemia, triggers lipid infiltration and immune activation within valve leaflets. Valve interstitial cells differentiate into osteoblast-like cells depositing calcium phosphate crystals, causing leaflet thickening and stiffening. Concomitant fibrosis limits leaflet mobility.[7] BAV-associated altered shear stress accelerates fibrocalcific remodeling, frequently resulting in earlier onset of severe AS.[8]

Left Ventricular Hemodynamic Overload and Remodeling

Valve narrowing imposes chronic pressure overload afflicting the LV. Compensatory concentric hypertrophy develops to normalize wall stress and maintain cardiac output initially.[9] However, sustained pressure overload induces:

- Myocardial ischemia secondary to disproportionate capillary supply and hypertrophic demand
- Diffuse interstitial and replacement myocardial fibrosis that stiffens the LV, impair relaxation, and predispose to arrhythmias
- Diastolic dysfunction with elevated LV filling pressures, left atrial enlargement, and pulmonary hypertension
- Progressive systolic dysfunction with contractile failure and declining ejection fraction (EF), heralding heart failure.[10,11]

Importantly, irreversible myocardial injury progresses silently during the asymptomatic stage, challenging symptom-based clinical management.

Clinical Staging

The 2020 ACC/AHA guidelines classify AS into stages reflecting valve abnormalities, symptoms, and LV function:[3]

- *Stage A:* At risk for AS (e.g., BAV without obstruction)
- *Stage B:* Mild-to-moderate AS, asymptomatic
- *Stage C:* Severe AS, asymptomatic, subdivided:
  - C1: Preserved EF
  - C2: Reduced EF (<50%)
- *Stage D:* Symptomatic severe AS

Stage C patients reflect a diverse population; some remain stable, others progress rapidly and face sudden death despite lack of symptoms.[12]

LIMITATIONS OF TRADITIONAL ASSESSMENT IN ASYMPTOMATIC AORTIC STENOSIS

Decision-making in asymptomatic AS relies on:

- *Transthoracic echocardiography (TTE):* Valve area, peak velocity, mean gradient, and LVEF
- *Symptom evaluation:* Clinical history for exertional dyspnea, angina, and syncope
- *Clinical and echocardiographic surveillance:* Periodic follow-ups every 6–12 months

  While essential, they present limitations.

Symptom Under Recognition

Symptoms are frequently underappreciated due to patient inactivity, comorbidities (e.g., COPD and arthritis), or cognitive decline. Patients adapt lifestyles to avoid exertion, masking symptoms. Studies show 20–30% of "asymptomatic" patients demonstrate objective exercise impairment on testing.[13]

Insensitivity of Left Ventricular Ejection Fraction

Left ventricular ejection fraction (LVEF) often remains preserved until late LV dysfunction because it reflects radial contraction; subclinical longitudinal fiber dysfunction is missed, delaying diagnosis of early myocardial injury.[14]

Flow-dependent Hemodynamic Parameters

Aortic valve area (AVA), V_{max}, and mean gradient depend heavily on LV stroke volume. Low-flow low-gradient AS may underestimate severity. Operator-dependent Doppler assessment introduces variability.[15]

Inadequate Prediction of Risk

Traditional parameters poorly predict rapid progression, sudden death, or heart failure. This results in delayed intervention for high-risk patients or premature intervention for low-risk patients.

Such knowledge motivates a *multiparametric approach* integrating more sensitive diagnostic modalities.

MULTIPARAMETRIC RISK STRATIFICATION: COMPONENTS

Advanced echocardiographic markers:

- *Global longitudinal strain (GLS):* It detects early myocardial dysfunction and strongly predicts symptom onset and mortality.
- *Valvuloarterial impedance (Zva):* It reflects total LV afterload from valve and arterial system.
- *Left atrial (LA) volume index:* Marker of chronically elevated LV filling pressure.

Multimodality Imaging

- *Cardiac MRI (CMR):* LGE identifies replacement fibrosis; T1 mapping quantifies diffuse interstitial fibrosis.

- *CT:* Quantifies valve calcification via Agatston scoring, predictive of disease acceleration.

Circulating Biomarkers

- *BNP/NT-proBNP:* Indicative of LV wall stress and prognosis
- *High-sensitivity troponin:* Indicates ongoing myocyte injury
- *Galectin-3:* Fibrosis and remodeling marker
- *Lipoprotein(a) [Lp(a)]:* Associated with accelerated calcification
- *Emerging markers:* Matrix metalloproteinases (MMPs) and oxidative stress indicators

Functional Testing

- *Exercise stress test:* Unmasks exertional symptoms, hypotension, and arrhythmia
- *Cardiopulmonary exercise testing (CPEX):* Assesses cardiorespiratory reserve and peak oxygen consumption

Advanced Echocardiographic Assessment

Echocardiographic parameters and clinical thresholds are as follows:

- V_{max} ≥4.4 m/s and mean gradient ≥40 mm Hg define severe AS; velocity progression >0.3 m/s/year indicates disease acceleration.[16]
- AVA ≤1.0 cm^2 confirms severe stenosis; body size indexing improves accuracy.
- GLS <–15.9% identifies preclinical myocardial dysfunction predictive of outcomes.[17]
- Zva exceeding 4.9 mm Hg/mL/m^2 correlates with mortality and heart failure risk.
- Indexed LA volume >12.2 cm^2/m^2 reflects elevated filling pressures.[3]

Advanced echocardiographic parameters for risk stratification are mentioned in **Table 1**.

Multimodality Imaging

Cardiac magnetic resonance provides accurate quantification of LV volumes and fibrosis:

- LGE detects replacement myocardial fibrosis that strongly predicts mortality and adverse remodeling.
- T1 mapping and ECV quantify diffuse fibrosis, potentially reversible by AVR.

Computed tomography calcium scoring of the aortic valve, with sex-specific thresholds (>2,000 AU men; >1,200 AU women), predicts rapid progression and poor outcomes.[18] 3D echocardiography and transesophageal echo complement structural evaluation.

Circulating Biomarker Assessment

Biomarkers offer dynamic molecular insight:

- Elevated BNP/NT-proBNP levels correlate with wall stress and adverse events.
- High-sensitivity troponin indicates subclinical cardiomyocyte injury.
- Galectin-3 levels relate to fibrosis and remodeling.
- Lp(a) influences calcific disease progression.
- Emerging markers such as MMPs provide additional prognostic information.

Key circulating biomarkers in asymptomatic AS are provided in **Table 2**.

TABLE 1: Advanced echocardiographic parameters for risk stratification.

Parameter	Threshold	Clinical relevance	References
Peak aortic jet velocity (V_{max})	≥4.4 m/s	Severe AS, symptom predictor	10,11,16
Mean pressure gradient	≥40 mm Hg	Validates severe stenosis	11,16
Aortic valve area (AVA)	≤1.0 cm^2	Severity quantification	11
Global longitudinal strain (GLS)	<–15.9%	Early LV dysfunction indicator	13,17
Valvuloarterial impedance (Zva)	>4.9 mm Hg/mL/m^2	Predictor of mortality/HF risk	12,14
Indexed left atrial volume	>12.2 cm^2/m^2	Chronic pressure overload marker	14

TABLE 2: Key circulating biomarkers in asymptomatic AS.

Biomarker	Threshold	Prognostic importance	References
BNP/NT-proBNP	Elevated/rising	Marker of myocardial stress	19-24
High-sensitivity troponin	Persistent elevation	Indicates subclinical injury	23,25
Galectin-3	Elevated	Fibrosis/remodeling surrogate	26
Lipoprotein(a) [Lp(a)]	High quartile	Valve calcification driver	
MMPs/TIMPs/oxidative markers	Elevated	Emerging risk markers	27

Functional Evaluation

Exercise stress testing objectively reveals occult symptoms, abnormal blood pressure profiles (hypotension), and arrhythmia that predict adverse events. Postexercise increases in BNP and worsening strain imaging reflect early LV impairment. Cardiopulmonary exercise testing quantifies anaerobic threshold, oxygen consumption, and ventilatory efficiency, enhancing functional risk assessment.[28]

Integrated Risk and Guideline Recommendations

Guidelines advocate AVR for asymptomatic severe AS patients exhibiting any of:

- LVEF <50%
- Very severe AS (V_{max} >5 m/s or mean gradient ≥60 mm Hg)
- Rapid V_{max} progression (>0.3 m/s/year)
- Elevated or rising BNP/NT-proBNP
- Reduced GLS (<–15.9%)
- Abnormal exercise response (symptom or hypotension)
- Fibrosis on CMR (LGE or elevated ECV)
- Elevated valvuloarterial impedance (Zva >4.9 mm Hg/mL/m^2).[25]

Multidisciplinary assessment integrates these to guide early AVR, balancing procedural risks and patient preferences.

Contemporary Management Strategies

Surveillance

Low-risk asymptomatic patients undergo clinical and echocardiographic follow-up every 6–12 months, with biomarker monitoring and exercise testing tailored to individual risk. Multidisciplinary clinics optimize detection and education.

TABLE 3: Landmark clinical trials.

Trial	Outcome summary	References
RECOVERY	Early surgery in very severe asymptomatic AS reduces mortality and heart failure hospitalization versus conservative management	16
AVATAR	Early AVR improves survival and reduces cardiac events in asymptomatic severe AS with preserved EF	17
EARLY TAVR	Ongoing RCT showing promising safety and efficacy of TAVR in asymptomatic high-risk AS	18

Early Intervention

High-risk patients benefit from early AVR. Surgical approaches remain first-line in younger or low surgical risk groups. Transcatheter aortic valve replacement (TAVR) extends options to elderly, frail, or high-risk patients with demonstrated safety and efficacy.[29,30]

Landmark clinical trials are mentioned in **Table 3**.

CONCLUSION

Asymptomatic AS is clinically heterogeneous with variable progression and risk profiles. Traditional symptoms and gradient-based assessments inadequately identify patients at risk. A multiparametric assessment integrating advanced echocardiography, multimodality cardiac imaging, circulating biomarkers, and exercise testing offers precise risk stratification to guide timely valve intervention. Contemporary evidence supports earlier AVR in selected asymptomatic patients, aligning with precision medicine objectives to improve survival and quality of life. Ongoing innovation in diagnostic and prognostic technologies promises further refinement of individualized management strategies.

REFERENCES

1. Lindman BR, Dweck MR, Lancellotti P, et al. Management of Asymptomatic Severe Aortic Stenosis: Evolving Concepts in Timing of Valve Replacement. JACC Cardiovasc Imaging. 2019;12(5):1055-69.
2. Banovic M, Iung B, Putnik S, et al. Asymptomatic Aortic Stenosis: From Risk Stratification to Treatment. Am J Cardiol. 2024;218:51-62.
3. Karampinos K, Ktenopoulos N, Apostolos A, et al. Navigating the silence: reconsidering treatment paradigms in asymptomatic severe aortic stenosis. Hellenic J Cardiol. 2025;S1109-9666(25)00146-0.
4. Siontis GC, Jüni P, Pilgrim T, et al. Meta-analysis of early surgery versus conventional treatment in asymptomatic severe aortic stenosis. Open Heart. 2022;9(1):e001982.
5. Clavel MA, Dumesnil JG, Capoulade R, et al. Impact of peak aortic jet velocity on outcome in asymptomatic aortic stenosis. Eur Heart J. 2019;40(7):573-82.
6. Clavel MA, Pibarot P. Imaging and Hemodynamics of Aortic Stenosis. Circ Cardiovasc Imaging. 2020;13(2):e009261.
7. Dweck MR, Chin CWL, Joshi S. Myocardial Fibrosis in Aortic Stenosis. Curr Cardiol Rep. 2020;22(2):8.
8. Clavel MA, Magne J, Pibarot P. Low-flow, low-gradient aortic stenosis: the diagnostic challenge. Eur Heart J. 2019;40(7):487-9.
9. Magne J, Donal E, Dijos M, et al. Exercise echocardiography for risk stratification of asymptomatic patients with aortic stenosis. J Am Coll Cardiol. 2020;62(4):362-70.
10. Pibarot P, Clavel MA. Diagnosis and Management of Paradoxical Low-Flow, Low-Gradient Aortic Stenosis. JACC Cardiovasc Imaging. 2019;12(4):883-5.
11. Lancellotti P, Magne J, Donal E, et al. Outcome prediction in asymptomatic severe aortic stenosis: the evolving role of multimodality imaging and biomarkers. Heart. 2019;105(18):1369-76.

12. Clavel MA, Capoulade R, Malouf J, et al. Impact of sex on the aortic valve calcium score to predict severe aortic stenosis. J Am Coll Cardiol. 2019;73(3):301-10.
13. Falk V, Baumgartner H, Bax JJ, et al. 2021 ESC/EACTS Guidelines for the management of valvular heart disease. Eur Heart J. 2021;42(36):3738-98.
14. Van Belle E, Clavel MA, Pibarot P, et al. Prognostic value of myocardial fibrosis in severe aortic stenosis undergoing surgery: the RELIEF study. J Am Coll Cardiol. 2021;77(26):3148-60.
15. Futier E, Vahanian A, Rosenkranz S, et al. Optimizing the timing of intervention in asymptomatic aortic stenosis: An expert consensus viewpoint. Eur Heart J. 2024;45(5):500-14.
16. Kang DH, Park SJ, Lee SA, et al. Early surgery or conservative care for asymptomatic aortic stenosis. N Engl J Med. 2020;382(2):111-9.
17. Nadji G, Mehdirad A, Détaint D, et al. The AVATAR study: Early surgery benefits in asymptomatic severe aortic stenosis patients. Circulation. 2022;145(3):123-35.
18. Carroll JD, Mack MJ, Vemulapalli S, et al. Early TAVR trial design and rationale. J Am Coll Cardiol. 2023;81(11):1215-25.
19. Marwick TH, Buccheri S, Le D, et al. Aortic stenosis and artificial intelligence: An update on imaging and risk stratification tools. Eur Heart J Cardiovasc Imaging. 2022;23:240-57.
20. Abdul Saboor Karim S, Helmy SM. Multimodality imaging and biomarkers in aortic valve stenosis and prediction of outcomes. Heart Views. 2022;23(1):22-9.
21. Kario K, Saito K, et al. Role of lipoprotein(a) in aortic valve disease: A review of mechanisms and clinical implications. Int J Mol Sci. 2025;26(5):1902.
22. Bhuva AN, Mitchell JD, Petrov G, et al. Artificial intelligence in cardiac imaging and risk stratification for aortic stenosis. Nat Rev Cardiol. 2023;20(4):265-79.
23. Bauer F, Pezel T, Dupuis C, et al. High-sensitivity cardiac troponin for risk prediction in aortic stenosis. JACC Cardiovasc Imaging. 2020;13(1):64-74.
24. Antony C. Imaging Modalities in the Diagnosis and Assessment of Aortic Stenosis Severity. J Heart Valve Dis. 2023;32(2):150-62.
25. Clavel MA, Burwash IG, Pibarot P. Early intervention in asymptomatic severe aortic stenosis: is it time now? Heart. 2016;102:1426-33.
26. Otto CM, Nishimura RA, Bonow RO, et al. 2020 ACC/AHA guideline for the management of valvular heart disease. J Am Coll Cardiol. 2021;77(4):450-503.
27. Magne J, Donal E, Dijos M, et al. Exercise echocardiography for risk stratification of asymptomatic patients with aortic stenosis. J Am Coll Cardiol. 2013;62:362-70.
28. Vahanian A, Beyersdorf F, Praz F, et al. 2021 ESC/EACTS guidelines for the management of valvular heart disease. Eur Heart J. 2021;42(36):3738-98.
29. Leon MB, Smith CR, Mack MJ, et al. Transcatheter or Surgical Aortic-valve Replacement in Intermediate-risk Patients. N Engl J Med. 2016;374(17):1609-20.
30. Mack MJ, Leon MB, Thourani VH, et al. Transcatheter Aortic-valve Replacement with a Balloon-expandable Valve in Low-risk Patients. N Engl J Med. 2019;380(18):1695-705.

CHAPTER 59

Secondary Mitral Regurgitation: Phenotypes, Proportionality, and Evolving Management

Arijit Ghosh, Arup Dasbiswas, Subhasis Roy Chowdhury, Mainak Mukhopadhyay

ABSTRACT

Secondary mitral regurgitation (SMR), caused by structural or functional changes in the left ventricle (LV), left atrium (LA), or mitral apparatus, accounts for ~65% of all mitral regurgitation and carries worse prognosis than primary MR.

SMR is heterogeneous, with two main phenotypes: ventricular SMR (vSMR), associated with LV dilation and HFrEF, and atrial SMR (aSMR), linked to LA enlargement and atrial fibrillation. The concept of proportionate versus disproportionate SMR—based on MR severity relative to LV size (EROA/LVEDV ratio)—helps explain variable treatment outcomes. Proportionate SMR reflects diffuse LV dysfunction and often improves with guideline-directed medical therapy (GDMT), whereas disproportionate SMR is less responsive to GDMT but benefits more from transcatheter edge-to-edge repair (M-TEER). Divergent results of MITRA-FR and COAPT highlight the importance of patient selection, MR quantification, and LV remodeling stage. Echocardiographic grading remains difficult, as methods like PISA are limited by dynamic orifice geometry and loading conditions, complicating treatment decisions.

GDMT is the cornerstone of therapy, improving MR in up to 60% of vSMR patients. Selected individuals may benefit from CRT, revascularization, or arrhythmia ablation. For non-responders, M-TEER offers durable MR reduction, improved survival, and symptom relief when performed in carefully chosen patients.

Surgical repair/replacement or annuloplasty may be considered, though recurrence is frequent.

SMR is a complex condition requiring phenotype-specific assessment and integration of proportionality concepts. Optimized medical therapy remains first-line, while M-TEER and emerging transcatheter technologies expand options for high-risk patients.

Keywords: Secondary mitral regurgitation, proportionate versus disproportionate MR, guideline-directed medical therapy (GDMT), mitral transcatheter edge-to-edge repair (M-TEER).

INTRODUCTION

Mitral regurgitation (MR) refers to retrograde flow of blood from the left ventricle (LV) into the left atrium (LA) during systole. MR can be classified into primary mitral regurgitation (PMR) (degenerative) and secondary (functional). PMR is characterized by leaflet prolapse or flail leading to loss of leaflet tip/edge coaptation.[1,2] SMR is common in heart failure and coronary artery disease, affecting about half of patients after MI and more than doubling the risk of death. It is a specific type of MR which arises not from primary valve leaflet pathology, but from structural/functional changes of the LV, LA, or mitral valve (MV) apparatus. It is increasingly recognized as a heterogeneous entity with distinct phenotypes, each with unique mechanisms, clinical implications, and management strategies. SMR is more common, accounting for 65% of all MR cases, and it conveys a worse prognosis (5-year survival, SMR vs. PMR, 46–50% vs. 66%).[3-5]

Despite therapeutic advances, SMR still leads to poor outcomes, making it a key clinical priority. SMR develops from an imbalance between leaflet tethering and LV closing force as shown in **Figure 1**. Besides apical displacement of the papillary muscles (PMs), mitral annular dilation and loss of the saddle-shaped geometry also contribute. Closing force comes from LV contraction, but in heart failure it is reduced due to systolic dysfunction and LV/PM displacement. Experimental data suggest that altered PM position is the main driver of SMR.[6,7] Secondary mitral regurgitation (SMR) may have a major health and economic burden

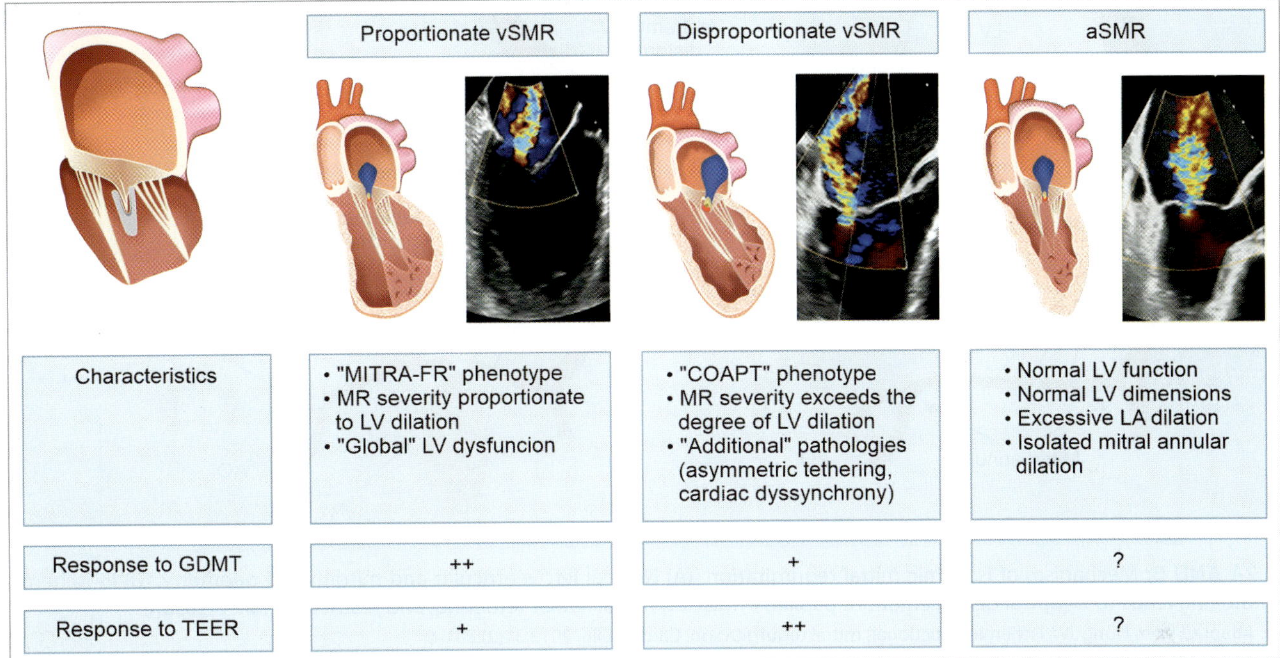

FIG. 1: Secondary mitral regurgitation phenotypes in the context of transcatheter mitral valve edge-to-edge repair.[10]

Source: Adapted from Stolz L, Doldi PM, Sannino A, et al. The Evolving Concept of Secondary Mitral Regurgitation Phenotypes: Lessons From the M-TEER Trials. JACC Cardiovasc Imaging. 2024;17(6):659-68.

along with varying clinical consequences and responses to its management. SMR is usually classified as ventricular secondary mitral regurgitation (vSMR) or atrial secondary mitral regurgitation (aSMR), but there is considerable overlap between the two entities. It often worsens over time, leading to structural and clinical changes. Understanding its causes and progression is important, as treatment should address the underlying mechanism.[8-10]

Ventricular secondary mitral regurgitation can result from many LV diseases that cause dilation, dysfunction, or geometric changes. Common causes include ischemic and nonischemic dilated cardiomyopathy, aortic valve disease, hypertensive or hypertrophic cardiomyopathy, as well as ventricular arrhythmias and conduction abnormalities.[11] vSMR is typically linked to HFrEF, while aSMR is associated with HFpEF and/or atrial fibrillation (AF). Management should target the underlying LV or LA disease, using guideline-directed medical therapy (GDMT) for all patients, and in selected cases, coronary revascularization, arrhythmia ablation, or cardiac resynchronization therapy (CRT).[11,12]

Not all patients with SMR respond equally to GDMT. Those without LV reverse remodeling or reduction in MR volume may benefit most from advanced interventions such as mitral transcatheter edge-to-edge repair (M-TEER) or MV surgery.[13]

This narrative review aims to summarize current knowledge on SMR phenotypes and their clinical relevance, especially in relation to M-TEER.

THEORY OF PROPORTIONATE AND DISPROPORTIONATE SECONDARY MITRAL REGURGITATION

Proportionate versus disproportionate SMR describes how severe the MR [measured by effective regurgitant orifice area (EROA) or regurgitant volume] is in relation to the size of the left ventricle (LVEDV). SMR is proportionate when the MR severity matches the degree of LV enlargement as shown in **Figure 2**. Proportionate MR happens when the whole LV is weak and dilated, causing symmetric MV distortion and symmetric MR jets. As the LV dilates more, MR gets worse. These patients often respond well to optimized medical therapy, which can improve LV size/function and reduce MR.[14,15]

Disproportionate MR occurs when MR is more severe than expected for the degree of LV dilation. This is often due to prior MI with asymmetric tethering or cardiac dyssynchrony. Such patients usually respond poorly to medical therapy because their LV has limited potential for reverse remodeling. Studies using the RegVol/LVEDV ratio show that in COAPT, disproportionate SMR resembled PMR and responded much better to M-TEER than to GDMT alone.[16,17]

In MITRA-FR, most patients had proportionate or even less-than-proportionate MR (large LVEDV with only moderate MR), explaining the lack of clear benefit from M-TEER. In contrast, COAPT patients had more severe MR relative to smaller LV size (disproportionate MR), and they showed significant benefit from M-TEER. This supports

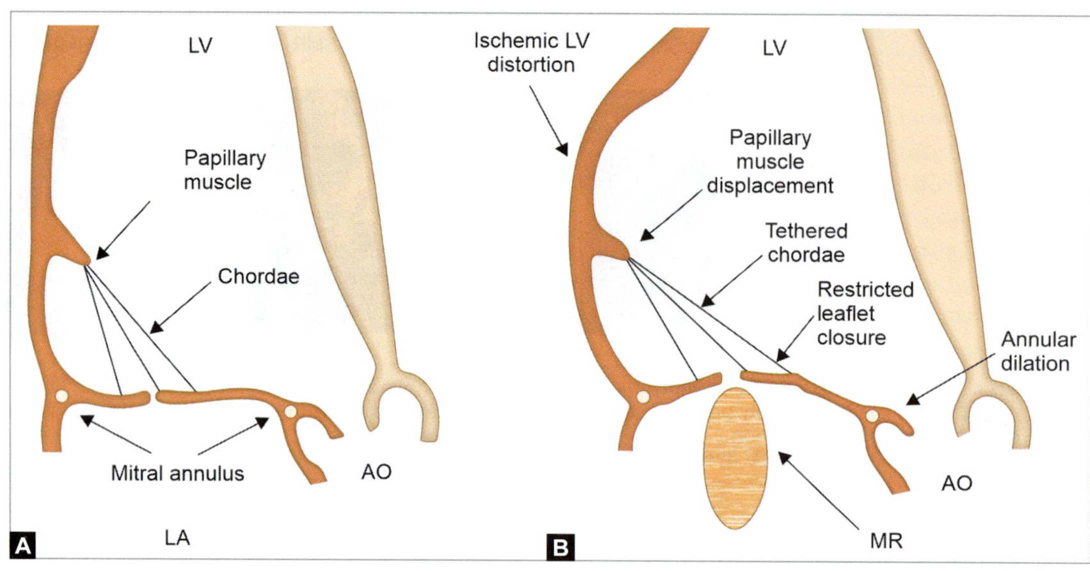

FIGS. 2A AND B: Mechanism of ischemic mitral regurgitation. (A) Normal left ventricular and mitral valve geometry. (B) In ischemic MR, LV remodeling leads to LV apical displacement of papillary muscles, mitral leaflet tethering, and restricted leaflet closure.
Source: Adapted from Hung JW. Ischemic (functional) mitral regurgitation. Cardiol Clin. 2013;31(2):231-6.

TABLE 1: MITRA-FR versus COAPT trials in secondary mitral regurgitation.[22-24]

Feature	MITRA-FR	COAPT
Definition of severe SMR	EROA >0.20 cm^2 (European guideline)	Multiparametric approach (EROA ≥ 0.30–0.40 cm^2, regurgitant volume, vena contracta, etc.)
LV characteristics	Very dilated LV (LVEDV ~252 mL)	Less dilated LV (LVEDV ~192 mL)
LVEF	Lower; included more severe LV dysfunction	Higher (but still reduced), excluded very low LVEF
RV dysfunction	Severe RVD allowed	Severe RVD excluded
MR severity relative to LV size	Proportionate/hypoproportionate	Disproportionate (MR more severe than expected for LV size)
Main result	No significant benefit of M-TEER over GDMT	Clear benefit of M-TEER on top of GDMT
Interpretation	MR mostly secondary to LV dilation → treating valve adds little	MR primary driver of pathology → valve repair helps
Lesson learned	EROA cutoff alone is insufficient; prognosis not equal to treatment response	Careful selection (high MR burden relative to LV size) identifies responders

(GDMT: guideline-directed medical therapy; LV: left ventricle; LVEF: left ventricular ejection fraction; MR: mitral regurgitation; M-TEER: mitral transcatheter edge-to-edge repair; SMR: secondary mitral regurgitation)

the idea that disproportionate MR responds better to valve intervention, though measuring LV size and MR severity precisely remains challenging in individual patients.[18,19]

The differences between COAPT and MITRA-FR were largely due to different inclusion criteria. MITRA-FR (following European guidelines) defined severe MR as EROA >0.2 cm^2 and included patients with very dilated LVs, lower left ventricular ejection fraction (LVEF), and even severe RV dysfunction. COAPT, in contrast, used a multiparametric definition of severe MR and stricter patient selection. This explains why COAPT showed benefit from M-TEER, while MITRA-FR did not. Importantly, EROA alone predicts prognosis but does not guarantee treatment response. Combining MR severity with LV size (EROA/LVEDV ratio) may better identify patients who improve with GDMT versus those needing valve intervention **(Table 1)**.[20,22-24]

The real-world applicability of COAPT and MITRA-FR differs. MITRA-FR included patients with very large LV volumes, representing advanced HFrEF, whereas most patients treated in current clinical practice have LV sizes similar to COAPT participants. Registries such as EuroSMR, EXPAND SMR, and COAPT PAS (>6,400 patients) confirm that real-world. M-TEER patients resemble the COAPT population more than MITRA-FR, supporting the generalizability of COAPT results.[24-26] The concept of SMR proportionality was initially developed to explain differential responses to M-TEER. Several retrospective analyses have stratified patients from registries or prior trials according to SMR proportionality and examined outcomes accordingly. A European multicenter registry, including over 1,000 patients with SMR, identified a subgroup with a LV-dominant pattern of SMR—termed proportionate MR—characterized by a mean EROA/LVEDV ratio of 0.0008 ± 0.0002 cm^2/mL. This subgroup was associated with higher 2-year mortality compared with patients with disproportionate SMR. Interestingly, symptomatic improvement following M-TEER appeared comparable across the spectrum of SMR proportionality.[27]

DIFFERENCES IN GUIDELINES AND COMPLICATED SMR QUANTIFICATION

Although current guidelines recommend a multiparametric approach to quantify SMR, obtaining precise and reliable grading—particularly using transthoracic echocardiography—remains highly challenging.[28] The most widely used parameters, regurgitant volume (RegVol) and EROA, are derived from the proximal isovelocity surface area (PISA) method. This technique is based on fundamental flow convergence principles but is subject to multiple limitations and pitfalls in SMR, leading to both overestimation and underestimation of MR severity.[29,30]

As because PISA radius is measured in a single systolic frame, selecting the largest convergence zone may overestimate EROA in SMR, given the dynamic variability of regurgitant flow throughout systole. Although three-dimensional PISA with frame-by-frame averaging can improve accuracy, this approach is labor-intensive and rarely used in routine practice. Conversely, if the regurgitant orifice is markedly elliptical, the PISA method may underestimate both EROA and RegVol due to under-sampling of the effective radius.[31]

Doppler volumetric quantification is also problematic in SMR owing to high measurement variability. Importantly, even small uncertainties in the PISA radius can introduce large errors, since the radius is squared in the calculation of EROA and RegVol.[32] A clinical example highlights these challenges: in a patient with an LVEDV of 200 mL and an LVEF of 35%, the total stroke volume is 70 mL. According to US guidelines, a RegVol ≥60 mL would define severe SMR. However, this implies a forward stroke volume of only 10 mL, translating to a cardiac output of just 0.7 L/min at a heart rate of 70 beats/min—a physiologically implausible scenario. This discrepancy raises the question of whether lower cutoffs for severe SMR should be considered in the context of reduced forward stroke volume, which is commonly seen in SMR.

GUIDELINE-DIRECTED MEDICAL THERAPY AND SMR RESPONSE

Guideline-directed medical therapy is the cornerstone of SMR treatment.[21] About 40–60% of patients with vSMR improve in MR severity when GDMT is properly adjusted.[33] In severe cases, however, low blood pressure, kidney problems, or electrolyte issues may prevent reaching target doses. In the MITRA-FR and COAPT trials, GDMT was optimized before enrollment, but these trials were conducted before sacubitril/valsartan and SGLT-2 inhibitors showed survival benefits. They also did not include patients whose SMR improved with GDMT alone. Recent evidence supports starting all four key HFrEF drug classes at once, rather than step by step, which helps to identify nonresponders sooner and allows earlier M-TEER treatment. Importantly, GDMT should be optimized not only before M-TEER but also after it. Data from the EuroSMR registry showed that M-TEER allowed further GDMT uptitration in 38% of patients, leading to better survival.[34,35]

In addition to echocardiographic assessment of SMR, LV fibrosis, scar, or infarction may also affect how patients respond to GDMT. Cardiac MRI can accurately measure chamber size, function, and scar burden. A recent study found MRI-detected fibrosis to be an important predictor of LV reverse remodeling, and myocardial scar has been linked to worse outcomes in heart failure with SMR. Whether the extent of fibrosis predicts treatment response still needs further study.[36-38]

ATRIAL SMR: DEFINITION AND PATHOPHYSIOLOGY

With the rising prevalence of HFpEF and AF, a new type of SMR—*aSMR*—has been recognized. Unlike vSMR, aSMR occurs with preserved LV size and function, and unlike PMR, the MV is structurally normal. The main cause is LA enlargement, which leads to dilation of the mitral annulus and changes in valve geometry. As because the subvalvular apparatus remains intact, annular dilation flattens the valve and shortens leaflet reserve, causing malcoaptation.[39,40]

While early studies did not show a clear link between AF and SMR, Gertz et al. found that persistent AF and larger annular size independently predicted significant MR. Notably, restoring and maintaining sinus rhythm reduced both the incidence of significant MR (24% vs. 82%, $p = 0.005$) and LA/annular dimensions.

Two phenotypes are seen:

1. *Central MR jet* (most common) due to poor leaflet coaptation
2. *Posterior eccentric jet* (20–30% of cases), caused by restriction of the posterior leaflet ("hamstringing") and often with anterior leaflet overriding

This posterior tethering results from marked LA dilation, especially in the posterior direction, which displaces the mitral annulus beyond the LV inlet. Since the LV and subvalvular structures are preserved, this mechanism is called atriogenic tethering. Whether posterior jet aSMR reflects progressive LA dilation or a distinct subtype remains uncertain.[41-44]

Atrial fibrillation has been shown to directly cause MR, leading to the definition of *atrial functional MR*

(AFMR)—significant MR with normal LV size and function. AFMR is found in about 13–19% of AF patients, both in trials and in the community. Compared to MR from LV remodeling, AFMR patients are typically older, more often female, and more likely to have hypertension or HFpEF. AFMR carries a poor outlook, with only approximately 50% 5-year survival—nearly double the mortality of matched controls.[45]

Annular dilation alone does not fully explain AFMR; atrial myopathy also plays a role. As the LA enlarges, the posterior annulus is pulled backward and upward, dragging the posterior leaflet and reducing leaflet coaptation ("atriogenic tethering"). This increases the papillary-annulus distance, tethers the posterior leaflet toward the apex, and flattens the anterior leaflet **(Figs. 3 and 4)**.[46]

ECHO FEATURES

- LA dilation
- Normal LV size and systolic function
- Central MR jet
- Frequent associated tricuspid/pulmonary regurgitation (bad prognosis)
- *Mitral annular changes:* Dilatation, flattening (loss of saddle shape), and reduced dynamic motion.

MANAGEMENT OF ASMR AND FUTURE PROGNOSIS

Current guidelines do not distinguish between aSMR and vSMR, despite their very different causes and outcomes. In aSMR patients with AF, restoring sinus rhythm can improve LA function and reduce MR. In HFpEF, SGLT-2 inhibitors lower hospitalization and mortality, but their effect on aSMR severity is still unknown.

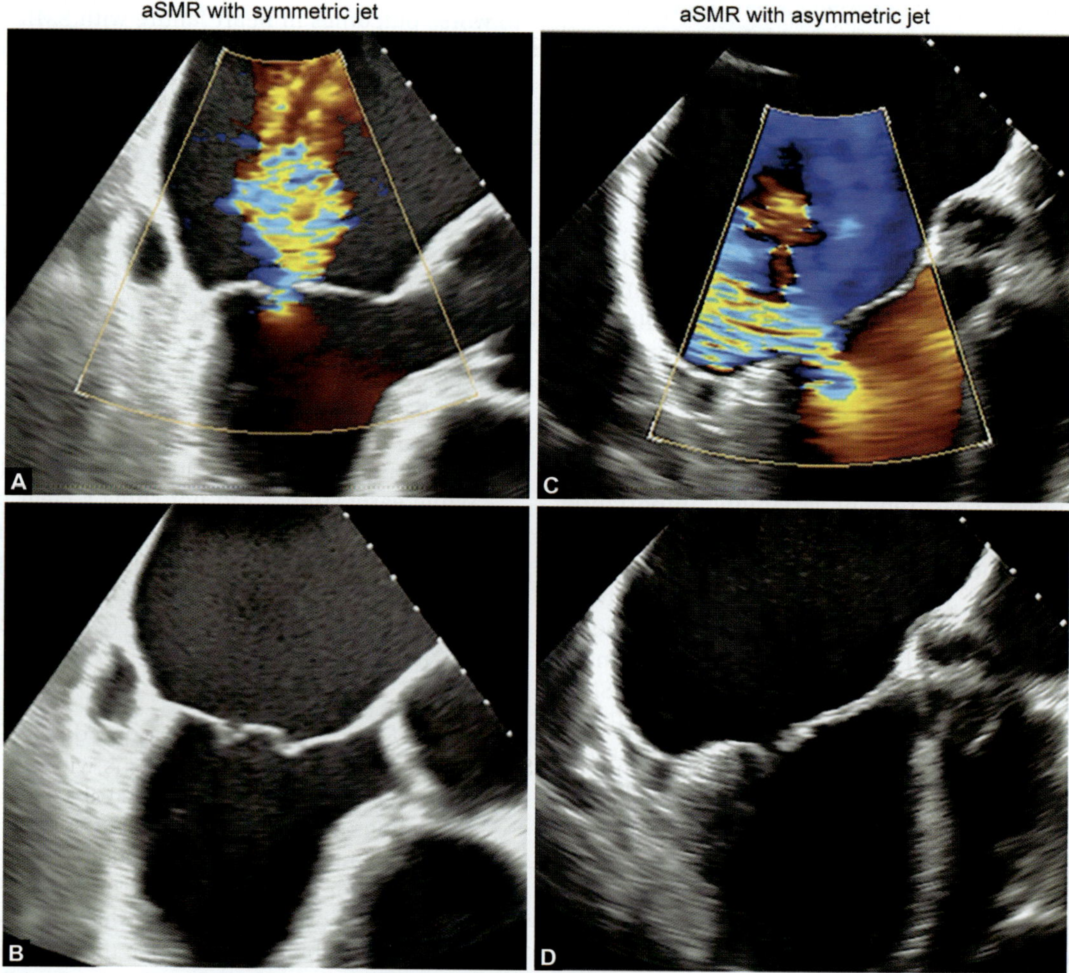

FIGS. 3A TO D: Phenotypes of atrial secondary mitral regurgitation (aSMR). (A and B) Most commonly, aSMR occurs with a central jet in the middle of the valve due to malcoaptation of the leaflets; (C and D) In a smaller subgroup of patients, eccentric mitral regurgitation (MR) jets are located posterior due to "hamstringing of the posterior mitral valve (MV) leaflet."

Source: Adapted from Stolz L, Doldi PM, Sannino A, et al. The Evolving Concept of Secondary Mitral Regurgitation Phenotypes: Lessons From the M-TEER Trials. JACC Cardiovasc Imaging. 2024;17(6):659-68.

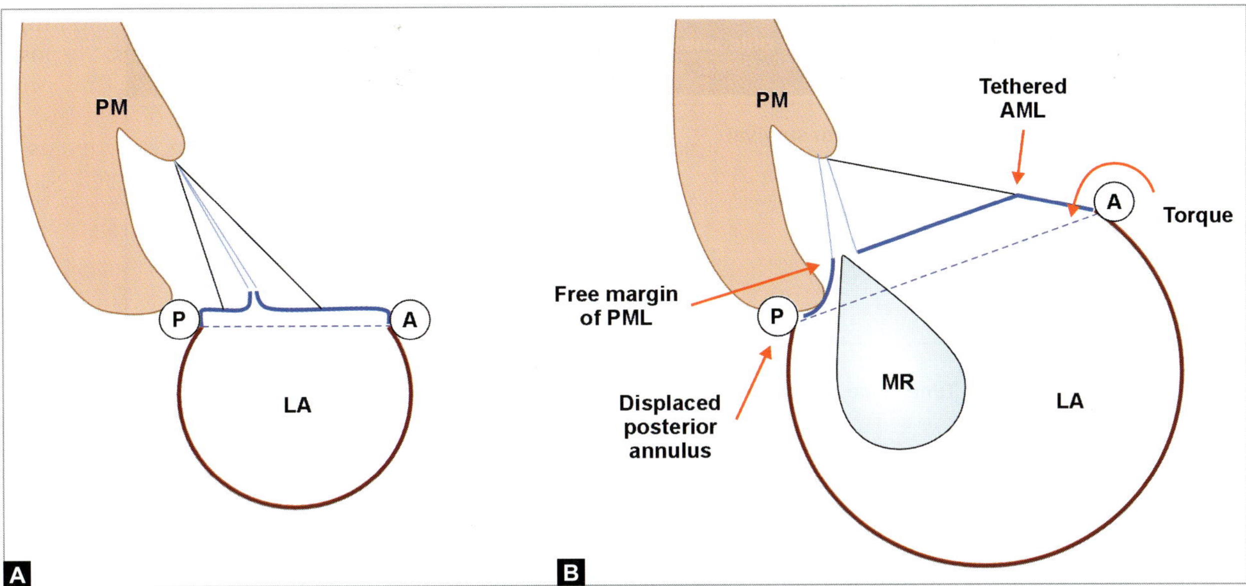

FIGS. 4A AND B: Proposed mechanism of atrial functional mitral regurgitation (AML). (A) Normal left atrial and mitral annulus geometry; (B) In atrial mitral regurgitation, left atrial dilation pulls the mitral annulus posteriorly onto the crest of the left ventricular (LV) inlet. This reduces the free edge/area of the posterior leaflet. The annulus displaces superiorly and "flattens" the anterior leaflet. This results in an increased distance between the annulus and papillary muscles, leading to restricted leaflet motion during systole.
Source: With permission from Silbiger JJ, et al. (2014).[44]

Although evidence is limited, small observational studies suggest that surgical mitral annuloplasty can be effective in aSMR. However, since AF and HFpEF are common in older patients, many are not good candidates for surgery. Retrospective studies of M-TEER in aSMR show high procedural success, improved symptoms, and better survival than vSMR, but worse survival than PMR. Data on transcatheter annuloplasty in aSMR are not yet available but eagerly awaited.

MEDICAL THERAPY

The goal of SMR therapy is to relieve symptoms, improve function, and lower morbidity and mortality. This requires treating reversible causes of LV dysfunction and heart failure, along with the MR itself. In particular, obstructive coronary artery disease should be revascularized to reduce LV ischemia.[47] Currently, there is little evidence and no formal guideline on the management of AFMR. Limited studies suggest that AF ablation may help reduce AFMR. The 2020 ACC/AHA Valvular Heart Disease Guideline strongly recommends GDMT for patients with chronic severe MR and reduced LVEF, supervised by a heart failure specialist. GDMT includes ACE inhibitors or ARBs, β-blockers, aldosterone antagonists, angiotensin receptor–neprilysin inhibitor (ARNI), and, when indicated, CRT. GDMT can reduce MR by reversing LV remodeling and improving LV function.[48]

In a randomized trial of 169 patients with dilated cardiomyopathy, MR improved in approximately 42% of those treated with metoprolol compared with 20% of controls. Another trial of 118 patients showed that an ARNI reduced MR more effectively than valsartan alone. For heart failure patients who remain symptomatic with LV dyssynchrony despite optimal medical therapy, CRT is recommended.[32,49]

Although guidelines differ on the exact criteria for CRT implantation (QRS duration, bundle branch pattern, and device type), CRT consistently reduces MR by lessening leaflet tethering and increasing LV closing force, which improves survival. After GDMT is optimized, patients should undergo echocardiography every 3–6 months to monitor LV remodeling and MR severity. MR improves in up to 40% of patients.[12,50-54]

SURGICAL THERAPY

Many patients do not respond to GDMT, and surgery may be considered for MR reduction, though its role in severe SMR remains uncertain.[55] In patients with moderate MR undergoing CABG, a randomized trial showed that adding MV repair reduced MR but did not improve 2-year survival or LV remodeling. In another trial of severe SMR, outcomes at 2 years were similar between MV repair and replacement, but >50% of the repair group developed recurrent MR and had more heart failure events and hospitalizations.[56,57] Guidelines recommend surgical repair for severe, symptomatic MR despite GDMT if the patient is already undergoing surgical revascularization, and it should also be considered in severe MR with LVEF >50%.[58]

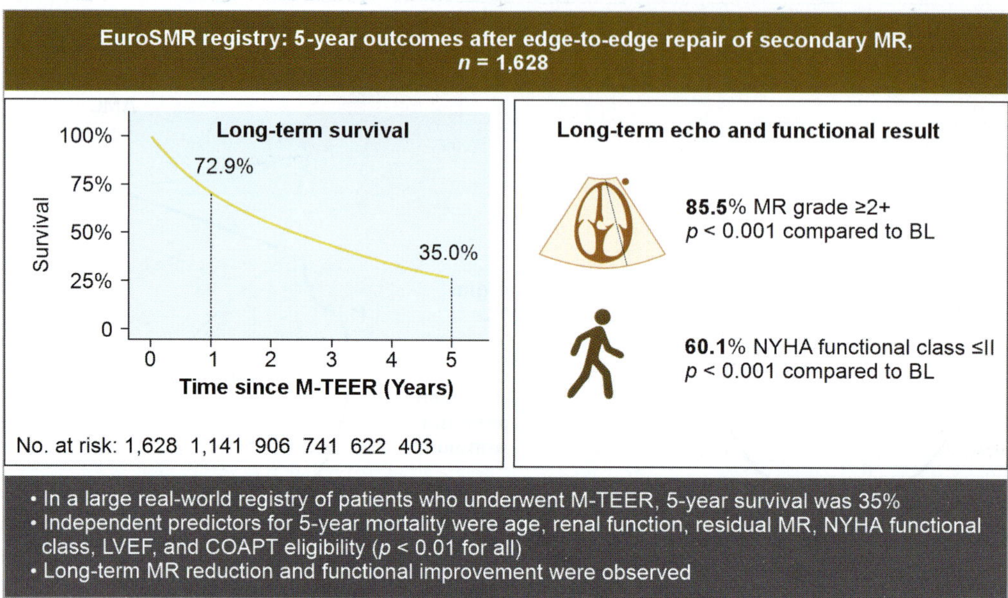

FIG. 5: Long-term outcomes after edge-to-edge repair of secondary mitral regurgitation.[67]
(LVEF: left ventricular ejection fraction; MR: mitral regurgitation; M-TEER: mitral transcatheter edge-to-edge repair)

TRANSCATHETER MITRAL EDGE-TO-EDGE REPAIR

Interest in treating SMR with transcatheter approaches has been growing. Transcatheter edge-to-edge repair (TEER) uses a clip (e.g., MitraClip) to bring the anterior and posterior mitral leaflets together, creating a double-orifice valve. Its safety and efficacy were tested in two major trials. In MITRA-FR (304 patients with symptomatic HF and severe SMR), TEER showed no benefit over medical therapy at 12 months for the combined endpoint of death or unplanned HF hospitalization (54.6% vs. 51.3%; p = 0.53).[59,60] At 2 years, *MITRA-FR* continued to show no benefit of TEER compared with medical therapy (63.8% vs. 67.1%; HR 1.01; 95% CI 0.77–1.34). In contrast, the *COAPT trial* (614 patients with symptomatic HF and at least moderate-to-severe SMR despite maximal GDMT) showed clear benefit. TEER significantly reduced HF hospitalizations at 24 months (35.8% vs. 67.9%; $p < 0.001$) and all-cause mortality (29.1% vs. 46.1%; $p < 0.001$).[61,62]

At 3 years, *COAPT showed durable MR reduction*, with continued improvement in outcomes compared to medical therapy. The different results between COAPT and MITRA-FR remain debated. Despite similar designs, key differences explain the contrast:[21,23,63-66]

- *Medical therapy:* COAPT ensured patients were on maximally tolerated GDMT supervised by HF specialists, while MITRA-FR reflected routine practice with less strict optimization.
- *MR severity:* COAPT enrolled patients with more severe MR (average EROA 41 ± 15 vs. 31 ± 10 mm^2).
- *LV size:* COAPT excluded patients with very large LV dilation (LVESD >7 cm), so its patients had less advanced remodeling and better potential for recovery.
- *Procedural outcomes:* COAPT had higher procedural success (5% vs. 17% residual MR at 1 year) and fewer complications (8.5% vs. 14.6%).

In a study by Stocker et al. which was a large, international, multicenter registry demonstrated long-term sustainability of MR reduction and symptomatic relief 5 years after M-TEER. Long-term survival rate 5 years after M-TEER was 35.0%. These findings and the identified predictors for long-term survival contribute valuable insights for optimizing patient selection in routine clinical practice and underscore the long-term efficacy of M-TEER **(Fig. 5)**.[67]

CONCLUSION

Secondary mitral regurgitation is a heterogeneous condition with multiple clinical phenotypes. Distinguishing between aSMR and vSMR subtypes can help to clarify treatment responses to both medical and interventional therapies. Ongoing research is needed to deepen our understanding of SMR and to optimize management strategies. In addition to currently available TEER, novel transcatheter technologies are at various stages of clinical trials. Assessing and grading the severity of SMR is often difficult and requires careful use of all available information. Before considering MV surgery or especially TEER, it is crucial to treat underlying heart failure with GDMT, and if needed, revascularization or CRT. Future advances in patient selection for TEER, therapies targeting MV leaflets, and new transcatheter treatments are expected to improve care for patients with SMR.

REFERENCES

1. Grayburn PA, Sannino A, Packer M. Proportionate and disproportionate functional mitral regurgitation: a new conceptual framework that reconciles the results of the MITRA-FR and COAPT Trials. JACC Cardiovasc Imaging. 2019;12(2):353-62.
2. Asgar AW, Mack MJ, Stone GW. Secondary mitral regurgitation in heart failure: pathophysiology, prognosis, and therapeutic considerations. J Am Coll Cardiol. 2015;65:1231-48.
3. Dziadzko V, Dziadzko M, Medina-Inojosa JR, et al. Causes and mechanisms of isolated mitral regurgitation in the community: clinical context and outcome. Eur Heart J. 2019;40:2194-202.
4. Bursi F, Enriquez-Sarano M, Nkomo VT, et al. Heart failure and death after myocardial infarction in the community: the emerging role of mitral regurgitation. Circulation. 2005;111:295-301.
5. Lamas GA, Mitchell GF, Flaker GC, et al. Clinical significance of mitral regurgitation after acute myocardial infarction. Survival and Ventricular Enlargement Investigators. Circulation. 1997;96:827-33.
6. Sannino A, Smith RL, Schiattarella GG, et al. Survival and Cardiovascular Outcomes of Patients With Secondary Mitral Regurgitation: A Systematic Review and Meta-analysis. JAMA Cardiol. 2017;2(10):1130-9.
7. Zoghbi WA, Adams D, Bonow RO, et al. Recommendations for noninvasive evaluation of native valvular regurgitation: a report from the American Society of Echocardiography developed in collaboration with the Society for Cardiovascular Magnetic Resonance. J Am Soc Echocardiogr. 2017;30:303-71.
8. Singh GK, Namazi F, Hirasawa K, et al. Extra mitral valvular cardiac involvement in patients with significant secondary mitral regurgitation. Am J Cardiol. 2022;162:143-9.
9. Stolz L, Doldi PM, Orban M, et al. Staging heart failure patients with secondary mitral regurgitation undergoing transcatheter edge-to-edge repair. JACC Cardiovasc Interv. 2023;16:140-51.
10. Vahanian A, Beyersdorf F, Praz F, et al. 2021 ESC/EACTS Guidelines for the management of valvular heart disease. Eur Heart J. 2022;43:561-632.
11. Grayburn PA, Packer M. The complex phenotypic expressions of functional mitral regurgitation. J Am Coll Cardiol. 2021;78:2422-4.
12. Ypenburg C, Lancellotti P, Tops LF, et al. Acute effects of initiation and withdrawal of cardiac resynchronization therapy on papillary muscle dyssynchrony and mitral regurgitation. J Am Coll Cardiol. 2007;50(21):2071-7.
13. Packer M, Grayburn PA. Contrasting effects of pharmacological, procedural, and surgical in terventions on proportionate and disproportionate functional mitral regurgitation in chronic heart failure. Circulation. 2019;140:779-89.
14. Adamo M, Tomasoni D, Stolz L, et al. Impact of transcatheter edge-to-edge mitral valve repair on guideline-directed medical therapy uptitration. JACC Cardiovasc Interv. 2023;16:896-905.
15. Stolz L, Orban M, Braun D, et al. Impact of asymmetric tethering on outcomes after edge-to edge mitral valve repair for secondary mitral regurgitation. Clin Res Cardiol. 2022;111:869-80.
16. Gaasch WH, Meyer TE. Secondary mitral regurgitation (part 1): volumetric quantification and analysis. Heart. 2018;104:634-38.
17. Grayburn PA, Sannino A, Packer M. Distinguishing proportionate and disproportionate subtypes in functional mitral regurgitation and left ventricular systolic dysfunction. JACC Cardiovasc Imaging. 2021;14:726-9.
18. Stone GW, Abraham WT, Lindenfeld J, et al. Five-year follow-up after transcatheter repair of secondary mitral regurgitation. N Engl J Med. 2023;388:2037-48.
19. Flachskampf FA, Grayburn PA. Who benefits from transcatheter edge-to-edge mitral valve repair and who does not: the enigma continues. JACC Cardiovasc Imaging. 2021;14:753-55.
20. Sannino A, Sudhakaran S, Milligan G, et al. Effectiveness of medical therapy for functional mitral regurgitation in heart failure with reduced ejection fraction. J Am Coll Cardiol. 2020;76:883-4.
21. Pibarot P, Delgado V, Bax JJ. MITRA-FR vs. COAPT: lessons from two trials with diametrically opposed results. Eur Heart J Cardiovasc Imaging. 2019;20(6):620-4.
22. Grinberg D, Donal E, Obadia JF. What do MITRA-FR and COAPT teach us about the percutaneous treatment of secondary mitral regurgitation? EuroIntervention. 2019;14(17):1713-5.
23. Atianzar K, Zhang M, Newhart Z, et al. Why Did COAPT Win While MITRA-FR Failed? Defining the Appropriate Patient Population for MitraClip. Interv Cardiol. 2019;14(1):45-7.
24. Orban M, Karam N, Lubos E, et al. Impact of proportionality of secondary mitral regurgita tion on outcome after transcatheter mitral valve repair. JACC Cardiovasc Imaging. 2021;14:715-25.
25. Kar S, von Bardeleben RS, Rottbauer W, et al. Contemporary outcomes following transcatheter edge-to-edge repair: 1-year results from the EXPAND study. JACC Cardiovasc Interv. 2023;16:589-602.
26. Koell B, Orban M, Weimann J, et al. Outcomes stratified by adapted inclusion criteria after mitral edge-to-edge repair. J Am Coll Cardiol. 2021;78:2408-24.
27. Hausleiter J, Stocker TJ, Adamo M, et al. Mitral valve transcatheter edge to-edge repair. EuroIntervention. 2023;18:957-76.
28. Grayburn PA, Thomas JD. Basic principles of the echocardiographic evaluation of mitral regurgitation. JACC Cardiovasc Imaging. 2021;14:843-53.
29. Thavendiranathan P, Liu S, Datta S, et al. Quantification of chronic functional mitral regurgitation by automated 3-dimensional peak and integrated proximal isovelocity surface area and stroke volume techniques using real-time 3-dimensional volume color Doppler echocardiography: in vitro and clinical validation. Circ Cardiovasc Imaging. 2013;1;6(1):125-33.
30. Simpson IA, Shiota T, Gharib M, et al. Current status of flow convergence for clinical appli cations: is it a leaning tower of "PISA"? J Am Coll Cardiol. 1996;27:504-9.
31. Grayburn PA, Sannino A, Lancellotti P. Redefining severe functional mitral regurgitation: can we reconcile guideline differences? JACC Cardiovasc Imaging. 2021;14:2316-8.
32. Kang DH, Park SJ, Shin SH, et al. Angiotensin receptor neprilysin inhibitor for functional mitral regurgitation. Circulation. 2019;139:1354-65.
33. Greene SJ, Fonarow GC, DeVore AD, et al. Titration of medical therapy for heart failure with reduced ejection fraction. J Am Coll Cardiol. 2019;73:2365-83.
34. Higuchi S, Orban M, Adamo M, et al. Guide line-directed medical therapy in patients under going transcatheter edge-to-edge repair for secondary mitral regurgitation. Eur J Heart Failure. 2022;24:2152-61.
35. Ajmone Marsan N, Delgado V, Shah DJ, et al. Valvular heart disease: shifting the focus to the myocardium. Eur Heart J. 2023;44:28-40.
36. Ikeda Y, Inomata T, Fujita T, et al. Cardiac fibrosis detected by magnetic resonance imaging on predicting time course diversity of left ventricular reverse remodeling in patients with idiopathic dilated cardiomyopathy. Heart Vessels. 2016;31:1817-25.

37. Tayal B, Debs D, Nabi F, et al. Impact of myocardial scar on prognostic implication of secondary mitral regurgitation in heart failure. JACC Cardiovasc Imaging. 2021;14:812-22.
38. Zoghbi WA, Levine RA, Flachskampf F, et al. Atrial functional mitral regurgitation: a JACC: cardiovascular imaging expert panel viewpoint. JACC Cardiovasc Imaging. 2022;15:1870-82.
39. Stolz L, Orban M, Braun D, et al. Anatomy and outcome of secondary mitral regurgitation sub types undergoing transcatheter mitral valve edge-to-edge repair. JACC Cardiovasc Interv. 2021;14:110-1.
40. Mesi O, Gad MM, Crane AD, et al. Severe atrial functional mitral regurgitation: clinical and echo cardiographic characteristics, management and outcomes. JACC Cardiovasc Imaging. 2021;14: 797-808.
41. Silbiger JJ. Mechanistic insights into atrial functional mitral regurgitation: far more complicated than just left atrial remodeling. Echocardiography. 2019;36:164-9.
42. Le Ruz R, Le Tourneau T, Guerin P. Type I Carpentier classification for aFMR definition: only one piece of the whole puzzle? JACC Cardiovasc Imaging. 2023;16:432-3.
43. Abe Y, Takahashi Y, Shibata T. A new disease entity: atrial functional mitral regurgitation. J Cardiol. 2021;77:565-9.
44. Silbiger JJ. Does left atrial enlargement contribute to mitral leaflet tethering in patients with functional mitral regurgitation? Proposed role of atriogenic leaflet tethering. Echocardiography. 2014;31:1310-1.
45. Ito K, Abe Y, Takahashi Y, et al. Mechanism of atrial functional mitral regurgitation in patients with atrial fibrillation: a study using three-dimensional transesophageal echocardiography. J Cardiol. 2017;70:584-90.
46. Gertz ZM, Raina A, Saghy L, et al. Evidence of atrial functional mitral regurgitation due to atrial fibrillation: reversal with arrhythmia control. J Am Coll Cardiol. 2011;58:1474-81.
47. Otto CM, Nishimura RA, Bonow RO, et al. 2020 ACC/AHA guideline for the management of patients with valvular heart disease: a report of the American College of Cardiology/American Heart Association Joint Committee on clinical practice guidelines. Circulation. 2021;143:e72-e227.
48. Waagstein F, Stromblad O, Andersson B, et al. Increased exercise ejection fraction and reversed remodeling after long-term treatment with metoprolol in congestive heart failure: a randomized, stratified, double-blind, placebo-controlled trial in mild to moderate heart failure due to ischemic or idiopathic dilated cardiomyopathy. Eur J Heart Fail. 2003;5:679-91.
49. Solis J, McCarty D, Levine RA, et al. Mechanism of decrease in mitral regurgitation after cardiac resynchronization therapy: optimization of the force-balance relationship. Circ Cardiovasc Imaging. 2009;2:444-50.
50. Solomon SD, Foster E, Bourgoun M, et al. Effect of cardiac resynchronization therapy on reverse remodeling and relation to outcome: multicenter automatic defibrillator implantation trial: cardiac resynchronization therapy. Circulation. 2010;122: 985-92.
51. Upadhyay GA, Chatterjee NA, Kandala J, et al. Assessing mitral regurgitation in the prediction of clinical outcome after cardiac resynchronization therapy. Heart Rhythm. 2015;12:1201-8.
52. Breithardt OA, Sinha AM, Schwammenthal E, et al. Acute effects of cardiac resynchronization therapy on functional mitral regurgitation in advanced systolic heart failure. J Am Coll Cardiol. 2003;41:765-70.
53. Ypenburg C, Lancellotti P, Tops LF, et al. Mechanism of improvement in mitral regurgitation after cardiac resynchronization therapy. Eur Heart J. 2008;29:757-65.
54. van Bommel RJ, Marsan NA, Delgado V, et al. Cardiac resynchronization therapy as a therapeutic option in patients with moderate-severe functional mitral regurgitation and high operative risk. Circulation. 2011;124:912-9.
55. Michler RE, Smith PK, Parides MK, et al. Two-year outcomes of surgical treatment of moderate ischemic mitral regurgitation. N Engl J Med. 2016;374:1932-41.
56. Smith PK, Puskas JD, Ascheim DD, et al. Surgical treatment of moderate ischemic mitral regurgitation. N Engl J Med. 2014;371: 2178-88.
57. Maggiore P, Anastasius M, Huang AL, et al. Transcatheter mitral valve repair and replacement: current evidence for intervention and the role of CT in preprocedural planning-a review for radiologists and cardiologists alike. Radiol Cardiothorac Imaging. 2020;2:e190106.
58. Feldman T, Kar S, Rinaldi M, et al. Percutaneous mitral repair with the MitraClip system: safety and midterm durability in the initial EVEREST (Endovascular Valve Edge-to-Edge REpair Study) cohort. J Am Coll Cardiol. 2009;54:686-94.
59. Stone GW, Lindenfeld J, Abraham WT, et al. Transcatheter mitral-valve repair in patients with heart failure. N Engl J Med. 2018;379:2307-18.
60. Mack MJ, Lindenfeld J, Abraham WT, et al. 3-Year outcomes of transcatheter mitral valve repair in patients with heart failure. J Am Coll Cardiol. 2021;77:1029-40.
61. Juilliere Y. Lessons from MITRA-FR and COAPT studies: can we hope for an indication for severe functional mitral regurgitation in systolic heart failure? Arch Cardiovasc Dis. 2019;112:370-3.
62. Pfister R, Hausleiter J, Boekstegers P, et al. Role of percutaneous edge-to-edge repair in secondary mitral regurgitation after MITRA-FR and COAPT: a comment by the section of AV-valve treatment of the Working Group of Interventional Cardiology (AGIK) of the German Society of Cardiology (DGK). Clin Res Cardiol. 2019;108:969-73.
63. Carabello BA. MitraClip and tertiary mitral regurgitation-mitral regurgitation gets Curiouser and Curiouser. JAMA Cardiol. 2019; 4:307-8.
64. Tang GHL, Verma S, Bhatt DL. Two randomized clinical trials on the treatment of secondary mitral regurgitation-contradictory or complementary? JAMA Cardiol. 2019;4:311-3.
65. Stocker TJ, Stolz L, Karam N, et al. Long-Term Outcomes After Edge-to-Edge Repair of Secondary Mitral Regurgitation: 5-Year Results From the EuroSMR Registry. JACC Cardiovasc Interv. 2024;17(21):2543-54.
66. Juilliere Y. Lessons from MITRA-FR and COAPT studies: can we hope for an indication for severe functional mitral regurgitation in systolic heart failure? Arch Cardiovasc Dis. 2019;112:370-3.
67. Pfister R, Hausleiter J, Boekstegers P, et al. Role of percutaneous edge-to-edge repair in secondary mitral regurgitation after MITRA-FR and COAPT: a comment by the section of AV-valve treatment of the Working Group of Interventional Cardiology (AGIK) of the German Society of Cardiology (DGK). Clin Res Cardiol. 2019;108:969-73.

CHAPTER 60

Mitral Annular Disjunction in Mitral Valve Prolapse

Biswaranjan Mishra

ABSTRACT

Mitral annular disjunction (MAD) is an anatomic–functional alteration in which the atrial hinge point of the mitral valve (MV) is displaced away from the left ventricular (LV) myocardium, creating a measurable gap that uncouples the posterior annulus from the ventricle during systole. MAD frequently coexists with myxomatous mitral valve prolapse (MVP) and may contribute to a substrate for ventricular arrhythmias (VAs) and, rarely, sudden cardiac death (SCD). Over the last decade, multimodality imaging especially echocardiography and cardiac magnetic resonance (CMR) has clarified how MAD, systolic curling of the posterior annulus, papillary muscle traction, and inferobasal LV fibrosis cluster with an "arrhythmogenic MVP (AMVP)" phenotype. Management is directed for associated MVP and mitral regurgitation with surgical and percutaneous intervention individualized. Malignant arrhythmia management includes its detection often by long-term ECG monitoring (Holter) and treatment by catheter ablation procedures and implantable cardioverter-defibrillator (ICD) implantation.

Keywords: Mitral annular disjunction, curling motion, mitral valve prolapse, ventricular arrhythmia, myocardial fibrosis.

INTRODUCTION

Mitral valve prolapse (MVP) is the most common primary valvular abnormality, traditionally viewed through the lens of degenerative mitral regurgitation (MR). However, in recent years, a renewed focus has emerged on its arrhythmic potential, particularly in a subset of patients who harbor structural and functional changes predisposing to ventricular arrhythmias (VAs) and, rarely, sudden cardiac death (SCD). Among these, mitral annular disjunction (MAD) has gained recognition as a distinct anatomic abnormality characterized by atrial displacement of the posterior mitral leaflet hinge point away from the ventricular myocardium.[1] Once considered an incidental echocardiographic curiosity, MAD is now understood as an important component of the arrhythmogenic MVP (AMVP) phenotype, often clustering with bileaflet prolapse, systolic curling of the annulus, and localized myocardial fibrosis.[2] With the advent of wide availability of echocardiography, long-term electrocardiography (ECG) monitoring, and cardiac magnetic resonance (CMR) imaging, MAD is being increasingly detected, risk stratified, and managed for mitral valve (MV) dysfunction and malignant VA.[3]

DEFINITIONS AND NOMENCLATURE

Mitral annular disjunction is defined as the atrial displacement of the mural leaflet hinge point away from the ventricular myocardium to the left atrial (LA) wall yielding a measurable separation between the ventricular myocardium and posterior mitral leaflet (PML) origin from the LA. Commonly ≥2–5 mm thresholds are used across modalities and studies.[4] MVP is commonly associated with MAD and is a marker of AMVP, at times the basal part of PML may abut the LA wall after a originating from a normally placed annulus known as pseudo-MAD, which should be differentiated from true MAD **(Fig. 1)**. AMVP denotes an MVP phenotype with a propensity to significant VAs and SCD, typically featuring some combination of myxomatous bileaflet prolapse, MAD, systolic curling, and basal/inferolateral fibrosis. The 2022 EHRA consensus standardized terminology and proposed a pragmatic risk-assessment framework.[5]

However, MAD may be seen without MVP. Significance of isolated MAD is unknown.[6]

EPIDEMIOLOGY AND PREVALENCE

In MVP cohorts, MAD is frequent but variably reported due to differences in modality, view selection, and cut-offs; CMR

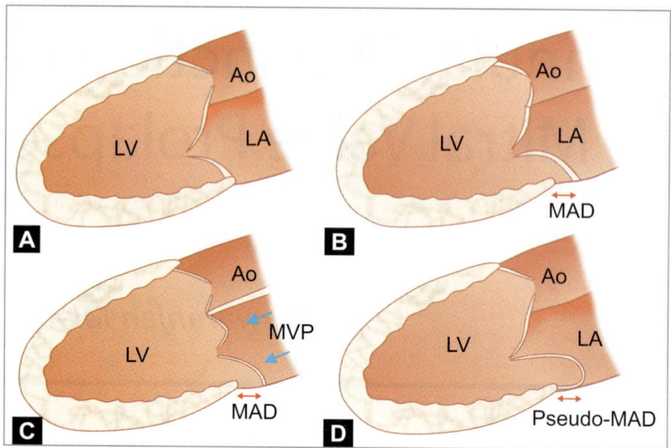

FIGS. 1A TO D: (A) Normal mitral annulus between left atrium (LA) and left ventricle (LV). (B) Double-headed arrow shows displacement of mitral annulus and origin of posterior mitral leaflet toward left atrium. (C) Arrows indicate presence of bileaflet mitral valve prolapse (MVP). (D) Double-headed arrow shows abutting of basal part of posterior mitral leaflet to left atrial wall causing pseudo-mitral annular disjunction (MAD).
(Ao: aorta)

and meticulous echo increase detection. Contemporary imaging series suggest prevalence ranging roughly from one-third to over one-half of MVP cases in specialized settings. A 2025 CMR study emphasizes that MAD may represent a spectrum from an anatomic variant to pathologic remodeling, depending on context.[7]

PATHOPHYSIOLOGY OF VENTRICULAR ARRHYTHMIA

The posterior annulus in MAD loses its normal saddle-shaped systolic contraction and paradoxically expands/uncouples during systole known as curling motion of the posterobasal LV wall. Abnormal motion and traction on long term is responsible for both substrate and trigger for Vas.[8] Hypermobility and repetitive traction on papillary muscles and the basal inferolateral myocardium may promote fibrosis, often seen in mid-wall or at papillary roots on late gadolinium enhancement (LGE) on CMR, potentiating triggered activity and reentry. MAD often coexists with diffuse myxomatous degeneration, redundant leaflets, and elongated chordae, amplifying mechanical stress.[9]

IMAGING THE MAD–MVP COMPLEX

Echocardiography

Transthoracic echocardiography (TTE) in parasternal long-axis view is the imaging of choice for diagnosis of MAD. MAD length is measured from ventricular crest to hinge point of posterior leaflet (usually P2–P3 scallops) in the LA wall.[10] The curling motion due to systolic annular expansion is also best seen in this view **(Fig. 2)**.[11] Tissue Doppler imaging of the lateral mitral annulus characteristically shows high velocity systolic motion due to structural abnormality of papillary-annular tissue. This tissue velocity resembles spike of historical German helmet, therefore when the lateral annular tissue velocity in midsystole is >16 cm/s, it called Pickelhaube sign **(Fig. 3)**.

Mitral valve prolapse defined as at least 2 mm systolic displacement of either mitral leaflet from the annular plane, which is also best seen in long-axis TTE.[12] Myxomatous thickening and bileaflet MVP are commonly associated with MAD. Variable degree of MR is caused by MVP.[13] MR is quantified by conventional methods such as vena contracta, proximal isovelocity surface area (PISA), and continuity equation.[14] Left ventricular (LV) function is also assessed by measurement of ejection fraction (EF) by a biplane Simpson's method. Assessment of pulmonary pressure and right ventricular function are also part of routine assessment in MVP and MAD.[15]

Left ventricular global longitudinal strain (GLS) should be measured to note some characteristic features like increased strain values of inferobasal segments.[16] From speckle-tracking-based GLS estimation, myocardial dispersion (MD) can be calculated automatically as standard deviation of time from onset of QRS complex to peak systolic strain of different segments.[17] Post-systolic shortening (PSS) or double-peak strain curve are sometime seen in MAD. Such strain parameters are associated with worse prognosis in MAD.[18]

Cardiac Magnetic Resonance

Cardiac magnetic resonance is more sensitive than echo for MAD length measurement along the posterior annulus and it has the unique ability to detect myocardial fibrosis. LGE to detect papillary muscle or inferolateral myocardial fibrosis indicates presence of substrate for VAs **(Fig. 4)**. CMR is more sensitive in assessing leaflet thickening, prolapse, LV volume, function, and quantification of MR.[6]

Computed Tomography

With excellent spatial resolution, CT has the ability to image detail annular geometry and leaflet–annulus relationships; emerging work suggests CT-derived metrics may help to plan ring size and posterior plication in repair strategies.[19]

Electrocardiography and Ambulatory Rhythm Monitoring

There are no specific ECG finding in cases of MAD. Inferior and lateral T-wave inversion and frequent premature ventricular contractions (PVCs) are common in AMVP.[20] Nonsustained ventricular tachycardia (NSVT) is occasional finding in routine ECG. Ambulatory ECG monitoring

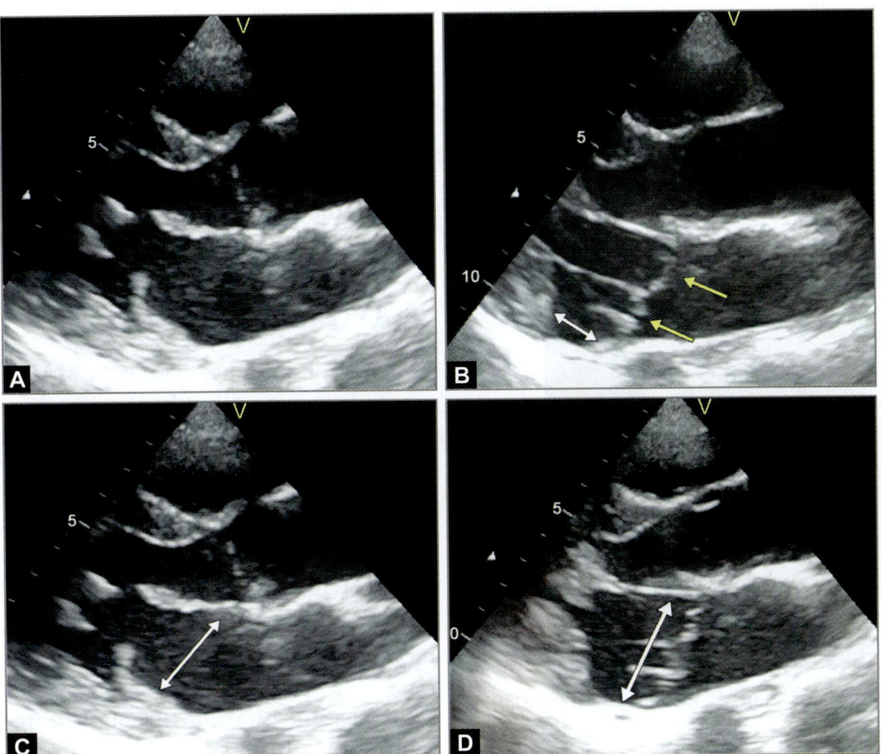

FIGS. 2A TO D: Transthoracic 2D echocardiography in parasternal long-axis view in a case of mitral annular disjunction (MAD). (A) Diastolic frame does not show MAD. (B) Systolic frame shows MAD (double arrow), yellow arrows show bileaflet mitral valve prolapse. (C) Double-headed arrow shows mitral annular dimension in diastole. (D) Mitral annular dimension (double-headed arrow) is more in systole indicating curling motion of posterior basal mitral annulus.

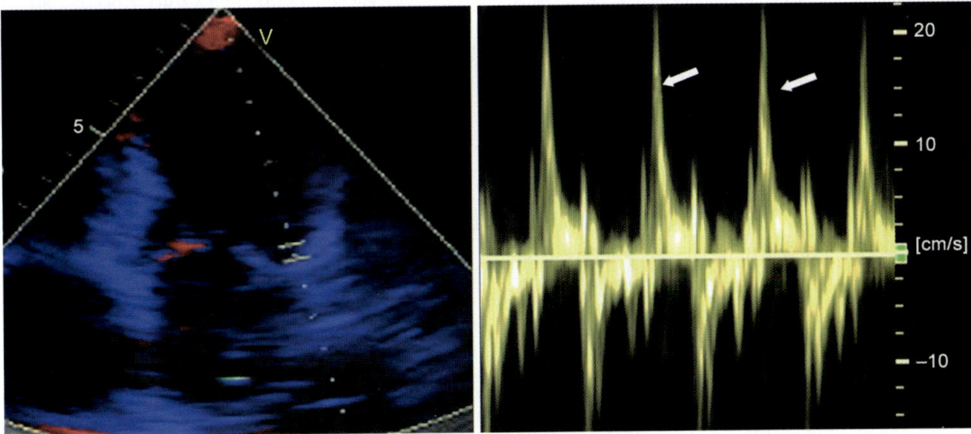

FIG. 3: Tissue Doppler imaging of the lateral annulus showing high velocity systolic waves >16 cm/s, indicating presence of Pickelhaube sign.

is advised in symptomatic patients such as those with history of syncope or palpitation. It may require repeated Holters, extended patch monitor or external loop recorder (ILR) for identification of VAs.[21] PVC morphology also sometime helps in identifying risk. QRS morphology consistent with origin from mitral annulus **(Fig. 5)** signals increased risk.[22]

RISK STRATIFICATION

No single variable identifies risk; instead, clustering of several of markers is considered in risk stratifying the individual. Several clinical, electrical, and morphological abnormalities are taken as risk determinants.[23] Those with unexplained syncope and family history of SCD are high-risk subsets.

Frequent and complex PVCs, NSVT, polymorphic VAs, and PVC origin from papillary or annular sites on ECG mapping pose high risk.[24] MAD with longer disjunction length, wider disjunction arc, systolic curling of the posterobasal wall, bileaflet myxomatous MVP, leaflet redundancy, flail leaflets, and severe MR particularly with LA enlargement and LV dysfunction are high-risk features. CMR fibrosis detected by LGE, particularly at papillary roots and inferolateral LV, is a feature of high risk.[25] The EHRA 2022 consensus proposes a staged approach—identify the phenotype, quantify arrhythmia burden, and escalate monitoring/therapy as markers accumulate. Validation data are emerging, and the framework is helpful for standardized practice even as thresholds continue to evolve.[2]

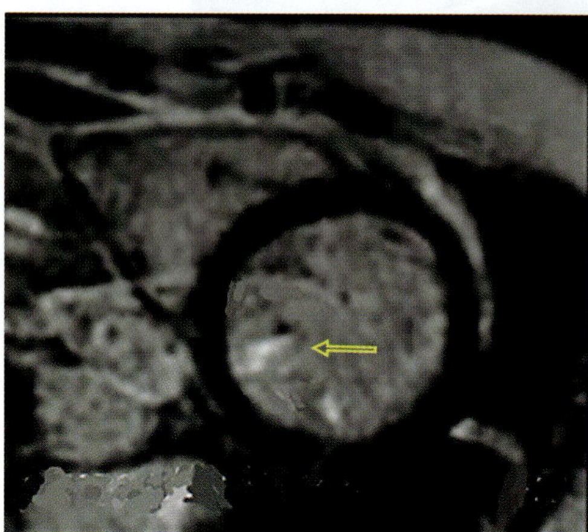

FIG. 4: Cardiac magnetic resonance imaging showing late gadolinium enhancement (arrow) in the posterior basal papillary muscle indicating presence of fibrosis.

NATURAL HISTORY

Most MVP patients even with MAD do well; risk is concentrated in a small subset with the AMVP phenotype. In observational series, MAD is associated with more frequent VAs and SCD compared with MVP without MAD, but effect sizes vary with selection, modality, and definitions; not all studies show independent risk after adjustment for cophenotypes. This underscores the importance of integrated phenotyping rather than "MAD-alone" decision-making.[26]

MANAGEMENT

Mitral regurgitation-directed therapy is to treat MR per guideline-directed care. In myxomatous disease, early

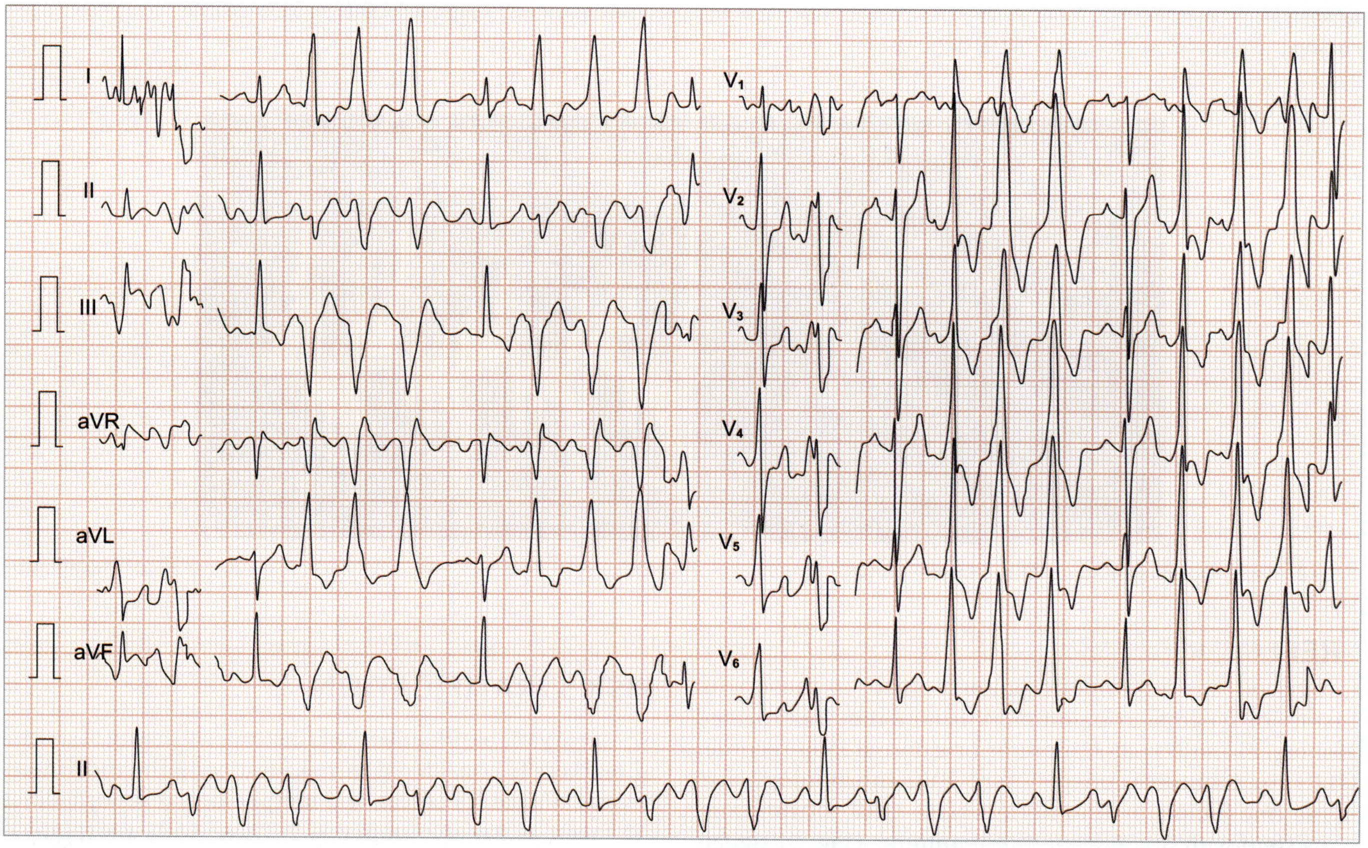

FIG. 5: Electrocardiography (ECG) in a case of mitral annular disjunction showing complex premature ventricular complexes (VPCs) in a ventricular quadrigeminy. Morphology of the VPCs with right bundle branch block and superior axis indicate origin in posterior mitral annulus.

repair at experienced centers improves outcomes and may secondarily reduce mechanical triggers of VAs by stabilizing the annulus and papillary stress. When MAD is present, surgeons should anticipate posterior annular instability and consider techniques that stabilize the disjunction (complete rigid/semirigid rings, targeted posterior annuloplasty, and selective plication). Limited series suggest VA reduction post-repair in some AMVP patients, but definitive prospective data are still limited.[12]

Arrhythmia surveillance and medical therapy should always be done in MAD particularly when symptoms such as palpitations, presyncope, or syncope are there, or complex ectopy is seen on baseline ECG or Holter. Serial ECGs and periodic ambulatory monitoring and also exercise testing to unmask exertional ectopy should be considered.[27]

Medical management includes β-blockers or antiarrhythmic drugs for symptomatic PVCs/NSVT. There is limited randomized data on medical management of arrhythmic MVP.[28]

For drug-refractory symptomatic VAs, catheter ablation at experienced centers can be effective. Recurrences may occur due to multifocal substrate or deep intramural foci. Preprocedural CMR to map fibrosis helps target substrate.[29]

IMPLANTABLE CARDIOVERTER-DEFIBRILLATOR

Implantable cardioverter-defibrillator (ICD) is indicated for secondary prevention after aborted SCD or sustained VT/VF without reversible cause. ICD for primary prevention in MVP and MAD is generally not recommended, however, with multiple high-risk markers such as extensive fibrosis, complex NSVT combined with history of syncope a heart-team may be consulted for consideration of ICD implantation.[15]

High-risk features warrant shared decision-making regarding high-intensity competitive sports.[30]

SURGICAL CONSIDERATIONS

Mitral annular disjunction implies posterior annular instability. Contemporary repair strategies include: (1) complete ring annuloplasty to restore saddle shape and restrain systolic annular expansion; (2) targeted posterior annular plication when the disjunction arc is focal; and (3) chordal repair for leaflet pathology. Early experiences suggest that annular stabilization may mitigate curling and triggers for VAs, but rigorous prospective trials are lacking. Preoperative CT/3D echo can assist with ring selection and plication planning.[31]

GENETICS AND FAMILY SCREENING

Most AMVP/MAD appears sporadic, although genes implicated in myxomatous MVP (e.g., DCHS1 and FLNA) and desmosomal/cytoskeletal variants have been reported in small series of VA-prone phenotypes. Consider family history and targeted genetic counseling where suspicion is high (early SCD and syndromic features).[32]

FUTURE DIRECTION

There are unmet needs which may be answered in future like standardization of modality-specific cut-offs for MAD length/arc that will robustly predict VA risk. Whether repair-mediated annular stabilization lowers arrhythmic events independent of MR correction is not yet known, further study may shed more light on this aspect. Optimal primary-prevention ICD criteria in MAD with MVP will be more clear as research advances.

CONCLUSION

Mitral annular disjunction represents more than a structural curiosity in MVP; it is a marker of altered valve–ventricular interaction that, in selected patients, contributes to an arrhythmogenic substrate. While most individuals with MVP and MAD remain at low risk, a subset with coexisting features such as bileaflet prolapse, systolic curling, myocardial fibrosis, and complex ventricular ectopy constitute the AMVP phenotype warranting closer surveillance. Advances in multimodality imaging and consensus-driven risk frameworks have improved our ability to identify and monitor such patients, although clear thresholds for intervention remain under active investigation. In clinical practice, careful phenotyping, individualized risk assessment, and multidisciplinary collaboration between imaging, electrophysiology, and valve teams are key to optimizing outcomes in this evolving field.

REFERENCES

1. Sabbag A, Essayagh B, Barrera JDR, et al. EHRA expert consensus statement on arrhythmic mitral valve prolapse and mitral annular disjunction complex in collaboration with the ESC Council on valvular heart disease and the European Association of Cardiovascular Imaging endorsed cby the Heart Rhythm Society, by the Asia Pacific Heart Rhythm Society, and by the Latin American Heart Rhythm Society. Europace. 2022;24(12):1981-2003.
2. Zugwitz D, Fung K, Aung N, et al. Mitral Annular Disjunction Assessed Using CMR Imaging: Insights From the UK Biobank Population Study. JACC Cardiovasc Imaging. 2022;15(11):1856-66.
3. Wunderlich NC, Ho SY, Flint N, et al. Myxomatous Mitral Valve Disease with Mitral Valve Prolapse and Mitral Annular Disjunction: Clinical and Functional Significance of the Coincidence. J Cardiovasc Dev Dis. 2021;8(2):9.

4. Constant Dit Beaufils AL, Huttin O, Jobbe-Duval A, et al. Replacement Myocardial Fibrosis in Patients With Mitral Valve Prolapse: Relation to Mitral Regurgitation, Ventricular Remodeling, and Arrhythmia. Circulation. 2021;143(18):1763-74.
5. Wang TKM, Kwon DH, Abou-Hassan O, et al. Strain evaluation for mitral annular disjunction by echocardiography and magnetic resonance imaging: A case-control study. Int J Cardiol. 2021;334:154-6.
6. Essayagh B, Mantovani F, Benfari G, et al. Mitral annular disjunction of degenerative mitral regurgitation: threedimensional evaluation and implications for mitral repair. J Am Soc Echocardiogr. 2022;35(2):165-75.
7. Essayagh B, Sabbag A, Antoine C, et al. Presentation and outcome of arrhythmic mitral valve prolapse. J Am Coll Cardiol. 2020;76(6):637-49.
8. Ignatowski D, Schweitzer M, Pesek K, et al. Pickelhaube spike, a high-risk marker for bileaflet myxomatous mitral valve prolapse: sonographer's quest for the highest spike. J Am Soc Echocardiogr. 2020;33(5):639-40.
9. Vaksmann G, Bouzguenda I, Guillaume MP, et al. Mitral annular disjunction and Pickelhaube sign in children with mitral valve prolapse: A prospective cohort study. Arch Cardiovasc Dis. 2023;116(11):514-22.
10. Vohra J, Morton JB, Morgan J, et al. Cryoablation of Papillary Muscles at Surgery for Malignant Ventricular Arrhythmias Due to Mitral Valve Prolapse. Heart Lung Circ. 2022;31(9):1285-90.
11. Zhou N, Zhao Q, Zeng X, et al. Association of mitral annular disjunction with premature cardiac mortality in a large series of autopsies. J Am Coll Cardiol. 2021;77:102-4.
12. Faletra FF, Leo LA, Paiocchi VL, et al. Morphology of mitral annular disjunction in mitral valve prolapse. J Am Soc Echocardiogr. 2022;35:176-86.
13. Putnam AJ, Kebed K, Mor-Avi V, et al. Prevalence of mitral annular disjunction in patients with mitral valve prolapse and severe regurgitation. Int J Cardiovasc Imaging. 2020;36:1363-70.
14. Toh H, Mori S, Izawa Y, et al. Prevalence and extent of mitral annular disjunction in structurally normal hearts: comprehensive 3D analysis using cardiac computed tomography. Eur Heart J Cardiovasc Imaging. 2021;22:614-22.
15. Mantegazza V, Volpato V, Gripari P, et al. Multimodality imaging assessment of mitral annular disjunction in mitral valve prolapse. Heart. 2021;107:25-32.
16. Essayagh B, Sabbag A, Antoine C, et al. The mitral annular disjunction of mitral valve prolapse: presentation and outcome. JACC Cardiovasc Imaging. 2021;14:2073-87.
17. Bennett S, Tafuro J, Duckett S, et al. Definition, prevalence, and clinical significance of mitral annular disjunction in different patient cohorts: A systematic review. Echocardiography. 2022;39:514-23.
18. van Wijngaarden AL, Kruithof BPT, Vinella T, et al. Characterization of degenerative mitral valve disease: Differences between fibroelastic deficiency and Barlow's Disease. J Cardiovasc Dev Dis. 2021;8:23.
19. Sa MP, Cavalcanti LRP, Van den Eynde J, et al. Respect versus resect approaches for mitral valve repair: A study-level metaanalysis. Trends Cardiovasc Med. 2022;S1050-1738:00007-X.
20. Hiemstra YL, Tomsic A, van Wijngaarden SE, et al. Prognostic value of global longitudinal strain and etiology after surgery for primary mitral regurgitation. JACC Cardiovasc Imaging. 2020;13(2 Pt 2):577-85.
21. Otto CM, Nishimura RA, Bonow RO, et al. 2020 ACC/AHA guideline for the management of patients with valvular heart disease: a report of the American College of Cardiology/American Heart Association Joint Committee on Clinical Practice Guidelines. Circulation. 2021;143:e72-e227.
22. Barman HA, Yıldız A, Güden M, et al. The disappearance of nonsustained ventricular tachycardia after surgical repair in a patient with mitral annular disjunction and mitral valve prolapse. Turk Kardiyol Dern Ars. 2021;49:419-23.
23. Freeman WK, Thibodeau J, Abuissa H. Unrecognized ventricular tachycardia in a patient with mitral annulus disjunction and syncope. Heart Rhythm Case Rep. 2020;6:646-51.
24. Demolder A, Timmermans F, Duytschaever M, et al. Association of mitral annular disjunction with cardiovascular outcomes among patients with marfan syndrome. JAMA Cardiol. 2021;6:1177-86.
25. Nagata Y, Bertrand PB, Baliyan V, et al. Abnormal mechanics relate to myocardial fibrosis and ventricular arrhythmias in patients with mitral valve prolapse. Circ Cardiovasc Imaging. 2023;16:e014963.
26. Biondi R, Ribeyrolles S, Diakov C, et al. Mapping of the myxomatous mitral valve: the threedimensional extension of mitral annular disjunction in surgically repaired mitral prolapse. Front Cardiovasc Med. 2022;9:1036400.
27. Aabel EW, Dejgaard LA, Chivulescu M, et al. Flecainide in patients with arrhythmic mitral valve syndrome: a case series. Heart Rhythm. 2023;20(4):635-6.
28. Vahanian A, Beyersdorf F, Praz F, et al. 2021 ESC/EACTS guidelines for the management of valvular heart disease. Eur Heart J. 2022;43:561-632.
29. Benfari G, Sorajja P, Pedrazzini G, et al. Association of transcatheter edge-to-edge repair with improved survival in older patients with severe, symptomatic degenerative mitral regurgitation. Eur Heart J. 2022;43:1626-35.
30. Chakrabarti AK, Bogun F, Liang JJ. Arrhythmic mitral valve prolapse and mitral annular disjunction: clinical features, pathophysiology, risk stratification, and management. JCDD. 2022;9:61.
31. Benito-González T, Freixa X, Godino C, et al. Ventricular arrhythmias in patients with functional mitral regurgitation and implantable cardiac devices: implications of mitral valve repair with Mitraclip R. Ann Transl Med. 2020;8:956.
32. Marano PJ, Lim LJ, Sanchez JM, et al. Long-term outcomes of ablation for ventricular arrhythmias in mitral valve prolapse. J Interv Card Electrophysiol. 2021;61:145-54.

CHAPTER 61

An Update on High-gradient Moderate Aortic Stenosis

Debika Chatterjee

ABSTRACT

Aortic stenosis (AS) is a common valvular heart disease (VHD) and a major cause of morbidity and mortality worldwide. Severity grading of AS typically relies on hemodynamic parameters derived from echocardiography (Echo). A subset of patients is newly identified who presents with discordant Echo parameters for diagnosis of severe AS where mean gradient (MG) across aortic valve (AV) is high (≥40 mm Hg) but aortic valve area (AVA) >1.0 cm². Echo parameters in this group of patients are posing diagnostic and therapeutic challenges. This emerging phenotype, which may be termed as high-gradient moderate AS, is underrecognized, not reported earlier and lacks dedicated recommendations. Potential contributors to this discrepancy include measurement errors, high stroke volume (SV), bicuspid aortic valve anatomy, and altered flow dynamics. Studies suggest that this subset of AS may not be truly moderate, and outcomes are comparable to severe AS. The absence of standardized classification criteria and management guidelines raises concerns regarding delayed aortic valve replacement (AVR) and adverse outcomes. Until prospective multicenter studies clarify its natural history, a meticulous echocardiographic assessment, comprehensive clinical evaluation, and individualized management are essential for this population.

Keywords: Aortic stenosis, echocardiography, mean gradient, stroke volume, aortic valve area, discordant parameters, high-gradient moderate aortic stenosis, aortic valve replacement.

INTRODUCTION

Aortic stenosis (AS) is one of the most prevalent valvular heart disease (VHD) and remains a leading cause of morbidity and mortality worldwide. For patients with severe AS, surgical or transcatheter aortic valve replacement (AVR) is the standard treatment. Echocardiography (Echo) with Doppler assessment is the primary imaging modality for diagnosing AS, quantifying its severity, and guiding the timing of intervention.

According to current American and European Echocardiographic guidelines, the assessment of AS severity primarily relies on two hemodynamic parameters: Mean gradient (MG) across AV and the aortic valve area (AVA). Severe AS is defined by a MG ≥ 40 mm Hg and an AVA ≤ 1 cm², a scenario where both parameters are concordant.[1-3]

However, in clinical practice, echocardiographic parameters are frequently discordant. A notable example is when the MG is ≥40 mm Hg, but the AVA is >1 cm². In this situation, one parameter indicates severe stenosis, while the other suggests moderate disease. This emerging clinical phenotype, where hemodynamic parameters indicating a picture of *high-gradient moderate aortic stenosis*, has gained increasing attention due to the diagnostic uncertainty it introduces. The presence of MG is ≥40 mm Hg, but the AVA is >1 cm² complicates disease severity assessment, prognostication, and decision-making regarding AVR.

ECHOCARDIOGRAPHIC ASSESSMENT OF AORTIC STENOSIS SEVERITY

Echocardiography plays a critical role in the clinical evaluation and decision-making for patients with AS. Therefore, before interpreting any discordance between echo parameters, it is essential to rule out potential sources of measurement error. A thorough understanding of principles, limitations, and potential pitfalls of Echo is crucial. All Echo studies should adhere to the standardized approach outlined in current echocardiographic guidelines for VHD. Special attention must be given to each step of image acquisition and analysis to minimize common errors.

AORTIC JET VELOCITY AND PRESSURE GRADIENTS

The initial hemodynamic parameter assessed during Echo in AS is the *aortic jet velocity*, obtained with continuous-wave (CW) Doppler.[4] Accurate measurement of the maximum pressure gradient requires alignment of the Doppler beam parallel to the direction of flow across the AV. To achieve this, multiple acoustic windows—including right parasternal and suprasternal views—should be routinely used in addition to the standard apical five-chamber (AP5CH) and apical long-axis (AP-LAX) views. Neglecting nonapical windows has been shown to increase misclassification of AS severity and cause discrepancies between mean pressure gradient and AVA[5]. Benfari et al. demonstrated that incorporating the right parasternal window is feasible in most patients with AS and can reclassify AS severity from moderate to severe in 13–26% of cases.[6]

While the *peak instantaneous gradient* derived from CW Doppler is not used for AS severity classification, the *mean pressure gradient (MG)* is preferred because it reflects the average systolic gradient and correlates better with peak-to-peak gradients obtained during cardiac catheterization. MG is measured by tracing the CW Doppler envelope.[7]

Since both Doppler velocities and pressure gradients are highly flow-dependent, interpretation of AS severity requires calculation of AVA, which provides a robust assessment of stenosis severity.[8]

CALCULATION OF AORTIC VALVE AREA

Aortic valve area (AVA) is derived utilizing continuity equation.[7,9] Principle of continuity equation is based on conservation of mass. In other words, it means that whatever goes in must come out. So, SV at left ventricular outflow tract (LVOT) should be equal to SV at AV. SV across any cardiac orifice is the product of its velocity time integral (VTI) and cross-sectional area (CSA). So, AVA can be calculated as follows: $AVA = (CSA_{LVOT} \times VTI_{LVOT})/VTI_{AV}$.

This requires three measurements:

1. *Left ventricular outflow tract diameter:* Measured in the parasternal long-axis (PLAX) view during mid-systole, 5–10 mm below the AV annulus, from the inner edge of the interventricular septum to the inner edge of the anterior mitral leaflet (AML).
2. *LVOT VTI:* Obtained by placing the pulsed-wave (PW) Doppler sample volume just below the AV in either the AP5CH or AP-LAX view, ensuring it is outside the zone of flow convergence across AV.
3. *AV VTI:* Measured by tracing CW Doppler signal of the AS jet in AP5CH or AP-LAX views.

MINIMIZING SOURCES OF MEASUREMENT ERROR

Errors in LVOT diameter measurement are the most frequent cause of AVA miscalculation because CSA is proportional to the square of the diameter, magnifying even minor inaccuracies. Careful optimization of the PLAX view, zooming, and selecting the systolic frame with the largest LVOT diameter are essential. Challenges include dense annular calcification extending to the base of AML, sigmoid shaped septum, or suboptimal transthoracic views. Transesophageal Echo should be considered if LVOT measurement is unreliable in transthoracic Echo.

When acquiring LVOT velocity with PW Doppler in AP5CH or AP-LAX view, the sample volume should be placed proximal to the AV but away from the high-velocity region of flow convergence. If placed too close to the region of flow convergence, the spectral Doppler signal may demonstrate dispersion. Adjusting the sample volume slowly toward the left ventricular apex until a smooth, narrow-velocity curve is achieved ensures accurate measurement. VTI should be traced along the modal velocity contour (brightest and strongest portion of the signal).

UPDATE ON SEVERITY OF AORTIC STENOSIS BY DOPPLER ECHOCARDIOGRAPHY

Over the years, the American College of Cardiology (ACC), American Heart Association (AHA), American Society of Echocardiography (ASE), and European Society of Cardiology (ESC) have provided comprehensive guidelines for the assessment of VHD. In the evaluation of AS, the traditional definition of severe AS is based on concordant Echo parameters: A transvalvular MG $\geq$ 40 mm Hg and an AVA $\leq$ 1.0 cm^2. However, recent updates have emphasized that not all patients present with these classical findings. Increasing attention has been directed toward patients with discordant Echo parameters, broadening the understanding of AS severity phenotypes.[1,2,10,11]

WELL ESTABLISHED PHENOTYPES OF SEVERE AORTIC STENOSIS WITH DISCORDANT ECHO PARAMETERS

Discordant findings with a MG < 40 mm Hg and an AVA $\leq$ 1.0 cm^2 are observed in approximately 30–40% of patients with severe AS.[12,13] There are two well-recognized phenotypes of severe AS with this discordance:

1. *Classical low-flow, low-gradient severe AS*: MG < 40 mm Hg, AVA $\leq$ 1.0 cm^2, with reduced left ventricular ejection fraction (LVEF < 50%).
2. *Paradoxical low-flow, low-gradient severe AS*: MG < 40 mmHg, AVA $\leq$ 1.0 cm^2, with preserved LVEF ($\geq$ 50%).

These two subgroups have been extensively studied, with robust literature supporting their prognostic and therapeutic implications.

EMERGING PHENOTYPE: HIGH-GRADIENT AORTIC STENOSIS WITH AVA > 1.0 cm²

A less commonly recognized discordant phenotype has been reported in the recent time in which patients exhibit a *high MG (≥ 40 mm Hg) but an AVA > 1.0 cm²*.[14] Although this presentation has been referred to as "high-gradient moderate AS," its true classification remains controversial. Current guidelines do not explicitly address this subgroup, creating uncertainty regarding severity assessment, prognosis, and management.[15] Published literature on this phenotype is limited,[16-19] and whether these patients should be classified as "severe," "moderate-severe," or "moderate" AS remains unresolved yet.

This phenotype appears to be relatively uncommon, representing approximately 5–7% of the overall AS population and 10–14% of high-gradient AS cases.[19,20] Prognostic data are inconsistent: Some studies report a more favorable outcome compared to concordant severe AS, whereas others suggest equivalent or even worse prognosis.[16,17] Misclassification as moderate AS may delay referral for AVR, despite the presence of high gradients, potentially leading to increased morbidity and mortality.[21] Notably, a high AV calcium score is frequently observed in these patients, suggesting disease progression and outcomes comparable to concordant severe AS.[22] These findings support a management approach that treats this group as severe AS rather than moderate disease.

INSIGHTS FROM RECENT STUDIES

A recent single-center retrospective study by Saki Ito et al. further examined this discordant subgroup, emphasizing the role of high flow status as a key contributor to the discrepancy in hemodynamic measurements.[23] Prior researches also have demonstrated that flow status significantly influences AVA measurement: Low flow tends to reduce AVA, whereas high flow may result in an AVA > 1.0 cm² despite severe obstruction.[24,25]

Saki Ito et al. reported that this phenotype is more common in men (86%), consistent with prior studies.[26,27] Larger body size, increased LVOT diameter, and higher SV in men may explain the elevated MG and larger AVA. Conditions associated with high output states—such as combined AS and regurgitation, anemia, hyperthyroidism, and intracardiac shunts—can further exaggerate gradients and AVA measurements.[19,28]

Notably, this phenotype is highly prevalent in *bicuspid AV* (40%), which itself is three times more common in men and is associated with altered LVOT geometry resulting in difficulty in measuring LVOT diameter and increased AVA measurements.[15,29,30]

Patients in this group tend to be younger, less symptomatic, and have fewer comorbidities, such as atrial fibrillation, heart failure, or diabetes. These factors may contribute to their relatively better prognosis.

CLINICAL IMPLICATIONS AND MANAGEMENT CONSIDERATIONS

No formal recommendations currently exist for this subgroup, as they do not fit neatly into existing "severe" or "moderate" AS classifications. Although Saki Ito et al. found that AVR was associated with reduced all-cause mortality in these patients, their findings are limited by the retrospective, single-center study design. Prospective, multicenter randomized trials are essential to define the optimal management strategy.

Given their high gradients with potential risk for adverse outcomes, *careful comprehensive evaluation* is warranted. This should include:

- Detailed Echo assessment for valve calcification, bicuspid morphology, and evidence of LV remodeling.
- Clinical assessment of symptoms, functional capacity, and comorbidities.
- Biomarker analysis (e.g., NT-proBNP) to identify early cardiac stress.

Until robust guidelines are available, early consideration for AVR may be appropriate in symptomatic patients with evidence of progressive cardiac remodeling, despite the AVA being >1.0 cm².[15]

CONCLUSION

A recently recognized entity within AS is high AV gradient (MG ≥ 40 mm Hg) but AVA > 1 cm². This phenotype, characterized by discordant Echo parameters, is not uncommon in the AS population. Because the AVA exceeds 1 cm², these patients are often classified as having moderate AS and are managed accordingly. However, the presence of a high transvalvular MG indicating severe AS cannot be overlooked, as it is associated with poor prognosis and adverse cardiovascular outcomes.

This discrepancy creates uncertainty regarding which hemodynamic parameter should be prioritized and thus presents a clinical dilemma in classifying the severity of AS and determining optimal management strategies, including the timing of AV intervention. Diagnosis of severity and therapeutic decision-making in AS rely heavily on Echo assessment. Careful attention must be paid to the accurate acquisition and interpretation of hemodynamic parameters by Echo to avoid measurement error. Additionally, the effect of underlying flow status on Doppler velocity, pressure gradient, SV, and AVA should be considered.

Currently, standardized recommendations and guidelines for this subset of AS are lacking, as it remains understudied. Prospective, large-scale, multicenter trials are warranted to guide clinical classification and therapeutic strategies in this population.

REFERENCES

1. Otto CM, Nishimura RA, Bonow RO, et al. 2020 ACC/AHA guideline for the management of patients with valvular heart disease: a report of the American College of Cardiology/American Heart, Association Joint Committee on Clinical Practice Guidelines. J Am Coll Cardiol. 2021;77(4):450-500.
2. Vahanian A, Beyersdorf F, Praz F, et al. 2021 ESC/EACTS Guidelines for the management of valvular heart disease. Eur Heart J. 2022;43:561-632.
3. Manzo R, Ilardi F, Nappa D, et al. Echocardiographic evaluation of aortic stenosis: a comprehensive review. Diagnostics (Basel). 2023;13:2527.
4. Currie PJ, Seward JB, Tajik AJ, et al. Continuous-Wave Doppler Echocardiographic Assessment of Severity of Calcific Aortic Stenosis: A Simultaneous Doppler-Catheter Correlative Study in 100 Adult Patients. Circulation. 1985;71:1162-9.
5. Thaden JJ, Nkomo VT, Lee KJ, et al. Doppler Imaging in Aortic Stenosis: The Importance of the Nonapical Imaging Windows to Determine Severity in a Contemporary Cohort. J Am Soc Echocardiogr. 2015;28:780-5.
6. Benfari G, Gori AM, Rossi A, et al. Feasibility and Relevance of Right Parasternal View for Assessing Severity and Rate of Progression of Aortic Valve Stenosis in Primary Care. Int J Cardiol. 2017;240:446-51.
7. Ring L, Shah BN, Bhattacharyya S, et al. Echocardiographic Assessment of Aortic Stenosis: A Practical Guideline from the British Society of Echocardiography. Echo Res Pract. 2021;8:G19-59.
8. Baumgartner H, Hung J, Bermejo J, et al. Recommendations on the Echocardiographic Assessment of Aortic Valve Stenosis: A Focused Update from the European Association of Cardiovascular Imaging and the American Society of Echocardiography. J Am Soc of Echocardiogr. 2017;30:372-92.
9. Baumgartner H, Hung J, Otto CM, et al. Recommendations on the Echocardiographic Assessment of Aortic Valve Stenosis: A Focused Update from the European Association of Cardiovascular Imaging and the American Society of Echocardiography. J Am Soc Echocardiogr. 2017;30:372-92.
10. Clavel MA, Magne J, Pibarot P, et al. Low-gradient aortic stenosis. Eur Heart J. 2016;37:2645-57.
11. Eleid MF, Sorajja P, Michelena HI, et al. Flow-gradient patterns in severe aortic stenosis with preserved ejection fraction: clinical characteristics and predictors of survival. Circulation. 2013;128:1781-9.
12. Minners J, Allgeier M, Gohlke-Baerwolf C, et al. Inconsistencies of echocardiographic criteria for the grading of aortic valve stenosis. Eur Heart J. 2008;29:1043-8.
13. Dumesnil JG, Pibarot P, Carabello B. Paradoxical low flow and/or low gradient severe aortic stenosis despite preserved left ventricular ejection fraction: implications for diagnosis and treatment. Eur Heart J. 2010;31(3):281-9.
14. Otto CM, Nishimura RA, Bonow RO, et al. 2020 ACC/AHA Guideline for the Management of Patients With Valvular Heart Disease: A Report of the American College of Cardiology/American Heart Association Joint Committee on Clinical Practice Guidelines. Circulation. 2021;143(5):e72-227.
15. Zoghbi WA. High-Gradient "Moderate Aortic Stenosis": Is it Moderate or Severe? JACC Cardiovasc Imaging. 2025;18(2): 177-9.
16. Vulesevic B, Burwash IG, Beauchesne LM, et al. Outcomes of patients with discordant high-gradient aortic valve stenosis. JACC Cardiovasc Imaging. 2020;13:1636-8.
17. Bohbot Y, Kubala M, Rusinaru D, et al. Survival and management of patients withdiscordant high-gradient aortic stenosis: a propensity-matched study. JACC Cardiovasc Imaging. 2021;14:1672-4.
18. Chew NWS, Ho YJ, Ngiam JHN, et al. Clinical, echocardiographic and prognostic outcomes of patients with concordant and discordant high-gradient aortic stenosis in an Asian cohort. Int J Cardiovasc Imaging. 2022;38:1351-60.
19. Unger P, Powers A, Le Nezet E, et al. Prevalence and outcomes of patients with discordant high-gradient aortic stenosis. J Am Coll Cardiol. 2024;83:1109-19.
20. Ito S, Oh JK, Michelena HI, et al. High-gradient aortic stenosis with valve area >1.0 cm2: the "forgotten" discordant hemodynamic phenotype. JACC Cardiovasc Imaging. 2025;18(2):166-76.
21. Crochan J, David O. Discordant High-Gradient Aortic Stenosis. Trust the Gradient JACC. 2024;83:1120-2.
22. Pawade T, Sheth T, Guzzetti E, et al. Why and how to measure aortic valvecalcification in patients with aortic stenosis. J Am Coll Cardiol Imaging. 2019;12:1835-48.
23. Saki Ito, Oh JK, Michelena HI, et al. High-Gradient Aortic Stenosis with Valve Area >1.0 cm^2. The "Forgotten" Discordant Hemodynamic Phenotype. JACC Cardiovasc Imaging. 2025;18(2): 166-76.
24. Burwash IG, Thomas DD, Sadahiro M, et al. Dependence of Gorlin formula and Continuity equation valve areas on transvalvular volume flow rate in valvular aortic stenosis. Circulation. 1994;89:827-35.
25. Namasivayam M, He W, Churchill TW, et al. Transvalvular flow rate determines Prognostic value of aortic valve area in aortic stenosis. J Am Coll Cardiol. 2020;75:1758-69.
26. Ito S, Miranda WR, Nkomo VT, et al. Sex differences in LV remodeling and hemodynamics in aortic stenosis: sex-specific criteria for severe stenosis? JACC Cardiovasc Imaging. 2022;15:1175-89.
27. Michelena HI, Margaryan E, Miller FA, et al. Inconsistent echocardiographic grading of Aortic stenosis: is the left ventricular out flow tract important? Heart. 2013;99:921-31.
28. Unger P, Clavel MA. Mixed aortic valve disease: a diagnostic challenge, a prognosticthreat. Structural Heart. 2020;4:468-74.
29. Disha K, Dubslaff G, Rouman M, et al. Evidence of subannular and left ventricular morphological differences in patients with bicuspid versus tricuspid aortic valve stenosis: magnetic resonance imaging-based analysis. Interact Cardiovasc Thorac Surg. 2017;24:369-76.
30. Siu SC, Silversides CK. Bicuspid aortic valve disease. J Am Coll Cardiol. 2010;55:2789-800.

CHAPTER 62

Comprehensive Risk Phenotyping in Aortic Stenosis

Dipankar Ghosh Dastidar

ABSTRACT

Aortic valve replacement is indicated only for symptomatic severe aortic stenosis or asymptomatic severe aortic stenosis with left ventricular dysfunction or with a plan for another open-heart surgery. Guidelines still advocate for watchful waiting in asymptomatic severe aortic stenosis or even symptomatic mild to moderate stenosis. Recent evidence suggests that long standing aortic stenosis causes left ventricular hypertrophy with fibrosis, atrial dilatation, pulmonary arterial hypertension, tricuspid regurgitation, and right ventricular dysfunction. The very presence of this cardiac damage even in mild to moderate aortic stenosis suggests that it might result from coexisting comorbidities such as hypertension, diabetes, ischemic heart disease, CKD, COPD. Valve replacement in symptomatic severe aortic stenosis as advocated by guidelines often gives suboptimal results because of this advanced cardiac damage, many of which such as obliterative pulmonary arterial hypertension and right ventricular dysfunction are irreversible. So comprehensive risk assessment in aortic stenosis is the need of the hour. A combination of advanced imaging modalities, biomarkers integrated with artificial intelligence can pick up cardiac damage even in mild aortic stenosis and advocate early remedial measures to prevent disease progression. This kind of personalized medicine can bring about a paradigm shift in aortic stenosis management.

Keywords: Aortic stenosis, symptomatic, asymptomatic, surgical aortic valve replacement (SAVR), transcutaneous aortic valve replacement (TAVR), cardiac damage, left ventricular hypertrophy.

INTRODUCTION

The prevalence of degenerative aortic stenosis (AS) is on the rise globally with increasing life expectancy and aging population.[1] Traditionally, the focus was only on valve damage as assessed by echocardiographic parameters such as peak aortic velocity (Vmax), mean transvalvular gradient, and calculated aortic valve area. For most guidelines, once severe AS is established, it is the presence of symptoms either spontaneously or on low-level stress test or a decline in left ventricular ejection fraction (LVEF) or there is a plan for another open-heart surgery that prompts consideration for valve replacement, either surgical aortic valve replacement (SAVR) or transcatheter (TAVI).[2]

However, this valve-centric approach has of late been questioned. The natural history of AS shows that valvular hemodynamics is not the only factor influencing morbidity and mortality. Rather, the degree of extravalvular involvement such as left ventricular hypertrophy (LVH), atrial dilatation, pulmonary arterial hypertension (PAH), tricuspid regurgitation (TR), and right ventricular (RV) dysfunction determines the outcomes and prognosis.[3] Généreux and associates has come forward with cardiac damage staging method classifying patients into four stages: Stage 0 (no damage) to stage 4 (right ventricular dysfunction).[4] The presence of these coexisting cardiac damage often accounts for the suboptimal results following SAVR or TAVI in symptomatic severe AS **(Fig. 1)**.

These changing concepts emphasize how cardiac damage starts earlier than is often thought, changes dynamically following intervention, and calls for a more comprehensive approach to risk assessment that goes beyond valvular gradients alone.

PATHOPHYSIOLOGY OF CARDIAC DAMAGE IN AORTIC STENOSIS

Traditionally, the concept was that AS causes chronic left ventricular (LV) pressure overload, which causes concentric LVH. This LVH was considered protective against the raised afterload preventing development of clinical heart failure.

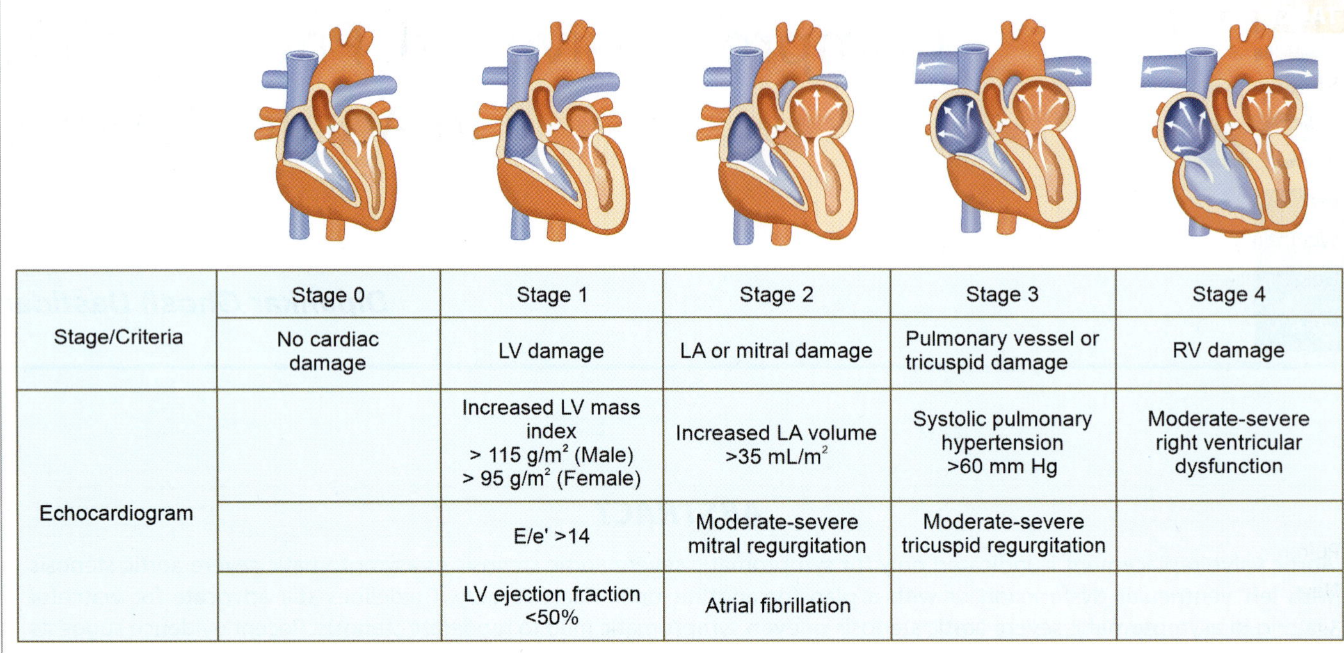

Stage/Criteria	Stage 0	Stage 1	Stage 2	Stage 3	Stage 4
	No cardiac damage	LV damage	LA or mitral damage	Pulmonary vessel or tricuspid damage	RV damage
Echocardiogram		Increased LV mass index > 115 g/m² (Male) > 95 g/m² (Female)	Increased LA volume >35 mL/m²	Systolic pulmonary hypertension >60 mm Hg	Moderate-severe right ventricular dysfunction
		E/e' >14	Moderate-severe mitral regurgitation	Moderate-severe tricuspid regurgitation	
		LV ejection fraction <50%	Atrial fibrillation		

FIG 1: Aortic stenosis staging classification based on extent of cardiac damage.

However, recent evidence shows that LVH invites fibrosis and myocardial dysfunction. Moreover, LVH with raised LV end diastolic pressure (LVEDP) invites left atrium (LA) dilation, atrial fibrillation, secondary mitral regurgitation (MR), pulmonary venous hypertension (PVH), reactive and ultimately obliterative pulmonary arterial hypertension (PAH), RV dysfunction and tricuspid regurgitation (TR) and ultimately to right heart failure (RHF).[5]

Following SAVR or TAVI, LVH may regress but other changes such as obliterative PAH and RV dysfunction often persist, influencing negative long-term outcomes.[6]

Existing Risk Scores

Society of Thoracic Surgeons (STS) is a risk assessment tool that predicts operative mortality in AVR patients. It takes into account factors such as age, gender, and comorbidities (e.g., diabetes and lung disease) **(Table 1)**.

Euroscore II is another useful for preoperative risk assessment **(Table 2)**.

TABLE 1: STS risk score.[7]

Variable	Preoperative score	Combined score
Age (for each 5 years over 55 years)	1	1
BMI 30–40 kg/m²	4	3
BMI 40 kg/m²	9	8
Diabetes	3	3
Renal failure	4	4
Congestive heart failure	3	3
Peripheral vascular disease	2	2
Female gender	2	2
Chronic lung disease	2	3
Cardiogenic shock	6	N/A
Myocardial infarction	2	N/A
Concomitant surgery	4	N/A
Perfusion time 100–200 minutes	N/A	3
Perfusion time 200–300 minutes	N/A	7
Intra-aortic balloon pump	N/A	5

(BMI: body mass index; STS: Society for Thoracic Surgeons).

CARDIAC DAMAGE IN EARLY AORTIC STENOSIS

Conventionally, moderate to severe AS was considered to have adverse hemodynamic consequences. However, Dahl et al. (2024) cast doubt on this concept thorough a retrospective investigation of 9,611 patients with mild AS (Vmax 2–3 m/s) in which he established 80% of mild AS patients had some form of cardiac damage.[9] Stage 1 accounted for 17% of patients, stage 2 for 50%, stage 3 for 9%, and stage 4 for 4%. So, half of all mild AS patients were already in stage 2, characterized by left atrial dilation, mitral regurgitation, and atrial fibrillation **(Fig. 2)**.

TABLE 2: Euroscore II calculator.[8]

Variable	Frequencies (%) or mean (SD) [range]
Patient-related factors	
Age (years)	64.6 (12.5) [18–95]
Female	6,919 (30.9%)
Weight (kg)	77.9 (15.9) [30–182]
Height (cm)	168.5 (9.6) [100–213]
BMI (calculated) (kg/m^2)	27.4 (4.8) [9.6–82.6]
Body surface area (calculated)	1.87 (0.21) [1.04–2.90]
Diabetes—no	16,783 (75.0%)
Diet only	803 (3.6%)
Oral therapy only	3,103 (13.9%)
Insulin	1,705 (7.6%)
Pulmonary disease	2,384 (10.7%)
Neurological dysfunction	713 (3.2%)
Serum creatinine (μmol/L)	96.4 (57.1)
Serum creatinine (mg/dL)	1.13 (0.92)
Serum creatinine > 200 μmol/L	562 (2.6%)
CC (calculated)	83.6 (50.9)
On dialysis	244 (1.1%)
Serum albumin (g/L)	31.6 (19.0)
Active endocarditis	497 (2.2%)
Critical preoperative state	924 (4.1%)
Preoperative VT/VF or aborted sudden death	137 (0.6%)
Preoperative cardiac massage	94 (0.4%)
Preoperative ventilation	251 (1.1%)
Preoperative inotropes	475 (2.1%)
Preoperative IABP	384 (1.7%)
Preoperative acute renal failure	108 (0.5%)

(IABP: intra-aortic balloon pump; VF: ventricular fibrillation; VT: ventricular tachycardia)

ROLE OF COMORBIDITIES VERSUS VALVE SEVERITY IN DETERMINATION OF PROGNOSIS

A surprising find in the work of Dahl et al. (2024) was that it is not the severity of AS that determines cardiac damage but many a time it is the presence of comorbidities such as hypertension, diabetes, ischemic heart disease, CKD, COPD that determines advanced cardiac damage.[9] This suggests age-related and systemic factors had significant influence in cardiac damage than only adverse hemodynamics. This implies patients conventionally labeled as "benign mild AS" may in fact be harboring greater cardiac damage and having a greater mortality risk.

EVOLUTION OF CARDIAC DAMAGE AFTER TAVI

Zhou et al. (2023) addressed this by studying 644 patients with severe AS undergoing TAVI and tracking changes in cardiac damage stage within the first 30 days and beyond.[10] Majority had advanced cardiac damage at baseline, which reflects the real-world cohort.

- *Stage 0–1:* 14%
- *Stage 2:* 66%
- *Stage 3–4:* 19%

Short-term Dynamics

About 22.2% of patients experienced a change in cardiac damage stage within 30 days post-TAVI. Majority showed reductions in MR, PAH, and TR severity. 19.9% improved by at least one stage with improvements in NYHA class and LVEF while 2.8% deteriorated due to periprocedural complications such myocardial infarction or acute kidney injury. However, for most (around 77%) cardiac damage remained unchanged, proving that TAVI may prevent but not reverse extravalvular damage **(Figs. 3 and 4)**.[10]

Long-term Prognosis

Long-term outcomes were highly influenced by preexisting cardiac damage. 2Y mortality was nearly three times higher in patients with advanced cardiac damage compared to those with lower stages (HR ~2.97). A subset of patients notably with COPD (OR ~4.3) and periprocedural MI (OR ~47) deteriorated acutely after TAVI and had 22 times higher mortality at 2Y.[10] So valve replacement stops continuous hemodynamic deterioration, but the progression of cardiac damage varies thus affecting survival.

MECHANISTIC INSIGHTS

This data classifies pathophysiological subsets into:

- *Reversible damage:* LVH, diastolic dysfunction, and functional MR/TR regress with afterload relief
- *Irreversible damage:* Established fibrosis, severe obliterative PAH, and RV dysfunction may persist despite successful TAVI.
- *Procedural insults:* Myocardial injury or acute kidney injury can exacerbate systemic stress, pushing patients into higher cardiac damage stages.

Risk Phenotyping beyond Valvular Severity

Fortuni and Grayburn (2024) argued risk of AS should not be judged solely on hemodynamics, but risk assessment should

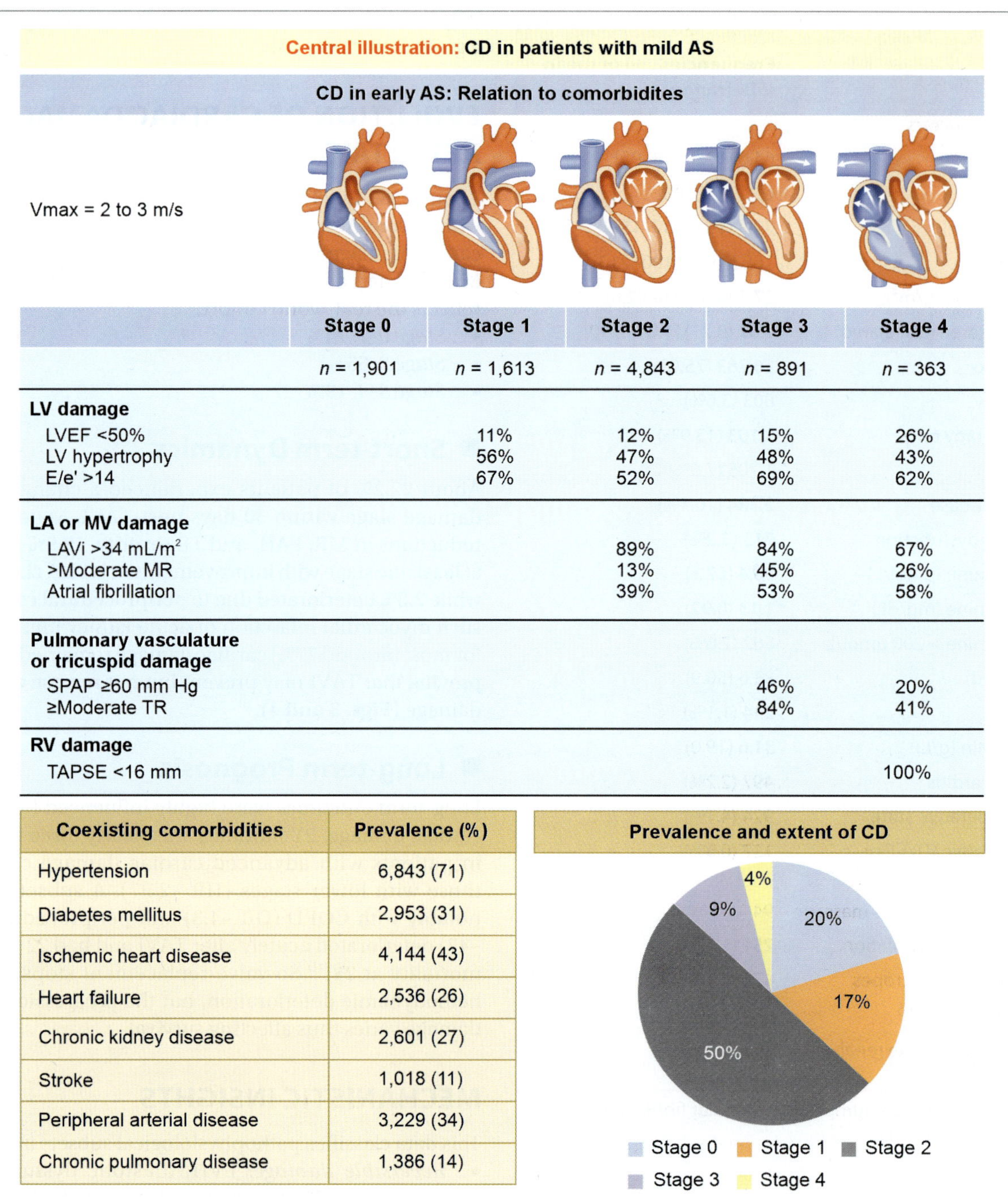

FIG. 2: Prevalence of various stages of cardiac damage in patients with mild aortic stenosis (AS).[9]
Source: With permission from Dahl JS, et al (2024).[9]

be comprehensive engulfing issues such as comorbidities and cardiac damage **(Fig. 5)**. They highlighted the limitations of Valve-Centric approach.

Risk phenotyping includes:

- *Valvular burden:* Pressure overload, concentric LVH, and afterload mismatch
- *Concomitant cardiac conditions:* Coronary artery disease, atrial fibrillation, cardiomyopathies, and secondary MR
- *Systemic comorbidities:* CKD, COPD, diabetes, hypertension, peripheral vascular disease, and inflammatory states

These features create phenotypes that extend beyond valve stenosis severity. Patients with mild AS can exhibit advanced cardiac damage due to comorbidities, while some with severe AS may remain with minimal cardiac damage. Changes such as LVH and secondary MR may be reversible

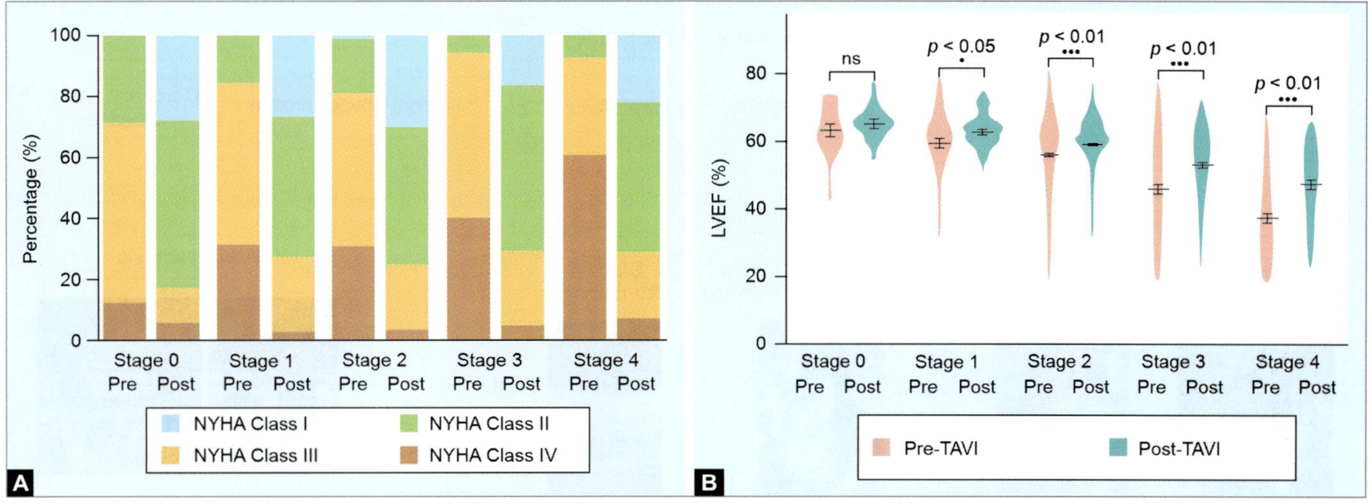

FIGS. 3A AND B: Changes in NYHA Functional Class and LVEF from baseline to 30 days after TAVI.[10]

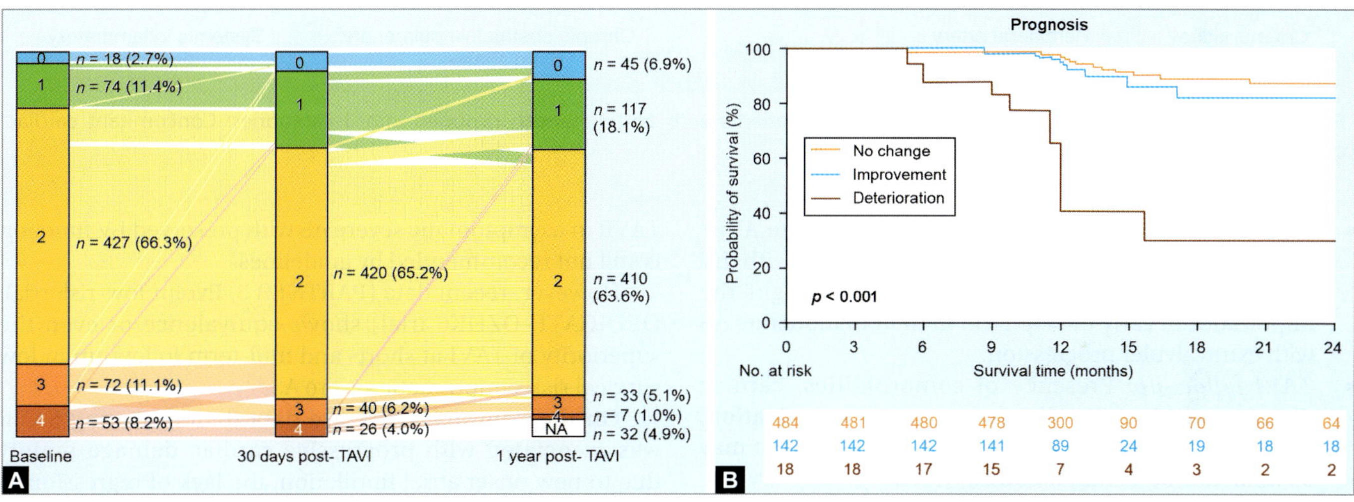

FIGS. 4A AND B: (A) Evolution of cardiac damage stage from baseline to 30 days and at 1 year after TAVI; (B) Kaplan–Meier estimates of all-cause mortality.[10]

following intervention but advanced cardiac damage such as obliterative PAH and RV dysfunction may be irreversible and cause relentless deterioration even after successful valve surgery.[12]

Integration of Imaging, Biomarkers, and Artificial Intelligence

- Echocardiography remains the cornerstone for diagnosis but may misclassify the severity of AS particularly in low-flow states.
- Cardiac MRI may provide information about fibrosis, chamber volumes, and flow dynamics. PET provides information about metabolic derangements. CT provides insight about valve calcification, aortic valve anatomy, aortic angle, coronary height, LVOT height, and membranous septum. Moreover, CT provides valuable information about access site anatomy.
- Biomarkers of heart failure such as NT-proBNP and myocardial damage such as troponins and systemic markers of renal function such as eGFR and inflammatory status such as CRP add to prognosis.
- Artificial intelligence can integrate these various parameters and detect hidden vulnerable phenotypes who might benefit from early intervention.

CLINICAL IMPLICATIONS

These emerging concepts are reshaping our clinical practice.[11]

- *Rethinking early disease:* Mild AS is no more benign if accompanied by comorbidities and cardiac damage.

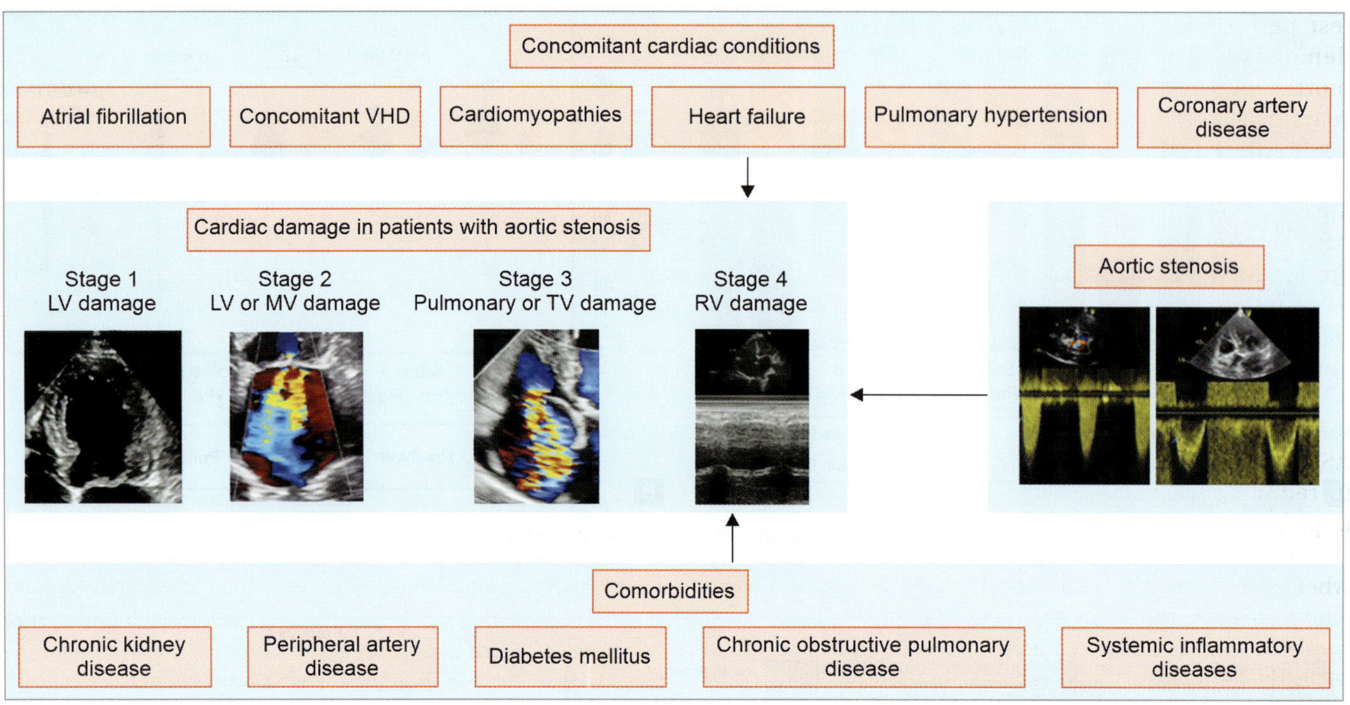

FIG. 5: Potential determinants of cardiac damage in patients with aortic stenosis grouped into 3 categories: Concomitant cardiac conditions, aortic stenosis, and comorbidities.[11]

- *Intervention timing:* Current guidelines advocate AVR/TAVI mainly in symptomatic severe AS or with LV dysfunction. However, recent findings highlight the importance of early intervention in mild to moderate AS with extravalvular progression.
- *TAVI follow-up:* Presence of comorbidities, cardiac damage, aortic valve phenotype, valve calcification, aortic angle, height of coronaries, and LVOT height may all influence outcomes following TAVI.
- *Personalized medicine:* Integrating comorbidities, biomarkers, and imaging creates phenotypic profiles with varying risks beyond just simple valve severity and hemodynamics.

ARE SURGICAL AORTIC VALVE REPLACEMENT AND TAVR AT EQUIPOISE?

Surgical aortic valve replacement/TAVR is meant for symptomatic severe AS or asymptomatic severe AS with LV dysfunction. The general notion is that TAVR is meant for older patients with high surgical risk, and certain anatomical features unsuitable for surgery. In contrast, SAVR is preferred for younger patients (<65 years old), those with a long life expectancy (>20 years), and patients with specific anatomies such as bicuspid aortic valves with aortic root dilatation, which may require additional root replacement.

There is an emerging indication for SAVR in asymptomatic very severe AS (peak velocity >5 m/s) thanks to the positive outcomes of RECOVERY and AVATAR trials. Performing TAVR in asymptomatic severe AS with preserved LV function is still not recommended by guidelines.

However, recent data (PARTNER 3, Evolut low-risk trial, DEDICATE-DZHK6 trial) shows equivalence or even the superiority of TAVI at short- and mid-term follow-up in low surgical risk symptomatic severe AS.[13]

On the contrary, there are data demonstrating SAVR was associated with progressive cardiac damage mainly due to new onset atrial fibrillation, the lack of regression of LVH (negative remodeling) and the occurrence of new RV dysfunction due to the on-pump phenomenon.[6]

The reduced invasiveness and safety of TAVI compared to SAVR have prompted many to advocate it as a pre-emptive strategy among asymptomatic severe AS with normal left ventricular function or even in moderate AS so as to prevent cardiac damage. However, others are cautious and prefer to wait for the results of more trials on this subject before advocating it in the guidelines.[13]

FUTURE DIRECTIONS

This paradigm shift in concept is being validated in several ongoing trials.

Recently, two small randomized trials of approximately 150 patients each demonstrated the benefits of SAVR among patients with asymptomatic critical aortic stenosis.

The randomized comparison of early surgery versus conventional treatment in very severe aortic stenosis (>65 years old, peak velocity >5 m/s, and no stress test performed) (RECOVERY) trial, published in 2019, demonstrated a reduction in the composite operative mortality or death from cardiovascular causes for up to 8 years in patients who underwent early surgical intervention.[14]

Similarly, the Aortic Valve Replacement Versus Conservative Treatment in Asymptomatic Severe Aortic Stenosis (>65 years old, peak velocity >4.5 m/s) (AVATAR) trial, published in 2021, supported a strategy of early surgical aortic valve replacement and showed a marked reduction in a composite collection of outcomes (death, acute myocardial infarction, stroke, and unplanned hospitalization for heart failure) at 3 years.[15]

The EARLY TAVR trial demonstrated promising results for patients undergoing TAVR in asymptomatic severe AS, proving TAVR was superior to clinical surveillance in reducing the composite endpoint of death, stroke, or unplanned hospitalization over 2 years.[16]

The PROGRESS trial (NCT04889872) aims to evaluate whether TAVR is superior to clinical surveillance in patients who have moderate, calcific aortic stenosis. The recruitment process is still on. The preliminary 2-year data shows promise for early TAVR in terms of survival, improved quality of life score, and possible reduction in severe adverse events.[17]

The Early Valve Replacement Guided by Biomarkers of Left Ventricular Decompensation in Asymptomatic Patients with Severe Aortic Stenosis (EVOLVED) trial failed to demonstrate benefits in early aortic valve intervention with SAVR/TAVR among patients with asymptomatic aortic stenosis, normal EF, and with evidence of LGE on CMR over a median duration of 42 months. The negative results that could have stemmed from asymptomatic status were based on physician assessment and not on exercise test, and the majority of patients received SAVR.[18]

The TAVR-UNLOAD study did TAVR in patients with moderate AS and HFrEF on GDMT. There was no improvement in primary endpoints such as all-cause death, disabling stroke, disease-related hospitalizations, and heart failure equivalents but demonstrated a reduction in symptoms from baseline in the Kansas City Cardiomyopathy Questionnaire Overall Summary Score.[19]

Danish National Randomized Study on Early Aortic Valve Replacement in Patients With Asymptomatic Severe Aortic Stenosis (DANAVR) (NCT03972644)—testing early AVR in patients with signs of elevated LV filling pressures may improve long-term outcome in patients with asymptomatic severe AS preserved LVEF, compared to conventional symptom-guided surgery.[20]

The Early Valve Replacement in Severe Asymptomatic Aortic Stenosis (EASY-AS) trial also aims to determine whether early aortic valve replacement improves clinical outcomes, quality of life, and cost-effectiveness compared to a guideline recommended strategy of "watchful waiting" in asymptomatic severe aortic stenosis.[21]

CONCLUSION

The last decade has witnessed a paradigm shift in AS management. From being a purely valvular condition, risk assessment of associated cardiac damage and comorbidities has shifted the focus to it being a systemic, multichamber cardiac disorder.

The need for comprehensive risk assessment is the way to go forward in all future aortic valve interventions. With advanced imaging studies, cardiac damage staging, and comorbidity assessment, we can now deliver personalized care to AS patients, thus moving beyond traditional risk assessments as predicted by Society of Thoracic Surgeons (STS) scores.

Key learning points include the presence of cardiac damage even in mild AS. TAVI alters the trajectory of cardiac damage, with some patients improving and others deteriorating with extremely poor outcomes. Comprehensive risk assessment beyond valvular severity, incorporating comorbidities, imaging, biomarkers, and dynamic reversibility is the approach to AS in future.

With growing evidence, clinical guidelines will likely incorporate cardiac damage staging and comprehensive risk phenotyping into decision-making. For now, the message is clear: In aortic stenosis, it is not just the valve, but the heart and the person as a whole matters.

REFERENCES

1. Yadgir S, Johnson CO, Aboyans V, et al. Global, regional, and national burden of calcific aortic valve and degenerative mitral valve diseases, 1990-2017. Circulation. 2020;141:1670-80.
2. Writing Committee Members, Otto CM, Nishimura RA, et al. 2020 ACC/AHA guideline for the management of patients with valvular heart disease: a report of the American College of Car diology/American Heart Association Joint Committee on Clinical Practice Guidelines. J Am Coll Cardiol. 2021;77:e25-197.
3. Fortuni F, Bax JJ, Delgado V. Changing the paradigm in the management of valvular heart disease: in addition to left ventricular ejection fraction, focus on the myocardium. Circulation. 2021;143:209-11.
4. Généreux P, Pibarot P, Redfors B, et al. Staging classification of aortic stenosis based on the extent of cardiac damage. Eur Heart J. 2017;38:3351-8.
5. Pibarot P, Iung B, Cavalcante JL. Risk Stratification in Patients With Aortic Stenosis. JACC Cardiovasc Interv. 2019;12:2169-72.
6. Généreux P, Pibarot P, Redfors B, et al. Evolution and prognostic impact of cardiac damage after aortic valve replacement. J Am Coll Cardiol. 2022;80:783-800.
7. The Society of Thoracic Surgeons. STS National Database Risk Calculator. [online] Available from http://www.sts.org/sections/stsnationaldatabase/riskcalculator [Last accessed October, 2025].

8. Nashef SA, Roques F, Sharples LD, et al. EuroSCORE II. Eur J Cardiothorac Surg. 2012;41:73444.
9. Dahl JS, Julakanti R, Ali M, et al. Cardiac damage in early aortic stenosis: is the valve to blame? JACC Cardiovasc Imaging. 2024;17(9):1031-40.
10. Zhou Y, Zhu Q, Lin X, et al. Impact of Early Changes in Cardiac Damage Following Transcatheter Aortic Valve Implantation. EuroIntervention. 2023;19:267-76.
11. Fortuni F, Grayburn PA. The Need for Comprehensive Risk Phenotyping in Aortic Stenosis. JACC Cardiovasc Imaging. 2024;17(9):1041-3.
12. Fukui M, Sorajja P, Hashimoto G, et al. Right ventricular dysfunction by computed tomography associates with outcomes in severe aortic stenosis patients undergoing transcatheter aortic valve replacement. J Cardiovasc Comput Tomogr. 2022;16:158-65.
13. Généreux P, Iung B. TAVI in asymptomatic patients with severe aortic stenosis: pros and cons. Eurointervention. 2022;18(10):793-5.
14. Kang DH, Park SJ, Lee SA, et al. Early surgery or conservative care for asymptomatic aortic stenosis. RECOVERY trial. N Engl J Med. 2020;382(2):111-9.
15. Banovic M, Putnik S, Penicka M, et al. Aortic valve replacement versus conservative treatment in asymptomatic severe aortic stenosis: the AVATAR trial. Circulation. 2022;145(9):648-58.
16. Généreux P, Schwartz A, Oldemeyer JB, et al. Transcatheter Aortic-Valve Replacement for Asymptomatic Severe Aortic Stenosis. N Engl J Med. 2025;392(3):217-27.
17. Edwards Lifesciences. Management of Moderate Aortic Stenosis by Clinical Surveillance or Transcatheter Aortic Valve Replacement. [online] Available from ClinicalTrials.gov.https://www.clinicaltrials.gov/study/NCT04889872.
18. Loganath K, Craig NJ, Everett RJ, et al; for the EVOLVED Investigators. Early Intervention in Patients With Asymptomatic Severe Aortic Stenosis and Myocardial Fibrosis: The EVOLVED Randomized Clinical Trial. JAMA. 2025;333(3):213-21.
19. Van Mieghem NM, Elmariah S, Spitzer E, et al. Transcatheter aortic valve replacement in patients with systolic heart failure and moderate aortic stenosis: TAVR UNLOAD. J Am Coll Cardiol. 2025;85(9):878-90.
20. Dahl J. Danish National Randomized Study on Early Aortic Valve Replacement in Patients With Asymptomatic Severe Aortic Stenosis (DANAVR). [online] Available from https://www.clinicaltrials.gov/study/NCT03972644 [Last accessed October, 2025].
21. Richardson C, Gilbert T, Aslam S. Rationale and design of the early valve replacement in severe asymptomatic aortic stenosis trial. Am Heart J. 2024;275:119-27.

CHAPTER 63

When to Treat Young and Low-risk Patients with Aortic Stenosis

Gopala Krishna Koduru, Raghuram Palaparti, Venkata RS Subrahmanya Sarma

ABSTRACT

Transcatheter aortic valve replacement (TAVR) has reshaped the management of severe aortic stenosis, moving from an option of last resort to a preferred intervention in selected younger and lower-risk patients. The shift reflects growing operator experience, refinement in valve design, and better patient selection aided by multimodality imaging. Yet, the enthusiasm is tempered by the need to understand long-term valve durability, the challenges of coronary access, and management of bicuspid anatomy. In the Indian context, TAVR programs are expanding rapidly, supported by improving infrastructure and trained teams. The focus is now on achieving durable results and defining lifelong strategies for valve care. The journey of TAVR continues to evolve from technical success toward ensuring sustained clinical benefit and quality of life.

Keywords: Transcatheter aortic valve replacement, aortic stenosis, surgical aortic valve replacement, low-risk patients, bicuspid aortic valve, valve durability, coronary access.

INTRODUCTION

Transcatheter aortic valve replacement (TAVR) has revolutionized the treatment of aortic stenosis (AS), emerging as a standard therapy across all surgical risk groups. Initially reserved for patients at high or prohibitive surgical risk, TAVR is now approved for individuals with severe symptomatic AS, irrespective of their calculated surgical risk scores.[1] This paradigm shift has been driven by numerous landmark trials demonstrating the noninferiority and in some cases superiority of TAVR compared to surgical aortic valve replacement (SAVR).

Aortic stenosis, a progressive valvular disorder, is increasingly being recognized not only in the elderly but also in younger, lower-risk populations. The expanded use of echocardiography and CT imaging, coupled with growing awareness, has led to earlier detection, including asymptomatic individuals. In this evolving landscape, the optimal timing and mode of intervention in young and low-risk patients with AS is a matter of ongoing clinical debate and research. This article explores the rationale for treating such patients, focusing on the nuances that influence procedural choice and timing.

DEFINITIONS

"Young" in the context of AS management typically refers to patients under 65 years of age, though clinical decisions are more often guided by biological age, comorbidities, and overall functional status. *"Low-risk"* patients are defined based on surgical risk scoring systems such as the Society of Thoracic Surgeons Predicted Risk of Mortality (STS-PROM) and EuroSCORE II, with a score of <4% indicating low operative risk.[2] Importantly, these patients should have no significant organ dysfunction or frailty that might influence postprocedural recovery.

EPIDEMIOLOGY

Among younger patients, bicuspid aortic valve (BAV) disease remains the predominant etiology of AS.[3] BAV occurs in approximately *1–2%* of the population and is responsible for nearly 50% of all valve replacements in patients younger than 70 years. It often leads to stenosis one to two decades earlier than trileaflet valves. In *India*, the uptake of *TAVI (transcatheter aortic valve implantation) procedures is rising rapidly*, with *3,900 procedures performed in 2022* alone.

Forecasts project a *compound annual growth rate (CAGR) of 24%* from 2024 to 2033. With an estimated *prevalence of 7.3%* for isolated AS, the *TAVI-eligible population in India* is estimated at *around 300,000 individuals*.[4] The widespread availability of *echocardiography and cardiac CT* has facilitated earlier detection of AS, even before symptoms manifest. However, challenges unique to the Indian setting include *streamlining procedural logistics, reducing costs,* and *addressing concerns over valve durability* in *younger low-risk individuals*. Sahu et al. found that *60%* of TAVI patients in India are *younger than 60 years*.[5] Moreover, a large single-center study indicated a *33% prevalence of bicuspid valve stenosis* in Indian TAVI candidates.[6] Interestingly, compared to the US and Europe, India tends to offer TAVI more frequently to younger patients, often due to *socioeconomic considerations, residual life expectancy, and patient preferences*. The *NOTION-2 trial*—a randomized study evaluating TAVI versus SAVR in *low-risk patients*, including those with BAV—reported *comparable clinical outcomes*.[7] As India's aging population grows and affordability improves, TAVI is poised to become a *transformative milestone* in the country's medical practice.

PATHOPHYSIOLOGY AND PROGRESSION IN YOUNG PATIENTS

The prevalence of *BAV* ranges from *0.5 to 1%*, frequently accompanied by *aortopathy*. Compared to trileaflet valves, BAV typically results in stenosis *a decade earlier*, making it the primary pathology in patients younger than 65 years. Studies suggest that such individuals face a *50% lifetime risk* of requiring aortic valve replacement.[3] In younger patients, calcification progresses rapidly due to abnormal flow dynamics associated with BAV. These patients often remain asymptomatic despite *left ventricular (LV) remodeling*, preserved *ejection fraction (EF)*, and *progressive subclinical myocardial dysfunction*. Research has shown that myocardial fibrosis and reductions in *GLS* can precede symptoms and serve as early indicators of adverse outcomes.[8]

DECISION-MAKING CONSIDERATIONS FOR TRANSCATHETER AORTIC VALVE REPLACEMENT IN LOW-RISK AND YOUNG PATIENTS

- *Age and life expectancy*: Age and projected life expectancy remain foundational in guiding treatment decisions. The *2020 American Heart Association (AHA)/American College of Cardiology (ACC)* guidelines[9] emphasize tailoring therapy based on life expectancy, patient preference, anticoagulation needs, and the likelihood of future interventions.
  - Patients under 65 years with a life expectancy exceeding 20 years are generally advised to undergo SAVR.
  - For patients younger than 50 years with no contraindications to anticoagulation, mechanical valves or the Ross procedure is preferred.
  - Those aged 50–65 years should engage in shared decision-making (SDM) to select between mechanical and biological prostheses.

The *2021 European guidelines 10* were more conservative, recommending *SAVR for all low-risk patients under 75 years*. The latest *ESC/EACTS Guidelines 2025* now support TAVI/TAVR for patients aged 70 years or older, regardless of their surgical risk, down from the previous cut-off of 75 years. This reflects expanded evidence showing safety and efficacy for TAVR in somewhat younger populations. For patients under 70, especially those at low surgical risk or with bicuspid valve anatomy, SAVR remains the preferred option.[28]

Despite these recommendations, registry data from the US show a *rapid increase in TAVR among patients younger than 65 years, with usage equalizing with SAVR* by 2021 in the *Vizient Database*.[11] As shown in **Figure 1**, life expectancy at birth in India was 71 in 2023 when compared to 77.8 in United States and 81.5 in Europe. Hence, residual life expectancy should also be taken into consideration while making clinical decisions for Indian patients.

- *High-risk surgical anatomy*: Anatomical considerations like prior coronary artery bypass grafting (CABG) or heavily calcified/porcelain aortas elevate the risks of surgery. These conditions often exclude patients from low-risk TAVR trials but may favor TAVR in real-world scenarios.[12]
- *Peripheral artery disease (PAD)*: SAVR is typically advised in patients with inadequate iliofemoral access or significant PAD.[13] Alternative access routes (e.g., transaxillary and transcarotid) may be pursued at high-volume centers equipped with hybrid ORs.
- *Annular dimension extremes*: Patients with very large or small annuli falling outside the device size range may be better suited for SAVR. In small annuli, aortic root enlargement during SAVR can facilitate future reintervention options like valve-in-valve TAVR.[12]
- *Anatomical risk factors for TAVR*: Several anatomical features predict TAVR-related complications,[14] including:
  - Left ventricular outflow tract (LVOT) calcification: It is a strong predictor of paravalvular leak (PVL).
  - Bulky leaflet or annular calcification: It is linked to annular rupture.
  - Low coronary heights, shallow sinuses, and narrow sinotubular junctions: It is associated with coronary obstruction
    - Paravalvular leak (PVL): Moderate to severe PVL increases 30-day mortality threefold and 1-year mortality 2.3-fold.[15] Incidence has dropped with newer-generation valves (e.g., 0.8% in PVT trials, 3.5% in Evolut Low Risk trial) thanks to sealing skirts and better sizing techniques.
    - Annular rupture: It occurs primarily with balloon-expandable valves and postdilatation.

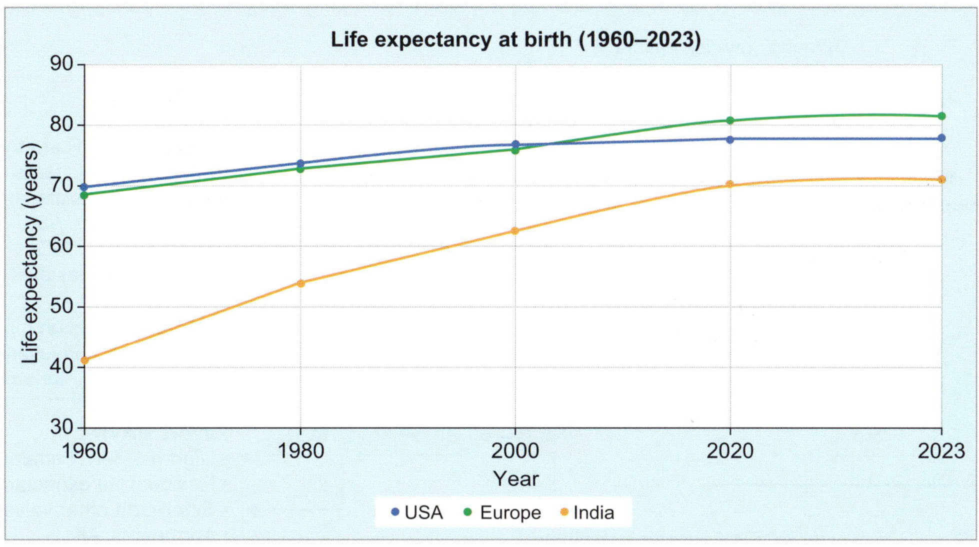

FIG. 1: Life expectancy at birth 1960–2023.

CT predictors include severe calcification, narrow aortic root, or oversizing beyond 20%.[16]

- Coronary obstruction: It occurs in 0.6% of native valve TAVRs, with mortality rates up to 50% despite bail-out percutaneous coronary intervention (PCI).[17] Predictors include coronary height <10 mm, valve-to-coronary distance <4 mm, and leaflet calcium volume >600 mm^3.
- Bicuspid anatomy: Challenges include large annuli, asymmetric or bulky cusp calcification, calcified raphe, and coronary anomalies. In the Nordic NOTION-2 trial,[7] bicuspid patients undergoing TAVR experienced worse mid-term outcomes, although the study was underpowered to reach definitive conclusions. However, Vijay Kumar et al. showed good procedural success rates and clinical outcomes at 2 years in Indian patients. The rates of PVL, pacemaker, and stroke were similar to that of many other studies and registries.[18]

- *Prosthesis-patient mismatch (PPM)*: PPM has been associated with worse outcomes in younger and particularly in patients with reduced LV function.[19] Supra-annular self-expanding valves tend to offer larger effective orifice areas (EOA), lower mean gradients, and lower PPM rates compared to balloon-expandable valves.
- *Coronary artery disease (CAD)*: While 20% of patients in low-risk trials had CAD, those with left main or multivessel disease were excluded. In patients with SYNTAX score >33: SAVR with CABG is preferred according to the guidelines. For lower SYNTAX scores, PCI + TAVR is an acceptable option.[20]
- *Concomitant mitral valve disease*: Primary mitral regurgitation in low-risk patients should be addressed via surgical repair or replacement. Secondary MR often improves post-AVR, but persistent MR is likely with significant mitral annular dilation and mitral annular calcification (MAC).[21]
- *Socioeconomic considerations*: In India, the adoption of TAVI is challenged by unique patient demographics and socioeconomic factors that differ significantly from Western populations. Working-age patients prefer faster recovery of TAVR. Limited social support and urgent noncardiac procedures favor TAVR. Multispecialty care requirements can influence timing and type of intervention. TAVR has shown lower rates of stroke, life-threatening bleeding, atrial fibrillation, and acute kidney injury.[22] Quality-of-life gains are more pronounced at 30 days, according to the Kansas City Cardiomyopathy Questionnaire (KCCQ). Many patients present at a younger age, often with BAVs, and overall life expectancy is lower, which influences long-term procedural planning and valve selection. Additionally, limited healthcare resources and variable insurance coverage make cost-effectiveness a critical consideration. These factors underscore the need for region-specific guidelines that address patient selection, procedural strategies, and device choice tailored to the Indian context, ensuring safe, effective, and equitable delivery of TAVI.
- *Lifetime management and durability*: Bioprosthetic valves deteriorate over time via structural valve deterioration (SVD), non-SVD mechanisms, thrombosis, and endocarditis. Younger patients, women, and those with diabetes mellitus are at higher risk for valve degeneration. Long-term outcomes data is available for SAVR bioprostheses and showed 1.9% reoperation at 10 years and 15% at 20 years. For TAVR, 10-year reintervention was 1.63% in Medicare data from USA.

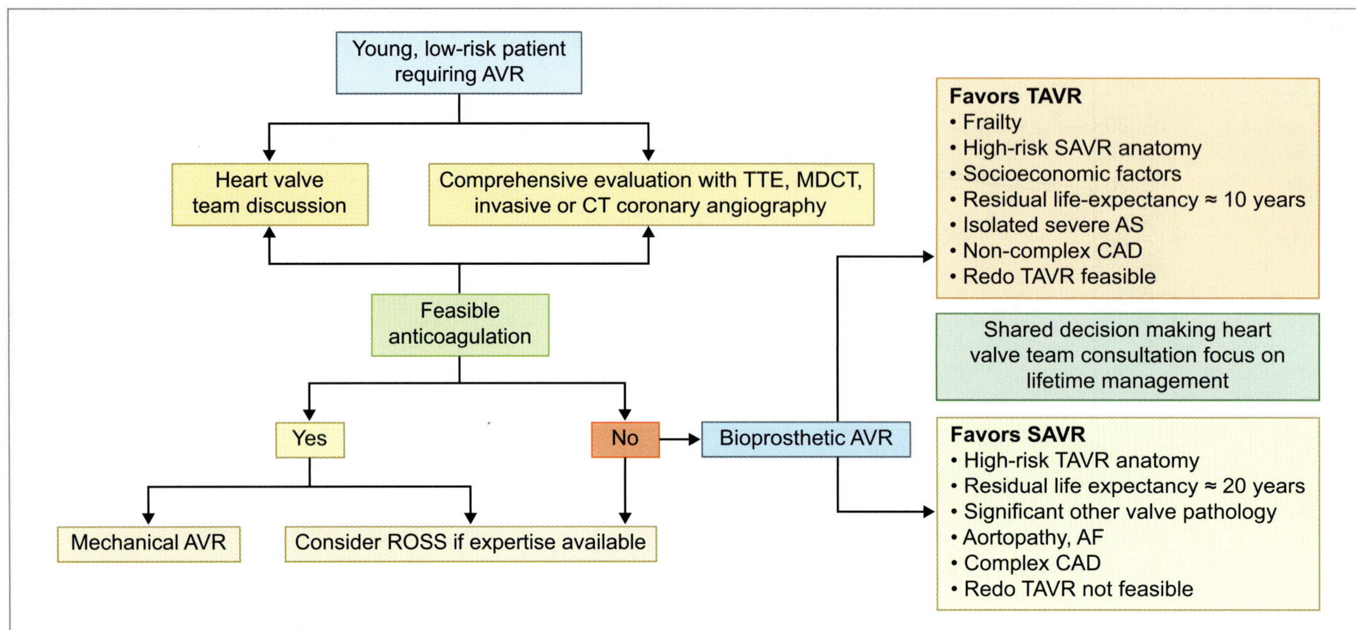

FLOWCHART 1: Approach to young and low-risk patient with severe AS.

Trials such as NOTION-2[7] (lower rates of severe SVD with CoreValve vs. SAVR), PARTNER 3[23] (comparable SVD rates at 5 years between SAPIEN 3 and SAVR), and Evolut Low-Risk trial[24] [4-year reintervention rates (1.3% TAVR vs. 1.7% SAVR)] showed comparable outcomes with SAVR. However, additional long-term data are needed to provide greater clarity.

- *Coronary access after TAVR*: After SAVR, access to coronaries and commissural alignment is ensured. However, in TAVR, spatial relationship between a TAV and the sinus of Valsalva, the position of the bioprosthetic leaflets, the commissural relationship with coronary ostia, and the valve design can limit access. ALIGN-ACCESS[25] and RE-ACCESS 2[26] studies show improved results with balloon-expandable valves and techniques promoting commissural alignment. However, implanting valves lower for better access raises PVL and pacemaker risks.
- *TAVR explantation risks*: Explantation of failed TAVR valves carries significantly higher mortality and morbidity than redo-SAVR, as shown in the EXPLANT-TAVR registry.[27] Patients often transition from low-risk to high-risk status, underscoring the need for judicious patient selection and long-term planning.

CONCLUSION

Choosing between TAVR and SAVR in young and low-risk patients with severe AS is a nuanced process, requiring careful consideration of *anatomy, durability, future intervention feasibility*, and *patient preferences*. While *low-risk trials* affirm TAVR's noninferiority, *long-term data* remain limited in younger populations. Given their *longer life expectancy*, younger patients must be counseled on valve longevity and the potential need for future interventions. A practical approach to young and low risk severe AS patients is summarized in **Flowchart 1**. Ultimately, a *multidisciplinary heart team* must engage in *SDM* to ensure optimal outcomes for the initial procedure while preserving options for future treatments. As clinical evidence continues to evolve, clearer guidance will emerge to shape treatment pathways for this growing demographic.

REFERENCES

1. Beerkens FJ, Tang GH, Kini AS, et al. Transcatheter aortic valve replacement beyond severe aortic stenosis: JACC state-of-the-art review. J Am Coll Cardiol. 2025;85(9):944-64.
2. Yerasi C, Rogers T, Forrestal BJ, et al. Transcatheter versus surgical aortic valve replacement in young, low-risk patients with severe aortic stenosis. Cardiovasc Interven. 2021;14(11): 1169-80.
3. Bulut HI, Arjomandi Rad A, Syrengela AA, et al. A Comprehensive Review of Management Strategies for Bicuspid aortic valve (BAV): exploring Epidemiology, Aetiology, Aortopathy, and interventions in light of recent guidelines. J Cardiovasc Develop Dis. 2023;10(9):398.
4. MD RD, Adivi S, Nukavarapu RR. TAVI in India–a Triumph. Indian J Clin Cardiol. 2024;5(2):113-4.
5. Sahu AK, Sagar P, Khanna R, et al. Etiology and distribution of isolated aortic stenosis in Indian patients–a study from a large tertiary care hospital in north India. Indian Heart J. 2020;72(4): 272-7.

6. Manjunath CN, Srinivas P, Ravindranath KS, et al. Incidence and patterns of valvular heart disease in a tertiary care high-volume cardiac center: a single center experience. Indian Heart J. 2014;66(3):320-6.
7. Jørgensen TH, Thyregod HG, Savontaus M, et al. Transcatheter aortic valve implantation in low-risk tricuspid or bicuspid aortic stenosis: the NOTION-2 trial. Eur Heart J. 2024;45(37):3804-14.
8. Le TT, Huang W, Singh GK, et al. Echocardiographic global longitudinal strain is associated with myocardial fibrosis and predicts outcomes in aortic stenosis. Front Cardiovasc Med. 2021;8:750016.
9. Otto CM, Nishimura RA, Bonow RO, et al. 2020 ACC/AHA guideline for the management of patients with valvular heart disease: executive summary: a report of the American College of Cardiology/American Heart Association Joint Committee on Clinical Practice Guidelines. J Am Coll Cardiol. 2021;77(4):450-500.
10. Vahanian A, Beyersdorf F, Praz F. 2021 ESC/EACTS Guidelines for the management of valvular heart disease: Developed by the Task Force for the management of valvular heart disease of the European Society of Cardiology (ESC) and the European Association for Cardio-Thoracic Surgery (EACTS). Euro Heart J. 2022;43(7):561-632.
11. Gupta T, DeVries JT, Huang HC, et al. Trends in Isolated and Combined Aortic Valve Replacement for Severe Aortic Stenosis in Patients Younger than 65 Years. Struct Heart. 2025;9(8):100684.
12. Gupta T, Malaisrie SC, Batchelor W, et al. Decision-making approach to the treatment of young and low-risk patients with aortic stenosis. Cardiovasc Interven. 2024;17(21):2455-71.
13. Tom S, Tully A, Kikuchi Y, et al. Peripheral intravascular lithotripsy to facilitate transfemoral transcatheter aortic valve replacement–Defining optimal treatable peripheral arterial disease burden. Cardiovasc Revascular Med. 2025;73:31-7.
14. Zou Q, Wei Z, Sun S. Complications in transcatheter aortic valve replacement: a comprehensive analysis and management strategies. Current problems in cardiology. 2024;49(5):102478.
15. Shimokawa A, Yoshitani K, Hayashi H, et al. Impact of Balloon Postdilation on Six-Year Mortality After Transcatheter Aortic Valve Replacement. J Cardiothorac Vasc Anesth. 2021;35(9):2626-30.
16. Tomii D, Pilgrim T, Okuno T, et al. Strategies for treatment of annular rupture complicating transcatheter aortic valve implantation: A retrospective analysis of the Bern TAVI registry. Circ Cardiovasc Interven. 2023;16(6):e012796.
17. Ojeda S, González-Manzanares R, Jiménez-Quevedo P, et al. Coronary obstruction after transcatheter aortic valve replacement: insights from the Spanish TAVI registry. Cardiovasc Interven. 2023;16(10):1208-17.
18. Kumar V, Sengottuvelu G, Singh VP, et al. Transcatheter aortic valve implantation for severe bicuspid aortic stenosis–2 years follow up experience from India. Front Cardiovasc Med. 2022;9:817705.
19. Dismorr M, Glaser N, Franco-Cereceda A, et al. Effect of prosthesis-patient mismatch on long-term clinical outcomes after bioprosthetic aortic valve replacement. J Am Coll Cardiol. 2023;81(10):964-75.
20. Stephan T, Thoma E, Rattka M, et al. Impact of extent of coronary artery disease and percutaneous revascularization assessed by the SYNTAX score on outcomes following transcatheter aortic valve replacement. BMC Cardiovasc Disord. 2021;21(1):568.
21. Mantovani F, Barbieri A, Albini A, et al. The common combination of aortic stenosis with mitral regurgitation: diagnostic insight and therapeutic implications in the modern era of advanced echocardiography and percutaneous intervention. J Clin Med. 2021;10(19):4364.
22. Avvedimento M, Nuche J, Farjat-Pasos JI, et al. Bleeding events after transcatheter aortic valve replacement: JACC state-of-the-art review. J Am Coll Cardiol. 2023;81(7):684-702.
23. Thourani VH, Leon MB, Makkar R, et al. Five-year outcomes in low-risk patients undergoing surgery in the PARTNER 3 trial. Ann Thorac Surg. 2025;119(3):555-66.
24. Forrest JK, Deeb GM, Yakubov SJ, et al. 4-Year outcomes of patients with aortic stenosis in the evolut low risk trial. J Am Coll Cardiol. 2023;82(22):2163-5.
25. Tarantini G, Nai Fovino L, Scotti A, et al. Coronary access after transcatheter aortic valve replacement with commissural alignment: the ALIGN-ACCESS study. Circ Cardiovasc Interven. 2022;15(2):e011045.
26. Costa G, Sammartino S, Strazzieri O, et al. Coronary cannulation following TAVR using self-expanding devices with commissural alignment: the RE-ACCESS 2 study. Cardiovasc Interven. 2024;17(6):727-37.
27. Bapat VN, Zaid S, Fukuhara S, et al. Surgical explantation after TAVR failure: mid-term outcomes from the EXPLANT-TAVR international registry. Cardiovasc Interven. 2021;14(18):1978-91.
28. Praz F, Borger MA, Lanz J et al. 2025 ESC/EACTS Guidelines for the management of valvular heart disease. Eur Heart J. 2025:ehaf194.

CHAPTER

64

Acute Rheumatic Fever and Rheumatic Heart Disease: A Continuum (Recent Advances)

Mohit D Gupta, Girish MP, Gaurav Sharma, Mayank Shami

ABSTRACT

Acute rheumatic fever (ARF) is an autoimmune response to group A streptococcal (GAS) infection leading to multisystem inflammation and, through recurrent episodes, chronic rheumatic heart disease (RHD). ARF–RHD forms a pathophysiologic continuum in which repeated or silent carditis causes progressive valvular fibrosis and stenosis. Though nearly eradicated in high-income countries, RHD persists in low- and middle-income nations—especially India—because of overcrowding, poverty, and poor antibiotic access. Echocardiography detects up to ten-fold more latent disease than clinical examination, redefining global and Indian prevalence estimates. Pathogenesis involves molecular mimicry and collagen-neoantigen mechanisms in genetically susceptible hosts (notably HLA class II and 11q24.1 variants). The 2015 Modified Jones Criteria incorporate echocardiographic detection of subclinical carditis and risk-stratified diagnostic thresholds. Major manifestations include arthritis, carditis, chorea, erythema marginatum, and subcutaneous nodules; carditis determines long-term outcomes. The 2023 World Heart Federation staging (A–D) emphasizes early, screen-detected "latent" RHD amenable to benzathine penicillin G prophylaxis, validated by the GOAL trial. Management spans anti-inflammatory therapy during ARF, guideline-directed percutaneous or surgical valvular intervention for established RHD, and comprehensive prevention—primordial (social), primary (sore-throat treatment), secondary (regular BPG prophylaxis), and tertiary (surgery and rehabilitation). Monthly intramuscular BPG remains the cornerstone; subcutaneous and implantable sustained-release formulations show promise to improve adherence. Global registries (REMEDY, Ina-RHD) and trials (INVICTUS) reveal ongoing gaps in anticoagulation, prophylaxis coverage, and access to intervention, underscoring the need for national surveillance, registry-based recall systems, and coordinated public-health programs to achieve eventual elimination of RHD. This chapter explores the shift from ARF to RHD along with different prevention and treatment strategies.

Keywords: Acute rheumatic fever, rheumatic heart disease, group A *Streptococcus*, secondary prophylaxis, echocardiographic screening, benzathine penicillin G.

INTRODUCTION

Acute rheumatic fever (ARF) is a multisystem autoimmune disorder occurring as a nonsuppurative complication of group A streptococcal (GAS) pharyngitis or impetigo. It affects the joints, heart, brain, skin, and subcutaneous tissues in varying combinations. Although most common in children and adolescents, ARF may occur at any age. Recurrent episodes in populations with limited healthcare access lead to cumulative valvular injury and progression to rheumatic heart disease (RHD) **(Fig. 1)**.

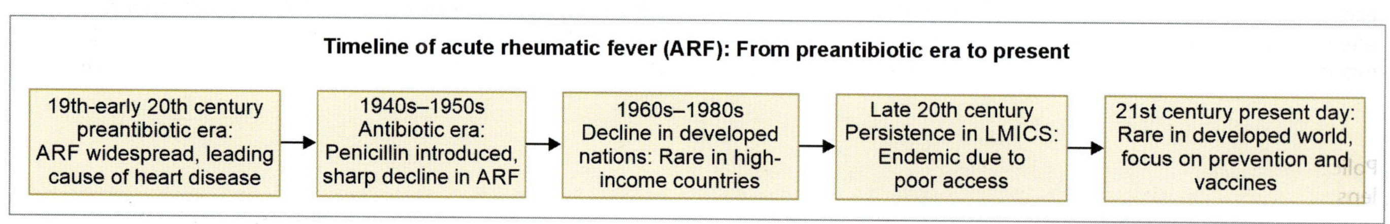

FIG. 1: ARF and RHD: A continuum.

Acute rheumatic fever and RHD represent a disease continuum[1]—ARF is the acute immune-mediated insult following GAS infection, while RHD reflects chronic valvular sequelae from recurrent or silent inflammation. ARF alone seldom causes death, but RHD remains a major cause of heart failure, stroke, and premature mortality in low- and middle-income countries.

Understanding this continuum underpins prevention at multiple levels—early antibiotic therapy for streptococcal infections, long-term secondary prophylaxis to prevent recurrences, and timely intervention for established valve disease. Despite available preventive strategies, RHD persists because of socioeconomic deprivation, overcrowding, and poor access to healthcare. This review summarizes recent advances in epidemiology, pathogenesis, diagnosis, and management, with emphasis on Indian data and key updates such as the 2015 Jones criteria and World Heart Federation classification.

EPIDEMIOLOGY

Acute rheumatic fever is the essential precursor to RHD, which continues to impose a major burden of morbidity and mortality in underprivileged regions.

Global Overview

In high-income countries, both ARF and RHD have nearly disappeared over the past five decades, attributed to improved living standards, early antibiotic therapy, and structured prevention programs. Nevertheless, sporadic outbreaks still occur, linked to emergent rheumatogenic GAS strains and evolving host susceptibility.

Conversely, in "low- and middle-income countries (LMICs)"[2,3] poverty, household overcrowding, and limited access to healthcare sustain ongoing transmission and recurrent infection, perpetuating the ARF–RHD cycle.

Global and Regional Burden

The 2021 Global Burden of Disease (GBD) study estimated approximately 55 million prevalent RHD cases worldwide, reflecting a 70% increase since 1990.[4] The incidence remains highly variable **(Table 1)**:

- *India*: 8.7 per 100,000 school-aged children (5–14 years)[5]
- *Australia (Northern territory, 1997–2010)*: 194 per 100,000[6]
- *New Zealand (2000–2018)*: 38.1 per 100,000 (Pacific), 16.8 (Māori), 0.86 (European)[7]

Indian Perspective

Indian data reveal a clinical RHD prevalence of 1–5.4 per 1,000 schoolchildren (Padmavati et al.),[8] with regional findings of "2.9 per 1,000 (ICMR)",[9] "4.54 per 1,000 (Kanpur)",[10] and "7.7 per 1,000 echocardiographically (RHEUMATIC study)".[11] Subclinical or silent disease remains common, emphasizing the need for echocardiographic screening and national surveillance to define the true burden of ARF and RHD in India.

CLASSIFICATION OF CARDITIS AND RHEUMATIC HEART DISEASE[18]

- Rheumatic cardiac involvement spans a spectrum from overt to silent disease **(Table 2)**. *Clinical carditis* presents with valvular lesions evident on examination. *Subclinical carditis* shows pathological mitral or aortic regurgitation on echocardiography despite normal clinical findings,

TABLE 1: Comparative burden of ARF, latent RHD in India and pitfalls.

Metric	Global	Indian	Why the change matters
ARF incidence	Classic global reviews report ~5–51 per 100,000-child-years; high-income settings typically <10/100,000[12]	Country-wide incidence not available; older North India estimate ~19/100,000 school-age (overall ~32/100,000) in the early 1990s[13]	Globally, we quote incidence; in India the "update" is that we still lack national ARF incidence surveillance
ARF incidence-high-risk pockets	*Surveillance shows very high rates in specific populations*: Australian First Nations 2013→2023 rose from 46.2 to 67.8 per 100,000 (peak 2021 higher)[14]	India almost certainly has high-risk pockets, but without a national notifiable-disease system for ARF[15]	Need for targeted Indian surveillance in tribal/rural and overcrowded urban communities
RHD prevalence by echocardiographic screening (proxy of missed ARF)	Meta-analyses and field studies in endemic settings commonly show ~5–20 per 1,000 schoolchildren by echo, far exceeding clinical detection	*India echo prevalence*: RHEUMATIC (Heart 2011) ~20.4/1,000 in rural North India; multi-site e-RHEUMATIC (2017) 7.7/1,000 by WHF criteria; newer single-site screens ~4–5/1,000 also reported—still many-fold above clinical pick-up[9,16]	The "update" is to present RHD echo prevalence as the more truthful burden indicator for India and to argue for school/community echo programs
Policy/Guidelines lens	WHO 2024 guideline modernizes prevention/diagnosis (including skin-infection pathways) and standardizes reporting	Indian analyses stress the absence of national registries and call for periodic, standardized surveys and registers[17]	Harmonize Indian data collection to the WHO 2024 so results can be compared and acted upon

TABLE 2: Taxonomy of RHD detection and estimated occurrence.

RHD classification	Operational definition in literature	Pooled prevalence (per 1,000)*
Clinical RHD	Audible murmur + echo evidence (clinically manifested)	2.7 (95% CI 1.6–4.4)[19]
"Missed clinical" RHD (i.e., cases missed by examination and found on echo)	Echo-detected without a murmur (clinically silent/latent)	21.1 (95% CI 14.1–31.4)[19]
Latent RHD Definite (WHF 2012)	Meets WHF "definite" criteria (echo)	11.4 (6.7–17.2)[20]
Latent RHD-borderline (WHF 2012)	Meets WHF "borderline" criteria (echo)	15.2 (10.5–20.7)[20]
Subclinical carditis in ARF (different denominator)	Echo evidence of valvulitis during ARF with no murmur	12–21%[21] *Pooled estimate*: 16.8% of ARF cases[21]

**Pooled prevalences are per 1,000 school-age children.*

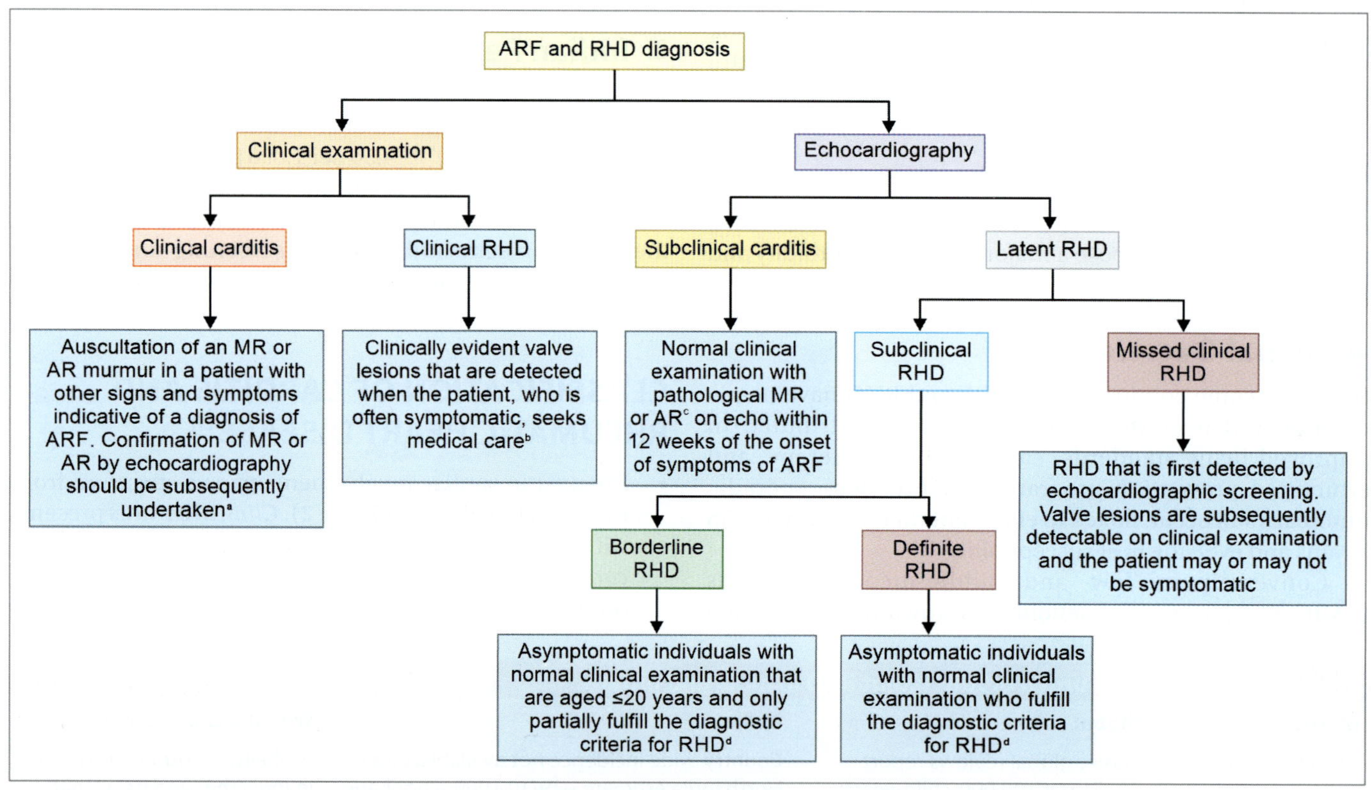

[a]Isolated pericarditis or myocarditis are not suf cient for a diagnosis of rheumatic carditis.
[b]Detection of a pathologic heart murmur without echocardiography is poorly sensitive and specic in echocardiographic screening studies for RHD.
[c]As de ned by the 2015 Jones criteria.
[d]As de ned by the 2012 World Heart Federation RHD diagnostic guidelines.

FLOWCHART 1: Proposed classification of rheumatic carditis and rheumatic heart disease (RHD).[18]
(AR: aortic regurgitation; ARF: acute rheumatic fever; MR: mitral regurgitation)

usually within 12 weeks of ARF onset. *Latent RHD* includes asymptomatic individuals fulfilling echocardiographic criteria, categorized as *definite* or *borderline* (≤20 years) **(Flowchart 1)**.*Missed clinical RHD* is first detected by screening echo, later clinically apparent.

- Echocardiography identifies about 10 times more RHD than auscultation in endemic regions; over two-thirds of patients recall no prior ARF. Latent disease progresses in 8% without prophylaxis versus 0.8% with regular 4-weekly benzathine penicillin.

PATHOPHYSIOLOGY OF ACUTE RHEUMATIC FEVER AND RHEUMATIC HEART DISEASE[18]

Acute rheumatic fever evolves through a defined sequence from *group A β-hemolytic Streptococcus* (GAS) infection to chronic valvular damage. Only 0.9–19% of sore throats are caused by GAS; among these, 0.3–3% progress to ARF after a latent interval, and 20–30% of ARF cases develop chronic RHD **(Flowchart 2)**.[5]

Initiation and Pathogen Factors

Group A streptococcal pharyngitis is the predominant trigger, though impetigo and scabies-associated skin infections also contribute, especially in high-risk indigenous and tropical populations.[20] Occasionally, *Group C* or *G streptococci* are implicated. Virulence relates to *M-protein* (emm-type) diversity rather than a single rheumatogenic strain.

Host Susceptibility

Disease expression depends on genetic and environmental factors—poverty, overcrowding, and limited antibiotic access. Many patients with established RHD recall no symptomatic ARF, highlighting the silent progression of subclinical carditis detectable only by echocardiography.

Immune Injury Mechanisms (Flowchart 3)

Two principal autoimmune pathways mediate valve injury:

- *Molecular mimicry:* Antibodies to GAS M-protein and N-acetyl-β-D-glucosamine cross-react with cardiac myosin, triggering endothelial activation (↑VCAM-1) and CD4+ T-cell infiltration; Th1 cytokines (IFN-γ, TNF-α) cause matrix injury and fibrosis.[18]
- *Collagen neoantigen theory:* M-protein PARF motifs bind type IV collagen (CB3 domain), forming neoantigens that provoke anti-collagen responses, worsening endothelial injury and valvular deformation.

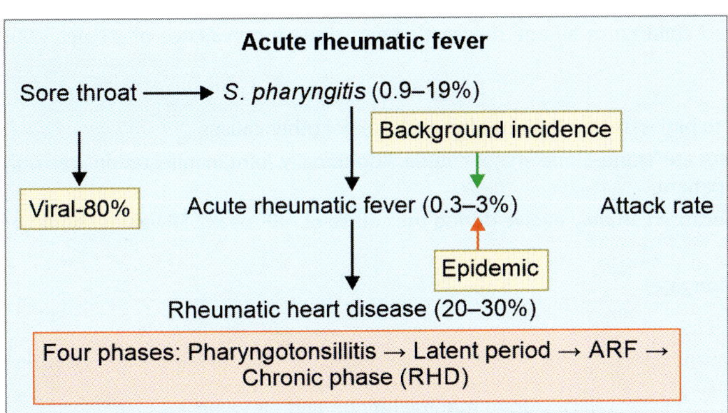

FLOWCHART 2: Natural history of sore throat.

Structural and Progressive Changes

Incomplete healing of carditis, or repeated subclinical episodes, produces leaflet thickening, commissural fusion, and chordal shortening. Early regurgitation often precedes eventual stenosis and multivalvular involvement.

Emerging Insights

Persistent inflammation shows a Th17/IL-17 bias with neo-angiogenesis, myofibroblast activation, and osteogenic remodeling driving stenosis. Valve proteomics reveals vimentin and lumican overexpression, confirming a chronic autoimmune process. Regular secondary prophylaxis halts immune reactivation and slows progression from latent to definite RHD.[22,23]

What are the Genetic Associations?

- Class 8 region of HLA (Indian and South African studies)
- HLA-DQA1, DQB1 (Australian study)
- 11q24.1 (RHD Gen Study)
- IGHV4-61*02 allele is strongly associated with an increased risk of RHD, with each copy of the allele increasing the risk by approximately 1.4-fold.

Point of care testing for GAS pharyngitis: *Gene expert*

- Good negative predictive value
- 100% sensitivity and 79% specificity
- False positive for dead DNA even after infection

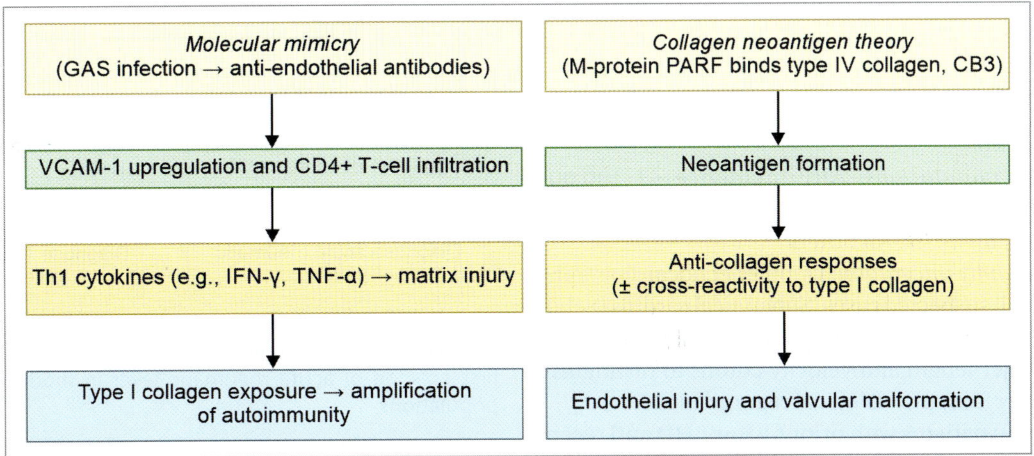

FLOWCHART 3: Two-pathway immune injury model of ARF carditis.[18]

TABLE 3: Modified jones criteria.[24]

A. For all patient populations with evidence of preceding group A streptococcal infection (other than chorea)	
Diagnosis: Initial ARF	Two major or one major plus two minor manifestations
Diagnosis: recurrent ARF	Two major or one major and two minor or three minor
B. Major criteria	
Low-risk populations[a]	Moderate- and high-risk populations
Carditis[b] (clinical and/or subclinical)	Carditis[b] (Clinical and/or subclinical)
Arthritis (polyarthritis only)	Arthritis (monoarthritis or polyarthritis or polyarthralgia[c])
Chorea	Chorea
Erythema marginatum	Erythema marginatum
Subcutaneous nodules	Subcutaneous nodules
C. Minor criteria	
Low-risk populations[a]	Moderate- and high-risk populations
Polyarthralgia	Monoarthralgia
Fever (≥38.5°C)	Fever (≥38°C)
ESR ≥60 mm/h and/or CRP ≥3 mg/dL[d]	ESR ≥30 mm/h and/or CRP ≥3 mg/dL[d]
Prolonged PR on ECG (for age) (unless carditis is a major criterion)	Prolonged PR on ECG (for age) (unless carditis is a major criterion)

*Prepared by utilizing the reference number 10.

[a]Low-risk populations are those with ARF incidence ≤2 per 100 000 school-aged children or all-age rheumatic heart disease prevalence of ≤1 per 1,000 population per year.

[b]Subclinical carditis is pathological echocardiographic valvulitis.

[c]Polyarthralgia should only be considered as a major manifestation in moderate- to high-risk populations after exclusion of other causes.

As in past versions of the criteria erythema marginatum and subcutaneous nodules are "stand-alone" major criteria. Additionally, joint manifestations can only be considered in either the major or minor categories but not both in the same patient.

[d]CRP value must be greater than upper limit of normal for the laboratory. Also, because ESR may evolve during the course of ARF, peak ESR values should be used.

(ARF: acute rheumatic fever; CRP: C-reactive protein; ESR: erythrocyte sedimentation rate)

THE MODIFIED JONES CRITERIA (2015)[24] (TABLE 3 AND FLOWCHART 4)

The 2015 Modified Jones Criteria offer a risk-based framework for diagnosing ARF, acknowledging its rarity in high-income countries and persistence in endemic, resource-limited areas.

Key Modifications

- *Risk stratification:*
  - *Low-risk populations:* ARF incidence ≤2/100,000 (ages 5–14) or all-age RHD prevalence ≤1/1,000
  - *Moderate/high-risk:* All others
- *Echocardiography integration*: Doppler echocardiography is advised in all suspected cases. Subclinical carditis (echo-only MR/AR) counts as a major criterion for all populations, with defined jet-length and velocity cutoffs to distinguish true pathology from physiological regurgitation.
- *Recurrences:* In patients with prior ARF or RHD and recent GAS infection, recurrence is diagnosed by two major, one major + two minor, or three minor criteria. Chorea and indolent carditis may be diagnosed even without GAS evidence.

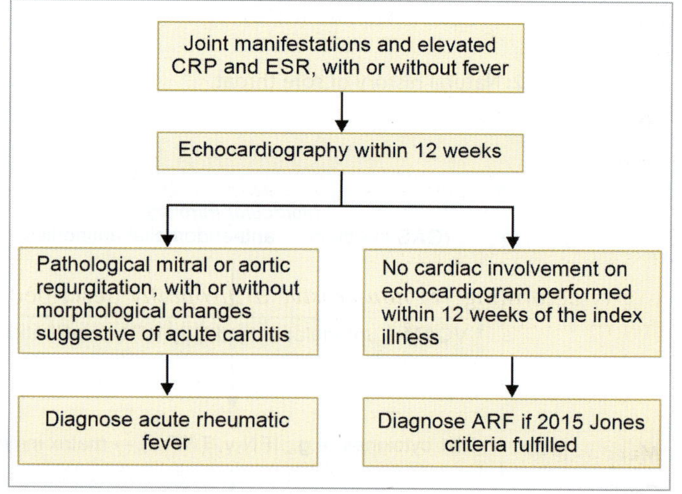

FLOWCHART 4: A simplified algorithm for the diagnosis of a first episode of acute rheumatic fever in moderate and high-risk populations.

- *Evidence of preceding GAS infection*: Documented by elevated ASO or anti-DNase B titers, positive throat culture, or rapid antigen testing—except in isolated chorea or indolent carditis.

- *Probable ARF:* When suspicion is strong but criteria are unmet, prophylactic *benzathine penicillin G* for 12 months and reassessment are advised.

Clinical Definitions

- *Relapse:* Worsening during therapy, usually due to active carditis—managed by escalating anti-inflammatory treatment.
- *Rebound:* Recurrence after steroid taper (4–6 weeks); prevented by gradual withdrawal.
- *Recurrent ARF:* A new episode after prior ARF/RHD, meeting recurrence criteria.

MAJOR MANIFESTATIONS OF ACUTE RHEUMATIC FEVER (FIRST EPISODE) (TABLE 4)

Arthritis[24]

Onset and Frequency

Arthritis typically appears 2–3 weeks after streptococcal pharyngitis and is the most common initial manifestation, occurring in 60–80% of patients. It is nonsuppurative, asymmetric, and migratory, predominantly affecting large joints—the knees, ankles, elbows, and wrists.

Clinical Features

The presentation is acute, with warmth, swelling, and severe tenderness but no pus formation. Characteristically, pain resolves rapidly—within 48–72 hours of aspirin or NSAID therapy. Lack of response should prompt reconsideration of the diagnosis; resistant cases may require a short steroid course.

Course and Outcome

Symptoms resolve spontaneously within 2–3 weeks and leave no residual joint deformity. Chronic damage is rare.

Jaccoud's Arthropathy

A rare, deforming yet *non-erosive arthropathy* described after rheumatic fever. It manifests as *ulnar deviation of the 2nd–5th fingers* with correctable metacarpophalangeal (MCP) subluxation and normal radiographs. Although historically linked to ARF, similar changes may occur in lupus, psoriatic arthritis, and inflammatory bowel disease.

TABLE 4: Major criteria of Modified Jone's criteria (2015).

Manifestation	Frequency
Carditis	50–70%
Arthritis	35–66%
Chorea	10–30%
Subcutaneous nodules	0–10%
Erythema marginatum	<6%
Subclinical carditis	12–21%

Carditis[24]

Frequency and Onset

Rheumatic carditis occurs in 50–80% of ARF cases, typically within 2–3 weeks of GAS infection. The severity has declined markedly in the antibiotic era.

Nature and Pathology

Usually presents as pancarditis, involving endocardium, myocardium, and pericardium. The disease may resolve completely or cause permanent valvular injury, particularly after recurrent episodes.

Clinical Findings

- *Tachycardia* and *new murmurs* are common.
- *Pericarditis* may present with a rub or effusion; tamponade and constriction are rare.
- *Myocarditis* produces LV dilatation and heart failure, with a soft S_1 and gallop rhythm.
- *Arrhythmias:* PR prolongation is typical; advanced blocks are rare.[21]

Valve Involvement[21]

- *Mitral valve*: 50–60%
- *Aortic*: ~20%
- *Tricuspid*: ~10%

Diagnostics

Echocardiography confirms MR/AR; chest X-ray shows cardiomegaly; ECG reveals PR prolongation.

Treatment and Outcome

- *Bed rest:* 4–12 weeks depending on severity.
- *Anti-inflammatory therapy:* Aspirin 100 mg/kg/day (mild), prednisolone 2 mg/kg/day (severe).
- *Heart failure management* as indicated.
- *Surgery:* Consider for persistent HF or severe valvular dysfunction after active inflammation subsides.

Recurrence and severity determine the transition to chronic rheumatic heart disease (RHD)—the most critical long-term complication of ARF **(Table 5)**.

SUBCLINICAL AND LATENT RHEUMATIC HEART DISEASE

Subclinical carditis and latent RHD represent silent rheumatic cardiac injury detectable only by echocardiography in the absence of murmurs. Subclinical carditis indicates valvulitis during ARF, whereas *latent RHD* refers to asymptomatic individuals fulfilling echocardiographic criteria for definite or borderline RHD without prior ARF.

A systematic RHD[18,26] review and meta-analysis reported a global pooled prevalence of latent at 1.3% and subclinical carditis at 16.8% (95% CI 11.9–21.6%).[27] In India, the RHEUMATIC study (Saxena et al., 2011) documented an echocardiographic prevalence of 20.4 per 1,000, with 4% worsening, 28% improving, and 68% stable on follow-up.[11] Approximately 12–21% of all RHD cases are subclinical at presentation.[18]

TABLE 5: Some important figures we must remember.[25]

Category	Frequency/Outcome
Carditis in the first episode	30–70%
Carditis in all attacks	73–99%
Prospective studies	33–46%
RHD in follow-up (5–10 years): Once RF	20–30%
RHD in follow-up (5–10 years): Once carditis	45–80%
RHD in follow-up (5–10 years): Chorea	20–34%

Progression from borderline to definite RHD occurs eightfold more frequently than in matched controls. Without secondary prophylaxis, recurrent or silent inflammation promotes cumulative fibrosis and mitral-predominant valvular deformity.

The World Heart Federation (WHF) 2023 classification redefined the disease continuum into stages A–D (at-risk → advanced) and established a two-tier echocardiographic approach, identifying stage B (subclinical/latent) as the key window for early intervention.[28]

The GOAL randomized trial (NEJM 2021) demonstrated that 4-weekly benzathine penicillin G for 2 years reduced progression of latent RHD from 8 to 0.8% (NNT = 13, 95% CI 10–21), proving that timely antibiotic prophylaxis can modify the natural history of screen-detected disease.[29]

Doppler Findings in Rheumatic Valvulitis

Refer to **Tables 6 to 8**.

Sydenham's Chorea

Epidemiology and Onset

Sydenham's chorea (SC) occurs in 10–30% of ARF cases, predominantly in girls aged 5–15 years.[6] Onset is delayed by

TABLE 6: WHF Screening criteria for echocardiographic detection of RHD.[26]

Lesion	Requirement	Criteria
MR	All	*MR jet length*: <30 kg → ≥1.5 cm; ≥30 kg → ≥2.0 cm; observed in at least one view; observed in at least two consecutive frames
AR	All	Any AR; observed in at least 1 view; observed in at least two consecutive frames
MS	–	Restricted leaflet with reduced valve opening
Positive screen	–	Presence of any of the defined MR, AR, or MS

TABLE 7: Confirmatory criteria for pathologic valve dysfunction.[26]

Lesion	Requirement	Criteria
Pathologic MR	All	Observed in at least two views; in at least one view MR jet length ≥1.5 cm (<30 kg) or ≥2.0 cm (≥30 kg); velocity ≥3.0 m/s for one complete envelope; pan-systolic jet in at least one envelope
Pathologic AR	All	Observed in at least two views; in at least one view AR jet length ≥1.0 cm; velocity ≥3.0 m/s in early diastole; pan-diastolic jet in at least one envelope
MS	All	Restricted leaflet motion with reduced valve opening; mean peak gradient ≥4.0 mm Hg

TABLE 8: RHD confirmatory morphologic criteria.[26]

Valve/Structure	Category	Criteria
Mitral valve	Valve apparatus thickening (either or both)	Anterior leaflet thickening; chordal thickening
Mitral valve	Valve mobility abnormalities (either or both)	Restricted anterior or posterior leaflet motion in diastole; excessive anterior leaflet tip motion during systole
Aortic valve	Morphologic changes	Cusp thickening; cusp prolapse; restricted cusp motion; coaptation defect in diastole

1-6 months after streptococcal infection and may occur as an isolated feature once other manifestations have resolved.

Pathophysiology and Clinical Features

Sydenham's chorea is an autoimmune disorder caused by molecular mimicry between GAS antigens and neuronal epitopes, leading to basal ganglia injury. It manifests as involuntary, irregular facial and limb movements that lessen during sleep, with features such as "milkmaid's grip," "darting tongue," dysarthria, and emotional lability.

Course and management: Diagnosis is clinical; most cases resolve in 2-6 months, though relapses occur. Valproate or carbamazepine are first-line, haloperidol for severe cases. Steroids are ineffective. SC causes no cardiac damage but signals high recurrence risk, necessitating long-term benzathine penicillin prophylaxis.

Erythema Marginatum

Epidemiology and Description

An uncommon manifestation (<6%), erythema marginatum usually appears early in ARF, more often in older children.[6] The rash is nonpruritic, evanescent, and composed of pink, annular macules with serpiginous margins and central clearing, affecting the trunk and proximal limbs while sparing the face, palms, and soles.

Diagnosis and Prognosis

Diagnosis is clinical. Lesions resolve spontaneously within hours to days and have no prognostic link with RHD, though they remain a major Jones criterion. Other transient skin eruptions—erythema multiforme, papulatum, urticaria, and erythema nodosum—may rarely occur.

Subcutaneous Nodules

Subcutaneous nodules occur in <10% of cases, usually late in disease and strongly associated with severe carditis.[6] They are small, firm, painless, and mobile, appearing symmetrically over extensor surfaces (elbows, knees, occiput, and spine).

Histology shows fibrinoid necrosis with surrounding inflammation. Lesions resolve within 1-2 weeks without sequelae but are highly specific for ARF, indicate severe cardiac involvement and a higher risk of chronic RHD.

Summary of Treatment

Refer to **Table 9**.

OTHER MANIFESTATIONS OF ACUTE RHEUMATIC FEVER

Occasional Systemic Features Lack Diagnostic Specificity

Abdominal pain (previous minor Jones criterion, 1956); transient fever, epistaxis, and hemoptysis (from 1944 criteria) need no specific therapy. Rheumatic pneumonitis presents as ARDS-like alveolitis managed with corticosteroids and ventilatory support, while glomerulonephritis causes mild hematuria or proteinuria with urinary casts.

RHEUMATIC HEART DISEASE

Clinical Spectrum

Rheumatic heart disease presents in adolescence or early adulthood with mitral regurgitation ± stenosis, evolving to atrial fibrillation (AF), pulmonary hypertension (PH), and right-heart failure. Echo shows leaflet thickening, commissural fusion, and chordal shortening. Recent cohorts highlight two patterns—(1) a reservoir of asymptomatic echo-only disease and (2) high-mortality symptomatic cases lacking intervention. Early anticoagulation, HF optimization, and percutaneous mitral valvotomy improve outcomes **(Table 10)**.

Multivalvular Rheumatic Heart Disease[25,26]

Concurrent involvement of ≥2 valves—typically mitral + aortic ± tricuspid—remains the leading cause of multivalvular

TABLE 9: Treatment summary of rheumatic fever.

Clinical	Drug	Dose	Schedule
Severe carditis	Prednisone	2 mg/kg/day (maximum 80 mg)	Once daily
Moderate carditis	Prednisone/aspirin	1–2 mg/kg/day, 75–100 mg/kg/day	Once daily divided into four doses
Mild carditis	Aspirin	50–60 mg/kg/day, maximum of 80–100 mg/kg	Divided into four doses
Polyarthritis	Aspirin Naproxen	75–100 mg/kg/day, 10–20 mg/kg/day	Divided into four doses. Divided into two doses
Chorea	Carbamazepine/valproic acid/haloperidol	4–10 mg/kg/day, 20–30 mg/kg/day, 2–6 mg/day	Divided into two doses/divided into two doses/ divided into two/three doses

TABLE 10: Indications for BMV.[33]

Recommendations	Class[a]	Level[b]
PMC is recommended in symptomatic patients in the absence of unfavorable characteristics for PMC	I	B
PMC is recommended in any symptomatic patients with a contraindication or at high risk for surgery	I	C
MV surgery is recommended in symptomatic patients who are not suitable for PMC	I	C
PMC should be considered as initial treatment in symptomatic patients with suboptimal anatomy but no unfavorable clinical characteristics for PMC	IIa	C
PMC should be considered in asymptomatic patients without unfavorable clinical and anatomical characteristics for PMC, and: • High thromboembolic risk (history of systemic embolism, dense spontaneous contrast in the LA, new-onset or paroxysmal AF), and/or • High risk of hemodynamic decompensation (sPAP >50 mm Hg at rest, need for major noncardiac surgery, pregnant or desire for pregnancy)	IIa	C
TMVI may be considered in symptomatic patients with extensive MAC and severe MV dysfunction at experienced heart valve centers with expertise in complex MV surgery and transcatheter interventions	IIb	C

[a]class of evidence.

[b]level of evidence.

disease in LMICs. Tricuspid lesions are usually functional, secondary to left-sided disease and AF; organic TR/TS occurs mainly with rheumatic MS. The Ina-RHD registry (n = 3,431) showed frequent AF, RV dysfunction, and underuse of secondary prophylaxis, underscoring the need for routine tricuspid evaluation.[30]

Indian Data (Manjunath et al., IHJ 2014)[31]

Among 136,098 echocardiograms, RHD = 64.3% of valvular disease.

- *Mitral:* 84.7%; *Aortic*: 35.8%; *Tricuspid*: 9.7%.
- *Isolated MS*: 97.4% rheumatic, female predominance, PH in 57.6%.
- *Isolated MR*: 25.6% of all cases; 41.1% rheumatic, 40.8% myxomatous.
- *Multivalvular RHD*: 36.8% of all VHD (MS + MR 46.6%; MS + AR 26.5%; MR + AR 23.3%; MS + AS 2.4%; MR + AS 0.9%; AS + AR 0.3%)
- *Organic tricuspid disease*: ≈ 10%.

Hemodynamics and Imaging[32]

Key interactions: MS + MR → ↑ LA pressure → PH/AF; MS + AR → masked AR severity; MR + AR → severe LV volume overload; MS ± MR + TR → RV dilation due to pulmonary hypertension and functional TR.

Accurate assessment demands multimodality imaging—CT for calcific AS, MRI for regurgitant quantification, and TEE for commissural anatomy and LA thrombus **(Table 11)**.

PREVENTION OF ACUTE RHEUMATIC FEVER AND RHEUMATIC HEART DISEASE

Prevention of RHD spans a continuum—from community measures limiting GAS transmission to antibiotic prophylaxis that halts progression after infection. Coordinated primordial, primary, secondary, and tertiary prevention remains the cornerstone for interrupting the infection-to-valve-damage pathway **(Flowchart 5)**.

Primordial Prevention[35]

This level targets the *social determinants* of GAS spread. Overcrowding, poor housing, inadequate ventilation, and poor sanitation are key drivers. Population-wide improvements in housing, school health, and hygiene education have sharply reduced ARF incidence to <1 per 100,000 in nations such as Cuba, Costa Rica, and Martinique following major public-health reforms.

Primary Prevention

The aim is to prevent the first ARF episode by prompt recognition and treatment of streptococcal pharyngitis or impetigo. Because most sore throats are viral, the Modified Centor (McIsaac) criteria (1998)[36,37] **(Fig. 2)** guide rational testing and therapy:

- *Score 0–1:* No testing or antibiotics
- *Score 2–3:* RADT or culture → treat if positive
- *Score ≥ 4:* empiric antibiotics

A single intramuscular dose of benzathine penicillin G lowers ARF risk by ≈ 80 %.[38] 10-day oral penicillin V or amoxicillin are alternatives; different drug regimens for primary prevention are described in **Table 12**.

Implementation Evidence

- A *cluster-randomized Nepal trial* validated school-based echocardiographic screening plus antibiotic therapy.[39]
- *Cuba and Costa Rica* virtually eliminated new ARF cases through systematic sore-throat programs.
- In *high-risk South-African communities*, algorithm-guided diagnosis with single-dose IM penicillin proved *more cost-effective* than laboratory confirmation.[40]

TABLE 11: Echocardiographic pitfalls and supportive measures in multivalvular heart disease.

	Valve lesion to be assessed			
Concomitant valve lesion	**AS**	**AR**	**MS**	**MR**
AS	—	PHT unreliable blunted ↑ LV volume (LVH, disproportionate diastolic LV pressure overload)	PHT unreliable Gradient ↓ (LF)	Regurgitant volume ↑ Jet area ↑ (↑ afterload and transmitral systolic pressure gradient)
AR	ΔG ↑ when LVOT velocity ↑	—	*PHT*: Unreliable *MVA by continuity*: Unreliable	Mitral-to-aortic VTI ratio is unreliable (increased transaortic flow)
MS	*AS*: LF–LG possible	Blunted ↑ in LV volume (preload ↓)	—	M-Ao VTI ratio unreliable (increased mitral VTI due to stenosis) Ca^{++} may shadow jet area
MR	*AS*: LF–LG AS Jet confused with MR jet	PHT unreliable Doppler volumetric method using net mitral forward flow invalid (↑ flow)	PHT unreliable (altered LA and LV compliance) Continuity equation unreliable (Transmitral flow ↑)	—
TR	*AS*: LF–LG	—	LF-LG PHT unreliable (impaired LV filling due to ventricular interdependence)	Regurgitant volume ↓ (preload ↓)
Robust echo measurements	AVA, DVI *In AS + AR*: V_{max} and ΔMG = Combined burden	EROA (PISA), VC	Planimetry/3D MVA (TOE) *MR + MS*: ΔMG = Combined burden	EROA (PISA), VC
Alternative imaging	*CT*: AV calcium score	*CMR*: Reg vol, %	—	*CMR*: Reg vol, %

[↑: increase; ↓: decrease; 3D: three-dimensional; Ao: aortic/aorta; AR: aortic regurgitation; AS: aortic stenosis; AV: aortic valve; AVA: aortic valve area; AVC: aortic valve calcium score; Ca^{++}: calcification (calcium deposits); CMR: cardiac magnetic resonance; CT: computed tomography; DVI: dimensionless velocity index; EROA: effective regurgitant orifice area; LA: left atrium; LF: low flow; LG: low gradient; LV: left ventricle; LVH: left ventricular hypertrophy; LVOT: left ventricular outflow tract; M/A VTI ratio: mitral-to-aortic VTI ratio; MR: mitral regurgitation; MS: mitral stenosis; MV: mitral valve; MVA: mitral valve area; PHT: pressure half-time; PISA: proximal isovelocity surface area; Reg: frac regurgitant fraction (%); Reg vol: regurgitant volume; RV: right ventricle; SMR: secondary mitral regurgitation; TOE: transoesophageal echocardiography; TR: tricuspid regurgitation; VC: vena contracta; VI: ventricular interdependence; V_{max}: peak jet velocity; VTI: velocity-time integral; ΔMG: mean transvalvular gradient]

Limitations

Up to one-third of ARF patients recall no sore throat, and asymptomatic GAS carriage may exceed 50% during outbreaks, limiting symptom-based screening alone. Integrated community and prophylactic approaches are therefore essential for durable RHD control.[41]

Vaccine Development

With GAS now classified by the World Health Organization (WHO) as a priority pathogen, vaccine development has gained renewed global impetus. Coordinated initiatives such as the Strep A Vaccine Global Consortium (SAVAC) and the Australian Strep A Vaccine Initiative (ASAVI) are advancing candidates targeting conserved GAS antigens. Successful immunization would prevent the first episode of ARF, offering the most sustainable, currently we have few vaccines in research long-term strategy to eliminate RHD in endemic regions **(Table 13)**.

Secondary Prophylaxis

Long-acting benzathine penicillin G (BPG) every 3–4 weeks remains the cornerstone of RHD control, preventing recurrences and valve damage. Oral regimens are less effective, while ≥80% adherence lowers recurrence risk four-fold (risk remains high until at least 40% doses are received).

Duration

- *Carditis:* ≥10 years or to age 25–40 years
- *Severe/Postsurgical*: Lifelong.
- *No carditis*: 5 years or to age 18–21 years (whichever longer).

Although different guidelines have different recommendations **(Table 14)**.

Sustained adherence to BPG prophylaxis remains the most proven, cost-effective strategy for long-term RHD prevention.

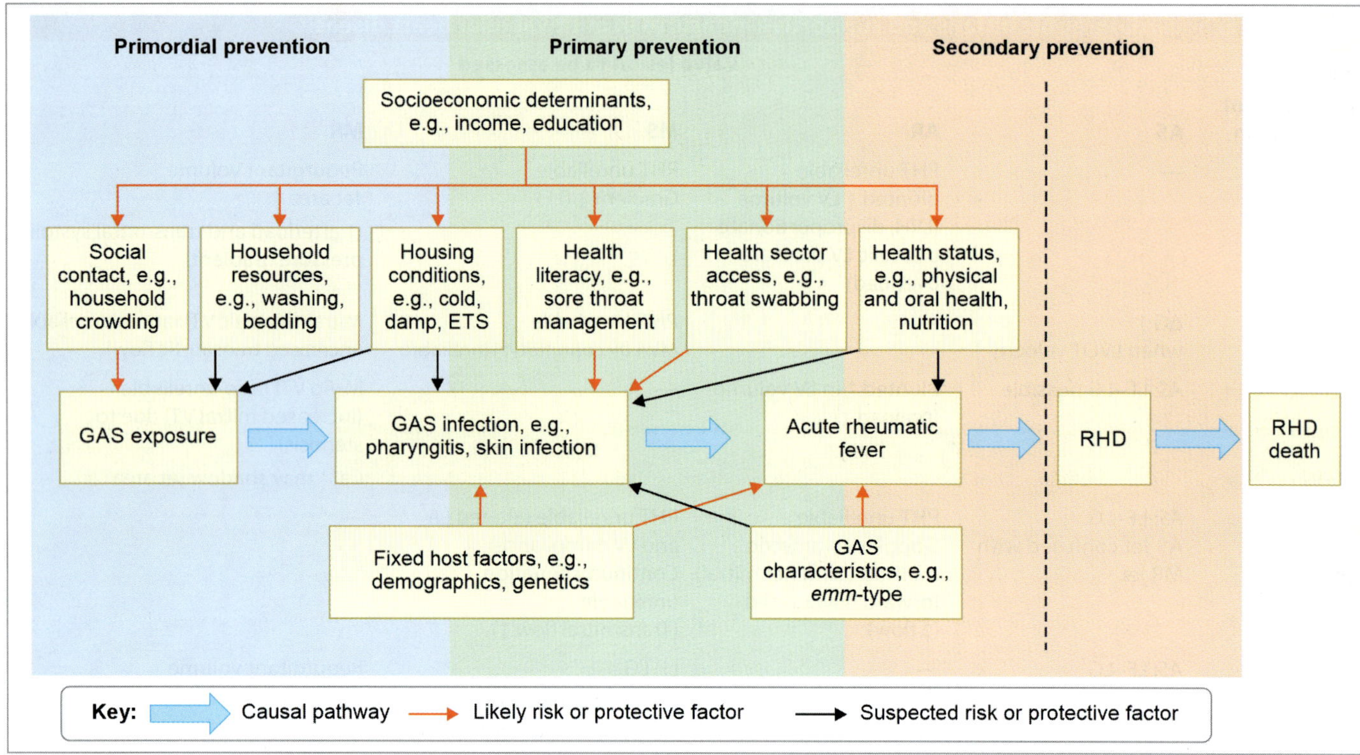

FLOWCHART 5: Levels of prevention of ARF and RHD.[34]

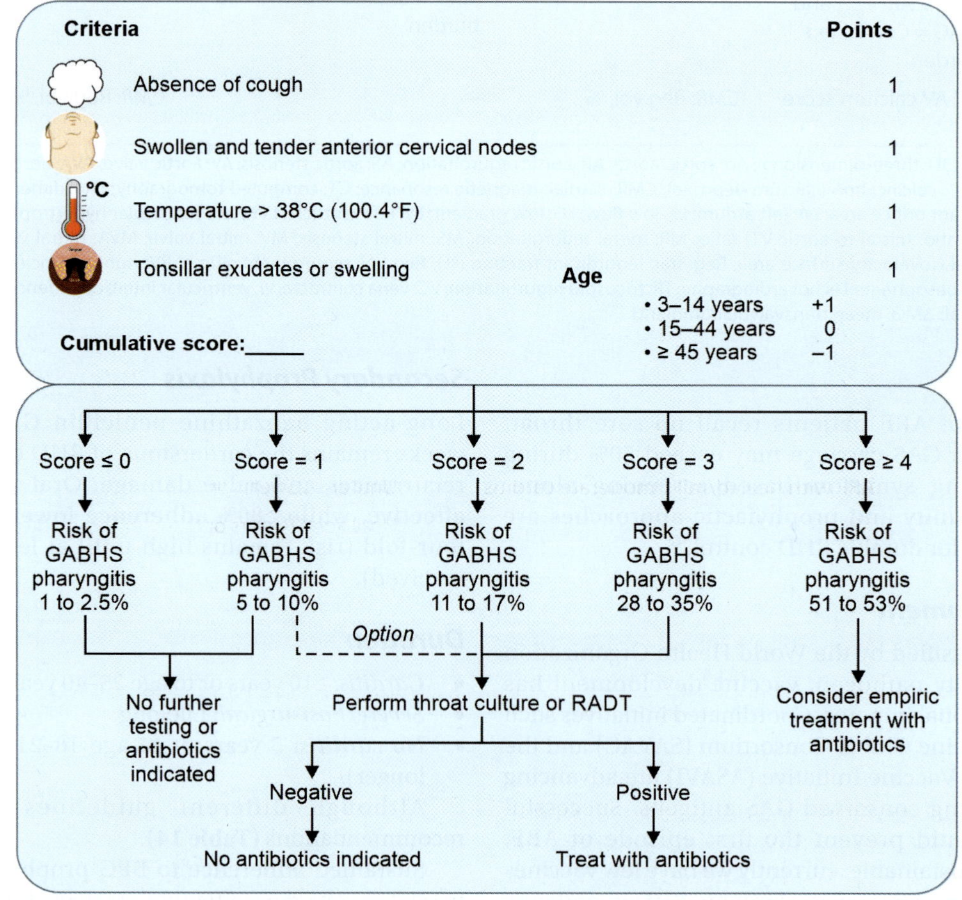

FIG. 2: Modified Centor Criteria.

TABLE 12: Drug regimens for primary prevention of rheumatic fever.

Agent	Dose	Route	Duration
Penicillin V (phenoxymethyl penicillin)	*Children ≤27 kg*: 250 mg 2–3 times daily *Children >27 kg*: 500 mg 2–3 times daily *Adolescents/adults*: 500 mg 2–3 times daily	Oral	10 days
Amoxicillin	50 mg/kg once daily (maximum 1 g)	Oral	10 days
Benzathine penicillin G	*≤27 kg*: 600,000 U IM once *>27 kg*: 1,200,000 U IM once	IM	Once
Narrow-spectrum cephalosporin (cephalexin, cefadroxil)*	Variable	Oral	10 days
Clindamycin	20 mg/kg/day in 3 doses (maximum 1.8 g/day)	Oral	10 days
Azithromycin	12 mg/kg once daily (maximum 500 mg)	Oral	5 days
Clarithromycin	15 mg/kg/day divided bid (maximum 250 mg bid)	Oral	10 days

*To be avoided in those with immediate (Type I) hypersensitivity reaction to a penicillin.

TABLE 13: Vaccines in research.

Platform	Candidate (example)	Key findings	Status
M-protein–based	*StreptNova (30-valent)*	Safe, immunogenic, no autoimmune cross-reactivity	Phase 1 completed[42]
	J8/S2 Combivax and P17/S2 Combivax	Strong preclinical immune response	Phase 1/2 underway[43]
	StrepInCor	Effective in animal models	Preclinical → phase 1 ready[44]
Non-M protein	*Combo5, Teevax*	Broad strain coverage	Preclinical[45]
Group A carbohydrate (GAC)	*VAX-A1* (modified GAC without GlcNAc side chains)	High immunogenicity without cross-reactivity	Preclinical[46]

TABLE 14: Recommended durations of secondary prophylaxis according to international guidelines.

Guideline	Scenario	Recommended duration
AHA (2009)[47]	ARF with carditis and residual heart disease	Until age 40 years or 10 years after last ARF (whichever longer); lifetime prophylaxis may be required
	ARF with carditis but no residual heart disease	Until age 21 years or 10 years after last ARF (whichever longer)
	ARF without carditis	Until age 21 years or 5 years after last ARF (whichever longer)
WHO Expert Consultation, Geneva (2004)[28]	Severe valvular disease/post-valve surgery	Lifelong prophylaxis
	ARF with carditis	10 years after last ARF or until age 25 years, whichever longer
	ARF without carditis	5 years after last ARF or until age 18 years, whichever longer
Indian Guidelines (2008)[48]	Severe disease/postintervention	Lifelong; may opt to continue until age 40 years
	ARF with healed/mild/moderate carditis	Until age 25 years or 10 years after last ARF (whichever longer)
	ARF without carditis	Until age 18 years or 5 years after last ARF (whichever longer)

AMERICAN HEART ASSOCIATION 2023–24 FRAMEWORK FOR SECONDARY PROPHYLAXIS OF ACUTE RHEUMATIC FEVER AND RHEUMATIC HEART DISEASE (FLOWCHART 6)

- Both American Heart Association (AHA) and WHO reaffirm BPG (IM) as the *first-line prophylaxis* for most patients.
- *Oral penicillin V* is reserved for elevated-risk or special subgroups (e.g., poor IM tolerance, cardiac decompensation).
- *Sulfadiazine/macrolides* are reserved for those with true hypersensitivity reactions.

EVIDENCE BASE AND ADVANCES IN SECONDARY PROPHYLAXIS[49,50]

Historic WHO penicillin programs (1950s–70s) achieved an ≈80% reduction in ARF recurrence and RHD progression.[49] In the landmark Tompkins et al. (1972) cohort of 115 children on monthly benzathine penicillin G (BPG), no deaths or new mitral stenosis occurred.[50] The GOAL trial

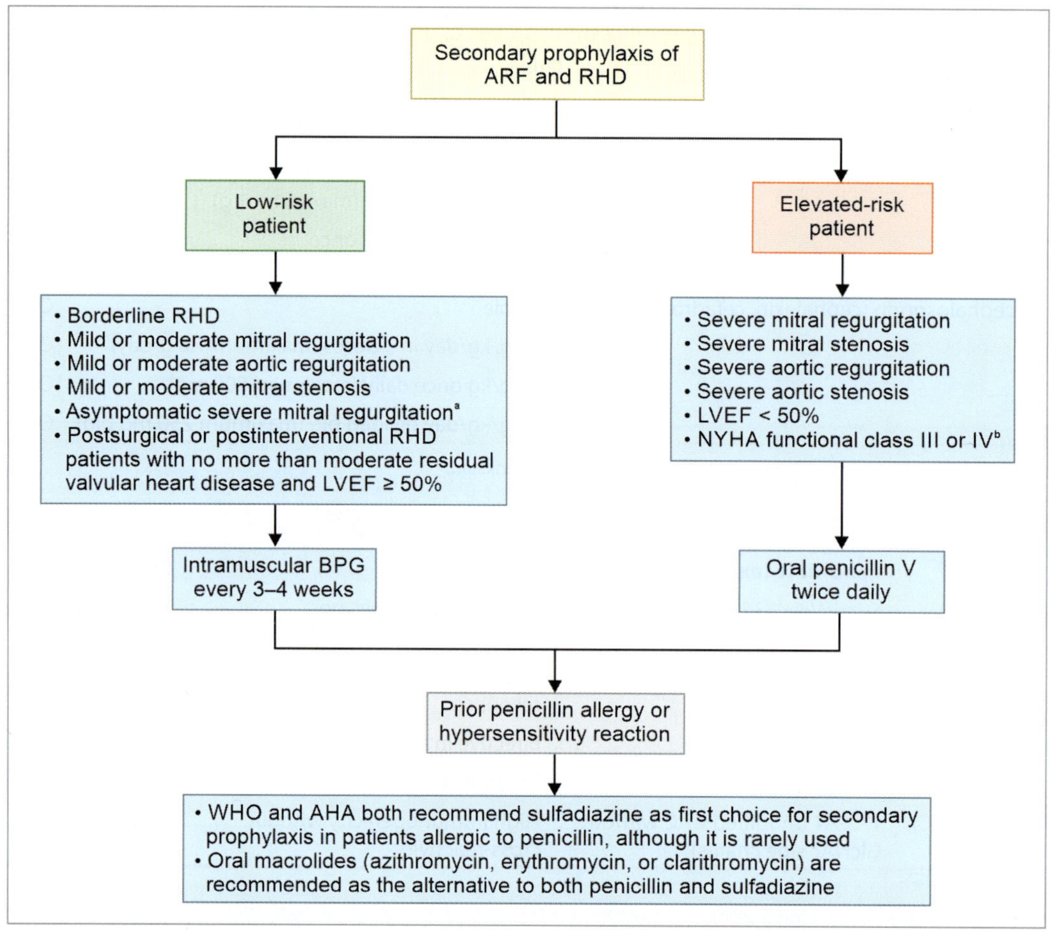

[a]Patients with isolated severe MR often move back and forth between low-risk and high-risk categories.

[b]Includes symptoms caused by nonstructural contributing factors such as atrial fibrillation and anemia.

FLOWCHART 6: American Heart Association (AHA) presidential advisory for prophylaxis of ARF and RHD.
(AHA: American Heart Association; BPG: benzathine penicillin G; LVEF: left ventricular ejection fraction; NYHA: New York Heart Association; WHO: World Health Organization)

(NEJM 2021) confirmed that 4-weekly BPG in latent RHD reduced 2-year progression from 8 to 0.8% (NNT = 13).[29]

Despite strict adherence, recurrence can occur because serum penicillin levels fall below 0.02 mg/L within 14 days, especially in higher BMI patients. Subcutaneous BPG shows a longer half-life, enabling potential extended-interval dosing.

Adherence can be improved through digital recall systems, registry tracking, outreach delivery, and reliable drug-supply chains. Programs like Uganda's decentralized mobile registry model enhance coverage and data quality.[51] The CHIP-GAS trial aims to redefine the minimal protective benzylpenicillin concentration, refining prophylaxis intervals and optimizing global RHD prevention frameworks.

STATUS OF ORAL AND SUBCUTANEOUS PENICILLIN IN SECONDARY PROPHYLAXIS

Intramuscular benzathine benzylpenicillin (BPG) every 3–4 weeks remains the global standard for secondary prevention of ARF and RHD. The 2024 WHO and 2023 AHA advisories reaffirm IM BPG as first-line due to its durable serum levels and superior efficacy over oral regimens. Oral penicillin V is reserved for selected cases where IM therapy is not feasible.

Evidence: Meta-analyses confirm IM BPG reduces recurrence rates up to tenfold compared with oral therapy. The GOAL trial demonstrated that 4-weekly IM BPG prevents latent RHD progression, while the ongoing GOALIE trial will test twice-daily oral penicillin's non-inferiority.[52]

Subcutaneous (SC) BPG shows promise—being less painful, with more sustained plasma levels. Modeling predicts that higher SC doses (10.4 million U) could maintain plasma concentration of ~20 ng/mL for 8–12 weeks in contrast to concentration of <20 for 9 days with IM, potentially improving adherence in endemic regions.[53]

National programs should prioritize uninterrupted IM BPG supply, adherence tracking, and registry-based recall systems to optimize RHD prevention.

SUSTAINED-RELEASE PENICILLIN/ IMPLANT (TABLE 15)

Long-acting depot preparations are being developed to overcome adherence barriers. Current evidence is summarized below:

"Future implementation research should focus on harmonizing pharmacokinetic optimization with real-world adherence strategies to achieve global elimination of rheumatic heart disease."

LANDMARK TRIALS AND REGISTRIES IN RHEUMATIC HEART DISEASE

- *WHO penicillin prophylaxis studies (1950s–70s)*: Large longitudinal and cluster trials among thousands of schoolchildren with ARF in India, Cuba, and South Africa compared monthly benzathine penicillin with no prophylaxis. Results showed an ≈80% reduction in ARF recurrences and markedly fewer new RHD lesions, yielding a number needed to treat ≈ 60. These data established 4-weekly intramuscular BPG as the cornerstone of secondary prevention.[49]
- *Tompkins et al. Circulation 1972*: At the Rainbow Rheumatic Fever Clinic (Cleveland), 115 children (mean age 8.6 years) with ARF were followed 9.3 years on strictly supervised monthly BPG. 69% had mitral regurgitation (MR), 13% MR + aortic regurgitation (AR), 30% no murmur. *Outcomes:* MR resolved in ≈70% (mean 1.8 years); AR persisted in 73% but remained mild; no new mitral stenosis or deaths occurred. Only one compliant patient had recurrent ARF. In contrast, nonadherent or orally treated patients developed endocarditis, deaths, and mitral stenosis in all six who received no prophylaxis.[50]
- *Bland and Jones (preprophylaxis era, ~1,000 patients)*: Only 20% of isolated MR resolved by 10 years; 30% mortality at 20 years (80% RHD-related). Among 347 who seemed "recovered," 24% developed MS within 10 years and 44% by 20 years, underscoring the transformative impact of sustained penicillin prophylaxis.[57]
- *Olesen KH, Br Heart J, 1962* **(Table 16)**[58]
- *Horstkotte D et al., Eur Heart J, 1991*[59]

  Cohort: >500 European patients with acquired mitral stenosis (MS), followed for ~25 years.

  Findings: Progressive fibrosis and calcification led to 50% requiring surgery; established that rheumatic MS is irreversible and ultimately demands intervention.
- *Inoue Balloon Valvotomy (1984, Japan)*[60]

  Cohort: ~50 symptomatic MS patients.

  Findings: Introduction of percutaneous transvenous mitral commissurotomy (PTMC) achieved immediate valve-area improvement and durable symptomatic relief equivalent to surgery—revolutionizing rheumatic MS management.
- *Kang DH et al., Eur Heart J, 2012*[61]

  Cohort: 244 asymptomatic patients with moderate MS (mean age ~40 years).

  Findings: Early PTMC reduced atrial fibrillation, heart failure, and need for surgery, favoring proactive intervention in selected moderate MS before symptom onset
- *REMEDY Registry, Circulation 2016*[62]
  The REMEDY study looked at the current state of rheumatic heart disease (RHD) across Africa, India, and Yemen. It followed more than 3,300 patients between 2010 and 2012. The average age of participants was only 28 years, and two out of three were women. This shows that RHD mainly affects young people in low- and middle-income countries.

Disease Burden and Complications

The majority of patients (about 64%) had serious, moderate-to-severe disease involving multiple heart valves. Complications were frequent and often severe:

- One in three had heart failure
- Almost three in 10 had pulmonary hypertension
- About one in five had atrial fibrillation
- 7% had suffered a stroke
- 4% developed infective endocarditis
- Nearly 3% experienced major bleeding

Adults were more likely than children to develop left ventricular dysfunction and chamber enlargement.

Gaps in Treatment and Prevention

Despite clear treatment guidelines, many patients were not receiving the care they needed:

- Only 55% were on secondary antibiotic prophylaxis
- Most eligible patients received oral anticoagulation, but fewer than one-third had therapeutic INR control

TABLE 15: Sustained-release penicillin/implant evidence summary.

Study type	Summary	Reference
Preclinical implant (sheep model)	PCL-coated implant → ~9 weeks release; size too large for human use	Barr RK et al. (2023)[54]
Phase I SCIP (healthy volunteers)	Safe/tolerable; modeling predicts up to 13-week dosing feasibility	Kado JH et al. (2023)[53]
Qualitative patient preference study	"Hurts less, lasts longer"; 95% preferred SCIP to monthly IM injections	Cooper J et al. (2024)[55]
Phase IIa SCIP (ARF patients)	Safe + favorable PK; improved penicillin exposure vs. IM BPG	Bennett J et al. (2025)[56]

- Among women of childbearing age, just 3.6% used contraception
- Access to valve repair or replacement procedures was very limited, especially in lower-income countries

Key Takeaways

The REMEDY study highlights that RHD remains a major cause of illness in young people from poorer regions. High rates of preventable complications and poor access to proven treatments are major concerns. Better use of antibiotics, improved anticoagulation monitoring, reproductive health support, and greater access to surgical options are urgently needed to improve outcomes.

TABLE 16: 10- and 20-year survival figures.

Subset	10-year survival	20-year survival
NYHA II	69%	49%
NYHA III	33%	0%
NYHA IV	All dead within 10 years	0%
AF	25%	0%
Sinus rhythm	46%	29%
Overall	34%	14%

- *Ina-RHD Registry (Indonesia, 2025)*[30]
  A total of 3,431 adults (median age 44 years; 64% female) from 21 hospitals. Dyspnea in 85.7%, NYHA III–IV in 25%. Isolated MS 39.6%, mitral–aortic 24.1%, mixed mitral 16.3%, triple-valve 12.7%. AF 62.5% (77% in mixed MS); PH and RV dysfunction in >50%. Only 37% on any prophylaxis; IM benzathine use 11.5%; INR control ≈32%.

India Comparison

Echo screening: 20.4/1000 (rural north) and 7.7/1000 (multisite WHF). *Indian REMEDY data*: AF 21.8%, HF 33%, PH 28.8%, prophylaxis 55%, INR therapeutic 28%. Similar gaps persist—under-anticoagulation, cost-related nonadherence, and limited access to valve intervention **(Table 17)**.

- The INVICTUS trial (2022)[63] reaffirmed vitamin K antagonists as standard in rheumatic AF, with DOACs ineffective. The INVICTUS trial (4,531 patients with rheumatic AF) compared rivaroxaban (n = 2,275) with vitamin K antagonists (VKA, n = 2,256). The primary composite endpoint (stroke, systemic embolism, MI, or vascular/non-vascular death) occurred in 8.21%/year with rivaroxaban versus 6.49%/year with VKA ($p < 0.001$), favoring VKAs. Stroke rates were 1.32%/year versus 0.94%/year, all-cause death 7.95%/year versus 6.55%/

TABLE 17: Comparison of Ina-RHD study with the Indian context.

Domain	Indonesia (Ina-RHD, adults)	India (recent evidence)	Update/Implication
Setting and period	3,431 adults; 21 hospitals; January 2020–June 2023	National incidence unknown; multiple cohorts and reviews, including REMEDY (India included)	Use recent multicenter cohorts + echo screening to quantify burden
Demography	Median age 44; 64% women	RHD peaks in young adults; female predominance is common	Women of reproductive age need dedicated care pathways
Predominant lesions	Isolated MS 39.6%, mixed MV 16.3%, multiple MV + AV 24.1%	Mixed lesions common; MS/MR dominate in many Indian series	Expect MS-heavy clinics; plan PBMV/surgery pathways
AF prevalence	62.5% overall; 77.3% in mixed MV; 70.4% in MS	~22% in REMEDY overall; higher with severe MV disease	Indonesia shows very late presentation; India should not assume low AF-screen proactively
Thromboembolism	Stroke ever 6.6%; intracardiac thrombus concentrated in MS	Stroke risk substantial in rheumatic-AF; INR control poor	Strengthen OAC pathways and INR access
PH and right heart	PH common (especially MS); right heart involvement ~50%	PH frequent with advanced MV disease	Echo surveillance and earlier referral are critical
Secondary prophylaxis	Any 37%; regular 23%; IM BPG only 11.5% of those on prophylaxis	Coverage variable; logistics and cost barriers documented	*Program fix*: Supply chains, pain-mitigation, reminder/reach models
Anticoagulation	VKA in 70%; only ~30% routinely check INR; ~32–35% of those reach INR > 2; DOAC ~0.5%	<80% on OAC; <30–40% therapeutic INR in many series	Build INR infrastructure; keep VKA-first (per INVICTUS)
Child/latent burden	Adult study	*Echo-screening*: 20.4/1000 (RHEUMATIC, 2011);[11] 7.7/1000 (e-RHEUMATIC, 2017)[16]	Justifies Indian school/community echo + fast-track prophylaxis

year, and major bleeding 0.67%/year versus 0.83%/year (p = 0.18). Thus, VKAs reduced stroke and mortality without more bleeding, remaining the standard of care for rheumatic AF.

CONCLUSION

Acute rheumatic fever and RHD form a preventable continuum driven by group A streptococcal infection, host susceptibility, and immune cross-reactivity. Early diagnosis using echocardiography, strict adherence to benzathine penicillin prophylaxis, and timely valvular intervention remain the pillars of control. Persistent disease in low-income regions reflects socioeconomic barriers rather than therapeutic gaps. Integration of WHO 2024 and AHA 2023 recommendations, registry-based follow-up, and emerging long-acting penicillin formulations can transform outcomes. Future elimination hinges on equitable healthcare access, surveillance, and Strep A vaccine development to break the infection-inflammation-fibrosis cycle underlying RHD.

REFERENCES

1. Hirani K, Rwebembera J, Webb R, et al. Acute rheumatic fever. Lancet. 2025;405(10495):2164-78.
2. Alberio AMQ, Pieroni F, Di Gangi A, et al. Toward the Knowledge of the Epidemiological Impact of Acute Rheumatic Fever in Italy. Front Pediatr. 2021;9:746505.
3. Egoroff N, Bloomfield H, Gondarra W, et al. An outbreak of acute rheumatic fever in a remote Aboriginal community. Aust N Z J Public Health. 2023;47(5):100077.
4. Ward ZJ, Goldie SJ. Global Burden of Disease Study 2021 estimates: implications for health policy and research. Lancet. 2024;403(10440):1958-9.
5. Carapetis JR, Steer AC, Mulholland EK, et al. The global burden of group A streptococcal diseases. Lancet Infect Dis. 2005;5(11): 685-94.
6. Gewitz MH, Baltimore RS, Tani LY, et al. Revision of the Jones Criteria for the diagnosis of acute rheumatic fever in the era of Doppler echocardiography: a scientific statement from the American Heart Association. Circulation. 2015;131(20):1806-18.
7. Kumar RK, Antunes MJ, Beaton A, et al. Contemporary Diagnosis and Management of Rheumatic Heart Disease: Implications for Closing the Gap: A Scientific Statement from the American Heart Association. Circulation. 2020;142(20):e337-57.
8. Padamavati S. Present status of rheumatic fever and rheumatic heart disease in India. Indian Heart J. 1995;47(4):395-8.
9. Negi PC, Sondhi S, Asotra S, et al. Current status of rheumatic heart disease in India. Indian Heart J. 2019;71(1):85-90.
10. Lalchandani A, Kumar HRP, Alam SM. Prevalence of rheumatic heart disease in rural and urban school children of district Kanpur (Abstract) Indian Heart J. 2000;52:672.
11. Saxena A, Ramakrishnan S, Roy A, et al. Prevalence and outcome of subclinical rheumatic heart disease in India: the RHEUMATIC (Rheumatic Heart Echo Utilisation and Monitoring Actuarial Trends in Indian Children) study. Heart. 2011;97(24):2018-22.
12. Koshi G, Benjamin V, Cherian G. Rheumatic fever and rheumatic heart disease in rural South Indian children. Bull World Health Organ. 1981;59(4):599-603.
13. Grover A, Dhawan A, Iyengar SD, et al. Epidemiology of rheumatic fever and rheumatic heart disease in a rural community in northern India. Bull World Health Organ. 1993;71(1):59-66.
14. Australian Institute of Health and Welfare. Acute rheumatic fever and rheumatic heart disease in Australia [Internet]. Canberra: Australian Institute of Health and Welfare, 2024. Available from: https://www.aihw.gov.au/reports/indigenous-australians/arf-rhd
15. Negi PC, Kanwar A, Chauhan R, et al. Epidemiological trends of RF/RHD in school children of Shimla in north India. Indian J Med Res. 2013;137(6):1121-7.
16. Saxena A, Desai A, Narvencar K, et al. Echocardiographic prevalence of rheumatic heart disease in Indian school children using World Heart Federation criteria—A multi-site extension of RHEUMATIC study (the e-RHEUMATIC study). Int Cardio. 2017;249:438-42.
17. Rothenbühler M, O'Sullivan CJ, Stortecky S, et al. Active surveillance for rheumatic heart disease in endemic regions: a systematic review and meta-analysis of prevalence among children and adolescents. Lancet Glob Health. 2014;2(12):e717-26.
18. Dougherty S, Okello E, Mwangi J, et al. Rheumatic Heart Disease. JACC. 2023;81(1):81-94.
19. Marangou J, Rwebembera J, Mwita J, et al. The Echocardiographic Diagnosis of Rheumatic Heart Disease: A Review of the Performance of the World Heart Federation Criteria 2012-2023. Glob Heart. 2024;19(1):47.
20. Noubiap JJ, Agbor VN, Bigna JJ, et al. Prevalence and progression of rheumatic heart disease: a global systematic review and meta-analysis of population-based echocardiographic studies. Sci Rep. 2019;9(1):17022.
21. Abernethy M, Bass N, Sharpe N, et al. Doppler echocardiography and the early diagnosis of carditis in acute rheumatic fever. Aust N Z J Med. 1994;24(5):530-5.
22. Jackson SJ, Steer AC, Campbell H. Systematic Review: Estimation of global burden of non-suppurative sequelae of upper respiratory tract infection: rheumatic fever and post-streptococcal glomerulonephritis. Trop Med Int Health. 2011;16(1):2-11.
23. Carapetis JR, Currie BJ, Mathews JD. Cumulative incidence of rheumatic fever in an endemic region: a guide to the susceptibility of the population? Epidemiol Infect. 2000;124(2):239-44.
24. Carapetis JR, Beaton A, Cunningham MW, et al. Acute rheumatic fever and rheumatic heart disease. Nat Rev Dis Primers. 2016;2(1):15084.
25. Vijayalakshmi IB. Acute Rheumatic Fever and Chronic Rheumatic Heart Disease. Jaypee Brothers Medical Publishers Pvt Limited; 2022. p. 340.
26. Rwebembera J, Marangou J, Mwita JC, et al. 2023 World Heart Federation guidelines for the echocardiographic diagnosis of rheumatic heart disease. Nat Rev Cardiol. 2024;21(4):250-63.
27. Ramakrishnan S. Echocardiography in acute rheumatic fever. Ann Pediatr Cardiol. 2009;2(1):61-4.
28. WHO Study Group on Rheumatic Fever and Rheumatic Heart Disease. Rheumatic fever and rheumatic heart disease: report of a WHO expert consultation, Geneva 2001.
29. Beaton A, Okello E, Rwebembera J, et al. Secondary Antibiotic Prophylaxis for Latent Rheumatic Heart Disease. N Eng J Med. 2022;386(3):230-40.

30. Soesanto AM, Almazini P, Ariani R, et al. Characteristics and Problems of Rheumatic Heart Disease in Indonesia. JACC. 2025;5(9):1171-83.
31. Manjunath CN, Srinivas P, Ravindranath KS, et al. Incidence and patterns of valvular heart disease in a tertiary care high-volume cardiac center: A single center experience. Indian Heart J. 2014;66(3):320-6.
32. Unger P, Pibarot P, Tribouilloy C, et al. Multiple and Mixed Valvular Heart Diseases. Circ Cardiovasc Imaging. 2018;11(8):e007862.
33. Praz F, Borger MA, Lanz J, et al. 2025 ESC/EACTS Guidelines for the management of valvular heart disease: Developed by the task force for the management of valvular heart disease of the European Society of Cardiology (ESC) and the European Association for Cardio-Thoracic Surgery (EACTS). Eur Heart J. 2025;ehaf194.
34. Watkins D, Baker MG, Kumar RK, et al. Chapter 1 - Epidemiology, Risk Factors, Burden and Cost of Acute Rheumatic Fever and Rheumatic Heart Disease. In: Dougherty S, Carapetis J, Zühlke L, et al. (Eds). Acute Rheumatic Fever and Rheumatic Heart Disease. San Diego (CA): Elsevier; 2021. pp. 1-18.
35. Monya-Tambi I, Robertson KR, Volmink JA, et al. Acute rheumatic fever. Lancet. 2005;366(9494):1355.
36. Centor RM, Witherspoon JM, Dalton HP, et al. The diagnosis of strep throat in adults in the emergency room. Med Decis Making. 1981;1(3):239-46.
37. McIsaac WJ, White D, Tannenbaum D, et al. A clinical score to reduce unnecessary antibiotic use in patients with sore throat. CMAJ. 1998;158(1):75-83.
38. Lennon D, Stewart J, Anderson P. Primary Prevention of Rheumatic Fever. Pediatr Infect Dis J. 2016;35(7):820.
39. Karki P, Uranw S, Bastola S, et al. Effectiveness of Systematic Echocardiographic Screening for Rheumatic Heart Disease in Nepalese Schoolchildren: A Cluster Randomized Clinical Trial. JAMA Cardiol. 2021;6(4):420-6.
40. Irlam J, Mayosi BM, Engel M, et al. Primary prevention of acute rheumatic fever and rheumatic heart disease with penicillin in South African children with pharyngitis: a cost-effectiveness analysis. Circ Cardiovasc Qual Outcomes. 2013;6(3):343-51.
41. Gordis L. Effectiveness of comprehensive-care programs in preventing rheumatic fever. N Engl J Med. 1973;289(7):331-5.
42. Pastural É, McNeil SA, MacKinnon-Cameron D, et al. Safety and immunogenicity of a 30-valent M protein-based group a streptococcal vaccine in healthy adult volunteers: A randomized, controlled phase I study. Vaccine. 2020;38(6):1384-92.
43. Reynolds S, Pandey M, Dooley J, et al. Preclinical safety and immunogenicity of Streptococcus pyogenes (Strep A) peptide vaccines. Sci Rep. 2021;11(1):127.
44. Postol E, Alencar R, Higa FT, et al. StreptInCor: a candidate vaccine epitope against S. pyogenes infections induces protection in outbred mice. PLoS One. 2013;8(4):e60969.
45. Burns K, Dorfmueller HC, Wren BW, et al. Progress towards a glycoconjugate vaccine against Group A Streptococcus. NPJ Vaccines. 2023;8(1):48.
46. Gao NJ, Uchiyama S, Pill L, et al. Site-Specific Conjugation of Cell Wall Polyrhamnose to Protein SpyAD Envisioning a Safe Universal Group A Streptococcal Vaccine. Infect Microbes Dis. 2021;3(2):87-100.
47. Gerber MA, Baltimore RS, Eaton CB, et al. Prevention of rheumatic fever and diagnosis and treatment of acute Streptococcal pharyngitis: a scientific statement from the American Heart Association Rheumatic Fever, Endocarditis, and Kawasaki Disease Committee of the Council on Cardiovascular Disease in the Young, the Interdisciplinary Council on Functional Genomics and Translational Biology, and the Interdisciplinary Council on Quality of Care and Outcomes Research: endorsed by the American Academy of Pediatrics. Circulation. 2009;119(11):1541-51.
48. Working Group on Pediatric Acute Rheumatic Fever and Cardiology Chapter of Indian Academy of Pediatrics, Saxena A, Kumar RK, et al. Consensus guidelines on pediatric acute rheumatic fever and rheumatic heart disease. Indian Pediatr. 2008;45(7):565-73.
49. Wood HF, Stollerman GH, Feinstein AR, et al. A controlled study of three methods of prophylaxis against streptococcal infection in a population of rheumatic children. I. Streptococcal infections and recurrences of acute rheumatic fever in the first two years of the study. N Engl J Med. 1957;257(9):394-8.
50. Tompkins DG, Boxerbaum B, Liebman J. Long-term prognosis of rheumatic fever patients receiving regular intramuscular benzathine penicillin. Circulation. 1972;45(3):543-51.
51. Minja NW, Pulle J, Rwebembera J, et al. Evaluating the implementation of a dynamic digital application to enable community-based decentralisation of rheumatic heart disease case management in Uganda: protocol for a hybrid type III effectiveness-implementation study. BMJ Open. 2023;13(10): e071540.
52. Rwebembera J, Ndagire E, Carvalho N, et al. Intramuscular versus enteral penicillin prophylaxis to prevent progression of rheumatic heart disease: Study protocol for a noninferiority randomized trial (the GOALIE trial). Am Heart J. 2024;275:74-85.
53. Kado JH, Salman S, Henderson R, et al. Subcutaneous administration of benzathine benzylpenicillin G has favourable pharmacokinetic characteristics for the prevention of rheumatic heart disease compared with intramuscular injection: a randomized, crossover, population pharmacokinetic study in healthy adult volunteers. J Antimicrob Chemother. 2020;75(10):2951-9.
54. Barr RK, Barber BW, Tait JR, et al. Development of a sustained release implant of benzathine penicillin G for secondary prophylaxis of rheumatic heart disease. Eur J Pharm Biopharm. 2023;189:240-50.
55. Cooper J, Enkel SL, Moodley D, et al. 'Hurts less, lasts longer'; a qualitative study on experiences of young people receiving high-dose subcutaneous injections of benzathine penicillin G to prevent rheumatic heart disease in New Zealand. PLoS One. 2024;19(5):e0302493.
56. Bennett J, Salman S, Moodley D, et al. High dose, subcutaneous injections of benzathine penicillin G (SCIP) to prevent rheumatic fever: A single arm, phase IIa trial of safety and pharmacokinetics. J Infect. 2025;91(1):106506.
57. Bland EF, Duckett Jones T. Rheumatic fever and rheumatic heart disease; a twenty-year report on 1000 patients followed since childhood. Circulation. 1951;4(6):836-43
58. Olesen KH. The Natural History of 271 Patients with Mitral Stenosis Under Medical Treatment. Br Heart J. 1962;24(3):349-57.
59. Horstkotte D, Niehues R, Strauer BE. Pathomorphological aspects, etiology and natural history of acquired mitral valve stenosis. Eur Heart J. 1991;12 Suppl B:55-60.
60. Inoue K, Owaki T, Nakamura T, et al. Clinical application of transvenous mitral commissurotomy by a new balloon catheter. J Thorac Cardiovasc Surg. 1984;87(3):394-402.
61. Kang DH, Lee CH, Kim DH, et al. Early percutaneous mitral commissurotomy vs. conventional management in asymptomatic moderate mitral stenosis. Eur Heart J. 2012;33(12):1511-7.
62. Zühlke L, Engel ME, Karthikeyan G, et al. Characteristics, complications, and gaps in evidence-based interventions in rheumatic heart disease: the Global Rheumatic Heart Disease Registry (the REMEDY study). Eur Heart J. 2015;36(18):1115-22.
63. Connolly SJ, Karthikeyan G, Ntsekhe M, et al. Rivaroxaban in Rheumatic Heart Disease–Associated Atrial Fibrillation. N Eng J Med. 2022;387(11):978-88.

CHAPTER 65

Comprehensive Approach to Aortic Valve Pathophysiology by Fibro-Calcific Imaging

Johann Christopher, Raja Ramesh Nukavarapu

ABSTRACT

Aortic stenosis is a progressive degenerative disorder. In the elderly, fibrocalcific disease is the commonest cause of aortic stenosis. The fibrous component predominates in women, while the calcific component dominates in men. Fibrosis increases leaflet thickening while calcium impairs leaflet mobility and causes narrowing. The pathogenesis is based on the disturbed flow and the biochemical milieu in the aortic valve–aorta interface. The disease is initially asymptomatic; however, over time, there is gradually increasing shortness of breath, angina, and syncope. The classic finding is the pulsus parvus et tardus. The key elements of the diagnosis are the ECG and ECHO, which will identify and quantify the stenosis. Additional tools such as MRI and CTA will refine the diagnosis and decrease the false negatives and positives. The initial plan is to control the comorbidities, as aortic stenosis alone is not amenable to medical management. The initial go-to option was surgical aortic valve replacement (metallic or prosthetic) based on the age and comorbidities. However, the last 10 years have demonstrated a rise of TAVER, a percutaneous approach which has revolutionized the management of patients with fibrocalcific aortic stenosis.

Keywords: Fibrocalcific, aortic stenosis, etiopathogenesis, management.

INTRODUCTION

Aortic stenosis (AS) is a progressive disease characterized by narrowing of the aortic valve opening, leading to obstruction of blood flow from the left ventricle to the aorta.[1] Fibrocalcific aortic valve disease (FCAVD), causing severe aortic valve stenosis, is the most common valve disease in the elderly population, with a significant increase in incidence after 65 years.[2] Morphologically, the FCAVD has two phenotypes—predominant fibrous, called fibrous aortic valve stenosis (FAS) and calcific aortic stenosis (CAS) with predominant calcium. The FAS and CAS differ in the relative content of fibrous and calcium tissue and the nature of lipid composition, with FAS containing mainly phospholipids and CAS having triacylglycerols.[3] The FAS is more common in females, with more fibrous and dense connective tissue in the aortic valve than in males **(Fig. 1)**.[4]

PATHOPHYSIOLOGY

Disease Mechanisms

Fibrous aortic valve stenosis is characterized by the accumulation of fibrous tissue and calcium deposits within the aortic valve **(Fig. 2)**. This dual process leads to leaflet thickening, reduced compliance, and ultimately, stenosis. Unlike pure CAS **(Fig. 3)**, FAS often features a prominent fibrotic component, especially in specific populations such as women. The interplay between fibrosis and calcification is

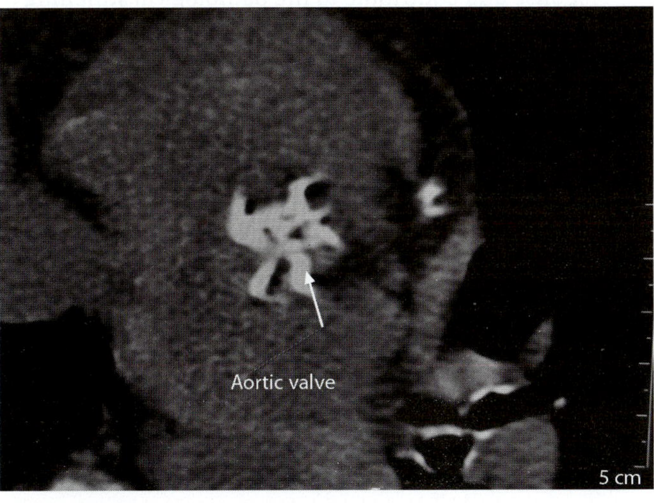

FIG. 1: Heavily calcified aortic valve.

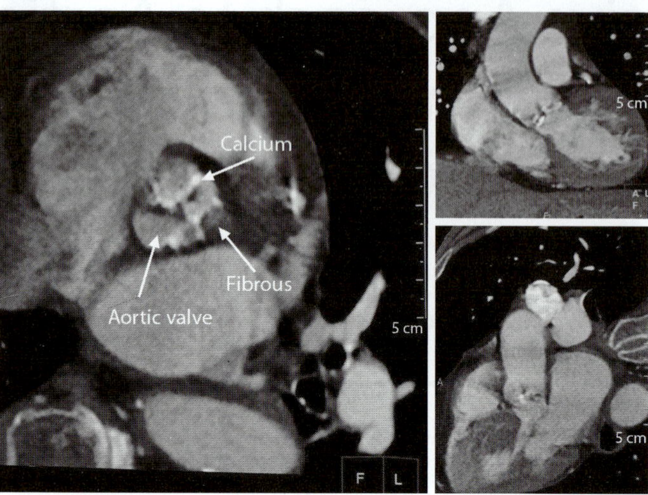

FIG. 2: Predominantly fibrosed aortic valve.

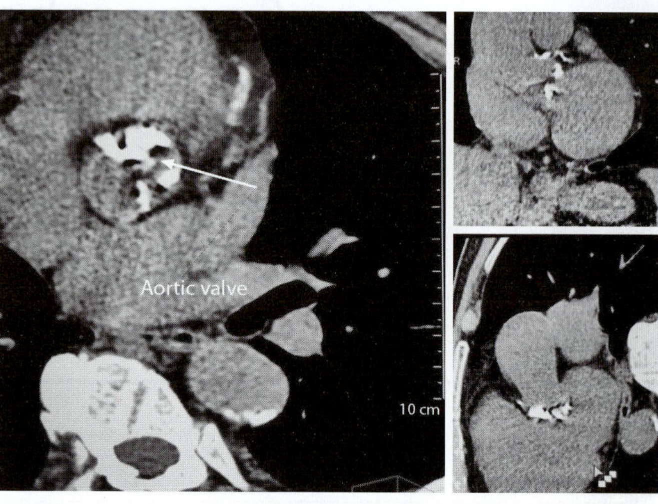

FIG. 3: Predominantly calcified aortic valve.

crucial—fibrosis increases leaflet stiffness, while calcification further impairs leaflet mobility and contributes to valve narrowing.[5]

Cellular and Molecular Changes

- *Endothelial dysfunction*: FAS typically begins on the aortic side of the valve cusps, where endothelial cells are exposed to disturbed flow and lower shear stress. This environment reduces the expression of inhibitors of osteogenic signaling (e.g., BMP antagonists), promoting osteogenic differentiation and calcification.[6]
- *Inflammation and matrix remodeling*: Proinflammatory mediators and growth factors (such as VEGF) contribute to matrix remodeling and neovascularization within the valve, facilitating inflammatory cell entry and promoting fibrosis and calcification.[7]
- *Myofibroblasts and pericytes*: Myofibroblasts, derived partly from pericytes near neovessels, play a pivotal role in the extracellular matrix production and the calcification process.[8] These cells drive the fibrotic response and contribute to the pathological stiffening of the valve.[9]

Hemodynamic Consequences

The mechanical interplay between calcium deposits and fibrotic tissue creates regions of increased stress within the valve leaflets. This not only impairs the opening and closing of the valve but also exacerbates the progression of stenosis. Computational models show that in FAS, elevated stresses develop particularly in the fibrotic areas between the belly and tips of the leaflets, further increasing leaflet stiffness and resistance to flow.[10] The result is a progressive narrowing of the aortic orifice, increased left **(Figs. 4A to D)** ventricular afterload, and eventual heart failure if left untreated.[11]

PATHOLOGY OF FIBROCALCIFIC AORTIC STENOSIS

Fibrocalcific AS is a degenerative process characterized by fibrosis and calcification of the aortic valve leaflets, leading to progressive narrowing of the valve orifice.

Key Pathological Features

- *Valve cusp changes:*
  - The aortic valve cusps become thickened, fibrosed, and calcified.
  - This results in increased valve stiffness, reduced cusp movement, and narrowing of the valve opening **(Figs. 5A and B)**.
- *Microscopic findings:*
  - Calcification predominantly affects the fibrosa layer of the valve.
  - Collagen deposition and fiber disorganization are prominent, contributing to leaflet rigidity.
  - Mineralization often arises near lipid deposits, reflecting an inflammatory response to injury.
  - Dense inflammatory infiltrates (mainly macrophages) may be present within the calcified tissue.
- *Fibrosis and calcification:*
  - Both fibrosis (collagen and extracellular matrix deposition) and calcification (calcium phosphate mineralization) work together to impair valve function.
  - Fibrosis increases leaflet stiffness and may serve as a scaffold for further calcification. This interplay accelerates disease progression.
- *Active cellular and molecular processes*:
  - The pathology is not just passive degeneration but involves active inflammation, cytokine signaling (e.g., TGF-β), and osteogenic metaplasia (occurrence of bone-like cells in some cases).

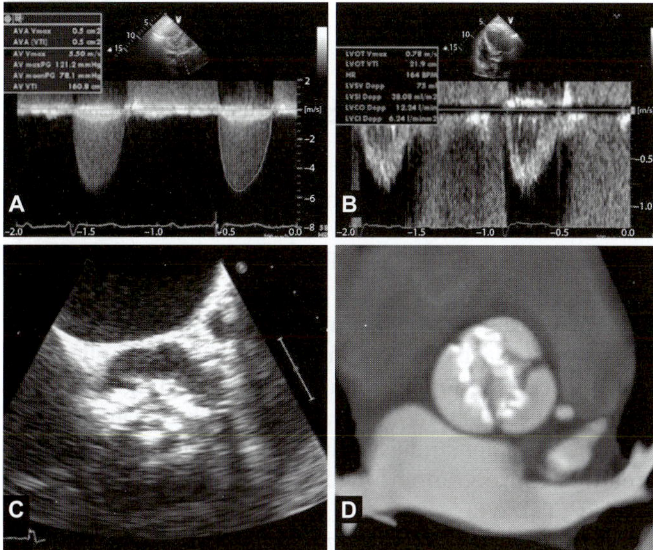

FIGS. 4A TO D: Calcified aortic valve-echo CT correlation.

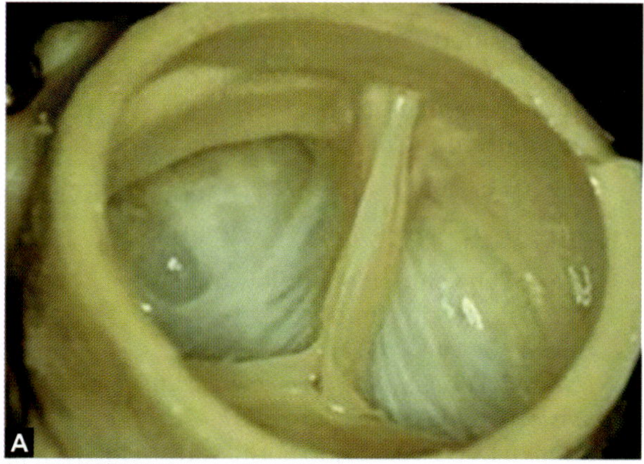

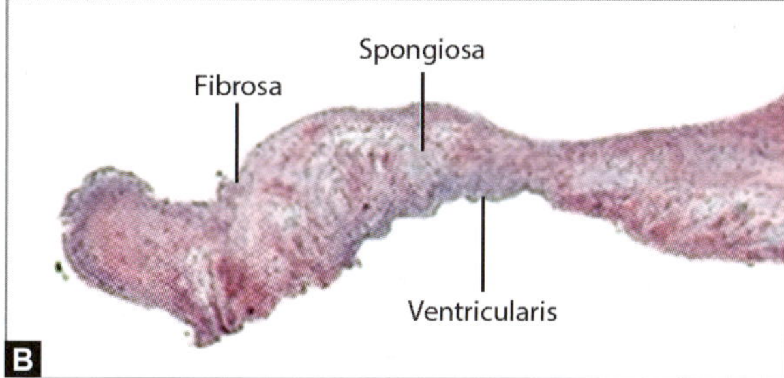

FIGS. 5A AND B: Fibrosed aortic valve pathology.

- Lipid deposition, oxidative stress, and chronic inflammation are central to disease initiation and progression.

- *Sex differences:*
    - There is evidence of sex-specific differences: Women may exhibit more fibrosis and less calcification compared to men, but both sexes suffer similar hemodynamic progression. Thus, fibrosis may be a more important contributor to valve dysfunction in women.

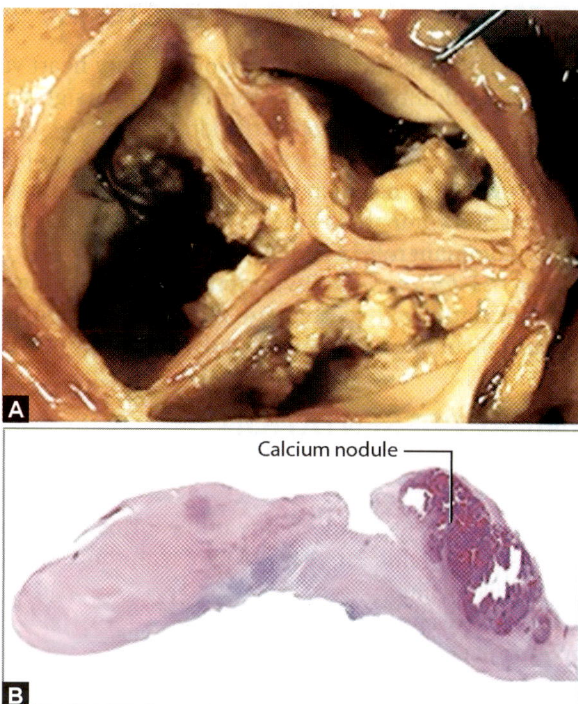

FIGS. 6A AND B: Calcified aortic valve pathology.

Histopathology

- *Valve leaflet changes*: Thickened, fibrosed, and calcified cusps.
- *Main pathological layers*: Fibrosa layer (site of calcification); collagen-rich fibrous tissue.
- *Cellular involvement*: Macrophages, T-lymphocytes; occasional osteoblast-like cells.
- *Molecular mechanisms*: Inflammation, oxidative stress, cytokines (e.g., TGF-β), lipid accumulation.
- *Sex differences*: Women more likely to have fibrosis; men more calcification, but similar stenosis.
- *Disease progression*: Both calcific and fibrotic processes drive valve narrowing and dysfunction.
    - Unlike rheumatic AS, fibrocalcific AS lacks commissural fusion, instead showing diffuse leaflet thickening and calcification.
    - The interaction of calcium deposits and fibrous tissue increases local mechanical stress, further exacerbating valve dysfunction **(Figs. 6A and B)**.

The pathogenesis of fibrocalcific AS is now understood as a biologically active process involving chronic injury, repair, inflammation, lipid accumulation, fibrosis, and calcification, rather than simple "wear and tear".

EPIDEMIOLOGY AND RISK FACTORS

- *Prevalence:* AS is the most common primary heart valve disease in adults, with FAS representing a significant subset, especially among elderly populations.
- *Sex differences:* Women are more likely to develop FAS with less severe calcification but similar hemodynamic progression compared to men, suggesting fibrosis plays a more dominant role in female patients.[12]
- *Other risk factors:* Age, hypertension, hyperlipidemia, chronic kidney disease, and genetic predisposition contribute to the development and progression of FAS.[13]

CLINICAL PRESENTATION

Symptoms

Fibrous aortic valve stenosis, like other forms of AS, may remain asymptomatic for years. When symptoms develop, they typically include:

- Exertional dyspnea class I to III
- Angina pectoris CCS Grade I to III
- Syncope and presyncope on exertion
- Heart failure symptoms (e.g., fatigue, orthopnea, paroxysmal nocturnal dyspnea)[14]

Physical Examination

Classic findings include:

- Systolic ejection murmur (crescendo-decrescendo) best heard at the right upper sternal border[15]
- Delayed and diminished carotid upstroke (pulsus parvus et tardus)
- Soft or absent second heart sound (S2)
- Prominent S4 best heard at the apex

Complications

- Left ventricular hypertrophy due to chronic pressure overload
- Heart failure (preserved ejection fraction)
- Arrhythmias (atrial fibrillation/ventricular tachycardia)
- Sudden cardiac death in advanced cases[16]

DIAGNOSIS

Imaging of fibrocalcific aortic valve stenosis relies on several complementary modalities, with echocardiography and contrast CT angiography being the most important for diagnosis and quantification.

Echocardiographic Evaluation in Aortic Stenosis

Echocardiography is the primary tool for diagnosing and grading the severity of AS. It provides information on valve anatomy, leaflet mobility, degree of calcification/fibrosis, and hemodynamic gradients. A comprehensive echocardiography assessment uses a multiparametric and stepwise approach to determine the severity and implications of AS on cardiac function. In FAS, echocardiography may reveal thickened, immobile leaflets with fibrotic and calcific changes. Doppler studies quantify the aortic valve area and mean pressure gradient, which are essential for grading severity **(Table 1)**.[17]

- *Key parameters assessed on echocardiography*:
  - *Aortic valve jet velocity (AV V_{max})*:
    - Measured with continuous wave (CW) Doppler.
    - *Severe AS*: Jet velocity >4.0 m/s.
  - *Mean pressure gradient (MPG)*:
    - Measured with CW Doppler.
    - *Severe AS*: Mean gradient >40 mm Hg.
  - *Aortic valve area (AVA)*:
    Calculated using the continuity equation:

$$\text{AVA} = (\text{LVOT area} \times \text{LVOT VTI})/\text{aortic VTIAVA}$$
$$= (\text{LVOT area} \times \text{LVOT VTI})/\text{aortic VTI}$$

    LVOT: Left ventricular outflow tract
    VTI: Velocity time integral
    Severe AS: AVA < 1.0 cm^2
    Indexed AVA for body surface area: <0.6 cm^2/m^2
- *Dimensionless index (velocity ratio)*:
  - Ratio of LVOT velocity to aortic valve velocity.
  - *Severe AS*: <0.25.
- *Assessment of valve morphology*:
  - Visual assessment for calcification and mobility
  - Identification of bicuspid, tricuspid, or rheumatic changes
- *Additional techniques and considerations*:
  - *Multiple echocardiographic windows*:
    - Optimal Doppler alignment is crucial; use apical, suprasternal, and right parasternal windows to avoid underestimating gradients.
    - At least three cardiac cycles should be averaged (more in atrial fibrillation).

TABLE 1: Grading severity of aortic stenosis.

Parameter	Mild	Moderate	Severe
Peak jet velocity (m/s)	<3.0	3.0–4.0	>4.0
Mean gradient (mm Hg)	<20	20–40	>40
Aortic valve area (cm^2)	>1.5	1.0–1.5	<1.0
Dimensionless index	>0.50	0.25–0.50	<0.25

- *Left ventricular (LV) assessment*:
    - LV size and function (ejection fraction, global longitudinal strain).
    - LV wall thickness and mass.
- *Doppler assessments:*
    - Color Doppler for turbulence and presence of aortic regurgitation.
    - Pulse-wave Doppler in LVOT for subvalvular assessment.
- *3D echocardiography*:
    - Provides accurate LVOT area and aortic annulus measurement, reducing underestimation from assuming a circular LVOT.
    - Useful in procedural planning and cases with elliptical LVOT anatomy.
- *Subclinical indicators and prognostic markers*:
    - Measurement of global longitudinal strain may detect early LV dysfunction.
    - Valvuloarterial impedance helps in assessing total LV afterload.
- *Stress echocardiography*: Used in low-flow, low-gradient, and unclear cases to differentiate actual severe from pseudo-severe AS.

Summary

Echocardiography in AS provides a structured, multi-parameter evaluation using Doppler and morphologic data to establish severity, guide management, and monitor disease progression. A stepwise protocol maximizes accuracy and clinical value. Emerging technologies such as 3D echocardiography and global longitudinal strain add precision and prognostic information.

Noncontrast computed tomography (CT) is endorsed as a guideline for quantifying the aortic valve calcium burden (Agatston score). This objectively assesses calcification, which is key in classic AS, but does not capture fibrosis.[18]

Contrast-enhanced CT angiography (CTA) allows simultaneous calcific and fibrotic (fibrocalcific) tissue quantification by analyzing the valve's attenuation characteristics. Recent techniques, such as Gaussian mixture modelling for tissue thresholds, have enabled the robust, automated, reproducible measurement of fibrocalcific volume. This approach correlates well with disease severity, progression, and underlying valve histology, especially in specific populations such as women and patients with bicuspid valves.[19]

Cardiac magnetic resonance imaging (MRI) provides valve morphology, quantifies valve thickening (fibrosis), and assesses cardiac function, though it is less sensitive for calcification than CT.[20]

Positron emission tomography (PET) with ^{18}F-NaF tracer can assess disease activity (calcification progression), particularly in native or bioprosthetic valves, but is not routinely used in native AS.[21]

Functional assessment (echocardiography) and tissue characterization (advanced CT or MRI) are crucial in detecting and grading fibrocalcific AS, as fibrosis and calcification contribute differently to disease progression in various patient groups. Quantifying fibrocalcific volume on CT may become increasingly important for diagnosis, risk stratification, and early detection of disease stages before heavy calcification appears.[22]

CATHETERIZATION EVALUATION OF AORTIC STENOSIS

Cardiac catheterization is an invasive procedure used to evaluate the severity of AS, particularly in cases where noninvasive tests (like echocardiography) provide inconclusive or conflicting results. Its central role is now mostly reserved for special situations, specifically when there is a discrepancy between clinical findings and noninvasive imaging, when echocardiographic data is technically suboptimal or does not clarify the severity of stenosis, or before valve surgery, typically to rule out concomitant coronary artery disease.

KEY HEMODYNAMIC MEASUREMENTS

During a catheterization evaluation for AS, the following parameters are directly measured:

- *Transvalvular pressure gradient*: This includes simultaneous measurement of the left ventricular (LV) and ascending aortic pressures.
- *Peak-to-peak systolic pressure drop (peak-to-peak gradient)*: Difference between the LV and aortic peak pressures.
- *Mean transvalvular pressure drop*: The average of instantaneous pressure drops during the ejection period.
- *Cardiac output (CO)*: Required for valve area calculation.

VALVE AREA CALCULATION (GORLIN EQUATION)

The aortic valve area (AVA) is estimated using the Gorlin equation:

$$\begin{aligned} AVA &= COHR \times SEP \times 44.3 \times \text{mean } \Delta PAVA \\ &= HR \times SEP \times 44.3 \times \text{mean } \Delta PCO \end{aligned}$$

Where:

- CO = Cardiac output
- HR = Heart rate
- SEP = Systolic ejection period
- mean ΔP = Mean systolic pressure gradient across the aortic valve

An AVA <1.0 cm^2 generally defines severe AS.

- *Procedural technique*:
    - Typically, a catheter is advanced from the femoral artery retrograde across the aortic valve into the LV.

  - Simultaneous pressures are measured using two separate catheters (one in LV, one in the aorta), a dual-lumen catheter, or pressure wire systems.
  - Accurate catheter placement is crucial—incorrect positioning can yield misleading gradients due to phenomena such as pressure recovery.
- *Pitfalls and technical considerations*:
  - Catheter type/size and position can affect measured gradients, especially in tight stenosis.
  - Pressure recovery can occur just distal to the valve, potentially underestimating the proper gradient if the aortic catheter is not placed far enough downstream.
  - Small errors in cardiac output measurement or misalignment of catheters can cause mistakes in calculated AVA.
- *Indications for catheterization evaluation*:
  - Invasive assessment is now not routine for all cases of AS. It is valuable primarily when noninvasive studies and clinical findings disagree, or when noninvasive imaging is inadequate.
  - It also plays a role before intervention to ensure accurate assessment and to check for associated coronary artery disease.

A comprehensive catheterization evaluation requires technical precision and is most useful when integrated with the overall clinical and echocardiographic picture.[23]

MANAGEMENT

Medical Therapy in Fibrocalcific Aortic Stenosis

Fibrocalcific AS is most common in older adults and is characterized by progressive thickening, fibrosis, and aortic valve calcification. The mainstay of treatment, especially for symptomatic severe cases, remains aortic valve replacement (AVR), either surgical or transcatheter.[24]

Medical Therapy: Current Evidence

No proven medical therapy exists that can halt or reverse the progression of fibrocalcific (calcific) aortic stenosis. Clinical trials and observational studies have investigated several pharmacological approaches, including:

- *Statins*: Despite their benefit in atherosclerosis, randomized controlled trials (RCTs) have not demonstrated an effect of statins on slowing the progression of aortic valve calcification.
- *Renin-angiotensin-aldosterone system (RAAS) inhibitors*: There is ongoing investigation, but conclusive evidence for their benefit in modifying AS progression is lacking.
- *Bisphosphonates and vitamin K2*: Agents modulating mineral metabolism and calcification have been explored, but thus far, have not proven effective in trials at slowing AS progression.
- *Other investigational agents*: Targets such as PCSK9 inhibitors, Lp(a) lowering drugs, DPP-4 inhibitors, and thiazolidinediones are under preclinical or early clinical investigation and are not standard therapy.

SYMPTOM MANAGEMENT

While no medical therapy can modify the natural course of valve calcification, some medications may be used to manage symptoms and comorbidities:

- *Diuretics*: For relief of heart failure or congestion symptoms.
- *Beta-blockers/ACE inhibitors/ARBs*: For coexistent hypertension or left ventricular dysfunction (usage may be cautious depending on AS severity).
- *Antiarrhythmic therapy*: Digoxin for atrial arrhythmias and Cordarone for ventricular arrhythmias.
- *General recommendations*: Heart-healthy lifestyle, blood pressure management, and careful monitoring.
- Medical therapy does not alter the course of fibrocalcific AS but is used to manage associated symptoms and conditions.
- Valve replacement remains the only definitive therapy.
- Clinical research is ongoing, but there are no licensed drugs to prevent or reverse valve calcification in AS.

Regular monitoring and risk factor management (blood pressure, cholesterol, etc.) are recommended for patients with mild or asymptomatic AS until or unless symptoms or severe stenosis develop.

SURGICAL INTERVENTION IN FIBROCALCIFIC AORTIC STENOSIS

Fibrocalcific AS is a progressive disease characterized by fibrosis and calcification of the aortic valve leaflets, leading to obstruction of blood flow from the heart. As the disease advances, surgical intervention becomes necessary because no medication has been proven to halt or reverse the progression of stenosis.

Definitive treatment: The mainstay of treatment for significant fibrocalcific AS is valve replacement through open surgical aortic valve replacement (SAVR) or the less invasive transcatheter aortic valve replacement (TAVR). Balloon valvuloplasty is rarely used in adults except as a temporary measure or in those at high surgical risk.

Symptomatic severe AS: Surgery is strongly recommended when symptoms such as exertional dyspnea, angina, syncope, or heart failure accompany severe AS. After symptom onset, survival drops dramatically, but valve replacement can provide substantial symptom relief and improved long-term survival.

Asymptomatic severe AS: Management is controversial. Most guidelines advise intervention if there is evidence of left ventricular systolic dysfunction (LVEF <50%) not due to another cause, abnormal exercise tests showing symptom provocation, very severe AS, rapid disease progression, severely elevated BNP, or pulmonary hypertension. Early intervention may also be considered in select high-risk patients, as some randomized trials suggest a potential survival benefit.

- *Surgical aortic valve replacement*:
  - Traditional open-heart surgery to replace the diseased valve with either a mechanical or biological prosthesis.
  - Mechanical valves last longer but require lifelong anticoagulation, while biological valves (from cow, pig, or human tissue) may eventually deteriorate and require reoperation.
  - Surgical aortic valve replacement (SAVR) is recommended for patients at low or moderate surgical risk.

TRANSCATHETER AORTIC VALVE REPLACEMENT

- Minimally invasive; performed via catheter through blood vessels.
- Typically used in intermediate or high surgical risk patients, but use is expanding as technology improves and more evidence accrues.
- Like SAVR, transcatheter aortic valve replacement (TAVR) uses biological valves.
- *Balloon valvuloplasty*: Rarely used in adults except as a bridge to surgery or nonsurgical candidates because the valve tends to re-narrow.
- *Valve repair*: Very rarely performed for stenosis, usually limited to separating fused leaflets in some instances.
- *Symptomatic patients*: Indication for surgery is clear and urgent to prevent rapid deterioration and death.
- *Asymptomatic patients*: Most can be safely observed; risk of sudden death is low but not negligible. Surgery may be considered earlier in patients with high-risk features such as rapid disease progression, severe calcification, reduced LV function, or evidence from risk stratification (e.g., high BNP, abnormal stress test).
- Operative risk is lower when performed before the onset of advanced symptoms or left ventricular dysfunction (<2% in NYHA class I/II vs. higher rates in more symptomatic patients).
- Long-term complications include prosthetic valve dysfunction, need for reoperation, bleeding (mechanical valves), and infection. These must be weighed against the risks of delaying surgery.

Fibrous aortic valve stenosis versus CAS may influence the hemodynamics and structural reactions during the treatment of aortic stenosis by TAVI (transcatheter aortic valve implantation), which is now the standard of care across the spectrum of surgical risk.

These two morphological forms of aortic stenosis behave differently during and after the TAVI. The anchoring forces for the TAVI stent frame differ between FAS and CAS. The CAS offers less contact area and greater contact pressure to the TAVI valve frame, whereas FAS provides greater contact area and less pressure.[25] This is why CAS patients are more prone to aortic root rupture during TAVI. The TAVI valve frame anchoring forces in FAS are mainly leaflets. In contrast, in CAS, the valve frame is detached due to bulky calcium deposits at leaflet edges, slightly reducing its anchoring. Due to the thicker leaflets in FAS, the chance of TAVI valve migration is higher during deployment. The pattern of paravalvular leak (PVL) also differs in these two entities due to the shape of the TAVI valve frame opening after deployment (triangular in FAS and circular in CAS). In CAS, there will be several PVL jets with higher velocities around the valve frame; in FAS, low velocity, fewer PVL jets at commissures may occur. The thrombogenicity of the TAVI valve frame is marginally elevated in CAS compared to FAS due to a difference in platelet activation.

The preprocedural CT scan analysis of the aortic valve for TAVI should focus on the morphology of the valve, along with other parameters, and quantify the fibrous and calcium components. Depending on the predominant element, the TAVI operators may choose the size and type of valve (self-expandable or balloon expandable). They can also plan the procedure, considering the valve migration (more with FAS) and the occurrence of PVL (more with CAS).[26] By recognizing the distinct characteristics of FAS and CAS, clinicians can provide more effective and personalized care for patients undergoing TAVI.[27]

Paravalvular leak (PVL): TAVR in FAS may result in lower PVL than highly calcified valves due to leaflet morphology and compliance.[28]

Thrombogenicity: FAS and CAS are associated with increased risk of thromboembolic events post-TAVR, but subtle differences in platelet activation may exist.

Untreated severe FAS carries a poor prognosis once symptoms develop, with high rates of morbidity and mortality. Timely valve replacement significantly improves survival and quality of life.[29,30]

CONCLUSION

Fibrocalcific aortic valve stenosis is a complex, multifactorial disease involving fibrosis and calcification of the aortic valve. It is associated with significant morbidity and mortality, particularly in older adults. Advances in understanding its pathophysiology, improved imaging, and evolving interventional strategies continue to enhance patient outcomes. However, challenges remain, particularly in the early detection and management of fibrotic disease, underscoring the need for ongoing research and innovation in this field.

REFERENCES

1. Lindman BR, Clavel MA, Mathieu P, et al. Calcific aortic stenosis. Nat Rev Dis Primers. 2016;2:16006.
2. Cosmi JE, Kort S, Tunick PA, et al. The risk of developing aortic stenosis in patients with "benign" aortic valve thickening. Arch Intern Med. 2002;162:2345-2.
3. Hughes BR, Chahoud G, Mehta JL. Aortic stenosis: is it a degenerative or active atherosclerotic process?. Clin Cardiol. 2005;28(3):111-4.
4. Rajamannan NM, Evans FJ, Aikawa E, et al. Calcific aortic valve disease: not simply a degenerative process: a review and agenda for research from the national heart and lung and blood institute aortic stenosis working group * executive summary: calcific aortic valve disease – 2011 update. Circulation. 2011;124:1783-91.
5. Iung B, Vahanian A. Degenerative calcific aortic stenosis: a natural history. Heart. 2012;98(Suppl 4):iv7-13.
6. Chen JH, Simmons CA. Cell-matrix interactions in the pathobiology of calcific aortic valve disease: critical roles for matricellular, matricrine, and matrix mechanics cues. Circ Res. 2011;108:1510-24.
7. Thanassoulis G, Campbell CY, Owens DS, et al. Genetic associations with valvular calcification and aortic stenosis. N Engl J Med. 2013;368:503-12.
8. Sánchez-Bayuela T, Peral-Rodrigo M, Parra-Izquierdo I. Inflammation via JAK-STAT/HIF-1α Drives Metabolic Changes in Pentose Phosphate Pathway and Glycolysis That Support Aortic Valve Cell Calcification. Arterioscler Thromb Vasc Biol. 2025;45(7):e232-49.
9. Weiss RM, Miller JD, Heistad DD. Fibrocalcific aortic valve disease: opportunity to understand disease mechanisms using mouse models. Circ Res. 2013;113(2):209-22.
10. Mathieu P, Boulanger MC. Basic Mechanisms of Calcific Aortic Valve Disease. Can J Cardiol. 2014;30:982-93.
11. Sverdlov AL, Ngo DT, Chapman MJ, et al. Pathogenesis of aortic stenosis: not just a matter of wear and tear. Am J Cardiovasc Dis. 2011;1(2):185-99.
12. Ferreira-González I, Pinar-Sopena J, Ribera A, et al. Prevalence of calcific aortic valve disease in the elderly and associated risk factors: a population-based study in a Mediterranean area. Eur J Prev Cardiol. 2013;20(6):1022-30.
13. Stewart BF, Siscovick D, Lind BK, et al. Clinical factors associated with calcific aortic valve disease. Cardiovascular Health Study. J Am Coll Cardiol. 1997;29:630-4.
14. Munt B, Legget ME, Kraft CD, et al. Physical examination in valvular aortic stenosis: correlation with stenosis severity and prediction of clinical outcome. Am Heart J. 1999;137(1999):298-306.
15. Levine SA. The systolic murmur: its clinical significance. JAMA. 1933;101:436-43.
16. Christensen NL, Carter-Storch R, Bakkestrøm R, et al. Sudden cardiac death in asymptomatic aortic stenosis: is the valve to blame? BMJ Case Rep. 2016;2016:bcr2015211473.
17. Baumgartner H, Hung J, Bermejo J, et al. Recommendations on the Echocardiographic Assessment of Aortic Valve Stenosis: A Focused Update from the European Association of Cardiovascular Imaging and the American Society of Echocardiography. Eur Heart J Cardiovasc Imaging. 2017;18(3):254-75.
18. Wanchaitanawong W, Kanjanavanit R, Srisuwan T, et al. Diagnostic role of aortic valve calcium scoring in various etiologies of aortic stenosis. Sci Rep. 2023;13(1):8019.
19. Chun EJ, Choi SI, Lim C, et al. Aortic Stenosis: Evaluation with Multidetector CT Angiography and MR Imaging. Korean J Radiol. 2008;9(5):439-48.
20. Grodecki K, Warniello M, Spiewak M, et al. Advanced Cardiac Imaging in the Assessment of Aortic Stenosis. J Cardiovasc Dev Dis. 2023;10(5):216.
21. Tzolos E, Kwiecinski J, Berman D, et al. Latest Advances in Multimodality Imaging of Aortic Stenosis. J Nucl Med. 2022; 63(3):353-8.
22. Nishimura RA, Otto CM, Bonow RO, et al. 2014 AHA/ACC guideline for managing patients with valvular heart disease: a report of the American College of Cardiology/American Heart Association Task Force on Practice Guidelines. J Am Coll Cardiol. 2014;63:e57-185.
23. Sung HW, Yu PS, Hsu CH, et al. Can cardiac catheterisation accurately assess the severity of aortic stenosis? An in vitro pulsatile flow study. Ann Biomed Eng. 1997;25(5):896-905.
24. Jain H, Goyal A, Khan ATMA, et al. Insights into calcific aortic valve stenosis: a comprehensive overview of the disease and advancing treatment strategies. Ann Med Surg (Lond). 2024;86(6): 3577-90.
25. Prabutzki P, Wölk M, Böttner J, et al. Sex-specific lipidomic signatures in aortic valve disease reflect differential fibro-calcific progression. Nat Commun. 2025;16(1):5163.
26. Morany A, Bardon RG, Lavon K, et al. Analysis of fibrocalcific aortic valve stenosis: computational pre- and post-TAVR haemodynamics behaviours. R Soc Open Sci. 2024;11(2):230905.
27. Karnibad M, Sharabi M, Lavon K, et al. The effect of the fibrocalcific pathological process on aortic valve stenosis in female patients: a finite element study. Biomed Phys Eng Express. 2022;8(2).
28. Synetos A, Ktenopoulos N, Katsaros O, et al. Paravalvular Leak in Transcatheter Aortic Valve Implantation: A Review of Current Challenges and Future Directions. J Cardiovasc Dev Dis. 2025;12(4):125.
29. Baumgartner H, Hung J, Bermejo J, et al. Recommendations on the Echocardiographic Assessment of Aortic Valve Stenosis: A Focused Update from the European Association of Cardiovascular Imaging and the American Society of Echocardiography; Baumgartner, Helmut et al. J Am Soc Echocardiogr. 2016;30(4):372-92.
30. Weiss RM, Miller JD, Heistad DD. Fibrocalcific aortic valve disease: opportunity to understand disease mechanisms using mouse models. Circ Res. 2013;113(2):209-22.

CHAPTER 66

Reimagining Valvular Heart Disease Management: Insights from the 2025 ESC/EACTS Guidelines

Mrinal Kanti Das

ABSTRACT

Valvular heart disease (VHD) management has rapidly evolved with the integration of advanced imaging, refined risk stratification, and expanded transcatheter therapies. This article attempts to reemphasize the 2025 European Society of Cardiology/European Association of Cardiothoracic Surgery (ESC/EACTS) Guidelines for the Management of Valvular Heart Disease to provide a clinician-focused framework for assessment, decision-making, and long-term care across aortic, mitral, and tricuspid diseases. The core emphasis was on a multidisciplinary valve-team approach, imaging-driven assessment, early referral for intervention in appropriate patients, and tailored medical therapy as an adjunct to definitive procedures. The outline of the practical algorithms for timing of interventions in aortic stenosis and regurgitation, mitral regurgitation and stenosis, and tricuspid disease has been discussed with changes based on contemporary data, including evolving indications for transcatheter therapies, durability considerations, and risk stratification refinements. Key takeaways were to prioritize timely valve intervention for severe disease, favor repair where feasible (notably in MV disease), and employ imaging and hemodynamics to guide timing and modality. The new ESC recommendations with class and level of recommendation have been presented for easy reckoning.

Keywords: European Society of Cardiology/European Association of Cardiothoracic Surgery (ESC/EACTS), transcatheter aortic valve replacement (TAVR), transcatheter mitral valve replacement (TMVR), transcatheter edge-to-edge repair (TEER), oral anticoagulation (OAC).

INTRODUCTION

Valvular heart disease (VHD) remains a leading cause of cardiovascular morbidity and mortality in developed and many developing regions. The European Society of Cardiology/European Association of Cardiothoracic Surgery (ESC/EACTS) guidelines established a comprehensive, anatomy- and physiology-driven framework for diagnosis, risk stratification, and intervention. The 2025 guidelines[1] expanded indications for transcatheter therapies [transcatheter aortic valve replacement (TAVR), transcatheter edge-to-edge repair (TEER), TAVR-in-valve, paravalvular leak closure, and transcatheter tricuspid interventions] and emphasized early specialist referral, multimodality imaging, and a patient-centered, shared-decision process. This chapter presents a clinically actionable synthesis for practicing cardiologists, focusing on decision-making workflows, terminology consistent with ESC language (class and level of evidence), and practical follow-up strategies. The whole exercise was based on the solid evidences gathered from different new and established trials and registries over the last few years and this article will also delve into the various intricacies of contemporary data, biopathological basis, and emerging technologies based on which the shifts have been driven.[1-13] Due to the space constraints, the chapter will focus mainly on the central points of interest.

KEY NEW RECOMMENDATIONS IN ESC 2025 VALVULAR HEART DISEASE GUIDELINES

- *Aortic stenosis (AS):* Intervention in asymptomatic patients with very severe AS (aortic velocity ≥5.5 m/s)—*IIa B.* The recommendation lowered threshold from previous guidelines to intervene earlier and prevent irreversible LV damage.
- Intervention in *asymptomatic patients with severe AS and rapid progression* (Vmax ≥0.3 m/s/year): *IIa C.*

It identified a high-risk subgroup that benefits from earlier intervention.

- Intervention should be considered in asymptomatic patients (confirmed by a normal exercise test, if feasible) with severe, high-gradient AS, and LVEF ≥50%, as an alternative to close active surveillance, if the procedural risk is low as *IIa A* recommendation. Transcatheter aortic valve implantation (TAVI) may be considered as *IIb B* recommendation for the treatment of severe bicuspid aortic valve (BAV) stenosis in patients at increased surgical risk if the anatomy is suitable.
- *Aortic regurgitation (AR):* Surgery for asymptomatic severe AR with LV systolic dysfunction (LVEF ≤55%): *I B.* It changed from LVEF ≤50% and recommended surgery at an earlier sign of LV impairment. However, TAVI may be considered as the *class IIb* recommendation for severe symptomatic AR.
- Surgical repair of mitral valve (MV) is recommended as class *I B* in low-risk asymptomatic patients with severe PMR without LV dysfunction (LVESD 60 mm) when a durable result is likely, if at least three of the criteria are fulfilled: (1) AF, (2) SPAP at rest >50 mm Hg, (3) LA dilatation (LAVI ≥60 mL/m^2 or LA diameter ≥55 mm), and (4) concomitant secondary TR ≥ moderate. Minimal invasive surgery may be considered as *IIb B* in experienced center.
- *Mixed aortic stenosis and regurgitation:* Intervention is recommended in symptomatic patients with mixed moderate AV stenosis and moderate regurgitation, and a mean gradient ≥40 mm Hg or Vmax ≥4.0 m/s: *I B.*
  Intervention is recommended in asymptomatic patients with mixed moderate AV stenosis and moderate regurgitation, with Vmax ≥4.0 m/s and LVEF <50% and due to other cause: *I C.*
- *Primary mitral regurgitation (PMR):* Intervention for symptomatic patients with severe PMR and LVEF >30%: *I C.*
  It strengthens the recommendation for intervention in symptomatic patients, even if not severely low LVEF.
- Intervention for *asymptomatic patients with severe PMR and signs of LV dysfunction* (LVEF ≤60% or LVESD ≥40 mm): *I B*
  It strengthened from class IIa to class I. Promotes earlier intervention to preserve LV function.
- *Secondary mitral regurgitation (SMR):* MV surgery, surgical AF ablation, if indicated, and left atrial appendage occlusion (LAAO) should be considered in symptomatic patients with severe atrial SMR under optimal medical therapy as *IIa B recommendation.*
  Transcatheter edge-to-edge repair may be considered in symptomatic patients with *severe atrial SMR* not eligible for surgery after optimization of medical therapy including rhythm control, when appropriate as *IIb B recommendation.*

  Mitral valve surgery may be considered in patients with moderate SMR undergoing CABG: *class IIb B.*

  Mitral valve surgery is recommended in patients with severe MR undergoing surgery for another valve: *I C.*

  Atrial SMR was defined by the presence of preserved LVEF (≥50%) without regional wall motion abnormalities or leaflet tethering and no or mildly dilated LV cavity (LV end-diastolic dimension of 35 mm) with enlarged LA (LAVI >34 mL/m^2).
- *Clinically severe rheumatic and degenerative mitral stenosis:* Transcatheter mitral valve implantation (TMVI) may be considered in symptomatic patients with extensive mitral annular calcification (MAC) and severe MV dysfunction at experienced heart valve centers with expertise in complex MV surgery and transcatheter interventions. Recommendation and level are *IIb C.*
- *Tricuspid regurgitation (TR):* Careful evaluation of TR etiology, stage of the disease (i.e., degree of TR severity, RV and LV dysfunction, and pulmonary hypertension), operative risk, and likelihood of recovery by a heart team (HT) is recommended in patients with severe TR prior to intervention. Recommendation and level are *I C.*
- A mechanical heart valve (MHV) should be considered in patients with an estimated long-life expectancy, if there are no contraindications for long-term oral anticoagulation (OAC): *IIa B.*
  Ross procedure was another consideration for surgical valve repair in very experienced center.
- Target INR for specific valve and education of the patients are *class I A* recommendation for OAC.
  Continuation of OAC is, in MHV, recommended as *class I A* in minimally invasive noncardiac surgery without bleeding risk. However, for bleeding risk patients, interruption for 3–4 days without bridging is *class IIb B* recommendation.
- Class *IIb C* recommendation for bioprosthetic valve or valve repair is lifelong; low-dose ASA (75–100 mg/day) 3 months after surgical implantation of an aortic or mitral positions without clear indication for OAC. It is *class IIb B* if there is high risk of bleeding.
- DAPT is not recommended to prevent thrombosis after TAVI, unless there is a clear indication for OAC: *III B.*
- OAC continuation is recommended in patients with a clear indication for OAC undergoing surgical BHV implantation as *I B.* Direct oral anticoagulant (DOAC) continuation may be considered after surgical BHV implantation in patients with an indication for DOAC: *IIb B.*
- Transesophageal echocardiography (TEE) and/or 4D-CT are recommended in patients with suspected valve thrombosis to confirm the diagnosis: *I C.*
- Reoperation has been recommended as *class I C* for failed MHV.
- Invasive coronary angiography may be omitted in TAVI candidates, if procedural planning CT angiography is of sufficient quality to rule out significant CAD: Recommendation class *IIa B.*

Percutaneous coronary intervention (PCI) should be considered in patients with a primary indication to undergo TAVI and ≥90% coronary artery stenosis in segments with a reference diameter ≥2.5 mm: Recommendation class *IIa B*.

- *HT discussion* is recommended for patients aged 65–75 years to decide between TAVI and surgical aortic valve replacement (SAVR): *I C*.

  It emphasizes shared decision-making based on individual patient factors such as anatomy, life expectancy, and preference. *HT decision is also must in complex heart diseases with valve dysfunction.*

Diagnostic approach for severity criteria and the determinants of the recommendations are as follows **(Fig. 1)**.

INITIAL EVALUATION AND IMAGING PATHWAY

- History, physical examination, and symptom assessment guide the diagnostic cascade
- TTE remains the primary tool for morphology, severity, and functional assessment; TEE provides enhanced anatomic detail for complex anatomy or planning interventions.
- 3D imaging augments assessment of repair feasibility (e.g., MV) and improves quantification of regurgitation fractions and valve area.

Advanced Imaging and Hemodynamics

- *Exercise echocardiography* is used for the assessment of LV global and segmental function, pulmonary artery pressure, and aortic and mitral pressure gradients. Apart from transthoracic approach, TEE plays an important role.
- *Cardiac CT* was recommended as essential for calcific burden assessment, annular sizing, and planning of TAVR (implant geometry, coronary access, and vascular access).
- *CMR*, the gold standard for volumetric quantification in MR and AR when echocardiography results are discordant or in complex regurgitation scenarios provides accurate LV and RV function measurements.
- *Right heart catheterization* was reserved for discordant hemodynamics, evaluation of pulmonary vasculopathy, or planning of high-risk anatomy where preciseness matters for intervention decisions.
- *Multimodality risk staging:* ESC 2025 emphasized a staging approach incorporating symptoms, LV function, pulmonary pressure, frailty, and comorbidity burden to identify patients who will benefit from valve intervention and to guide surveillance.
- *Pulmonary valve disease* was not a central focus of the 2025 guidelines and pulmonary valve management is addressed in congenital heart disease protocols. Key points include:
  - Percutaneous pulmonary valve implantation (PPVI) for RVOT dysfunction
  - Surgical replacement in complex congenital anatomies
  - Multidisciplinary care is essential for long-term outcomes.

INDICATIONS FOR REFERRAL TO SPECIALIST CENTERS

- Severe disease with symptoms attributable to the lesion or with objective LV dysfunction or pulmonary hypertension
- Asymptomatic severe disease with adverse remodeling or anatomy that favors repair/intervention
- Complex valve pathology, consideration of transcatheter options, or need for surgical planning in high-volume centers with valve teams

Explanation of classes and levels

Class I: Evidence and/or general agreement that a given treatment or procedure is beneficial, useful, effective. (Recommended/indicated)

Class IIa: Weight of evidence/opinion is in favor of usefulness/efficacy. (Should be considered)

Class IIb: Usefulness/efficacy is less well established by evidence/opinion. (May be considered)

Class III: Evidence or general agreement that the treatment/procedure is not useful/effective and may be harmful. (Not recommended).

Level A: Data derived from multiple randomized clinical trials or meta-analyses

Level B: Data derived from a single randomized clinical trial or large nonrandomized studies

Level C: Consensus of opinion of the experts and/or small studies, retrospective studies, registries

FIG. 1: Classes and levels of recommendation.

Medical therapy across VHD types (as adjunct to intervention) is mandatory in all patients. Special focus was on patients with *atrial fibrillation*. In patients with MV disease like mitral stenosis, rate control and rhythm management are keys; SMVR with left atrial appendectomy and management for atrial fibrillation simultaneously were adequately covered.

INTERVENTIONAL AND SURGICAL MANAGEMENT—SHARED DECISION-MAKING FRAMEWORK

A multidisciplinary HT approach was emphasized time and again. The cardiologists, cardiac surgeons, imaging specialists, interventionalists, anesthesiologists, and heart failure experts must collaborate on anatomy-based decisions, risk assessment, and shared goals with patients. The task force used the standard recommendation class and level as per prevailing practice. These are shown in **Figure 1**.

Special Scenarios

- Bicuspid aortic valve was recommended with special planning for coronary access and individualized planning for aortic intervention.
- For valve-in-valve and degenerated bioprostheses, preprocedural planning to address coronary obstruction risk and valve sizing were recommended as the prerequisites.
- Mixed valvular disease warranted integrated management prioritizing the dominant lesion and hemodynamic impact.

Follow-up, Surveillance, and Outcomes: Postintervention Surveillance

- Recommendations for structured early postdischarge follow-up with clinical and imaging assessment were reemphasized with periodic imaging to monitor valve function, ventricular remodeling, and hemodynamics.
- Antithrombotic management was of utmost priority to tailor to prosthesis type, rhythm status (AF vs sinus), and bleeding risk. The periodical reassessment for anticoagulation needs and risks were warranted.

Endocarditis risk and prophylaxis: Prosthetic valve endocarditis risk varies. It was recommended to adhere to guidelines on antibiotic prophylaxis and patient education regarding infection prevention.

Special Populations and Considerations

Elderly and frailty: Frailty assessment informs risk–benefit calculations; the general recommendation is to consider less invasive options where appropriate and align care with patient goals and expected benefit.

Pregnancy: VHD management requires multidisciplinary coordination; some interventions may be staged to postpartum if feasible, and maternal-fetal risk must be weighed in planning. CT imaging was not recommended due to the risk of radiation.

Chronic kidney disease (CKD) and comorbidity burden: Renal function impacts contrast use, imaging choices, and intervention strategies. It is therefore recommended to optimize CKD management in collaboration with nephrology when possible.

Sports and activity: Postintervention activity recommendations vary by valve type and recovery. It needs to be tailored to patient status and device-specific guidelines.

CONCLUSION

The European Society of Cardiology 2025 emphasized the following for practical takeaways:

- Early specialist referral for severe valve disease with symptoms or adverse remodeling, and even for certain asymptomatic cases where anatomy favors repair or transcatheter strategies
- *Greater integration of multimodality imaging:* Emphasizing the role of CT, CMR, and advanced echocardiography throughout the diagnostic and management pathway.
- *Earlier intervention:* A clear trend toward recommending intervention at an earlier stage of disease to preserve left ventricular function and improve long-term outcomes.
- *Expansion of minimally invasive options:* Refining the indications for TAVI and TEER based on newer evidence.
- Repair-first philosophy, particularly for MR, to maximize durability and outcomes
- TAVR expansion into broader populations remains feasible but requires careful consideration of durability, anatomy, and coronary access
- A dedicated valve team with standardized imaging and decision workflows improves consistency and outcomes
- Use ESC severity criteria and LV functional markers to guide timing and modality coupled with patient preferences and frailty status
- In SMR, TEER with MitraClip recommendation is class I A, based on strong evidence from recent trials for selected patients.
- For TR, transcatheter tricuspid valve intervention (TTVI) for severe symptomatic TR in inoperable/high-risk patients, recommendation was IIa B reflecting the arrival and efficacy of new transcatheter technologies.
- Surgery for isolated severe symptomatic TR without severe RV dysfunction had IIa C recommendation encouraging earlier intervention for isolated TR before right ventricular failure develops.
- General TAVI is the preferred option over SAVR for patients ≥75 years; I A reflects the accumulation of data

on TAVI outcomes in older populations where lifetime durability is less a concern.

- HT discussion is recommended for patients aged 65–75 years to decide between TAVI and SAVR; *I C* emphasizes shared decision-making based on individual patient factors such as anatomy, life expectancy, and preference.
- *Focus on lifetime management:* Particularly for younger patients, considering the entire patient journey and potential future reinterventions.

REFERENCES

1. Praz F, Borger MA, Lanz J, et al. 2025 ESC/EACTS Guidelines for the management of valvular heart disease. Eur Heart J. 2025:ehaf194.
2. Mack MJ, Leon MB, Thourani VH, et al. Transcatheter aortic-valve replacement with a balloon-expandable valve in low-risk patients. N Engl J Med. 2019;380(18):1695-705.
3. Reardon MJ, Van Mieghem NM, Popma JJ, et al. Surgical or transcatheter aortic-valve replacement in intermediate-risk patients. N Engl J Med. 2017;376(14):1321-31.
4. Obadia JF, Messika-Zeitoun D, Leurent G, et al. Percutaneous repair or medical treatment for secondary mitral regurgitation. N Engl J Med. 2018;379(24):2297-306.
5. Stone GW, Lindenfeld J, Abraham WT, et al. Transcatheter mitral-valve repair in patients with heart failure. N Engl J Med. 2018;379(24):2307-18.
6. Otto CM, Nishimura RA, Bonow RO, et al. 2020 ACC/AHA guideline for the management of patients with valvular heart disease. J Am Coll Cardiol. 2021;77(4):e25-197.
7. Vahanian A, Beyersdorf F, Praz F, et al. 2021 ESC/EACTS Guidelines for the management of valvular heart disease. Eur Heart J. 2021;43(7):561-632.
8. Généreux P, Piazza N, Alu MC, et al. Valve Academic Research Consortium 3: updated endpoint definitions for aortic valve clinical research. J Am Coll Cardiol. 2021;77(3):336-69.
9. Collet JP, Berti S, Cequier A, et al. Antithrombotic therapy after transcatheter aortic valve implantation in patients with an indication for oral anticoagulation: a randomized controlled trial. Lancet. 2022;399(10327):1380-9.
10. Lauck SB, Gulati M, Lewis KB, et al. A path forward for the implementation of shared decision-making in valvular heart disease: global joint recommendations from clinicians, patients and researchers. Health Res Policy Syst. 2025;23:136.
11. Thyregod HGH, Jørgensen TH, Ihlemann N, et al. Transcatheter or surgical aortic valve implantation: 10-year outcomes of the NOTION trial. Eur Heart J. 2024;45(13):1116-24.
12. Poletti E, Backer OD, Scotti A, et al. Transcatheter aortic valve replacement for pure native aortic valve regurgitation. JACC Cardiovasc Interv. 2023;16:1974-85.
13. De Backer O, Dangas GD, Jilaihawi H, et al. Reduced Leaflet Motion after Transcatheter Aortic-Valve Replacement. N Engl J Med. 2020;382(2):130-9.

CHAPTER 67

Rheumatic Heart Disease in India: An Imperative Tale to Tell

Sanjeev Asotra, Vinay Bhardwaj, Preetam Thakur

ABSTRACT

Rheumatic fever and rheumatic heart disease (RHD) are autoimmune sequelae of Group A *Streptococcus* (GAS) infection. There is an apparent decline in RHD in India, but there is huge heterogeneity in epidemiological data, and poorly developed states still carry a significant burden of disease. The World Heart Federation aims to eliminate rheumatic fever and reduce the burden of RHD by 2025. India contributes to 40% of the world's burden of RHD, accounting for 3.7 million disability-adjusted life years and more than 100,000 deaths every year. A multipronged approach is needed, combining public awareness, advocacy, education, continuous surveillance, easy access to penicillin prophylaxis, and strengthening of territory care service to provide cost-effective surgery.

Keywords: RHD in India, subclinical RHD, prevention of RHD, surgery in RHD, streptococcal vaccine.

INTRODUCTION

Rheumatic heart disease (RHD) remains a significant preventable cause of cardiovascular death and disability and is an important global health problem. Acute rheumatic fever (ARF) begins with Group A streptococcal infection. Patients with prolonged untreated ARF can develop RHD, which may result in severe valve damage, significant cardiac morbidity, and premature death, creating a serious medical burden on society.[1]

Driven by poverty, poor access to health services, and other health system weaknesses, the majority of people with RHD live in low- and middle-income countries, with the remainder in vulnerable communities of wealthy nations. "Eliminate rheumatic fever (RF) and minimize the burden of RHD by 2025" is the goal of the World Heart Federation (WHF).[2]

Rheumatic heart disease is the most common acquired heart disease occurring in the young population. Subclinical RHD refers to the presence of a valvular lesion diagnosed by echocardiography in an individual with no clinical manifestations of RHD. Its prevalence is substantially higher than that of clinical RHD, thereby contributing to the burden of cardiovascular disease.[3]

Group A *Streptococcus* (GAS) is a significant pathogen responsible for a wide range of diseases, including severe complications like RHD. GAS infections impact over 800 million individuals annually, resulting in approximately 639,000 deaths due to RHD and its complications. The development of an effective vaccine against GAS has been recognized as a critical global health priority, particularly in light of the World Health Assembly's resolution on ARF and RHD adopted in 2018.[4]

GLOBAL BURDEN OF RHEUMATIC HEART DISEASE

Rheumatic heart disease is a critical public health issue worldwide, and its epidemiological patterns have changed over the decades.

A systematic review of the global burden of RHD, comparing several studies from 1990–2013 from all across the globe, estimated that there are 33 million prevalent cases of RHD, causing more than 9 million disability-adjusted life years (DALYs) lost and 275,000 deaths each year **(Table 1 and Fig. 1)**.[5]

A meta-analysis of the 48 South Asian countries reveals that inequalities in the distribution of the RHD burden in the Asian Region remain significant, with the burden generally higher in economically disadvantaged areas, such as Pakistan, the Philippines, Laos, Bhutan, and India.[7]

TABLE 1: Rheumatic heart disease morbidity [disability adjusted life years (DALYs) and mortality in high burden countries (1990, 2005, 2017)].

Country	Total DALYs (thousands) 1990	Total DALYs (thousands) 2005	Total DALYs (thousands) 2017	DALY rate/100,000 1990	DALY rate/100,000 2005	DALY 2017
Global	12372.6	10318.3	9393.5	229.4	156.4	122.9
India	3438.6	3634.5	3733.3	394.6	315.7	270.4
Pakistan	226.4	292.7	296.2	208.6	182.7	138.2
Bangladesh	146.5	159.3	135.0	134.5	116.3	86.0
Myanmar	105.5	77.5	51.1	260.9	169.7	102.4
Afghanistan	36.2	55.4	54.1	362.2	245.6	164.5
Uzbekistan	64.0	84.7	68.6	305.2	314.8	212.9
Nepal	67.0	49.1	52.4	345.8	189.6	175.3
Madagascar	44.2	38.2	45.9	369.8	207.7	175.6
Iraq	34.5	36.5	25.1	162.2	129.5	72.5
Angola	32.2	28.1	25.4	354.9	225.3	118.9
Mozambique	28.4	24.8	31.1	197.0	124.7	103.4
Kazakhstan	31.9	27.2	30.3	397.9	200.1	141.8
Niger	40.9	44.4	19.8	242.9	292.7	118.6
Tajikistan	12.6	13.8	11.7	202.3	197.9	126.6
Turkmenistan	8.4	9.9	7.2	225.6	226.6	145.0

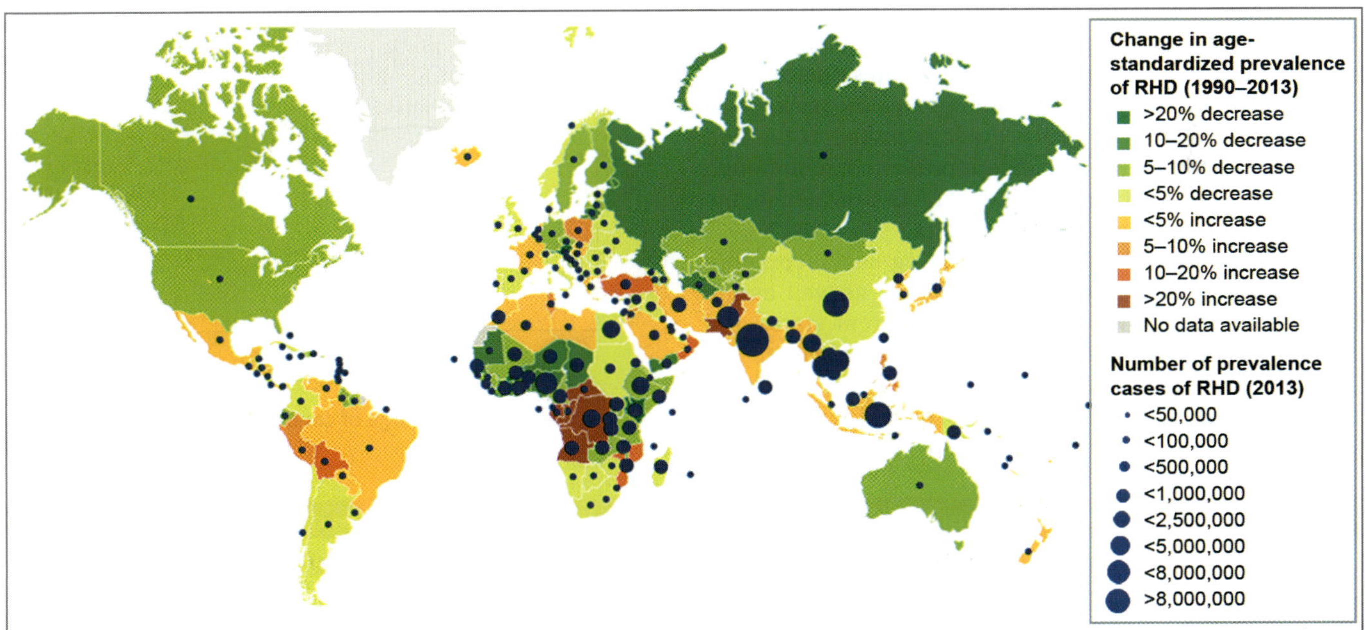

FIG. 1: Global burden of RHD.

Data on the burden of RHD were explored in the Global Burden of Disease Study 2019. Trends of the RHD burden were estimated using the estimated annual percentage change (EAPC) and age-standardized rate (ASR) **(Fig. 1)**. It showed increasing trends in the ASR of RHD incidence and prevalence worldwide. The largest increasing trends in the ASR of incidence and prevalence were seen in Fiji. The largest decreasing trend in deaths was observed in Thailand.[6]

BURDEN OF RHEUMATIC HEART DISEASE IN INDIA

Rheumatic heart disease remains a major public health problem in India. India contributes to nearly 50% of the global burden of RHD. According to WHO estimates, nearly 1.33 lakh deaths occur from RF/RHD annually in Southeast Asia compared with 10,000 and 30,000 deaths in the Americas and Europe, respectively.[8]

Rheumatic heart disease mortality rate trends from the Global Health Data between 2010 and 2014, the global mortality linked to RHD from India increased from 45.23% to 46.94%, then decreased gradually to 44.47% in 2021 owing to the multiple health initiatives like "Jai Vigyan Mission Mode Project", The National Programme for Prevention and Control of Cancer, Diabetes, Cardiovascular Diseases and Stroke (NPCDCS), and Rashtriya Bal Swasthya Karyakram (RBSK) programs **(Tables 2 and 3)**. This study also predicted that India will contribute around 40.96% of global RHD deaths by 2030, and the overall death rate per 100,000 population is estimated to reach 9.23% **(Fig. 2)**.[9]

STATE-LEVEL BURDEN OF RHEUMATIC HEART DISEASE

There is a wide diversity in state-level RHD burden (DALY and mortality rates) in India, with Bihar, Assam, and Chhattisgarh topping the charts for DALY rates due to RHD, while Arunachal Pradesh, Mizoram, and Goa are at the bottom of the same list. When it came to mortality rates due to RHD, Orissa, Bihar, Chhattisgarh, and Manipur led the pack, while Mizoram, Goa, and Arunachal Pradesh trailed at the end **(Table 4)**.[10] The data are still underrepresented, so although the figures indicate a significant decline in prevalence, the actual national burden may be substantial.

The wide diversity is due to varying socioeconomic statuses and access to quality healthcare, as well as the Human Development Index, among different states and various regions or districts within the states themselves.

There is a limitation to the GBD data in India, as it relies on indirect estimates and is based on epidemiological modeling. There is a significant absence of a comprehensive population-based registry. There is huge heterogeneity among states and within a state. RHD is a clinical diagnosis that requires confirmation by comprehensive echocardiography, which may not be readily available in all areas. The data regarding the burden of disease have been obtained from hospital records, school-based surveys conducted earlier through clinical examinations, and later through survey studies utilizing echocardiography.

Unfortunately, no data are available from an active surveillance study in a representative sample of a country or state.

Hospital-based data had shown a significant decline in admission rates of RHD over a time period. The emerging epidemic of coronary artery disease and waning interest of cardiologists in RHD and decline in prevalence of RF and RHD may be all contributory factors. A population-based survey can provide us with reliable data, but there have been no active surveillance studies conducted in recent times.

TABLE 3: Anticipated trend of mortality rate contribution from India.

Year	2010	2014	2021	2030
Mortality % contribution from India	45.23%	46.94%	44.47%	40.96%

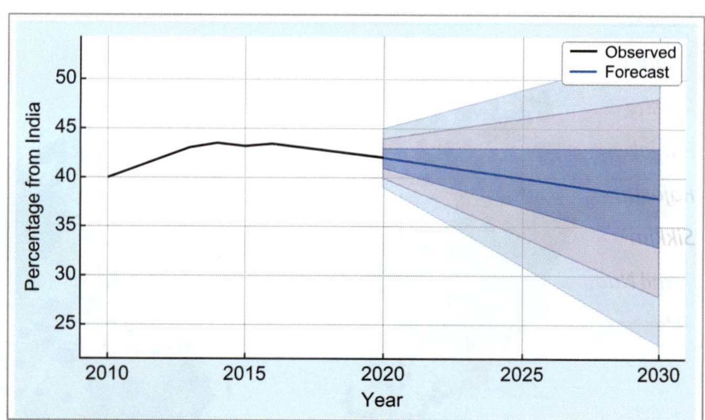

FIG. 2: Forecast of percentage of cases from India.

TABLE 2: Secular trends in rheumatic heart disease-related burden in India (Global Burden of Disease Study 2017).

Years	DALY (thousands)	DALY rate/100,000	Mortality (thousands)	Death rate/100,000
1990	3438.6	394.6	80.5	9.23
1995	3429.5	357.9	81.3	8.49
2000	3841.1	315.7	94.1	8.94
2005	3634.5	364.8	92.2	8.01
2010	3940.1	315.3	105.1	8.41
2015	3773.3	279.9	108.4	8.04
2017	3733.3	270.4	108.5	7.86

TABLE 4: State-level rheumatic heart disease burden (India, 2016).

State (alphabetic)	DALY (thousands)	DALY rate/100,000	Deaths (n)	Death rate/100,000
Andhra Pradesh	152.3	291.8	4,304	8.3
Arunachal Pradesh	2.2	150.4	60	4.0
Assam	124.2	354.8	3,398	9.7
Bihar	422.2	384.9	12,240	11.2
Chhattisgarh	97.1	351.0	2,812	10.2
Delhi	49.7	240.9	1,325	6.6
Goa	1.5	99.0	46	3.0
Gujarat	170.6	254.1	4,895	7.2
Haryana	70.4	246.0	2,017	7.0
Himachal Pradesh	13.1	178.9	411	5.6
Jammu and Kashmir	29.3	237.6	816	6.6
Jharkhand	101.1	295.7	2,870	8.4
Karnataka	195.4	295.0	5,544	8.4
Kerala	59.8	161.1	1,991	7.2
Madhya Pradesh	53.3	319.8	7,368	9.3
Maharashtra	271.1	218.8	8,095	5.5
Manipur	7.5	232.5	212	10.2
Meghalaya	4.4	208.8	114	6.4
Mizoram	1.1	91.4	35	3.0
Nagaland	4.6	176.7	132	5.0
Odisha	173.8	379.9	5,316	11.6
Punjab	196.4	263.9	5,633	7.0
Rajasthan	196.4	263.9	5,633	7.0
Sikkim	1.2	158.3	38	7.1
Tamil Nadu	173.2	232.5	5,304	7.3
Telangana	90.5	242.9	2,712	7.3
Tripura	14.9	329.6	374	7.3
Uttarakhand	30.5	242.5	868	7.1
Uttar Pradesh	687.5	315.9	19,782	8.1
West Bengal	297.6	290.2	8,382	8.2

The school surveys conducted earlier were based on clinical screening in the 1990s and later by echocardiography, revealing a constant decline in the prevalence of RHD **(Tables 5 to 7)**. The decline is real and requires further clarification. There is a clear lack of data from the most underdeveloped states and regions within the states. The improvement in the human development index, education, and better availability of quality healthcare has shown a marked reduction in the prevalence of most diseases in other southern states in India.[11-18]

According to a cross-sectional study conducted in the south Indian states of India, the age-standardized RHD prevalence rate was 9.7/1,000 population, more common in younger age groups (<44 years) and relatively high among females, concluding that RHD rates are still high in rural India among populations covered through the governmental health insurance scheme.[11]

There are expected to be more than 3.6 million patients of RHD estimated from the 2011 census. Almost 44,000 patients are added every year, and the expected mortality is 1.5–3.3% per year.[12]

TABLE 5: Population-based studies for RHD prevalence in India.

Author	Time	Place	Population	Age	Prevalence
Roy et al.	1969	Haryana	4,847	5–30	2.2
Mathur et al.	1971	Agra	7,953	5–30	1.8
Berry et al.	1972	Chandigarh	19,768	5–30	1.87
Grover et al.	1988–1991	Haryana	31,200	5–15	2.1
Agarwal et al.	1991–1992	Uttar Pradesh	3,760	0–15	6.4
Lalchandani et al.	2000	Kanpur	3,963	7–15	4.5
SriHaribabu et al.	2007–2012	Andhra Pradesh	44,164	>15	9.7

TABLE 6: School-based studies of RHD based on clinical screening.

Author	Year of survey	Area	Population	Age group	Prevalence/1,000
ICMR	1972–1975	Agra, Alleppy, Delhi, and Hyderabad	133,000	–	6–11
Koshi et al.	1975–1978	Vellore	3,890	4–16	4.4
ICMR	1982–1990	Delhi	13,509	5–15	2.9
ICMR	1984–1987	Delhi, Varanasi, and Vellore	52,793	–	1.0–5.7
Patel et al.	1986	Anand	11,346	8–18	2.03
Avasthi	1987	Ludhiana	6,005	6–16	1.3
Padamavati	1984–1994	Delhi	40,000	5–10	3.9
Kumar et al.	1992	Churu	10,168	5–15	3.34
Gupta et al.	1991	Jammu	10,263	6–16	1.4
Thakur et al.	1992–1993	Shimla	15,080	5–16	1.98–4.8
Jose	2001–2002	Vellore	229,829	6–18	0.68
ICMR	2002–2005	Kochi, Vellore, Chandigarh, and Indore	100,269	–	0.43–1.47
Misra et al.	2003–2006	Gorakhpur	118,212	4–18	0.5
Periwal et al.	2006	Bikaner	3,292	5–14	0.67
Bharani et al.	2009	Indore	25,676	5–15	0.46
Soman et al.	2010	Kochi	25,033	5–16	0.1
Negi et al.	2013	Shimla	15,145	5–15	0.6
Rama et al	2013	Andhra Pradesh	4,213	5–16	8.3

TABLE 7: School-based studies based on clinical screening followed by echocardiography.

Author	Year	Region	Sample	Age	Prevalence
Gupta et al.	1992	Jaipur	213	3–12	4.7
Bhaya et al.	2010	Bikaner	1,059	6–16	51
Saxena et al.	2011	Delhi	6,270	5–15	20.4
Ramakumari et al.	2013	Andhra Pradesh	4,213	5–16	7.6
Nair et al.	2015	Kerala	2,060	5–15	5.6
Saxena et al.	2017	Multisite	16,294	5–15	7.7
Panwar et al.	2018	Bikaner	1,508	10–15	35.2
Chaudhary et al.	2021	Bikaner	3,000	10–15	9
Kapoor et al.	2025	Meghalaya	4,039	5–15	5.19

SUBCLINICAL RHEUMATIC HEART DISEASE

Subclinical RHD is the presence of a valvular lesion diagnosed by echocardiography in a person with no clinical manifestation of RHD, and it still adds to the burden of cardiovascular diseases.[3]

A study done in 229,829 rural school children between 6 and 18 years reported the prevalence of subclinical RHD to be 0.68 per 1,000 children.[19]

A prevalence and outcome study of subclinical RHD in India estimated the prevalence of clinical RHD to be 0.8/1,000 school children. The study found that the prevalence of RHD was several-fold higher using echocardiographic screening compared with clinical examination. The prevalence is higher among girls and children of lower socioeconomic status.[20]

A study was conducted among school children in South India using echocardiographic criteria, which revealed that RHD was detected in 7.6 cases per 1,000 school children. Cases were detected several times more often using echocardiographic screening than by clinical examination alone.[21]

Chaudhary et al. (2021) conducted a study based on the WHF echocardiography criteria in school students of Rajasthan and observed a high prevalence of subclinical RHD.[22] An echocardiographic study in school children of Meghalaya identified subclinical RHD in 4.7/1,000, and subclinical RHD prevalence was significantly higher than clinical RHD.[23,24]

Progression in Subclinical Rhematic Heart Disease

The 2023 WHF guidelines provided a concise and updated resource for clinical and research applications in regions endemic to RHD. The current guidelines are designed to provide diagnostic guidance for healthcare practitioners and researchers conducting active case-finding programs, for opportunistic case detection in clinical settings, and for healthcare practitioners who detect possible RHD cases as part of routine care.

NEW FEATURES OF THE WORLD HEART FEDERATION 2023 GUIDELINES[25] (TABLE 8)

- *Introduction of two sets of echocardiographic criteria for RHD*: (1) Screening criteria are designed principally for nonexperts to apply in appropriate settings for detecting suspected cases of RHD; (2) Confirmatory criteria are designed for experts to use to confirm a diagnosis of RHD.
- Classification of RHD into stages A, B, C, and D based on the risk of progression to more advanced valvular heart disease; the terms "borderline", "definite", and "latent" RHD are no longer recommended.
- Weight-based measurements for valvular regurgitation jet length
- Recommendations for the management of the early stages of RHD

PREVENTION OF RHEUMATIC HEART DISEASE

Rheumatic heart disease is a preventable noncommunicable condition that disproportionately affects the poorest and most vulnerable populations. It is driven by poverty, poor access to health services, and other health system weaknesses. The diversity of "Eliminate rheumatic fever (RF) and minimize the burden of RHD by 2025" is the goal of the WHF.[2]

TABLE 8: Revised classification of RHD.

	Stage A	Stage B	Stages C and D
Definition	Minimum echocardiographic criteria for RHD achieved; patient might be at risk of disease progression	Mild RHD; patient is at risk of developing clinical symptoms of valvular heart disease	Advanced RHD; patient is at high risk of developing clinical complications (stage C) or already has clinical complications (stage D) and is needing medical or surgical intervention (in addition to SAP)
Risk of progression	Low risk on the basis of risk score	Moderate or high risk of RHD progression on the basis of risk score	Patients with stage C disease are at high risk of progression to stage D and/or death
Initial care	Enrolment in an RHD registry; SAP initiation is reasonable (class 2A recommendation); re-review using echocardiogram data in 1–2 years (class 1 recommendation)	Enrolment in RHD registry; SAP is recommended (class 1 recommendation)	Enrolment in RHD registry; SAP (class 1A recommendation) per local guidelines, and specialized care per local, regional, or international guidelines
Prophylaxis duration	Cessation of SAP could be considered if echocardiographic findings are normal after 1–2 years (class 2B recommendation)	Per local guidelines, or WHO guidelines if local guidelines are unavailable	Per local guidelines, or WHO guidelines if local guidelines are unavailable

India plays a crucial and important role in achieving this goal, as it contributes to nearly one-third of the global burden of disease, despite showing a decreasing trend in prevalence.

Primordial Prevention

Primordial prevention measures for RHD are categorically defined as improved socioeconomic and living conditions, as well as well-organized and effective health systems. Although there has been a constant decline in the incidence of RHD since the 1950s, largely due to improvements in economic status, the link between enhanced housing and hygiene, reduced household crowding, improved nutrition, and declining rates of ARF are evident. Social and economic improvements coupled with better healthcare systems and access to effective antibiotic treatment for GAS infections have led to ARF becoming a rare disease in almost all high-income countries.[26]

Historically, community-based prevention programs, such as those implemented in countries like Cuba and Martinique, have led to community sensitization, education, and continuous surveillance, resulting in a significant reduction in the incidence of ARF. Negi et al. demonstrated a significant five-fold reduction in the prevalence of RHD, from 2.98/1,000 in the early 1990s to 0.59/1,000 among schoolchildren in Shimla, attributed to improved socioeconomic status, better healthcare delivery, and higher human development indices.[27]

There is a clear association between ARF and socio-economic deprivation even in developed countries. The Deprivation Index, which combines nine variables including income, education, employment, accommodation, and access to car and/or telephone, strongly correlates with ARF.[28]

SCOPE OF THE *STREPTOCOCCUS* VACCINE IN INDIA

Group A *Streptococcus* infections impact over 800 million individuals annually, resulting in approximately 639,000 deaths due to RHD complications. The development of an effective vaccine against GAS has been recognized as a critical global health priority, particularly in light of the World Health Assembly's resolution on ARF and RHD adopted in 2018.[4]

Recent vaccine research has focused on both M protein-based and non-M protein-based vaccines, with several candidates showing promising results. However, current vaccines only address 50% of the prevalent types in India, highlighting the need for further research and development **(Table 9)**.[29]

Primary Prophylaxis

Acute rheumatic fever is a delayed autoimmune response to untreated Group A streptococcal pharyngitis. There is only a 0.3–3% chance of developing ARF in sporadic and epidemic GAS pharyngitis. The development of RF following GAS pharyngitis is considered a natural selection, and its pathogenesis is not well understood, as there is no successful animal model for RF.

Apart from the agent and host factors, environmental conditions that influence the development of ARF include overcrowding, low socioeconomic status, and inadequate healthcare facilities.[5] A meta-analysis underscored the importance of various preventive interventions in reducing the incidence and burden of GAS pharyngitis, ARF, and RHD. The findings indicate that school-based primary prevention services targeting the early detection and treatment of GAS pharyngitis infection with penicillin have the potential to reduce the incidence of *Streptococcus* pharyngitis and ARF.[30,31]

A study reviewed the concepts of national strategy working toward prevention of RHD with special reference to the utility of penicillin in the prophylaxis of ARF/RHD, the utility of echocardiography as the early marker of RHD, the concept of elimination or eradication of ARF/RHD, and the current scenario of prevention and control of ARF/RHD in India and concluded that adherence to these measures will bring the India down from its leading position in RHD/ARF.[32,33]

Administration of a 10-day course of penicillin for suspected streptococcal pharyngitis results in a 90% reduction in the incidence of first attacks of RF.[34]

TABLE 9: Practical issues with Group A *Streptococcus* (GAS) vaccine development.

Problem identified	Specific issues
Orphan status	Vaccine has not been wholeheartedly accepted by the industry or larger governmental or nongovernmental research bodies
Focus on strains in developed nations	The vaccine in the most advanced stage of development focuses on common strains in developed nations. GAS strains are completely different in the developing world
Paucity of clinical trials	Only one vaccine appears to have undergone clinical trials of any kind. Most candidate vaccines have not yet been tested for safety and efficacy
Cost of vaccine	Many current candidate vaccines depend on expensive technologies; their products could potentially be nonaffordable in developing countries with high disease burden

However, challenges remain in patients having mild symptoms not seeking medical attention, which undermines the effectiveness of efforts for primary prevention. Sensitizing school teachers and integrating chapters on streptococcal sore throat, ARF, and RHD into the school curriculum can lead to increased awareness and improved sore throat management in the school clinic, ultimately resulting in effective and early treatment of streptococcal sore throat. A randomized controlled trial conducted in New Zealand of a school-based sore throat intervention involving approximately 22,000 students determined the efficacy of active sore throat surveillance, accompanied by throat swab confirmation and antibiotic treatment of GAS-positive cases, and found a 28% reduction in ARF incidence in schools where the intervention was implemented.[35]

The primary prevention coverage, as shown by the African model, can reduce the projected age-standardized incidence of RHD in 2030 by 7.6% preventing 187,200 new RHD cases from 2022 to 2030.

Secondary Prevention

An important secondary preventive measure is to identify cases in the early stage of disease and facilitate interventions to avert subsequent complications. Recurrence of RF can be prevented by effective secondary prophylaxis, which includes either oral penicillin twice daily or a long-acting BPG injection every 3 weeks for a period of up to 18 years or until the age of 25 years, depending on the time of illness onset.[36-38]

Lack of awareness, nonavailability of penicillin, poor patient adherence to long-term penicillin due to various reasons, limited access to healthcare facilities, and out-of-pocket expenses are the major challenges. In a prospective study based on registry data from a tertiary care center in North India, self-reported data on drug- and transportation-related issues were collected. It concluded that RHD patients receiving BPG prophylaxis incur substantial out-of-pocket costs, causing less adherence to completing the prophylaxis.[39]

A review study on adherence to secondary prophylaxis identified a range of demographic, clinical, sociocultural, and healthcare delivery factors that influence adherence globally.[40]

The GOAL study was a randomized, controlled trial of secondary antibiotic prophylaxis in Ugandan children and adolescents 5–17 years of age with latent RHD. Among 102,200 children and adolescents who had screening echocardiograms, 3,327 were initially assessed as having latent RHD, out of which 916 with latent RHD were confirmed by echocardiogram. It concluded that secondary antibiotic prophylaxis reduced the risk of disease progression at 2 years.[41]

Penicillin administration is generally safe, and life-threatening allergic reactions are very rare in patients on long-term intramuscular BPG for secondary prevention of RHD, with the incidence of adverse events being 0.03% of injections and 0.28% of patients.[42]

A cohort model was used to estimate lifetime health outcomes and resulting costs among a cohort of 1,000 healthy children for seven intervention scenarios, namely primary prevention, secondary prevention, tertiary prevention, primary and secondary prevention, secondary and tertiary prevention, primary and tertiary prevention, and primary, secondary, and tertiary prevention. A combination of secondary and tertiary prevention strategies, with an incremental cost of ₹ 23,051 per QALY gained, was the most cost-effective strategy for the prevention and control of RF and RHD in India.[43]

Cytokine plasma levels in patients with RHD can be possible markers of disease severity, and high levels of cytokines are associated with the severity of RHD. The co-regulated expression of IL-6 and TNF-α is associated with severe valve dysfunction, whereas high levels of IL-10 and IL-4 predict a subsequent adverse outcome.[44]

Use of benzathine penicillin in patients with RHD has lower levels of IL-1β and may play a role in modifying the progression of RHD.[45]

SURGERY IN RHEUMATIC HEART DISEASE

The majority of patients with ARF will progress to develop RHD and will have involvement of the mitral and/or aortic valve. The degree and progression of valve involvement greatly depend on the inflammatory milieu, mechanical shear, and recurrence of ARF. Unfortunately, no effective medical therapy has shown evidence in modifying the rate of progression or limiting the injury to the valvular apparatus.[46]

A significant percentage of RHD patients eventually require intervention, mainly at a young age. Those with severe functional valvular changes and dilated ventricles have progressive cardiac deterioration. Timely and appropriately performed surgery and perioperative care will be required.

Late diagnosis, poverty, difficult access to quality healthcare, poor compliance with prophylaxis, and difficulty in long-term anticoagulation and its regular monitoring are significant challenges in our country, and the availability of trained cardiac surgeons compounds the problem. The available treatment options include repair and replacement, using either mechanical or bioprosthetic valves. Although valve repair significantly reduces early mortality and the mechanical valve-related complications, there is no difference in late mortality. The surgical setups are generally available in big towns and have long waiting lists of months to years, and not many cardiac surgeons have the skillset for valve repairs.[47]

NEGLECTING THE NEGLECTED

Rheumatic heart disease is a disease of poverty, and largely it is preventable. Though it is showing a decline in our country, unfortunately, a poor understanding of disease has led to limited opportunities in exploring newer prevention strategies for the progression of disease. RHD continues to receive little attention in terms of funding and research among researchers in India and globally. According to the GBD study and funding data from the G-Finder database, RHD secured the least funding relative to its disease burden, with a DALYs index of 3.83 among 16 major tropical diseases. Much remains to be done, particularly in primary prevention, the development of safe vaccines against GAS, the availability and development of safer and longer-acting penicillin, understanding the mechanisms of disease progression, the role of immunomodulation, and developing therapies that modify the natural history of valvular stenosis and regurgitation. Nonavailability of quality healthcare access to these patients leads to increased morbidity and mortality.

THE PATH TO WAY FORWARD

- A comprehensive national strategy is needed for the prevention and control of ARF and RHD in India.
- Comprehensive and robust population-based surveillance is necessary, involving active surveillance in high-risk communities and states with endemicity.
- As the enrolment rate in schools in India is high, mandatory cardiac evaluation at entry and exit can be an effective screening strategy.
- Declaring ARF and RHD to be a notifiable disease and developing a national registry.
- Using echocardiography as a robust tool to detect latent, subclinical RHD and extending this tool to noncardiologists for its diagnosis by upscaling their knowledge and skill in high-risk and remote settings. Nonecho experts can add real data transmission for expert review to prevent overdiagnosis or false positives.
- Modification is needed in the PCPNDT Act, which hinders the portability of echo machines for schools and mass screening.
- Developing tools in artificial intelligence for automatic detection and diagnosis of RHD can help to reduce the workload of medical professionals and facilitate large-scale screening.
- Evaluation of a new smartphone-based digital stethoscope for resource-crunching settings can offer an effective and accessible method as a screening tool.
- Investing in newer research, genomics, mechanistic pathways, role of immunomodulation, newer therapeutic targets in ARF, latent RHD, and in the progression of valvular heart lesions.
- Strengthening secondary prevention by ensuring the easy availability of BPG and reducing multiple barriers at both the individual and system levels.
- The Strep A vaccine presents numerous challenges, including scientific, technical, safety, regulatory, and commercial hurdles. The indigenous scientific research groups need to collaborate with the Strep A vaccine Global Consortium (SAVAC) and develop a clear roadmap for the development of an effective vaccine.
- Regional center of research and excellence of developing low-cost indigenous effective valves, surgery for valve repair, replacement, research, training for surgeons to reduce cost, early repair, and reduce waiting list for surgery in existing tertiary care centers.
- Sustained public health campaign generating public awareness of Strep A sore throat, ARF, and RHD.

CONCLUSION

Rheumatic heart disease is a disease that is a physical manifestation of poverty. There is a significant interplay of GAS infection with a susceptible host residing in a conducive environment. There has been a significant decline in RHD in India due to improvements in human development indices, enhanced socioeconomic status, improved living conditions, and increased access to healthcare. There is a strong need for a population-based surveillance system to assess the magnitude and extent of the problem, and to formulate a structured program for the prevention and control of RF/RHD.

REFERENCES

1. Lv M, Jiang S, Liao D, et al. Global burden of rheumatic heart disease and its association with socioeconomic development status, 1990-2019. Eur J Prev Cardiol. 2022;29(10):1425-34.
2. Palafox B, Mocumbi AO, Kumar RK, et al. The WHF Roadmap for Reducing CV Morbidity and Mortality Through Prevention and Control of RHD. Glob Heart. 2017;12(1):47-62.
3. Kazahura PT, Mushi TL, Pallangyo P, et al. Prevalence and risk factors for Subclinical Rheumatic Heart Disease among primary school children in Dar es Salaam, Tanzania: a community based cross-sectional study. BMC Cardiovasc Dis. 21021;21:610.
4. Moses V, Joel B, Sahni RD, et al. Group A *Streptococcus* vaccine Development: An Indian public health imperative. Indian J Med Microbiol. 2025;55:100855.
5. Carapetis JR, Beaton A, Cunningham MW, et al. Acute rheumatic fever and rheumatic heart disease. Nat Rev Dis Primers. 2016;2:15084.
6. Ou Z, Yu D, Liang Y, et al. Global burden of rheumatic heart disease: trends from 1990 to 2019. Arthritis Res Ther. 2022;(24)128:5-13.
7. Guan C, Xu W, Wu S, et al. Rheumatic heart disease burden, trends, and inequalities in Asia, 1990-2019. Glob Health Action. 2023;16(1):2215011.

8. World Health Organization. Rheumatic fever and rheumatic heart disease: report of a WHO expert consultation, Geneva, 29 October-1 November, 2001. World Health Organization; 2004 Feb 4.
9. Kamleshun R, Singh k, Goswami g, et al. Abstract 4144731: Trends in Rheumatic Heart Disease Mortality in India (2010-2021) and Projections to 2030. Circulation. 2024;150 Suppl_1.
10. Gupta R, Panwar RB, Sharma A, et al. Continuing Burden of Rheumatic Heart Disease in India. J Assoc Physicians India. 2020;68(10):60-5.
11. Sriharibabu M, Himabindu Y, Kabir Z. Rheumatic heart disease in rural south India: A clinico-observational study. J Cardiovasc Dis Res. 2013;4(1):25-9.
12. Negi PC, Sondhi S, Asotra S, et al. Current status of rheumatic heart disease in India. Indian Heart J. 2019;71(1):85-90.
13. Roy SB. Indian council of Medical Research. Prevalence of Rheumatic Fever and Rheumatic Heart Disease in Ballabhgarh; Annual Report. ICMR; 1968-1969. p. 52.
14. Mathur KS, Banerji SC, Nigam DK, et al. Rheumatic heart disease and rheumatic fever-prevalence in a village community of Bichpuri Block Agra. J Assoc Phys India. 1971;19:151-6.
15. Berry JN. Prevalence survey of chronic rheumatic fever in Northern India. Br Heart J. 1971;34:134-49.
16. Grover A, Dhawan A, Iyenger SD, et al. Epidemiology of rheumatic fever and rheumatic heart disease in rural community in northern India. Bull World Health Organ. 1993;71:59-66.
17. Agarwal AK, Yunus M, Ahmad J, et al. Rheumatic heart disease in India. JR Soc Health. 1995;115:303-4.
18. Lalchandani A, Kumar HRP, Alam SM. Prevalence of rheumatic heart disease in rural and urban school children of district Kanpur. Indian heart J. 2002;52(suppl):672.
19. Jose VJ, Gomathi M. Declining prevalence of rheumatic heart disease in rural schoolchildren in India: 2001-2002. Indian Heart J. 2003;55(2):158-60.
20. Saxena A, Ramakrishnan S, Roy A, et al. Prevalence and outcome of subclinical rheumatic heart disease in India: the RHEUMATIC (Rheumatic Heart Echo Utilisation and Monitoring Actuarial Trends in Indian Children) study. Heart. 2011;97(24):2018-22.
21. Rama Kumari N, Bhaskara Raju I, Patnaik AN, et al. Prevalence of rheumatic and congenital heart disease in school children of Andhra Pradesh, South India. J Cardiovasc Dis Res. 2013;4(1):11-4.
22. Choudhary D, Panwar SR, Gupta BK, et al. Prevalence and follow-up of subclinical rheumatic heart disease among asymptomatic school children in a north-western district of India based on the World Heart Federation echocardiographic criteria. Echocardiography. 2021;38(7):1173-8.
23. Kapoor M, Lyngdoh WV, Gunasekaran AK, et al. Prevalence of rheumatic heart disease in school going children of Meghalaya - An echocardiographic study from Northeast of India. Indian Heart J. 2025:S0019-4832(25)00165-8.
24. Karthikeyan G. Measuring and reporting disease progression in subclinical rheumatic heart disease. Heart Asia. 2016;8(2): 74-5.
25. Rwebembera J, Marangou J, Mwita JC, et al. 2023 World Heart Federation guidelines for the echocardiographic diagnosis of rheumatic heart disease. Nat Rev Cardiol. 2024;21(4):250-63.
26. Ali SKM, Engel ME, Zühlke L, et al. Primary prevention of acute rheumatic fever and rheumatic heart disease. In: Dougherty S, Carapetis J, Zühlke L, Wilson N (Eds). Acute Rheumatic Fever and Rheumatic Heart Disease. Elsevier; 2020.
27. Negi PC, Mahajan K, Rana V, et al. Clinical Characteristics, Complications, and Treatment Practices in Patients With RHD: 6-Year Results From HP-RHD Registry. Glob Heart. 2018;13(4):267-74.e2.
28. Salmond C, Crampton P. Deprivation and health. In: Howden-Chapman P, Tobias M (Eds.). Social Inequalities in Health. New Zealand, Wellington: Ministry of Health; 1999.
29. Karthikeyan G, Mayosi BM. Is primary prevention of rheumatic fever the missing link in the control of rheumatic heart disease in Africa? Circulation. 2009;120(8):709-13.
30. Balaji K, Thenmozhi R, Prajna L, et al. Comparative analysis of emm types, superantigen gene profiles and antibiotic resistance genes among *Streptococcus pyogenes* isolates from ocular infections, pharyngitis and asymptomatic children in south India. Infect Genet Evol. 2013;19:105-12.
31. Shimanda PP, Shumba TW, Brunström M, et al. Preventive Interventions to Reduce the Burden of Rheumatic Heart Disease in Populations at Risk: A Systematic Review. J Am Heart Assoc. 2024;13(5):e032442.
32. Bhargav BR, Sivasankaran S. Prevention and Control of Rheumatic Fever in India: An Achievable Health Target. Indian J Cardiovasc Dis Women. 2024;10(3);216-24.
33. Kumar R, Paul M, Paul F. RHD in India: are we ready to shift from secondary prophylaxis to vaccinating high-risk children? Curr Sci. 2009;97(3):397-404.
34. Markowitz M. The decline of rheumatic fever: role of medical intervention. Lewis W. Wannamaker Memorial Lecture. J Pediatr. 1985;106(4):545-50.
35. Lennon D, Stewart J, Farrell E, et al. School-based prevention of acute rheumatic fever: a group randomized trial in New Zealand. Pediatr Infect Dis J. 2002;28:787-94.
36. Silwa K, Watkins DA, et al. An investment case for the prevention and management of Rheumatic heart disease in Africa union2021-30: A modelling study. Lancet Glob Health. 2021;9(7): e957-66.
37. Gandhi GD, Krishnamoorthy N, Motal UMA, et al. Towards developing a vaccine for rheumatic heart disease. Glob Cardiol Sci Pract. 2017;2017(1):e201704.
38. Aalbers J, O'Brien KK, Chan WS, et al. Predicting streptococcal pharyngitis in adults in primary care: a systematic review of the diagnostic accuracy of symptoms and signs and validation of the Centor score. BMC Med. 2011;9:67.
39. Vasudevan J, Mannu A, Ganavi G, et al. Modification of Centor Score in Diagnosis of Streptococcal Pharyngitis and Antibiotic Sensitivity Pattern of Beta-hemolytic Streptococci in Chennai, India. Indian Pediatr. 2019;56(1):49-52.
40. Balaji A, Saxena A, Kazi DS, et al. Out-of-pocket expenditure for administration of benzathine penicillin G injections for secondary prophylaxis in patients with rheumatic heart disease: A registry-based data from a tertiary care center in Northern India. Ind Heart J. 2020;73:169-73.
41. Kevat PM, Reeves BM, Ruben AR, et al. Adherence to Secondary Prophylaxis for Acute Rheumatic Fever and Rheumatic Heart Disease: A Systematic Review. Curr Cardiol Rev. 2017;13(2):155-66.
42. Beaton A, Okello E, Rwebembera J, et al. Citation: Secondary Antibiotic Prophylaxis for Latent Rheumatic Heart Disease. N Engl J Med. 2021;386:230-40.
43. Bhat P, Shivashankarappa AB, Krishnappa RB, et al. Safety and concerns of secondary prophylaxis for rheumatic heart disease with benzathine penicillin: A tertiary care cardiac centre experience. J Clin Prev Cardiol. 2021;10:129-32.

44. Dixit J, Panja S, Jyani G, et al. Evaluating efficiency and equality of prevention and control strategies for rheumatic fever and rheumatic heart disease in India: an extended cost effectiveness analysis. The Lancet Global Health. 2023;11(3):e445 -e455.
45. Diamantino Soares AC, Araújo Passos LS, Sable C, et al. Circulating cytokines predict severity of rheumatic heart disease. Int J Cardiol. 2019;289:107-9.
46. Kumar S, Negi PC, Asotra S, et al. Inflammatory cytokine levels in rheumatic heart disease and their association with use of benzathine penicillin: A case-control pilot study. Indian Heart J. 2025;77(2):59-62.
47. Antunes M, Finucane K, Kumar A, et al. Surgical management of rheumatic valvular heart disease. In: Dougherty S, Carapetis J, Zühlke L, Wilson N (Eds). Acute Rheumatic Fever and Rheumatic Heart Disease. Elsevier; 2020. pp. 147-70.

SECTION

9

Cardio-Obstetrics

Section Outline

68. Cardiac Interventions during Pregnancy
S Anne Princy, R Archana, G Justin Paul

69. Antepartum Cardiovascular Risk Assessment and Management of High-risk Cardiac Delivery
Monika Bhandari, Saket Ramraika

70. Understanding and Managing Heart Failure during Pregnancy—What is New in Peripartum Cardiomyopathy?
Roopali Khanna, Sumang Mohan, Harshit Khare

71. Hypertensive Disorder of Pregnancy and Long-term Cardiovascular Outcome
S Anne Princy, G Justin Paul

72. Understanding and Managing Anticoagulant during Pregnancy in Women with Heart Valves
Abhishek Garg, Shibba Takkar Chhabra

CHAPTER 68

Cardiac Interventions during Pregnancy

S Anne Princy, R Archana, G Justin Paul

ABSTRACT

With advancing maternal age, more women are entering pregnancy with the background risk for various cardiovascular conditions. Among these, valvular heart disease, congenital heart disease, and thromboembolic disease are of particular concern. Though rare, pregnant women may require various cardiac interventions in the catheterization laboratory. Optimal management depends on preconception counseling, risk stratification, multidisciplinary care, and cardiac interventions when indicated. The choice of intervention, surgical, or catheter-based depends on the balance between maternal benefit against fetal safety. This document highlights the common indications, the need for interventions, and multidisciplinary decision-making in various cardiac conditions.

Keywords: Cardiac interventions, radiation, balloon valvotomy, percutaneous coronary interventions.

INTRODUCTION

Heart disease complicating pregnancy is a leading cause of maternal deaths in the developing nations. Over the past few decades, the number of pregnancies in women with cardiovascular disease has been rising due to improved survival in congenital and rheumatic heart diseases, advancing maternal age with associated cardiovascular risk factors. Cardiovascular disease now accounts for about one-third of pregnancy-related deaths[1] with rates increasing from 7.2 to 17.2 per 100,000 live births between 1987 and 2017.[2] With the expanding gambit of interventional cardiology, more and more critical heart diseases are now-a-days being managed with nonsurgical cardiac interventions. However, the use of percutaneous interventions during pregnancy requires careful balancing of maternal benefit and fetal risk. In high-income countries, valvular heart disease is predominantly of congenital origin, and congenital heart disease is the most frequent indication for cardiac interventions during pregnancy while in low- and middle-income countries (LMICs), rheumatic heart disease, especially mitral stenosis (MS), predominates. Selected arrhythmias may require electrophysiological procedures or device therapy, and cardiomyopathies can occasionally necessitate mechanical circulatory support. Timing of intervention often aligns with clinical deterioration—arrhythmia management in the second trimester and valve or mechanical support interventions during late pregnancy or postpartum. Involvement of a dedicated pregnancy heart team is essential for managing complex cardiovascular disease.

PHYSIOLOGICAL CHANGES DURING PREGNANCY[3]

The hemodynamic adaptations of pregnancy may worsen preexisting cardiac disease or unmask previously undiagnosed conditions as highlighted in **Figure 1**.

These changes necessitate timely cardiac interventions/surgery in appropriately chosen patients who remain symptomatic despite optimal medical therapy to improve pregnancy outcomes. Recognition of the hemodynamic burden is, therefore, critical in deciding the type, timing, and urgency of intervention, with the goal of preventing adverse maternal and fetal outcomes.

KEY CONSIDERATIONS WHEN PLANNING CARDIAC INTERVENTIONS IN PREGNANT PATIENTS

Interventional Cardio-obstetrics Team Care

A multidisciplinary cardiovascular team approach is essential for planning and performing interventions during

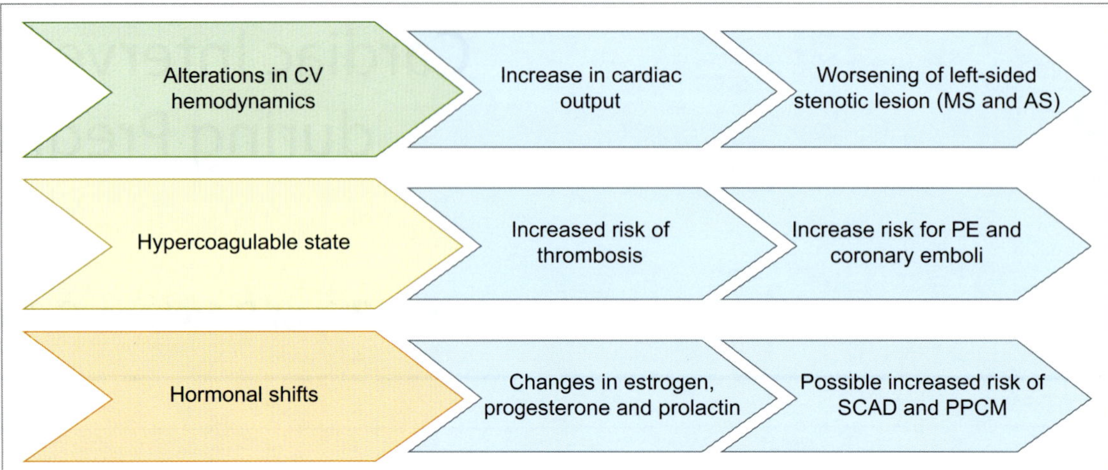

FIG. 1: Maternal changes in pregnancy and risk of CV conditions. Significant changes during pregnancy can increase the risk of various cardiovascular conditions.

(AS: aortic stenosis; CV: cardiovascular; MS: mitral stenosis; PE: pulmonary embolism; PPCM: peripartum cardiomyopathy; SCAD: spontaneous coronary artery dissection.

Source: Adapted from Park K, et al. (2022).[3]

pregnancy. This includes interventional cardiologists, cardiac surgeons, obstetricians, anesthesiologists, neonatologists, and specialized nursing staff. Such collaboration ensures careful planning of timing, choice of intervention, and periprocedural care, balancing maternal benefit with fetal safety.

Shared Decision-making and Consent

Prior to any cardiac intervention in pregnancy, patients should undergo comprehensive counseling regarding maternal risks, potential fetal implications, procedural alternatives, and the consequences of no intervention. Discussion should include the likelihood of complications, radiation exposure, and possible obstetric outcomes such as preterm delivery. Informed written consent must be obtained after ensuring that the patient has understood the information and had the opportunity to ask questions.

Radiation Exposure

Radiation exposure to the fetus is always a concern, considering interventional procedures. Most interventional procedures can be done under 5-rad, and no single diagnostic study exceeds this maximum.[4] The risk of birth defect is highest during the period of organogenesis, the first trimester and decreases with advancing gestational age. Consideration for intervention should be deferred until after the first trimester, but not at the cost of maternal health. Measures to minimize radiation like collimation of windows, avoiding angulated views, optimal table height, decreasing the fluoroscopy frame rates, and utilizing "fluoroscopy-save" features instead of cineangiography should be considered. Shielding is meant to reduce radiation, but in this case, it can trap scattered radiation inside the body that can lead to higher fetal exposure to radiation.[5]

Use of Pharmacological Agents during Cardiac Intervention

Most drugs used in the cardiac catheterization laboratory are compatible with pregnancy. Intravenous heparin is the anticoagulant of choice, with standard ACT monitoring to allow real-time procedural adjustment. Iodinated contrast agents do cross the placenta and may transiently suppress fetal thyroid function; however, this risk should not delay or prevent a necessary procedure. Their excretion in breast milk is minimal, and no interruption of breastfeeding is required.

Indications for Cardiac Interventions during Pregnancy

Whenever feasible, cardiac interventions in women with heart disease should be optimally planned and performed before pregnancy. During pregnancy, interventions are reserved for emergencies or situations where maternal/fetal life is at risk and medical therapy has failed. General indications for intervention do not differ much for pregnant women and nonpregnant patients **(Table 1)**.

CATHETER-BASED INTERVENTIONS

When medical therapy fails, interventions in the form of surgery or catheter-based interventions are required to preserve maternal life and fetal viability. In view of the high fetal loss risk associated with surgery, catheter-based interventions have become a preferred alternative.

TABLE 1: Indications for cardiac interventions during pregnancy.

Indication	Intervention	
Mitral stenosis	Severe, symptomatic, and refractory to medical therapy (pulmonary edema/NYHA III–IV)	Percutaneous mitral balloon commissurotomy
Aortic stenosis	Severe, symptomatic with syncope/angina/HF, and unresponsive to therapy	• Balloon aortic valvotomy • TAVR (rare and selected inoperable cases)
Pulmonary stenosis	Usually tolerate well Severe and symptomatic with right ventricular dysfunction	Balloon pulmonary valvotomy
Tachyarrhythmias	Refractory and life-threatening despite drugs	Catheter ablation (selected cases)
Bradyarrhythmia	Symptomatic complete heart block and symptomatic severe bradycardia	Permanent pacemaker
High-risk cardiac arrhythmias	Risk of sudden cardiac death	Implantable cardioverter-defibrillator (ICD)
Acute myocardial infarction	Ongoing ischemia, shock, and failed thrombolysis	Percutaneous coronary intervention (PCI)
Aortic dissection (Type A)	Acute dissection with rupture risk	Emergency aortic surgery
Pulmonary embolism (PE)	Massive/submassive PE with shock, thrombolysis contraindicated	Catheter-directed thrombolysis

(NYHA: New York Heart Association; TAVR: transcatheter aortic valve replacement)

Percutaneous Mitral Balloon Commissurotomy

In LMICs, rheumatic heart disease remains the most common cardiac disorder in pregnancy. MS is the predominant lesion, making percutaneous mitral balloon commissurotomy (PMBC) the most frequently performed intervention. Data from the European Registry on Pregnancy and Cardiac Disease (ROPAC) show that native MS, either isolated or with MR, accounted for about 70% of cases, with 39.2% moderate and 19.8% severe MS.[6] Heart failure complicating MS remains a major contributor to maternal morbidity and mortality in developing countries, underscoring need for timely intervention.

Indications: Patients with severe MS with New York Heart Association (NYHA)-III/IV and/or systolic PAP > 50 mm Hg, despite medical therapy in the absence of contraindication.

Patient selection: Symptomatic patients with critical MS (MVA ≤ 1.0 cm^2) favorable valve morphology with less than moderate (2b) MR and absence of LA thrombus should be considered for PBMV. Patients with severe MS (MVA ≤ 1.5 cm^2) and moderate-to-severe symptoms (NYHA functional class II–IV) with pulmonary hypertension may also be offered PBMV.

Valve suitability is assessed according to the preference of the intervention team, and it is advisable to involve senior and experienced operators in the procedure. In general, patients with an Echo-Score ≥ 12 are less likely to achieve favorable immediate or long-term outcomes with PBMV, whereas those with a score ≤ 8 typically have good results. Favorable procedural outcomes are associated with a pliable mitral valve, minimal leaflet thickening, absence of commissural calcification, limited subvalvular disease, and nil to mild mitral regurgitation.[7]

Timing: PMBC is usually performed after 20 weeks' gestation, preferably between 24 and 28 weeks' gestation. PMBC in minimally symptomatic patients may be performed around 28 weeks to ensure fetal viability in case of early onset labor postintervention. Advancing hardware from the groin to the heart for BMV can be more difficult after 30 weeks with a gravid uterus pressing on the iliac veins and inferior vena cava.

Technique: The primary aim during pregnancy is to achieve a reasonable valve area sufficient to relieve symptoms and allow safe progression of pregnancy. Hence, it is preferable to underdilate using a balloon size 1–2 mm less than that calculated by Hungs formula. A conservative approach is advised—begin with a smaller balloon size and gradually increase as necessary. Underdilatation can minimize complications, importantly, acute severe mitral regurgitation requiring emergency surgery which carries high maternal mortality and fetal risk.

Maternal outcomes: The risk of maternal events was higher if women were symptomatic prior to pregnancy; however, maternal mortality was low (0.5%).[8] Raoui et al. have recently reported PMBC in 246 pregnant women (mean age: 28 ± 5 years) with severe symptomatic MS performed at mean gestational age of 28 ± 4 weeks. The procedural complication rate was 1.8%. Pregnancy reached full term in 95% of the cases with a low fetal morbidity or mortality; spontaneous labor began at 38 ± 1 weeks, and 85% of the women underwent vaginal deliveries with an average birth weight of 2,800 ± 250 g.[8]

Percutaneous Balloon Aortic Valvuloplasty

Bicuspid aortic valve (BAV) remains the most common cause of aortic stenosis, followed by RHD. Severe symptomatic AS (mWHO-IV) is poorly tolerated in pregnancy, resulting in arrhythmia, syncope, and heart failure. In view of the high-risk nature of the disease, termination is advised if associated with left ventricular (LV) dysfunction. Because surgical aortic valve replacement (SAVR) carries higher maternal and fetal risk, PBAV is the preferred first-line option when valve morphology is favorable. Flowchart showing decision-making for aortic stenosis intervention before pregnancy based on ESC/AHA-ACC Guidance and ROPAC data.

Indications: Based on stenosis severity, LV function, aortic root size, and symptom burden. The ACC/AHA guidelines recommend PBAV or SAVR only for patients with hemodynamic deterioration despite medical therapy or persistent NYHA class III–IV symptoms. BNP levels and invasive hemodynamic assessment help to distinguish true deterioration, since echocardiographic PA pressures may be overestimated.

Timing: Reports of PBAV in pregnancy (14–36 weeks) show >50% reduction in peak gradients with minimal maternal or fetal complications.

Technique:[8] In pregnancy, the primary aim of PBAV is to enable the pregnancy to continue safely to term while minimizing maternal complications, making a conservative strategy preferable. Balloons should not exceed the dimensions of the aortic annulus or sinotubular junction to prevent acute regurgitation. Techniques such as antegrade or retrograde approaches, ultrasound-guided vascular access, smaller sheaths or radial entry, and TTE/TEE-based balloon sizing help to limit both radiation exposure and vascular injury. The procedural target is a moderate gradient reduction sufficient for maternal stabilization, rather than maximal dilation, thereby avoiding overexpansion and the risk of severe AR that might necessitate urgent surgery. The use of percutaneous preclosure devices is recommended to minimize bleeding complications.

Transcatheter Aortic Valve Replacement

Data on TAVR during pregnancy are extremely limited, with only seven case reports[9] published to date—six involving deteriorated bioprosthetic valves and one involving a native BAV. TAVR compared to SAVR carries a lower fetal risk, avoids open-heart surgery and sternotomy, eliminates the need for cardiopulmonary bypass, imposes less physiological strain on the mother, and involves minimal radiation exposure. In contrast, SAVR during pregnancy requires cardiopulmonary bypass and has been associated with a 20–29% risk of fetal demise.[9] However, performing TAVR at a young age complicates lifetime management of aortic valve disease, as it often entails the need for multiple reinterventions and carries a higher cumulative risk of complications over time. However, in patients with aortic dilatation or aneurysm, surgical intervention remains the preferred option to allow simultaneous repair of the aorta along with valve replacement. In patients associated with dilatation of aorta, surgical intervention is preferred in view of simultaneous repair of aneurysm associated with valve repair.

Percutaneous Balloon Pulmonic Valvuloplasty

Valvular PS with normal RV function is usually well tolerated in pregnancy, and PBPV is not required and can be delayed and be performed after the delivery. In severe PS with symptoms or right ventricular dysfunction, percutaneous valvuloplasty is considered if the patients do not respond to medical therapy.[10]

Percutaneous Pulmonic Valve Implantation

In pregnancy, pulmonary conduit or homograft stenosis with RV dysfunction carries higher maternal–fetal risk compared with isolated PS. In selected symptomatic women, percutaneous pulmonic valve implantation (PPVI) may be considered to stabilize hemodynamics and support pregnancy continuation, but published case reports[11] are few and highlight variable maternal and fetal outcomes. Hence, a cautious and individualized approach is essential.

Percutaneous Coronary Interventions

Pregnancy-associated myocardial infarction (PAMI) differs from the general population in that spontaneous coronary artery dissection (SCAD) is the most common cause, particularly in late pregnancy or the early postpartum period. In a recent series of 132 women, SCAD accounted for 43% of cases, followed by atherosclerosis (27%) and coronary thrombosis without atherosclerosis (17%).[12] The latter likely reflects the hypercoagulable state of pregnancy.

The management plan for PAMI should follow usual guideline recommendations. Radial approach is preferred over femoral in view of restricting direct pelvic radiation.

PCI in SCAD is technically challenging and carries a high risk of procedure related complications. Deep guide catheter engagement during coronary cannulation and high-pressure contrast injections can result in propagation of the dissections and thereby expand infarction. Coronary guidewires may inadvertently enter a false lumen, making stent placement potentially disastrous **(Flowchart 1)**.[13]

According to ESC guidelines, primary PCI is the preferred reperfusion strategy in pregnancy. When acute MI is due to coronary thrombus, stent implantation is appropriate. In the absence of evidence for fetal harm, drug-eluting stents (DES) are preferred.[13] The DES are generally favored in the first two

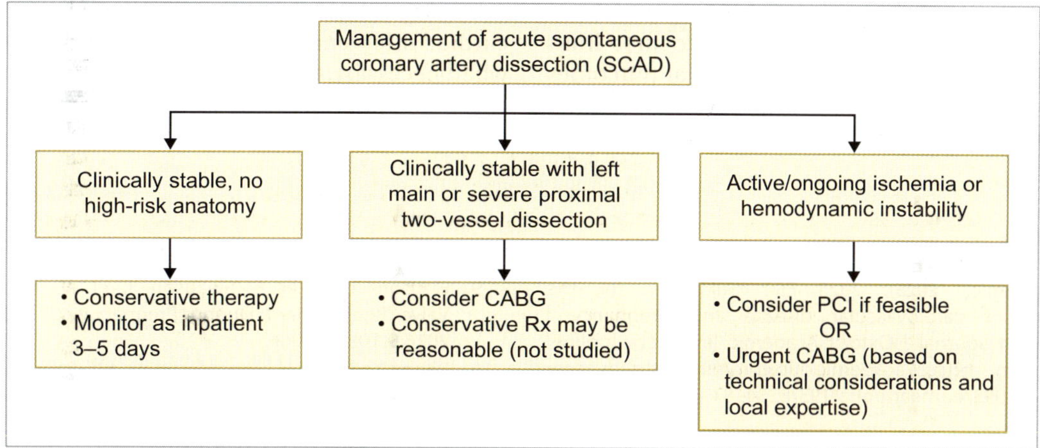

FLOWCHART 1: Management of SCAD during pregnancy.
(CABG: coronary artery bypass grafting; PCI: percutaneous coronary intervention)

trimesters, whereas in the third trimester either a bare-metal stent or DES may be reasonable, taking into account the need for dual antiplatelet therapy.

Pacemaker Implantation in Pregnancy

Sinus node dysfunction and AV block are the most common reasons for pacemaker implantation in women of reproductive age group. Only limited number of case reports were published in pregnant women with pacemaker/ bradyarrhythmia. For women paced before pregnancy, pacemaker is well tolerated in patients without structural heart disease. Beyond 8 weeks, permanent pacemaker implantation can be safely performed, if deemed necessary. Nonfluoroscopic transvenous pacemaker implantation in pregnant women with congenital heart disease, using electroanatomic mapping to visualize the RV lead and its apical placement to avoid radiation exposure has been reported.[14]

Radiofrequency Ablation during Pregnancy

Catheter ablation for focal atrial tachycardia and SVT emerges as an efficacious treatment, particularly when it is refractory to medical treatment or associated with tachycardia-induced cardiomyopathy. With the development and adoption of nonfluoroscopic three-dimensional (3D) mapping technology[15] (e.g., CARTO and EnSite), fetal exposure to radiation can be avoided. Recommendation is to postpone the procedure until after delivery whenever possible.

Catheter-directed Pulmonary Thrombectomy/Thrombolysis

The mortality rate for pregnant women with PE is about 3%, significantly higher than that for nonpregnant women with PE.[16] Catheter-based thrombectomy and thrombolysis have not been systematically evaluated in pregnancy, and current knowledge is derived solely from isolated case reports. For massive or high-risk acute pulmonary embolism, systemic thrombolysis is indicated. Percutaneous treatment is considered for high-risk PE when systemic thrombolysis is contraindicated or has failed.[10] Percutaneous procedures are more relevant in the early postpartum period, where the risk of postpartum hemorrhage is high with systemic thrombolysis.

Advanced Hemodynamic Support in Pregnancy

Peripartum cardiogenic shock carries maternal mortality rates up to 30–50%, with most cases linked to peripartum cardiomyopathy, acute myocardial infarction, or massive pulmonary embolism. Use of venoarterial ECMO (VA-ECMO) has been associated with maternal survival rates of 50–80%, while fetal survival is lower (30–50%) due to frequent preterm delivery and hemodynamic instability. IABP and Impella are reported mainly as adjuncts for LV unloading in combination with ECMO, though evidence is limited to case series and registries. Timely initiation of mechanical circulatory support before onset of multiorgan failure is a key determinant of outcome. Pregnancy should not be a reason for deferring the use of Implella, ECMO, or VADs, etc., when indicated. Device selection must be carefully tailored to the patient's hemodynamic profile and anatomical considerations, with management guided by a multidisciplinary cardio-obstetric team to optimize maternal stabilization while safeguarding fetal outcomes.[17]

CONCLUSION

Cardiac interventions during pregnancy remain a delicate balance between maternal rescue and fetal safety. Although advances in catheter-based techniques have expanded treatment options, the risks of radiation, procedural complications, and uncertain long-term outcomes limit their use to carefully selected patients. Optimal outcomes depend on individualized decision-making, timing interventions to minimize maternal and fetal harm, and involving a multidisciplinary cardio-obstetric team. While cardiac interventions can be performed during pregnancy when necessary, the real cornerstone is optimizing maternal cardiac conditions with appropriate interventions before conception whenever possible.

REFERENCES

1. Oxford Academic. (2025). 2025 ESC Guidelines for the management of cardiovascular disease and pregnancy | European Heart Journal | Oxford Academic [Internet]. [online] Available from https://academic.oup.com/eurheartj/advance-article/doi/10.1093/eurheartj/ehaf193/8234487 [Last accessed Oct., 2025].
2. Mehta LS, Warnes CA, Bradley E, et al. Cardiovascular Considerations in Caring for Pregnant Patients: A Scientific Statement From the American Heart Association. Circulation. 2020;141(23):e884-903.
3. Park K, Bortnick AE, Lindley KJ, et al. Interventional Cardiac Procedures and Pregnancy. J Soc Cardiovasc Angiogr Interv. 2022;1(5):100427.
4. Davis MB, Arendt K, Bello NA, et al. Team-Based Care of Women With Cardiovascular Disease From Pre-Conception Through Pregnancy and Postpartum: JACC Focus Seminar 1/5. J Am Coll Cardiol. 2021;77(14):1763-77.
5. Toppenberg KS, Hill DA, Miller DP. Safety of radiographic imaging during pregnancy. Am Fam Phys. 1999;59(7):1813-8, 1820.
6. Sayed YG. (2025). Mitral stenosis in pregnant patients [Internet]. [online] Available from https://www.escardio.org/Journals/E-Journal-of-Cardiology-Practice/Volume-16/Mitral-stenosis-in-pregnant-patients# [Last accessed Oct., 2025].
7. Oxford Academic. (2025). Percutaneous mitral balloon valvuloplasty - state of the art [Internet]. [online]] Available from https://www.oaepublish.com/articles/2574-1225.2020.72. [Last accessed Oct., 2025].
8. Elkayam U, Bansal P, Mehra A. Catheter-Based Interventions for the Management of Valvular Heart Disease During Pregnancy. JACC Adv. 2022;1(2):100022.
9. Hodson R, Kirker E, Swanson J, et al. Transcatheter Aortic Valve Replacement During Pregnancy. Circ Cardiovasc Interv. 2016;9(10):e004006.
10. Regitz-Zagrosek V, Roos-Hesselink JW, Bauersachs J, et al. 2018 ESC Guidelines for the management of cardiovascular diseases during pregnancy. Eur Heart J. 2018;39(34):3165-241.
11. Detzner AA, Hopkins KA, Kay WA, et al. Successful TPV Implantation in a Pregnant Patient With Right Ventricle to Pulmonary Artery Conduit Obstruction. JACC Case Rep. 2020;2(1):135-8.
12. JACC. (2025). High-Risk Cardiac Disease in Pregnancy: Part I | JACC [Internet]. [online] Available from https://www.jacc.org/doi/10.1016/j.jacc.2016.05.048. [Last accessed Oct., 2025].
13. American Heart Association. (2025). Pregnancy-Associated Myocardial Infarction | Circulation: Cardiovascular Interventions [Internet]. [online] Available from https://www.ahajournals.org/doi/10.1161/CIRCINTERVENTIONS.120.008687. [Last accessed Oct., 2025].
14. Hartz J, Clark BC, Ito S, et al. Transvenous nonfluoroscopic pacemaker implantation during pregnancy guided by 3-dimensional electroanatomic mapping. Hear Case Rep. 2017;3(10):490.
15. Hartz J, Clark BC, Ito S, et al. Transvenous nonfluoroscopic pacemaker implantation during pregnancy guided by 3-dimensional electroanatomic mapping. Hear Case Rep. 2017;3(10):490-2.
16. Cueto-Robledo G, Cervantes-Naranjo FD, Gonzalez-Hermosillo LM, et al. Pulmonary Embolism During Pregnancy: An Updated Review With Case Series Description. Curr Probl Cardiol. 2023;48(7):101683.
17. Botti G, Thirunavukarasu S, Ziviello F, et al. Peripartum Cardiogenic Shock and Mechanical Circulatory Support. Interv Cardiol Rev Res Resour. 2023;18:e28.

CHAPTER 69

Antepartum Cardiovascular Risk Assessment and Management of High-risk Cardiac Delivery

Monika Bhandari, Saket Ramraika

ABSTRACT

Cardiovascular disease is a major contributor to maternal morbidity and mortality during pregnancy. This chapter reviews antepartum cardiovascular risk assessment, hemodynamic adaptations, and evidence-based management strategies. It emphasizes multidisciplinary cardio-obstetric teamwork, individualized delivery planning, and updated global and Indian guideline perspectives for high-risk cardiac pregnancies.

Keywords: Pregnancy, cardiovascular disease, risk assessment, cardio-obstetrics, heart failure, valvular disease, cardiomyopathy, arrhythmia, aortic disease, anticoagulation, high-risk delivery, maternal outcomes.

INTRODUCTION

Pregnancy is a complex physiological state that presents substantial challenges to the maternal cardiovascular system. These challenges arise from a series of hemodynamic, hormonal, and structural changes that accommodate the growing fetus and prepare the mother for labor and delivery. While healthy women adapt to these changes seamlessly, those with pre-existing cardiovascular disease (CVD) or a predisposition to cardiac dysfunction may experience serious complications. The field of *cardio-obstetrics* has evolved to meet this need, emphasizing the integration of obstetricians, cardiologists, anesthesiologists, and neonatologists into a multidisciplinary team. This collaborative model has demonstrated improved outcomes in high-risk pregnancies, particularly when risk stratification, pharmacologic optimization, and delivery planning are conducted proactively. This chapter provides a comprehensive framework for the antepartum cardiovascular risk assessment and the management of high-risk cardiac delivery.

EPIDEMIOLOGY AND ITS CLINICAL SIGNIFICANCE

Among developed countries, the United States has the highest maternal mortality rate. Cardiovascular (CV) disease complicates 1–4% of pregnancies and remains the leading cause of maternal mortality in many developed countries. As symptoms of normal pregnancy like fatigue, shortness of breath, and swelling often overlap that of CVD, *diagnosis of CVD is often challenging during pregnancy.* Thus, many patients are often not identified during pregnancy, delivery, hospitalization, or even during the postpartum period leading to increased maternal loss.[1] Therefore, the primary reasons of adverse maternal outcomes related to CVD are delay in recognition and timely management of maternal cardiac disease. There is an alarming increase in maternal deaths to 32.9 from 23.8 per 100,000 births in 2020 in a recent report by the Centres for Disease Control calls.[2] Due to increase in the mortality rate from 12.6 to 28 per 100,000 live births from 2019 to 2021 in US, a CVD toolkit was developed through California Maternal Quality Care Collaborative (CMQCC) and Cardiac Conditions in Obstetrical Care (CCOC) which involved obstetricians, cardiologists, anesthetist, and others.[3,4] This alliance was an innovation to improve these worsening outcomes.[5] CVD is responsible for including for one-quarter of maternal deaths.[4] The American College of Obstetrics and Gynaecology provides guidance for the evaluation of symptoms suggestive of CVD and the urgency for additional evaluation if needed.[6] The *CMQCC cardiovascular risk assessment* algorithm and other methodologies which use physical examination and electrocardiograms as screening tests for CVD detection in pregnant patients are helpful in identifying pregnant patients at increased risk of CVD.[7] The role of a "*Pregnancy Heart Team*" also known as the Cardio-Obstetric Team is integral to the care of this high-risk group of patients.[6]

ANTEPARTUM CARDIOVASCULAR RISK ASSESSMENT: PROMPT RECOGNITION OF CARDIOVASCULAR DISEASE

- History and functional status assessment
- Clinical examination
- *Biomarkers*: Brain natriuretic peptide (BNP) and NT-proBNP

Risk stratification tools: *Modified WHO* classification *CARPREG II* score *ZAHARA* score.

Similarly, the *AIM CCOC bundle* is another obstetric care which involves a Change Package where there is transitions of care, especially in the "fourth" trimester, involving care at the time of discharge from the birthing facility to home and transition from postpartum care to ongoing primary and specialty care along with the resources and tools for institutions to utilize and implement in various healthcare settings.[8] A *CVD risk assessment algorithm* has been postulated that stratifies pregnant and postpartum patients into the categories of "low risk" and "high risk" for CVD **(Fig. 1)**.[9] Benefits of risk assessment can be demonstrated over immediate, short, and long-term benefits **(Fig. 2)**.[10]

PHYSIOLOGICAL CARDIOVASCULAR CHANGES IN PREGNANCY

Pregnancy induces substantial cardiovascular adaptations necessary to meet the metabolic and oxygenation demands of the developing fetus. These adaptations begin early in gestation and peak during the second and early third trimesters.

- *Hemodynamic adaptations*: Cardiac output increases by 30–50% during pregnancy. Initially, this is due to an increase in stroke volume, but later, heart rate also rises (by 10–20 bpm). The increase in output begins as early as 5 weeks of gestation and peaks around 28–32 weeks.
- *Blood volume and plasma changes*: Plasma volume increases by 40–50%, while red blood cell mass increases by only about 20–30%, leading to a dilutional anemia known as the *"physiological anemia of pregnancy."* This state enhances placental perfusion but may also mask anemia or overestimate volume status in women with heart failure.
- *Structural and functional cardiac changes*: The left atrium and left ventricle undergo eccentric hypertrophy, with increased chamber size and mass. *While these changes are physiological, they may mimic or exacerbate pre-existing conditions like dilated cardiomyopathy or valvular regurgitation.*
- *Autonomic and respiratory effects*: Pregnancy results in heightened sympathetic tone and increased sensitivity to catecholamines, contributing to palpitations and increased arrhythmogenic potential. Tidal volume increases, leading to mild respiratory alkalosis. *Dyspnea* is a common symptom even in healthy women, which can confound the evaluation of heart failure.
- *Labor and delivery considerations*: Uterine contractions result in autotransfusion of 300–500 mL of blood into the central circulation with each contraction. This volume load can stress the cardiovascular system, particularly in patients with limited cardiac reserve. The postpartum period is marked by diuresis, vasoconstriction, and reversal of the placental shunt, all of which challenge the maternal heart **(Fig. 3 and Table 1)**.[11]

CLASSIFICATION OF MATERNAL CARDIOVASCULAR RISK

Classification of maternal cardiovascular risk is pivotal to planning antenatal surveillance, delivery, and postpartum care. Several systems have been developed, but the most used are the modified WHO classification, CARPREG II score, and ZAHARA model.

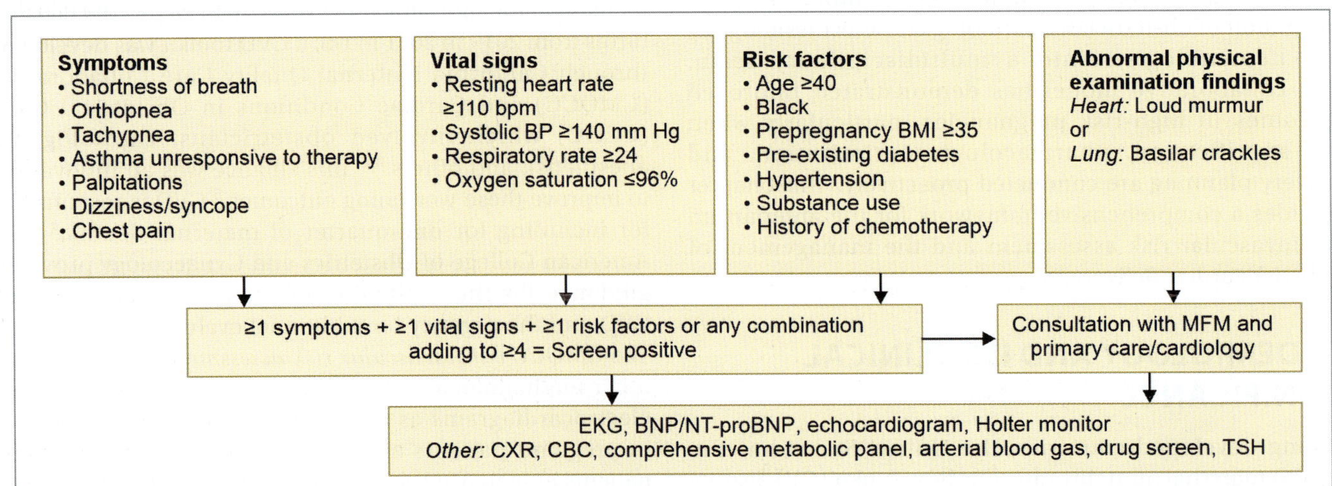

FIG. 1: CVD risk assessment algorithm during pregnancy and postpartum.
(CVD: cardiovascular disease)

Modified WHO classification (mWHO): This system classifies cardiac conditions into four groups:

1. *Class I*: Minimal risk (e.g., small ASD, MVP without regurgitation)
2. *Class II*: Mild risk (e.g., repaired tetralogy of Fallot)
3. *Class III*: Significant risk (e.g., mechanical valve, EF <40%)

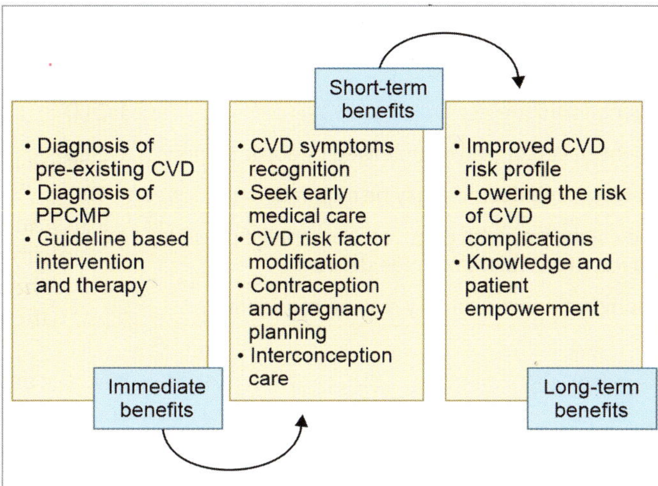

FIG. 2: Benefits of risk cardiovascular risk assessment in pregnancy.

4. *Class IV*: Contraindication to pregnancy (e.g., PAH, Eisenmenger)

Studies show that women in mWHO Class III–IV are at 25–70% risk of adverse maternal events, including death.

CARPREG II score:
This model incorporates:

- Prior cardiac events (3 points)
- Cyanosis/NYHA III–IV (3 points)
- EF < 40% (2 points)
- Obstructive lesions (2 points)
- Use of anticoagulants (1.5 points)

Scores correlate with escalating risk:

- 0 points—5% complication risk
- ≥4 points—up to 75% risk

ZAHARA score (for congenital heart disease): Derived from a large European cohort, it assigns weights to—surgical history, cyanosis, pulmonary hypertension, and ventricular dysfunction.

SPECIFIC LESIONS

- Valvular heart disease
- Native valve disease
- Stenotic lesions

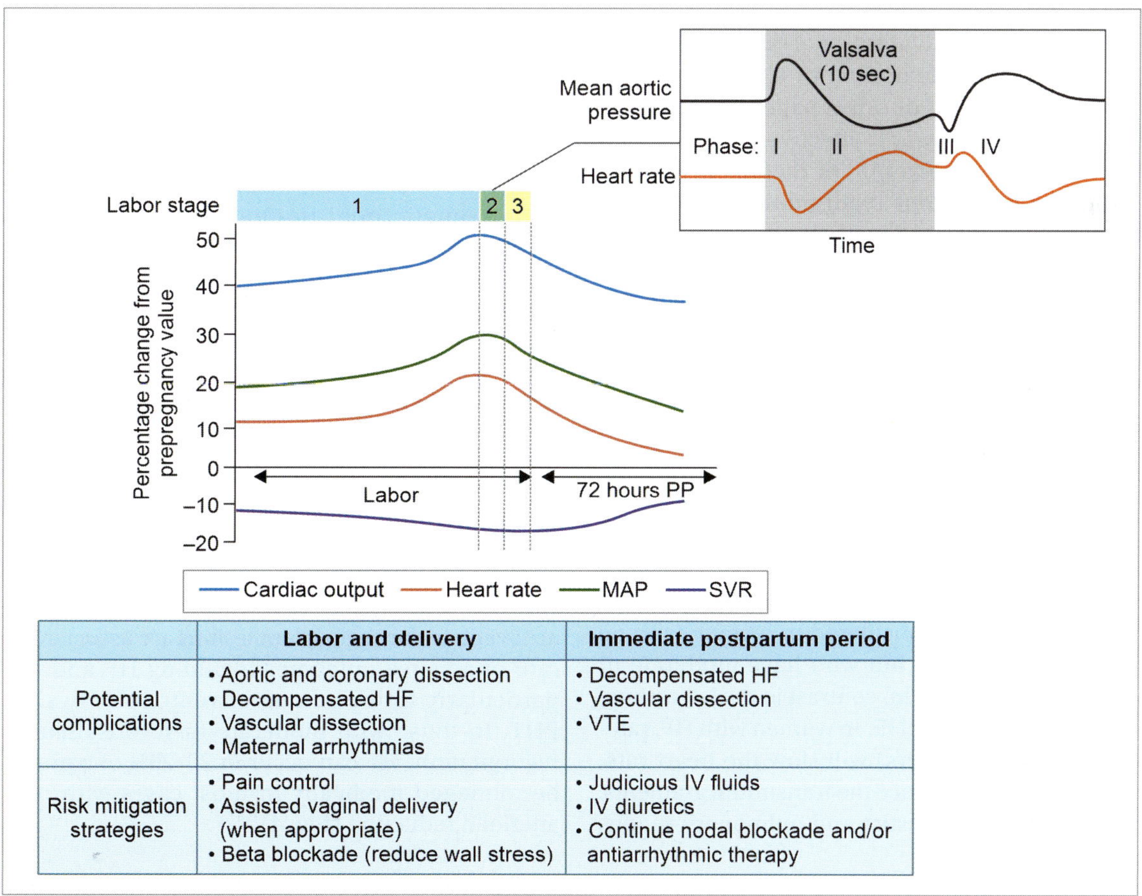

	Labor and delivery	Immediate postpartum period
Potential complications	• Aortic and coronary dissection • Decompensated HF • Vascular dissection • Maternal arrhythmias	• Decompensated HF • Vascular dissection • VTE
Risk mitigation strategies	• Pain control • Assisted vaginal delivery (when appropriate) • Beta blockade (reduce wall stress)	• Judicious IV fluids • IV diuretics • Continue nodal blockade and/or antiarrhythmic therapy

FIG. 3: Hemodynamic changes during pregnancy and labor.

TABLE 1: Mode of delivery in patient with aortopathies based on aortic diameter.

Condition	Aortic diameter	Delivery mode	COR LOE
Aorta[a] not significantly dilated	<4 cm	Vaginal[b]	1 C-EO
Aortic enlargement[a]	4–4.5 cm	Vaginal reasonable[c]	2b C-EO
Syndromic (Marfan syndrome, Ehler–Danlos, Loeys–Dietz syndromes) or ns-HTAD	4–4.5 cm	Cesarean reasonable[d]	2a C-EO
Aortic diameter	≥4.5 cm	Cesarean reasonable	2a C-EO
Chronic aortic dissection	NA	Cesarean recommended	1 C-EO
Acute type A dissection T1–T2	—	Urgent aortic surgery[e]	1 C-LD
Acute type A dissection T3	—	Urgent cesarean delivery followed by aortic surgery	1 C-LD
Acute type A dissection 24–28 weeks	—	Individualized decision may be required	
Type B dissection	—	Medical therapy with endovascular repair if possible and required. Cesarean mode delivery	1 C-LD
Progressive aortic growth	—	Prophylactic aortic surgery may be considered	2b C-EO

[a]Aortic root diameter, ascending aortic diameter, or both.
[b]In absence of obstetric indication for cesarean mode of delivery.
[c]With regional anesthesia, expedited second stage, assisted delivery.
[d]Patients with vascular Ehlers–Danlos syndrome should always undergo cesarean delivery due to risk of uterine rupture with labor.
[e]Surgery should be performed with fetal monitoring and modification of bypass to reduce fetal loss.

Note: For all patients with aortopathy, beta-blockade therapy titrated to maximum tolerated dose is recommended.

(COR: class of recommendation; EO: expert opinion; LD: limited data; LOE: level of evidence; ns-HTAD: nonsyndromic heritable)

Percutaneous balloon valvuloplasty (PBV) as a bridge to surgery or as a therapeutic option for stenotic valvular disease should be considered during a patient's pregnancy when pharmacologic therapy is ineffective for those with severe congenital aortic stenosis (AS) or rheumatic MS with less than moderate concurrent regurgitation. PBV using fluoroscopic guidance should ideally be performed after 15 weeks' gestation and the completion of organogenesis. PBV may be performed using transesophageal echocardiography guidance to reduce or obviate the need for ionizing radiation.[12]

Mitral Stenosis

Three percent mortality risk, 37% risk of developing pulmonary edema, and a 16% risk of developing new or recurrent arrhythmias in pregnant women with severe MS. Women with MS and atrial fibrillation or a previous thromboembolic episode should be anticoagulated. Anticoagulation can also be considered in women with no documented atrial fibrillation but who have moderate or greater MS with spontaneous echo contrast in the left atrium, a large left atrium (60 cc/m^2), or HF. In women with HF, rate-slowing medications (β-blockers) will slow the heart rate, extend diastolic filling time, reduce the transmitral gradients, and decrease the left atrial pressure and pulmonary venous congestion. Diuretics can also be used to treat HF refractory to adequate rate control.[13]

Aortic Valve Stenosis

Pregnancy is usually well-tolerated in women with asymptomatic mild-to-moderate AS. In a recent meta-analysis, the risks of death, pulmonary edema, and new or recurrent arrhythmias were 2%, 9%, and 4%, respectively, in pregnant women with severe AS and 0%, 8%, and 2%, respectively, in pregnant women with moderate AS.[13] Women with severe AS who develop HF should be treated with diuresis. If women remain symptomatic or have HF despite medical therapy, consideration should be given to relief of the AS either with a PBV or surgical aortic valve replacement.

Regurgitant Lesions

Aortic and pulmonary regurgitant lesions are usually well tolerated during pregnancy. However, moderate-to-severe atrioventricular regurgitant lesions are associated with a 15% rate of adverse outcomes including HF and arrhythmias, particularly in the setting of ventricular dysfunction and PHT. In those with moderate-to-severe rheumatic mitral regurgitation, HF can occur in 20–25% of patients. This can be managed medically in most cases with diuretics and afterload reduction **(Fig. 4)**.[14]

PROSTHETIC VALVES AND ANTICOAGULATION

Anticoagulation for women with a mechanical valve may be achieved with warfarin, low molecular weight heparin, or full-dose unfractionated heparin. With all of this in mind, there are three potential strategies: (1) warfarin throughout pregnancy, particularly if the required dose is < 5 mg daily; (2) heparin throughout pregnancy; and (3) sequential therapy, with heparin during the first trimester and warfarin during the second and third trimesters **(Table 2)**.[15]

Cardiomyopathy: In women with a known cardiomyopathy, a major component of preconception counseling involves reviewing regular medications because many standard HF therapies are contraindicated in pregnancy. *Assessing left ventricular (LV) function without such medications improves risk stratification before pregnancy.* Diuretics and β-blockers should be continued and hydralazine and nitrates are alternatives to the contraindicated medications **(Fig. 5)**.[16]

Acute HF: Effort intolerance, fatigue, and ankle edema are common findings during normal pregnancy and, therefore, similar signs and symptoms of HF can be missed. Suspicion should be high with new onset of orthopnea and paroxysmal nocturnal dyspnea and persistent tachycardia. Presentation during pregnancy occurs generally in the second or third trimester or in the postpartum period. The assessment and

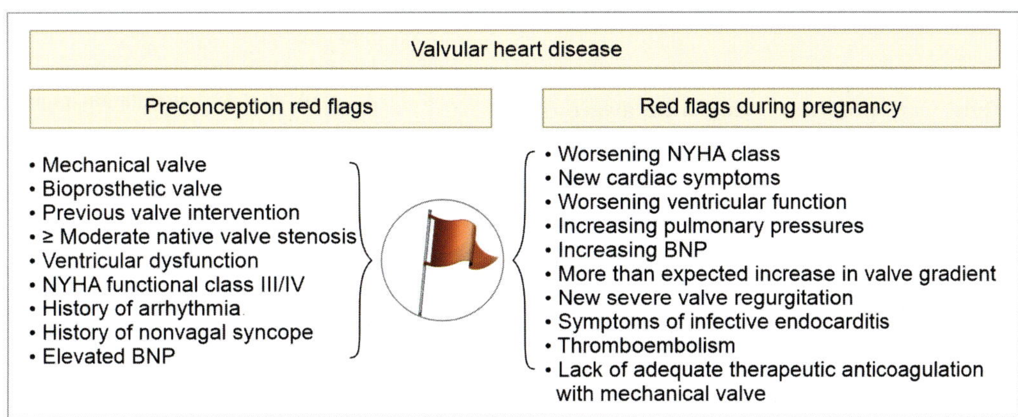

FIG. 4: Red flags in valvular heart disease for pregnancy.

TABLE 2: Pros and cons of various methods of anticoagulation during pregnancy.

Pros	Cons
VKA: • Lowest risk of valve thrombosis and thromboembolism • Lowest maternal mortality and morbidity • Oral administration	*VKA*: • Crosses the placenta • Warfarin embryopathy and fetopathy • Highest risk for miscarriage/fetal loss • Close INR monitoring • Dose adjustments during pregnancy
LMWH: • Does not cross the placenta • No embryopathy and fetopathy • Most live births • Reduced risk of valve thrombosis and thromboembolism with meticulous anti-Xa monitoring	*LMWH*: • Twice daily injections • Expensive • Close anti-Xa monitoring • Dose adjustments during pregnancy • Higher risk of valve thrombosis compared with VKA
UFH: • Does not cross the placenta • No embryopathy and fetopathy	*UFH*: • Highest risk of valve thrombosis and thromboembolism • Highest maternal mortality and morbidity • Highest risk of fetal complications • Close PTT monitoring • Dose adjustments during pregnancy

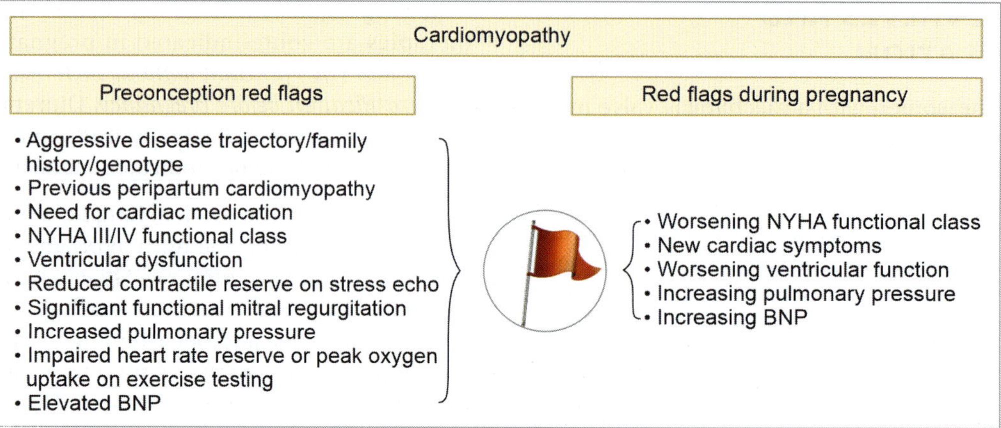

FIG. 5: High-risk features for pregnancy with cardiomyopathies.

treatment of acute HF follow the same principles as for the nonpregnant patient. Care providers should be aware of red flags indicative of women particularly at higher risk of complications **(Fig. 6)**.[17]

Peripartum cardiomyopathy (PPCM): It is an idiopathic condition with LV systolic dysfunction [ejection fraction (EF) < 45%] occurring toward the end of pregnancy or within 5 months after delivery, when no other cause is found. [Pregnancy in women with severe LV systolic dysfunction (EF < 30%) is very high risk and counseling about the potential significant complications to mother and fetus should occur. If already pregnant, early termination should be offered] put in cardiomyopathy section). Patients with previous PPCM and normalization of LV function with good contractile reserve on stress echocardiography can consider future pregnancy after thorough risk stratification and understanding that there is a risk of recurrent PPCM.[18,19]

Hypertrophic cardiomyopathy: Most patients with familial hypertrophic cardiomyopathy do well-during pregnancy. Exceptions are women with prepregnancy symptoms despite optimal medical treatment, moderate or greater LV dysfunction, diastolic dysfunction, PHT, and/or severe LV outflow tract obstruction.[20]

Ischemic heart disease: Pregnancy is associated with a three- to fourfold increase in acute coronary syndrome (ACS) risk compared with age-matched nonpregnant women. It is most commonly related to coronary atherosclerotic plaque rupture, dissection, or myocardial infarction in the absence of coronary artery disease (thrombosis, vasospasm, microvascular dysfunction). Incidence of ACS ranges between 3 and 8 cases per 100,000 deliveries with mortality upward of 7%. Acute ST-segment elevation myocardial infarction (STEMI) or high-risk non-STEMI due to plaque rupture or thrombosis requires a timely invasive strategy. Thrombolysis can be considered in women with STEMI because it does not cross the placenta, but it is not a preferred option because coronary dissection is a leading cause of myocardial infarction in pregnant women. ACS presentation

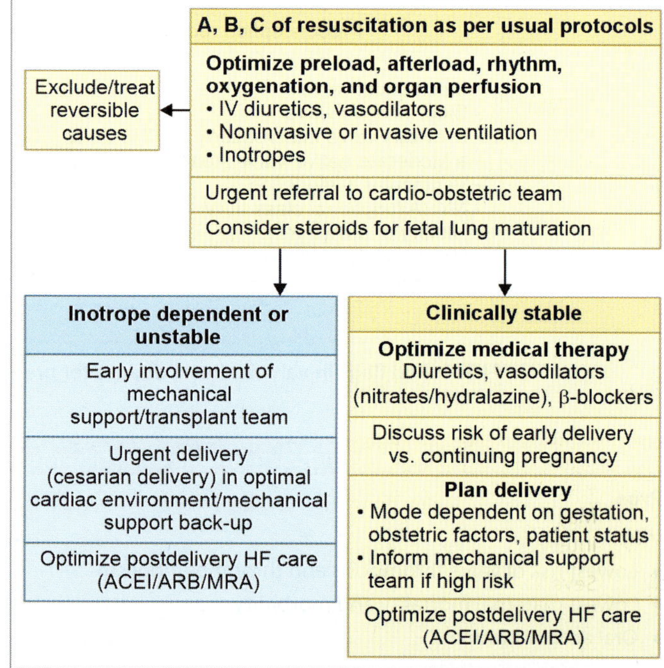

FIG. 6: Algorithm for management of acute heart failure in pregnancy.

due to pregnancy-associated spontaneous coronary artery dissection (p-SCAD) is commonly associated with left main, left anterior descending, or multivessel involvement and thus is associated with ventricular dysfunction and life-threatening maternal complications. Pharmacologic management consists of β-blockers and antiplatelet therapy. PCI can propagate the dissection and should only be considered if high-risk features are present.[21]

Arrhythmias in pregnancy: Supraventricular tachycardias (SVTs) in pregnancy are common (atrioventricular nodal re-entry and atrioventricular re-entrant tachycardia). Atrial fibrillation or flutter is most commonly seen in women with structural heart disease and there are various therapeutic options to consider including cardioversion.

Anticoagulation should be initiated with a congestive heart failure, hypertension, age 75, diabetes, and prior stroke/ transient ischemic attack (doubled) (CHADS2) risk factor score 1 in the absence of structural heart disease. Catheter ablation should be considered for significant ventricular arrhythmias (VAs) detected before pregnancy. Alternatively, medical stabilization, followed by catheter ablation postpartum can be considered. Lead shielding can reduce the dose of radiation to the fetus but does not eliminate exposure. Although cardiac arrest is rare in pregnancy, emergent cesarean delivery for fetal rescue is indicated if there is no return of spontaneous circulation after 4 minutes of resuscitation. Emergent cesarean delivery might also be performed as a part of the maternal resuscitation.[22]

Aortic disease: There is an increased risk of progressive aortic dilation and dissection due to associated hemodynamic and hormonal changes. The need for prophylactic aortic root surgery for the prevention of aortic dissection should be considered before pregnancy. Prophylactic aortic surgery to facilitate safe pregnancy should be considered at an ascending aortic diameter >50 mm. In Marfan's, pregnancy should be avoided in the setting of an ascending aortic diameter 45 mm and prophylactic aortic surgery should be considered; however, the risk of type B dissection remains. In Turner's syndrome, pregnancy has been thought to be higher risk among those with aortic size indexed of 2.5 cm/m^2 or aortic size index of 2.0 cm/m^2 with at least 1 of hypertension, bicuspid aortic valve, aortic coarctation, or transverse arch elongation is present and requires close surveillance.[23] The approach to stratify the risk for fetal loss and a framework for planning delivery management for those who are high risk for neonatal hemodynamic compromise **(Table 3)**.[24]

TABLE 3: Pregnancy and delivery plan in congenital heart disease.

LOC	Complexity and concerns	Example CHD	Prenatal planning	Delivery planning	Post-delivery recommendations
1	Mild complexity CHD. No physiologic instability in first weeks of life	• Septal defects (e.g., ASD, VSD, AVSD) • Benign arrhythmias	No specific planning. Phone call from fetal cardiology × 1 in pregnancy	Spontaneous vaginal delivery	Nursery or NICU (if extracardiac concerns). Routine perinatal management. Postnatal cardiac testing as per fetal cardiology to confirm diagnosis
2	Moderate complexity CHD. Possible physiologic instability in first weeks of life. May require early intervention	• Possible ductal dependency (e.g., "pink" TOF, possible coarctation of aorta) • No sustained or controlled tachyarrhythmia	Prenatal evaluation at JHACH Fetal Care Program. Delivery at location with pediatric cardiology support available	Spontaneous vaginal delivery	CVICU/NICU. Early postnatal cardiology consult. Prostaglandins readily available but do not start without discussing with cardiology first
3	Severe complexity CHD with physiologic stability. Requires postnatal intervention/ surgery before discharge	Ductal dependent lesions or lesions with complex physiology (e.g., HLHS, PA/IVS, "blue" TOF, truncus arteriosus, unbalanced AVSD)	Prenatal evaluation at JHACH Fetal Care Program. Delivery at BBFP	Spontaneous vaginal delivery vs. induction at 39 weeks gestation	• CVICU admission. Umbilical catheters. • Prostaglandins for ductal dependent lesions
4	• Severe complexity CHD with expected instability • Requires postnatal intervention/ surgery before discharge, and possibly urgently	• Severe Ebstein's anomaly or TOF/APV • D-TGA, HLHS with restrictive PFO/intact atrial septum • *Palliative care*: Possible instability leading to death shortly after delivery or may be stable for several hours to several days before death. Family has chosen comfort care • Significant cardiomyopathy • Hydrops	Prenatal evaluation at JHACH Fetal Care Program delivery at BFBP. Predelivery team meeting with CVICU, cardiology, neonatology, and MFM. Interventional/surgical team on standby	• Planned induction at 39 weeks with daytime delivery • NICU contacts CVICU and cardiology when mother arrives for delivery to arrange predelivery huddle. Consideration of planned C-section to ensure coordinated daytime delivery in the most severe cases	• CVICU admission <1 hour of age. Umbilical catheters. Prostaglandin for ductal dependent lesions. Stabilizing medication/ equipment predetermined by care plan • High acuity rapid transport protocol (Code Hart)

Peripartum antithrombotic therapy: Judicious monitoring to ensure therapeutic anticoagulation must occur [target anti-Xa levels 0.8–1.2 U/mL at 4–6 hours post-LMWH dose or activated partial thromboplastin time (aPTT) 2–3 times control for IV UFH]. for patients on therapeutic anticoagulation for mechanical heart valves using LMWH, bridging with IV UFH (starting 36 hours prior to planned delivery until 4–6 hours before delivery) is recommended by expert consensus by both the European Society of Cardiology and the American College of Cardiology/American Heart Association. For patients on antiplatelet monotherapy with aspirin, aspirin may be continued throughout delivery. For pregnant patients on dual antiplatelet therapy, discontinuation of P2Y12 inhibitor is recommended in anticipation of labor and need for neuraxial anesthesia **(Table 4)**.[25]

RECENT GUIDELINES AND RECOMMENDATIONS

Over the last decade, several professional societies have published comprehensive guidelines on the management of cardiovascular disease during pregnancy. These evidence-based recommendations standardize care, guide clinical decisions, and encourage multidisciplinary collaboration.

- *European Society of Cardiology (ESC) 2022 guidelines*: Highlight the importance of specialized cardio-obstetrics teams for women in mWHO Class II–IV. Strongly advise against pregnancy in women with pulmonary hypertension or severe aortic disease. Offer algorithms for mechanical valve management using LMWH, warfarin, or combined protocols with anti-Xa and INR monitoring.
- *American College of Obstetricians and Gynecologists (ACOG) practice bulletin 2023*: Emphasizes the use of the CARPREG II risk model in prenatal counseling. Recommends aspirin prophylaxis for preeclampsia prevention in women with cardiac disease.
- *American Heart Association (AHA) 2020 scientific statement*: Calls for early detection of maternal CVD and routine postpartum follow-up. Emphasizes racial disparities in maternal outcomes and the need for equitable care access. Recommends universal cardio-obstetric training in residency programs.
- *International Society for Adult Congenital Heart Disease (ISACHD)*: Offers lesion-specific care models and pregnancy compatibility guidance for congenital lesions. Supports individualized delivery plans and preconception counseling.
- *Federation of Obstetric and Gynecological Societies of India (FOGSI) and Cardiological Society of India (CSI)*: Joint guidelines promote the establishment of cardio-obstetrics clinics in tertiary hospitals. Recommend echocardiographic screening in all women with prior rheumatic fever or undiagnosed murmurs. Provide risk classification adapted to the Indian context (e.g., high burden of RHD).
- WHO Safe Motherhood Initiative and Global Goals

TABLE 4: Anticoagulation management during peripartum and postpartum in patients on anticoagulant treatment.

	Before placing a neural anesthetic	Before initiating or resuming anticoagulation
UFH SC low dose (≤5,000 U twice or 3 times daily)	Consider holding the dose >4–6 h or assessing coagulation status	Wait ≥1 h after neuraxial procedure (if no signs of postpartum hemorrhage) and ≥1 h after epidural catheter removal
UFH SC intermediate dose (7,500 or 10,000 U twice daily, ≤20,000 U)	Consider holding the dose ≥12 h and assessing coagulation status	
UFH SC high dose (individual doses >10,000 U per dose, total daily dose >20,000 U)	Consider holding the dose ≥24 h since last dose and assessing coagulation status	
UFH IV	Consider stopping the infusion 4–6 h and assessing coagulation status	Wait ≥1 h after neuraxial block (if no signs of postpartum hemorrhage)
Low-dose LMWH SC (e.g., enoxaparin <40 mg once daily or 30 mg twice daily, or dalteparin ≤5,000 U once daily)	Consider holding the dose ≥12 h	Wait ≥12 h after neuraxial procedure and ≥4 h after epidural catheter removal
Intermediate-dose LMWH SC (e.g., enoxaparin >40 mg once daily or 30 mg twice daily and <1 mg/kg twice daily or 1.5 mg/kg once daily or dalteparin >5,000 U once daily and <120 U/kg twice daily or 200 U/kg once daily)	Insufficient published data to recommend a specific interval between 12 and 24 h to delay neuraxial anesthesia. *Expert panel recommends: Consider holding the dose ≥24 h (in keeping with recommendations for therapeutic dose LMWH)*	Wait ≥24 h after neuraxial procedure and ≥4 h after epidural catheter removal
High-dose LMWH SC (e.g., enoxaparin ≥1 mg/kg twice daily or 1.5 mg/kg once daily or dalteparin: ≥120 U/kg twice daily or 200 U/kg once daily)	Consider holding the dose ≥24 h	

FUTURE DIRECTIONS AND RESEARCH GAPS

Despite advances in cardio-obstetrics, multiple research and implementation gaps remain. Bridging these will enhance patient outcomes, improve equity, and inform future guidelines. *Personalized risk models*: Existing models (mWHO, CARPREG II) are not individualized and may overestimate or underestimate risk. Machine learning algorithms integrating clinical, echocardiographic, and biomarker data may improve predictive accuracy. Integration of AI into EHR systems can assist with automated alerts and tailored recommendations. *Pharmacologic safety data*: Most drugs used during pregnancy lack robust safety data from randomized trials due to ethical barriers. Pregnancy-specific drug registries and observational cohorts (e.g., EURObservational Research Program) are key to filling this gap. Future research should explore dosing adjustments, pharmacokinetics, and fetal exposure profiles.

CONCLUSION

Pregnancy in women with cardiovascular disease presents a complex interplay of physiology, pathology, and risk. It is a leading cause of maternal mortality worldwide and requires a systematic, multidisciplinary approach for effective management. Early and accurate risk stratification through tools like mWHO classification, CARPREG II, and ZAHARA lays the foundation for safe, tailored care. This is complemented by evidence-based pharmacologic management, meticulous monitoring, and individualized delivery planning. The emergence of cardio-obstetrics as a formal specialty has brought critical improvements in care coordination, outcomes, and patient education. Despite these advances, challenges remain. The future of cardio-obstetrics lies in precision care, patient empowerment, and global collaboration ensuring that every heartbeat counts, from the first trimester to beyond the fourth.

REFERENCES

1. Hameed AB, Tarsa M, Graves CR, Chang J, Billah M, Hatfield T, Thiel de Bocanegra H. Cardiovascular Risk Assessment as a Quality Measure in the Pregnancy and Postpartum Period. JACC Adv. 2023;2(1):100176.
2. The Commonwealth Fund. (2023). Maternal mortality and Maternity care in the United States compared to 10 other developed countries. [online] Available from https://www.commonwealthfund.org/publications/issue-briefs/2020/nov/maternal-mortality-maternity-care-us-compared-10-countries. [Last accessed November, 2025]
3. Hoyert DL. (2022). Maternal mortality rates in the United States, 2020. [online] Available from https://www.cdc.gov/nchs/data/hestat/maternal-mortality/2020/maternal-mortality-rates-2020.htm. [Last accessed November, 2025]
4. Hoyert DL. (2023). Maternal mortality rates in the United States, 2021. [online] Available from https://www.cdc.gov/nchs/data/hestat/maternal-mortality/2021/maternal-mortality-rates-2021.htm. [Last accessed November, 2025]
5. Hameed AB, Lawton ES, McCain CL, et al. Pregnancy-related cardiovascular deaths in California: beyond peripartum cardiomyopathy. Am J Obstet Gynecol. 2015;213:379.e1-10.
6. American College of Obstetricians and Gynecologists' Presidential Task Force on Pregnancy and Heart Disease and Committee on Practice Bulletins—Obstetrics. ACOG Practice Bulletin No. 212: Pregnancy and Heart Disease. Obstet Gynecol. 2019;133(5):e320-e356.
7. Black A, Gute J, Kindschuh A. Implementing a cardiovascular screening tool for high-risk pregnant women in a hospital setting. Nurs Womens Health. 2022;26(1):38-43.
8. McCucheon A, Wolfe DS, Institute for Healthcare Improvement. (2022). Cardiac Conditions in Obstetric Care Chage Package. [online] Available from https://saferbirth.org/wp-content/uploads/CCOC_CP_Final_V1_2022.pdf. [Last accessed November, 2025]
9. Pearson GD, Veille JC, Rahimtoola S, et al. Peripartum cardiomyopathy: National heart, lung and blood Institute and Office of Rare diseases (National Institutes of Health) workshop recommendations and review. JAMA. 2000;283(9):1183-8.
10. Pearson GD, Veille JC, Rahimtoola S, et al. Peripartum cardiomyopathy: national heart, lung and blood Institute and Office of Rare diseases (national Institutes of health) workshop recommendations and review. JAMA. 2000;283(9):1183-8.
11. Lau ES, Aggarwal NR, Briller JE, Crousillat DR, Economy KE, Harrington CM, et al. (2024). Recommendations for the Management of High-Risk Cardiac Delivery: ACC Cardiovascular Disease in Women Committee Panel. [online] Available from https://www.jacc.org/doi/10.1016/j.jacadv.2024.100901. [Last accessed November, 2025]
12. Kultursay H, Turkoglu C, Akin M, et al. Mitral balloon valvuloplasty with transesophageal echocardiography without using fluoroscopy. Cathet Cardiovasc Diagn. 1992;27:317-21.
13. Ducas RA, Javier DA, D'Souza R, et al. Pregnancy outcomes in women with significant valve disease: a systematic review and meta-analysis. Heart. 2020;106:51.
14. Pfaller B, Javier A, Grewal J, et al. Risks associated with valvular regurgitation during pregnancy. J Am Coll Cardiol. 2021;77:2656-64.
15. Elkayam U. Anticoagulation therapy for pregnant women with mechanical prosthetic heart valves: how to improve safety? J Am Coll Cardiol. 2017;69:2692-5.
16. Windram J, Grewal J, Bottega N, Sermer M, Spears D, Swan L, et al. Canadian Cardiovascular Society: Clinical Practice Update on Cardiovascular Management of the Pregnant Patient. Can J Cardiol. 2021;37(12):1886-901.
17. Ruys TP, Roos-Hesselink JW, Hall R, et al. Heart failure in pregnant women with cardiac disease: data from the ROPAC. Heart. 2014;100:231-8.
18. Grewal J, Siu SC, Ross HJ, et al. Pregnancy outcomes in women with dilated cardiomyopathy. J Am Coll Cardiol. 2009;55:45-52.
19. Davis MB, Arany Z, McNamara DM, et al. Peripartum cardiomyopathy: JACC State-of-the-Art Review. J Am Coll Cardiol. 2020;75:207-21.
20. Ommen SR, Mital S, Burke MA, et al. 2020 AHA/ACC guideline for the diagnosis and treatment of patients with hypertrophic cardiomyopathy: a report of the American College of Cardiology/American Heart Association Joint Committee on Clinical Practice Guidelines. Circulation. 2020;142:e558-631.

21. James AH, Jamison MG, Biswas MS, et al. Acute myocardial infarction in pregnancy: a United States population-based study. Circulation. 2006;113:1564-71.
22. Regitz-Zagrosek V, Roos-Hesselink JW, Bauersachs J, et al. 2018 ESC guidelines for the management of cardiovascular diseases during pregnancy. Eur Heart J. 2018;39:3165-241.
23. Januzzi JL, Isselbacher EM, Fattori R, et al. Characterizing the young patient with aortic dissection: results from the International Registry of Aortic Dissection (IRAD). J Am Coll Cardiol. 2004;43:665-9.
24. Donofrio MT, Levey RJ, Schuette JJ, et al. Specialized Delivery room planning for Fetuses with Critical Congenital Heart Disease. Am J Cardiol. 2013;111:737-47.
25. Douketis JD, Spyropoulos AC, Murad MH, et al. Perioperative management of antithrombotic therapy: an American College of Chest Physicians Clinical Practice Guideline. Chest. 2022;162:e207-e243.

CHAPTER

70

Understanding and Managing Heart Failure during Pregnancy—What is New in Peripartum Cardiomyopathy?

Roopali Khanna, Sumang Mohan, Harshit Khare

ABSTRACT

Peripartum cardiomyopathy (PPCM) is an uncommon but potentially life-threatening condition characterized by heart failure (HF) in late pregnancy or early postpartum, without other identifiable causes. Its pathogenesis involves genetic, inflammatory, and hormonal factors, with clinical presentations often overlapping with normal pregnancy symptoms. Early diagnosis, multidisciplinary care, and cautious HF management are critical. Emerging therapies like bromocriptine show promise but remain under investigation. Long-term follow-up and counseling are essential, particularly regarding subsequent pregnancies due to relapse risk.

Keywords: Peripartum cardiomyopathy, heart failure in pregnancy, left ventricular dysfunction, PPCM management, subsequent pregnancy, maternal mortality.

INTRODUCTION

The 2019 European Society of Cardiology (ESC) working group used the following criteria to define peripartum cardiomyopathy:[1]

- Development of heart failure (HF) toward the end of pregnancy or in the postpartum period
- Absence of another identifiable cause of HF
- Left ventricular (LV) systolic dysfunction with a LV ejection fraction <45%; LV may or may not be dilated.

According to the initial definition, the peripartum cardiomyopathy (PPCM) onset period ranged from the last month of pregnancy to the 5th month postpartum; however, due to similar cases being documented before and after this time frame, the definition has been made time-independent.[2]

EPIDEMIOLOGY

The worldwide incidence is 1 in 2,000 births, which varies depending on geographic region, socioeconomic factors, and ethnicity, with an incidence ranging from 1 to 4 per 1,000 births in the United States of America and 4.5–10 per 1,000 births in Nigeria.[3-5]

The incidence in India is reported to be around 1 in 1,340 live births,[6] with the worldwide lowest incidence in Japan.[7]

PATHOPHYSIOLOGY

Recent evidence suggests a multiple-hit theory for the development of PPCM, with the accumulation of genetic and environmental factors that converge on a common pathway **(Fig. 1)**. Genetic variants (TTN, FLNC, BAG3, and DSP) are comparable to those found in DCM cohorts, supporting similarity between PPCM and dilated cardiomyopathy (DCM). Approximately 15% of patients with PPCM have genetic variants similar to those identified in nonischemic DCM. Other proposed causes include viral etiology, abnormal immune response to pregnancy, malnutrition, and activation of apoptotic pathways.[8]

CLINICAL MANIFESTATIONS

Women with PPCM present with symptoms of HF, including fatigue, dyspnea, paroxysmal nocturnal dyspnea, and pedal edema.[9,10] Clinical signs include tachypnea, tachycardia, elevated JVP, pedal edema, and inspiratory rales on chest examination. The most frequent presentation is acute decompensated HF, with NYHA III/IV symptoms. Mild to moderate symptomatic cases may be mistaken for physiological changes during pregnancy.

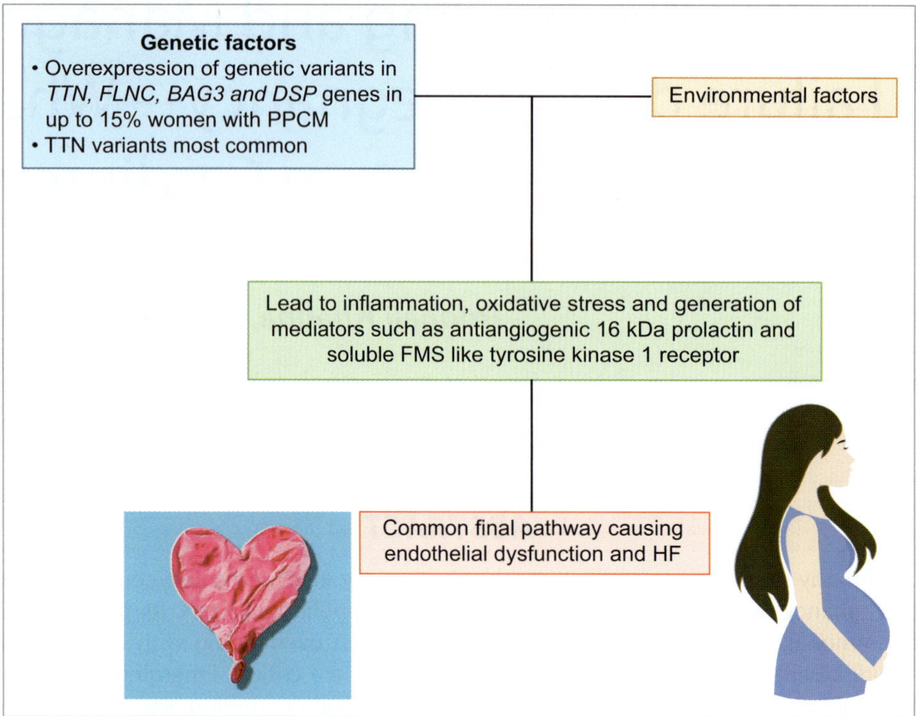

FIG. 1: Pathogenesis of peripartum cardiomyopathy (PPCM).

DIFFERENTIAL DIAGNOSIS

Peripartum cardiomyopathy is a diagnosis of exclusion, and the following are the differential diagnoses that need to be ruled out in women presenting with LV dysfunction:

- Myocarditis
- Acute exacerbation or worsening of symptoms in preexisting structural heart disease
- Pulmonary embolism
- Preeclampsia-induced pulmonary edema without LV dysfunction
- Spontaneous coronary artery dissection
- Takotsubo cardiomyopathy
- Aortic dissection

INVESTIGATIONS AND WORKUP

Workup includes:

- *ECG:* It may show nonspecific changes, sinus tachycardia, and ST/T changes. ECG may be particularly useful to rule out ST-segment elevation MI.[3]
- *Cardiac biomarkers:* Natriuretic peptides are normal in pregnancy and slightly elevated in preeclampsia. Serum BNP and NT-pro-BNP are usually elevated in PPCM, with elevations in cardiac troponin.[10,11] The possible diagnostic and prognostic roles of additional biomarkers, such as soluble fms-like tyrosine kinase 1 and specific microRNA, require further investigation.[12,13]
- *Echocardiography:* To assess the degree of LV dysfunction, RV involvement, if any, AV valve regurgitation, and LV apical thrombosis.[14]
- *CMR:* Gadolinium administration is not advisable during pregnancy; it should be considered in the postpartum period in specific cases.
- *Endomyocardial biopsy:* Not diagnostic of PPCM, may be considered when other etiologies are suspected, such as giant cell myocarditis.[14]

MANAGEMENT

Management can be broadly divided into three clinical scenarios, as summarized in **Table 1**.

Heart Failure Medication

There is a dearth of data and no randomized controlled trials assessing the effect of drugs in patients with PPCM. Ensuring drug safety is of the utmost importance while treating HF in pregnancy. Oral diuretics, including furosemide, and bumetanide, and β-blockers, excluding atenolol, are deemed safe during pregnancy.[15,16] Drugs acting on RAAS, including ACE inhibitors, ARBs, and MRA, are contraindicated during pregnancy, along with SGLT2 inhibitors.[16] If vasodilation is needed, hydralazine-nitrate combination should be considered.[15]

During the postpartum period, diuretics and β-blockers are continued. ACE inhibitor and MRAs are considered safe

TABLE 1: Management of peripartum cardiomyopathy (PPCM) according to severity of disease and clinical status.

	Mild PPCM	Moderate PPCM	Severe PPCM
Clinical presentation	Subacute heart failure	Acute heart failure	Cardiogenic shock
Hemodynamics	Stable	Stable	Unstable
Echocardiography	LVEF 35–45%	LVEF 20–35%	LVEF ≤ 20%
Management	*Oral HF medication*: • Diuretics, if needed • Bromocriptine × 1 week (postpartum) • Beta blockers	*Oral HF medications*: • Beta blockers • IV diuretics • NIV, if needed • Vasodilators • Bromocriptine × 8 weeks (postpartum) • Anticoagulation if LVEF < 25%	*Inotropes*: • IV diuretics • Invasive ventilation • MCS • Anticoagulation • Bromocriptine × 8 weeks • Oral HF medication

(HF: heart failure; IV: intravenous; LVEF: left ventricle ejection fraction; MCS: mechanical circulatory support; NIV: noninvasive ventilation)

during breastfeeding, but data are lacking for SGLT2 inhibitor and ARNI.

Inotropes and Mechanical Circulatory Support

Norepinephrine is the preferred inotrope. Levosimendan, although safe, has no proven benefit.[17] Dobutamine should be avoided due to increased propensity for β-agonist-mediated side effects in pregnancy.[18] In inotrope-dependent HF, MCS should be considered, with a lower threshold. Long-term MCS may be required in up to 7% PPCM as a bridge to recovery.[13] As LV function improvement in PPCM is usually delayed, the heart transplant threshold should be high and should be delayed as much as possible.

Management during Delivery

Vaginal delivery is advisable, in the absence of obstetric contraindications, with epidural anesthesia, to prevent a sudden increase in BP. In case of hemodynamic instability, an emergent cesarean section should be performed.[14]

Postpartum Management

Immediately after delivery, due to the removal of caval compression and placental blood autotransfusion, there is a risk of fluid overload and precipitating HF, and it should be managed accordingly with diuretics.

Breastfeeding is deemed safe in mild and moderate PPCM and should be continued. However, in severe PPCM, a tailored approach is needed, as breastfeeding equates to increased metabolic demands.[14]

EXPERIMENTAL THERAPY FOR PERIPARTUM CARDIOMYOPATHY

Bromocriptine

Peripartum cardiomyopathy patients exhibit elevated levels of prolactin, accompanied by a high proapoptotic 16-kDa prolactin fragment, which is implicated in the pathogenesis of PPCM. Bromocriptine is a dopamine D2 receptor agonist that suppresses prolactin secretion.[19] The ESC guidelines suggest that bromocriptine may be considered for the treatment of PPCM *(IIb)*.[2] Bromocriptine 2.5 mg BD for 8 weeks in moderate or severe PPCM and for 1 week in mild PPCM. Main concerns are the prothrombotic effects of bromocriptine and suppression of lactation. Clinical data regarding efficacy in PPCM is limited, although meta-analysis of observational studies suggests significantly higher survival rates with greater improvement in LVEF.[20] In the recently published ESC EURObservational Research Programme (EORP) PPCM registry, the bromocriptine group had fewer patients with severe LV dysfunction at 6 months, but it did not affect hospital admission rates or mortality.[21] The results of the ongoing Randomized Evaluation of Bromocriptine in Myocardial Recovery for Peripartum Cardiomyopathy (REBIRTH) study are expected in 2029, and shall address the uncertainty regarding the usage of bromocriptine in PPCM.

Anticoagulation

Patients with PPCM with severely decreased LVEF are at increased risk of apical thrombosis. Anticoagulation is recommended in patients with LVEF < 35%, as per the ESC guidelines.[2] LMWH is the preferred anticoagulant (class IIa), although VKA can be taken beyond the first trimester. UFH is preferable in patients on MCS with aPTT monitoring. NOACs are contraindicated during pregnancy and breastfeeding.

Hilfiker-Kleiner D, et al. proposed the *acronym "BOARD"* enclosing the main pharmacologic therapies in PPCM, i.e., bromocriptine, oral HF agents, anticoagulants, IV relaxants, and diuretics in patients with PPCM with LVEF < 35%.[22]

Implantable Cardioverter-defibrillator

There is a risk of developing ventricular arrhythmias in these cases, and they should be monitored. Approximately 50% of women with PPCM have recovered LVEF; routine implantable cardioverter-defibrillators (ICDs) are not recommended. Wearable cardioverter-defibrillators may be considered *(IIb)* in selected cases (LVEF < 35%) as a bridge to recovery or a definite indication for ICD implantation.[2]

The prognosis of PPCM is variable and depends on the geographical distribution, with mortality rates ranging from 2% in developed countries to 19% in underdeveloped countries.[22-24] Risk factors associated with increased risk of complications include LVEF < 30%, LV end-diastolic diameter > 60 mm, biventricular dysfunction, ECG QT interval prolongation, delayed diagnosis, and Middle Eastern or African ethnicity and/or geography.[25] Age (>40 or <20 years), antepartum diagnosis, hemodynamic parameters at presentation, and cardiac biomarkers can further refine risk stratification.

Left Ventricular Function Recovery

The IPAC study showed improvement in LVEF to >50% in most women at the end of 6 months, but in some women, it may take longer. In some subset of women, there is never a full recovery of LVEF.[24] Several factors influence the recovery of LVEF. The European Society of Cardiology (ESC) EORP PPCM Registry proposed a predictive model for LV function recovery.[26] It was derived from 752 women with PPCM enrolled from 51 countries. Six-month postpartum echocardiography was available in 465 patients. LV function was recovered in 216 (46.5%) patients. The ESC EROP PPCM recovery score consisted of six components, including baseline LVEF, baseline LV end-diastolic diameter, human development index (a summary measure of a country's social and economic development), duration of symptoms, QRS duration, and preeclampsia **(Tables 2A and B)**.

Data on long-term follow-up are limited, and the duration of HF medications in patients with recovered LVEF is unclear. Recent data suggest weaning from HF medications gradually with continuation of β-blockers for the long term.

Subsequent Pregnancy

There is a significant concern of relapse in patients with recovered LVEF in subsequent pregnancy. The preconception counseling is very crucial in assessing the risk of relapse and counseling for close follow-up.[27] Stress echocardiography may be helpful in risk stratification of women with mild LV dysfunction and planning a new pregnancy. There are chances of 20% relapse in women with recovered LVEF, and about 50% of women without LVEF recovery may have deterioration in the LV function. Close monitoring of clinical symptoms, echocardiography, and biomarkers (such as BNP) should be performed in these cases at the end of the first and second trimesters, 1 month prior to delivery, postdelivery, and 1 month

TABLES 2A AND B: Integer score for left ventricular recovery (A) and predicted probability of left ventricular recovery for each score (B). ESC EROP PPCM recovery score.[26]

(A)

Parameters	Score
LVEF:	
• <35%	0
• >35%	1
LV end diastolic diameter (mm):	
• ≥62	0
• 53–61	1
• <53	4
Human developmental index:	
• Low	0
• Medium	0
• High	1
Duration of symptoms:	
• >10 days	0
• ≤10 days	1
QRS duration (ms):	
• ≥110	0
• 81–109	2
• ≤80	3
Preeclampsia:	
• No	0
• Yes	1

(B)

Total score	Predicted recovery at 6 months
≤1	6%
2	14%
3	23%
4	35%
5	49%
6	65%
7	75%
8	83%
9	90%
≥10	95%

postpartum. Beta-blockers may be beneficial in women with subsequent pregnancy, irrespective of the LV function.[28]

CONCLUSION

Peripartum cardiomyopathy is one of the major causes of maternal morbidity and mortality. The pathogenesis is unclear and considered to be multifactorial. Early diagnosis and multidisciplinary management are essential in patients, especially those with severe LV dysfunction and hemodynamically unstable. Guideline-directed medical therapy of HF with reduced ejection fraction cannot be started in these cases, as most HF medications are fetotoxic and are contraindicated during pregnancy (ACE inhibitor, ARB, MRA, and SGLT2 inhibitor). The role of bromocriptine is still controversial and needs more data to be prescribed regularly. Lifelong follow-up and preconception counseling are essential in these cases. The risk of a subsequent pregnancy is complex, depending on LVEF, and requires shared decision-making.

REFERENCES

1. Bauersachs J, Konig T, van der Meer P, et al. Pathophysiology, diagnosis and management of peripartum cardiomyopathy: a position statement from the Heart Failure Association of the European Society of Cardiology Study Group on peripartum cardiomyopathy. Eur J Heart Fail. 2019;21(7):827-43.
2. De Backer J, Haugaa KH, Hasselberg NE, et al. 2025 ESC Guidelines for the management of cardiovascular disease and pregnancy. Eur Heart J. 2025:ehaf193.
3. Mielniczuk LM, Williams K, Davis DR, et al. Frequency of peripartum cardiomyopathy. The American journal of cardiology. 2006;97(12):1765-8.
4. Brar SS, Khan SS, Sandhu GK, et al. Incidence, mortality, and racial differences in peripartum cardiomyopathy. The American journal of cardiology. 2007;100(2):302-4.
5. Karaye KM, Ishaq NA, Sa'idu H, et al. Incidence, clinical characteristics, and risk factors of peripartum cardiomyopathy in Nigeria: results from the PEACE Registry. ESC Heart Fail. 2020;7(1):235-43.
6. Agarwal R, Baid R, Sinha DP. Peripartum cardiomyopathy in Indian population: A pooled analysis. J Clin Prev Cardiol. 2021;10(2): 54-7.
7. Isogai T, Kamiya CA. Worldwide incidence of peripartum cardiomyopathy and overall maternal mortality. Int Heart J. 2019;60(3): 503-11.
8. Arany Z. Peripartum cardiomyopathy. New Engl J Med. 2024;390(2):154-64.
9. Iannaccone G, Graziani F, Kacar P, et al. Diagnosis and management of peripartum cardiomyopathy and recurrence risk. Int J Cardiol Congenit Heart Dis. 2024;17:100530.
10. Elkayam U. Clinical characteristics of peripartum cardiomyopathy in the United States: diagnosis, prognosis, and management. J Am Coll Cardiol. 2011;58(7):659-70.
11. Jackson AM, Macartney M, Brooksbank K, et al. A 20-year population study of peripartum cardiomyopathy. Eur Heart J. 2023;44(48):5128-41.
12. Gentry MB, Dias JK, Luis A, et al. African-American women have a higher risk for developing peripartum cardiomyopathy. J Am Coll Cardiol. 2010;55(7):654-9.
13. Halkein J, Tabruyn SP, Ricke-Hoch M, et al. MicroRNA-146a is a therapeutic target and biomarker for peripartum cardiomyopathy. J Clin Invest 2013;123(5):2143-54
14. Regitz-Zagrosek V, Roos-Hesselink JW, Bauersachs J, et al. ESC Guidelines for the management of cardiovascular diseases during pregnancy. Eur Heart J. 2018;39(34):3165-241.
15. McDonagh TA, Metra M, Adamo M, et al. ESC Guidelines for the diagnosis and treatment of acute and chronic heart failure. Eur Heart J. 2021;42(36):3599-726.
16. Halpern DG, Weinberg CR, Pinnelas R, et al. Use of Medication for Cardiovascular Disease During Pregnancy: JACC State-of-the-Art Review. J Am Coll Cardiol. 2019;73(4):457-76.
17. Biteker M, Duran NE, Kaya H, et al. Effect of levosimendan and predictors of recovery in patients with peripartum cardiomyopathy, a randomized clinical trial. Clin Res Cardiol. 2011;100(7):571-7.
18. Stapel B, Kohlhaas M, Ricke-Hoch M, et al. Low STAT3 expression sensitizes to toxic effects of β-adrenergic receptor stimulation in peripartum cardiomyopathy. Eur Heart J. 2017;38(5):349-61.
19. Hilfiker-Kleiner D, Kaminski K, Podewski E, et al. A cathepsin D-cleaved 16 kDa form of prolactin mediates postpartum cardiomyopathy. Cell. 2007;128(3):589-600.
20. Trongtorsak A, Kittipibul V, Mahabir S, et al. Effects of bromocriptine in peripartum cardiomyopathy: a systematic review and meta-analysis. Heart Fail Rev. 2022;27:533-43.
21. Van der Meer P, van Essen BJ, Viljoen C, et al. Bromocriptine treatment and outcomes in peripartum cardiomyopathy: the EORP PPCM registry. Eur Heart J. 2025;46(11):1017-27.
22. Hilfiker-Kleiner D, Haghikia A, Berliner D, et al. Bromocriptine for the treatment of peripartum cardiomyopathy: a multicentre randomized study. Eur Heart J. 2017;38:2671-9.
23. Karaye K, Sa'idu H, Balarabe S, et al. Clinical Features and Outcomes of Peripartum Cardiomyopathy in Nigeria. J Am Coll Cardiol. 2020;76(20):2352-64.
24. McNamara DM, Elkayam U, Alharethi R, et al. Clinical outcomes for peripartum cardiomyopathy in North America: results of the IPAC study (Investigations of Pregnancy- Associated Cardiomyopathy). J Am Coll Cardiol. 2015;66:905-14.
25. Sliwa K, Bauersachs J, Arany Z, et al. Peripartum cardiomyopathy: from genetics to management. Eur Heart J. 2021;42:3094-102.
26. Jackson AM, Goland S, Farhan HA, et al. A novel score to predict left ventricular recovery in peripartum cardiomyopathy derived from the ESC EORP Peripartum Cardiomyopathy Registry. Eur Heart J. 2024;45(16):1430-9.
27. Davis MB, Arany Z, McNamara DM, et al. Peripartum Cardiomyopathy: JACC State-of-the-Art Review. J Am Coll Cardiol. 2020;75(2):207-21.
28. Sliwa K, Jackson A, Viljoen C, et al. Pregnancies in women after peri-partum cardiomyopathy: the global European Society of Cardiology EuroObservational research programme peri-partum cardiomyopathy registry. Eur Heart J. 2025;46:1031-40.

CHAPTER

71

Hypertensive Disorder of Pregnancy and Long-term Cardiovascular Outcome

S Anne Princy, G Justin Paul

ABSTRACT

Hypertensive disorders of pregnancy (HDPs) are a major cause of maternal and fetal morbidity and mortality worldwide, accounting for a substantial proportion of maternal deaths in both high-income and low- and middle-income countries. Beyond their immediate obstetric implications, HDPs have profound long-term consequences on cardiovascular health. Rightfully, as they are now well recognized as predictors of future cardiovascular disease (CVD) and premature cardiovascular mortality. The physiological adaptations of pregnancy are crucial to maintain adequate uteroplacental perfusion and support fetal growth. When these adaptations are disrupted, HDP may develop. The hemodynamic implications of HDP can persist for years after delivery, contributing to elevated lifelong risk of hypertension, ischemic heart disease, heart failure, and stroke. Identifying women with a history of HDP during pregnancy and the postpartum period offers a unique window for early risk stratification and implementing preventive strategies. Integrating lifestyle measures, structured follow-up, and timely therapeutic interventions is therefore crucial to reduce long-term cardiovascular morbidity and improve outcomes in this high-risk population.

Keywords: Preeclampsia, cardiovascular risk, maternal morbidity and mortality, long-term outcomes, follow-up plans.

INTRODUCTION

Hypertensive disorders of pregnancy (HDPs) are among the leading contributors to maternal and perinatal mortality worldwide. Globally, preeclampsia affects an estimated 2–8% of all pregnancies.[1] These conditions account for about 16% of maternal deaths in high-income countries and nearly one-quarter of maternal deaths in low- and middle-income countries.[2] The effects of HDP extend well beyond the pregnancy itself, serving as a powerful predictor of long-term cardiovascular (CV) health. Women with a history of HDP have nearly twice the risk of developing cardiovascular disease (CVD) and experiencing premature CVD-related mortality compared with those who had normotensive pregnancies.[3]

Hypertensive disorders of pregnancy represent a spectrum of conditions with distinct diagnostic criteria and varying implications for maternal and fetal health.

Definitions/diagnostic criteria for the HDP are given in **Table 1**.

Hypertensive disorders of pregnancy vary from mild gestational hypertension to severe conditions such as eclampsia and HELLP syndrome, with differing risks for short-term maternal/fetal complications and long-term CVD.

PATHOGENESIS OF HYPERTENSIVE DISORDERS OF PREGNANCY

The maternal systemic response, involving immune and inflammatory pathways, ultimately results in clinical manifestations such as hypertension, preeclampsia, HELLP syndrome, and eclampsia.[4]

Pathophysiological cascade leading to HDPs are given in **Figure 1**.

MATERNAL CARDIOVASCULAR ADAPTATIONS DURING NORMAL PREGNANCY AND HYPERTENSIVE DISORDERS OF PREGNANCY

Pregnancy is associated with hemodynamic and physiological changes to accommodate the physiological needs of the growing fetus. These CV changes begin in the first 5–8 weeks

TABLE 1: Definitions/diagnostic criteria for the hypertensive disorders in pregnancy.

Disorder	Diagnostic criteria
Gestational hypertension (HTN)	• New-onset SBP ≥140 mm Hg and/or DBP ≥90 mm Hg on ≥2 occasions, 4 hours apart, after 20 weeks in a previously normotensive woman *and* • No proteinuria • No end-organ dysfunction (e.g., thrombocytopenia, acute kidney injury, ↑ LFTs, pulmonary edema, and cerebral/visual symptoms)
Preeclampsia	• New-onset SBP ≥140 mm Hg and/or DBP ≥90 mm Hg on ≥2 occasions ≥4 hours apart after 20 weeks *and* • Proteinuria (≥300 mg/24 h or protein creatinine ratio ≥0.3, or urine dipstick ≥2+)
Preeclampsia with severe features	• Diagnosis of preeclampsia *and* Any of the following features of severe disease • BP ≥160/110 mm Hg on two occasions ≥4 hours apart • Thrombocytopenia (<100,000/μL). • Impaired liver function (LFTs ≥2 × normal or severe RUQ/epigastric pain) • Acute kidney injury (Cr >1.1 mg/dL or doubling of baseline) • Pulmonary edema • Persistent cerebral or visual disturbances
Eclampsia	• Generalized seizure in a patient with preeclampsia, not attributable to other causes
HELLP syndrome	• *H*emolysis, *E*levated *L*iver enzymes, *L*ow *P*latelets • HTN may or may not be present • Often considered a variant of preeclampsia
Chronic (preexisting) HTN	• HTN present before pregnancy or diagnosed before 20 weeks • HTN first detected in pregnancy that persists ≥12 weeks postpartum *BP cutoffs:* ○ *Pregnancy:* SBP ≥140 or DBP ≥90 mm Hg ○ *Prepregnancy/12 weeks postpartum:* – Stage 1 (130–139/80–89 mm Hg) – Stage 2 (≥140/≥90 mm Hg)
Chronic HTN with superimposed preeclampsia	In a woman with chronic HTN, any of following: • Sudden ↑ in BP or need to escalate therapy • New proteinuria or sudden ↑ in proteinuria (if already present) • New end-organ dysfunction consistent with preeclampsia (after 20 weeks or postpartum)
Chronic HTN with superimposed preeclampsia: Severe features	In addition to above, presence of any of the following: • BP ≥160/110 mm Hg despite treatment • Thrombocytopenia (<100,000/μL) • Impaired liver function (LFTs ≥2 × normal or severe RUQ/epigastric pain) • New/worsening renal insufficiency • Pulmonary edema • Persistent cerebral/visual symptoms

Source: Adapted from Gestational hypertension and preeclampsia: ACOG Practice Bulletin, Number 222. Obstet Gynecol 2020;135:e237-60; Report of the National High Blood Pressure Education Program Working Group on high blood pressure in pregnancy. Am J Obstet Gynecol 2000;183:S1. Jones DW, Ferdinand KC, Taler SJ, et al. 2025; AHA/ACC/AANP/AAPA/ ABC/ACCP/ ACPM/AGS/ AMA/ASPC/NMA/PCNA/SGIM Guideline for the Prevention, Detection, Evaluation and Management of High Blood Pressure in Adults: A Report of the American College of Cardiology/American Heart Association Joint Committee on Clinical Practice Guidelines. Hypertension 2025;82(10):e212-316.

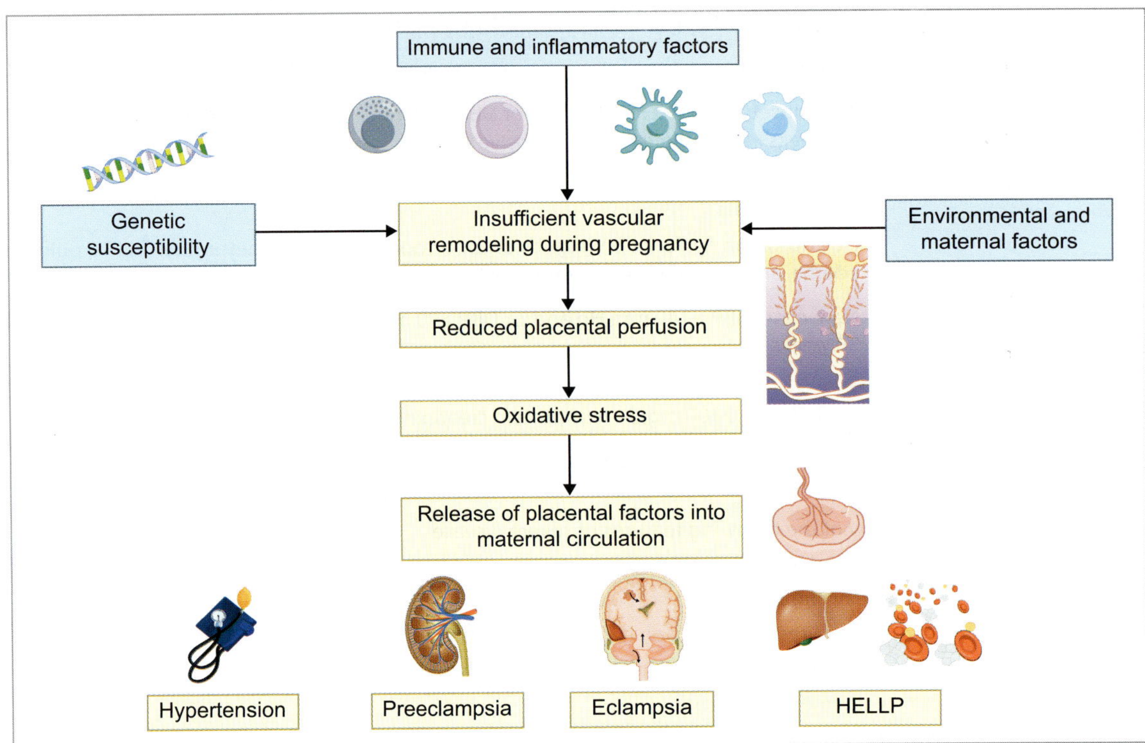

FIG. 1: Pathophysiological cascade leading to hypertensive disorders of pregnancy.
Source: Modified form Deer. et al. (2023).[4]

of gestation. In pregnancy, optimal CV adaptation involves an increase in blood volume and left ventricular mass, accompanied by higher stroke volume, heart rate, and cardiac output. Although plasma volume expands significantly, the fall in systemic vascular resistance (SVR) more than compensates, leading to a slight reduction in blood pressure.[5]

In HDP, the maternal CV system shows maladaptation characterized by increased left ventricular mass, concentric hypertrophy, and elevated systemic vascular resistance. The hemodynamic alterations seen in HDP are thought to result from preexisting CV impairment and/or chronic increases in CV load during pregnancy. These changes, which reflect disease severity, begin as early as the first trimester and can often be detected before HDP becomes clinically evident. Women with chronic hypertension often have reduced intravascular volume expansion, while preeclampsia is marked by decreased stroke volume, impaired myocardial performance, and cardiac dysfunction in up to 45% of cases,[6] with more severe effects in early-onset or severe disease. The mechanisms that account for an increased risk of CVD in women with a history of preeclampsia are not yet well understood, but endothelial dysfunction, which has been linked to atherosclerosis, persists in women with a history of preeclampsia many years after an affected pregnancy. Importantly, these alterations may persist beyond pregnancy, significantly increasing long-term CVD and mortality risk.

Cardiovascular changes during normal pregnancy versus HDPs are listed in **Table 2**.

LONG-TERM MATERNAL RISKS OF PREGNANCY-ASSOCIATED HYPERTENSION

Women with HDPs are predisposed to future CVD, partly due to the so-called "metabolic syndrome of pregnancy", which serves as a "failed stress test" unmasking latent endothelial and metabolic dysfunction.

Early evidence from the landmark meta-analysis by Bellamy et al.[7] demonstrated that women with a history of preeclampsia have significantly higher long-term CV risks, with approximately twofold increased risk of ischemic heart disease (RR 2.16), stroke (RR 1.81), and venous thromboembolism (RR 1.79), within 4–12 years postpartum. These findings were further reinforced by a 2017 meta-analysis,[8] which reported a four-fold increased risk of heart failure and a two-fold increased risk of coronary heart disease, stroke, and CV death among women with prior preeclampsia. Together, these studies highlight the strong and consistent evidence linking preeclampsia to adverse CV outcomes later in life.

Thus, women with HDP have a higher likelihood of developing long-term complications, including hypertension, CVD (coronary heart disease, stroke, heart failure, and atrial fibrillation), as well as venous thromboembolism, chronic kidney disease, and an increased risk of both all-cause and cause-specific mortality (particularly from ischemic heart disease, stroke, and diabetes). The risk is especially elevated in cases of recurrent affected pregnancies, early-onset

TABLE 2: Cardiovascular changes during normal pregnancy versus HDPs.

Parameter	Normal pregnancy (adaptive physiology)	HDP's (pathological adaptation)
CO	↑ 30–50% due to ↑ stroke volume and ↑ heart rate	Variable; in preeclampsia, stroke volume ↓ and CO may be reduced
SVR	↓ due to vasodilation and hormonal changes	↑ SVR (persistent in chronic HTN, markedly ↑ in preeclampsia)
BP	Slight ↓ in early/mid-pregnancy and returns to baseline in third trimester	↑ BP (gestational HTN and preeclampsia) and persistent HTN
LV remodeling	Eccentric hypertrophy/mild LV mass ↑ (adaptive)	Concentric hypertrophy, ↑ LV mass, and impaired relaxation
Intravascular volume	Marked plasma volume expansion	Reduced expansion (especially chronic HTN and preeclampsia)
SV	↑ due to ↑ preload	↓ in preeclampsia
Myocardial performance	Preserved	Impaired (↑ MPI in preeclampsia)
Long-term CV risk	Usually returns to baseline postpartum	Persistent vascular/cardiac dysfunction; ↑ lifetime risk of HTN, CVD, stroke, heart failure, and mortality

preeclampsia requiring delivery before 34 weeks, or when conventional CV risk factors are also present.[9]

CARDIOVASCULAR RISKS AND HYPERTENSIVE DISORDER OF PREGNANCY

The American Heart Association (AHA) now considers preeclampsia and pregnancy-induced hypertension as significant CV risk factors,[10] a conclusion reinforced by evidence from large case-control and cohort studies. The long-term CV risk is shaped by the severity of preeclampsia, the gestational age at delivery, and whether the condition recurs[11] in subsequent pregnancies. Women who develop early-onset severe preeclampsia requiring preterm delivery face the greatest risk of future cardiovascular disease, even before menopause **(Table 3)**. Since many patients and their primary care providers may not recognize the long-term CV implications of preeclampsia—including heightened risk of myocardial infarction, left ventricular dysfunction, and mortality—it is important for obstetricians to counsel patients about these risks during the postpartum period.

Multiple meta-analyses have demonstrated a strong association between preeclampsia and long-term CVD. A large meta-analysis including 50 studies with over 10 million women found that those with a history of preeclampsia in their first pregnancy had significantly higher risks of CV and metabolic complications compared with women with normal pregnancies **(Table 4)**. The risks were particularly elevated in women with early-onset preeclampsia (delivery <34 weeks) compared to late-onset cases **(Table 5)**.[12]

TABLE 3: Deaths from cardiovascular causes.

Population	Relative hazard rate (95% CI)
No preeclampsia, term delivery	1
No preeclampsia, preterm delivery	2.95 (2.12–4.11)
Preeclampsia, term delivery	1.65 (1.01–2.70)
Preeclampsia, preterm delivery	8.12 (4.31–15.33)

Source: Irgens HU, Reisaeter L, Irgens LM, et al. Long-term mortality of mothers and fathers after preeclampsia: Population based cohort study. BMJ. 2001;323:1213.

TABLE 4: Long-term risks after preeclampsia versus normal pregnancy.

Outcome	Preeclampsia (%)	Normal pregnancy (%)	Adjusted odds ratio (OR, 95% CI)
Composite adverse CV event	2.57	0.97	1.99 (1.79–2.22)
Cardio- or cerebro-vascular disease	1.20	0.56	1.79 (1.61–2.01)
Cardiovascular death	2.39	1.12	2.18 (1.79–2.66)
Hypertension	8.84	3.32	3.74 (2.87–4.87)
Type-2 diabetes	3.55	1.88	2.28 (1.58–3.28)
Kidney disease/ESKD	0.38	0.15	3.35 (2.25–5.00)
Metabolic syndrome	20.6	4.2	4.05 (2.42–6.77)
Dyslipidemia	66.3	54.6	2.54 (0.81–2.95)

TABLE 5: Early versus late-onset preeclampsia and CVD risk.

Outcome	Early-onset preeclampsia (<34 weeks)	Normal pregnancy	OR (95% CI)	Late-onset preeclampsia (≥34 weeks)	Normal pregnancy	OR (95% CI)
Composite CVD outcome	3.22%	1.44%	3.79 (2.70–5.31)	3.77%	1.51%	1.89 (1.53–2.33)
Cardiovascular death	1.77%	0.92%	5.12 (3.22–8.12)	1.06%	0.49%	1.65 (1.46–1.86)

Preeclampsia is a recognized risk factor for cardiomyopathy, both peripartum and later in life. Women with a history of preeclampsia or gestational hypertension have a higher likelihood of developing cardiomyopathy for over 5 years postpartum, with 11% of cases in the cohort occurring in this group—about half attributable to chronic hypertension—though the absolute risk remains low (14.6–17.3 per 100,000 person-years).[13]

CARDIOVASCULAR RISK ASSESSMENT IN WOMEN WITH A HISTORY OF HYPERTENSIVE DISORDER OF PREGNANCY

Several international guidelines now recognize pregnancy and HDPs as key opportunities to detect and address a woman's CV risk. Thus, pregnancy and the postpartum period represent a critical early window to assess lifetime CV risk and initiate preventive interventions. Following a pregnancy complicated by HDP, women should undergo CV and metabolic risk screening in the first year postpartum.[14]

Interventions for Minimizing Cardiovascular Health Risks

Multidisciplinary Postpartum Team Approach[2]

Postpartum follow-up is best conducted through a multidisciplinary team approach, involving healthcare and allied professionals who can provide both medium- and long-term care **(Box 1)**. Despite potential challenges, recent evidence supports the creation of structured postpartum CV risk screening programs for women after complicated pregnancies.[15]

Postpartum Hypertensive Clinics: A Comprehensive Approach[16]

Postpartum hypertensive clinics are specialized care models designed to monitor and manage women who have experienced HDPs. These clinics aim to provide comprehensive follow-up care to mitigate the risk of persistent hypertension and associated CV complications.

Key components include:

- Timely blood pressure monitoring
- Cardiovascular risk assessment
- Multidisciplinary care team
- Patient education and support

BOX 1: Key members of the multidisciplinary postpartum team.

Short term care:
- Obstetric care providers
- Maternal–fetal medicine specialist

Identify women requiring follow-up and advise on strategies to minimize adverse pregnancy outcomes in future pregnancies

Medium and long-term care:
- Cardiologist
- Gynecologist
- General practitioner
- Family physician
- Internist

Provide ongoing medical follow-up and CV risk assessment; contraception, counseling and management of subsequent pregnancy

Allied health professionals:
- Dietician
- Social worker
- Physiotherapist

Support lifestyle and behavioral interventions

Implementing such specialized clinics can significantly improve maternal health outcomes by ensuring timely detection and management of postpartum hypertension, thereby reducing the risk of long-term CVDs.

Postpartum Follow-up: Key Assessment Parameters[17]

- *History and physical examination:* Review of maternal history and evaluation of current health status
- *Blood pressure monitoring:* Local hypertension guidelines for measurement and management
- *Anthropometrics:* BMI and waist circumference
- *Investigations:*
  - Oral glucose tolerance test/HbA1c
  - Lipid profile
  - Urine albumin-to-creatinine ratio

Short-term Interventions and Follow-up Plans (0–12 Weeks Postpartum) (Fig. 2)

- *Breastfeeding:* Encourage and support breastfeeding to improve cardiometabolic health. A recent meta-analysis of 1,192,700 women found that breastfeeding is linked to a significantly lower maternal risk of CVD [hazard ratio

Short-term interventions and follow-up plans (0–12 Weeks postpartum)

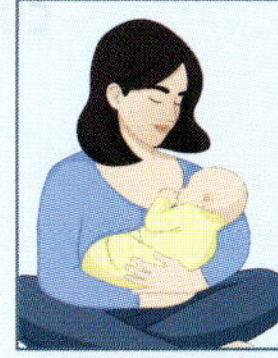

Breastfeeding
Encourage and support breastfeeding to improve cardiometabolic health

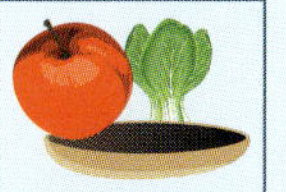

Lifestyle modifications
Heart-healthy diet, DASH diet has been demonstrated to reduce the 10-year Framingham risk score (FRS) for CVD b 13%

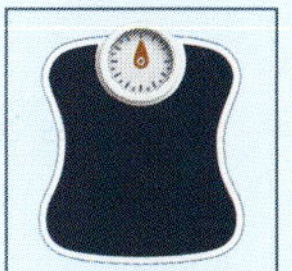

Weight management
Monitor and manage postpartum weight gain or retention, as it increases the risk of future pregnancy complications

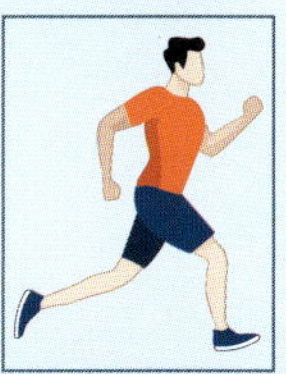

Physical activity
It is recommended that women engage in at least 150 minutes of moderate-intensity exercise (such as brisk walking, cycling) or over 75 minutes of high-intensity exercise (like jogging, running) each week to lower the risk of future CVD

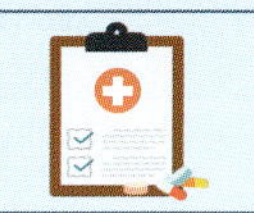

Antihypertensives
Titration of medications

FIG. 2: Short-term interventions for cardiovascular health after HDP.

(HR) 0.89; 95% CI 0.83–0.95], coronary artery disease (HR 0.86; 95% CI 0.78–0.95), stroke (HR 0.88; 95% CI 0.79–0.99), and CV-related maternal mortality (HR 0.83; 95% CI 0.76–0.92).[18]

- *Lifestyle modifications:* Heart-healthy diet and DASH diet has been demonstrated to reduce the 10-year Framingham risk score (FRS) for CVD by 13%.
- *Weight management:* Monitor and manage postpartum weight gain or retention, as it increases the risk of future pregnancy complications.
- *Physical activity:* It is recommended that women engage in at least 150 minutes of moderate-intensity exercise (such as brisk walking and cycling) or over 75 minutes of high-intensity exercise (such as jogging and running) each week to lower the risk of future CVD.[19]
- *Antihypertensives:* Titration of medications
- *Follow up:* Monitor blood pressure and CV risk markers *(discussed above in Postpartum Follow-up)* at 6 and 12 weeks.

Medium-term Interventions and Follow-up Plans (3–12 Months Postpartum)

- *Cardiovascular screening:* Monitor blood pressure and CV risk markers *(discussed above in Postpartum Follow-up)* at 6 and 12 months.
- *Integration with newborn care:* The WHO recommends newborn immunizations at birth, 6 weeks, 6 months, and 12 months, providing an opportunity to align maternal CV follow-up with these visits to improve postpartum care adherence.

Long-term Interventions and Follow-up Plans (beyond 12 Months Postpartum)

- *Periodic cardiovascular risk assessment:* Assess CV risk factors at least every 4–6 years for all women aged 20 years and older, as recommended by the AHA.
- *Cardiovascular risk reduction program:* Women with preexisting cardiovascular risk factors (e.g., hypertension and diabetes) should engage in a long-term risk reduction program, maintaining a healthy lifestyle through diet, exercise, and weight management.
- *Secondary prevention efforts:* Implement aggressive CV risk modification and secondary preventive efforts to reduce CV events.
- *Pharmacological strategies:*[2]
  - *Antiplatelets:* Low-dose aspirin can reduce the risk of preeclampsia and small-for-gestational-age births, but in women with prior HDP, it showed a nonsignificant reduction in stroke risk before age of 60 years (adjusted HR 0.8, 95% CI 0.4–1.7) compared with higher risk if not used (adjusted HR 1.5, 95% CI 1.0–2.1), and carries a 46% increased risk of major bleeding; therefore, it is not recommended for primary CVD prevention in this population.
  - *Statins:* These have not shown benefits in reducing this risk. High-quality evidence confirming these findings is limited, and the effects of aspirin on other CV outcomes in women with a history of HDP remain unclear.

Timing of CVD risk factor follow-up within the first year postpartum is given in **Figure 3**.

CONCLUSION

Hypertensive disorders of pregnancy are not only a major cause of maternal and perinatal morbidity but also a significant predictor of long-term CVD. The postpartum period represents a critical window for early identification, risk stratification, and preventive interventions. Structured follow-up through multidisciplinary postpartum clinics, incorporating lifestyle modification, CV screening, and patient education, can significantly reduce long-term CV risk in women with a history of HDP. Integration of maternal follow-up with routine new-born care enhances adherence and ensures comprehensive care. While pharmacological interventions such as low-dose aspirin may have specific indications, lifestyle measures remain the cornerstone of CV risk reduction. Overall, proactive, evidence-based postpartum management provides a unique opportunity to improve lifelong CV health for this high-risk population.

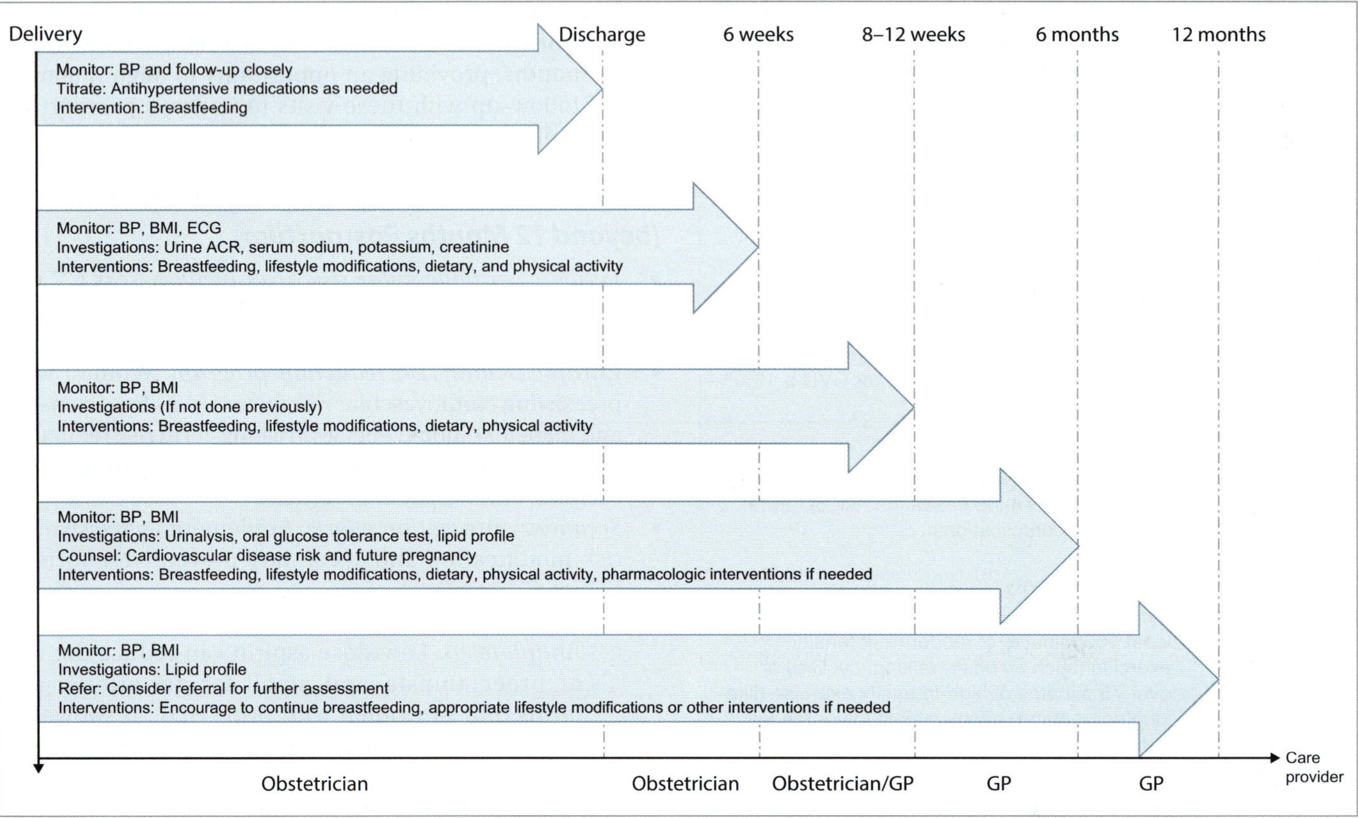

FIG. 3: Timing of CVD risk factor follow-up within the first year postpartum.
Source: Modified from Parikh et al. and Graves et al.[20,21]

REFERENCES

1. Gestational Hypertension and Preeclampsia: ACOG Practice Bulletin, Number 222. Obstet Gynecol. 2020;135(6):e237-60.
2. Poon LC, Nguyen-Hoang L, Smith GN, et al. Hypertensive disorders of pregnancy and long-term cardiovascular health: FIGO Best Practice Advice. Int J Gynaecol Obstet. 2023;160 Suppl 1:22-34.
3. Grandi SM, Vallée-Pouliot K, Reynier P, et al. Hypertensive disorders in pregnancy and the risk of subsequent cardiovascular disease. Paediatr Perinat Epidemiol. 2017;31(5):412-21.
4. Deer E, Herrock O, Campbell N, et al. The role of immune cells and mediators in preeclampsia. Nat Rev Nephrol. 2023;19(4):257-70.
5. Sanghavi M, Rutherford JD. Cardiovascular physiology of pregnancy. Circulation. 2014;130(12):1003-8.
6. Bamfo JE, Kametas NA, Chambers JB, et al. Maternal cardiac function in normotensive and pre-eclamptic intrauterine growth restriction. Ultrasound Obstet Gynecol. 2008;32(5):682-6.
7. Bellamy L, Casas JP, Hingorani AD, et al. Pre-eclampsia and risk of cardiovascular disease and cancer in later life: Systematic review and meta-analysis. BMJ. 2007;335(7627):974.
8. Wu P, Haththotuwa R, Kwok CS, et al. Preeclampsia and future cardiovascular health: A systematic review and meta-analysis. Circ Cardiovasc Qual Outcomes. 2017;10(2):e003497.
9. Voskamp LW, Verdonk K, van Lennep JER, et al. Blood pressure patterns during pregnancy and early postpartum in preeclampsia with severe features: Predictors of chronic hypertension. Pregnancy Hypertens. 2025;41:101240.
10. Mosca L, Benjamin EJ, Berra K, et al. Effectiveness-based guidelines for the prevention of cardiovascular disease in women--2011 update: A guideline from the American Heart Association. Circulation. 2011;123(11):1243-62.
11. Kessous R, Shoham-Vardi I, Pariente G, et al. Long-term maternal atherosclerotic morbidity in women with pre-eclampsia. Heart. 2015;101(6):442-6.
12. Dall'Asta A, D'Antonio F, Saccone G, et al. Cardiovascular events following pregnancy complicated by pre-eclampsia with emphasis on comparison between early- and late-onset forms: systematic review and meta-analysis. Ultrasound Obstet Gynecol. 2021;57(5):698-709.
13. Behrens I, Basit S, Lykke JA, et al. Association between hypertensive disorders of pregnancy and later risk of cardiomyopathy. JAMA. 2016;315(10):1026-33.
14. Smith GN, Louis JM, Saade GR. Pregnancy and the postpartum period as an opportunity for cardiovascular risk identification and management. Obstet Gynecol. 2019;134(4):851-62.
15. Spaan J, Peeters L, Spaanderman M, et al. Cardiovascular risk management after a hypertensive disorder of pregnancy. Hypertension. 2012;60(6):1368-73.
16. Countouris M, Mahmoud Z, Cohen JB, et al. Hypertension in pregnancy and postpartum: Current standards and opportunities to improve care. Circulation. 2025;151(7):490-507.
17. American College of Obstetricians and Gynecologists' Presidential Task Force on Pregnancy and Heart Disease and Committee on

Practice Bulletins—Obstetrics. ACOG Practice Bulletin No. 212: Pregnancy and Heart Disease. Obstet Gynecol. 2019;133(5): e320-56.

18. Tschiderer L, Seekircher L, Kunutsor SK, et al. Breastfeeding is associated with a reduced maternal cardiovascular risk: Systematic Review and meta-analysis involving data from 8 studies and 1 192 700 parous women. J Am Heart Assoc. 2022;11(2):e022746.
19. Arnett DK, Blumenthal RS, Albert MA, et al. 2019 ACC/AHA Guideline on the Primary Prevention of Cardiovascular Disease: A Report of the American College of Cardiology/American Heart Association Task Force on Clinical Practice Guidelines. Circulation. 2019;140(11):e596-646.
20. Parikh NI, Gonzalez JM, Anderson CAM, et al. Adverse pregnancy outcomes and cardiovascular disease risk: unique opportunities for cardiovascular disease prevention in women: a scientific statement from the American Heart Association. Circulation. 2021;143:e902-e916.
21. Graves M, Howse K, Pudwell J, Smith GN. Pregnancy-related cardiovascular risk indicators: Primary care approach to postpartum management and prevention of future disease. Can Fam Physician. 2019;65:883-9.

CHAPTER 72

Understanding and Managing Anticoagulant during Pregnancy in Women with Heart Valves

Abhishek Garg, Shibba Takkar Chhabra

ABSTRACT

Managing anticoagulation in pregnant women with prosthetic heart valves (PHV) remains a significant clinical challenge, requiring a careful balance between maternal and fetal risks. Available strategies include continued use of vitamin K antagonists (VKAs; e.g., warfarin) throughout pregnancy, transitioning to unfractionated heparin (UFH) or low-molecular-weight heparin (LMWH) during early gestation followed by resumption of warfarin in the second trimester, or using heparin-based therapies for the entire pregnancy. While warfarin offers superior protection against maternal thromboembolic complications, it poses considerable danger to fetal development, including teratogenic effects and pregnancy loss. In contrast, UFH and especially LMWH offer a safer fetal profile but are less effective in preventing maternal valve thrombosis. Determining what constitutes an acceptable balance of risks for both mother and fetus is often subjective, varying across both clinicians and patients. Therefore, a clear, evidence-based, and empathetic discussion of all therapeutic options is essential to guide shared decision-making and ensure that women are empowered to make informed choices during this high-risk clinical scenario.

Keywords: Pregnant, anticoagulation, prosthetic heart valves.

INTRODUCTION

Cardiovascular disorders remain among the foremost contributors to maternal mortality and morbidity during pregnancy. Pregnancy poses dual challenges in such patients due to the physiologic hypercoagulable state and altered hemodynamics, increasing the risk of valve thrombosis and thromboembolic events. This hypercoagulability presents a grave concern for women with mechanical heart valves, where the risk of valve thrombosis carries a mortality rate approaching 20%.[1] Achieving effective anticoagulation is vital in such cases, yet it comes with the competing danger of bleeding complications. Historically, the likelihood of an uneventful pregnancy resulting in a live birth among women with mechanical valves was as low as 58%.[2] Various anticoagulation protocols have been adopted in clinical practice, each with inherent limitations. Regimens based on vitamin K antagonists (VKAs) are generally more effective in protecting the mother but increase the risk of fetal harm. In contrast, therapies using low-molecular-weight heparin (LMWH) or unfractionated heparin (UFH) tend to be safer for the fetus but raise maternal thrombotic risk.[3,4]

Evidence suggests that maintaining effective anti-coagulation through meticulous monitoring can help reduce complications. Current clinical guidelines recommend strict surveillance using the international normalized ratio (INR), anti-Xa levels, and activated partial thromboplastin time (aPTT) to ensure therapeutic efficacy.[1] However, there is limited robust data directly correlating these monitoring targets with actual reductions in thromboembolic events. As a result, both the ideal anticoagulation regimen and the most effective monitoring strategies remain areas of uncertainty. In this chapter, we explore the complex and high-risk domain of anticoagulation management in pregnant women with prosthetic heart valves (PHV), with a focus on mechanical valve prostheses.

MATERNAL AND FETAL COMPLICATIONS ASSOCIATED WITH PROSTHETIC HEART VALVES IN PREGNANCY

Pregnancy poses a significant thrombotic risk for women with mechanical heart valves, classified as WHO risk category III, indicating a high probability of serious maternal complications.[1] Data from the ROPAC registry reveal that only 58% of pregnancies in women with mechanical PHV resulted in live births without major events—substantially lower than the outcomes seen in women with bioprosthetic valves (79%) or those with heart disease without valve prostheses (78%).[2] During pregnancy, the likelihood of developing valve thrombosis rises significantly, but maintaining optimal anticoagulation can help reduce this risk. Several factors contribute to this, including the mechanical valve's design and placement, the effectiveness of anticoagulation therapy, and individual patient characteristics. According to the ROPAC registry, valve thrombosis occurred in 4.7% of cases, with a maternal mortality rate of 20%.[2] Similarly, a UK study noted 9% maternal mortality due to thrombotic or valve-related complications and a striking 41% severe morbidity, including 16% with thromboembolic events.[5]

In women with bioprosthetic heart valves, the overall risk of maternal cardiovascular complications during pregnancy is generally low—provided the prosthesis is functioning well and left ventricular function remains preserved. However, when significant structural or functional deterioration of the bioprosthetic valve is present, the likelihood of adverse outcomes can increase substantially.

Moreover, due to anticoagulants, an increased likelihood of miscarriage, postpartum hemorrhage, and retroplacental bleeding may contribute to preterm delivery or even intrauterine fetal demise. The M-PAC registry (Maternal Prosthetic Valve and Anticoagulation Registry), the largest prospective single-center study of pregnant women with heart disease (PWWHD) conducted in a low- and middle-income country (LMIC), was carried out in India and enrolled 1,029 pregnancies over a 3-year period.[6] Among women with PHVs, adverse outcomes were significant.[6] Women with mechanical prosthetic valves remain highly vulnerable to prosthetic valve thrombosis (PVT), both during gestation and in the postpartum period. In the MPAC series, 12 patients (17.1%) experienced valve thrombosis, with eight cases occurring during pregnancy and four after delivery. Most episodes were observed during the transition from oral anticoagulants to heparin.[6] This incidence is considerably greater than the 7% reported in the ROPAC registry. Many affected women had independently discontinued anticoagulation soon after confirming pregnancy, motivated by concerns about fetal malformations. Overall, maternal mortality in this group was 8.6%.[6] These findings emphasize the substantial maternal and fetal risks associated with PHVs during pregnancy, especially in resource-limited settings, and highlight the urgent need for individualized care and optimized anticoagulation strategies.

MATERNAL AND FETAL OUTCOMES ACROSS ANTICOAGULANT THERAPIES

The continuation of VKAs throughout pregnancy has been correlated with a relatively lower incidence of PVT, estimated at 0–4%.[2] Evidence from two major systematic reviews indicates that the likelihood of fetal loss under VKA therapy is strongly dose-dependent. The fetal loss rate with low-dose VKAs (warfarin <5 mg/day, acenocoumarol <2 mg/day) ranges from 13.4 to 19.2%, while the overall fetal loss rate with VKAs may be as high as 32.5%.[4,7] In comparison, regimens involving heparin followed by VKA result in a fetal loss rate of 22.7%, whereas, LMWH throughout pregnancy shows the lowest risk at 12.2%.[4,7] However, differences in study design and outcome reporting limit the direct comparability of these figures, and the safety of low-dose VKAs remains a subject of debate. A major concern with VKAs during organogenesis (6–12 weeks) is embryopathy, including limb abnormalities and nasal hypoplasia, reported in 0.6–10% of cases.[4,7] This risk also demonstrates a dose-dependent pattern, with low-dose warfarin therapy showing a comparatively reduced incidence of embryopathy, ranging between 0.45 and 0.9%.[4,7] During the second and third trimesters, however, continued exposure to VKAs may result in fetopathy, including ocular abnormalities, central nervous system defects, and intracranial hemorrhage, with an estimated prevalence of 0.7–2%.[4,7] Data from the ROPAC registry indicate that VKAs, when used during the first trimester, are associated with a significantly higher rate of miscarriage (28.6%) compared to LMWH or UFH (9.2%), along with lower live birth rates.[2]

On the other hand, UFH—especially when used either in the first trimester or throughout pregnancy—has been linked to a much higher thrombosis rate (9–33%), along with other risks such as thrombocytopenia and osteoporosis.[4] LMWH also carries a risk of valve thrombosis, particularly if dosing is not adjusted carefully. Due to enhanced renal clearance during pregnancy, dose requirements often increase, necessitating close monitoring of anti-Xa levels. Studies suggest that using LMWH with anti-Xa-guided dose adjustments throughout pregnancy still results in a thrombosis risk of 4.4–8.7%.[4] Moreover, even when peak anti-Xa levels (1.0–1.2 IU/mL) fall within the recommended range, valve thrombosis has been reported.[8] These findings suggest that trough levels (predose levels) may also be important but are under-monitored in current practice. Limiting the use of LMWH to the first trimester results in a PVT rate of 5.8–7.4%, which is similar to the incidence observed when LMWH is administered throughout the entire pregnancy.[3] The UK registry study showed particularly high thrombotic risk with LMWH-based regimens, raising concerns about its safety profile.[9] Subtherapeutic trough levels—despite seemingly adequate peaks—may explain some of these failures. Yet, evidence regarding dual (peak and trough) anti-Xa monitoring is limited and mostly comes from case reports.[9]

Unlike VKAs, UFH and LMWH do not cross the placenta, and replacing VKAs with heparins during this critical period significantly lowers the risk of embryopathy. Although cases of fetopathy have been occasionally reported with UFH, such complications have not been documented with the continuous use of LMWH throughout pregnancy. Hemorrhagic complications in the mother may occur with

TABLE 1: Maternal and fetal outcomes on various anticoagulation regimes.[3]

Anticoagulation regimen	Maternal mortality			Thromboembolism			Livebirth rate			Anticoagulant-related fetal/neonatal adverse events		
	Studies	Events	Estimate (%)	Studies	Events	Estimate (%)	Studies	Events	Estimate (%)	Studies	Events	Estimate (%)
VKAs (INR target 2.5–3.5)	11	7/581	0.9 (0.1–1.6)	11	22/581	2.7 (1.4– 4.0)	10	369/531	64.5	11	12/407	2.0
Sequential treatment	20	11/530	2.0 (0.8–3.1)	20	44/530	5.8 (3.8–7.7)	18	381/475	79.9	19	5/431	1.4
LMWH alone	10	1/132	2.9 (0.2–5.7)	9	13/127	8.7 (3.9–13.4)	7	68/74	92.0	8	0/103	NA
UFH alone	4	2/64	3.4 (0.7–7.7)	3	7/52	11.2 (2.8–19.6)	3	33/51	69.5	4	4/44	7.6

Note: This table highlights the balance between maternal and fetal outcomes across different anticoagulation regimens in pregnancy with mechanical heart valves. VKAs offer the lowest maternal thromboembolic risk but are associated with adverse fetal outcomes. Sequential therapy and LMWH provide improved live birth rates, though at the cost of higher maternal thromboembolic risk. UFH alone shows the poorest maternal protection with relatively higher adverse outcomes.

(LMWH: low-molecular-weight heparin; UFH: unfractionated heparin; VKAs: vitamin K antagonists)

all anticoagulant regimens. **Table 1** summarizes the number of studies reviewed and the maternal and fetal complications associated with different anticoagulant regimens.

Hence, significant uncertainties remain regarding the use of LMWH in pregnant women with mechanical valves, including optimal anti-Xa targets, the role of peak versus trough levels, the appropriate monitoring frequency, and the safest duration of use. These unresolved questions highlight the need for individualized management and closer clinical monitoring in this high-risk population.

LOW-DOSE ASPIRIN IN PROSTHETIC VALVE MANAGEMENT DURING PREGNANCY

The concomitant use of low-dose aspirin with either VKAs or heparin during pregnancy has not shown consistent evidence of reducing the incidence of PVT.[2,4] On the contrary, it is linked with a significantly increased incidence of maternal bleeding complications, including life-threatening hemorrhagic events.

MANAGEMENT OF THE HEART VALVES DURING PREGNANCY

Choice of Heart Valve

Selecting the most appropriate valve type in women of childbearing age poses a significant clinical challenge. While mechanical valves provide superior durability and hemodynamic performance, their requirement for lifelong anticoagulation substantially increases the risk of maternal and fetal complications during pregnancy, including thromboembolic events and bleeding. In contrast, bioprosthetic valves eliminate the need for long-term anticoagulation, making them a safer option during pregnancy. However, in younger women, these valves are more prone to early structural degeneration, raising the possibility of valve dysfunction during a future pregnancy and the likelihood of reintervention or reoperation.[10] Alternative surgical options, such as transcatheter valve implantation (particularly in pulmonary positions) and the Ross procedure (where the pulmonary valve is used to replace the aortic valve), may be considered in select patients.[11] Although data on pregnancy outcomes after the Ross procedure are limited, existing evidence suggests a relatively low-risk profile—especially in the absence of aortic dilatation.[12]

For women who express a strong desire to conceive in the future, implantation of a bioprosthetic valve is a Class IIa recommendation.[13] The pregnancy heart team should be actively involved in decision-making, ensuring that the woman is fully informed about the benefits and limitations of each option, with shared decision-making guiding the final choice.

During Pregnancy

Before conception, women with PHV should receive a thorough cardiovascular evaluation. This includes evaluating for any clinical symptoms, performing echocardiography to assess heart function, and examining the condition and performance of both prosthetic and remaining native valves. Furthermore, factors including the type of prosthetic valve (mechanical vs. bioprosthetic), its anatomical location (aortic, mitral, or multiple valve positions), and any history of PVT must be thoroughly evaluated. These elements are critical in estimating the risk of complications during pregnancy.[10]

For women at high risk, especially those with mechanical valves and a history of complications, preconception counseling should explore the potential maternal and fetal risks associated with pregnancy. In some cases, based on clinical judgment, the option of deferring or avoiding pregnancy altogether should be openly discussed to protect maternal health.

Medical Therapy

As per the 2025 European Society of Cardiology guidelines,[14] before conception, it is essential to have a thorough discussion with the patient regarding the pros and cons of various anticoagulation options. The woman must be informed that VKAs offer the most reliable protection against PVT, making them the safest option for maternal health. However, the use of VKAs—especially in the first trimester—is associated with significant fetal risks, including embryopathy, fetal bleeding, miscarriage, and developmental toxicity, which are influenced by the dose of VKA used. LMWH, while associated with reduced fetal complications, carries a higher maternal risk for valve thrombosis. Therefore, the woman's prior adherence to anticoagulation therapy should be evaluated, and it must be emphasized that strict compliance with whichever regimen is selected is critical for both maternal and fetal safety. In the preconception phase, VKAs should be continued until pregnancy is confirmed. If pregnancy is achieved and the required VKA dose is low (<5 mg/day warfarin), some guidelines support continuing VKAs throughout pregnancy, since the risks of fetal harm (embryopathy <2% and fetal loss <20%) remain relatively low. The protection against valve thrombosis remains superior.[4,15] INR should be managed according to established clinical targets, with weekly or biweekly monitoring, and self-INR monitoring may be appropriate for selected patients **(Table 2)**. Alternatively, for women requiring lower VKA doses, a switch to LMWH between 6 and 12 weeks of gestation may be considered after providing comprehensive counseling **(Flowchart 1)**.[10]

In women needing higher VKA doses (>5 mg/day warfarin), transitioning from VKAs during this critical window to either adjusted-dose intravenous UFH or dose-adjusted LMWH twice daily is a reasonable option **(Flowchart 2)**.[10] Peak anti-Xa levels should guide LMWH dosing, and in certain cases, trough anti-Xa monitoring (target ≥ 0.6 IU/mL) may be considered, although data supporting this approach are limited **(Table 3)**.

Initial LMWH doses include enoxaparin at 1 mg/kg or dalteparin at 100 IU/kg, both administered twice daily subcutaneously.[10,14] These doses should be titrated daily based on anti-Xa levels until therapeutic targets are met, then reassessed weekly. Routine addition of aspirin is not advised in this context. When UFH is selected, therapy should aim for a stable aPTT, ideally greater than twice the baseline, with weekly monitoring thereafter.[10,14] In the second and third trimesters, VKAs are generally the preferred anticoagulant, as the teratogenic risk declines while their efficacy in preventing valve thrombosis remains unmatched.[10,14]

Pregnant patients with mechanical heart valves should receive care under the supervision of a dedicated pregnancy

TABLE 2: Target for INR in case of VKAs use for the mechanical valves.

	Patient-related risk factors INR Target	
Thrombogenicity	**None**	**≥ 1**
Low	2.5	3.0
Medium	3.0	3.5
High	3.5	4.0

Note:
- *Patient-related risk factors:* Mitral or tricuspid valve replacement, previous thromboembolism, atrial fibrillation, mitral stenosis of any degree, or low-molecular-weight heparin (LVEF) <35%.
- *Low thrombogenicity:* Carbomedics, Medtronic Hall, ATS, or Medtronic Open-Pivot, St Jude Medical, On-X, or Sorin Bicarbon.
- *Medium thrombogenicity:* Bileaflet valves
- *High thrombogenicity:* Lillehei-Kaster, omniscience, Starr-Edwards (ball-cage), Björk-Shiley and other tilting-disc valves; any pulmonary valve prosthesis.

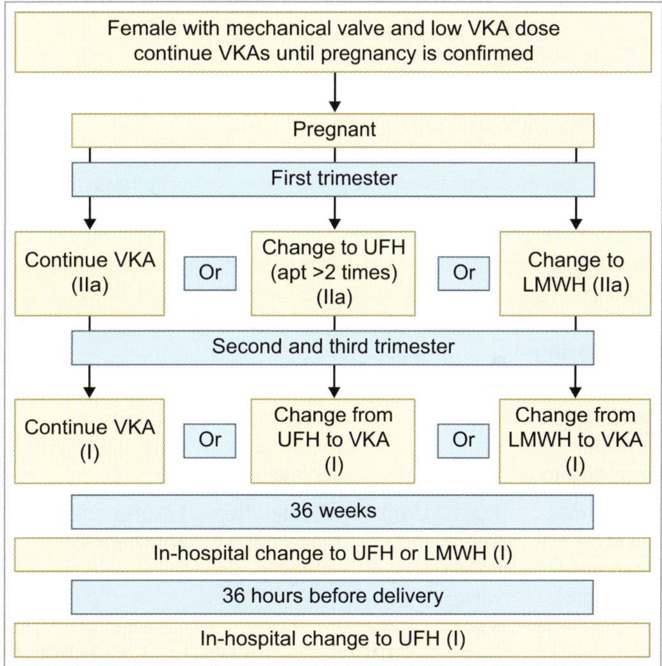

FLOWCHART 1: Management of mechanical valve during pregnancy with requiring a low dose of VKAs.

Note: Low-dose VKAs—warfarin <5 mg/day and acenocoumarol <2 mg/day.

(LMWH: low-molecular-weight heparin; UFH: unfractionated heparin; VKA: vitamin K antagonist)

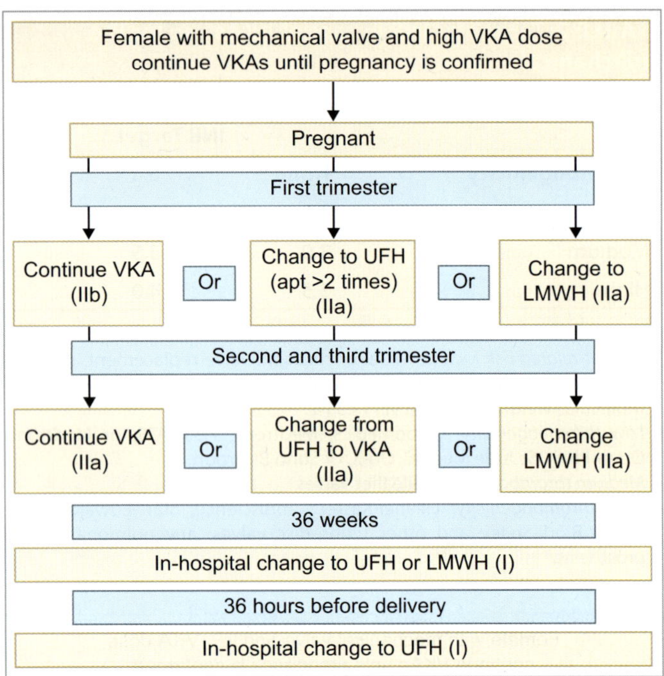

FLOWCHART 2: Management of mechanical valve during pregnancy with requiring high dose of VKAs.

Note: High-dose VKAs—warfarin ≥5 mg/day and acenocoumarol ≥2 mg/day.
(LMWH: low-molecular-weight heparin; UFH: unfractionated heparin; VKA: vitamin K antagonist)

TABLE 3: Anti-Xa monitoring targets in pregnancy for mechanical heart valves.

Monitoring step	Target levels	Frequency	Remarks
In-hospital anti-Xa monitoring	–	Daily, until the target is achieved	Initiate after starting LMWH
Peak-anti-Xa level (4–6 hours postdose)	1.0–1.2 U/mL (mitral and right-sided valves) 0.8–1.2 U/mL (aortic valves)	Weekly, after the target is achieved	Ensures adequate anticoagulation
Predose (trough) anti-Xa level	> 0.6 U/mL	Weekly, after the target is achieved	Helps detect subtherapeutic levels due to rapid clearance

heart team within a specialized center experienced in managing high-risk cardiac pregnancies. The chosen anticoagulation strategy must be closely monitored, with INR or anti-Xa levels checked weekly or biweekly, depending on the anticoagulant used. Regular clinical evaluations, including echocardiographic assessment, should be carried out at least once a month to ensure maternal and fetal well-being and detect any valve-related complications early.[10]

SPECIAL CASE

Valve Thrombosis

If a pregnant woman presents with dyspnea or signs of systemic embolism, an urgent transthoracic echocardiogram should be performed to assess for valve thrombosis, often followed by transesophageal echocardiography for better visualization. Fluoroscopy can also aid in diagnosis and is generally considered safe with minimal fetal radiation exposure.[10] Treatment approaches for PVT in pregnancy largely mirror those in nonpregnant individuals. In noncritical cases with recent subtherapeutic anticoagulation, initiating intravenous UFH and resuming oral anticoagulants may suffice. However, in patients with obstructive thrombosis or clinical deterioration, surgery is indicated when medical therapy fails.[13] Fibrinolytic therapy is a potential option in patients who are critically ill or when surgery is not immediately accessible.[10] Alteplase (tPA), characterized by its high molecular weight and minimal placental transfer, is considered the preferred fibrinolytic agent.[10] Though the use of thrombolytics carries risks, including embolism and subplacental bleeding, it may be considered over surgery, especially in stable patients or those with right-sided PVT. Given the high fetal mortality associated with surgery (up to 30%), thrombolysis may offer a safer alternative in select cases.[16] Patients must be thoroughly counseled regarding potential maternal and fetal risks before proceeding with any intervention.

Delivery

A planned approach to delivery is essential in women with mechanical heart valves. For those aiming for vaginal delivery, a prior transition to intravenous heparin is required to minimize thrombotic risk.[10,14] However, the use of epidural anesthesia poses challenges, as it necessitates a prolonged cessation of anticoagulation, making it unsuitable for patients on mechanical prostheses.[10,14] In such cases, particularly for women at high risk of valve thrombosis, a scheduled cesarean section may be a safer option, as it allows better control of anticoagulation and minimizes the duration without VKAs.[10] Furthermore, if labor begins while the patient is still on VKA therapy, an immediate cesarean section is recommended to avoid complications related to maternal and fetal bleeding **(Table 4)**.[10,14]

Restarting Anticoagulation after Delivery

Restarting anticoagulation after childbirth is a complex decision that requires balancing the competing risks of thromboembolism and postpartum bleeding.[14] This process demands coordination among multiple specialties—including anesthesiology, cardiology, hematology, and obstetrics—with the patient's preferences also playing a central role. Delayed obstetric bleeding beyond 24 hours

TABLE 4: Recommendations by 2025 ESC Guidelines for Anticoagulants in Heart Valves.

Recommendations	Class	Level
In mitral stenosis, therapeutic anticoagulation with heparins or VKAs is indicated in pregnant patients with atrial fibrillation, left atrial thrombus, or a history of embolic events	I	C
It is recommended to manage pregnancy in women with mechanical valves in a center with a pregnancy heart team		
If delivery starts while on a VKA or in <2 weeks after discontinuation of a VKA, cesarean section is recommended		
It is recommended to discontinue VKAs and start adjusted-dose intravenous UFH (aPTT ≥ 2× control) or adjusted-dose LMWH at the 36th weeks' gestation		
In pregnant women on LMWH or UFH, it is recommended to perform weekly anti-Xa level monitoring or aPTT monitoring with dose adjustment (within 36 hours)		
In pregnant women on a VKA, it is recommended to perform INR monitoring weekly or every 2 weeks		
In pregnant women with LMWH, it is recommended to target anti-Xa levels 4–6 hours postdose at 0.8–1.2 U/L (aortic valve prosthesis) or 1.0–1.2 IU/mL (mitral and right-sided valve prostheses)		
It is recommended to replace LMWH with intravenous UFH (aPTT ≥ 2× control) at least 36 hours before planned delivery. UFH should be continued until 4–6 hours before planned delivery and restarted 4–6 hours after delivery if there are no bleeding complications		
It is recommended to anticipate the timing of delivery to ensure safe and effective peripartum anticoagulation		
Immediate echocardiography is recommended in women with mechanical valves presenting with dyspnea and/or an embolic event		
It is recommended to implement changes in the anticoagulation regimen during pregnancy in a hospital		
During the second and third trimesters until the 36th week, VKAs are recommended in women needing a low dose		

(aPTT: activated partial thromboplastin time; LMWH: low-molecular-weight heparin; UFH: unfractionated heparin; VKAs: vitamin K antagonists)

is relatively frequent, as highlighted by recent findings from the ROPAC III registry,[14] where bleeding events were observed around an average of 3.6 days after delivery. These episodes often coincided with the period when UFH was being administered alongside the reintroduction of VKAs. Acceptable approaches for reinitiating therapy include UFH titrated to achieve an aPTT at least twice the control, or low-to-intermediate doses of LMWH.[14] Strategies to minimize bleeding risk include active management of the third stage of labor, particularly with oxytocin.[14] One study demonstrated that supplementing a standard low-dose oxytocin infusion with an additional 2 IU bolus over 10 minutes significantly reduced blood loss without causing adverse cardiovascular effects.[17] Given the elevated risk of delayed hemorrhage, VKAs are best resumed no earlier than 7–14 days postpartum.

CONCLUSION

The management of anticoagulation in pregnancy with PHV demands an individualized, multidisciplinary approach. Mechanical valves, though durable, require long-term anticoagulation and are associated with increased maternal and fetal risks, while bioprosthetic valves offer a safer profile in pregnancy but carry a risk of structural degeneration. Anticoagulant selection must be carefully tailored throughout each trimester, balancing thrombotic and hemorrhagic risks. Regular monitoring, timely dose adjustments, and structured delivery planning are essential to minimize complications. In all cases, prepregnancy counseling and involvement of a specialized pregnancy heart team are vital to optimize maternal and fetal outcomes.

REFERENCES

1. van der Zande JA, Ramlakhan KP, Sliwa K, et al. Pregnancy with a prosthetic heart valve, thrombosis, and bleeding: the ESC EORP Registry of Pregnancy and Cardiac disease III. Eur Heart J. 2025:ehaf265.
2. van Hagen IM, Roos-Hesselink JW, Ruys TP, et al. Pregnancy in women with a mechanical heart valve: data of the European Society of Cardiology Registry of Pregnancy and Cardiac Disease (ROPAC). Circulation. 2015;132:132-42.
3. D'Souza R, Ostro J, Shah PS, et al. Anticoagulation for pregnant women with mechanical heart valves: a systematic review and meta-analysis. Eur Heart J. 2017;38:1509-16.
4. Xu Z, Fan J, Luo X, et al. Anticoagulation regimens during pregnancy in patients with mechanical heart valves: a systematic review and meta-analysis. Can J Cardiol. 2016;32:1248.e1-9.
5. Vause S, Clarke B, Tower CL, et al. Pregnancy outcomes in women with mechanical prosthetic heart valves: a prospective

descriptive population-based study using the United Kingdom Obstetric Surveillance System (UKOSS) data collection system. BJOG. 2017;124:1411-9.

6. Justin Paul G, Anne Princy S, Anju S, et al. Pregnancy outcomes in women with heart disease: the madras medical college pregnancy and cardiac (M-PAC) registry from India. Eur Heart J. 2023;44(17):1530-40.
7. Hassouna A, Allam H. Limited dose warfarin throughout pregnancy in patients with mechanical heart valve prosthesis: a meta-analysis. Interact Cardiovasc Thorac Surg. 2014;18: 797-806.
8. Basude S, Hein C, Curtis SL, et al. Low-molecular-weight heparin or warfarin for anticoagulation in pregnant women with mechanical heart valves: what are the risks? A retrospective observational study. BJOG. 2012;119:1008-13.
9. Goland S, Schwartzenberg S, Fan J, et al. Monitoring of anti-Xa in pregnant patients with mechanical prosthetic valves receiving low-molecular-weight heparin: peak or trough levels? J Cardiovasc Pharmacol Ther. 2014;19:451-6.
10. Regitz-Zagrosek V, Roos-Hesselink J. 2018 ESC guidelines for the management of cardiovascular diseases during pregnancy. Russ J Cardiol. 2019;24(6):151-228.
11. Elkayam U, Goland S, Pieper PG, et al. High-risk cardiac disease in pregnancy: part I. J Am Coll Cardiol. 2016;68:396-410.
12. Yap SC, Drenthen W, Pieper PG, et al. Outcome of pregnancy in women after pulmonary autograft valve replacement for congenital aortic valve disease. J Heart Valve Dis. 2007;16:398-403.
13. Baumgartner H, Falk V, Bax JJ, et al. 2017 ESC/EACTS guidelines for the management of valvular heart disease. Eur Heart J. 2017;38:2739-91.
14. De Backer J, Haugaa KH, Hasselberg NE, et al. 2025 ESC Guidelines for the management of cardiovascular disease and pregnancy: developed by the Task Force on the Management of Cardiovascular Disease and Pregnancy of the European Society of Cardiology (ESC), endorsed by the European Society of Gynecology (ESG). Eur Heart J. 2025:ehaf193.
15. Abildgaard U, Sandset PM, Hammerstrom J, et al. Management of pregnant women with mechanical heart valve prosthesis: thromboprophylaxis with low molecular weight heparin. Thromb Res. 2009;124:262-7.
16. Ozkan M, Cakal B, Karakoyun S, et al. Thrombolytic therapy for the treatment of prosthetic heart valve thrombosis in pregnancy with low-dose, slow infusion of tissue-type plasminogen activator. Circulation. 2013;128:532-40.
17. Cauldwell M, Steer PJ, Swan L, et al. The management of the third stage of labour in women with heart disease. Heart. 2017;103(12): 945-51.

SECTION

10

Coronary Artery Disease

Section Outline

73. Sarcopenia and Coronary Microvascular Dysfunction
Nakul Sinha

74. Spontaneous Coronary Artery Dissection
Prakas Chandra Mondal

75. Platelet Biology and Function: Plaque Erosion versus Rupture
Ranjit K Nath, MD Asif Iqbal, Shreya Gupta

76. Coronary Artery Aneurysm: A Therapeutic Dilemma
Ramesh Thakur, Kumar Himanshu

77. Atherosclerosis, Aortic Dissection, and Peripheral Artery Disease: New Therapeutic Targets
Akhilesh Kumar, Suman Bhandari

CHAPTER 73

Sarcopenia and Coronary Microvascular Dysfunction

Nakul Sinha

ABSTRACT

Sarcopenia which signifies a low muscle strength or mass or muscle quality, is a progressive skeletal muscle disorder associated with adverse outcomes, including frailty, disability, hospitalization and death. Its prevalence can be up to 20–30% in elderly patients with an increased propensity to heart failure, especially with preserved ejection fraction. Sarcopenia, at the cell level, features muscle protein homeostasis dysregulation with a pro-inflammatory state resulting in endothelial and mitochondrial dysfunction. Screening tests comprise of strength assessment parameters or by computed tomography and MR imaging aided by bioelectrical impedance analysis. Sarcopenia is also a component of cardiorenal cachexia syndromes. Coronary microvascular dysfunction in the absence of significant large vessel obstruction, is a common accompaniment with multiple interactive pathophysiological mechanisms. Such patients having both these components are at risk for more adverse events, especially amongst young females and obese individuals. Sarcopenia as an established parameter needs to be subclassified for more elaborate studies in assessment in elderly patients specially those with heart failure.

Keywords: Sarcopenia, heart failure with preserved ejection fraction, muscle wasting, coronary microvascular dysfunction, cardiorenal cachexia.

INTRODUCTION

Sarcopenia was first described by Irwin Rosenberg in 1989 as age-related loss of muscle mass. Gradually, over time, this also now includes muscle strength and physical performance. It has now been labelled as a distinct disease entity by the ICD-10 codes. It also forms a component of frailty. European Working Group on Sarcopenia in Older People (EWGSOP)[1] clinically defines it as the presence of low muscle strength and mass or muscle quality with a shift toward the function-related model. Later, the definition has expanded to signify it as a progressive skeletal muscle disorder associated with adverse outcomes, including frailty, disability, hospitalization, and death. This has also been acknowledged by the Asian working group on sarcopenia.[2] Skeletal muscle is now recognized as a major endocrine organ, releasing bioactive molecules that can influence endothelial function. Oxidative stress and platelet activity which are all key mediators of coronary microvascular dysfunction (CMVD). Sarcopenia has traditionally been investigated in geriatric and metabolic disorders. Perhaps there is more of a bidirectional relationship between muscle integrity and cardiovascular health.

The prevalence of sarcopenia can be up to 5–13% in the general population above 60 years of age, going up to even 20–30% in elderly hospitalized patients. Up to 50% of patients with heart failure (more in heart failure with preserved ejection fraction) can have sarcopenia.[3]

The diagnosis of sarcopenia includes low muscle strength, low muscle mass, and impaired muscle performance. Besides aging, sarcopenia is often associated with other chronic conditions, such as diabetes, obesity, and heart disease. At the cellular level, the key features may include muscle protein homeostasis dysregulation, a proinflammatory state leading to endothelial and mitochondrial dysfunction. Other mechanisms may include anabolic resistance together with activation of catabolic pathways, causing a disbalance. Chronic low-grade inflammation, often referred to as "inflammaging," can also lead to the release of bioactive cytokines, which may affect protein synthesis in the muscle. Age-related loss of motor neurons can also be an important contributory factor.

Objective methods to measure skeletal muscle mass are based on computed tomography and magnetic resonance imaging. Dual energy X-ray absorptiometry and bioelectrical impedance analysis also determine the body composition, including the lean body mass, while the hand grip dynamometer and the isokinetic dynamometer can measure muscle strength. Physical performance can be seen by a simple 6-minute walk test. Supplementary estimations of inflammatory cytokines or hormones can be added to the information. A few screening tests, such as SARC-F (Strength, Assistance with walking, Rise from a chair, Climb stairs, Falls) and SARC-Calf, can assess strength parameters, walking efficiency, or a tendency to falls, aided by the calf muscle circumference.[4,5] The EWGSOP suggests that sarcopenia be diagnosed based on objective parameters of low muscle mass: <8.90 kg/m^2 for males and <6.37 kg/m^2 for females, a low handgrip strength <30 kg for males and <20 kg for females, together with a gait speed of <0.8 m/s. The Asian working group for sarcopenia (AWGS) has proposed updated cutoff values in Asians: (1) muscle mass measurements of <7 kg/m^2 for males and <5.4 kg/m^2 for females using dual X-ray absorptiometry or <7 kg/m^2 for males and <5.7 kg/m^2 for females using bioimpedance analysis (2) muscle strength of <28 kg for males and <18 kg for females by handgrip strength and (3) physical performance of <1 m/s gait speed in a 6-minute walk test.[6]

Classically, metabolically healthier obesity is associated with increased subcutaneous adipose tissue (SAT), better insulin sensitivity, a lower waist-hip ratio, and relatively better vascular function. The unhealthier obesity is associated with increased visceral adipose tissue (VAT), lower insulin sensitivity, higher waist-hip ratio, and worse vascular function.[7]

Sarcopenia is a recognized component of the cardiorenal-cachexia syndrome, which is seen in patients with heart failure due to reduced muscle perfusion, anabolic resistance, and catabolic activation. This is more common in patients with heart failure with preserved ejection fraction. Reduced physical activity postmyocardial infarction or cardiac surgery contributes to a rapid muscle loss, which correlates with reduced cardiac reserve. Influencing rehabilitation outcomes. Sarcopenia has also been correlated with vascular aging since arterial stiffness is negatively associated with muscle quality and affects oxidative stress pathways.

Coronary microvascular dysfunction involves small coronary vessels less than 150 microns and is characterized by abnormalities in coronary blood flow and myocardial perfusion, in the absence of significant large vessel obstruction. CMVD is a multifactorial disorder influenced by endothelial dysfunction, smooth muscle dysregulation, oxidative stress, and platelet activation. This process is further aided by reduced nitric oxide bioavailability, increased endothelin-1 activity, promoting vasoconstriction, and heightened oxidative stress from mitochondrial dysfunction. Coronary microvascular dysfunction (CMD) is more than an isolated cardiac condition—it reflects systemic microvascular involvement, which is particularly relevant in patients with sarcopenia. Skeletal muscles harbor large capillary networks, and capillary rarefaction in sarcopenic patients mirrors the microvascular abnormalities observed in CMD. Myopathic changes in the skeletal muscles may predispose the coronary microcirculation to similar histopathological results.

Sarcopenia and CMVD share some common pathophysiological pathways, which include chronic inflammation mediated by interleukin 6, oxidative stress, and reactive oxygen species accumulation leading to vascular stiffening and capillary dysfunction, endothelial dysfunction due to less bioavailability of nitric oxide, and insulin resistance, which impairs the microvascular muscle perfusion. Hyperactivation of the renin–angiotensin–aldosterone system (RAAS) and sympathetic system also promotes muscle catabolism via oxidative stress and inflammatory cascades.[8]

TYPES OF CORONARY MICROVASCULAR DYSFUNCTION

This can be either a "Classical type" with reduction of myocardial flow reserve. Predominantly due to impaired hyperemic flow, or the "Endogenic type" with reduced myocardial flow reserve, predominantly related to increases in resting flow, as seen in women, arterial hypertension, and advanced obesity.[9]

Souza et al., in a study with a 6-year follow up demonstrated that sarcopenia was an independent predictor for CMVD. Both worse CMD and skeletal mass, but not higher SAT or VAT, were independently associated with adverse events, particularly heart failure hospitalization. Additionally, patients with both CMVD and sarcopenia were at the highest risk for adverse events, especially amongst young, female, and obese individuals, and this group can be considered a new phenotype.[10]

CONCLUSION

Sarcopenia is a significant but often overlooked comorbidity in cardiovascular patients, especially those with heart failure, coronary disease, and hypertension. In older adults, particularly those with multiple comorbidities, comprehensive geriatric assessment can guide individualized treatment and integrate sarcopenia screening into cardiology care pathways, e.g., during cardiac rehabilitation. Sarcopenia can also be incorporated in heart failure clinics by routine use of hand grip testing and gait speed, and in cardiac rehabilitation by incorporating resistance training as a component of post-MI and postoperative care, which will aid early mobilization. Ultimately, outpatient hypertension and diabetes clinics can also include these parameters into the routine components of assessment. Early identification and a multidimensional management strategy-focusing on resistance training, nutrition, and comorbidity control, has the potential to substantially improve outcomes. Cardiologists must embrace sarcopenia screening and treatment as part of comprehensive cardiovascular care to reduce frailty, improve quality of life, and enhance longevity.

KNOWLEDGE GAPS

Despite the advancement in understanding of the correlation between sarcopenia and CMVD, many knowledge gaps remain, which can provide opportunities for seminal research. The variability in diagnostic tools and thresholds limits consistency across studies. Standardization across guidelines, particularly for cardiovascular settings, is needed. Emerging biomarkers, e.g., growth differentiation factor-15 (GDF-15), myostatin, and interleukin-6 (IL-6), require further validation at different stages. Remote monitoring of gait speed and activity levels can be a reality by deploying smartwatches and accelerometers. Direct prospective studies to specifically assess whether sarcopenia independently predicts CMVD [measured by positron emission tomography (PET)/coronary flow reserve (CFR) or invasive CFR/index of microcirculatory resistance (IMR)] are limited. Mechanistic human studies tying endothelial signaling to both muscle perfusion and coronary microvascular integrity are emerging but require further translation. Interventional trials testing whether improving the muscle mass and function can reduce CMVD or affect related cardiac outcomes in the short and long run are still to be designed. More prospective imaging studies in predefined subgroups are the need of the hour.

FUTURE DIRECTIONS

Sarcopenia, now being an established parameter with far-reaching implications, especially for the cardiovascular syndromes in the geriatric population, needs to be further subclassified for its effect in various situations. Sarcopenic heart failure perhaps merits more discussion and classification, along with the addition of sarcopenia assessment in routine heart failure and drug evaluation studies. The glucagon-like peptide-1 (GLP-1) receptor agonists, with their wide-ranging effects and momentous implications, need to be correlated and protocols tried out for finding the usefulness of muscle testing studies in patients using this class of drugs. However, still the most important advancement that is still lacking is a reliable, quick, reproducible, and accurate noninvasive quantification of coronary microvasculature, which can serve as a measurable target for future interventional studies.

REFERENCES

1. Cruz-Jentoft AA, Bahat G, Bauer J, et al. Sarcopenia Revised European consensus on definition and diagnosis. Age Ageing. 2019;48(1):16-31.
2. Chen LK, Liu LK, Woo J, et al Sarcopenia in Asia: Consensus report of the Asian Working Group for sarcopenia. J Am Med Dir Assoc. 2014;15(2):95-101.
3. Von Haehling S, Morley JE, Anker SD, An overview of sarcopenia: Facts and numbers on prevalence and clinical impact. J Cachexia Sarcopenia Muscle. 2010;1(2):129-33.
4. Malmstrom TK, Morley JE. SARC-F. A simple questionnaire to rapidly diagnose sarcopenia. J Am Med Dir Assoc. 2013;14(8): 531-2.
5. Barbosa-Silva TG, Menezes AM, Bielemann RM, et al. Enhancing SARC-F: improving sarcopenia screening in the clinical practice. J Am Med Dir Assoc. 2016;17(12):1136-41.
6. Chen LK, Woo J, Assantachai P, et al. Asian Working Group for Sarcopenia 2019 consensus update on sarcopenia diagnosis and treatment. J Am Med Dir Assoc. 2020;21(3):300-7.
7. Koenen M, Hill MA, Cohen P, Sowers JR. Obesity , adipose tissue and vascular dysfunction. Circ Res. 2021;128(7):951-68.
8. Frederick BR, Bettina TE, Frances MF, et al. J Asean Fed Endoc Soc. 2024;39(1):69-78.
9. Schindler TH, Fearon WF, Pallatie-Galarneau M, et al. PET for detection and reporting coronary microvascular dysfunction. A JACC Cardiovascular Imaging Expert Panel Statement. J Am Coll Cardiol Img. 2023;16(4):536-48.
10. Souza ACdoAH, Rosenthal MH, Moura FA, et al. Body composition, coronary microvascular dysfunction, and future risk of cardiovascular events including heart failure. J Am Coll Cardiol Img. 2024; 17(2):179-91.

CHAPTER

74

Spontaneous Coronary Artery Dissection

Prakas Chandra Mondal

ABSTRACT

Spontaneous coronary artery dissection (SCAD) is an uncommon cause of acute coronary syndrome (ACS) but involves whole clinical spectrum of ACS including sudden cardiac arrest. It predominantly affects younger females usually without traditional coronary atherosclerotic risk factors but linked with hormonal influences and triggered by physical or emotional stresses. Genetic predisposition and associations with connective tissue disorders are increasingly recognized. Fibromuscular dysplasia screening is now routine and beta blocker therapy should be prescribed to all patients with SCAD to prevent recurrence. Advanced coronary imaging such as intravascular ultrasound (IVUS) and optical coherence tomography (OCT) along with invasive coronary angiography are needed for specific diagnosis and to guide therapy. Noninvasive imaging modalities such as coronary CT angiography (CCTA) and cardiac magnetic resonance imaging are emerging as great supporting tools without risk for iatrogenic extension of dissections. Cardiac rehabilitations including psychosocial supports are needed for all patients to improve outcomes and quality of life.

Keywords: Spontaneous coronary artery dissection, acute coronary syndrome, intravascular ultrasound, optical coherence tomography (OCT), atherosclerotic, ischemia.

INTRODUCTION

Spontaneous coronary artery dissection (SCAD) is defined pathologically as a nonatherosclerotic, noniatrogenic, nontraumatic dissection of coronary artery resulting in intimal tear or an intramural hematoma causing luminal narrowing or occlusion with resultant jeopardized coronary perfusion. Spontaneous coronary dissection is an important cause of whole spectrum of acute coronary syndrome (ACS), namely, unstable angina, non-ST-elevation myocardial infarction (NSTEMI), acute ST-elevation myocardial infarction (STEMI), and even sudden cardiac death. It is often underdiagnosed and historically thought to be a rare condition. With greater awareness and improved imaging techniques, it is getting identified more.

Spontaneous coronary artery dissection affects primarily young individuals without traditional atherosclerotic risk factors. SCAD affects predominantly females (up to 90%).[1] SCAD accounts for a significant proportion of ACS patients in young and middle-aged females with strong association with pregnancy, fibromuscular dysplasia (FMD), and connective tissue diseases.[2] Its true demographic data is limited due to lack of dedicated global registries and epidemiological data.

PATHOPHYSIOLOGY

Formation of a false lumen within the coronary arterial wall is the basic pathophysiology of SCAD. Formation of intramural hematoma can be due to two basic mechanisms, either an intimal tear that allows luminal blood to enter the vessel wall—"inside-out" model or a spontaneous rupture of the vasa vasorum leading to intramural hematoma formation—"outside-in" model.[3] But the precise sequence of events whether an intimal tear initiates the hematoma or primary intramural hematoma causes intimal tear is still unresolved. Body of evidence based on imaging and histologic studies favor "outside-in" model, i.e., initial spontaneous rupture of vasa vasorum with consequent primary intramural hematoma, which may subsequently tear the overlying intima and communicate with the coronary arterial lumen. In up to two-thirds of cases, no communication exists between intramural hematoma and coronary arterial lumen.[4] Serial angiographic studies demonstrate that intramural hematoma precedes intimal tear.[5] Both the mechanisms are conceivable and possible, and it may be possible that SCAD is actually two closely related pathological entities having common clinical sequelae.

SPONTANEOUS CORONARY ARTERY DISSECTION TYPES

The Yip-Saw angiographic classification: Phenotypic recognition of SCAD:[6]

- *Type 1:* Classic double lumen appearance with an intimal flap
- *Type 2a:* Long diffuse narrowing with a segment of the artery returning to normal caliber distally with no improvement following intracoronary nitroglycerin
- Type 2b: Long diffuse narrowing extending to the distal end without returning to normal caliber with no improvement following intracoronary nitroglycerin
- Type 3: Mimics focal atherosclerotic disease presenting as a focal stenosis; needs IVUS or OCT for diagnosis
- Type 4: Total occlusion of the vessel often misinterpreted as thrombotic occlusion

EPIDEMIOLOGY OF SPONTANEOUS CORONARY ARTERY DISSECTION

Overall Demography

Studies indicate that SCAD accounts for 1–4% of ACS but given the high burden of ACS, SCAD represents a significant global absolute burden.[6] SCAD most characteristically affects young and middle aged individuals with 80–90% female preponderance across the globe.[7] In the large Canadian SCAD registry (n = 1,173, prospective recruitment from 22 sites across Canada and United states), females accounted for 89.5% of SCAD patients.[8] In the Australian–New Zealand registries (n = 505, retrospective and prospective patients of ACS-related SCAD from 23 hospital sites), females accounted for 88.7% of the cohort.[9] Similar high female preponderance (95.6%) was noted in the multicentre Mayo Clinic SCAD Registry.[10] Contradictory finding was observed in a study from Persian Gulf area with only 50.6% females in the study cohort (n = 83).[11] This curious finding may be due to a lack of core laboratory confirmation and chance inclusion of atherosclerotic or iatrogenic dissection. UK SCAD registry includes 2.9% Indians in their study cohort and found 94.2% female preponderance.[12]

Spontaneous coronary artery dissection can also occur in males, approximately 10% of SCAD patients. In Canadian SCAD registry, males were found to present at younger age (mean age 49.4 ± 9.6 years vs. 52.0 ± 10.6 years in females) and more likely relate isometric physical stress as a trigger for their SCAD events (25.6% vs. 7.1% $p < 0.001$). Males have less likelihood of underlying FMD (27.8% vs. 52.7% $p = 0.001$), heightened emotional stress (3.5% vs. 11%. $p < 0.05$), and depression (9.8% vs. 20.2%, p +0.005).[13] No significant differences were found in angiographic types of SCAD between sexes but male were more likely to have dissection of left circumflex artery and less likely to have right coronary artery involvement.[13]

Ethnic Demography

Ethnicity data was more rigorously collected in the Australian–New Zealand SCAD Registry (n = 505 patients, both prospective and retrospective recruitment). The ethnic proportions in patients with SCAD more closely resembled the general populations: 78.6 % Caucasians, 5% East/South Asians, 1% Aboriginal or Torres Strait Islander people, 5% Maori, 1.3% Pacific Islander, and 9.6% other.[14] Data on SCAD in low- and middle-income countries are very sparse because of limited access to coronary angiography and advanced imaging techniques.

SPONTANEOUS CORONARY ARTERY DISSECTION IN PREGNANCY

Spontaneous coronary artery dissection is the leading cause of pregnancy-related myocardial infarction and accounts for 5–10% of maternal cardiovascular-related mortality. Heightened risk of SCAD has been associated with multiparity that is evident from the Mayo Clinic Registry (n = 323 women), which reported higher rates of multiparity among pregnancy-associated SCAD patients compared to both nonpregnancy SCAD and the general population (91% vs. 76%, respectively, $p = 0.018$).[15]

In contrast to nonpregnant counterparts, patients with pregnancy-related SCAD have a higher rate of STEMI, left ventricular dysfunction, and cardiogenic shock.[16] Pregnancy-associated SCAD has been related to proximal coronary artery involvement and a more severe disease phenotype.

RISK FACTORS AND ASSOCIATED CONDITIONS WITH SPONTANEOUS CORONARY ARTERY DISSECTION

Risk factors and associated conditions:

- *Female sex hormones:* It is not yet clear whether female dominance in SCAD is related to hormonal factors or a complex interplay of sex and gender-based variables such as nonhormonal physiological differences, psychological stressors, and coexistent condition such as FMD. Estrogen may influence vascular physiology such as autonomic regulation, angiogenesis, and vessel dynamicity.[17] Besides pregnancy, exogenous hormone exposure might have causal relation, especially use of contraception, assisted reproductive technologies, breast cancer treatments, pregnancy termination, and hormone replacement therapy.[18]
- *Genetic predisposition:* True hereditary clustering is rare and no SCAD-specific genetic testing is available.

Heritable collagen type-III deficiency (COL3A1), thoracic aortic aneurysm-associated genes (LOX and FLNA), and monogenic polycystic kidney disease (PKD1) have been linked to SCAD.[19] Clinical SCAD presentations have also been observed in Ehlers–Danlos syndrome, Marfan syndrome (FNB1) and Loeys–Dietz syndrome (TGFBR1, TGFBR2, SMAD2, SMAD3, TGFB2, and TGFB3) in the context of advanced vascular abnormalities.[20]

An allele in the PHACTR1 (phosphatase and actin regulator-1) on chromosome 6p24 (rs9349379-A) was implicated in susceptibility to both SCAD and FMD, explaining their common clinical associations.[19]

- *Fibromuscular dysplasia and systemic inflammatory onnective tissue diseases:* FMD and SCAD share a common pathophysiological mechanism primarily involving vascular smooth muscle cells and extracellular matrix. Both the conditions are at heightened risk of extracoronary vascular abnormalities such as aneurysms, pseudoaneurysms, dissections, and vessel tortuosity.[21] For these associations, screening for FMD is recommended at the time of diagnosis of SCAD. Systemic lupus and polyarteritis nodosa are also associated with SCAD.
- *Lifestyle risk factors:* Precipitating stressors are reported in 66% of SCAD cases. Common stressors include intense emotional stress, extreme physical exertion, and heavy isometric activities. Activities that increase intrathoracic pressure such as Valsalva-like maneuvers, for example, coughing, sneezing, and vomiting have been related to onset of SCAD.[22] Smoking and cocaine abuse have also implicated.

CLINICAL PRESENTATIONS

There are wide variations of clinical spectrum of presentations and a high index of suspicion is needed, especially in young females presenting with ACS, especially during pregnancy and postpartum period in absence of coronary risk factors. In the Canadian SCAD study, 69.9% of patients presented with (NSTEMI) and 29.7% had STEMI but chest discomfort has been reported by 91.5% of the patients.[11] A small percentage (8.1%) presented with ventricular tachycardia or fibrillation[1] and <1% presented with cardiogenic shock or sudden cardiac death.[13]

DIAGNOSIS

Accurate diagnosis of SCAD is based on strong clinical suspicion and advanced imaging. Proper differentiation from atherosclerotic causes of ACS are of great importance as clinical management and evaluations are substantially different. Diagnostic tools such as invasive coronary angiography, intravascular ultrasound (IVUS), and OCT can be essential to differentiate SCAD from coronary vasospasm, Takotsubo cardiomyopathy, myocardial bridging, coronary embolism, and atherosclerotic vascular disease.[6]

Coronary Angiography

Coronary angiography remains the gold standard for diagnosis and also for recognition of high-risk features such as left main, proximal vessel involvement, and multivessel involvement. Specific angiographic features of SCAD include long diffuse narrowing (45–48 mm) longer than those typically observed in atherosclerotic lesions, a "double lumen" appearance, and increased vessel tortuosity defined as three or more consecutive vessel curvatures of 90–180°. Tortuosity is most commonly seen in left circumflex artery.

Intravascular Ultrasound and Optical Coherence Tomography

To resolve any diagnostic ambiguity, imaging tools such as IVUS and OCT are invaluable in detecting the presence of intimal dissection, detection of intramural hematoma, false lumen, and fenestrations. The use of contrast during OCT has the potential to increase dissection and further vessel injury but its superior resolution can identify planes of dissection and intramural pathology.[23] Despite their utility, these invasive imaging techniques are underutilized due to safety concerns, cost, availability, and absence of specific recommendations of their use in SCAD.

Noninvasive Adjunctive Imaging

Cardiac MRI and coronary CT angiography (CCTA) play an emerging role specifically in situations of inconclusive invasive coronary angiography and evaluation of extracoronary vascular abnormalities such as FMD. CCTA findings suggestive of SCAD are abrupt stenosis, intramural hematoma, tapered stenosis over 50%, and dissection flaps.[24] Limitations of CCTA include potential for motion artifacts and lower spatial resolutions but minimizes iatrogenic dissection risk. Main role of cardiac MRI is in detection of myocardial infarction through late gadolinium enhancement and also in assessing fibromuscular dysplasia.

SPONTANEOUS CORONARY ARTERY DISSECTION MANAGEMENT

Two consensus statements (2018) from American College of Cardiology (ACC)/American Heart Association (AHA) and the European Society of Cardiology (ESC) supported a conservative approach for stable patients.[25] The rationale for a conservative approach is due to high likelihood of spontaneous healing over time. Percutaneous interventions are associated with high rates of complications including slow/no flow, iatrogenic dissections and long-term stent malposition. Urgent revascularization with PCI or coronary bypass grafting is needed in the presence of high-risk anatomy (left main stem or proximal double vessel involvement) or hemodynamic instability with cardiogenic shock, arrhythmias, and ongoing ischemia.[25]

Use of antiplatelets therapy in SCAD remains under debate and dual antiplatelet therapy (DAPT) may not be beneficial rather may be harmful with potent P2Y12 inhibitors. Use of statins is also not routinely indicated unless there are concomitant atherosclerotic risk factors. Beta blockers reduce recurrence of SCAD and is recommended for all patients with SCAD.[26]

The long-term management of SCAD should emphasize cardiac rehabilitation and psychosocial support to improve patient outcomes and quality of life. Long-term management should also include screening for FMD.

The mortality risk rate of ACS caused by SCAD was generally lower than atherosclerotic ACS with 3% mortality over 3 years and recurrence between 2 and 5% to 5.7%.[27]

CONCLUSION

Spontaneous coronary artery dissection is an uncommon cause of ACS that affects younger age groups, predominantly females. There is lack of robust epidemiological data regarding its true prevalence among different ethnic groups. Global adoption of the WHO's proposed ICD-11 codes that include a code for coronary artery dissection (BA82) could allow a more accurate understanding of SCAD prevalence. Raising awareness among general public, especially in high-risk groups is crucial for early detection and medical interventions with consequent improved outcomes.[28] Further research is needed to guide exercise and physical activity re-engagement and mental health management.

REFERENCES

1. Tweet MS, Hayes SN, Pitta SR, et al. Clinical features, management, and prognosis of spontaneous coronary artery dissection. Circulation 2012;126(5):579-88.
2. Hayes SN, Kim ESH, Saw J, et al. Spontaneous coronary artery dissection: Current state of the science: A scientific statement from the American Heart Association. Circulation. 2018;137:e523-57.
3. Dang Q, Burgess S, Psaltis PJ, et al. Spontaneous coronary artery dissection: A clinically oriented narrative review. NPJ Cardiovasc Health. 2024;1:1-9.
4. Jackson R, Al-Hussaini A, Joseph S, et al. Spontaneous coronary artery dissection: Pathophysiological insights from optical coherence tomography. JACC Cardiovasc Imaging. 2019;12(12):2475-88.
5. Adlam D, Maas A, Vrints C, et al. Spontaneous coronary artery dissection: No longer a rare disease. Eur Heart J. 2019;40:1198-201.
6. Saw J, Starovoytov A, Aymong E, et al. Canadian Spontaneous coronary artery dissection cohort study: 3-year outcomes. J. Am Coll Cardiol. 2022;80(17):1585-97.
7. Nishiguchi T, Tanaka A, Ozaki Y, et al. Prevalence of spontaneous coronary artery dissection in patients with acute coronary syndrome. Eur Heart J Acute Cardiovasc Care. 2016;5(3):263-70.
8. McAlister C, Alfadhel M, Samuel R, et al. Differences in demographics and outcomes between men and women with spontaneous coronary artery dissection. JACC Cardiovasc Interv. 2022;15(20):2052-61.
9. Clare R, Duan L, Phan D, et al. Characteristics and clinical outcomes of patients with spontaneous coronary dissection. J Am Heart Assoc. 2019;8(10):e012570.
10. Sumner JA, Kim ESH, Wood MJ, et al. Post traumatic stress disorder after spontaneous coronary artery dissection Registry. J Am Heart Assoc. 2024;13(7):e032819.
11. Daoulah A, Al-Faifi SM, Hurley WT, et al. Spontaneous coronary artery dissection: Does being unemployed matter? Insights from the GASCAD Registry. Curr Cardiol Rev. 2021;17:328-39.
12. Persu A, Lopez-Sublet M, Al-Hussaini A, et al. Prevalence and disease spectrum of extraordinary arterial abnormalities in spontaneous coronary artery dissection. JAMA Cardiol. 2022;7:159-66.
13. Elkayam U, Jalnapurkar S, Barakkat MN, et al. Pregnancy-associated acute myocardial infarction: A review of contemporary experience in 150 cases between 2006 and 2011. Circulation. 2014;129:1695-702.
14. Kim SK, Wing-Lun E, Chandrasekhar J, et al. The Australian New Zealand Spontaneous coronary artery dissection (ANZ-SCAD). Registry—A Multi-center cohort study: Protocol, background, and significance. Heart Lung Circ. 2022;31:1612-8.
15. Cerrato E, Giacobbe F, Quadri G, et al. Antiplatelet therapy in patients with conservatively managed spontaneous coronary artery dissection from the multicenter "DISCO Registry". Eur Heart J. 2021;42(33):3161-71.
16. Tweet MS, Hayes SN, Codsi E, et al. Spontaneous coronary artery dissection associated with Pregnancy. J Am Coll Cardiol. 2017;70:426-35.
17. Tweet MS, Miller VM, Hayes SN. The evidence on estrogen, progesterone, and spontaneous coronary artery dissection. JAMA Cardiol. 2019;4:403-4.
18. Crousillat D, Sarma A, Wood M, et al. Spontaneous coronary artery dissection: Current knowledge, research gaps and innovative Research initiatives: JACC advances Expert Panel. JACC Adv. 2024;3(12):101385.
19. Adlam D, Berrandou TE, Georges A, et al. Genome-wide association meta-analysis of spontaneous coronary artery dissection identifies risk variants and genes related to artery integrity and tissue-mediated coagulation. Nat Genet. 2023;55:964-72.
20. Kaadan MI, MacDonald C, Ponzini F, et al. Prospective cardiovascular genetics evaluation in spontaneous coronary artery dissection. Circ Genom Precis Med. 2018;11:e001933.
21. Adlam D, Olson TM, Combaret N, et al. Association of the PHACTR1/EDN1 genetic locus with spontaneous coronary artery dissection. J Am Coll Cardiol. 2019;73(1):58-66.
22. Bouchard K, Lalande K, Coutinho T, et al. Spontaneous coronary artery dissection across the health care pathway: A national, multicenter, patient-informed investigation. J Am Heart Assoc. 2023;12:e032141.
23. Franco C, Eng L, Saw J. Optical coherence tomography in the diagnosis and management of spontaneous coronary artery dissection. Interv Cardiol Clin. 2015;4(3):309-20.

24. Pergola V, Continisio S, Mantovani F, et al. Spontaneous coronary artery dissection: The emerging role of coronary computed tomography. Eur Heart J Cardiovasc. Imaging. 2023;24:839-50.
25. Adlam D, Alfonso F, Maas A, et al. European Society of cardiology, acute cardiovascular care association, SCAD study group: A position paper on spontaneous coronary artery dissection. Eur Heart J. 2018;39:3353-68.
26. Kidess GG, Brennan MT, Harmouch KM, et al. Spontaneous Coronary artery dissection: A review of medical management approaches. Curr Pronl Cardiol. 2024;49:102560.
27. Dang QM, Psaltis PJ, Burgess S, et al. The Australian–New Zealand spontaneous coronary artery dissection cohort study: Predictors of major adverse cardiovascular events and recurrence. Eur Heart J. 2025;7:ehaf097.
28. Bollati M, Ercolano V, Mazzarotto P. Spontaneous coronary dissection review: A complex picture. Rev Cardiovasc Med. 2024;25:448.

CHAPTER

75

Platelet Biology and Function: Plaque Erosion versus Rupture

Ranjit K Nath, MD Asif Iqbal, Shreya Gupta

ABSTRACT

Atherosclerotic plaque disruption by rupture or erosion triggers acute coronary syndromes (ACS) via arterial thrombosis. Platelets are central to this process but contribute differently depending on plaque phenotype. Ruptured plaques—characterized by thin fibrous caps overlying large lipid cores with abundant macrophages—expose tissue factor and collagen, driving high thrombin and fibrin formation. Thrombi here are often "red," rich in fibrin and red blood cells, reflecting robust coagulation. In contrast, eroded plaques feature an intact cap, abundant vascular smooth muscle cells (VSMCs), proteoglycans, and hyaluronan, with sparse macrophages. Endothelial denudation predominates, yielding "white" platelet-rich thrombi. Plaque erosion is associated with neutrophil activation and neutrophils extracellular traps (NET) formation. These pathobiological differences influence clinical presentation and outcomes—erosions often cause NSTEMI in younger patients with fewer risk factors and better prognosis, while ruptures more commonly cause STEMI with larger infarcts. Therapeutically, dual antiplatelet therapy (DAPT) remains standard after ACS, but recent trials (e.g., P2Y12 inhibitor monotherapy after brief DAPT aim to balance ischemic protection with bleeding risk. Novel targets (PAR4, GPVI inhibitors) are under study to inhibit platelet-driven thrombosis without excessive hemorrhage. Understanding the divergent roles of platelets in plaque erosion versus rupture may enable more tailored antithrombotic strategies.

Keywords: Atherothrombosis, platelet activation, plaque rupture, plaque erosion, thrombus composition, antiplatelet therapy.

INTRODUCTION

Atherothrombosis occurs when an atherosclerotic plaque destabilizes, provoking intraluminal thrombosis and ischemia. Under physiological hemostasis, platelets rapidly adhere to exposed vascular subendothelium via von Willebrand factor (vWF) and collagen, become activated, and recruit additional platelets by secreting ADP, thromboxane A2, and other autocrine mediators.[1] Thrombin generated via tissue factor and coagulation cascades then forms fibrin mesh, stabilizing the clot.[1] In ACS, however, this process is pathologically triggered by plaque injury, leading to occlusive thrombi rather than normal hemostasis.[2] Both plaque rupture and erosion expose thrombogenic material to flowing blood, but the upstream plaque biology differs markedly.[2,3] Rupture of a thin fibrous cap over a large necrotic core releases tissue factor-rich lipid debris and collagen, eliciting intense platelet adhesion and thrombin generation.[4] In contrast, superficial plaque erosion involves endothelial denudation over largely proteoglycan-and VSMC-rich intima with intact cap, provoking platelet aggregation via alternative mechanisms.[2,5] These divergent plaque morphologies shape the ensuing thrombus: rupture tends to produce "red" erythrocyte- and fibrin-rich clots, whereas erosion yields "white" platelet-rich thrombi.[1,2]

PATHOPHYSIOLOGY

Ruptured and eroded plaques both initiate platelet adhesion to exposed matrix. In rupture, collagen (types I/III) and vWF in the necrotic core bind platelet GPVI and GPIbα, triggering robust activation.[1,2] Tissue factor (TF) from the plaque core also drives massive thrombin production, amplifying platelet activation via PAR1/PAR4 receptors.[1] This generates a dense fibrin network—a hallmark of rupture thrombi.[2,4] By contrast, erosion leaves the fibrous cap largely intact; instead, proteoglycans (versican, hyaluronic acid) and VSMCs underlie the exposed endothelium.[2,5] Platelet adhesion in

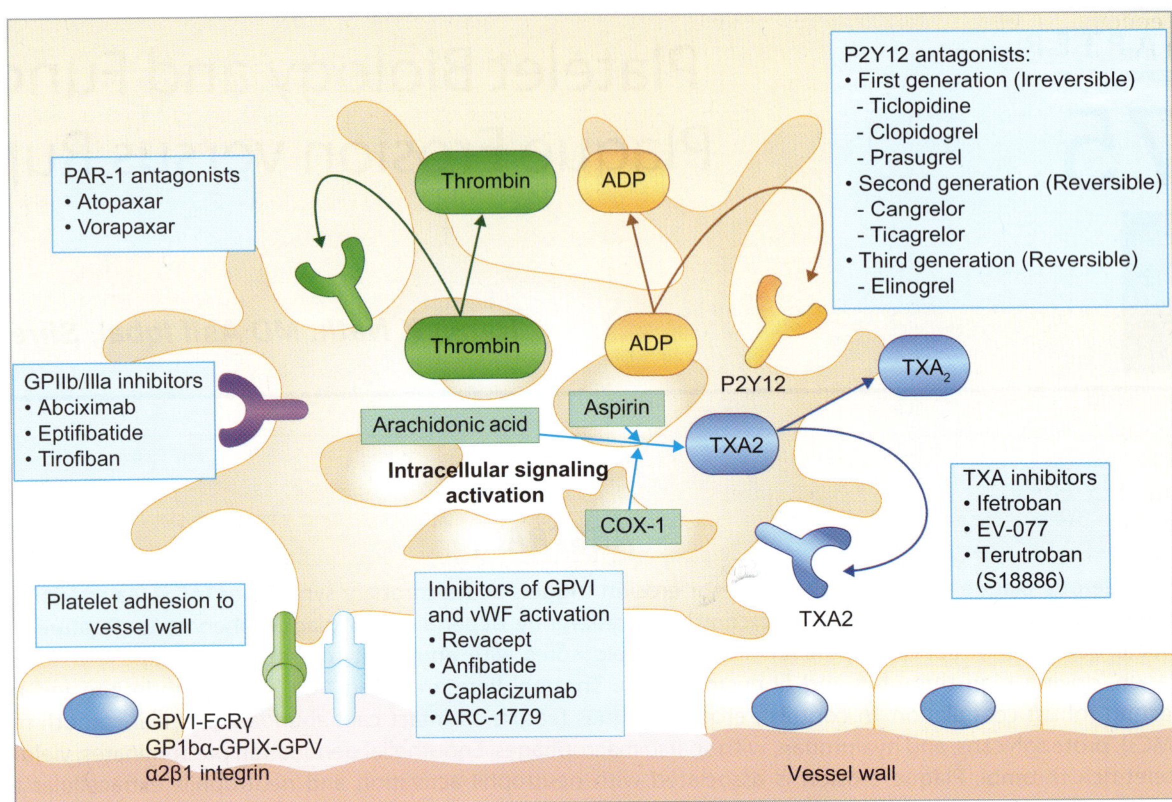

FIG. 1: Platelet receptors and drugs acting on them to prevent platelet aggregation.

erosion relies more on vWF and stromal factors than TF. For example, high shear at stenotic sites and reduced endothelial ADPase lead to platelet P2Y12/TXA2-driven aggregation in erosion.[2,3] Eroded lesions also exhibit neutrophil extracellular traps (NETs) and innate immune activation.[5] It releases DNA and proteases that directly activate platelets and coagulation.[2,5] Toll-like receptor-2 signaling (linked to hyaluronan fragments) may further stress endothelium in plaque erosion **(Fig. 1)**.[2]

PLAQUE MORPHOLOGY

Advanced plaques evolve divergent compositions. Ruptured plaques are thin-cap fibroatheromas with large necrotic lipid cores and heavy macrophage/foam cell infiltration at the cap shoulders.[4,6] Histologically, ruptures lack VSMCs at the tear site due to collagen degradation by macrophage-derived enzymes.[4] These lesions often show extensive calcification and intraplaque hemorrhage.[4] In contrast, eroded plaques have minimal lipid core and are rich in VSMCs, proteoglycans (versican) and hyaluronan at the luminal surface.[1,2,5] Inflammation (macrophages, T cells) is sparse in erosion compared to rupture,[2,5] but neutrophil aggregates and NETs are prominent at the site of endothelial loss.[5] The increasing use of statins and risk-factor control appears to shift ACS phenotypes toward erosion: modern imaging shows approximately 40% of culprit lesions are erosions.[2] Better primary prevention (lower LDL, smoking) is linked to this trend.[5,6] Importantly, plaque erosion tends to produce smaller culprit lesions and preserves vessel lumen better than rupture.[2,3] Intravascular imaging and transcriptomic studies reveal that eroded plaques have gene signatures of extracellular matrix and VSMC phenotypes, whereas ruptures align with lipid and inflammation pathways.[5-7]

THROMBUS COMPOSITION

The histology of arterial thrombi differs markedly between erosion and rupture. Plaque rupture exposes thrombogenic core material that generates large fibrin-rich clots. Aspirated thrombi from ruptures (often STEMI) exhibit a red appearance: high fibrin and erythrocyte content with relatively fewer platelets.[4] A dense fibrin network and embedded red cells make these clots stiff and resistant to lysis.[4,8] Over time, ischemic duration further accentuates this: longer time from onset is associated with more fibrin and fewer platelets in aspirated clots.[4] Plaque erosion, by contrast, yields white platelet-rich clots. With platelets at the core and scant erythrocytes,[2,3] erosive thrombi are less densely fibrinous and often nonocclusive.[1,2] Imaging and pathological studies show erosion thrombi are loosely structured, often with prominent platelet aggregates at the site of endothelial denudation.[2,3] Neutrophil NETs have been found interwoven in erosive clots, potentially contributing to local platelet activation.[5] In mixed thrombi (e.g., those from rupture), platelets and fibrin tend to line the outer shell while red cells occupy the core.[4] Clinically, these differences matter: platelet-rich (erosion) clots may respond better to antiplatelet agents, whereas red cell-fibrin clots (rupture) may require more intensive therapy with antiplatelets and added anticoagulation.[2]

CLINICAL OUTCOMES

Patients with plaque erosion and rupture clinically present differently. Plaque rupture classically causes ST-elevation MI (STEMI) due to abrupt vessel occlusion, whereas erosion more often causes non-ST elevation MI (NSTEMI) or unstable angina.[2,4] Epidemiologically, erosions account for approximately 30–40% of ACS cases.[1,2] Patients with erosive lesions are typically younger, more often female, and have fewer traditional risk factors (lower LDL, triglycerides, and CRP) than rupture patients.[2,5] Prognostically, plaque erosion carries a more favorable short-term outcome. In OCT studies, erosion-ACS patients had smaller infarcts and lower infarct-related artery complexity.[3] A cohort with intact fibrous caps (erosions) had significantly fewer major adverse cardiovascular events (MACE) during follow-up than those with ruptures.[3,4] In the multicenter OCT registry, erosion was independently associated with lower 1-year MACE compared to rupture.[3] This better prognosis is attributed to smaller thrombus burden and lower overall atherosclerotic burden in erosion.[2,3] Given these differences, identifying plaque phenotype may guide therapy. For example, emerging OCT-based algorithms aim to detect erosion in vivo so that some patients might avoid immediate stenting. In the EROSION pilot study, ACS patients with OCT-confirmed erosion received intensive DAPT without stent implantation; at 1 month, 92.5% were free of MACE and most showed marked thrombus resolution.[3] Over longer follow-up, revascularization rates rose modestly (~23% at 4 years).[3] These findings suggest that in select erosion cases, medical therapy alone may suffice, though larger trials are needed **(Table 1)**.[9]

TABLE 1: Differences between plaque erosion and plaque rupture.

Characteristics	Plaque erosion	Plaque rupture
Cap	Intact cap with endothelial denudations	Ruptured thin fibrous cap
Composition	Abundant VSMCs, proteoglycans, hyaluronan with sparse macrophages	Large lipid cores with abundant macrophages. High thrombin and fibrin formation.
Thrombi type	"White," platelet-rich thrombi	"Red," rich in fibrin and RBCs
Pre-event	Neutrophil activation, NET formation	Inflammation
Event pattern	NSTEMI, young patients, better prognosis	STEMI, larger infarct, worst prognosis
OCT image of plaque[9]	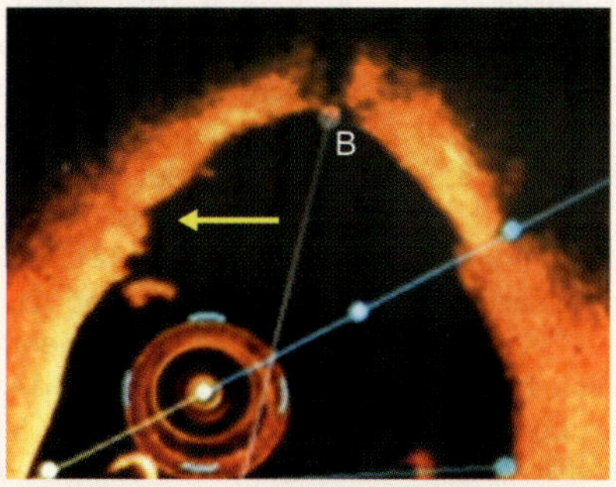	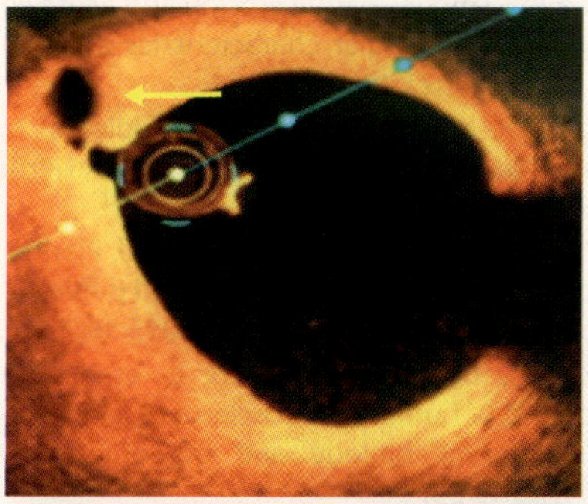
OCT image of thrombi[9]	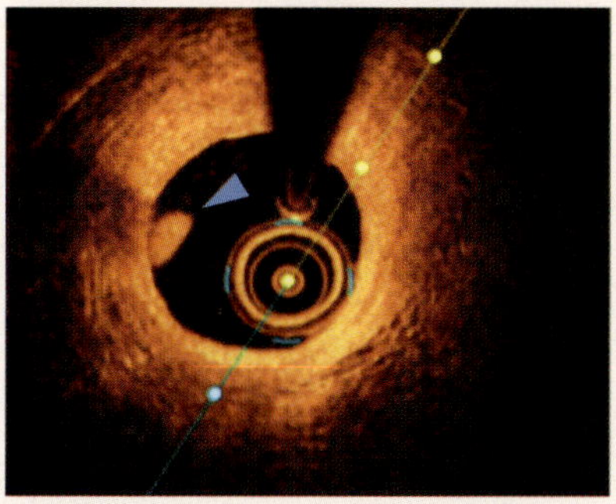	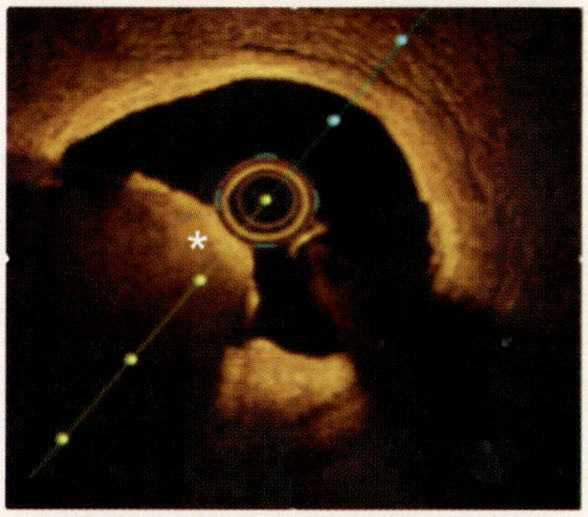

(NET: neutrophil extracellular traps; VSMC: vascular smooth muscle cells)

THERAPEUTIC IMPLICATIONS

Current ACS treatment emphasizes DAPT (aspirin plus a $P2Y_{12}$ inhibitor) as the foundation of care.[10-12] ESC guidelines (2023) recommend 12 months of DAPT after ACS (shorter duration in high-bleed-risk patients).[10] However, prolonged DAPT increases bleeding risk, prompting trials of de-escalation.[10,11] Recent meta-analyses (cumulative ~24,000 patients) show that switching to $P2Y_{12}$-inhibitor monotherapy after 1–3 months of DAPT cuts major bleeding by ~50% without raising ischemic events.[10,11] Ticagrelor monotherapy, in particular, maintains efficacy while reducing hemorrhage, whereas clopidogrel monotherapy was associated with slightly higher ischemic rates compared to full DAPT.[10-12] Despite these advances, recurrent thrombosis remains a challenge, especially after plaque rupture. Novel strategies are under investigation. One focus is on thrombin and protease-activated receptors: even on DAPT, thrombin generation is high post-ACS and PAR4 signaling on platelets remains active.[1,2] Because PAR1 antagonism (vorapaxar) caused bleeding, attention has turned to PAR4 inhibitors.[1] Another target is platelet collagen signaling via GPVI. GPVI-blocking agents (revacept, glenzocimab/ACT017) have shown safety and promising effects on platelet function.[1] PAR4 and GPVI inhibitors exemplify attempts to block atherothrombosis more selectively. Other exploratory approaches target platelet-leukocyte interactions (CD40L-CD40, P-selectin) or inflammation (IL-1β, colchicine).[2,5] Finally, antithrombotic therapy may increasingly be tailored to plaque phenotype.[3] Intensifying platelet inhibition along with anticoagulation might be particularly useful in large ruptures, whereas in erosion, very potent antiplatelet regimens (with minimal anticoagulation) might suffice.[3] Clinical trials are needed to test phenotype-guided strategies.

CONCLUSION

Plaque rupture and erosion represent distinct pathobiological pathways to ACS. Rupture exposes a thrombogenic necrotic core, promoting fibrin-rich clots and high-risk events, while erosion involves endothelial denudation over proteoglycan-rich intima, yielding platelet-rich thrombi with relatively better short-term prognosis. Platelets lie at the nexus of both processes, but the triggers and clot architecture differ. Recognizing these differences is clinically important: It may explain variations in ACS presentation and outcomes, and it opens avenues for tailored therapy. Current management relies on DAPT for all ACS, but emerging evidence supports personalized adjustments (shorter DAPT, P2Y12 monotherapy) and novel agents targeting platelet-collagen or PAR receptors.[10-12]

REFERENCES

1. Baaten CCFMJ, Nagy M, Bergmeier W, et al. Platelet biology and function: plaque erosion vs. rupture. Eur Heart J. 2024;45(1):18-31.
2. Fahed AC, Jang IK. Plaque erosion and acute coronary syndromes: phenotype, molecular characteristics and future directions. Nat Rev Cardiol. 2021;18(10):724-34.
3. Vergallo R, Jang IK, Crea F. New prediction tools and treatment for ACS patients with plaque erosion. Atherosclerosis. 2021;318:45-51.
4. Niccoli G, Montone RA, Di Vito L, et al. Plaque rupture and intact fibrous cap assessed by OCT portend different outcomes in acute coronary syndrome. Eur Heart J. 2015;36(22):1377-84.
5. Mokry M, Boltjes A, Slenders L, et al. Transcriptomic-based clustering of human atherosclerotic plaques identifies subgroups with different biology and outcomes. Nat Cardiovasc Res. 2022;1:1140-55.
6. Fernandez DM, Rahman AH, Fernandez NF, et al. Single-cell immune landscape of human atherosclerotic plaques. Nat Med. 2019;25(10):1576-88.
7. Depuydt MAC, Prange KHM, Slenders L, et al. Microanatomy of the human atherosclerotic plaque by single-cell transcriptomics. Circ Res. 2020;127(11):1437-55.
8. Kramer MCA, Rittersma SZH, de Winter RJ, al. Relationship of thrombus healing to underlying plaque morphology in sudden coronary death. J Am Coll Cardiol. 2010;55(2):122-32.
9. Watanabe H, Domei T, Morimoto T, et al. Effect of 1-month dual antiplatelet therapy followed by clopidogrel vs 12-month therapy on cardiovascular and bleeding events in patients receiving PCI. JAMA. 2019;321(24):2414-27.
10. Mehran R, Cao D, Baber U, et al. Ticagrelor monotherapy after PCI in patients at high bleeding risk. J Am Coll Cardiol. 2020;75(19):2403-14.
11. Storey RF, James SK, Siegbahn A, et al. Lower mortality with ticagrelor compared with clopidogrel in patients with acute coronary syndromes: PLATO trial. Lancet. 2010;376(9749):1320-8.
12. Gupta A, Shrivastava A, Nath RK, et al. Optical coherence tomography: An eye into the coronary artery. Frontiers in Cardiovascular Medicine. 2022;9:1-22.

CHAPTER

76

Coronary Artery Aneurysm: A Therapeutic Dilemma

Ramesh Thakur, Kumar Himanshu

ABSTRACT

In modern times with the easy availability of CT angiography, the diagnosis of coronary artery aneurysms has become ultra-simple. However, strategizing an optimal management continues to haunt the human mind. An appropriate treatment essentially depends on the age of the patient, number, size, location, and etiology of the coronary artery aneurysm.

Keywords: Coronary artery aneurysm, complications, percutaneous management, covered stenting, coiling.

INTRODUCTION

Coronary artery aneurysm (CAA) continues to perplex the cardiologists and patients alike and still remains an enigma. While much is now known about the pathogenesis of these aneurysms, the treatment is still an Achilles' heel. The entity is not always benign and often leads to significant adverse cardiovascular outcomes from limitation of functional capacity to even death. In fact, many suggest, and not wrongly, that the advent of percutaneous angioplasty itself might have led to an increase in the incidence of aneurysms. Many of the aneurysms that we deal these days are iatrogenic in nature. This is all the more a reason why the condition has to be addressed. The future will only see a rise in aneurysm cases, and therefore, young cardiologists should be well-versed with its etiopathogenesis and approach to treating it.[1,2]

In a large retrospective study carried out by Khubber et al.,[3] it was reported that the incidence of aneurysm was nearly 0.7%. The study also evaluated the outcome of medical, percutaneous, and surgical treatment and found no difference between them. The use of oral anticoagulants was also not found to have any significant effect on cardiovascular outcomes. Though the study was limited by its small sample size, it is reflective of the dilemma that cardiologists face about aneurysms.

DEFINITION

Coronary artery aneurysms are defined as abnormal focal dilatation of coronary artery exceeding 1.5 times of the normal diameter. A similar term "coronary ectasia" is also occasionally used but it refers to diffuse involvement of the coronary artery to abnormal dimensions rather than a focal one.

Broadly, we have two anatomical types of aneurysms: (1) Saccular and (2) fusiform as can be seen in **Figure 1**.

INCIDENCE

While there have been varied reports about the incidence, it is now accepted that the incidence is nearly 1%.[1,4] The right coronary artery is most commonly involved followed by the left descending anterior, left circumflex and left main artery have a lower incidence of aneurysms. There is a male predilection that aligns with the etiological causes as well.

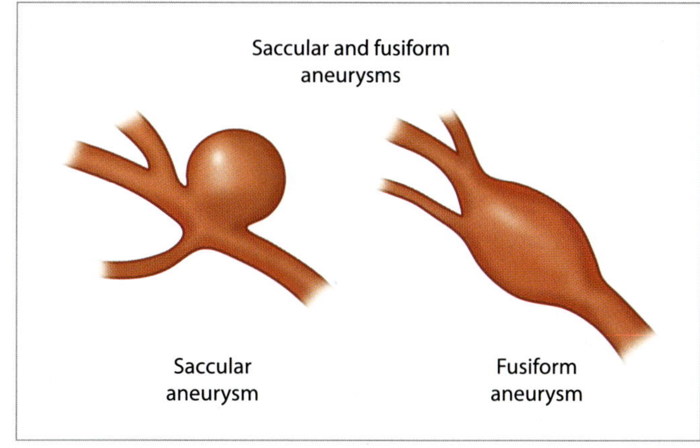

FIG. 1: The two different types of aneurysms.

RISK FACTORS

There are certain well-identified etiologies and risk factors that lead to aneurysm formation and have been summarized in **Box 1**.[3,5]

PATHOPHYSIOLOGY

- The one thing common to all the etiologies leading to CAA formations is inflammation coupled with a high level of matrix metalloproteinase. Inflammation triggered by Kawasaki, mycotic infections, etc. also increase the level of these proteinase enzymes along with release of nitric oxide. The raised enzymes result in degradation of the arterial wall that leads to aneurysm formation.[1,2]
- Poststent implantation, especially when the stent is oversized, or high-pressure balloon dilatations have been done across the artery; the artery at edges of the stent undergoes a similar process eventually leading to aneurysm formation.
- Mycotic aneurysms are bane in the days of intervention. Though uncommon, they are challenging to treat as their sizes are usually much larger and the propensity to rupture is usually higher and the systemic symptoms are very prominent. They are largely avoidable with thorough asepsis.

DIAGNOSIS

- While invasive angiography continues to be the gold standard, there is an increasing role of CT angiography. It delineates the anatomy better and also sheds light on the surrounding structures.
- For pediatric populations, especially when dealing with Kawasaki disease, there is a role for MRI-based angiography to avoid the exposure to radiation.
- While performing invasive angiography, intravascular ultrasound may be used to study the morphoanatomy of the aneurysm.
- When dealing with mycotic aneurysms, it is advisable to take targeted blood cultures using the microcatheter to increase the diagnostic yield.

BOX 1: The risk factors leading to coronary artery aneurysm formation.

- *Hereditary*:
  - Marfan's syndrome
  - Ehler–Danlos syndrome
  - HLA DR 13 and 16 genes
- *Acquired disease*:
  - Coronary artery disease
  - Kawasaki disease
  - Takayasu arteritis
  - SLE and rheumatoid arthritis
- *Iatrogenic*:
  - Post stent implantation
  - Mycotic aneurysms

COMPLICATIONS

While the most dreaded complication has always been rupture, coronary aneurysms are known to cause other complications such as thrombosis, compression, and angina. These complications have been summarized in **Box 2**.

MANAGEMENT

Medical Management

- When aneurysms are associated with coronary artery disease, they should be treated like CAD. Statins and ACE inhibitors have been hypothesized to show some benefit in a few small studies.
- The use of high-intensity statins after PCI may help prevent the formation and progression of aneurysms as they have been shown to inhibit metalloproteinase enzymes in studies carried out in-vitro.
- The role of anticoagulation is still debatable. The risk of thrombosis has to be balanced against the long-term risk of bleeding. Still a larger size and the presence of aneurysms in critical positions such as the left main artery or ostioproximal involvement of other arteries justify the use of anticoagulants.
- In a large study carried out by D'Ascenzo et al. of nearly 1,200 patients , it was found that use of oral anticoagulants decreased the composite endpoint of acute coronary syndrome, myocardial infarction, and aneurysm thrombosis in patients with CAA.[5]
- Early initiation of intravenous immunoglobulin (IVIG) has been shown to decrease the rate and size of aneurysm

BOX 2: Possible complications arising from aneurysm.

- *Thrombosis*: Aneurysms present a site for flow stasis and thus, become a source of de novo thrombosis and distal embolism
- *Perforation*:
  - While not very common unless the size is very large, it is a potentially life-threatening complication
  - Larges aneurysms, i.e., >8 cm are usually excised surgically to circumvent this risk
- *Compression*:
  - Very large aneurysms may compress adjacent structures such as the right atrium ventricle and pulmonary artery
  - Large aneurysms arising from the left main coronary artery many end up compressing the same artery as well
- *Spasm and angina*: While traditionally, it was speculated that aneurysm did not have enough smooth muscle to cause spasm, it is now accepted that it is one of the reasons for spasms leading to recurrent episodes of angina. The mechanism is, however, poorly understood

formed in Kawasaki disease. Similarly, treating the inflammation associated with Takayasu arteritis and other inflammatory disorders is likely to help.

- In a case series of 24 patients of Kawasaki disease with giant coronary aneurysm reported by Dummer et al., the use of oral anticoagulants was found to be safe and feasible.[5]

Surgical Management

- Surgical management is reserved for very large aneurysm, especially involving the left main coronary artery or aneurysms that are very large in size and likely to rupture.
- The ideal surgical technique is a subject of debate, but marsupialization is the usual go-to method. Rarely, if the size and neck are large, aneurysectomy is performed.
- Of late, surgical management is usually reserved for cases where transcatheter interventions are not feasible or avoidable.
- Mycotic aneurysms should preferably be treated surgically.

Transcatheter Management

While percutaneous management of aneurysms is a relatively new thing, it is now standard practice for small- and moderate-sized aneurysms. Larger aneurysms still warrant surgical closure. There are no clear guidelines regarding how to approach the aneurysms and which method to use, so the techniques vary. There are, however, three major ways to close the aneurysm percutaneously and are described in **Figure 2**.

- *Covered stenting:*
  - This has been the traditional method to close aneurysms.
  - It is easy to perform and entails delivery of a covered stent, i.e., stent with an additional biocompatible layer of polytetrafluoroethylene (PTFE) or Dacron over a coronary wire.
  - It has its own limitations though. It is bulkier than the normal stents and difficult to deliver if the aneurysm is associated with tortuosity or calcifications.
  - In addition, it leads to side vessel closure, which may lead to an unnecessary side-branch compromise. This becomes important when the lesion is located proximally.
  - Also, the covered stents are associated with higher incidences of in-stent restenosis, which may cause future morbidity.
  - **Figure 3** shows a case of an aneurysm of right coronary artery. It was treated by transcatheter covered stenting; the postprocedure result can be seen in **Figure 4**.

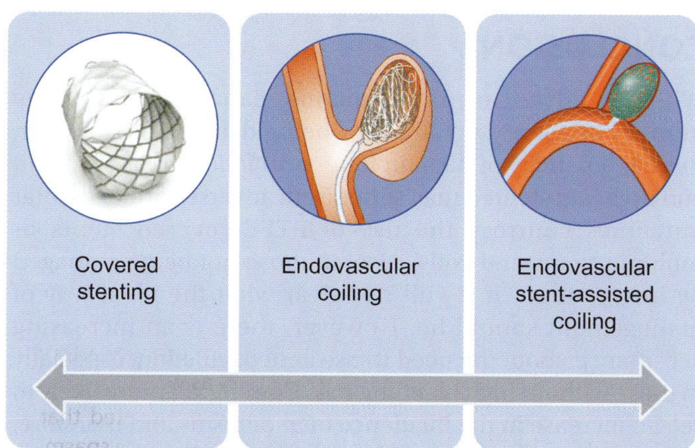

FIG. 2: Techniques employed for transcatheter management of aneurysms.

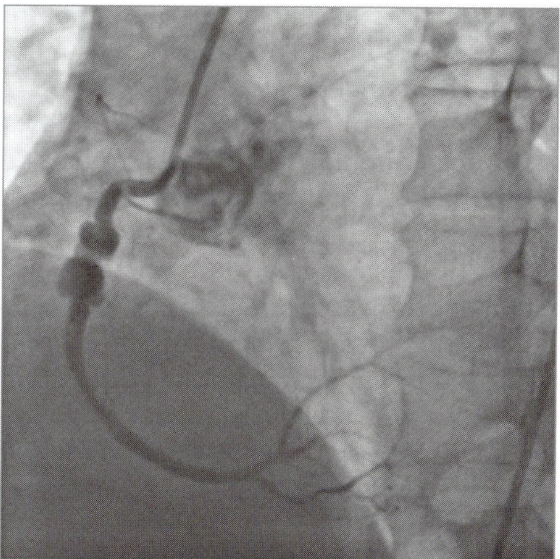

FIG. 3: Coronary aneurysm of the right coronary artery.

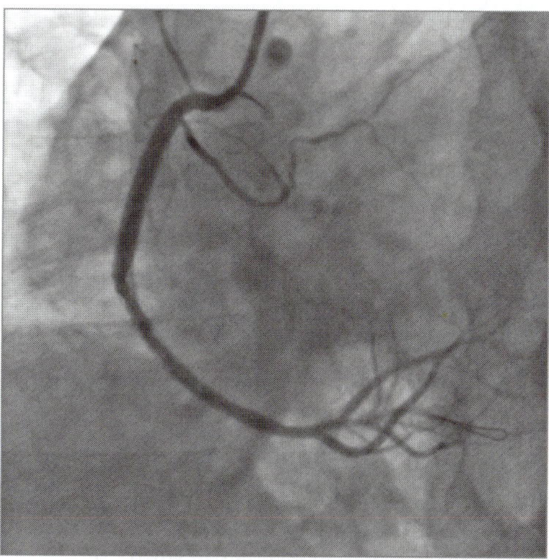

FIG. 4: The same patient depicted in **Figure 3** after closure of aneurysm using a PTTE covered stent.

- *Endovascular coiling:*
  - The method of endovascular coiling was initially developed for closing bleeding peripheral arterial aneurysms or tumors by interventional radiologists and neurologists. Gradually, it has found its use in cardiology as well.
  - It is a targeted delivery of coils, made of platinum or steel mesh, into the aneurysm leading to stasis thrombosis and eventual closure.
  - The technique is easy and entails delivery of coils through a microcatheter, which has been inserted into the aneurysm over a coronary wire.
  - It addresses certain shortcomings of covered stenting, i.e., there is no side branch occlusion, and coils can easily be delivered even across calcific and tortuous arteries.
  - It has its own limitations though with a failure rate of nearly 1–5 %. Such patients may end up requiring another procedure. The failure is usually due to inadequate or undersized coil usage.
  - Also, rarely, using oversized coils may lead to aneurysm perforation or rarely, the coil may dislodge into the main artery, these conditions are catastrophic.
- *Stent assisted coiling:*
  - The technique was devised by neurologists while treating cerebrovascular aneurysms and is gradually finding its way in our domain as well.
  - The procedure entails initial delivery of a drug-eluting stent across the artery from which the aneurysm arises. This stent then acts as a base for delivery of coils using a microcatheter. The advantages include decreased possibility of stent dislodgement in main vessel as well as narrowing of neck due to stent placement.

Treatment of Mycotic Coronary Aneurysms

- With an ever-increasing number of PCI being performed, mycotic aneurysms are not rare these days. They are multiple, usually large, and may be associated with infective endarteritis. They are devastating if left untreated. **Figures 5 and 6** show multiple mycotic aneurysms in the left anterior descending artery post angioplasty.
- The empirical treatment is usually IV antibiotics (cephalosporin + vancomycin) for a duration of 4–6 weeks. Culture may help guide the therapy.
- Surgical management is reserved for large aneurysm with impending rupture or failure of medical therapy.
- Percutaneous management is usually avoided in these cases and should only be only attempted as a lifesaving procedure if the surgical risk is too high.

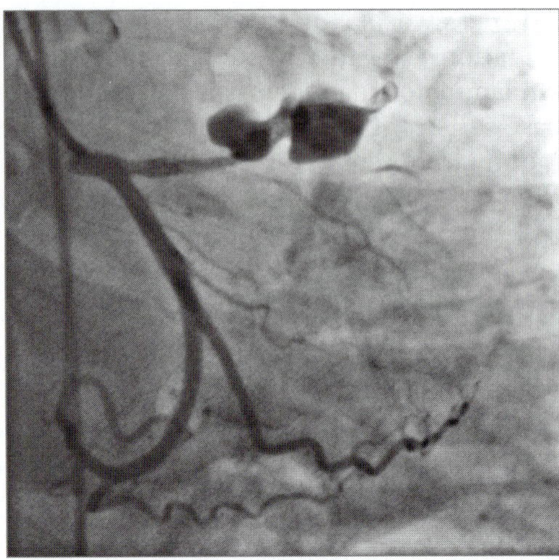

FIG. 5: Post PCI large aneurysms of the left anterior descending artery. The stent is also visualized with the aneurysm.

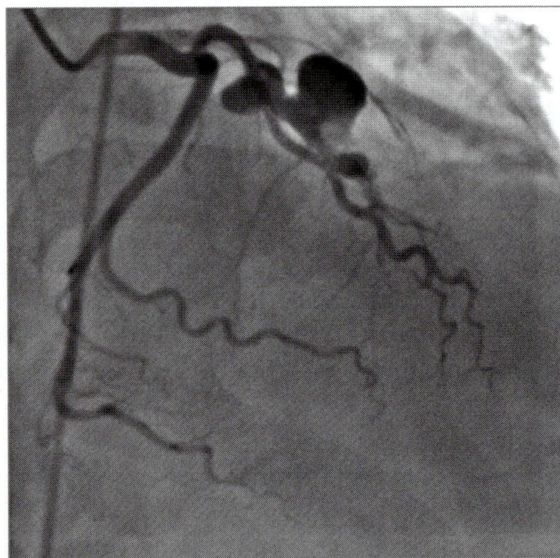

FIG. 6: Post PCI mycotic aneurysm of left anterior descending artery. Multiple aneurysms can be seen with associated flow occlusion in the artery as well.

CONCLUSION

With the advent of percutaneous management, a large number of aneurysms are now being dealt with. However, there is a paucity of data on long-term follow up. Many who end up being stented may suffer from adverse cardiovascular outcomes courtesy the use of PTFE-covered stents or multiple stents and coils. Also, in those not being managed by intervention, it is still not clear what the ideal way of management should be. However, there is an increasing acceptance about the need to use anticoagulation, especially in those without high bleeding risk. Coming years are likely to see an increase in the incidence of aneurysms and therefore, prospective cohort studies are warranted.

REFERENCES

1. Dummer KB, Miyata K, Shimizu C, et al. DOACs in patients with giant coronary artery aneurysms after Kawasaki disease. JAMA Netw Open. 2023;6(11):e2343801.
2. Sharma R, Ruia AV, Mahant TS. Case series of coronary artery aneurysms after Everolimus eluting stent implantation and comparison with Sirolimus eluting stents. BMC Cardiovasc Disord. 2022;22(1):60.
3. Khubber S, Chana R, Meenakshisundaram C, et al. Coronary artery aneurysms: Outcomes following medical, percutaneous interventional and surgical management. Open Heart. 2021;8(1): e001440.
4. Lu CH, Fang CW, Chen HM, et al. Prescribing patterns of coronary artery aneurysm in Taiwan. BMC Cardiovasc Disord. 2019;19(1):188.
5. D'Ascenzo F, Saglietto A, Ramakrishna H, et al. Usefulness of oral anticoagulation in patients with coronary aneurysms: Insights from the CAAR registry. Catheter Cardiovasc Interv. 2021;98(5):864-71.

CHAPTER 77

Atherosclerosis, Aortic Dissection, and Peripheral Artery Disease: New Therapeutic Targets

Akhilesh Kumar, Suman Bhandari

ABSTRACT

Cardiovascular diseases remain the leading cause of mortality worldwide, with atherosclerosis, aortic dissection, and peripheral artery disease (PAD) constituting major contributors to morbidity and healthcare burden. While traditional therapies such as lipid lowering, blood pressure control, and surgical or endovascular repair remain cornerstones, residual cardiovascular risk persists. Over the past decade, the therapeutic landscape has expanded beyond conventional paradigms, with novel targets emerging across lipid metabolism, inflammation, thrombosis, and vascular wall biology. In atherosclerosis, therapies directed at inflammatory pathways (colchicine, IL-1β, and IL-6 inhibitors), lipoprotein(a)-lowering strategies, and dual-pathway inhibition have shown significant promise in reducing residual cardiovascular events. PAD management has evolved with the introduction of low-dose rivaroxaban combined with aspirin, PCSK9 inhibitors, and exploration of regenerative therapies.

This review provides a practical, clinician-oriented update on these evolving therapies, highlighting trial evidence, mechanistic insights, and implications for practice.

Keywords: Atherosclerosis, aortic dissection, peripheral artery disease, novel therapeutics, anti-inflammatory therapy, lipoprotein(a), dual-pathway inhibition.

INTRODUCTION

Cardiovascular diseases (CVDs) account for approximately one-third of all deaths globally.[1,2] Despite significant advances in preventive cardiology, interventional therapies, and surgical techniques, the burden of atherosclerotic disease, aortic pathology, and peripheral artery disease (PAD) remains high. Current standard therapies—statins, antiplatelets, β-blockers, antihypertensives, and surgical interventions—have dramatically improved outcomes but fail to address residual risk.[3,4]

Several factors underlie this residual burden. First, atherosclerosis is increasingly recognized as a chronic inflammatory disease, not merely a lipid storage disorder.[5] Second, inherited and acquired abnormalities of the aortic wall are only partially mitigated by blood pressure control, with a need for targeted therapies that modulate vascular remodeling.[6] Third, PAD continues to be underdiagnosed and undertreated, with event rates comparable to or higher than coronary disease.[7]

In this context, the search for *new therapeutic targets* has become central to contemporary cardiovascular medicine. These targets include:

- *Inflammation* (targeting IL-1β, IL-6, and NLRP3 inflammasome)
- *Residual lipoprotein risk* (lipoprotein(a), remnant cholesterol)
- *Thrombosis beyond platelets* (dual-pathway inhibition with factor Xa blockade)
- *Vascular extracellular matrix remodeling* (MMPs and TGF-β signaling)

This review summarizes key advances across three interrelated entities—atherosclerosis, aortic dissection, and PAD—with emphasis on clinical trial data, mechanistic rationale, and practical implications for the clinician.

ATHEROSCLEROSIS: PATHOBIOLOGY RECAP

Atherosclerosis arises from a complex interplay between lipid accumulation, endothelial dysfunction, immune cell infiltration, and maladaptive remodeling.[8] Modified lipoproteins LDL, Lp(a) trigger chronic inflammation, leading to plaque formation and eventual clinical sequelae including myocardial infarction and stroke.[9]

Steps in Plaque Formation

Consequent to the initial lesion to the endothelium, both innate and adaptive immune responses are triggered (**Fig. 1**, initial lesion). Circulating monocytes infiltrate subendothelial regions upon binding to adhesion molecules upregulated on the endothelial cells, leading to the accumulation of intimal macrophages.[10] Furthermore, disturbed endothelial homeostasis facilitates the transportation and entrapment of low-density lipoprotein LDL) into the subendothelial space, where it undergoes oxidation and is subsequently taken up by macrophages, leading to the development of foam cells (**Fig. 1**, initial lesion). Additionally, foam cells derived from vascular smooth muscle cells (VSMCs) exacerbate the vascular inflammatory response.[11]

The accumulation of necrotic foam cells, cholesterol crystals, and cellular debris forms the lipid core of the atherosclerotic plaque. The consequent upregulation of multiple chemokines and cytokines stimulates VSMCs to undergo proliferation and migration toward the intima, resulting in the synthesis of extracellular matrix components such as collagen and elastin.[12] This process contributes to the formation of the fibrous cap and thickening of the arterial wall.

Subsequently, the plaques expand as fibrous tissues proliferate, thereby restricting blood flow. In some cases, the fibrous cap thins because there is a decrease in the synthesis of extracellular matrix macromolecules, while in other cases, plaques may progress to accumulate a higher proportion of matrix and a lower proportion of lipid over time.[13] Both

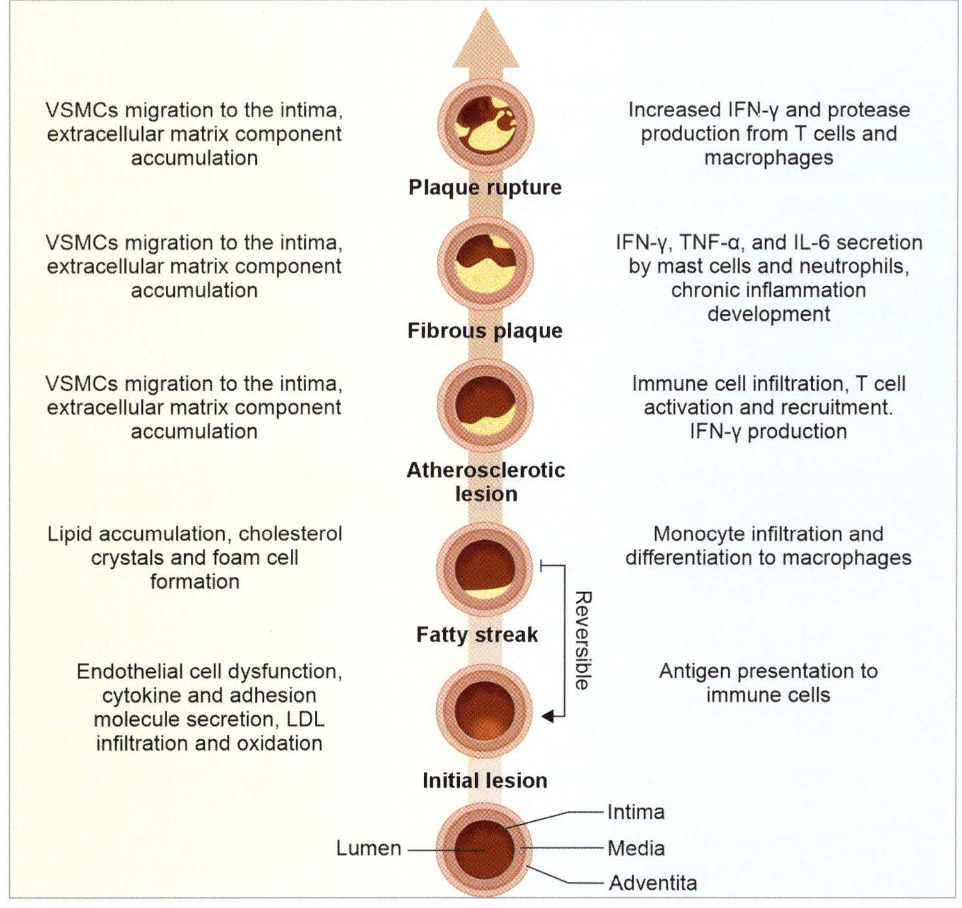

FIG. 1: Atherosclerosis as a metabolic and chronic inflammatory disease. Damage to endothelial cells results in the release of adhesion molecules and the accumulation of intimal macrophages. The oxidation of LDL and the subsequent formation of foam cells intensify inflammation and the development of plaques. Plaque advancement occurs through lipid accumulation and production of extracellular matrix components, resulting in arterial wall thickening and the formation of fibrous caps. Concurrently, chronic inflammation ensues, as immune cells are recruited to the plaque site, secreting elevated levels of inflammatory mediators. Finally, plaque rupture leads to clinical complications.

(IFN-γ: interferon-gamma; IL-6: interleukin 6; LDL: low-density lipoprotein; TNF-α: tumor necrosis factor alpha; VSMCs: vascular smooth muscle cells)

types of plaques eventually culminate in thrombosis, either through plaque rupture or superficial erosion, consequently leading to ST elevated myocardial infarction STEMI) or non-ST elevated myocardial infarction NSTEMI.[14]

Plaque formation and vulnerability are not solely propelled by lipids but also by inflammation. Changes in the composition of numerous immune cells, including macrophages, dendritic cells, T cells, B cells, mast cells, and neutrophils, as well as the modified release of cytokines, chemokines, and other bioactive molecules, disrupt the balance between inflammation and anti-inflammation at plaque formation sites.[15] For instance, vulnerable plaques have fewer regulatory T cells and more effector T cells compared with stable plaques.[16]

■ Current Standard Therapies

- *Lipid lowering*: Statins remain first-line, achieving ≈25 35% reduction in events.[17] Ezetimibe and PCSK9 inhibitors add incremental benefits.[3,4]
- *Antithrombotic therapy*: Aspirin and P2Y12 inhibitors reduce recurrent ischemic events, though bleeding risk persists.[18]
- *Lifestyle and risk factor control*: Smoking cessation, diabetes management, and hypertension control remain essential.[19]

Despite aggressive therapy, patients continue to experience residual cardiovascular events, fueling research into new mechanisms.

ATHEROSCLEROSIS NEWER CONCEPTS

The past decade has seen an integration of immunology, hematology, microbiology, and systems biology into cardiovascular science. Today, atherosclerosis is described as a *chronic maladaptive inflammatory and immune-metabolic disease of the arterial wall* rather than a static lipid storage disorder.[12] It is a dynamic ecosystem of immune cells, vascular cells, lipoproteins, extracellular matrix, and microbiota-derived signals. Newer concepts in atherosclerosis and their mechanisms are summarized in **Table 1**.

■ Immunity and Inflammation: The Core Driver

The Inflammatory Hypothesis

Pathological and experimental studies consistently demonstrate that inflammation, not just lipid retention, drives lesion initiation and progression.[20] LDL particles undergo oxidative modification, acting as neoantigens that stimulate both innate and adaptive immune responses. Activated endothelial cells upregulate adhesion molecules VCAM-1, ICAM-1, facilitating leukocyte recruitment.[21] Monocytes differentiate into macrophages that ingest modified lipids, generating foam cells. The inflammatory milieu perpetuates further leukocyte recruitment, extracellular matrix degradation, and necrotic core expansion.[10]

Clinical Validation

The CANTOS trial (2017) provided definitive proof-of-principle—*canakinumab*, an IL 1β inhibitor, reduced recurrent cardiovascular events by 15% independent of lipid lowering.[22] Similarly, colchicine COLCOT, LoDoCo2 reduced events by broadly dampening inflammatory responses, with hazard ratios of 0.69 (95% CI 0.57–0.83) in LoDoCo2 and 0.77 (95% CI 0.61–0.96) in COLCOT.[23,24] However, anti-inflammatory therapy is not universally effective—increased

TABLE 1: Newer concepts in atherosclerosis and their mechanisms.

Concept	Key mechanism	Translational relevance
Trained immunity	Epigenetic/metabolic reprogramming of innate cells	Explains residual inflammatory risk
Clonal hematopoiesis (CHIP)	Somatic mutations in HSCs → proinflammatory myeloid clones	Genetic risk marker; potential target for inflammasome blockade
Immunometabolism	Glycolysis vs. OXPHOS balance in immune cells	Druggable pathways; links diabetes/obesity to CVD
VSMC plasticity	Dedifferentiation into foam-like, osteogenic, fibroblast-like cells	Drivers of calcification, instability
EndoMT	Endothelial cells → mesenchymal-like cells under TGF-β, shear stress	Contributes to fibrosis, restenosis
Gut microbiome	TMAO, bile acids, SCFAs	Dietary and microbiota-targeted therapies
Lipoprotein(a)	Prothrombotic, pro-inflammatory, carries oxidized phospholipids	RNA therapies in late-phase trials
Plaque ecosystem	Interacting multicellular system	Imaging-based risk stratification

(CHIP: clonal hematopoiesis of indeterminate potential; CVD: cardiovascular disease; EndoMT: endothelial-to-mesenchymal transition; HSCs: hematopoietic stem cells; OXPHOS: oxidative phosphorylation; SCFAs: short-chain fatty acids; TMAO: trimethylamine N-oxide; VSMC: vascular smooth muscle cells)

infection risk, cost, and lack of broad applicability highlight the need for precision immunomodulation.[25]

Trained Immunity: Memory in Innate Cells

Traditionally, immunologic memory was attributed only to adaptive cells T and B lymphocytes). However, it is now clear that innate immune cells—monocytes, macrophages, NK cells—can undergo epigenetic reprogramming after exposure to stimuli such as oxidized LDL, β-glucan, or microbial products.[26]

- *Mechanism:* Epigenetic marks (e.g., histone methylation/acetylation) and metabolic rewiring (shift to glycolysis, mevalonate pathway activation) prime progenitor cells in bone marrow to generate hyperresponsive monocytes/macrophages.[27]
- *Impact in atherosclerosis:* Even after clearance of the initial insult, trained cells maintain heightened inflammatory capacity, perpetuating vascular inflammation.[28]
- *Clinical relevance:* This explains residual inflammatory risk in patients who achieve LDL C goals but continue to suffer events. It also provides rationale for therapies targeting metabolic checkpoints (e.g., mevalonate pathway, glycolysis inhibitors).[29]

Clonal Hematopoiesis of Indeterminate Potential

Concept

Clonal hematopoiesis of indeterminate potential (CHIP) refers to the age-related expansion of hematopoietic stem cell clones carrying mutations in genes such as *TET2, DNMT3A, ASXL1, JAK2.*[30] While initially described as a precursor state to hematologic malignancy, CHIP is now firmly linked to cardiovascular disease.[31]

Mechanism

Mutant clones produce monocytes/macrophages with heightened inflammatory responses, increased IL-1β, IL-6, and NLRP3 inflammasome activation.[32] Animal models of TET2 deficiency show accelerated atherosclerosis.[32]

Clinical Implications

- *Risk magnitude:* CHIP carriers have two-fold higher risk of coronary heart disease and all-cause mortality.
- *Independence from traditional risk factors:* The association persists after adjusting for LDL C, hypertension, smoking, etc.[33]
- *Future directions:* Screening for CHIP may refine risk stratification, and therapies aimed at mutant clone suppression (e.g., hypomethylating agents, inflammasome inhibitors) are under exploration.[34]

Immunometabolism: Metabolic Control of Immunity

Immune cells dynamically adjust their metabolism to suit function.[35]

- *Pro-inflammatory macrophages M1:* Shift to glycolysis, succinate accumulation, and ROS generation.
- *Anti-inflammatory macrophages M2:* Rely on oxidative phosphorylation and fatty acid oxidation.

This metabolic plasticity intersects with trained immunity, diabetes, and obesity—linking systemic metabolic disorders to vascular inflammation.[36] Drugs modulating metabolism (e.g., metformin, glutamine antagonists, statins beyond lipid lowering) may exert anti-atherosclerotic effects partly via immunometabolic pathways.[37,38]

Vascular Smooth Muscle Cells Phenotypic Switching

Vascular smooth muscle cells, traditionally viewed as contractile structural cells, can adopt diverse phenotypes under stress.[39,40]

- *Foam cell-like phenotype*: Express macrophage markers and ingest lipids.[41,42]
- *Osteogenic phenotype*: Promote vascular calcification.[39,43]
- *Fibroblast-like phenotype*: Contribute to fibrous cap and matrix deposition.

This plasticity underlies plaque calcification and instability. Importantly, *lineage tracing studies* demonstrate that a substantial proportion of plaque "macrophage-like cells" originate from VSMCs, not monocytes.[44]

Endothelial-to-mesenchymal Transition

Endothelial cells exposed to inflammatory cytokines, disturbed shear stress, or TGF-β signaling can lose endothelial markers (VE-cadherin, CD31) and gain mesenchymal markers (α-SMA, vimentin).[45,46] Endothelial-to-mesenchymal transition (EndoMT) contributes to intimal thickening, fibrosis, and neointimal hyperplasia.[47] Therapeutically, inhibiting EndoMT or stabilizing endothelial identity may limit early lesion development and restenosis after interventions.[48]

Gut Microbiome and Atherosclerosis

Trimethylamine N-oxide (TMAO) Pathway

Gut bacteria metabolize dietary choline, carnitine, and phosphatidylcholine into trimethylamine (TMA), converted by hepatic Flavin-containing monooxygenase 3 (FMO3) into trimethylamine N-oxide (TMAO).[49,50]

Elevated trimethylamine N-oxide promotes:[51,52]

- Enhanced platelet reactivity
- Impaired cholesterol transport and bile acid metabolism
- Endothelial dysfunction and vascular inflammation

Other Microbial Metabolites

- *Short-chain fatty acids (SCFAs):* Generally protective, improve gut barrier integrity and anti-inflammatory tone.[53-55]
- *Secondary bile acids:* Can signal through FXR/TGR5, influencing lipid metabolism and vascular inflammation.[54,55]

Therapeutic Approaches

Microbiome-targeted interventions (dietary modulation, pre/probiotics, antibiotics, enzyme inhibitors of TMA lyase) are being explored, though translation into human benefit remains preliminary.[49,50,52]

Lipoprotein(a) and Oxidized Phospholipids

Lipoprotein(a) [Lp(a)] is a genetically determined LDL-like particle with apolipoprotein(a).[56] Its atherogenicity stems from:[57,58]

- Carriage of oxidized phospholipids
- Structural homology to plasminogen, impairing fibrinolysis and promoting thrombosis.
- Induction of inflammatory responses in vascular cells.

Residual risk: Elevated Lp(a) explains why some patients with optimal LDL-C still develop premature coronary disease.

The "Plaque Ecosystem" Model

Plaques are not homogeneous—they are *ecosystems* where immune cells, VSMCs, endothelial cells, lipids, extracellular matrix, and microcalcifications interact dynamically.[59]

The fate of a plaque (stable vs. vulnerable) depends less on size/stenosis and more on ecosystem balance:

- Necrotic core versus fibrous cap integrity
- Inflammatory versus reparative macrophages
- Microcalcification versus macrocalcification
- Intraplaque angiogenesis and hemorrhage

Advanced intravascular imaging (OCT, NIRS-IVUS) and molecular PET tracers (targeting inflammation, protease activity, and microcalcification) allow in vivo characterization of these features, paving the way for biology-driven risk stratification.[60,61]

NOVEL THERAPEUTIC TARGETS

The contemporary management of atherosclerotic cardiovascular disease has entered an unprecedented era of molecular precision, marked by the emergence of innovative therapeutic agents that transcend traditional lipid-lowering paradigms. While statins remain foundational therapy, achieving substantial reductions in cardiovascular events, the persistent residual risk observed in optimally treated patients has catalyzed the development of next-generation therapeutics targeting distinct pathophysiological mechanisms underlying atherosclerosis. These novel interventions represent a paradigm shift from conventional "one-size-fits-all" approaches to precision medicine strategies that address the complex interplay between lipid metabolism, chronic inflammation, immune dysregulation, and emerging pathways such as clonal hematopoiesis and microbiome modulation. The clinical pipeline features groundbreaking agents such as olpasiran and lepodisiran for lipoprotein(a) reduction, ziltivekimab for interleukin-6 inhibition, and evinacumab for ANGPTL3 blockade, each representing first-in-class mechanisms with the potential to address previously "untreatable" cardiovascular risk factors.

Lipoprotein Metabolism

- *PCSK9 inhibitors (monoclonal antibodies)*:
  - *Evolocumab, alirocumab* → inhibit PCSK9, ↑ LDL receptor recycling → ↓ LDL C.[62]
  - *Clinical evidence:* FOURIER[63] (HR 0.85; 95% CI 0.79–0.92), ODYSSEY OUTCOMES[64] (HR 0.85; 95% CI 0.78–0.93).
- *PCSK9 siRNA*:
  - *Inclisiran* → blocks PCSK9 synthesis RNA interference) → LDL C lowering with twice- yearly dosing.[65]
- *Lp(a) targeted agents*:
  - *Pelacarsen (antisense oligonucleotide):* Lowers Lp(a) ~80%.[66]
  - *siRNA therapies (olpasiran, lepodisiran, and zerlasiran):* Durable reductions >90%.[67]
  - *Outcome trials:* Ongoing [Lp(a)HORIZON and OCEAN(a)-DOSE trial] to prove cardiovascular benefit.
- *ANGPTL3 inhibitors*:
  - *Evinacumab* (mAb) → inhibits ANGPTL3, ↓ LDL, TG, HDL.

Approved for homozygous familial hypercholesterolemia.[68]

Inflammation and Immunomodulation

- *IL-1β inhibition*:
  - *Canakinumab* → neutralizes IL-1β; landmark CANTOS trial[22] showed MACE reduction independent of lipid levels.
- *IL-6 pathway blockade*:
  - *Ziltivekimab* → anti-IL-6 ligand mAb; RESCUE-2 trial[69] (hs-CRP lowering); (ZEUS trial for CV outcomes ongoing).
  - *Tocilizumab* (anti-IL-6R, approved for rheumatology) under investigation in ACS.[70]
- *NLRP3 inflammasome inhibitors*:
  - *Dapansutrile (oral), MCC950* (experimental) → directly block inflammasome activation.[71]
- *Colchicine (repurposed)*:
  - Low dose (0.5 mg daily) → broad anti-inflammatory effects; LoDoCo2 and COLCOT showed CV benefit.[23,24]

TABLE 2: Novel therapeutic targets.

Molecular target	Mechanism	Key drugs	Trial status
PCSK9	Prevents LDLR degradation → ↓ LDL-C	Evolocumab, alirocumab, andinclisiran	Approved, large RCTs (FOURIER, ODYSSEY, and ORION)
Lipoprotein(a)	Silencing apo(a) → ↓ Lp(a)	Pelacarsen, olpasiran, and lepodisiran	Phase 2–3 [OCEAN(a)-DOSE, HORIZON, ALPACA]
ANGPTL3	Inhibition of ANGPTL3 → ↓ LDL, TG	Evinacumab, ANGPTL3 siRNA	Approved for HoFH; early siRNA in Phase 2
IL-1β	Neutralizes IL-1β → ↓ vascular inflammation	Canakinumab	Phase 3 (CANTOS, positive outcomes)
IL-6 pathway	Blocks IL-6/IL-6R signaling	Ziltivekimab and tocilizumab	Phase 2–3 (RESCUE, ZEUS ongoing)
NLRP3 inflammasome	Blocks inflammasome activation	Dapansutrile, MCC950	Phase 2 (early development)
Inflammation (broad)	Broad anti-inflammatory action	Colchicine	Approved (LoDoCo2, COLCOT)
Endothelial dysfunction/ oxidative stress	Restores NO, reduces ROS	NADPH oxidase inhibitors, eNOS enhancers	Preclinical/Early clinical
Clonal hematopoiesis (CHIP)	Reduces cytokine-driven inflammation from mutant clones	IL-1/IL-6 blockers (precision use)	Conceptual/Early translational
Platelet activation	Inhibits platelet PAR-1 and dual pathway	Vorapaxar and novel antiplatelets	Phase 3 (vorapaxar), new agents in Phase 2
Metabolism and microbiome	Targets TMAO, bile acid, and metabolic signaling	FXR agonists, TMAO inhibitors, and probiotics	Preclinical/Early translational

Endothelial Dysfunction and Oxidative Stress

- *Endothelial nitric oxide synthase (eNOS) enhancers/NO donors* (experimental)
- *NADPH oxidase inhibitors* (preclinical)
- *Antioxidant mimetics* (limited translation to CV endpoints so far)

Clonal Hematopoiesis of Indeterminate Potential

- *Targeting pro-inflammatory cytokines* (IL-1β, IL-6 blockade particularly relevant in TET2/ASXL1 mutations).
- *Future: Clone-directed therapies* under investigation (precision immunotherapy).

Metabolic and Microbiome Modulation

- *FXR agonists, bile acid sequestrants* → improve lipid/inflammatory signaling.
- *Gut microbiome-targeted therapies* (e.g., inhibitors of TMAO generation, probiotics) are experimental but promising.

CONCLUSION

- *Established and late-stage*: PCSK9 inhibition, Lp(a)-lowering (ASO/siRNA), IL-1β, and IL-6 blockade.
- *Emerging*: NLRP3 inhibitors, NETosis modulators, CHIP-directed immunotherapies, microbiome interventions.
- The field is *moving beyond lipid lowering* to *multi-target molecular therapy*, integrating lipid, inflammatory, immune, and thrombotic pathway. Novel therapeutic targets have been summarized in **Table 2**.

Aortic Dissection: Targeting the Vascular Wall

- *Pathophysiology*: Acute aortic dissection results from medial degeneration, elastin fragmentation, and abnormal matrix turnover. Genetic syndromes [Marfan, Loeys–Dietz, vascular Ehlers–Danlos syndrome (vEDS)] and hypertension are key contributors.
- *Current management*:
  - *Medical therapy:* Blood pressure and shear stress reduction with β-blockers and ARBs.
  - *Surgical/Endovascular repair:* Indicated for type A and complicated type B dissections.

Novel Therapeutic Targets (Table 3)

TGF-β Pathway Modulation

- The ARB-TGF-β interaction demonstrates tissue-specific therapeutic effects:
  - *Cardiac tissue:* Reduced myocardial fibrosis and improved cardiac function
  - *Vascular tissue:* Prevention of adverse vascular remodeling and aortic dilatation
- *ARBs (losartan and irbesartan):* The AIMS trial[72] showed irbesartan reduced aortic root dilatation versus placebo in Marfan syndrome (difference of 0.22 mm/year, $p = 0.013$). Meta-analyses confirm ARBs reduce aortic growth rate by 50% compared to placebo. Ongoing evidence supports ARBs as standard in heritable aortopathies.

β-blockade with Vasodilating Properties

Celiprolol: The BBEST trial[73] demonstrated reduced rupture/dissection in vEDS patients. Celiprolol is recommended where available, though not globally approved.

Matrix Metalloproteinase Inhibition

Doxycycline: Early promise as a matrix metalloproteinase (MMP) inhibitor was not confirmed in randomized AAA trials. Not recommended in practice.[74]

Peripheral Artery Disease: Expanding Horizons

- *Burden and clinical challenge*: Peripheral artery disease affects >200 million people worldwide. Morbidity includes claudication, chronic limb-threatening ischemia, and high rates of cardiovascular events. Event rates often rival those of CAD.
- *Current therapies*:
  - Antiplatelet therapy (aspirin or clopidogrel)
  - Statin plus ezetimibe
  - Exercise therapy and smoking cessation
  - Antihypertensive [angiotensin-converting enzyme (ACE) inhibitors/angiotensin receptor blockers (ARB) preferred][75]

Novel Therapeutic Targets (Table 4)

Dual-pathway Inhibition

- *VOYAGER-PAD trial:* Rivaroxaban 2.5 mg bid + aspirin reduced acute limb ischemia and MACE after lower extremity revascularization.[76]
- *COMPASS PAD subset:* Similar benefit in stable PAD.[77]

PCSK9 Inhibitors

Peripheral artery disease subanalyses of FOURIER[78] and ODYSSEY[64] showed reduced limb events and MACE.

Inflammation and Lipoprotein(a)

Mechanistic rationale for colchicine and Lp(a) lowering in PAD; definitive trials awaited.

Regenerative Approaches

Stem-cell and angiogenic therapies under exploration but not yet established in clinical practice.

TABLE 3: Medical strategies in aortic syndromes.

Target pathway	Agent	Evidence/Trials	Clinical role
Hemodynamic load	β-blockers	Reduced mortality in dissection	First-line
TGF-β modulation	Losartan and irbesartan	Slowed aortic root growth in Marfan/LDS	Preferred in heritable aortopathy
Vascular wall strength	Celiprolol	BBEST: ↓ rupture in vEDS	For vEDS patients (where available)
MMP inhibition	Doxycycline	Failed AAA trials	Not recommended

TABLE 4: Landmark PAD trials with novel therapies.

Trial	Intervention	Population	Outcome
COMPASS (PAD subset)	Rivaroxaban 2.5 mg + ASA	Stable PAD	↓ MACE, ↓ limb events
VOYAGER-PAD	Rivaroxaban 2.5 mg + ASA	Post lower-extremity revascularization PAD	↓ acute limb ischemia, ↓ MACE
FOURIER PAD sub study	PCSK9i (evolocumab)	PAD patients	↓ MACE, ↓ limb events
ODYSSEY OUTCOMES PAD sub study	PCSK9i (alirocumab)	PAD + ACS	↓ MACE, limb events

REFERENCES

1. Roth GA, Mensah GA, Johnson CO, et al. Global Burden of Cardiovascular Diseases and Risk Factors, 1990-2019: Update from the GBD 2019 Study. J Am Coll Cardiol. 2020;76(25):2982-3021.
2. Virani SS, Alonso A, Aparicio HJ, et al. Heart Disease and Stroke Statistics-2021 Update: A Report from the American Heart Association. Circulation. 2021;143(8):e254-e743.
3. Cannon CP, Blazing MA, Giugliano RP, et al. Ezetimibe Added to Statin Therapy after Acute Coronary Syndromes. N Engl J Med. 2015;372(25):2387-97.
4. Sabatine MS, Giugliano RP, Keech AC, et al. Evolocumab and Clinical Outcomes in Patients with Cardiovascular Disease. N Engi J Med. 2017;376(18):1713-22.
5. Libby P, Ridker PM, Hansson GK. Progress and challenges in translating the biology of atherosclerosis. Nature. 2011;473(7347):317-25.
6. Milewicz DM, Prakash SK, Ramirez F. Therapeutics Targeting Drivers of Thoracic Aortic Aneurysms and Acute Aortic Dissections: Insights from Predisposing Genes and Mouse Models. Circ Res. 2017;121(9):1055-9.
7. Fowkes FG, Rudan D, Rudan I, et al. Comparison of global estimates of prevalence and risk factors for peripheral artery disease in 2000 and 2010: a systematic review and analysis. Lancet. 2013;382(9901):1329-40.
8. Hansson GK, Hermansson A. The immune system in atherosclerosis. Nat Immunol.2011;12(3):204-12.
9. Nordestgaard BG, Chapman MJ, Ray K, et al. Lipoprotein(a) as a cardiovascular risk factor: current status. Eur Heart J. 2010;31(23):2844-53.
10. Moore KJ, Sheedy FJ, Fisher EA. Macrophages in atherosclerosis: a dynamic balance. Nat Rev Immunol. 2013;13(10):709-21.
11. Allahverdian S, Chehroudi AC, McManus BM, Abraham T, Francis GA. Contribution of intimal smooth muscle cells to cholesterol homeostasis and inflammatory responses in atherosclerosis. Circ Res. 2014;114(9):1400-9.
12. Libby P, Buring JE, Badimon L, et al. Atherosclerosis. Nat Rev Dis Primers. 2019;5(1):56.
13. Bentzon JF, Otsuka F, Virmani R, Falk E. Mechanisms of plaque formation and rupture. CircRes. 2014;114(12):1852-66.
14. Davies MJ. Stability and instability: two faces of coronary atherosclerosis. The Paul Dudley White Lecture 1995. Circulation. 1996;94(8):2013-20.
15. Hansson GK, Libby P. The immune response in atherosclerosis: a double-edged sword. Nat Rev Immunol. 2006;6(7):508-19.
16. Ait-Oufella H, Salomon BL, Potteaux S, et al. Natural regulatory T cells control the development of atherosclerosis in mice. Nat Med. 2006;12(2):178-80.
17. Cholesterol Treatment Trialists' (CTT) Collaboration; Baigent C, Blackwell L, et al. Efficacy and safety of more intensive lowering of LDL cholesterol: a meta-analysis of data from 170,000 participants in 26 randomised trials. Lancet. 2010;376(9753):1670-81.
18. Antithrombotic Trialists' (ATT) Collaboration; Baigent C, Blackwell L, et al. Aspirin in the primary and secondary prevention of vascular disease: collaborative meta-analysis of individual participant data from randomised trials. Lancet. 2009;373(9678):1849-60.
19. Piepoli MF, Hoes AW, Agewall S, et al. 2016 European Guidelines on cardiovascular disease prevention in clinical practice: The Sixth Joint Task Force of the European Society of Cardiology and Other Societies on Cardiovascular Disease Prevention in Clinical Practice. Eur Heart J. 2016;37(29):2315-81.
20. Libby P, Ridker PM, Maseri A. Inflammation and atherosclerosis. Circulation.2002;105(9):1135-43.
21. Davies MJ, Gordon JL, Gearing AJ, et al. The expression of the adhesion molecules ICAM-1, VCAM-1, PECAM, and E-selectin in human atherosclerosis. J Pathol. 1993;171(3):223-9.
22. Ridker PM, Everett BM, Thuren T, et al. Antiinflammatory Therapy with Canakinumab for Atherosclerotic Disease. N Engl J Med. 2017;377(12):1119-31.
23. Nidorf SM, Fiolet ATL, MosterdA, et al. Colchicine in Patients with Chronic Coronary Disease. N Engl J Med. 2020;383(19):1838-47.
24. Tardif JC, Kouz S, Waters DD, et al. Efficacy and Safety of Low-Dose Colchicine after Myocardial Infarction. N Engl J Med. 2019;381(26):2497-2505.
25. Ridker PM, MacFadyen JG, Thuren T, et al. Effect of interleukin-1B inhibition with canakinumab on incident lung cancer in patients with atherosclerosis: exploratory results from a randomised, double-blind, placebo-controlled trial. Lancet. 2017;390(10105):1833-42.
26. Netea MG, Dominguez-Andrés J, Barrero LB, et al. Defining trained immunity and its role in health and disease. Nat Rev Immunol. 2020;20(6):375-88.
27. Bekkering S, Quintin J, Joosten LA, et al. Oxidized low-density lipoprotein induces long-term proinflammatory cytokine production and foam cell formation via epigenetic reprogramming of monocytes. Arterioscler Thromb Vasc Biol. 2014;34(8):1731-8.
28. Christ A, Günther P, Lauterbach MAR, et al. Western Diet Triggers NLRP3-Dependent Innate Immune Reprogramming. Cell. 2018;172(1-2):162-75.e14.
29. Bekkering S, Arts RJW, Novakovic B, et al. Metabolic induction of trained immunity through the mevalonate pathway. Cell. 2018;172(1-2):135-46.e9.
30. JaiswalS, Fontanillas P, Flannick J, et al. Age-related clonal haematopoiesis associated with adverse outcomes. N Engl J Med. 2014;371(26):2488-98.
31. Jaiswal S, Natarajan P, Silver AJ, et al. Clonal Haematopoiesis and Risk of Atherosclerotic Cardiovascular Disease. N Engl J Med. 2017;377(2):111-21.
32. Fuster JJ, MacLauchlan S, Zuriaga MA, et al. Clonal haematopoiesis associated with TET2 deficiency accelerates atherosclerosis development in mice. Science. 2017;355(6327):842-7.
33. Dorsheimer L, Assmus B, Rasper T, et al. Association of Mutations Contributing to Clonal Hematopoiesis of Indeterminate Potential with Prognosis in Chronic Ischemic Heart Failure. JAMA Cardiol. 2019;4 (1):25-33.
34. Wang Y, Sano S, Yura Y, et al. CHIP promoting cardiac dysfunction and arrhythmias. Basic Res Cardiol. 2020;115(1):8.
35. O'Neill LA, Kishton RJ, Rathmell J. A guide to immunometabolism for immunologists. Nat Rev Immunol. 2016;16(9):553-65.
36. Viola A, Munari F, Sánchez-Rodriguez R, et al. The Metabolic Signature of Macrophage Responses. Front Immunol. 2019; 10:1462.
37. Shirakawa K, Endo J, Kataoka M, et al. IL (Interleukin)-10-STAT3-Galectin-3 Axis Is Essential for Osteopontin-Producing Reparative Macrophage Polarization After Myocardial Infarction. Circulation. 2018;138(18):2021-35.
38. Salnikova D, Orekhova V, Grechko A, et al. Mitochondrial Dysfunction in Vascular Wall Cells and Its Role in Atherosclerosis. Int J Mol Sci. 2021;22(16):8990.
39. Zhang F, Guo X, Xia Y, et al. An update on the phenotypic switching of vascular smooth muscle cells and its implications in atherosclerosis. Cell Mol Life Sci. 2021;78(20):6703-28.

40. Sorokin V, Vickneson K, Kofidis T, et al. Role of Vascular Smooth Muscle Cell Plasticity and Interactions in Vessel Wall Inflammation. Front Immunol. 2020;11:599415.
41. Li Y, Zhu H, Zhang Q, et al. Smooth muscle-derived macrophage-like cells contribute to multiple cell lineages in the atherosclerotic plaque. Cell Discov. 2021;7(1):109.
42. Zhao L, Zhao L, Liu D, et al. Vascular Smooth Muscle Cells: A Therapeutic Target in Atherosclerosis. Int J Mol Sci. 2025;26(12):6703.
43. Grootaert MOJ, Bennett MR. Vascular smooth muscle cells in atherosclerosis: time for a re-assessment. Cardiovasc Res. 2021;117(11):2326-39.
44. Bentzon JF, Majesky MW. Lineage tracking of origin and fate of smooth muscle cells in atherosclerosis. Cardiovasc Res. 2017;114(4):492-500.
45. Souilhol C, Harmsen MC, Evans PC, et al. Endothelial-mesenchymal transition in atherosclerosis. Cardiovasc Res. 2018;114(4):565-77.
46. Evrard SM, Lecce L, Michelis KC, et al. Endothelial to mesenchymal transition is common in atherosclerotic lesions and is associated with plaque instability. Nat Commun. 2016;7:11853.
47. Huang Q, Gan Y, Yu Z, et al. Endothelial to Mesenchymal Transition: An Insight in Atherosclerosis. Front Cardiovasc Med. 2021;8:734550.
48. Chen PY, Schwartz MA, Simons M. Endothelial-to-Mesenchymal Transition, Vascular Inflammation, and Atherosclerosis. Front Cardiovasc Med. 2020;7:53.
49. Zhu Y, Li Q, Jiang H. Gut microbiota in atherosclerosis: focus on trimethylamine N-oxide. APMIS. 2020;128(4):353-66.
50. Oktaviono YH, Dyah Lamara A, Saputra PBT, et al. The roles of trimethylamine-N-oxide in atherosclerosis and its potential therapeutic aspect: A literature review. Biomed Pharmacother. 2023;167:115563.
51. Nam HS. Gut Microbiota and Ischemic Stroke: The Role of Trimethylamine N-Oxide. J Stroke. 2019;21(2):151-9.
52. Wang BY, Qiu J, Lian J, et al. Gut Metabolite Trimethylamine-N-Oxide in Atherosclerosis: From Mechanism to Therapy. Front Cardiovasc Med. 2021;8:723886.
53. Callender C, Attaye I, Nieuwdorp M. The Interaction between the Gut Microbiome and Bile Acids in Cardiometabolic Diseases. Nutrients. 2022;14(2):411.
54. Fogelson KA, Dorrestein PC, Zarrinpar A, et al. The Gut Microbial Bile Acid Modulation and Its Relevance to Digestive Health and Diseases. Gastroenterology. 2023;165(4):1074-85.
55. Zhang Z, Lv T, Wang X, et al. Role of the microbiota–gut–heart axis between bile acids and cardiovascular disease. Biomed Pharmacother. 2024;174:116567.
56. Rehberger Likozar A, Zavrtanik M, Šebeštjen M. Lipoprotein(a) in atherosclerosis: from pathophysiology to clinical significance and treatment options. Wien Klin Wochenschr. 2020;132(15-16):439-50.
57. Gilliland TC, Liu Y, Mohebi R, et al. Lipoprotein(a), Oxidized Phospholipids, and Coronary Artery Disease Severity and Outcomes. J Am Coll Cardiol. 2023;81(18):1780-92.
58. Mohammadnia N, van Broekhoven A, Bax WA, et al. Interleukin-6 modifies Lipoprotein(a) and oxidized phospholipids associated cardiovascular risk. Atherosclerosis. 2025;408:118122.
59. Eligini S, Gianazza E, Mallia A, et al. Macrophage Phenotyping in Atherosclerosis by Proteomics. Int J Mol Sci. 2023;24(3):2613.
60. Hammad B, Evans NR, Rudd JHF, et al. Molecular imaging of atherosclerosis with integrated PET imaging. J Nucl Cardiol. 017;24(3):938-43.
61. Grandjean CE, Pedersen SF, Christensen C, et al. Imaging of atherosclerosis with [64Cu]Cu-DOTA-TATE in a translational head-to-head comparison study with [18F]FDG, and Na[18F]F in rabbits. Sci Rep. 2023;13(1):9249.
62. Ma H, Ma W, Liu Y, et al. Effects of Alirocumab and Evolocumab on Cardiovascular Mortality and LDL-C: Stratified According to the Baseline LDL-C Levels. Rev Cardiovasc Med. 2025;26(4):26980.
63. Kang YM, Giugliano RP, Ran X, et al. Cardiovascular Outcomes and Efficacy of the PCSK9 Inhibitor Evolocumab in Individuals With Type 1 Diabetes: Insights From the FOURIER Trial. Diabetes Care. 2025;48(9):1512-6.
64. Schwartz GG, Gabriel Steg P, Bhatt DL, et al. Clinical Efficacy and Safety of Alirocumab After Acute Coronary Syndrome According to Achieved Level of Low-Density Lipoprotein Cholesterol: A Propensity Score-Matched Analysis of the ODYSSEY OUTCOMES Trial. Circulation. 2021;143(11):1109-22.
65. Di Giacomo-Barbagallo F, Andreychuk N, Scicali R, et al. Inclisiran, Reasons for a Novel Agent in a Crowded Therapeutic Field. Curr Atheroscler Rep. 2025;27(1):25.
66. Bhatia HS, Bajaj A, Goonewardena SN, et al. Pelacarsen: Mechanism of action and Lp(a)-lowering effect. J Clin Lipidol. 2025:S1933-2874(25)00322-8.
67. Kanbay M, Ozbek L, Guldan M, et al. siRNA-based therapeutics for lipoprotein (a) lowering: A path toward precision cardiovascular medicine. Eur J Clin Invest. 2025;55(9):e70079.
68. Sosnowska B, Adach W, Surma S, et al. Evinacumab, an ANGPTL3 Inhibitor, in the Treatment of Dyslipidemia. J Clin Med. 2022;12(1):168.
69. Wada Y, Jensen C, Meyer ASP, et al. Efficacy and safety of interleukin-6 inhibition with ziltivekimab in patients at high risk of atherosclerotic events in Japan (RESCUE-2): A randomized, double-blind, placebo-controlled, phase 2 trial. J Cardiol. 2023;82(4):279-85.
70. d'Aiello A, Filomia S, Brecciaroli M, et al. Targeting Inflammatory Pathways in Atherosclerosis: Exploring New Opportunities for Treatment. Curr Atheroscler Rep. 2024;26(12):707-19.
71. Chhunchha B, Kubo E, Lehri D, et al. NLRP3 Inflammasome and Inflammatory Response in Aging Disorders: The Entanglement of Redox Modulation in Different Outcomes. Cells. 2025;14(13):994.
72. Mullen M, Jin XY, Child A, et al. Irbesartan in Marfan syndrome (AIMS): a double-blind, placebo-controlled randomised trial. Lancet. 2019;394(10216):2263-70.
73. Baderkhan H, Wanhainen A, Stenborg A, et al. Celiprolol Treatment in Patients with Vascular Ehlers-Danlos Syndrome. Eur J Vasc Endovasc Surg. 2021;61(2):326-31.
74. Gouveia E Melo R, Rodrigues M, Caldeira D, et al. Doxycycline is not Effective in Reducing Abdominal Aortic Aneurysm Growth: A Mini Systematic Review and Meta-Analysis of Randomised Controlled Trials. Eur J Vasc Endovasc Surg. 2021;61(5):863-4.
75. Abraham AT, Mojaddedi S, Loseke IH, et al. Hypertension in Patients with Peripheral Artery Disease: An Updated Literature Review. Cureus. 2024;16(6):e62246.
76. Bauersachs RM, Szarek M, Brodmann M, et al. Total Ischemic Event Reduction With Rivaroxaban After Peripheral Arterial Revascularization in the VOYAGER PAD Trial. J Am Coll Cardiol. 2021;78(4):317-26.
77. Steffel J, Eikelboom JW, Anand SS, et al. The COMPASS trial. Circulation. 2020;142(1):40-8.
78. Bonaca MP, Nault P, Giugliano RP, et al. Low-Density Lipoprotein Cholesterol Lowering With Evolocumab and Outcomes in Patients With Peripheral Artery Disease: Insights From the FOURIER Trial (Further Cardiovascular Outcomes Research With PCSK9 Inhibition in Subjects With Elevated Risk). Circulation. 2018;137(4):338-50.

SECTION

11

Cardiac Arrhythmia

Section Outline

78. **VT Ablation as Stand Alone Procedure without ICD in Stable Scar VT in Mild or Moderate LV Dysfunction**
Anees Thajudeen

79. **Atrial Fibrillation and Long-term CV Outcome**
Bhuban Majhi, Rajarshi Halder

80. **Effect of Left Atrial Dyssynchrony on Long-term Clinical Outcomes during Cardiac Resynchronization Therapy**
Anil Mishra

81. **Divergence from Guideline Directed Management of Cardiac Implantable Electronic Device Infections**
Ashish Nabar, Amit Vora

82. **Leadless Pacing: Past, Present, and Future**
Aftab Khan, Navanil Biswas, Arif Nabi Bhat

83. **Atrial Fibrillation in Heart Failure: Role of Catheter Ablation**
Sharath K Kumar, Calambur Narasimhan

84. **Ventricular Tachycardia Ablation in the Emergency Setting**
Aditya Mulgaonkar, Deepak Padmanabhan

85. **Prevention of Sudden Cardiac Death beyond Automated External Defibrillators and Implantable Cardioverter Defibrillators**
Girish B Navasundi

86. **Pulsed Field Ablation—in Present Perspective**
Vadivelu Ramalingam, Atul Verma, KK Talwar

87. **Para-Hisian Ventricular Arrhythmias**
Sathish S Reddy, Priyanka Agarwal

CHAPTER 78

VT Ablation as Stand Alone Procedure without ICD in Stable Scar VT in Mild or Moderate LV Dysfunction

Anees Thajudeen

ABSTRACT

Implantable cardioverter-defibrillator (ICD) implantation has not been shown to be of benefit in patients with hemodynamically tolerated ventricular tachycardia (VT) in the various ICD trials till date. In patients with mild or moderate LBV dysfunction, post-MI and VT could be treated with VT ablation procedure with marked mid- and long-term benefits. Data, though limited, is currently available which suggests that VT ablation alone provides long-term benefits in such patients and that implanting an ICD is unlikely to benefit this group.

Keywords: Implantable cardioverter-defibrillator, ventricular tachycardia, VT ablation, left ventricular dysfunction, postmyocardial infarction, arrhythmia management, long-term outcomes.

INTRODUCTION

It has been routine practice, based on very limited evidence from the various implantable cardioverter-defibrillator (ICD) trials for secondary and primary prevention, to recommend ICD implantation in patients who had a sustained ventricular tachycardia (VT) in the setting of old myocardial infarctions. While ICD implantation significantly reduces risk of sudden death and all-cause mortality in this group of patients, the benefit is demonstrated only in patients with severe left ventricular dysfunction. The important ICD studies of secondary prevention like AVID trial did not include patients with hemodynamically tolerated VT. The primary prevention trials specifically included patients with EF < 40 (MUSTT and MADIT 1) or 30% (MADIT 2).

RISK OF SUDDEN DEATH AFTER MI

The risk of SCD, after MI with or without primary PCI is maximum in the first month, the risk plateaus after around 6–12 months to lower values dependent on the ejection fraction (EF). In many patients, the LVEF improves to mid-range EF level when rechecked months after revascularization. A few of these patients can still have appropriate ICD treatment or sudden death. The current patient profile is also different from the late 1990s when data for secondary prevention was sought from various trials. Mortality in patients without severe LV dysfunction is mostly from noncardiac causes. Among cardiac mortality, around 50% are SCD (presumed sudden arrhythmic death—SAD). The PRE-DETERMINE study[1] showed that 4-year incidence of SAD is 4.9% for EF 30–39 and 3.1% for EF 40–49. The study looked at 4-year risk of SAD and based on EF, the number needed to prevent sudden death (NNT) with ICD would be 51 for EF between 40 and 49, and 34 for patients with EF between 30 and 39. It has to be remembered that these are not data from randomized trials and not all sudden deaths are prevented by ICD implants. The VALIANT trial showed that when SCD is suspected, if patients actually had autopsy only 51% SCD were definitely arrhythmic. The PRE-DETERMINE study also showed that the annualized risk of SCD was several times lower than in the patient groups studied in the primary prophylaxis ICD trials. The risk of SCD is clearly high with lower EF and since proportional risk of SCD, compared to non-SCD mortality is lower as the subjects age increases, the benefit of ICD may be much stronger in younger patients.

The presence of a tolerated VT is often considered a high-risk marker for arrhythmia in post-MI patients with EF > 35%, but ICD trials of such patients are not available and data from primary prevention trials show that ICD has no significant benefit when EF is >35%.

The VALIANT trial follow-up showed that more than half of all SCD occur with initial post-MI EF > 30%. This is because of the higher number of patients who have EF > 30%. Recent studies show that only 12% of patients in the current era end up with long-term EF < 40%, mainly attributed to widespread use of primary angioplasty and optimal medical treatment for ventricular remodeling. The PARADISE MI trial data showed that only 2,6% post-MI patients had sudden death in 22 months, 30% of SCD happened in first month post-MI. The SCD rate/year was 1.4% in this trial, much lower than the high rates experienced in the older trials.[2]

The risk of sudden death for which ICD implantation is recommended, and has also changed with updated treatment options for heart failure. The recent analysis of SCD risk in HF trials, including the PARADIGM trial, for instance, had shown that guideline-directed medical treatment with sacubitril/valsartan along with other medications for heart failure can significantly reduce risk of sudden death and all-cause mortality.[3]

Ventricular tachycardia ablation has a significantly benefited patients with ischemic cardiomyopathy and VT. In clinical practice, successful VT ablation is most gratifying when it helps to prevent recurrent VT in the setting of an electrical storm. Patients with recurrent cardiac arrest episodes or incessant VT requiring repeated cardioversions make remarkable recovery with a successful VT ablation procedure. This brings into question utility of VT ablation, without ICD implantation to reduce risk of cardiac events and sudden death in select groups of patients.

VENTRICULAR TACHYCARDIA ABLATION IN ISCHEMIC CARDIOMYOPATHY: CURRENT RECOMMENDATIONS

The current guidelines recommend VT ablation as class I in patients with IHD and VT when there is recurrence of VT on amiodarone or after failed AAD. VT ablation as first option, in lieu of antiarrhythmic drugs is given a class IIa recommendation.[4] The guidelines however do not consider IHD patients in the absence of an implanted ICD or without consideration of ICD implantation after VT ablation. Studies in this group clearly showed that VT ablation had significant benefit over escalation of antiarrhythmic medications such as higher dosage of amiodarone or addition of mexiletine (VANISH trial). Other prospective cohort studies has clearly shown a very marked reduction in the incidence of recurrent VT or ICD shocks in medium term follow-up after VT ablation.

For patients with first episode of VT, who have not been on AAD, VT ablation as first-line strategy has been studied in various RCTs. The trials targeting first episode of VT mostly were restricted to patients with an AICD or planned for AICD implant for VT. The studies in general showed a significant reduction in ICD therapies when VT ablation was employed as first-line strategy. The most recent VANISH2 trial showed that arrhythmia outcomes, especially appropriate ICD shocks and treated sustained VT was significantly reduced with a first-line ablation approach; the primary outcome of all-cause death, sustained VT requiring intervention, appropriate ICD shock, and VT storm showed an absolute reduction of 9.8%.[5] These trials show that early VT ablation improves outcomes mainly by reducing the recurrence of ventricular arrhythmia, much more than antiarrhythmic drugs without increasing the risk of complications from treatment.[6]

An updated meta-analysis of all the RCTs for VT ablation, with analysis from individual patient level data showed that VT ablation significantly reduced the incidence of all-cause mortality at 24 and 48 months (HR 0.73; CI 0.53–1.0), compared to antiarrhythmic therapy. This means VT ablation has mortality reduction benefits, not just reduction of ICD treatment or VT storm episodes.[7]

LONG-TERM SUCCESS AFTER VENTRICULAR TACHYCARDIA ABLATION

Ventricular tachycardia ablation is a complex procedure and is mostly performed in a high-risk group of patients who are at risk for SCD and heart failure mortality. In general, with the latest armamentarium VT-free survival at 2 years is between 60 and 70%.[7] In the more recent PARTITA trial,[8] 96% VT-free survival was noted at 1 year in a small group of patients. However, based on preprocedural risk, completeness of procedure and results of VT induction testing after procedure, the long-term success is highly variable. The long-term benefits depend on the baseline risk of sudden death and cardiac death. The risk of death at 1 year can vary between negligible to >60% in the highest risk cohort, e.g., patients with EF < 20%, electrical storm, and poor functional class. Greater reduction in ICD shocks and events was noted in patients who had EF > 35% and who had VT ablation early after their first ventricular arrhythmia event.[9]

VENTRICULAR TACHYCARDIA ABLATION AS DEFINITIVE TREATMENT FOR VT, WITHOUT ICD IMPLANTATION

Although not part of standard recommendation, in many instances patients with VT often cannot get an ICD implanted—either due to financial reasons or because of physician or patient reluctance. It is also the case that the evidence for benefit from ICD is not proven in trials for patients in the low-risk group—patients with hemodynamically tolerated VT or patients with EF > 35%. The VT trials also showed that greater reduction in VT recurrence or ICD shock was seen in patients with EF > 30%, with mortality benefits in meta-analysis (see above).

People have looked at factors predicting adverse outcomes after VT ablation. A pooled analysis of retrospective data from 1,251 patients showed that EF is an important prognostic factor. An EF of 30% or more showed a lower risk of VT recurrence, especially in the group who had no ICD implanted (hazard ratio of 0.38). The group with the lowest risk of VT recurrence at 1 year was those with a combination of ischemic cardiomyopathy, EF > 30% and absence of ICD. In the same analysis, the 1-year risk of death was very low (0.86%) in VT ablation subjects who had EF > 30% and had no previous VT ablation.[9] Patients with electrical storm had a high risk of mortality after VT ablation, compared to those who had ablation for tolerated VT. After ablation, these patients were found to have a higher VT recurrence risk. Risk stratification can also be obtained by the results of final programmed stimulation after ablation. If programmed electrical stimulation induced clinical VT or if PES was not done for VT induction, the patients were found to have high risk.

In effect, ablation success as demonstrated by non-inducibility of any VT, EF > 30–35% and hemodynamically tolerated VT as indication for ablation may indicate a group of patients with low risk of SCD.

Maury et al. studied VT ablation as standalone treatment, without ICD in 160 patients with well-tolerated sustained monomorphic ventricular tachycardia (SMVT) and LVEF over 30%.[10] A group of similar patients who had ICD served as controls. The mean EF in the group was 50 ± 10%. The study showed that the risk of VT recurrence was low and while 12% of patients required an ICD, only four patients out of the 160 died suddenly. All-cause mortality was not different from the group which received ICD (control group). The four patients who died had actually presented with some symptoms of hemodynamic compromise, like near syncope before the index procedure. Evaluation for residual ischemia was not reported in the study and the follow-up duration was limited. Another study of 31 patients with EF > 40%, published in 2015, showed that VT recurrence was considerably reduced by VT ablation with no incidence of SCD without an ICD. In this group when VT remained inducible, ICD was recommended, but ICD did not influence survival.[11]

In a more recent observational study published in 2024, Rademaker et al. demonstrated the effect of VT ablation alone in a group of patients who had tolerated VT and EF > 35%.[12] In these patients ICD implantation was offered if any VT was inducible after ablation. In the 37 patients who had no VT inducible, ICD was not offered as a recommendation and only five patients had ICD. None of these patients had VT recurrence or SCD after 39 months. Those who had VT inducible after ablation (14 patients) had ICD implanted. VT recurrence was seen in 4 out of the 14 patients. None in this group had sudden cardiac death. This latest observational study buttresses the benefit of VT ablation alone as a stand-alone treatment in this setting.

These remarkable observational data suggests that VT ablation can significantly reduce cardiac events and may serve as the only treatment option needed in this group of patients who are at low risk of sudden death. Thus, ICD implantation may be avoided in these groups of hemodynamically tolerated VT patients.

ACHIEVING LONG-TERM SUCCESS WITH VENTRICULAR TACHYCARDIA ABLATION

Ventricular tachycardia ablation is a complex interventional procedure. Achieving lasting benefits from this requires a good understanding of the principles of VT mapping, the electrical properties of the VT substrate and dedicated operators with technical skills willing for repeated mapping and VT induction in each patient. The patient themselves may have significant risk of hemodynamic deterioration during procedure and are at risk of complications such as stroke and cardiac perforation from the procedure.

A detailed description of the procedure is beyond the scope of this chapter. The following points are relevant to achieving good results in the contemporary setting; especially when VT ablation is offered without ICD in the patients with low risk.

- *The end point of VT ablation is often a combination of:*
    - *Complete elimination of the VT substrate:* This includes mapping the slow conducting areas (sometimes called the deceleration zones) in the substrate to eliminate late potentials which represent late activating discrete near field signals from muscle bundles which may serve as conducting channels during VT. After ablation procedure, remapping is often done in the same area to show that the discrete late potentials are eliminated. The deceleration zone fragmented or late potentials may sometimes be masked by local EGM from more viable tissue and may require special procedures like decremental evoked potential mapping (progressive extra stimulus testing to bring out late potentials which decrement and gets separated from the main EGM).
    - VT induction (PES testing) at end of procedure to show that no VT is inducible. Aggressive stimulation from RV and LV with triple extra stimulation is consistently pursued. In patients with EF > 35% and tolerated VT, induction can be safely done without much risk of hemodynamic collapse. The best results are when no VT is inducible at the end of procedure. If any VT is inducible (unless they are very fast, e.g., CL < 250 ms), the VT is again mapped, or substrate ablation is again pursued to achieve a better result.
- Recurrence of clinical or nonclinical VT is often the result of incomplete mapping and ablation and repeat studies for recurrence show that critical sites of ablation for VT are intact slow conducting zones which are spatially adjacent to the previous ablation site.
- *Deep myocardial or epicardial critical sites have to be looked for:*
    - All the critical sites for conducting channels for VT circuit are not located in the endocardium. The VT

circuit is a three-dimensional structure. Discrete nearfield potentials represent local activation from under the mapping catheter. Deeper critical sites should be suspected when activation mapping during VT, even when meticulously done, fails to identify diastolic potentials in a significant portion of the diastolic interval.

   - The diastolic interval is best considered as the duration between VT QRS ending to VT QRS (next beat) onset. VT QRS onset corresponds to VT exit into viable myocardium from the VT conducting channel. During the diastolic interval, slow conduction of electrical activity spreads through the critical channel of the VT located in scar tissue. Detailed high density mapping should ideally pick up diastolic potentials representing this activation. When a significant chunk of diastolic interval potentials is missing, the circuit is considered deep—mid-myocardial or epicardial.
   - Epicardial mapping should be done when remapping procedures are done for failed cases, especially when the initial procedure was meticulously done or when features suggested deeper circuits in the initial procedure.
- *VT mapping in tolerated VT:*
   - In many cases of VT ablation, VT mapping is done mainly focusing on substrate mapping. However, when VT is well tolerated, detailed activation mapping can be done. With high density mapping during VT, the opportunity to get information about critical potentials spanning the diastolic interval of VT can be more easily obtained. Combining this information—the location of diastolic potentials crowded together in areas of closely spaced isochrones, with entrainment mapping can identify critical sites of the clinical VT. Ablation here may terminate the VT within a few ablations. This makes VT ablation for tolerated VT much more lucid, complete, and meticulous. Elucidation of diastolic pathway with activation mapping will significantly improve long-term success of VT ablation with VT-free survival above 80% **(Fig. 1)**.[13]
   - After targeting the late potentials and fragmented signals around the critical site (where ablation was successful), the following should be done:
      - Further ablation based on substrate characteristics—late potentials deep within scar/ in the deceleration zones identified in sinus rhythm and in the border zones of scar
      - VT induction—anticipating the induction of another VT which may indicate another critical site within the same scar or another dense scar, which requires again detailed mapping during the second VT.
   - Studies have clearly shown that when ablation procedure is limited to ablation and successful termination of a clinical VT only, without targeting late potentials which may be targeted in sinus rhythm (substrate modification), the long-term recurrence risk is high.

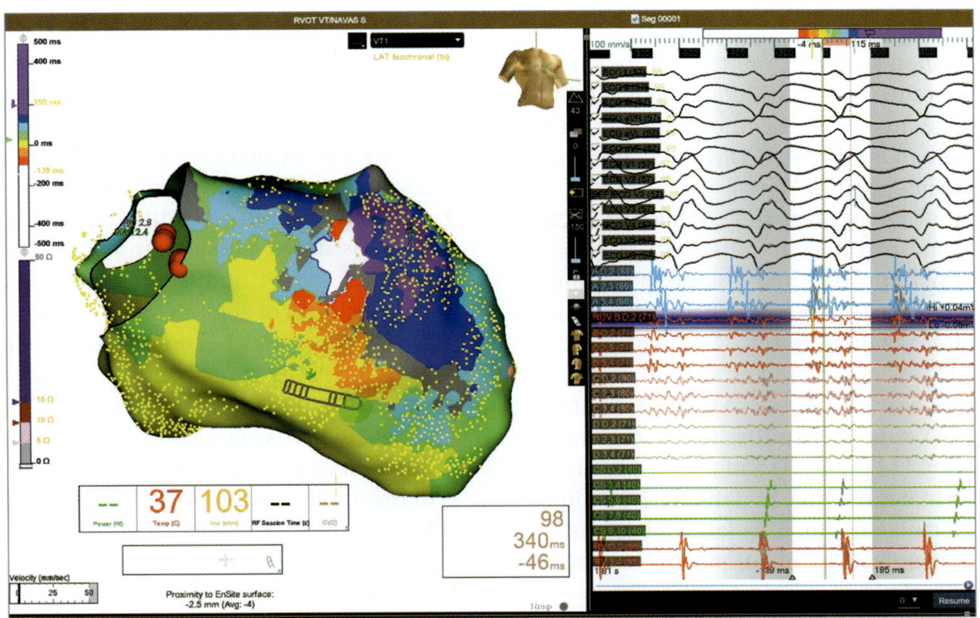

FIG. 1: An activation map created during ongoing ventricular tachycardia with a high-definition (HD) grid catheter: The diastolic interval is being mapped and the electrogram in the HD grid catheter shows fragmented near field signals corresponding to critical pathway activation at the area of slow conduction. Note that diastolic signals immediately after the QRS ending (initial part of the mapping window) are missing—indicating the need for further meticulous mapping or possible deep myocardial critical channels.

CONCLUSION

There is no clear evidence that ICD seriously impacts morbidity or mortality in patients with hemodynamically tolerated VT and mild or moderate LV dysfunction.

Ventricular tachycardia ablation has now been shown to have significant impact on VT-free survival and has shown promise in reducing hospitalizations, and perhaps death in patients with post-MI VT. Based on current evidence, VT ablation could be considered as a class 1 therapeutic option in patients with structural heart disease and VT.

Recent observational studies have shown that in patients with tolerated VT and EF > 35%, VT ablation alone can be perused as a therapeutic option without ICD implantation. When a good VT ablation and evaluation protocol is followed, in this group of patients, VT recurrence in the medium term is significantly reduced with no adverse impact on sudden arrhythmic mortality.

REFERENCES

1. Chatterjee NA, Moorthy MV, Pester J, et al. Sudden Death in Patients With Coronary Heart Disease Without Severe Systolic Dysfunction. JAMA Cardiol. 2018;3(7):591-600.
2. Curtain JP, Pfeffer MA, Braunwald E, et al. Rates of Sudden Death After Myocardial Infarction-Insights From the VALIANT and PARADISE-MI Trials. JAMA Cardiol. 2024;9(10):928-33.
3. Shen L, Jhund PS, Petrie MC, et al. Declining Risk of Sudden Death in Heart Failure. N Engl J Med. 2017;377(1):41-51.
4. Cronin EM, Bogun FM, Maury P, et al. 2019 HRS/EHRA/APHRS/LAHRS expert consensus statement on catheter ablation of ventricular arrhythmias. Europace. 2019;21(8):1143-4. Erratum in: Europace. 2019;21(8):1144. Erratum in: J Arrhythm. 2020;36(1):214. Erratum in: Europace. 2020;22(3):505.
5. Sapp JL, Tang ASL, Parkash R, et al. Catheter Ablation or Antiarrhythmic Drugs for Ventricular Tachycardia. N Engl J Med. 2025;392(8):737-47.
6. Maan A, Waseem M, Carter A, et al. Early vs. deferred catheter ablation of ventricular tachycardia in patients of ischaemic substrate: systematic review and meta-analysis of clinical outcomes. Eur Heart J Open. 2025;5(4):oeaf076.
7. Reddy RK, Samways JW, Howard JP, et al. Catheter Ablation for Ventricular Tachycardia After Myocardial Infarction: An Updated Meta-Analysis of Randomized Controlled Trials. JACC Clin Electrophysiol. 2025;11(5):1047-50.
8. Della Bella P, Baratto F, Vergara P, et al. Does Timing of Ventricular Tachycardia Ablation Affect Prognosis in Patients With an Implantable Cardioverter Defibrillator? Results From the Multicenter Randomized PARTITA Trial. Circulation. 2022; 145(25):1829-38.
9. Vergara P, Tzou WS, Tung R, et al. Predictive Score for Identifying Survival and Recurrence Risk Profiles in Patients Undergoing Ventricular Tachycardia Ablation: The I-VT Score. Circ Arrhythm Electrophysiol. 2018;11(12):e006730.
10. Maury P, Baratto F, Zeppenfeld K, et al. Radio-frequency ablation as primary management of well-tolerated sustained monomorphic ventricular tachycardia in patients with structural heart disease and left ventricular ejection fraction over 30%. Eur Heart J. 2014;35(22):1479-85.
11. Clemens M, Peichl P, Wichterle D, et al. Catheter Ablation of Ventricular Tachycardia as the First-Line Therapy in Patients With Coronary Artery Disease and Preserved Left Ventricular Systolic Function: Long-Term Results. J Cardiovasc Electrophysiol. 2015;26(10):1105-10.
12. Rademaker R, de Riva M, Piers SRD, et al. Excellent Outcomes After First-Line Ablation in Post-MI Patients With Tolerated VT and LVEF >35. JACC Clin Electrophysiol. 2024;10(11): 2303-11.
13. Hadjis A, Frontera A, Limite LR, et al. Complete Electroanatomic Imaging of the Diastolic Pathway Is Associated With Improved Freedom From Ventricular Tachycardia Recurrence. Circ Arrhythm Electrophysiol. 2020;13(9):e008651.

CHAPTER 79

Atrial Fibrillation and Long-term CV Outcome

Bhuban Majhi, Rajarshi Halder

ABSTRACT

Atrial fibrillation (AF) is the most common sustained cardiac arrhythmia worldwide and is associated with a large spectrum of long term cardiovascular (CV) harms including ischemic stroke, heart failure (HF), myocardial infarction (MI), cognitive decline, and increased mortality. Large registry data, most notably the REACH Registry, shows that AF co-existing with atherothrombosis roughly doubles the 4-year risk of CV-related death, MI or stroke, but still guideline-recommended anticoagulation remains underused in many settings. Population-based analyses from Denmark quantify age-specific risks and estimate life-years lost after AF diagnosis, revealing that younger patients may lose the greatest number of potential life years. Evidence from randomized trials and meta-analyses indicates that anticoagulation prevents stroke across a wide range of AF presentations, while rhythm-control strategies (including catheter ablation) and aggressive risk-factor management can reduce AF burden and, in selected populations, improve hard outcomes. Closing treatment gaps, refining risk stratification (including AF burden and age at diagnosis), and integrating multimodal care are main stay to reduce AF's long-term CV burden.

Keywords: Atrial fibrillation, thromboembolic stroke, tachycardia-induced cardiomyopathy, heart failure, catheter ablation, atrial remodeling.

INTRODUCTION

Atrial fibrillation (AF) is marked by chaotic electrical activation in the atria, resulting in ineffective contractions, irregular responses in the ventricles, and gradual changes in the structure and electrical function of the atria. This condition exhibits a range of variations (paroxysmal, persistent, and permanent) and can present in different ways (symptomatic, asymptomatic, and subclinical).

The occurrence of AF significantly increases with age, but it can also be seen in younger patients, particularly when there are accompanying health issues such as hypertension, coronary artery disease, diabetes, obesity, chronic kidney disease, and obstructive sleep apnea. Furthermore, it is becoming more commonly identified in active individuals (such as endurance athletes), those recovering from surgery, and individuals with a genetic inclination to cardiomyopathies.[1]

In addition to causing discomfort and diminishing quality of life, AF considerably heightens the risk of:

- Thromboembolic incidents (notably ischemic stroke)
- Heart failure (HF; which can be both a cause and an outcome)
- Myocardial infarction (MI)
- Cognitive impairment and dementia
- Overall mortality

As the global population ages, with advancements in arrhythmia detection and a rise in cardiometabolic health issues, AF presents a significant public health concern. Assessing its long-term effects and identifying modifiable risk factors are crucial for effective patient management and health system strategies.[2]

DISCUSSION

Epidemiology and Absolute Burden

The global prevalence of AF is currently estimated to be in the tens of millions, with forecasts indicating it could double by the year 2050. In certain regions, particularly in middle-income countries undergoing significant lifestyle and demographic changes, the age-adjusted incidence is on the rise.

As per *sex differences* concerned, women with AF face a heightened risk of stroke and a more significant impact on their quality of life, whereas men exhibit a higher overall prevalence of the condition.

According to *ethnic variations*, AF is more common in Caucasian populations, but its prevalence is rapidly increasing in Asian populations, with some studies suggesting that Asian patients may experience a greater risk of stroke.

Socioeconomic factors play a role as well, with lower socioeconomic status associated with inadequate AF detection, underutilization of anticoagulation treatments, and elevated complication rates.

Subclinical AF, frequently identified through devices such as pacemakers, implantable loop recorders, or wearable technology, has become a notable contributor to the disease burden. Research indicates that even brief episodes of AF (lasting minutes to hours) may increase thromboembolic risk, although this risk is lower compared to that of persistent AF.

The high prevalence of *comorbid conditions* such as hypertension, HF, chronic kidney disease, and diabetes amplifies both the overall cardiovascular (CV) risk and the complexity of management.[3]

Atrial Fibrillation and Long-term Cardiovascular Outcomes—Registry and Population Evidence

The REACH registry, which is an international cohort of outpatients with established atherothrombotic disease or multiple risk factors, found baseline AF in approximately 10% of participants and demonstrated an adjusted approximately 2 times higher 4-year risk of CV death, MI or stroke in patients with AF versus those without AF (18.9% vs. 9.4%).[4] Importantly, despite elevated risk, only approximately 50% of AF patients were anticoagulated at 4 years, indicating a critical treatment gap. These findings underscore that AF in the context of systemic atherothrombosis identifies a particularly vulnerable population.

More recently, national register analyses from Denmark have measured age-specific links between AF diagnosis and later CV events and deaths. These studies show that AF carries significant extra risks at all ages. The median age for an AF diagnosis was 72.2 years. When life expectancy is factored in the loss of expected life years is highest in patients diagnosed at younger ages. As per the entire cohort, the loss of life years by age at AF diagnosis was as follows: Those diagnosed at or before 30 years lost approximately 11.3 years (95% CI 11.0–11.6). Those diagnosed at or before 60 years lost about 7.4 years (95% CI 7.3–7.5). These findings highlight that early-onset AF is serious and that looking at population-level measures, such as life years lost, offers important insights beyond just relative risk metrics.[2]

Mechanisms Linking Atrial Fibrillation to Adverse Outcomes

Thromboembolism

Disruption of organized atrial contraction results in blood stasis, particularly in the left atrial appendage, which promotes the formation of clots.

Heart Failure

Increased rapid and irregular ventricular rates, along with the absence of atrial contribution to ventricular filling, can trigger or exacerbate HF. Persistent AF can lead to tachycardia-induced cardiomyopathy, which may improve with rhythm or rate management.[2] Moreover, AF induces AF.[5]

Worsening Valvular Heart Disease

Chronic AF alters the structure of the atria and their annulus, leading to mitral and tricuspid regurgitation (MR/TR) even when the leaflets appear nearly normal and left ventricular size is often maintained—referred to as atrial functional mitral regurgitation (AFMR) and atrial functional tricuspid regurgitation (A-FTR). The underlying mechanisms involve atrial cardiomyopathy, dilation of the annulus (resulting in the loss of saddle shape/planarity in MR and an increase in the anterior-posterior dimension for TR) and compromised atrial contraction; pulmonary hypertension and increased right-sided volume load further exacerbate TR.

Pulmonary hypertension—AF contributes to group 2 pulmonary hypertension due to left heart disease through several mechanisms:

- Loss of the atrial contraction, known as "atrial kick," leads to decreased left ventricular filling efficiency and increased left atrial pressure.
- An irregular ventricular rhythm causes fluctuating filling of the left ventricle, resulting in congestion in the pulmonary veins.
- Atrial remodeling and dilation of the annulus create functional mitral regurgitation or tricuspid regurgitation, leading to volume and pressure overload in the pulmonary circuit.
- An increase in right ventricular afterload occurs due to chronic pulmonary venous hypertension, which can eventually result in right-sided HF.

If the pulmonary vasculature undergoes remodeling due to sustained high pressures, this ongoing postcapillary pulmonary hypertension may evolve into a combination of precapillary and postcapillary pulmonary hypertension.

Atherosclerosis and Inflammation

Atrial fibrillation is linked to systemic inflammation, impaired endothelial function, and a prothrombotic environment. These factors play a role in the onset and advancement of coronary artery disease and other vascular complications.

Impaired Coronary Microcirculation/ Microvascular Angina

Atrial fibrillation disrupts the coronary microcirculation by causing irregular ventricular rhythms and the absence of atrial systole, both of which decrease the necessary perfusion time and pressure gradient for optimal subendocardial blood flow. Experimental models confirm the rapid onset of microvascular dysfunction and oxidative stress, highlighting the immediate hemodynamic effects of AF.

The simultaneous activation of the sympathetic nervous system and increased levels of vasoactive mediators further intensify microvascular constriction. At a molecular level, AF triggers endothelial dysfunction through inflammation and thromboinflammatory processes, which hinder nitric oxide-mediated vasodilation. These interrelated factors significantly reduce coronary flow reserve, leading to subclinical ischemia, exacerbating the progression of HFpEF, and deteriorating long-term CV outcomes.

Peripheral Artery Disease Progression

Atrial fibrillation is linked to a greater occurrence and quicker advancement of peripheral artery disease (PAD), probably because of common atherosclerotic risk factors and overall inflammation in the body. In patients with AF, PAD leads to a poorer outlook, heightening the likelihood of ischemic and bleeding complications.

Neurocognitive Decline

Asymptomatic cerebral infarcts and microvascular damage associated with AF are connected to a heightened risk of dementia, even among individuals without clear stroke symptoms.

Sudden Cardiac Death

Although AF typically is not the primary factor leading to sudden cardiac death (SCD), it indicates an arrhythmogenic environment in individuals with cardiomyopathy or structural heart conditions. Research indicates that patients with AF have an increased risk of SCD, particularly those with HF or left ventricular (LV) dysfunction.

Atrial Fibrillation Phenotype and Burden: Prognostic Importance

Atrial fibrillation is heterogeneous. Paroxysmal, persistent, and permanent patterns differ in arrhythmic burden and prognostic implications. Device-based studies show a link between AF burden, which includes the percentage of time in AF or the length of the longest episodes, and the chances of stroke, HF, and death. Progression from paroxysmal to persistent or permanent AF leads to higher event rates. Therefore, measuring AF burden and preventing its progression are key goals for better long-term outcomes.[6,7]

Interventions that Modify Long-term Outcome

Anticoagulation and Stroke Prevention

Randomized trials, meta-analyses, and guidelines consistently show that oral anticoagulants (OACs) reduce ischemic stroke risk in nonvalvular AF compared with no anticoagulation or antiplatelet therapy. Direct oral anticoagulants (DOACs) are generally preferred over vitamin K antagonists (VKAs) for their equal or superior efficacy, better safety, and ease of use. Trials in device-detected (subclinical) AF—ARTESiA and NOAH-AFNET 6—show that OACs lower stroke risk but increase bleeding, requiring individualized decisions.[8] Real-world data (e.g., REACH) indicates underuse of OACs in eligible patients.

The 2024 ESC guidelines highlight:

- Avoid switching between DOACs or from DOAC to warfarin for secondary stroke prevention if already anticoagulated.
- In patients >75 years tolerating therapy with stable INR, warfarin may be preferred over DOACs (FRAIL-AF).
- Anticoagulation is recommended for all patients with hypertrophic cardiomyopathy and AF, regardless of CHA_2DS_2-VASc score.

Rhythm Control and Catheter Ablation

Historically, using antiarrhythmic drugs to control rhythm did not consistently lower mortality compared to rate control. However, recent evidence indicates that early rhythm control and catheter ablation can reduce AF burden and may improve severe outcomes in certain groups of patients. The CASTLE-AF trial showed that ablation led to fewer composite death or HF hospitalizations compared to medical therapy. Other trials and meta-analyses also showed improved quality of life, fewer HF hospitalizations, and in some cases, lower mortality. Large pragmatic trials, such as CABANA,[9] produced mixed results, but post-hoc analyses and pooled data suggest benefits for specific patient groups. Overall, ablation is increasingly seen as a treatment that can change outcomes for carefully chosen patients, particularly those with HF or early symptomatic AF, but there is no proof of universal benefits for all AF patients.[10]

Risk Factor Management and Guideline-directed Medical Therapy

Aggressive treatment of hypertension, obesity, diabetes, sleep apnea, and alcohol intake lowers the incidence, recurrence, and progression of AF. Current HF therapies, such as SGLT-2 inhibitors and angiotensin-neprilysin inhibitors, seem to improve arrhythmia burden and outcomes. Care models that include stroke prevention, symptom control, ablation when needed, and management of other comorbidities show promise for better long-term results.[11]

Special Considerations—Age at Diagnosis and Young Atrial Fibrillation

The studies from Denmark and related editorials indicate that AF diagnosed at a younger age carries considerable long-term risks and results in a significant number of life-years lost. A comprehensive study revealed that the incidence of AF grows with advancing age, beginning at around 0.9 cases per 1,000 person-years among people aged 40 to 49, and escalating to 17.7 cases per 1,000 person-years in individuals aged 70 and older.[12] Potential factors include a genetic predisposition to cardiomyopathy in those with early-onset AF, increased lifetime exposure to AF burden, and the possibility of undiagnosed comorbidities in some young patients. This information emphasizes the importance of timely evaluation and customized care for younger patients with AF. Nevertheless, the screening methods and overall advantages of early invasive treatments for asymptomatic young individuals still need further investigation.[13]

Gaps, Challenges, and Research Priorities

Despite the existence of effective treatments, there are various gaps which limit the conversion of trial advantages into improved population outcomes.

Inadequate Use of Anticoagulation and Unsuitable Combinations

Registry studies, including REACH and others, indicate insufficient use of anticoagulation and a common tendency to prescribe antiplatelet medications simultaneously. Current guidelines highlight the preference for DOAC and advise reducing unnecessary combinations of OACs and antiplatelets.[14]

Lack of Diverse Representation in Clinical Trials

Numerous randomized trials fail to sufficiently include patients with multivessel atherothrombosis, recent acute coronary syndrome (ACS), or complex health conditions, limiting their direct relevance to high-risk real-world populations.[4]

Limitations in Risk Stratification Accuracy

The CHA_2DS_2-VASc and HAS-BLED scores are practical yet have shortcomings. A research study conducted in the UK demonstrated the predictive effectiveness of the CHA_2DS_2-VA score when compared to CHA_2DS_2-VASc in pinpointing AF patients who truly have a low risk of stroke and therefore do not need oral anticoagulation. The guidelines also noted that the application of CHA_2DS_2-VASc excludes individuals who identify as nonbinary, transgender, or are receiving sex hormone therapy.[15] Innovative models and machine-learning approaches show potential for improved personalized risk assessment but require validation and implementation in future prospective studies.

CONCLUSION

Atrial fibrillation is not simply a harmless rhythm irregularity; it is a complex, progressive disorder that indicates a greater CV risk. The long-term effects of AF go well beyond mere palpitations or temporary discomfort and include a wide range of serious outcomes, such as ischemic stroke, HF, MI, cognitive decline, dementia, the progression of chronic kidney disease, and an increase in overall mortality rates. The Danish nationwide cohort study revealed important age-related patterns in absolute and excess CV risks. For cardiomyopathy of any type, younger patients had higher absolute risks than older patients—1.81% (95% CI 1.57–2.05) at ≤50 years versus 0.63% (95% CI 0.55–0.70) at >80 years. Dilated cardiomyopathy occurred in 1.02% of those ≤50 years and 0.31% of those >80 years, while hypertrophic cardiomyopathy rates were 0.36% and 0.19%, respectively. HF risk rose sharply with age (6.69% in ≤50 years to 22.2% in >80 years), as did ischemic stroke (1.59% to 6.92%) and mortality. In terms of excess risk compared with matched controls, cardiomyopathy showed the greatest relative excess in the youngest group, while HF and mortality excesses increased with age; ischemic stroke excess peaked in the 50–60-year age group.

Data from major registries, randomized controlled trials, and real-world studies have shifted our perception of AF from being solely an arrhythmia issue to a systemic condition with extensive implications for hemodynamics, thromboembolism, inflammation, and the neurohormonal system. The finding that younger individuals with AF may lose more years of life compared to older patients underscores the need for early diagnosis and proactive management to alleviate symptoms and prevent a series of long-term complications.

Looking ahead, the use of wearable technology, ongoing rhythm monitoring, AI-based risk assessment, and genomic profiling offers the potential for a more individualized and proactive strategy for managing AF. Future health policies must emphasize equitable access to these innovations, reduce disparities in diagnosis and treatment, and promote extensive prevention initiatives targeting population-level risk factor management.

Ultimately, effectively tackling AF calls for a shift in perspective—moving from viewing it purely as an electrical issue to acknowledging it as a sign of systemic CV illness. A coordinated, multidisciplinary, and patient-centered approach, grounded in both precision medicine and public health principles, has the potential to significantly lessen the global impact of AF and its severe downstream effects.

REFERENCES

1. Van Gelder IC, Rienstra M, Bunting KV, et al. 2024 ESC Guidelines for the management of atrial fibrillation developed in collaboration with the European Association for Cardio-Thoracic Surgery (EACTS). Eur Heart J. 2024;45:3314-414.
2. Paludan-Müller C, Vad OB, Stampe NK, et al. Atrial fibrillation: age at diagnosis, incident cardiovascular events, and mortality. Eur Heart J. 2024;45:2119-29.

3. Vinter N, Cordsen P, Paaske Johnsen S, et al. Temporal trends in lifetime risks of atrial fibrillation and its complications between 2000 and 2022: Danish, nationwide, population based cohort study. BMJ. 2024;385:e077209.
4. Ruff CT, Bhatt DL, Steg PG, et al. Long-term cardiovascular outcomes in patients with atrial fibrillation and atherothrombosis in the REACH Registry. Int J Cardiol. 2014;170:413-8.
5. Wijffels MC, Kirchhof CJ, Dorland R, et al. Atrial fibrillation begets atrial fibrillation. A study in awake chronically instrumented goats. AHAJ. 1995;92(7):1954-68.
6. Isabelle CVG, Michiel R, Karina VB, et al. 2024 ESC Guidelines for the management of atrial fibrillation developed in collaboration with the European Association for Cardio-Thoracic Surgery (EACTS). Eur Heart J. 2024;45(36):3314-414.
7. Jeanne EP, Tristram DB, Kristi HM, et al. Recurrence of Atrial Fibrillation After Catheter Ablation or Antiarrhythmic Drug Therapy in the CABANA Trial. JACC. 2020;75:20.
8. Schnabel RB, Benezet-Mazuecos J, Becher N, et al. Anticoagulation in device-detected atrial fibrillation with or without vascular disease: a combined analysis of the NOAH-AFNET 6 and ARTESiA trials. Eur Heart J. 2024;45(46):4902-16.
9. Poole JE, Bahnson TD, Monahan KH, et al. Recurrence of Atrial Fibrillation After Catheter Ablation or Antiarrhythmic Drug Therapy in the CABANA Trial. J Am Coll Cardiol. 2020;75(25):3105-18.
10. Marrouche NF, Brachmann J, Andresen D, et al. Catheter Ablation for Atrial Fibrillation with Heart Failure. New England Journal of Medicine. 2018;378(5):417-27.
11. Rienstra M, Tzeis S, Bunting KV, et al. Spotlight on the 2024 ESC/EACTS management of atrial fibrillation guidelines: 10 novel key aspects. Europace. 2024;26(12):euae298.
12. Morseth B, Geelhoed B, Linneberg A, et al. Age-specific atrial fibrillation incidence, attributable risk factors and risk of stroke and mortality: results from the MORGAM Consortium. Open Heart. 2021;8(2):e001624.
13. Steinberg BA. Atrial fibrillation and long-term cardiovascular outcomes: bringing the whole picture into focus. Eur Heart J. 2024;45:2130-2.
14. Dan GA, Martinez-Rubio A. The 2024 European Society of Cardiology Atrial Fibrillation Guidelines: A Moving Goalpost. Eur Cardiol Rev. 2025;20:e01.
15. Boriani G, Vitolo M, Mei DA. CHA_2DS_2-VA instead of CHA_2DS_2-VASc for stroke risk stratification in patients with atrial fibrillation: not just a matter of sex. EP Europace. 2024;26(11).

CHAPTER 80

Effect of Left Atrial Dyssynchrony on Long-term Clinical Outcomes during Cardiac Resynchronization Therapy

Anil Mishra

ABSTRACT

Left atrial (LA) mechanical dyssynchrony—temporal dispersion of mechanical activation within the left atrium—is increasingly recognized as an important marker of atrial remodeling and a potential mediator of adverse clinical outcomes in heart failure (HF). Cardiac resynchronization therapy (CRT) is a proven therapy for selected patients with heart failure with reduced ejection fraction (HFrEF) and electrical ventricular dyssynchrony, improving mortality, heart failure hospitalizations, and ventricular remodeling. However, up to 30% of patients do not respond to therapy. Recent data suggest CRT can modify LA mechanics and dyssynchrony, and that baseline LA dyssynchrony and its change after CRT are associated with long-term outcomes. This chapter tries to summarize current knowledge on mechanisms linking LA dyssynchrony to outcomes, methods for quantifying LA dyssynchrony (with emphasis on speckle-tracking echocardiography), and clinical evidence connecting LA dyssynchrony to CRT response and long-term prognosis.[1-5]

Keywords: Left atrial dyssynchrony, cardiac resynchronization therapy, speckle tracking echocardiography, heart failure, atrial strain, CRT response, long-term outcomes.

INTRODUCTION

Heart failure remains a leading cause of morbidity and mortality worldwide. Cardiac resynchronization therapy (CRT) improves outcomes in appropriately selected patients with HFrEF with LVEF (≤35%) and ventricular conduction delay QRS (≥150 ms LBBB), by restoring more coordinated left ventricular (LV) contraction and improving hemodynamics.[6] Unfortunately, one-third of patients fail to demonstrate LV reverse remodeling after CRT.[7] This warrants improved patient selection using other means available. MADIT CRT trial had shown that a smaller baseline LA volume is independently associated with response to CRT therapy.[8,9] Speckle-tracking echocardiography (STE) allows a more comprehensive analysis of LA function that could be of additional value to predict CRT response. The effects of CRT on the left atrium (LA)—a chamber central to LV filling, atrial transport function, and arrhythmogenesis—have received increasing attention because LA structure and function are tightly coupled to LV diastolic function and filling pressures. LA mechanical dyssynchrony refers to regional timing differences in LA contraction/relaxation across atrial segments and can be measured noninvasively, typically using STE or tissue Doppler techniques. Growing evidence indicates that LA dyssynchrony may reflect both electrical and mechanical atrial remodeling and be prognostically important for arrhythmia (especially atrial fibrillation) and overall cardiovascular outcomes. Importantly, CRT may reduce LA dyssynchrony in responders, suggesting LA mechanical behavior is modifiable and may mediate some of the long-term benefits (or lack thereof) of CRT.[5]

PHYSIOLOGY AND MECHANISMS LINKING LEFT ATRIAL DYSSYNCHRONY TO OUTCOMES

Atrial Mechanics and Ventricular Coupling

The LA serves three functional phases: Reservoir (during LV systole), conduit (during early LV diastole), and booster pump (atrial contraction contributing to late diastolic LV filling).[10] The ejection of blood therefore takes place in three phases. In early diastole by passive contraction (elastic recoil), in late diastole by active contraction (booster pump) and conduit phase starting after mitral valve opening until active LA contraction **(Fig. 1)**. The first two can be measured by LA strain imaging (STE) but conduit function cannot be measured by strain imaging.[11]

Disruption in the timed activation or relaxation of atrial regions perturbs these phases, reduces effective atrial contribution to ventricular filling, and increases atrial and pulmonary venous pressures. Chronic elevations in LA pressure and volume stimulate structural remodeling (fibrosis and myocyte hypertrophy) and electrical heterogeneity, creating a substrate for atrial tachyarrhythmias and further mechanical inefficiency.

Origins of Left Atrial Dyssynchrony

Left atrial dyssynchrony may arise from several interrelated processes:

- *Electrical conduction abnormalities:* Interatrial conduction delay (e.g., interatrial block) or regional conduction slowing (fibrosis) causes time dispersion of atrial activation.
- *Mechanical coupling to ventricular dyssynchrony:* Mechanistically, LA reservoir strain (LARS) is tightly coupled to LV longitudinal shortening, since the two chambers are anatomically connected, and in systole, the LV thereby exerts a direct stretching effect on the atrium. LV conduction delay (e.g., LBBB) and resultant mechanical discoordination alter left-sided filling patterns and transmit abnormal load to the LA. Recent mechanistic work shows LBBB can cause LA dyssynchrony via altered LV–LA interactions. LA strain is a mirror image of LV strain.[12]

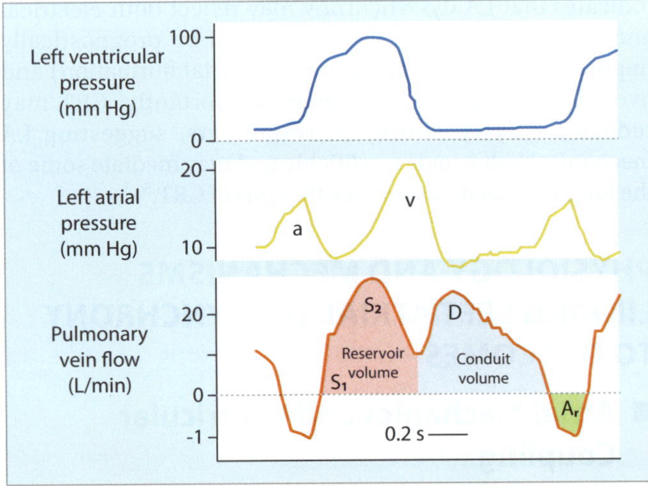

FIG. 1: Intraoperative recordings of LV and LA pressures (by micromanometers) and pulmonary venous flow (by flowmeter) in a patient prior to coronary artery bypass surgery. Red and blue colored areas represent volumes entering the LA as reservoir and conduit volumes, respectively. The area labeled Ar marks flow reversal during LA contraction.

(LA: left atrium; LV: left ventricle)

Source: With permission from Smiseth OA, Baron T, Marino PN, et al(2022).[2]

- *Structural remodeling and fibrosis:* Atrial fibrosis produces heterogeneity in contraction and relaxation kinetics, worsening mechanical dyssynchrony and promoting arrhythmia.
- *Intrinsic atrial cardiomyopathy:* Progressive atrial myopathy in HF impairs synchronous mechanics even without predominant conduction defects.

Pathophysiologic Consequences

Left atrial dyssynchrony reduces effective atrial pump function (decreased booster contribution) and reservoir efficiency, promoting elevated pulmonary venous pressure, symptoms of congestion, exercise intolerance, and risk of AF—all contributors to poorer long-term outcomes. Because LA dysfunction both reflects and contributes to LV diastolic dysfunction, LA dyssynchrony is plausibly a marker and mediator of adverse prognosis.[12]

METHODS TO QUANTIFY LEFT ATRIAL DYSSYNCHRONY

Imaging Modalities

- *Speckle-tracking echocardiography:* Two-dimensional STE-derived longitudinal strain is widely used to quantify regional atrial deformation and timings (time to peak strain for different segments), allowing calculation of a standard deviation or range of times to peak as a dyssynchrony metric. STE is angle independent, validated for myocardial deformation assessment, and practical for atrial analysis with contemporary software.[13] In addition, STE systolic strain could be used to identify area of scar.[14] LA strain typically is measured using a nonforeshortened apical four-chamber view **(Fig. 2)**. Due to presence of LA

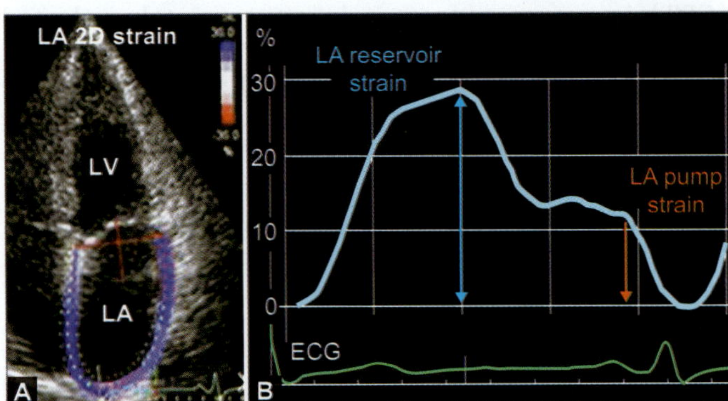

FIGS. 2A AND B: Left atrial strain by speckle tracking echocardiography. (A) echocardiographic image (apical four-chamber view) showing the left ventricle (LV) and left atrium (LA) with color-coded region of interest for LA strain. (B) LA strain trace along with ECG. Reservoir strain is indicated by the blue arrow and pump strain by the red arrow.

(ECG: electrocardiogram)

Source: With permission from Smiseth OA, Baron T, Marino PN, et al (2022).[2]

appendage and pulmonary veins, assessment of proximal third (roof) of LA is challenging and not used routinely. Key parameters include peak atrial longitudinal strain (PALS), time-to-peak strain (TPS) across LA segments, and standard deviation or range of TPS as a dyssynchrony index. Typically, 12 LA segments are analyzed from apical views. Dyssynchrony is defined as the standard deviation of TPS across these segments. A higher value indicates greater temporal dispersion. Corresponding to three functional phases of LA, reservoir phase, conduit phase, and contraction phase (booster pump) on STE there are three strain phases—LA reservoir strain, conduit strain, and LA contraction (pump) strain on STE **(Fig. 2)**. Though LA reservoir strain (LARS/LASr) and LA contraction (LACS/LASp) strain can be measured easily, the conduit strain cannot be measured easily. LARS is calculated from LV-end diastole and LA pump strain after onset of the p-wave in the electrocardiogram at the sharp downslope of the strain trace, as recommended in the American Society of Echocardiography/European Association of Cardiovascular Imaging consensus report and most recent expert statement.[15,16] LARS is closely linked to LV longitudinal shortening, since the two chambers are anatomically connected. LA pressure as reflected in pulmonary capillary wedge pressure, contractility of LA, and LA volume (LAV) are other independent determinants of LARS **(Fig. 3)**.

- *Tissue doppler imaging (TDI):* It measures regional myocardial velocities and timing. Its application is limited by its inability to differentiate active from passive motion, and it is angle-dependent and therefore less widely favored for atrial dyssynchrony than STE.[17,18]
- *Three-dimensional echocardiography (3DE):* Emerging for LA volumetry and regional timing but limited by spatial/temporal resolution for detailed dyssynchrony measures[19]
- *Cardiac MRI:* It offers excellent tissue characterization (fibrosis via late gadolinium enhancement) and can infer dyssynchrony; In the study by Kowallick et al.,[20] they sought to evaluate the efficacy and reproducibility of CMR

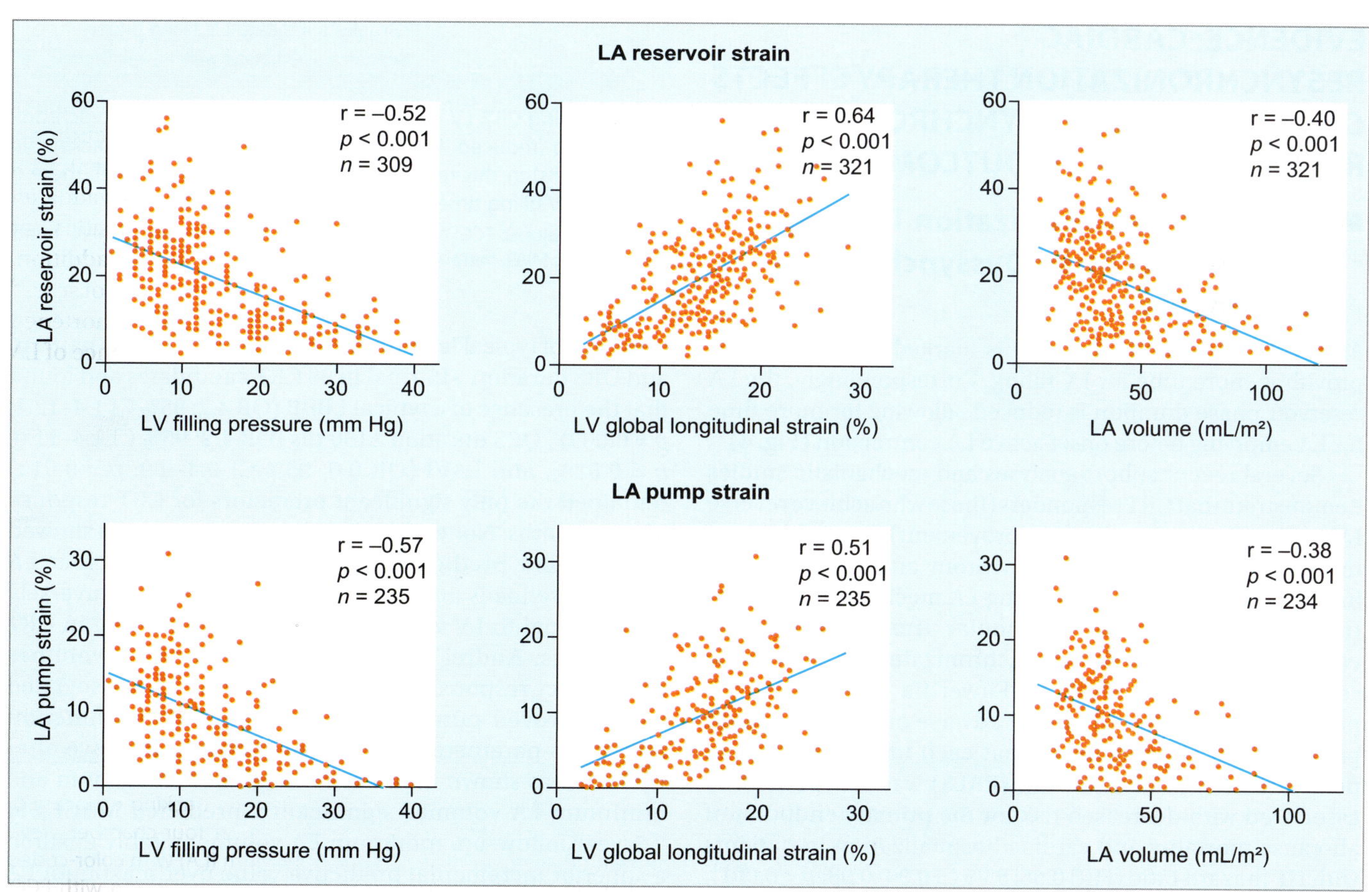

FIG. 3: Determinants of left atrium (LA) strain: relationships between LA reservoir strain (upper panels) and pump strain (lower panels) and their determinants. Data from a multicenter study of 322 patients with cardiovascular disease of different etiologies.

Source: Reproduced with permission from Inoue K, Khan FH, Remme EW, et al. Determinants of left atrial reservoir and pump strain and use of atrial strain for evaluation of left ventricular filling pressure. Eur Heart J Cardiovasc Imaging. 2021;23(1):61-70.

in appraising LA strains and strain rates. They showed that CMR is able to accurately assess LA longitudinal strain and strain rates using standard cine-CMR images. However, routine use for dynamic timing metrics is less established.

- *Cardiac CT:* It gives excellent spatial and satisfactory temporal resolution, useful for planning of percutaneous procedures such as TAVI, LA appendage closure, and AF ablation. Its use in detecting LA dyssynchrony is limited, because of radiation and need for iodinated contrast and its role in clinical evaluation is not established.[21]

Practical Considerations and Reproducibility

Measurement of LA dyssynchrony demands high frame rates, careful delineation of atrial endocardium, and consistent timing reference (commonly QRS onset or onset of LV systole). Intervendor variability and software algorithms produce heterogeneity among studies. Nevertheless, STE-based measures have acceptable reproducibility in experienced labs and are used in contemporary research.[13]

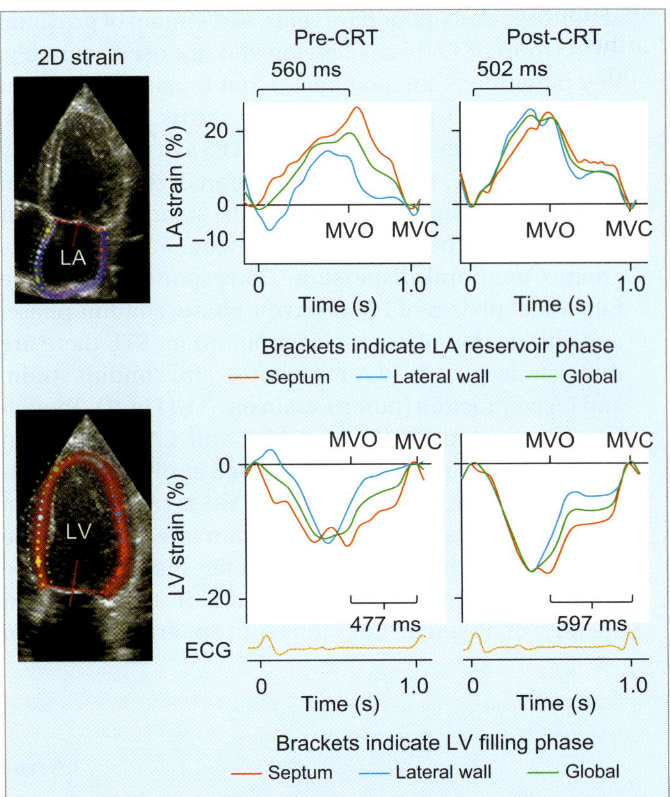

FIG. 4: During CRT, LV resynchronization results in LA resynchronization with reduced LA reservoir phase duration (brackets in upper panels) in this representative responder. In parallel, there is increased LV filling time (brackets in lower panels).

(2D: 2-dimensional; ECG: electrocardiogram; LV: left ventricular; MVC: mitral valve closure; MVO: mitral valve opening)

EVIDENCE: CARDIAC RESYNCHRONIZATION THERAPY EFFECTS ON LEFT ATRIAL DYSSYNCHRONY AND RELATIONSHIP WITH OUTCOMES

Cardiac Resynchronization Therapy Reduces Left Atrial Dyssynchrony in Responders

After CRT, LV systolic duration is markedly reduced, thus providing more time for LV filling. Correspondingly, the LA reservoir phase duration is reduced, allowing for more time for LA emptying before onset active LA contraction **(Fig. 4)**.

Several recent cohort analyses and mechanistic studies demonstrate that CRT responders (those who achieve reverse LV remodeling or functional improvement) frequently show marked reductions in LA dyssynchrony and improvements in atrial strain indices, suggesting LA mechanical behavior tracks with improved ventricular timing and filling conditions after effective resynchronization. A systematic review and meta-analysis by Fuwei Jia et al.[22] of 7,787 patients in 17 studies to predict adverse outcomes in adult patients with HF concluded that each unit increment of peak atrial longitudinal strain (PALS) was independently associated with decreased risk for the primary endpoint of all-cause mortality and cardiac hospitalization in patients with HF [hazard ratio (HR) 0.96; 95% CI 0.94–0.98; $p < 0.001$]. A study by Sjoerd Bouwmeester et al.[23], studied Indexed LA volume (LAVI), LA reservoir strain (LASr), LV end-diastolic volume, and LV ejection fraction along with other known predictors of CRT response (gender, etiology of heart failure, presence of typical left bundle branch block (LBBB) pattern, and QRS duration >150 ms) in 99 CRT candidates and found that the presence of a typical LBBB (OR 4.2; 95% CI 1.4–12.1; $p = 0.009$), QRS duration ≥150 ms (OR 4.2; 95% CI 1.4–11.0; $p = 0.029$), and LAVI (OR 0.6; 95% CI 0.4–0.9; $p = 0.012$) remained the only significant predictors for CRT response after 3 months. None of the baseline LV parameters showed independent predictive value. They concluded that LA size at baseline is an independent predictor and inversely proportional to LV volumetric reverse remodeling in CRT candidates. Andrei Dan Radu et al.[5] found LA volumes can predict responsiveness to CRT, being also associated with improved outcome in these patients. LA function and strain parameters have been shown to improve after CRT.[5] It was shown that, even though both maximum and minimum LA volumes significantly predicted MACEs at 2.5-year follow-up, minimum LA volume notably ensured a superior incremental predictive value over maximum LA volume. A baseline indexed maximum LA volume of under 34 mL/m^2 predicted positive response to CRT.[24] Russo et al.[25] proved that 3D echocardiography-based LA volumes significantly predicted MACEs, while minimum LA volume was superior to other parameters and performed best. Further studies by Badran et al.,[26] Rossi et al.,[27] Koruth et al.,[28] and Lupu et al.[29] could all corelate maximum or minimum LA volumes to CRT response. The STAR (Speckle Tracking and Resynchronization) study[4] was the first prospective, multicenter study on association of speckle tracking strain dyssynchrony and EF response and long-term survival after CRT. It showed that speckle tracking short-axis radial strain and transverse strain from apical views were associated with favorable EF response to CRT and long-term outcome, while longitudinal and circumferential strains were less sensitive in detecting dyssynchrony; and that a lack of baseline radial or transverse dyssynchrony before CRT was significantly associated with serious unfavorable events. The association of dyssynchrony by speckle tracking radial strain with long-term outcome was also reported by Gorcsan et al.[30] in another study of 229 patients wherein a lack of dyssynchrony by radial strain was associated with unfavorable outcome in patients with shorter QRS duration of 120–150 ms. The study by Donal et al.[31] showed the positive impact of CRT on LA remodeling by improving left atrial total emptying fraction (LATF) and LAS-r (LARS) after implantation. A recently published study this year by Hammersboen et al.[32] showed that in CRT responders, reduction in LA dyssynchrony was substantially larger than in nonresponders (70 ± 99 ms versus 32 ± 94 ms; p <0.05). LA dyssynchrony before CRT was significantly associated with LV reverse remodeling after CRT in univariable analysis ($r = 0.27$; $p < 0.001$) **(Fig. 5)**.

However, in multivariable analysis including predictors of CRT response like LV dyssynchrony, QRS duration, and QRS morphology, LA dyssynchrony was not independently associated with LV reverse remodeling ($p = 0.068$) It further showed that combination of LARS ≥ 18% (preserved reservoir strain)and LA dyssynchrony ≤ 53 ms (resolved LA dyssynchrony) or LARS ≥ 18% with LA reservoir phase duration ≤ 516 ms after 6 months, identified patients with excellent long term survival HR 0.11(95% CI 0.03–0.42) **(Figs. 6A to D)**.

Study by Dokuni et al.[33] proved that, at 6 months after CRT implantation, patients who had a LARS of over 14.6% at follow-up had considerably better prognosis compared to others. Another study by Feneon et al.[34] followed to assess the predictive ability of LARS for LV reverse remodeling. They found that LARS was an independent predictor for positive response to CRT. In the study by Huntjens et al. conducted in patients who received CRT, increased values in LARS were correlated with event-free survival, while lower LARS was associated with MACEs.[35] In a study by Jan Stassen et al.,[36] the study cohort could finally be divided into three groups where the LARS and LVGLS could together predict the response to CRT: (i) No significant reverse remodeling (change in LVGLS <20% and change in LARS <5%; (ii) Incomplete reverse remodeling (change in LVGLS ≥ 20% or change in LARS ≥ 5%, but not both); and (iii) complete reverse modeling (change in LVGLS ≥ 20% and change in LARS ≥ 5%;

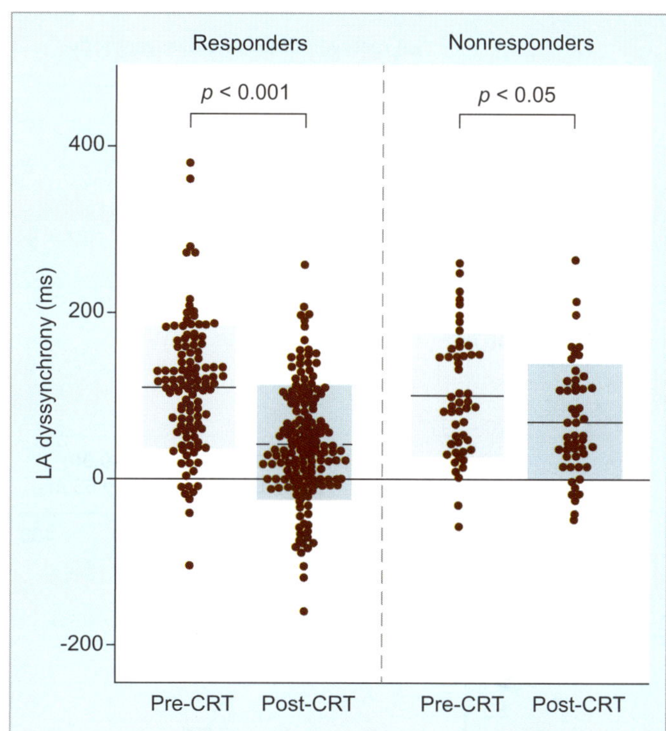

FIG. 5: LA dyssynchrony before and after CRT in responders and nonresponders.

Note: CRT response was associated with market reduction in LA dyssynchrony (left boxes). In contrast, in CRT nonrespnders there was only a modest reduction in LA dyssynchrony (right boxes). The central lines indicate the mean and the upper and lower edges of the SD.

(CRT: cardiac resynchronization therapy; LA: left artial)

Figs. 7A and B). A recent study in JACC Cardiovascular Imaging (2024) mechanistically linked LBBB-induced atrial dyssynchrony to ventricular conduction abnormalities and found that CRT responders had a pronounced decrease in LA dyssynchrony whereas nonresponders had little improvement, suggesting LA dyssynchrony is modifiable and associated with CRT response.[1]

Clinical Implications

Clinical application of LA mechanics by STE may be used to detect high-risk patients and predict prognosis in heart failure patients undergoing CRT. Improvement in LAVI, LVGLS, and/or LARS at 6 months post-CRT is independently associated with a lower risk of mortality. Patients with complete reverse remodeling have the lowest mortality risk when compared with patients showing incomplete or no significant reverse remodeling. This supports the use of integrated LA and LV deformation imaging to assess CRT response and may aid in the refinement of risk-stratification of patients treated with CRT. The assessment of LARS and LVGLS after CRT implantation may allow the identification of a subgroup of CRT recipients who might otherwise be

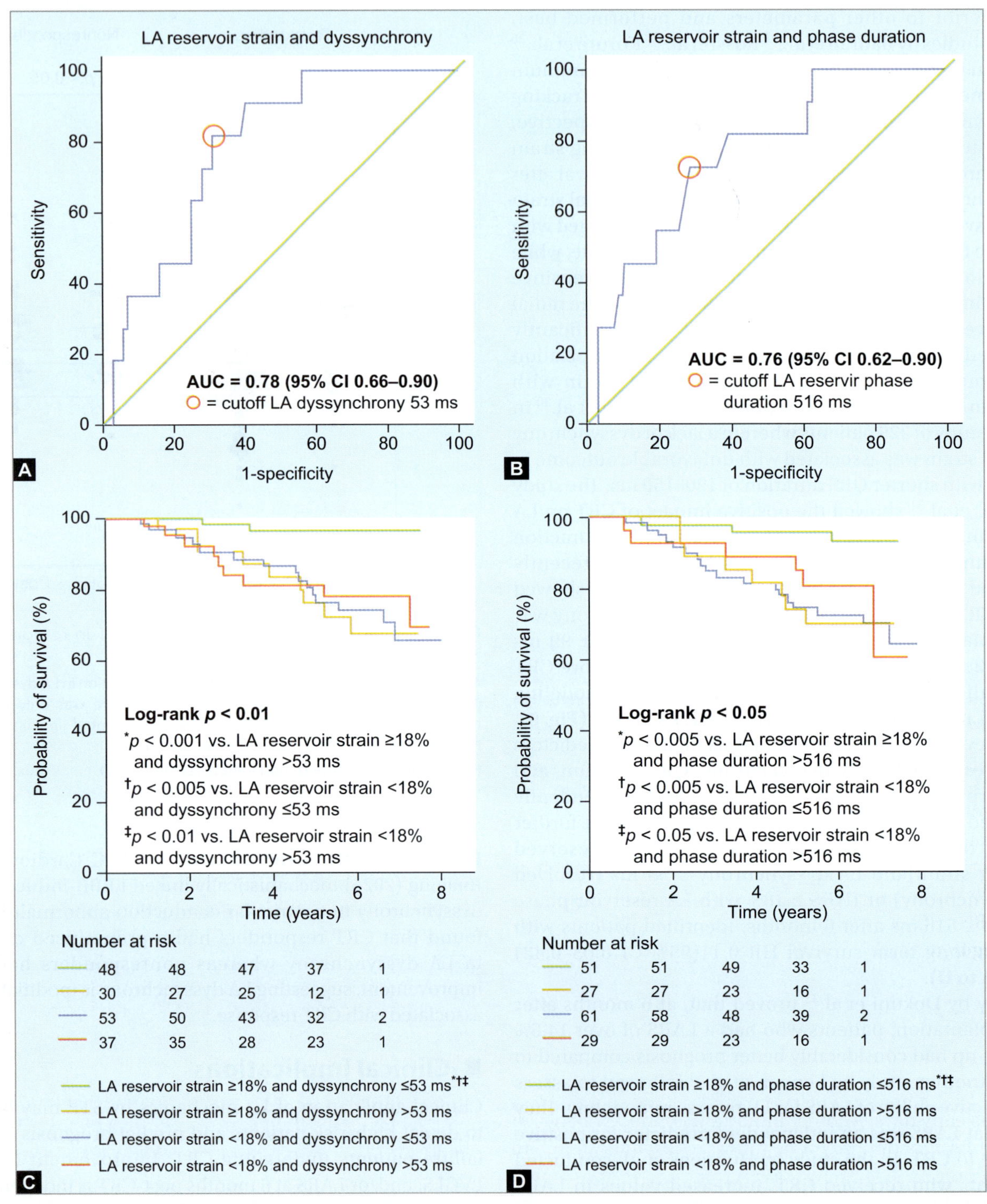

FIGS. 6A TO D: The figures shown are a under the receiver operating characteristic curves and Kaplan–Meier curves for long-term survival after CRT using LARS together with measures of LA dyssynchrony and reservoir phase duration. (A and B) Combination of LARS and LA dyssynchrony. (C and D) Combination of LARS and LA reservoir phase duration. The analysis used LARS ≥ 18%, LA dyssynchrony ≤ 53 ms, and LA reservoir phase duration ≤516 as cutoffs. Please note that results were essentially similar for LARS combined with LA dyssynchrony and LARS combined with reservoir phase duration. Both combinations identified patients with excellent long-term survival.

(AUC: area under the curve)

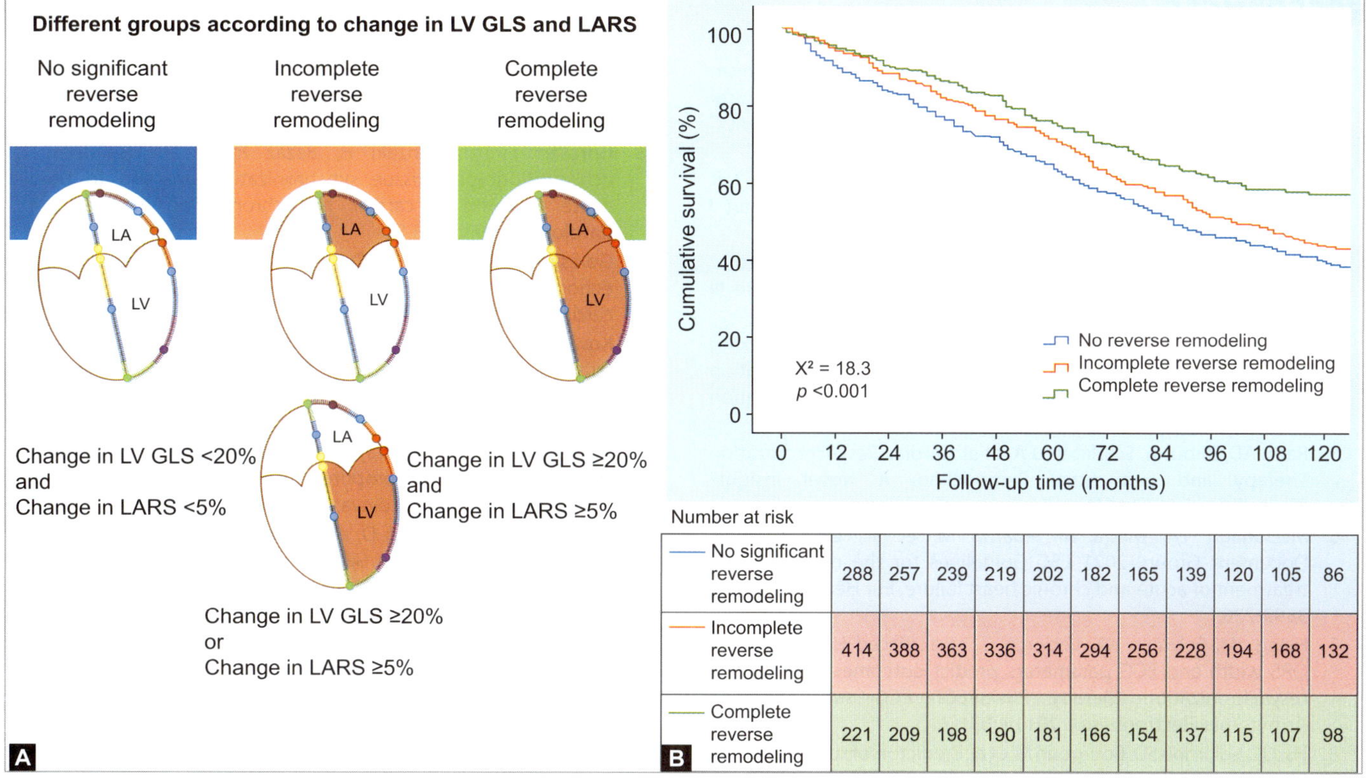

FIGS. 7A AND B: Patients showing complete reverse remodeling (improvement in LARS and LVGLS both) have better outcomes than those showing incomplete reverse remodeling (improvement in LARS or LVGLS, but not both) or no significant reverse remodeling (no improvement in LARS and LVGLS).

classified as responders by conventional criteria, but who will nevertheless experience suboptimal outcomes. The identification of such patients may argue for more intensive follow-up and allow the institution of therapies to optimize the effects of CRT, especially on LA and LV mechanics, e.g., use of ARNi, SGLT-2 inhibitors, treating atrial fibrillation, or mitral regurgitation.[13,37,38]

FUTURE CONSIDERATIONS

Emerging data report promising results regarding the link between CRT and LA remodeling, even though research is only in its early days. Another important connector between CRT and LA function might be mitral regurgitation, due to its impact on LA size, shape, and function. It is known that CRT might become useful in managing functional mitral regurgitation due to the fact that cardiac dyssynchrony aggravates the severity of regurgitation.[12] Further studies should assess whether reducing mitral regurgitant volume and fraction by CRT might lower the burden on LA volumes and functioning and possibly improve LV diastolic dysfunction.

CONCLUSION

Left atrial dyssynchrony is a newly emerging tool to predict and assess response to CRT. Speckle tracking echocardiography (STE) is easy to use, widely available, inexpensive, reproducable, and reliable means of measuring this dyssynchrony. Together with LAVI and LV GLS, LARS has proven to be important parameter to predict outcome and assess response to CRT. LA dyssynchrony, when resolved post-CRT and accompanied by preserved reservoir strain, is associated with significantly improved long-term outcomes. These findings underscore the importance of atrial mechanics in CRT response and survival. Restoring cardiac synchrony by CRT has positive impact on LA remodeling. In patients who are CRT responders, it reduces LA volumes, and it improves LA phasic functions and strain. Conversely, increased LA volumes and impaired LA strain are able to predict CRT responsiveness and outcome in these patients. Use of LA dyssynchrony by STE may help better selection of candidates for CRT and identify subjects who are likely to be partial responders or nonresponders and to initiate more intensive medical therapy and other interventions to address atrial fibrillation and or mitral regurgitation, which could both be contributing significantly to LA and LV dyssynchrony.

REFERENCES

1. Hammersboen LR, Stugaard M, Puvrez A, et al. Mechanism and Impact of Left Atrial Dyssynchrony on Long-Term Clinical Outcome During Cardiac Resynchronization Therapy. JACC Cardiovasc Imaging. 2025;18(4):421-32.
2. Smiseth OA, Baron T, Marino PN, et al. Imaging of the left atrium: pathophysiology insights and clinical utility. Eur Heart J Cardiovasc Imaging. 2022;23(1):2-13.
3. Cleland JG, Daubert JC, Erdmann E, et al. The Effect of Cardiac Resynchronization on Morbidity and Mortality in Heart Failure. N Engl J Med. 2005;352:1539-49.
4. Tanaka H, Nesser HJ, Buck T, et al. Dyssynchrony by speckle tracking echocardiography and response to cardiac resynchronization therapy: results of the Speckle Tracking and Resynchronization (STAR) study. Eur Heart J. 2010;31:1690-700.
5. Radu AD, Zlibut A, Scarlatescu A, et al. Cardiac Resynchronization Therapy and Left Atrial Remodeling: A Novel Insight? Biomedicines. 2023;11(4):1156.
6. McDonagh TA, Metra M, Adamo M, et al.; ESC Scientific Document Group. 2021 ESC Guidelines for the diagnosis and treatment of acute and chronic heart failure. Eur Heart J. 2021;42: 3599-726.
7. Hsing JM, Selzman KA, Leclercq C, et al. Paced left ventricular QRS width and ECG parameters predict outcomes after cardiac resynchronization therapy PROSPECT ECG substudy. Circ Arrhythmia Electrophysiol. 2011;4:851-7.
8. Hsu JC, Solomon SD, Bourgoun M, et al. Predictors of super-response to cardiac resynchronization therapy and associated improvement in clinical outcome: the MADIT-CRT (multicenter automatic defibrillator implantation trial with cardiac resynchronization therapy) study. J Am Coll Cardiol. 2012;59:2366-73.
9. Kuperstein R, Goldenberg I, Moss AJ, et al. Left atrial volume and the benefit of cardiac resynchronization therapy in the MADIT-CRT trial. Circ Heart Fail. 2014;7:154-60.
10. Blume GG, Mcleod CJ, Barnes ME, et al. Left atrial function: Physiology, assessment, and clinical implications. Eur J Echocardiogr. 2011;12:421-30.
11. Smiseth OA, Baron T, Marino PN, et al. Imaging of the left atrium: pathophysiology insights and clinical utility. Eur Heart J Cardiovasc Imaging. 2021;23:2-13.
12. Hammersboen LR, Stugaard M, Puvrez A, et al; Mechanism and Impact of Left Atrial Dyssynchrony on Long-Term Clinical Outcome During Cardiac Resynchronization Therapy. JACC Cardiovasc Imaging. 2025;18(4):421-32.
13. Zhang X, Ha S, Wang X, et al. Speckle tracking echocardiography: clinical applications in cardiac resynchronization therapy. Int J Clin Exp Med. 2015;8(5):6668-76.
14. Becker M, Hoffmann R, Kühl HP, et al. Analysis of myocardial deformation based on ultrasonic pixel tracking to determine transmurality in chronic myocardial infarction. Eur Heart J. 2006;27:2560-6.
15. Badano LP, Kolias TJ, Muraru D, et al. Standardization of left atrial, right ventricular, and right atrial deformation imaging using two dimensional speckle tracking echocardiography: a consensus document of the EACVI/ASE/industry task force to standardize deformation imaging. Eur Heart J Cardiovasc Imaging. 2018;19:591-600.
16. Voigt JU, Malaescu GG, Haugaa K, et al. How to do LA strain. Eur Heart J. Cardiovasc Imaging. 2020;21:715-7.
17. Bax JJ, Bleeker GB, Marwick TH, et al. Left ventricular dyssynchrony predicts response and prognosis after cardiac resynchronization therapy. J Am Coll Cardiol. 2004;44:1834-40.
18. Gorcsan J 3rd, Kanzaki H, Bazaz R, et al. Usefulness of echocardiographic tissue synchronization imaging to predict acute response to cardiac resynchronization therapy. Am J Cardiol. 2004;93:1178-81.
19. Gorcsan J III, Oyenuga O, Habib PJ, et al. Relationship of echocardiographic dyssynchrony to long-term survival after cardiac resynchronization therapy. Circulation. 2010;122:1910-8.
20. Kowallick JT, Kutty S, Edelmann F, et al. Quantification of left atrial strain and strain rate using Cardiovascular Magnetic Resonance myocardial feature tracking: A feasibility study. J Cardiovasc Magn Reson. 2014;16:60.
21. Szilveszter B, Nagy AI, Vattay B, et al. Left ventricular and atrial strain imaging with cardiac computed tomography: validation against echocardiography. J Cardiovasc Comput Tomogr. 2020;14:363-9.
22. Fuwei J, Chen A, Zhang D, et al. Prognostic Value of Left Atrial Strain in Heart Failure: A Systematic Review and Meta-Analysis. Front Cardiovasc Med. 2022;9:935103.
23. Bouwmeester S, Mast T, Prinzen F, et al. Predictive Value of Left Atrial Remodeling for Response to Cardiac Resynchronization Therapy. J Ultrason. 2022;22(90):e168-73.
24. Bytyçi I, Bajraktari G, Henein M. Left atrial volume index predicts response to cardiac resynchronisation therapy: A systematic review and meta-analysis. Arch. Med. Sci. 2020;18:930-8.
25. Russo C, Jin Z, Homma S, et al. LA Phasic Volumes and Reservoir Function in the Elderly by Real-Time 3D Echocardiography. JACC Cardiovasc. Imaging. 2016;10:976-85.
26. Badran HA, Abdelhamid M, Ibrahim MT, et al. Left atrium in cardiac resynchronization therapy: Active participant or innocent bystander. J Saudi Heart Assoc. 2017;29:259-69
27. Rossi L, Malagoli A, Piepoli M, et al. Indexed maximal left atrial volume predicts response to cardiac resynchronization therapy. Int J Cardiol. 2013;168:3629-33.
28. Koruth J, Shen X, Holmberg MJ, et al. The predictive value of left atrial volume in patients with wide QRS, left ventricular Dyssynchrony and cardiac resynchronization therapy. Chest. 2007;132:579A.
29. Lupu S, Mitre A, Sus I, et al. Changes in left atrial size and function early after cardiac resynchronization therapy as assessed by conventional two-dimensional echocardiography. Med. Ultrason. 2018;20:362.
30. Gorcsan J III, Oyenuga O, Habib PJ, et al. Relationship of echocardiographic dyssynchrony to long-term survival after cardiac resynchronization therapy. Circulation. 2010;122:1910-8.
31. Donal E, Tan K, Leclercq C, et al. Left Atrial Reverse Remodeling and Cardiac Resynchronization Therapy for Chronic Heart Failure Patients in Sinus Rhythm. J Am Soc Echocardiogr. 2009;22:1152-8.
32. Hammersboen LR, Stugaard M, Puvrez A, et al. Mechanism and Impact of Left Atrial Dyssynchrony on Long-Term Clinical Outcome During Cardiac Resynchronization Therapy. JACC: Cardiovasc Imaging 2025;18(4):421-32.
33. Dokuni K, Matsumoto K, Tatsumi K, et al. Cardiac resynchronization therapy improves left atrial reservoir function through resynchronization of the left atrium in patients with heart failure with reduced ejection fraction. Int J Cardiovasc Imaging. 2020;36:1203-12.

34. Feneon D, Behaghel A, Bernard A, et al. Left atrial function, a new predictor of response to cardiac resynchronization therapy? Heart Rhythm. 2015;12:1800-6.
35. Huntjens P, Sugahara M, Soyama, et al. Abstract 15815: Left Atrial Strain Characterizes the Atrio-ventricular Substrate Responsive to Cardiac Resynchronization Therapy in Patients with Intermediate Electrocardiographic Criteria. Circulation. 2020;142:A15815.
36. Stassen J, Galloo X, Chimed S, et al. Clinical implications of left atrial reverse remodelling after cardiac resynchronization therapy. Eur Heart J Cardiovasc Imaging. 2022;23:730-40.
37. Mazzetti S, Scifo C, Abete R, et al. Short-term echocardiographic evaluation by global longitudinal strain in patients with heart failure treated with sacubitril/valsartan. ESC Heart Fail. 2020;7:964-72.
38. Tsang TSM, Barnes ME, Abhayaratna WP, et al. Effects of quinapril on left atrial structural remodeling and arterial stiffness. Am J Cardiol. 2006;97:916-20.

CHAPTER

81

Divergence from Guideline Directed Management of Cardiac Implantable Electronic Device Infections

Ashish Nabar, Amit Vora

ABSTRACT

Cardiac implantable electrical device (CIED) infection occurs immediately or late in the postimplantation period. This can be in the form of pocket infection, lead endocarditis, or symptomatic bacteremia. While CIED extraction should be the standard of care, this is not uniformly offered, alternate and suboptimal management strategies are often followed. This can be disastrous due to the associated morbidity and mortality. In this chapter, various reasons for divergence from guideline-directed management of CIED infection are discussed. Imaging (transesophageal echocardiogram and FDG-PET/CT) and cultures (from blood, CIED pocket, and extracted hardware) supplement the clinical judgement for making a diagnosis of CIED infection. The bottom line is that early CIED extraction is the key and antibiotic cover is to be continued thereafter for 2–6 weeks depending on the nature of infection.

Keywords: Cardiac implantable electrical device, endocarditis, lead extraction.

INTRODUCTION

In the present-days cardiac implantable electrical devices (CIED) are implanted for bradyarrhythmias, prevention of sudden cardiac death (SCD) and heart failure. Further, patients with CIEDs outlast the battery longevity of their devices, thus needing repeat procedures, commonly for generator change, lead revision, or device upgrade. The risk of CIED infection in the early post-implant days and in the long-term are small but finite (1.2–3.4%), slightly more during repeat procedures.[1,2] CIED infection may be minor like suture line infection or major like pocket infection, lead/valve endocarditis and persistent bacteremia. Unfortunately, contemporary practice patterns, world over and in India, related to diagnosis and treatment of major CIED infections are inadequate and not in line with the guidelines.[3] A positive step in this regard would be to disseminate the recommendation from the EHRA consensus document[4] and refer to the published Indian registry data.[5] This chapter deals with the various reasons for inadequacies in management of CIED infections and dwells on methods to mitigate them.

INADEQUATE RECOGNITION OF INDICATION FOR CIED EXTRACTION

The extent and severity of CIED infection needs to be judged carefully and could be a continuous process requiring reassessments on outpatient basis or after a hospital admission. Only a suture line infection, in the early post-implant days, could heal well by wound management, including local debridement, as required, or by repeated sterile dressings at closer follow-ups. This is best handled by the implanting cardiologist and done with aseptic precautions in dedicated outpatient areas or operating suites intended for minor procedures. Another early post-implant scenario is a discharging pocket, where often times it gets difficult to decide if the extruded fluid is sterile serosanguinous or pus-like. A wound assessment for swelling, redness, pain/tenderness and sending the extruded material for culture would help.[6] An immediate discontinuation of anti-thrombotic, if not mandatory, would settle a serosanguinous discharge. However, a frankly purulent discharge or an exposed device/generator should be considered as a pocket infection and attempts to avert a CIED explantation/

extraction would eventually be futile. Similarly, a late device extrusion, even in absence of purulent discharge, should be assumed to be CIED infection warranting extraction. Echocardiography (to rule out lead vegetation-endocarditis) and blood cultures (to rule out bacteremia) should be the next step in a suspected CIED infection, a positive finding demands CIED extraction without delay.

CONFOUNDING CLINICAL SCENARIO

Even in a recipient of CIED implant, particularly in the tropics, endemic infections such as malaria, dengue, or viral infections are the provisional diagnosis in a febrile patient. On occasions, symptoms such as solitary fever spikes, chills, and night sweats may not get due attention from the patient or treating physician and thus delay suspicion of CIED infection. If the CIED pocket shows no signs of infective process, transthoracic echocardiogram (TTE) is unrevealing for a lead vegetation and blood cultures are negative; CIED infection may not be included as a differential diagnosis of fever. It is possible that in an elderly patient with comorbidities who is prone to other systemic infections, culture positive respiratory and urinary tract infections may be treated as the only cause of recurring fever. Small infective emboli from the CIED leads may be treated as pneumonia. I am aware of a CIED patient with unresolving fever who had a pet cat and positive immunology tests for *Bartonella*, this patient was treated for cat-scratch fever—a rare disease, while the CIED-related fever went undiagnosed for a while. In a hospitalized CIED patient, iatrogenic infections—like central or peripheral line infections may be incriminated as the cause of recurring fever and investigations directed at diagnosing endocarditis further delayed. Anorexia, weight loss, elevated procalcitonin levels, unrelenting risen CRP, low complement levels, thrombocytopenia, and microscopic hematuria should lead to investigations to rule out CIED infection.

COMORBIDITIES—A DAMPENER IN DECISION-MAKING

Higher age (octa- and nonagenarians) and higher frailty-index would induce reluctance to perform lead extraction procedures. Morbidity of the CIED extraction procedure is likely to be higher when the indication is pocket infection or device-related infection, as compared to lead extraction planned for an abandoned lead. Coexisting diabetes and renal insufficiency can respectively double and triple the CIED extraction procedure risk. It is important to remember the bottom-line in CIED infections; the morbidity and mortality is higher, irrespective of the baseline risk assessment, when CIED extraction is delayed or only long-term suppressive antibiotic therapy is used. Further, only a complete CIED system removal reduces the risk of relapsing infection to a low 0–4.2%; any partial removal or antibiotic treatment alone has a relapse rate of 50–100%.

PERSISTENT CULTURE-NEGATIVE STATUS

While culture positivity helps to confirm the diagnosis and make a most-appropriate antibiotic choice, a culture negative status can compel treatment with empiric broad spectrum antibiotic cover. If fever remains indolent in a culture-negative patient, despite the clinical scenario suspicious of CIED infection, decision-making regarding lead extraction can be delayed. Conversely, according to the EHRA consensus statement, if there is persistent bacteremia with alpha-or beta-hemolytic *Streptococcus* species, *Enterococcus* species, non-pseudomonal/*Serratia* gram-negative bacteria or *Pneumococcus* species in a CIED patient, extraction should be performed. This might seem a bold step in clinical settings where pocket is not infected and leads have no demonstrable vegetation. A close communication and guidance from an infectious disease specialist and clinical microbiologist is important. All possible samples should be cultured, including pus from the pocket and blood samples - particularly the latter samples should be sent multiple times and spaced out in time, collected during fever spikes and prior to or after a short discontinuation of antibiotic therapy. Longer incubation periods (>48–72 hours, for 1 week) and use of biomolecular techniques are some important tips to detect the culprit organism, particularly when fastidious microorganisms, e.g., HACEK are involved. Even a single positive culture with coagulase-negative staphylococci (CoNS) or gram-positive bacteria should be interpreted as specific for CIED infection.

EQUIVOCAL IMAGING DIAGNOSIS

In the early postimplantation days, distinguishing a pocket hematoma versus infection using ultrasound may be challenging. A 4–7 MHz probe showing echo-septation in the pocket and Doppler suggestive of increased vascularity would favor abscess formation. While small hematomas are a distinct present-day possibility related to scheduling CIED implants during continued, at times mandatory, use of antiplatelets, operating with therapeutic anticoagulation status, suboptimal surgical skills related to achieving good hemostasis and insistence on early discharge; distinguishing from a brewing pocket infection may need time.[7] TTE can easily miss a lead vegetation, particularly at blind-spots such as superior vena cava—right atrium junction. Trans-esophageal echocardiogram (TEE), initially and if required after a 1-week interval, would be more sensitive to localize lead or an associated native/prosthetic valve endocarditis **(Fig. 1)**. Again, there can be a difficulty in assigning the lead mass as thrombus versus vegetation, clinical profile of patient will provide the clue. Intracardiac echocardiogram is a still superior imaging modality, but its use may be restricted by

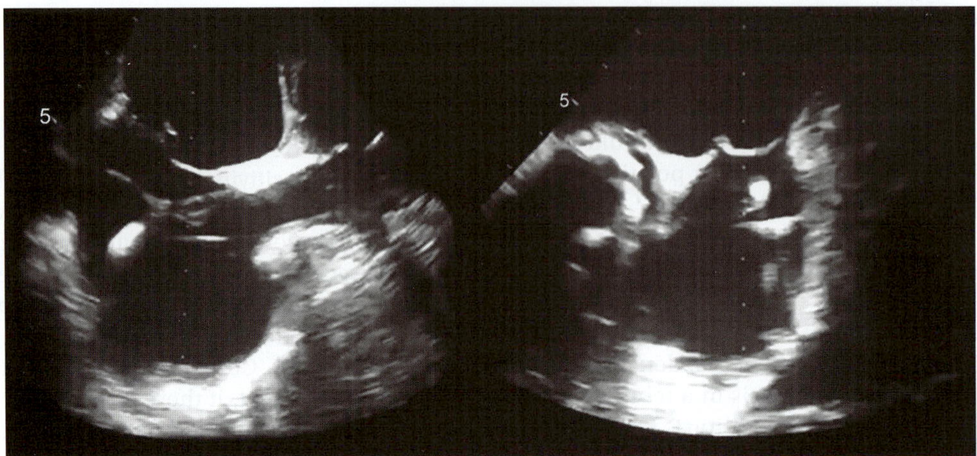

FIG. 1: Biplane transesophageal echocardiogram (TEE) showing vegetation of the atrial lead in a patient with dual chamber pacemaker.

very limited availability. Fluorine-18-fludeoxyglucose (FDG) positron emission tomography/computerized tomography (PET/CT) scanning, beyond the immediate postimplant 6-week period, may help to diagnose different aspects of CIED infection—pocket infection, lead/valve endocarditis, embolic/metastatic infection or entry site of infection. FDG PET/CT scan has a 93% specificity and 98% sensitivity for diagnosis but requires adequate preparation with a low carbohydrate—high fat diet to be interpreted correctly.

LACK OF FAMILIARITY WITH PUBLISHED GUIDELINES

The readers of this chapter are referred to the EHRA consensus paper published in the Europace journal (2020) and endorsed by multiple Heart Rhythm Societies.[4] This document updates knowledge regarding investigation and management of CIED infections beyond what was published in the Novel 2019.

INTERNATIONAL CIED INFECTION CRITERIA

It includes clear instructions for diagnosis of CIED infections by clinical findings, microbiology, and imaging. The consensus document advises to refer the patient to centers with CIED infection/extraction expertise. CIED extraction within 7 days of diagnosis followed by antibiotic therapy for an appropriate duration is uniformly advised for (A) isolated pocket infection with negative blood culture (2 weeks) or (B) Pocket + systemic infection with or without lead/valve endocarditis (4–6 weeks). It is important to disseminate this protocol to the implanting cardiologists and physicians responsible for follow-up care of the patient, thereby avoiding divergence from the recommendations. At times, there are divergences on certain points within the societal guidelines and therefore geography-specific registries should be one of the future considerations. One such Indian experience is the recently published—The Srinagar extraction registry—by Lone et al. **(Flowchart 1)**.

ATTENDING PHYSICIAN'S SPECIALTY—A REASON FOR LOW REFERRAL?

CIED infections are best managed by a cardiac electrophysiologist who can steer a multidisciplinary team by seeking opinions and choosing different diagnostic modalities to reach a diagnosis of definite or most probable CIED infection and then firmly counsel CIED extraction without undue delays.[8] The converse often happens. The generator pocket may be aspirated with a needle to draw the suspected pus collection for culture when it is strictly avoidable to vitiate the sterility of the implant site. Patients are often treated with multiple antibiotic regimens, simultaneously or serially, whether culture positive or empirically, with the hope of avoiding intervention; thus, working against the principle of source control. A pocket infection may progress to lead endocarditis, large vegetations would then contraindicate transcatheter lead extraction (TLE). Some cardiologists might consider salvage by pocket debridement and reimplantation of the device in the subpectoral plane, ultimately these patients require CIED extraction. In the contemporary era it would be a "step for the worse" to explant the generator and cut the leads hoping to have cleared the pocket of infected material.[9] These implant sites may develop a chronic-infected discharging sinus and TLE with cut lead(s) is now a technically difficult procedure. In the considered view of this author, in elderly patients, the delays worsen their nutritional and mental status irreparably.

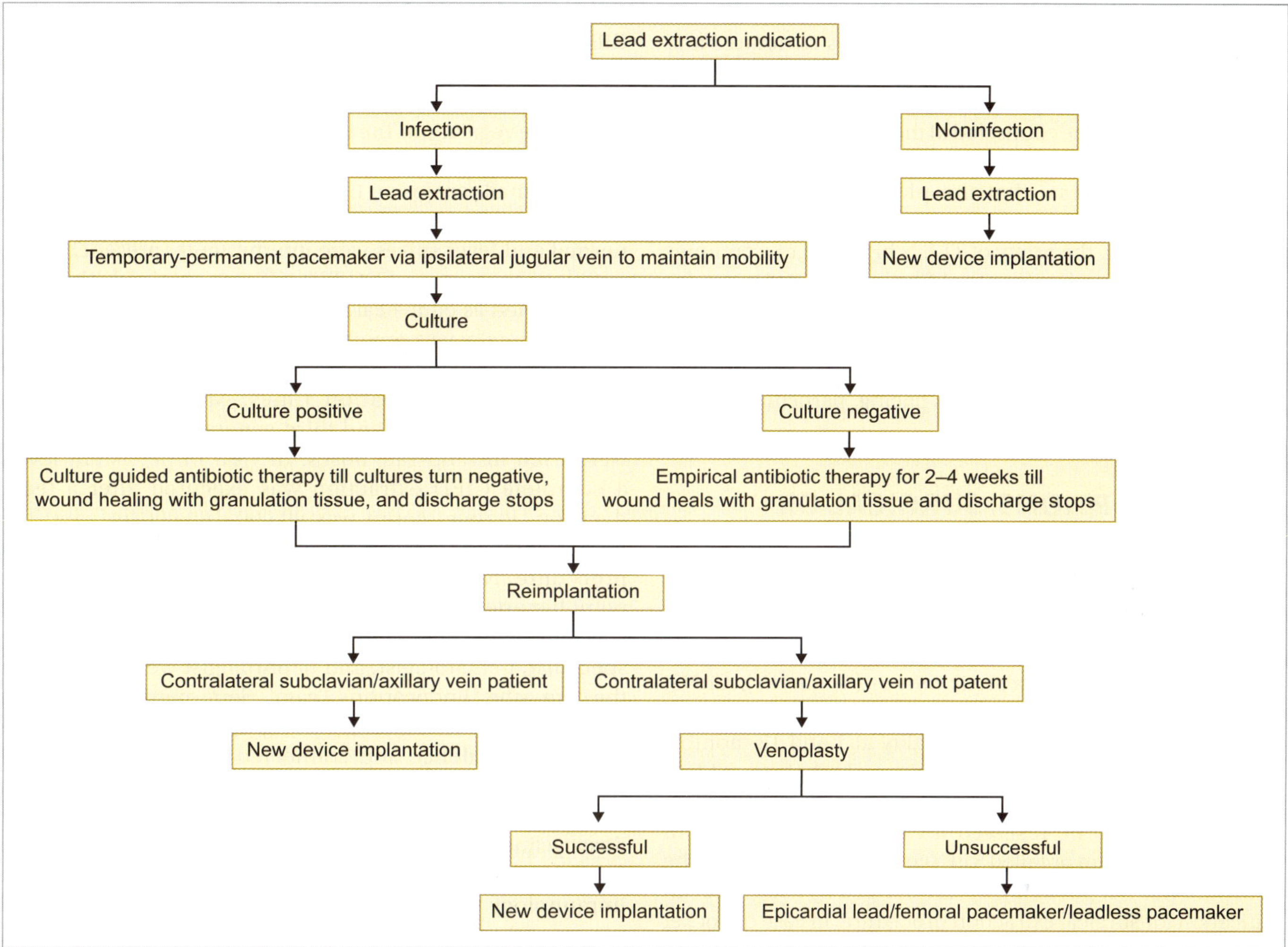

FLOWCHART 1: Cardiac implantable electrical device (CIED) infection management protocol of the Srinagar extraction registry.
Source: Reproduced with permission from Lone AA, et al. (2025).[5]

CIED EXTRACTION—SKILLS AVAILABLE?

No two CIED extractions are the same and complete system removal is the goal.[10] Considering this a minimum operator volume of 50 CIED procedures/year is recommended. If such an expertise is not available in the local hospital, then referral to an expert in the region should be considered. These procedures are best done by forming a working group involving cardiologists (possibly two with experience in TLE), cardiac surgeon providing on-site stand-by and anesthesia team. Intra-procedure imaging involves venogram and continuous TEE monitoring. Patient (gender, BMI, diabetes, renal insufficiency, and previous sternotomy) and CIED (type and number of leads and implant duration) characteristics should be recognized. Between 2017 and 2024, our group has performed TLE in 35 patients involving extraction of 85 leads (unpublished data). Almost all lead extractions were for pocket infection or lead endocarditis. Average age of patients was 58 years with an average lead dwell time of 6 years (range 1–15 years). CIED pocket and lead preparation are important surgical skills to learn before the extraction device can be used. Our modest experience involved use of rotational mechanical extraction device and complete removal was achieved in 28 patients. Two post procedure deaths were not related to the procedure. Dr Osswald's editorial advises, "here there is no place for ego and arrogance".[11]

CIED EXTRACTION—RISKS OVERESTIMATED?

Many a referral for CIED extraction gets delayed or do not happen at all because CIED extraction is perceived as a risky procedure (>6% risk). Real world figures suggest that only 11% CIED infections undergo the extraction procedure, despite the fact that it is a life-saving procedure and that a delay beyond 7 days increases in-hospital mortality. Fibrous binding of the lead to - each other, venous structures and cardiac tissue is the real difficulty which cannot be completely judged pre-procedure by any existing risk score; and patients (and families) must be counseled of the risk related to vascular laceration and life-threatening emergency therefrom. Lexicon data suggests that the physician perception of major adverse events and mortality of TLE is higher than it actually is. In fact, the safety of TLE is higher than a complex angioplasty or ablation for atrial fibrillation. Of course, for want of large experience, more difficulties could be expected with certain active fixation leads implanted in the coronary sinus (Attain Starfix 4195) and lumenless leads (SelectSecure 3830) used for conduction system pacing, particularly when they have a longer dwell time.

THERAPY OPTIONS: SURGICAL OR INTERVENTIONAL CIED EXTRACTION?

It must be disseminated among the physicians and cardiologists caring for patients with CIED that in event of pocket infection, lead endocarditis or occult bacteremia/ fungemia [with *Staphylococcus aureus* (*S. aureus*), CoNS, *Cutibacterium* species or *Candida* species]; TLE is associated with less adverse events and mortality at 1 and 12 months, than a surgical extraction procedure. Therefore, TLE is preferred over surgical extraction procedure. Surgical extraction should be reserved for lead endocarditis with vegetations >20 mm or failed TLE (complete extraction of the hardware was not possible). Epicardial lead by itself is not an indication for surgical extraction procedure, in case of pocket infection with an epicardial lead, the proximal part of the lead can be cut short through a separate incision away from the pocket.

IS A MULTIDISCIPLINARY TEAM AVAILABLE IN THE HOSPITAL?

Here is a brief presentation of an exemplary real-life scenario recently encountered by the author. It is representative of how a multidisciplinary team can work and is a must to manage a patient with CIED infection. A septuagenarian hypertensive diabetic lady with creatinine of 1.4 mg% was following with her referring physician after a dual chamber permanent pacemaker implantation (7 years ago) and bioprosthetic aortic valve (AV) replacement (3 years ago for aortic stenosis). Left ventricular (LV) function improved postoperatively and the epicardial LV lead implanted at the time of surgery for a possible biventricular pacer upgrade was not required later in the follow-up. She was referred to the nephrologist for anemia and rising creatinine (1.9 mg%). She received injection erythropoietin for anemia. Subsequently, her constellation of occasional fever spike, thrombocytopenia, microscopic hematuria, and reduced complement levels prompted her referral back to the implanting EP cardiologist to rule out CIED-related infection. She had a dental extraction 1 month ago under antibiotic cover. Her CRP was 43 mg/L. The CIED implant site was clinically unremarkable and TTE ruled out lead/valve vegetation. The prosthetic AV had normal function with a calcific spur seen on one leaflet. TEE done the next day showed small masses on the right atrial lead and no evident prosthetic AV endocarditis. Since the leukocyte counts were normal and fever spikes were intermittently present despite antibiotic therapy, an FDG PET/CT was obtained. The latter was reported as equivocal for the uptake in the region of AV ring. No uptake was reported elsewhere in the heart, at the implant site or in the body. Blood cultures remained negative despite longer incubation times. Multiple antibiotics including vancomycin and third generation cephalosporin were used in reno-safe doses. In view of persistent fever, a complete CIED extraction was executed after a team decision. Platelet count was 90,000–100,000/mL and the hematologist had given the go-ahead for the extraction procedure. No implant hardware was left behind. At this point her attending physician, cardiac EP, infectious disease specialist, clinical microbiologist, cardiac surgeon, imaging specialist, hematologist, and nephrologist were involved in the care—the "Endocarditis Team". Semi-permanent pacing lead was introduced through the right jugular vein to mitigate pacing dependence and connected to an extracorporeal pacer. Postextraction her fever spikes continued. Antibiotics were changed to vancomycin and minocycline (and later doxycycline) based on three positive cultures—lead culture for CoNS, sputum culture for *Klebsiella pneumoniae* and an immunology which was positive for *Bartonella* (she had a pet cat and cat scratch fever was suspected). Multiple blood cultures drawn on different days and during fever were negative. Other sources of fever such as multiple intravenous line change, loose motions in the interim and possibility of urinary tract infection were probed and if required treated. Similarly, early heart failure due to single chamber pacing, respiratory worsening—exacerbation of pre-existing obstructive airway disease, acute kidney injury (AKI) with creatinine elevation was treated appropriately. Repeat imaging done due to intermittent fever spikes with chills, now a month later was not different—TEE did not reveal AV endocarditis and the ghost residua seen on table after the extraction procedure had disappeared, FDG PET/CT showed equivocal (and reduced) uptake around the AV prosthesis without any uptake elsewhere. A change of antibiotic to levonadifloxacin seemed to restore afebrile status for 6 days when a right-sided reimplant of the pacemaker was contemplated. This plan was aborted at first scheduling due to intermittent recurrence of low-grade fever, occurrence of a new maculopapular rash and a further drop in platelet count to 40,000–53,000/mL. A shared decision-making was done wherein the dermatologist considered antibiotic hypersensitivity-related rash and advised observation under anti-allergic medications, the hematologist considered that dropped platelet count could be related to poly-pharmacy and was not a strict contraindication to the reimplantation procedure and the infectious disease specialist was of the view that the present febrile status in presence of a further reduced CRP (=7) and a negative procalcitonin was antibiotic-related fever. There was no evidence of infection at the semipermanent pacing-lead insertion site, and she was on oral medications (avoiding intravenous lines) for the last 10 days. The clinical equipoise here was whether the normally functioning aortic valve prosthesis needs explantation (as the only possible source of infection left with an equivocal FDG PET/CT reporting) and whether the permanent pacemaker implantation should be epicardial? A 3rd TEE, by an experienced echocardiographer ruled out any evidence of AV prosthesis endocarditis and the pacemaker reimplantation was finally scheduled from the contralateral site. A protracted hospital stay brings along with issues of physical deconditioning and mental well-being where a supportive family helps.

TIMING THE CIED EXTRACTION

The EHRA consensus document strongly recommends doing the CIED extraction within 3 days of hospital admission to an enabled center. Lin et al.[12] found lower complication rates such as acute kidney injury, respiratory failure, prolonged antibiotic therapy, and mortality, when the procedure was performed within 7 days. Yet, after establishing a diagnosis of CIED infection, delays occur, some of the reasons for which may be (1) assumption that infection restricted to the pocket is less urgent than confirmed bacteremia, (2) multiple physician opinions, (3) discussion over lead vegetation size cutoff to prefer surgical over TLR, (4) delays in transfer to extraction enabled center, and (5) difficulty in coordinating a date for the extraction procedure with the surgical team.

AVAILABILITY OF SURGICAL STANDBY

On site cardiothoracic surgery standby implies having the designated surgeon available and involved in the steps of the procedure, patient prepped with a possibility of quick sternotomy, operating room on alert, units for blood transfusion available in the catheterization laboratory and bridge balloon available for rescue.[13] Surgeon can also help with pocket management. This level or preparedness requires scheduling of the extraction procedure after a close communication with the surgical team. The availability of the surgical team might induce delays. In fact, at some international centers, cardiothoracic surgeons are primary operators for TLE. The dictum is despite all the successful TLE procedures behind you, the first complication is waiting to happen, and overconfidence should at no point lead to exclusion of the surgeon from the interdisciplinary team.

PATIENT FACTORS

Often patients are not adequately instructed at discharge to recognize early signs of pocket infection and seek immediate attention of the implanting cardiologist. An outstation patient may often engage a local surgeon, not accustomed to CIED management, to inspect and do dressings at the implantation site—leading to delays. Many patients would resist reintervention and request for maximal conservative approach using antibiotics and surgical intervention restricted to pocket management. Adequate treatment of the entry site of infection, uncontrolled diabetes, AKI, or pneumonia resulting from lead vegetation emboli may be required to obtain better patient status prior to TLE. Some patients might be unwilling for prolonged intensive care unit stay/hospitalization and delay decision-making. General frailty of the patient may discourage the family/caregiver personnel from consenting to undergo TLE.

NONAVAILABILITY OF CIED EXTRACTION HARDWARE

The versatility of mechanical rotational TLE technique is achieved by using lead locking stylet, Sightrail and the Tightrail devices. These can often be in short supply with the solitary vendor, understandably this can be a region-specific problem. Laser extraction sheaths have their advantages but most centers in India lack the availability of the laser console on-site.

FINANCIAL CONCERNS

The costs of lead extraction hardware are very high,[14] even from the perspective of a middle-class Indian patient. It is still optional in India to have a health insurance policy for oneself and for their entire family. With a low penetration of health insurance coverage, still a larger section of the society ends up spending a significant amount of their savings on rising healthcare services as they are not insured enough. The national and state health schemes may not code for this procedure rendering them unavailable to the underprivileged. With this background, the cost and recommendation of early TLE for CIED infection comes as a rude shock and early intervention can seem utopic. A big chunk of finances may already be exhausted on antibiotics hoping to avoid CIED extraction. Prolonged hospitalization (2–4 weeks), especially if in an intensive care unit, consumes resources. In pacemaker-dependent patients, post extraction, using semi-permanent pacing lead with an extracorporeal pulse generator, permits nursing in the rooms and saves cost. Wearable defibrillator, to be used after an AICD explantation, is not available in India. CIED reimplantation with new leads and generator is recommneded; however in our country at times the previously explanted and re-sterilized generator is used, to reduce the overall cost, a blatant divergence.

Use of antibacterial envelopes at reimplantation is a valid consideration but may be limited by cost. The financial burden itself spurs alternate and non-effective strategies. It is definitely time to liaise with the industry to innovate and manufacture medical devices locally.

CIED REIMPLANTATION PLAN—WHAT IS THE EXIT PLAN?

Finally, the appropriate date for reimplantation after CIED extraction has to be individualized. Explant pocket site wound healing by secondary intention takes longer, a well debrided wound without any device material residua therein may be suitable for primary closure. Total duration of post explant antibiotic therapy should be for 2 weeks for CIED pocket infection and for 4–6 weeks for CIED endocarditis, no divergence from this recommendation is wise. Clinical judgement to conclude eradication of bacteremia based on; afebrile status, CRP, and blood counts reassessment, culture negativity, and discussion within the "Endocarditis Team" should help to plan reimplantation. Before reimplantation, think through the following—the type of new CIED device, value of incorporating newer advances such as leadless pacemaker, conduction system pacing to minimize the leads used or extravascular ICD to reduce the risk of recurrence of infection, clinical status (such as hemodynamics, AKI, respiratory status, and preanesthesia evaluation), presence of a continued indication for the device reimplant (pacing dependence and secondary SCD prevention would be compelling), comorbidities, quality of life to accrue and the financial burden.[15]

CONCLUSION

Despite publications and recommendations from various Heart Rhythm Societies regarding expeditious management of CIED infection, divergent paths are taken toward reaching a definite diagnosis and planning CIED extraction procedure. CIED infection is life-threatening, and salvage is possible only after an extraction procedure followed by antibiotic therapy. Therefore, without undue delay, diagnosis in suspected circumstances should be achieved using cultures and imaging. Multispeciality consults under the umbrella of "Endocarditis Team" can be better steered by a practicing cardiac electrophysiologist who is also an expert in TLE. Following adequate treatment of bacteremia and source control, on definite persistence of CIED indication, reimplantation procedure should be considered on the contralateral site. Costs of this exercise often exceed the initial implant costs and can be a serious barrier to follow the guidelines.

REFERENCES

1. Biffi M, Ammendola E, Menardi E, et al. Real-life outcome of implantable cardioverter-defibrillator and cardiac resynchronization defibrillator replacement/upgrade in a contemporary population: observations from the multicentre decode registry. Europace. 2019;21:1527-36.
2. Clementy N, Carion PL, de Leotoing L, et al. Infections and associated costs following cardiovascular implantable electronic device implantations: a nationwide cohort study. Europace. 2018;20:1974-80.
3. Traykov V, Bongiorni MG, Boriani G, et al. Clinical practice and implementation of guidelines for the prevention, diagnosis and management of cardiac implantable electronic device infections; results of a worldwide survey under the auspices of the European Heart Rhythm Association. Europace. 2019;21:1270-9.
4. Blomstrom-Lundqvist C, Traykov V, Erba PA, et al. European Heart Rhythm Association (EHRA) international consensus document on how to prevent, diagnose, and treat cardiac implantable electronic device infections — endorsed by the Heart Rhythm Society (HRS), the Asia Pacific Heart Rhythm Society (APHRS), the Latin American Heart Rhythm Society (LAHRS), International Society for Cardiovascular Infectious Diseases (ISCVID) and the European Society of Clinical Microbiology and Infectious Diseases (ESCMID) in collaboration with the European Association for Cardio-Thoracic Surgery (EACTS). Europace. 2020;22:515-49.
5. Lone AA, Dar MI, Sheikh JM, et al. Transvenous lead extraction: Experience from a Northern state of India – The Srinagar Extraction registry. Indian Pacing Electrophysiol J. 2025;25:58-66.
6. Hussein AA, Baghdy Y, Wazni OM, et al. Microbiology of cardiac implantable electronic device infections. JACC: Clin Electrophysiol. 2016;2:498-505.
7. Essebag V, Verma A, Healey JS, et al. BRUISE CONTROL Investigators. Clinically significant pocket hematoma increases long term risk of device infection: BRUISE CONTROL INFECTION study. J Am Coll Cardiol. 2016;67:1300-8.
8. Al-Khatib SM, Greiner MA, Peterson ED, et al. Patient and implanting physician factors associated with mortality and complications after implantable cardioverter-defibrillator implantation, 2002-2005. Circ Arrhythm Electrophysiol. 2008;1:240-9.
9. Pokorney SD, Mi X, Lewis RK, et al. Outcomes associated with extraction versus capping and abandoning pacing and defibrillator leads. Circulation. 2017;136:1387-95.
10. Bongiorni MG, Burri H, Deharo JC, et al. 2018 EHRA expert consensus statement on lead extraction: recommendations on definitions, endpoints, research trial design, and data collection requirements for clinical scientific studies and registries: endorsed by APHRS/HRS/LAHRS. Europace. 2018;20:1217-17.
11. Osswald B. Expect the unexpected. Lead extraction – a perfect example? Indian Pacing Electrophysiol J. 2025;25:67.
12. Lin AY, Saul T, Aldaas OM, et al. Early Versus Delayed Lead Extraction in Patients with Infected Cardiovascular Implantable Electronic Devices. JACC Clin Electrophysiol. 2021;7(6):755-63.
13. Tułecki Ł, Czajkowski M, Targońska S, et al. The role of cardiac surgery in transvenous lead extraction. A high-volume center experience with 3207 procedures. Kardiochir Torakochirurgia Pol. 2022;19(3):122-9.
14. Pokorney SD, Zepel L, Greiner MA, et al. Impact of timing of treatment for cardiac implantable electronic device infections on healthcare utilization and expenditures. Europace. 2025;27(8):euaf146.
15. Deharo JC, Bongiorni MG, Rozkovec A, et al. European Heart Rhythm Association. Pathways for training and accreditation for transvenous lead extraction: a European Heart Rhythm Association position paper. Europace. 2012;14:124-34.

CHAPTER 82

Leadless Pacing: Past, Present, and Future

Aftab Khan, Navanil Biswas, Arif Nabi Bhat

ABSTRACT

Leadless pacemakers (LPMs) represent one of the most transformative innovations in cardiac rhythm management since the advent of the first permanent pacemaker in 1958. By eliminating leads and device pockets—the primary sources of complications in conventional systems—LPMs have redefined the safety and feasibility of long-term pacing. This chapter traces their remarkable journey, from early visionary concepts and the rise and fall of the Nanostim, to the global success of the Micra and the re-emergence of Abbott's AVEIR platform. It explores the evolution from single-chamber devices to AV-synchronous pacing with Micra AV, culminating in the breakthrough dual-chamber leadless system, AVEIR DR. Real-world registry data and meta-analyses confirm their superiority over transvenous pacemakers (TVMs) in reducing reinterventions and complications, while ongoing refinements are expanding indications across age groups and clinical scenarios. The chapter also examines frontiers at the horizon: Integration with subcutaneous ICDs, leadless CRT systems, conduction system pacing (CSP), self-rechargeable devices, and bioresorbable pacemakers. Together, these advances underscore not just the present impact of leadless pacing but its transformative potential to reshape the future of electrophysiology toward safer, smarter, and more physiologic therapies.

Keywords: Leadless pacemaker, Micra, AVEIR.

INTRODUCTION

Since the first human implantation of a permanent Pacemaker in 1958 on *Arne Larrson* by cardiac surgeon *Ake Senning* and engineer *Rune Elmqvist*, pacemaker technologies have grown by leaps and bounds. Notable advances have been made with respect to battery longevity, device size, pacing algorithms, and transvenous lead mechanics. In spite of these advances, the "Achilles Heel" of transvenous pacemakers (TVMs) have been the leads and the subcutaneous pacemaker pocket. Together, they account for >90% of TVM-related complications. It was to address these two important limitations, the leadless pacemaker (LPM) or the *"bullet" pacemaker*, as fondly called by some, was conceptualized by *Dr Jeffrey Spickler* as early as 1970. Indeed, he is regarded as the "intellectual founder" of the LPMs.

LOOKING BACK AT THE PAST: THE PATHFINDER IS NO MORE

The main advantage of the LPM remains the significant reduction in complications, by >50%, compared to its transvenous counterparts. Though the complications concerning leads and pockets, such as infection, hematoma, pneumothorax, lead fracture, and lead dislocation declined, LPM has been associated with more vascular complications and pericardial effusions. The first trials to prove the efficacy and safety of the LPMs were the *LEADLESS I trial* (involving only 33 patients) and the *LEADLESS II trials* (slightly larger, with 526 patients from 56 centers).

They evaluated the *Nanostim device* (founded in Sunnyvale, California by Dr Randall Wolf and team in 2011 and later acquired by Abbott). *It was the first LPM to be implanted in humans*, and achieved the CE mark approval in 2013, but however was never FDA approved. From December 2012 to March 2017, this Nanostim device, operating in the VVI(R) mode, was implanted 1,423 times worldwide. A medical device advisory was issued in 2016, when seven of these devices reported early premature battery failures (within 2 years). However, later reports indicated that around 37% of these devices suffered the same problem, and hence, this resulted in a recall of all Nanostim devices, and future implantation was cancelled. So, the pathfinder of LPMs, the Nanostim device, was permanently retired.

The legacy of LPMs was continued by the *Micra VR* (Medtronic), which received CE mark in 2015 and FDA approval in 2016, and recently by the AVEIR VR (Abbott), the successor of the Nanostim device, which achieved FDA approval in 2022, and CE mark in 2023. They were all single-chamber models, MRI compatible, and were extensively used worldwide. Their comparing features are illustrated in **Figure 1**.

The first Micra LPM device was implanted in December 2013, in Linz, Austria. Since then, >20,000 Micra VR Devices have been implanted worldwide.[1] The Micra VR was evaluated and established by the *Micra Investigational Device Exemption (IDE) study* (n = 725), *Micra Post-Approval Registry (PAR)* (n = 1,809), and the *Micra MAP EMEA study* (n = 928). All of them demonstrated a very high implantation success rate of around 98%, and declining complication rates (<3%). Most of the complications consisted of pacing issues, including pacemaker syndrome and pacing-induced cardiomyopathy. The *Micra Longitudinal Coverage with Evidence Development (CED) study* involving 5,746 medicare patients revealed an acute complication rate of 8.4%, with perforation making up 0.8%, and a chronic complication rate of 5% with dislodgment reported in only 0.4%.

Though RV apical septum and apex were initially the preferred site for Micra LPM implantations, it was seen to cause higher risk of complications, like perforations and pericardial effusions. Accordingly, the RV septal area became the chosen site, with higher septal locations, like *RV mid-septum and RV outflow tract (RVOT) being associated with lesser complications and also the narrowest paced QRS complexes.* This device used a lithium-hybrid CFx silver vanadium oxide battery having a battery longevity of 12 years with 100% ventricular pacing.

The *AVEIR* was the Abbott's successor to the Nanostim, which was approved by the FDA in 2022 and received CE mark in 2023. This device, the AVEIR VR, was actually evaluated in the LEADLESS phase II trials (n = 210). They reported a 98% implant success rate over 14 months. It has a lithium carbon-monofluoride battery with an expected longevity of about 17.6 years. Besides battery longevity, AVEIR also improved its docking design (direct attachment to the LPM) and retrieval capability. However, *the main advantage was the option to map the local electrical signal before selecting the final site for screwing the LPM.*

Two studies that comparing the AVEIR (n = 67) and Micra (n = 50) LPMs demonstrated longer procedure time and fluoroscopy duration with AVEIR, possibly due to lack of experience with this new device. Complication rates remained same, and AVEIR had a longer projected battery life at 6 months interrogation **(Fig. 2)**.

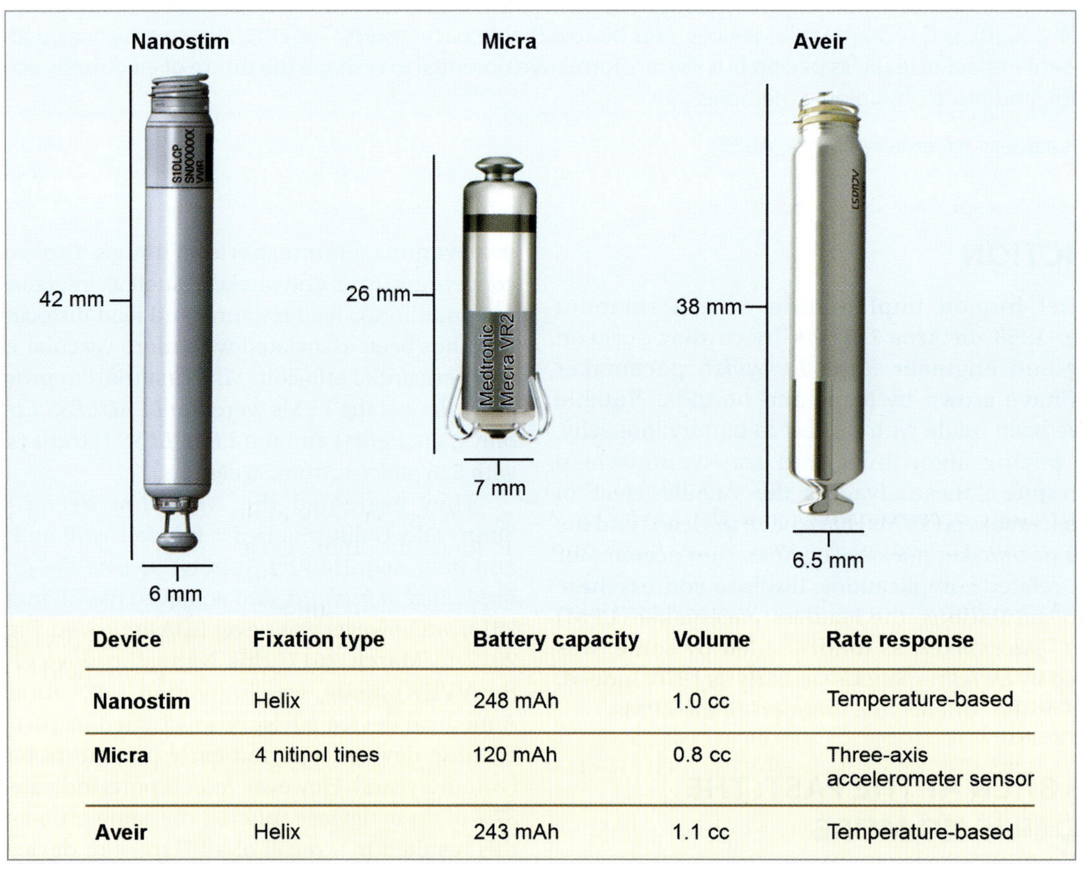

Device	Fixation type	Battery capacity	Volume	Rate response
Nanostim	Helix	248 mAh	1.0 cc	Temperature-based
Micra	4 nitinol tines	120 mAh	0.8 cc	Three-axis accelerometer sensor
Aveir	Helix	243 mAh	1.1 cc	Temperature-based

FIG. 1: First-generation leadless pacemakers.

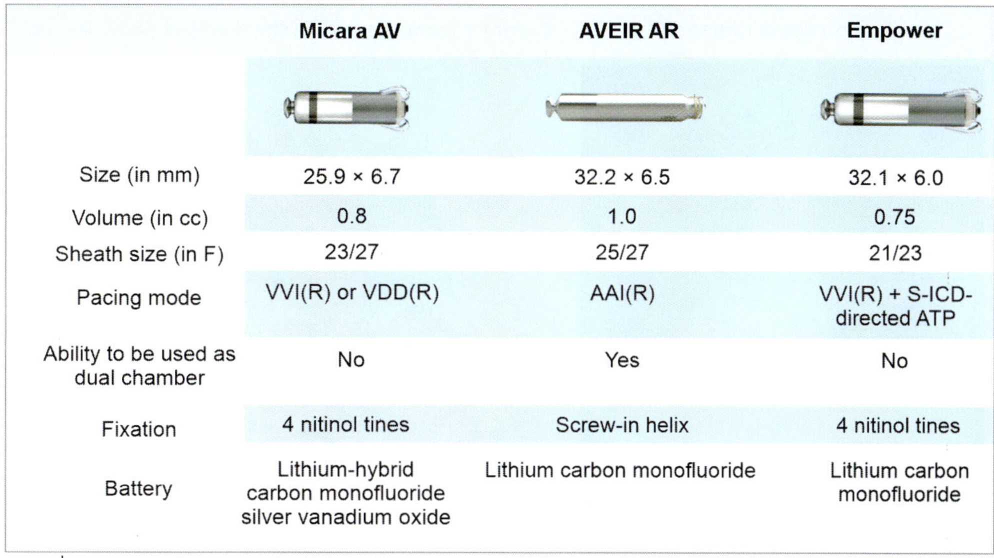

	Micara AV	AVEIR AR	Empower
Size (in mm)	25.9 × 6.7	32.2 × 6.5	32.1 × 6.0
Volume (in cc)	0.8	1.0	0.75
Sheath size (in F)	23/27	25/27	21/23
Pacing mode	VVI(R) or VDD(R)	AAI(R)	VVI(R) + S-ICD-directed ATP
Ability to be used as dual chamber	No	Yes	No
Fixation	4 nitinol tines	Screw-in helix	4 nitinol tines
Battery	Lithium-hybrid carbon monofluoride silver vanadium oxide	Lithium carbon monofluoride	Lithium carbon monofluoride

FIG. 2: Newer generation of leadless devices.

LEADLESS PACEMAKERS: CURRENT SCENARIO

Currently, both Micra VR and AVEIR VR are being implanted frequently around the world in a specific subgroup of patients. LPMs are a suitable option for most patients who are in need of single-chamber pacing only. But, the same problems with TVMs capable of only single-chamber pacing and sensing resurfaced in these LPS too—notably the loss of AV synchrony resulting in various forms of pacemaker syndrome. To overcome this challenge, atrial sensing algorithms were incorporated in these devices.[2,3]

This was possible in the Micra LPM, where the new model came to be known as the *Micra AV*, and was actually introduced in 2020. The AV synchronous pacing is achieved by a three-axis accelerometer algorithm, which detects mechanical vibrations of cardiac motion, especially the atrial kick (last rapid filling phase) and times ventricular pacing accordingly. Though the device remained the same, it was the software incorporated that was upgraded. This was tested by the *MARVEL 1 (Micra Atrial tRacking using a Ventricular accelerometer) and the MARVEL 2 trials,* which demonstrated an AV synchrony of 87 and 89.2%, respectively. However, there remained a problem in achieving AV synchrony with higher heart rates (HR > 100). Considering everything, Micra AV has expanded the patient indications for LPS, and can be reliably used in those with sinus rhythm with significant AV conduction disease. Updated versions of both Micra devices have been released, the Micra *VR_2* and the *Micra AV_2*, which received FDA approval in 2023, and CE mark in 2024. The improvements reported were increased battery longevity, software updates, and increased propensity to achieve AV synchrony at higher heart rates for the Micra AV_2 device.

Dual-chamber LPMs—it is here: Though the Micra AV LPM offers synchronous pacing, the major limitation lies in its inability to pace the atrium when required. To overcome this shortcoming, *AVEIR has introduced its atrial module, which incorporates a separate LPM for the atrium, and is combined with a ventricular LPM for dual-chamber leadless pacing.* This has been named the *AVEIR DR* **(Fig. 3)** and this device has also been approved by the FDA in 2023 and achieved CE mark in 2024, along with the Micra AV_2 device.

The feasibility of this device was demonstrated in the *AVEIR-i2i study*, which was the first in-human trial of dual-chamber leadless pacing. 300 patients across three countries were enrolled, and complete system implantation was achieved in 98.3% of patients. The rate of complications was 9.7% at 3 months, comparable to transvenous systems. The rate of cardiac perforation was low (0.7%, both involving the atrial LPM), which was again similar to transvenous atrial lead (0.8%). Coming to lead dislodgment, atrial LPMs showed a higher dislodgment rate of 3.3% compared to ventricular LPM (0.3%). Studies revealed that the base of the right atrial appendage was the preferred implant location, compared to middle or distal right atrial appendage as it lead to lower dislodgment rates as well as better device-device communication, a finding supported by anatomic review and 3D modeling in human cadavers.

The parameters acceptable of atrial pacing, as evaluated in this study, was an atrial pacing threshold of <3 V at 0.4 ms and sensing of P wave ≥ 1 mV, which was achieved in 90.2% of patients. AV synchrony was achieved 96.5% of the time, even in multiple postures and during fast walking. However, the continuous implant to implant communication was shown to adversely impact battery longevity, with projected battery life of 6.4 years for atrial LPM and 11.3 years for the ventricular LPM only.

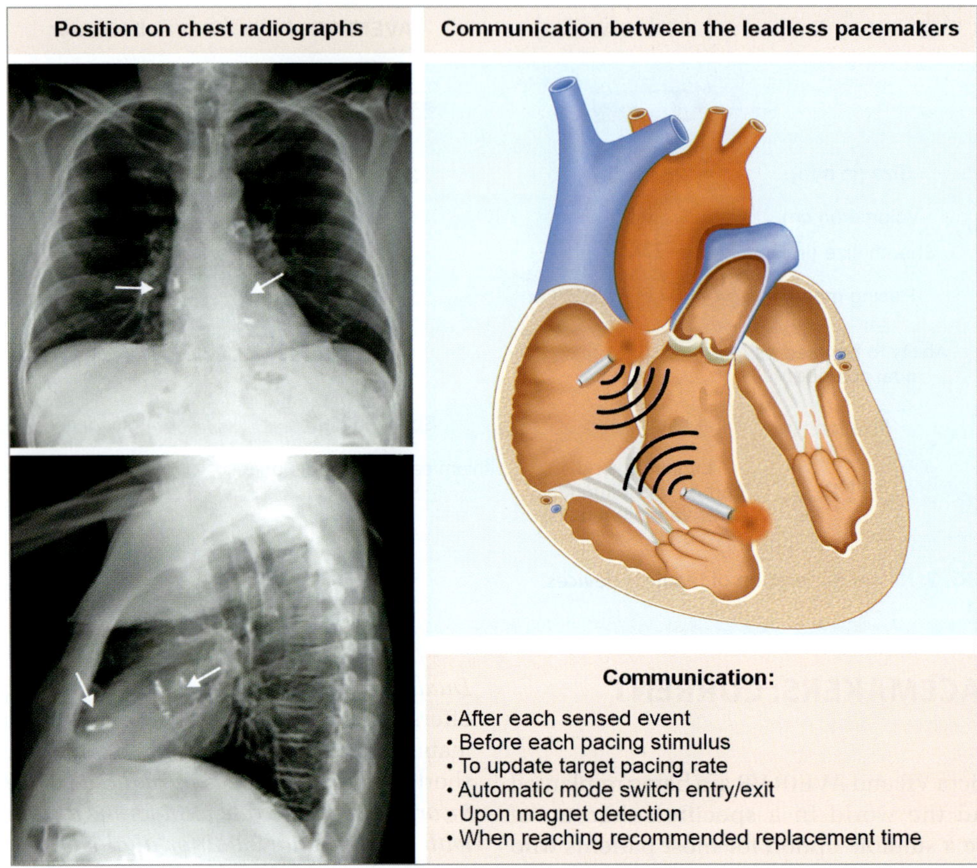

FIG. 3: Dual-chamber leadless pacemakers—imaging, anatomy, and communication.

CURRENT PERSPECTIVES ON LEADLESS PACEMAKERS

With increasing number of LPMs being implanted worldwide, it gives the opportunity to conduct large-scale trials comparing LPMs with traditional TVM. *The Micra CED* study did just that, comparing 6,219 LPMs with 10,212 TVM patients with a long-term follow-up of 3 years. It revealed a 41% lower system revision rate and a 43% lower complication rate in the leadless population. However, the 3-year mortality rate was same for both the cohorts.

This finding was echoed in other studies, such as the meta-analysis by Shtembari et al., which demonstrated a 42% lower complication rate in LPM ($n = 8,340$) versus TVPM ($n = 15,008$), as well as 46% lower rate of reintervention. The meta-analysis by Ngo et al., comparing five studies showed a 51% lower complication rate with Micra LPMs ($n = 1,030$) compared to TVPM ($n = 2,959$). Besides proving undoubtedly the superiority of LPMs, a number of other important perspectives were brought forward by these studies and are discussed here:

Patient selection: The 2021 ESC guidelines have given a *class IIa indication* for LPM, only as an *alternative* to TVPM when there is *no/difficult upper extremity venous access or when risk of device pocket infection is high*. This includes patients on hemodialysis or history of pacemaker infection. It is important to note that LPM implantation before or even simultaneously with the extraction of infected pacemakers is feasible and has been done. This is very useful in pacing-dependent patients as it excludes requirement of temporary pacing. Patients who require only single-chamber pacing, like those with bradyarrhythmia and AF, or those with low expected pacing burden also are indicated for LPM (*ESC guidelines class IIb*).

Leadless pacemaker implantation in the very young and very old: LPM insertion has been proven to be safe and effective in the elderly, with complication rates remaining the same when compared to the normal population. The tortuousness of the lower extremity veins might present a problem while introducing the device, which might make jugular venous approach more favorable. Studies have also been done on the pediatric patients receiving LPM by Siddeek et al. and Shah et al., both of which proved LPMs in this age group were feasible and associated with stable electrical parameters during follow-up.

Approach—femoral or jugular?: The most common route of LPM insertion is femoral, without any doubt. However, various studies and case reports have explored the *internal jugular vein (IJV) as an alternative implantation route.* The main advantage of the jugular approach seems to be the shorter route to the right atrium, bypassing the tortuous femoral veins, easier manipulation of the device and a less painful procedure. Also, such patients could be ambulated immediately, reducing pain and discomfort of lying still, especially in the elderly with joint and back issues, and same day discharges.

Pericardial effusion and cardiac perforation: These two remain the main drawbacks of LPM insertion procedures, being considerably higher than the TVPMs. However, with newer studies the complication rates seem to be on the decline. Factors responsible might be the better learning curve, advancement in the implantation procedure recommendations, and preference for RV septal implantation rather than apical. Still, *LPM insertion is always recommended to be done in centers with back-up cardiothoracic surgery department on site.*

LOOKING AT THE FUTURE: WHAT IS IN STORE IN THE FIELD OF LEADLESS PACEMAKER?

In just a few years since LPMs have come into the market, their use and potentials have exploded. The significant reduction in complications, as well as the increasing ease of implantation due to technological advances has greatly made it into a welcome addition to the device armamentarium. Now further advancements are being made, and even more are being planned, to make use of the yet untapped potential of this novel device.

Leadless pacemaker and subcutaneous ICDs: In the field of heart failure and ventricular arrhythmia, the patients with difficult venous access, or other contraindications to implanted devices, subcutaneous ICDs were the only option to provide vasculature free defibrillator therapy. However, it lacked pacing capabilities. Combining a LPM with a subcutaneous ICD will provide backup bradycardia pacing options as well as the ability to provide antitachycardia pacing for terminating suitable VTs. Boston Scientific has in this regard developed a modular cardiac rhythm management system involving a novel LPM, the *Empower LPM* combined with S-ICD (Model A209 Emblem, or Model A219 Emblem). This was tested in the *MODULAR ATP study* (n = 293), which had a very low LMP-related complication rate of 2.5%, successful device-to-device communication of 98.8%, and good ventricular pacing threshold (≤2 V at 0.4 ms) in 97.4% subjects.

LPM and CRT: Wise CRT—the EBR systems group developed the *Wise CRT device* **(Fig. 4)** for patients who failed conventional CRT. It consists of a wireless left ventricular electrode, implanted endocardially in the LV by an antegrade trans-septal approach or retrograde aortic approach, which was then connected to a subcutaneous transmitter and battery, and needed a transvenous right-sided system to achieve biventricular synchronization. Studies proving the efficacy of this device was the *SELECT-LV study* (n = 35), and the pivotal *SOLVE-CRT trial* (n = 31), which demonstrated an implant success rate of 95.5%, with appreciable improvements in reverse remodeling, QRS shortening, as well as in functional outcomes (NYHA class, KCCQ scores), with a low acute complication rate of 5.9%. This device achieved FDA approval in April 2025, and also has been designated a "*breakthrough device*". Though the original Wise CRT system

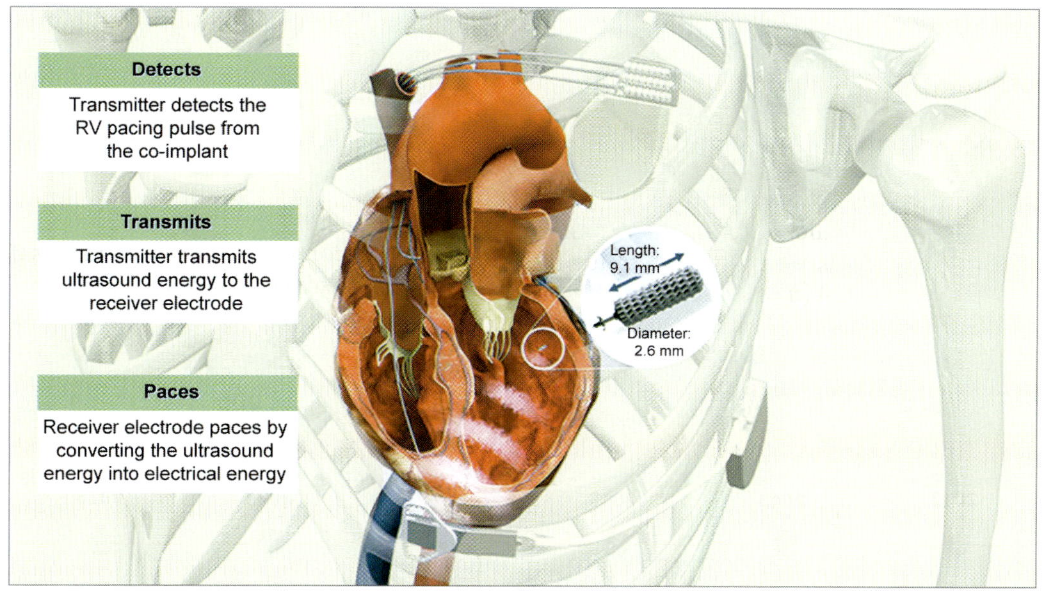

FIG. 4: Leadless Wise CRT system.

is not completely leadless, as it involves transvenous leads in RA and RV, methods are being explored to combine Wise CRT systems with Micra LPM to achieve a totally leadless CRT system.

Leadless conduction system pacing (CSP): It is well known that RV pacing is associated with ventricular dyssynchrony, and consequently increased incidences of atrial fibrillation, heart failure, and mortality. To overcome this shortcoming, CSP gained prominence. Currently, left bundle branch area pacing (LBBAP) is preferred over His-bundle pacing (HBP) due to various reasons including shorter procedure time, larger anatomical area and more stable electrical parameters. To bring CSP into the domain of leadless pacing, smaller devices with more advanced fixation mechanisms are required and are currently in development.

Leadless self-rechargeable devices: A major limitation of LPMs is the limited battery longevity. Though recent devices have been able to extend the battery life using advanced technology (the Micra AV_2 and Micra VRx have a projected battery life of 15.6 and 16.7 years, respectively), yet the problem of extraction of such devices, as well as hosting two or more such devices in the RV requires further consideration. The advent of the *triboelectric nanogenerators*, which provide high power density, excellent output performance, and dependable durability, might solve this problem.[4] This device *harvests kinetic energy from the intrinsic motion of the heart and converts it into kinetic energy* which can be used for cardiac pacing. Such self-rechargeable devices seem more feasible when data from recent studies are considered, where the energy harvested from one cardiac cycle was seen to be 0.495 mJ, while the energy required for endocardial pacing is only 0.377 mJ.

Leadless bioresorbable pacemakers: Bioresorbable LPMs are an emerging class of *temporary* pacing systems designed to deliver postoperative or bridge pacing and then disappear, eliminating leads, batteries, extraction procedures, and their attendant risks. The foundational 2021 Nature Biotechnology work demonstrated a fully implantable, *battery-free*, and wirelessly powered (13.56 MHz inductive) epicardial device built from resorbable materials (e.g., Mg/PLGA with W-coated Mg conductors). Most recently (2025), a millimeter-scale, *light-activated, syringe-injectable* pacemaker—smaller than a grain of rice—was reported with a dissolvable implant powered via a galvanic cell and controlled by an external chest patch that delivers optical pulses through the chest. However, these systems remain *preclinical* (no routine human trials reported), but they provide enormous potential in scenarios of postcardiotomy pacing, temporary support after structural interventions, and neonatal/postcongenital surgery scenarios.

Looking further into the future: Though appreciable advancements have been made in the field of leadless pacing, more research is needed in many areas. One very important field is the LPM extraction procedure, as large-scale trials on safety of extraction of endothelialized LPM is still absent. Also, more studies regarding presence of simultaneous devices in the RV need to be undertaken. *Currently, up to 3 Micra LPMs could be implanted in RV without device-device interaction, as demonstrated in cadaveric studies.* However, in humans, reports of a maximum of two simultaneous LPMs in the RV septum exist **(Fig. 5)**.[5]

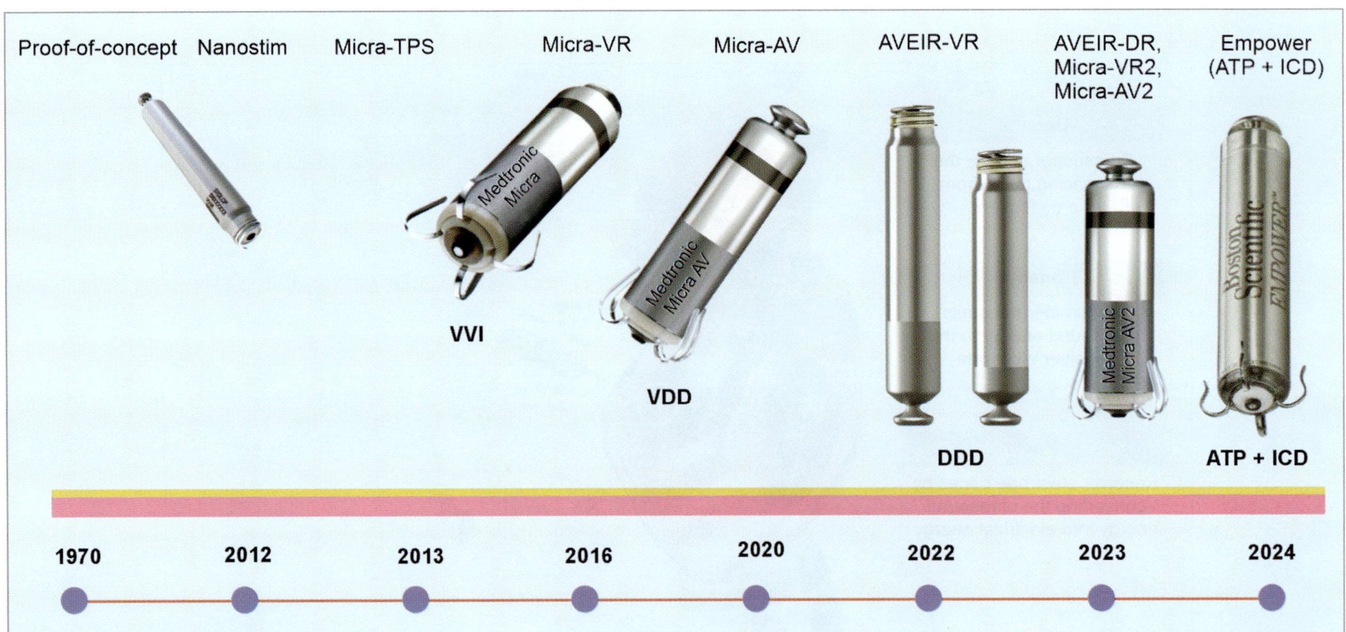

FIG. 5: Timeline of leadless pacing.

CONCLUSION

Leadless pacemakers have rapidly evolved from a visionary concept into a clinically established technology that has fundamentally changed the way bradyarrhythmias are managed. Early limitations of bulky experimental devices gave way to the successful commercial introduction of single-chamber systems such as Micra and AVEIR, proving the feasibility, safety, and efficacy of transcatheter leadless pacing while dramatically reducing lead- and pocket-related complications. Subsequent advances with AV-synchronous platforms (Micra AV) and the pioneering dual-chamber leadless system (Aveir DR) have expanded physiologic pacing possibilities, addressing the long-standing gap of atrioventricular coordination. Parallel innovations, such as modular approaches to cardiac resynchronization (e.g., Wise CRT), subcutaneous ICDs, and CSP underline the adaptability of wireless pacing to complex indications. Together, these milestones reflect not only how far leadless pacing has come but also how much further it may transform cardiac rhythm management—toward a future where devices are smaller, smarter, more physiologic, and potentially even transient, leaving behind no foreign material.

REFERENCES

1. Breeman KTN, Tjong FVY, Miller MA, et al. Ten Years of Leadless Cardiac Pacing. J Am Coll Cardiol. 2024;84(21):2131-47.
2. Beurskens NEG, Breeman KTN, Dasselaar KJ, et al. Leadless cardiac pacing systems: current status and future prospects. Expert Rev Med Devices. 2019;16(11):923-30.
3. Vouliotis AI, Roberts PR, Dilaveris P, et al. Leadless Pacemakers: Current Achievements and Future Perspectives. Eur Cardiol. 2023;18:e49.
4. Vardas PE. Leadless and scarless pacing: towards symbiotic nanogenerators. Eur Heart J. 2024;45(14):1252-4.
5. Saleem-Talib S, Hoevenaars CPR, Molitor N, et al. Leadless pacing: a comprehensive review. Eur Heart J. 2025;46(21):1979-90.

CHAPTER

83

Atrial Fibrillation in Heart Failure: Role of Catheter Ablation

Sharath K Kumar, Calambur Narasimhan

ABSTRACT

Atrial fibrillation (AF) commonly coexists with heart failure (HF), worsening symptoms and outcomes. Catheter ablation (CA) has shown superior results over medical therapy, particularly in heart failure with reduced ejection fraction (HFrEF), by improving left ventricular function, reducing hospitalizations, and lowering mortality. Evidence in heart failure with preserved ejection fraction (HFpEF) indicates symptomatic and functional improvement with comparable safety. Early ablation and newer energy sources such as cryoballoon and pulsed-field ablation enhance success and safety. CA is now a key therapeutic option to break the AF–HF cycle and improve overall prognosis.

Keywords: Atrial fibrillation, heart failure, catheter ablation, HFrEF, HFpEF, pulmonary vein isolation, rhythm control, cryoballoon, pulsed-field ablation, left ventricular function.

INTRODUCTION

Heart failure (HF) and atrial fibrillation (AF) frequently coexist, which can lead to a negative cycle of worsening hemodynamics, more hospital stays, and higher death rates. Atrioventricular dyssynchrony, tachycardia-induced cardiomyopathy, and elevated filling pressures are some of the ways that AF worsens HF, while HF increases the risk of AF by four to six times.[1] In HF, the prevalence of AF varies greatly, ranging from 10% in moderate cases to more than 50% in severe cases. A meta-analysis of over 248,000 patients showed that AF is more prevalent with higher ejection fraction and is strongly associated with increased mortality and hospitalization in heart failure with mildly reduced ejection fraction (HFmrEF) and heart failure with preserved ejection fraction (HFpEF), but not consistently in heart failure with reduced ejection fraction (HFrEF).[2] Management is complex; rhythm control techniques, particularly catheter ablation (CA), have been shown to improve left ventricular (LV) function and reduce hospitalizations and mortality in certain HFrEF patients. Rate control frequently proves inadequate.[3] Despite advancements, there are still gaps in our understanding of AF in HFpEF, proper screening techniques, and early rhythm regulation therapies.[4]

PATHOPHYSIOLOGY

Atrial fibrillation and HF are interconnected through a vicious cycle of hemodynamic stress, neurohormonal activation, and structural remodeling. In HF, elevated LV filling pressures raise left atrial (LA) pressure and stretch, often worsened by mitral regurgitation. AF further impairs diastolic filling by eliminating atrial contraction and shortening LV filling time due to irregular and rapid ventricular rates, especially during exertion.[5] Chronic elevations in pressure drive ventricular remodeling and chamber dilatation, which in turn propagate abnormal left-sided pressures and predispose to worsening AF and HF. Restoration of sinus rhythm has been shown to reverse this process, improving LV diameters and ejection fraction.

At the myocardial level, AF-induced cardiomyopathy develops through three major mechanisms: (1) Tachycardia-related cardiac dysfunction, with sustained high rates causing ventricular dilatation, contractile dysfunction, and fibrosis;[6] (2) rhythm irregularity, which disrupts calcium cycling, reduces contractile efficiency, and triggers oxidative stress and neurohormonal activation;[6] and (3) atrial myopathy, characterized by LA dilatation, interstitial fibrosis, myofibrillar loss, and structural remodeling.[7] Together, these overlapping mechanisms establish a self-reinforcing cycle: AF worsens hemodynamics and remodeling, while HF alters atrial and ventricular substrate to promote AF. This interplay highlights the need for early rhythm control, risk factor control, and neurohormonal modulation to prevent irreversible remodeling and progression to refractory AF-HF overlap.

EVIDENCE FROM RANDOMIZED CONTROLLED TRIALS

Atrial Fibrillation Ablation in Heart Failure with Reduced Ejection Fraction (Table 1)

The landmark CASTLE-AF randomized controlled trial enrolled patients with symptomatic AF and an LVEF of 35% or less, most with paroxysmal or persistent arrhythmia. Subjects were randomized to receive either CA or optimal medical therapy. Over a median 5-year follow-up, CA led to a significant reduction in the composite endpoint of all-cause mortality or HF hospitalization [hazard ratio (HR) 0.62; 95% confidence interval (CI): 0.43–0.87]. Moreover, patients undergoing ablation experienced marked improvement in LV function (absolute increase of 8%), symptom burden, and quality of life (QoL).[14] The AMICA trial enrolled patients with advanced HF: Persistent AF, very low LVEF (≤35%), and a high prevalence of CRT devices. This sicker population showed similar improvement in LVEF between ablation and medical management, with neither group outperforming the other. The authors of AMICA cite factors such as lower baseline function, more persistent AF, and shorter follow-up (1 year) as possible reasons for the lack of demonstrable benefit with CA in their cohort.[15] The CAMERA-MRI trial contributed a unique perspective by targeting patients with idiopathic LV dysfunction—excluding those with significant coronary artery disease. These subjects were randomized to CA or rate control, and the results showed a robust, 14% greater improvement in LVEF following ablation.[13] Restoration of sinus rhythm was even associated with regression of diffuse ventricular fibrosis on cardiac MRI, supporting the notion that AF-induced cardiomyopathy can be partially reversible through ablation in selected cases. The AATAC trial randomized patients with persistent AF, LVEF ≤40%, and ICD/CRT-D devices to CA or amiodarone. Ablation was markedly more successful, with 70% freedom from arrhythmia recurrence versus only 34% with amiodarone over three years.[12]

Meta-analyses **(Table 2)** incorporating these trials and others uniformly reinforce these findings showing that CA leads to lower all-cause mortality, fewer HF hospitalizations, higher arrhythmia-free survival, and greater improvements in ventricular function and QoL in HFrEF populations.[20-23] For example, pooled risk ratios for all-cause mortality with CA versus medical therapy are as low as 0.31–0.52, and CA outperforms drugs in sustaining sinus rhythm and reversing HF symptoms.[20,21] The CASTLE-HTx trial further extends these results to patients with end-stage HF, finding that ablation even in advanced cases lowers the risk of death, need for LV assist device, or urgent transplantation compared to medical management.[19] Other studies, such as RAFT-AF and CABANA subanalyses, corroborate that improvements in LV function, symptoms, and hospitalizations are most pronounced in patients with reduced ejection fraction—although benefits may also extend to those with preserved EF. The RAFT-AF trial randomized 411 patients with AF and NYHA Class II–III HF, regardless of LV function, to ablation-based rhythm control or to optimized rate control. Although the primary end point was not met, the secondary outcomes consistently favored ablation, with significant improvements in LV ejection fraction, 6-minute walk distance, QoL, and serum BNP levels for the ablation group.[16]

Prospective Evidence for Arrhythmia-Induced Cardiomyopathy

An arrhythmia-induced cardiomyopathy is a variety of dilated cardiomyopathy, which is purely attributed to an arrhythmia. But, in clinical practice, it is difficult to establish a clear causal relationship at patient presentation with the majority having a diagnosis retrospectively. The CAMERA-MRI study showed a greater improvement in LV function in the absence of fibrosis on MRI, making it one of the features of an AIC.[13] Schach et. al. (TACHY-HF pilot trial) showed that in patients with new LV systolic dysfunction and tachyarrhythmia, AIC was highly prevalent (82%) and most showed rapid, substantial recovery of LVEF within 2–6 months after rhythm control. A smaller baseline LV end-diastolic diameter (<56.5 mm) predicted reversibility, while biomarkers and scar imaging were not useful.[24] The WITHDRAW-AF trial showed that in carefully selected patients (no late gadolinium enhancement on MRI and low NT proBNP) with AF-mediated cardiomyopathy and normalized LVEF after rhythm control, withdrawal of HF therapy was safe, with ~90% maintaining LVEF ≥ 50% at 6 months and sustained recovery at long-term follow-up. Relapses were rare, asymptomatic, and reversible with therapy reinitiation.[25]

The greatest improvement in LVEF typically occurs within the first 2 months after restoration of sinus rhythm, with further recovery up to 6 months. Accordingly, most studies assess improvement at 6 months, defining recovery as either an absolute increase in LVEF ≥ 15%, or an increase of ≥10% with normalization of LVEF to ≥50% within this time frame.

Evidence Supporting Catheter Ablation in Heart Failure with Preserved Ejection Fraction (Table 3)

The data supporting CA in HFpEF are less robust and the guidelines suggest CA as a Class IIa recommendation in

TABLE 1: Trials of AF ablation in heart failure with reduced.

Trial (Year)	N	Population (EF threshold)	AF type	Intervention vs. Control	Primary outcome	Result (direction)	LVEF change (approximately)	Key notes
PABA-CHF (2008)[8]	81	AF with symptomatic HF; LVEF ≤ 40%	Persistent/ long-standing	Pulmonary vein isolation vs. AV-node ablation + BiV pacing	Functional capacity, LVEF, QoL at 6 months	PVI superior (↑LVEF, ↑6-MWT, ↑QoL)	↑ ~8–13% absolute (vs. smaller with AVN + BiV). The mean absolute change in EF was an increase of 8 ± 8% with ablation compared with a decrease of 1 ± 4% with AVN ablation + biventricular pacing ($p < 0.001$)	First RCT showing superiority of AF ablation over AVN + BiV for symptoms/LVEF in CHF
MacDonald (2011)[9]	41 (22 ablation, 19 medical)	Advanced HF; LVEF <35%; persistent AF	Persistent	Radiofrequency AF ablation vs. Rate control (medical therapy)	Change in LVEF by CMR at 6 months	Neutral (no CMR LVEF improvement; ↑ radionuclide EF modestly)	4.5% (CMR, NS) vs. +8.2% radionuclide ($p = 0.03$)	50% in sinus rhythm at follow-up; high complication rate (≈15%); small single-center trial
ARC-HF (2013)[10]	52	Symptomatic HF; LVEF ≤ 35%	Persistent	Catheter ablation vs. rate control	Change in peak VO_2 at 12 months	Positive (↑ exercise capacity, QoL, BNP improvement). The primary endpoint, peak oxygen consumption, showed no significant change at 3 months but improved significantly at 12 months in the ablation arm (mean difference +3.07 mL/kg/min, $p = 0.018$)	Approximate 8% increase in LVEF compared with rate control	First RCT powered for functional capacity (rate vs. rhythm control); significant VO_2 improvement. Ablation was also associated with significant improvements in the Minnesota Living with Heart Failure score, reductions in BNP levels

Continued

Continued

Trial (Year)	N	Population (EF threshold)	AF type	Intervention vs. Control	Primary outcome	Result (direction)	LVEF change (approximately)	Key notes
CAMTAF (2014)[11]	50	Symptomatic HF; LVEF < 50%	Persistent	Catheter ablation vs. medical rate control	Change in LVEF at 6 months	Positive (Ablation superior)	Ablation +8.1% vs. −3.6% with rate control	Improved VO_2, BNP, NYHA, and QoL with ablation
AATAC (2016)[12]	203	Symptomatic HFrEF; LVEF ≤ 40%; ICD/CRT-D common	Persistent	Catheter ablation vs. Amiodarone (rhythm-control)	Freedom from AF at 24 months	Ablation superior (≈70% vs. 34%)	↑ with ablation	Lower HF hospitalization (≈31% vs. 57%) and all-cause mortality (≈8% vs. 18%) with ablation
CAMERA-MRI (2017)[13]	66	Idiopathic cardiomyopathy; LVEF ≤ 45%	Persistent	Catheter ablation vs. Rate-control strategy	Change in LVEF at ~6 months	Ablation markedly ↑LVEF (especially without LGE)	↑ ~18% absolute (no-LGE subgroup)	Supports AF-mediated (tachycardia) cardiomyopathy reversibility with ablation
CASTLE-AF (2018)[14]	363	Symptomatic HF (NYHA II–IV); LVEF ≤35%; ICD/CRT-D	Paroxysmal or persistent	Catheter ablation vs. Medical therapy (rate/ antiarrhythmic)	All-cause death or HF hospitalization	Ablation significantly reduced the primary EP compared with medical therapy (28.5% vs. 44.6%, $p = 0.006$. Reduced composite with ablation (HR ~0.62); ↓death (HR ~0.53)	↑ ~8% absolute with ablation	Landmark positive hard-outcome trial in HFrEF
AMICA (2019)[15]	140 randomized; 68 vs. 72 analyzed	Persistent/ longstanding AF; LVEF ≤35%; ICD/ CRT-D required	Persistent/ longstanding persistent	Catheter ablation vs. Best medical therapy (rate/ rhythm control)	Change in LVEF at 1 year	Neutral (LVEF ↑ in both groups, no difference)	Ablation +8.8% vs. BMT +7.3% (NS)	Terminated early for futility; advanced HF patients; no clinical benefit. Underpowered; early termination limits inference

Continued

Continued

Trial (Year)	N	Population (EF threshold)	AF type	Intervention vs. Control	Primary outcome	Result (direction)	LVEF change (approximately)	Key notes
RAFT-AF (2021)[16]	411	HF (HFrEF ≤ 45% or biomarker-defined HF), NYHA II/III on OMT This trial included HFpEF patients too and reported outcomes separately	High burden paroxysmal, persistent/long-standing	Ablation-based rhythm control vs. Rate control	Death or HF events. FU 37 months	Primary endpoint occurred less frequently with ablation (23.4%) than with rate control (32.5%), though the difference did not reach statistical significance	↑ with ablation In prespecified analyses, patients with *LVEF ≤45%* showed a clear benefit with ablation (HR: 0.63, 95% CI: 0.41–0.96), while those with preserved EF did not	Stopped early; improved QoL and LVEF; more procedure-related AEs
CABANA HF subgroup (2021)[17]	778	HF (mixed EF; HF history)	Paroxysmal/persistent	Catheter ablation vs. Drug therapy	CABANA primary composite (death, disabling stroke, serious bleeding, CA arrest)	Benefit signal in HF subgroup; not HF-specific primary	Most patients had preserved EF at baseline, and ablation did *not* produce a significant overall change in EF	Subgroup; open-label; not limited to HFrEF. EF was available in 73% of patients: 9.3% <40%, 11.7% 40–49%, and ~80% ≥50%
Zakeri et. al.: ARC-HF and CAMTAF (combined long-term follow-up)[18]	102 (52 ER-CA, 50 RC)	Symptomatic HFrEF (NYHA II–III), mean LVEF ~31%, median AF duration 24–36 months	Persistent or long-standing persistent AF	Early routine catheter ablation (ER-CA) vs. pharmacological rate control (RC; some later had delayed selective ablation, DS-CA)	All-cause mortality (ITT); secondary: death + CV hospitalization	ITT: No significant difference (mortality 32.7% ER-CA vs. 34% RC; HR 0.89, $p = 0.73$). Treatment-received: CA associated with reduced all-cause mortality (HR 0.43, $p = 0.028$) and death/CV hospitalization (HR 0.48, $p = 0.031$)	At 12 months: ER-CA improved LVEF by median +8.4% vs. RC −2.0% ($p = 0.0003$)	Longest follow-up (~8 years). >50% of RC patients eventually crossed to ablation. Recurrent AF ~40% after CA. ER-CA vs. DS-CA showed similar long-term survival, but ablation overall linked to better outcomes
CASTLE-HTx (2023)[19]	194	Advanced HF (LVAD/HTx candidates); reduced EF typical	Paroxysmal/persistent	Catheter ablation vs. Medical therapy	Composite of mortality/advanced HF endpoints. FU 18 months	Ablation lowered primary events (8% vs. 30%) and mortality (6% vs. 20%) compared with medical therapy	N/A or not primary	Advanced HF cohort; contemporary management

TABLE 2: Major meta-analyses of AF Ablation in HFrEF.

First author/year	N (studies/patients)	Population	Comparison	Follow-up	Key findings
Chen et al. 2020 (Eur Heart J)[20]	11 RCTs of rate vs. rhythm control trials, 3,598 patients (1,112 CA vs. medical) 7 trials of ablation	AF + HF (HFrEF)	CA vs. medical therapy	0.5–3.2 years	CA ↓ mortality (OR 0.51), ↓ rehospitalization (OR 0.44), improved LVEF (+6.8%), lower arrhythmia recurrence
Pan et al. 2021 (Int J Med Sci)[21]	6 RCTs, 775 patients	AF + HFrEF	CA vs. medical therapy	6–38 months	CA ↓ all-cause mortality (RR: 0.52), ↓ HF hospitalization (RR: 0.56), improved LVEF, 6MWT, QoL
Pasqualotto et al. 2024 (Heart Rhythm)[22]	6 RCTs, 1,055 patients	AF + HFrEF (LVEF ≤40%)	CA vs. medical therapy	6 months to 60 months	CA ↓ HF hospitalization (RR: 0.57), ↓ CV mortality (RR: 0.46), ↓ all-cause mortality (RR: 0.53), ↑ LVEF (+3.8%), ↑ QoL
Zhang et al. 2024 (ESC Heart Failure)[23]	9 RCTs, 2,293 patients	AF + HF (mostly HFrEF). All trials had low EF, except the CABANA-HF which had higher EF	CA vs. medical therapy	0.5–7.8 years	CA ↓ all-cause mortality (RR: 0.60), ↓ HF rehospitalization (RR 0.65), improved LVEF (+6.3%), ↑ QoL, ↓ AF recurrence

appropriate symptomatic HFpEF patients. **Table 3** enlists all the studies of HFpEF and rhythm control strategies for AF.

Historically, rhythm control in HFpEF has presented challenges, as antiarrhythmic drugs have limited efficacy and may cause adverse effects, while rate control alone does not address the hemodynamic burden of AF.[43] Clinical studies and meta-analyses **(Table 4)** have increasingly shown that CA is effective and safe in the HFpEF population, with efficacy and safety broadly comparable to outcomes seen in AF with HFrEF.[2,44-46] Several cohort and matched studies demonstrate that recurrence rates, freedom from arrhythmia, and safety profiles after ablation in HFpEF are similar to those in patients without HF or with HFrEF.[29,43] Prospective and retrospective studies also report significant improvements in QoL, New York Heart Association (NYHA) class, mitral inflow parameters, and functional capacity after restoration of sinus rhythm with CA.[16,35] One large matched analysis including tens of thousands of patients found that ablation did not significantly affect 1-year HF readmission or mortality when compared to conventional therapy but did substantially reduce the risk of AF-related readmissions.[31] Other studies, such as Fukui et al,[26] found that CA independently reduced HF rehospitalization compared to drug therapy, and Rattka et al.[34] observed that both HF hospitalization and mortality were lower after ablation. Randomized pilot studies (e.g., Chieng et al[37] and STALL AF-HFpEF[32]) further demonstrate that effective rhythm control with ablation lowers pulmonary capillary wedge pressure, improves exercise tolerance, and alleviates HFpEF symptoms and biomarkers compared to medical therapy. In the CABANA trial subgroup of 778 patients with clinically stable HF, CA compared with drug therapy was associated with a 36% relative reduction in the primary composite outcome and a 43% reduction in all-cause mortality over 48.5 months. It must be noted that only 9.3% of patients in this trial had EF < 40%, making this predominantly a study of HFpEF patients.[42]

Despite these promising results, most data are from nonrandomized or observational studies, and ongoing multicenter randomized trials are evaluating **(Table 5)** hard outcomes like mortality, HF hospitalization, and QoL in HFpEF with AF.

CATHETER ABLATION: RATIONALE AND TECHNIQUES

Pulmonary vein isolation (PVI) is the cornerstone of AF ablation, whether the addition of substrate-based ablation or trigger-based ablation confers benefit is unclear.

Substrate Ablation

Voltage-guided Substrate Modification

Meta-analyses show that ablating LVAs along with PVI improves freedom from arrhythmia in patients with persistent AF, without increasing adverse event rates. Compared to PVI alone, voltage-guided substrate ablation leads to higher rates of long-term arrhythmia suppression and fewer postablation

TABLE 3: Recent studies of rhythm control and atrial fibrillation ablation trials in HFpEF.

Trial (Year)	N	Population	AF type	Primary outcome	Follow-up	Result	Notes
Fukui et al. (2020, Japan)[26]	85 (35 ablation vs. 50 medical)	AF + HFpEF (EF ≥50%, prior HF hospitalization)	60% persistent	HF rehospitalization	~2 years	Positive—ablation ↓ rehospitalization (9% vs. 48%)	Retrospective single center
Krishnamurthy et al. (2022, NRD US)[27]	50,299 AF ablation cases (HFpEF subset)	Real-world AF + HFpEF	Mixed	30-day readmissions, complications	30 days	30 day readmission after AF ablation was high in HFpEF patients. (18.3%)	National readmissions database
Zylla et al. (2022, Circulation HF)[28]	102 (24 HFpEF vs. 78 no-HF)	AF + HFpEF (LVEF ≥ 50%)	Mixed	Functional/QoL, AF recurrence, Echo parameters	12 months	Negative—HFpEF patients had more recurrence and rehospitalization. (Compared to no HF)	Cryoballoon ablation, prospective observational
Aldaas et al., 2020 (UCSD Registry)[29]	51 HFpEF, 40 HFrEF, 456 no HF	Retrospective study of patients who underwent de novo ablation enrolled in the UC San Diego AF Ablation Registry	Mixed	Primary recurrence of atrial arrhythmia Others: in-hospital adverse events, all-cause hospitalization and mortality	5 years	Arrhythmia-free survival (off AAD at 5 years): 71% HFpEF vs. 34% HFrEF vs. 49% no HF ($p = 0.053$). No significant mortality difference	Retrospective cohort study with long FU. HFpEF outcomes comparable to no HF and better than HFrEF
Zhang et al. (2020)[30]	447	AF + HFpEF	Newly diagnosed AF and HF. Rate control vs. rhythm control with medications and/or ablation	Mortality	12–24 months	Rhythm control offered no benefit in HFpEF	Observational
Arora et al. (2020)[31]	56,395	AF + HFpEF	Mixed	Composite of HF readmission and mortality at 1 year	184 days	Primary outcome was not significant (ablation 10.4% vs. 11.4% without ablation)	Regardless of HF phenotype, ablation failed to reduce death or HF readmission at 1 year, though it was effective in lowering AF-related hospitalizations
Sugumar et al., 2021 (STALL AF-HFpEF, Australia)[32]	N = 54 (35 HFpEF, 20 underwent ablation)	Symptomatic AF, preserved EF (≥50%), HFpEF by invasive exercise RHC	Paroxysmal and persistent AF	Hemodynamic (PCWP), BNP, QoL, and symptom scores	12 ± 6 months	45% no longer met HFpEF criteria postablation; improved PCWP, BNP, and MLHF scores in arrhythmia-free patients	Prospective observational; invasive hemodynamics; small sample size

Continued

Continued

Trial (Year)	N	Population	AF type	Primary outcome	Follow-up	Result	Notes
EAST-AFNET4 HF subgroup (Rillig et al. 2021)[33]	798 HF patients, 442 (56%) HFpEF and 211 patients had HF midrange EF	AF diagnosed ≤12 months, NYHA II–III or LVEF <50%	Early AF (paroxysmal or persistent)	Composite of CV death, stroke, or hospitalization for HF/ACS	Median 5.1 years	Early rhythm control (ablation or AAD) reduced primary outcome: HR: 0.74 (95% CI: 0.56–0.97, $p = 0.03$). Effect consistent across HFpEF, HFmrEF, and HFrEF	Intervention not limited to ablation—~20% had ablation, rest on AADs. Shows benefit of systematic early rhythm control in HFpEF
Rattka et al., 2021 (Ulm, Germany)[34]	86 (43 CA vs. 43 medical)	Symptomatic HFpEF (NYHA ≥ II), confirmed by echo + NT-proBNP, AF	Paroxysmal and persistent AF	Composite of death or HF hospitalization	Mean 35 ± 22 months	CA reduced composite endpoint (HR 0.30, $p = 0.003$), fewer HF hospitalizations, ↓ AF recurrence (HR 0.47), improved diastolic function and NYHA class, HFpEF resolution 35% vs. 9%	Single-center, nonrandomized, PS matched. Patients receiving CA progressed from paroxysmal to persistent AF significantly less frequently than medically treated patients
Yamauchi et al., 2021 (Ogaki, Japan)[35]	502 (293 HFpEF, 84 HFmrEF + HFrEF, 125 no HF)	Nonparoxysmal AF patients undergoing index ablation; subgroup with HFpEF (LVEF ≥50%, BNP ≥ 100 pg/mL or HF hospitalization)	Nonparoxysmal AF only (persistent and long-standing persistent)	AF recurrence at 1 year, changes in function, BNP, and NYHA class	12 months	In HFpEF: AF recurrence 16.4%; 95% sinus rhythm; BNP ↓ significantly; NYHA and LVEF improved; HF remission (BNP < 100) in 79.6%	Large single-center observational; compared HFpEF vs. HFrEF vs. no HF; freedom from AF recurrence predicted HF remission
Swedish HF Registry (von Olshausen et al. 2022)[36]	434 ablation vs. 868 matched nonablation (of ~44,000 registry patients)	AF + HF across EF spectrum; subgroup: HFpEF (≥50%)	Real-world AF (paroxysmal and persistent)	Composite: All-cause mortality + first HF hospitalization	Median 2.6 years (up to 14 years)	Ablation ↓risk of primary outcome: HR: 0.78 (95% CI: 0.65–0.94). In HFpEF: Also ↓ recurrent HF hospitalization (IRR: 0.17, 95% CI: 0.07–0.42)	Large unselected national cohort; confirms ablation benefit in HFpEF in real-world practice
RAFT-AF Trial 2022 (Canada and international RCT)—HFpEF category[16]	411 (214 ablation-based rhythm vs. 197 rate control). 171 patients with HFpEF (Rate control = 81 patients vs. Ablation = 90 patients)	Symptomatic HF (NYHA II–III), AF (high-burden paroxysmal or persistent), NT-proBNP elevated; included HFpEF (LVEF > 45%)	High-burden paroxysmal or persistent AF	Composite of all-cause mortality + HF events	Median 37 months (trial stopped early for futility)	Primary endpoint: (HFpEF category) 24.4% ablation vs. 25.9% control (HR 0.71, $p = 0.066$). Secondary: ↑LVEF, ↑6MWD, ↓NT-proBNP, better QoL. (Nonsignificant)	First large RCT including HFpEF. Did not reach significance due to early stop, but trends favored ablation

Continued

Continued

Trial (Year)	N	Population	AF type	Primary outcome	Follow-up	Result	Notes
Chieng et al. (2023, RCT JACC HF)[37]	31 (16 ablation vs. 15 medication)	AF + HFpEF (PCWP ≥ 15/25)	81% persistent	Peak PCWP exercise	6 months	Positive – ↓ PCWP, ↑VO_2, ↓NT-proBNP, QoL ↑	First RCT in HFpEF
Tsuda et al. 2023 (Japan)[38]	212 (106 ablation vs. 106 medical therapy)	AF with HFmrEF (40–49%) or HFpEF (≥50%), mean age 68 years	Mixed AF types (paroxysmal and persistent)	Composite of CV death + HF hospitalization	Median 24.6 months	Ablation reduced events: HR: 0.32 (95% CI: 0.13–0.70, $p = 0.004$)	Multicenter registry, robust PS-matching
Xie et al. (2024, Europace)[39]	1,034 (392 ablation vs. 642 medication)	AF + HFpEF	Mixed	Death or HF hospitalization	Median 39 months	Positive—ablation ↓ primary (HR 0.55) and rehospitalization	Cohort, large Chinese series
DeLuca et al. (2024, TriNetX US)[40]	23,419 (1,959 CA vs. 7,689 AAT). After matching, each group had 1,816 patients, with a total of 3,632 patients for outcomes analysis	AF + HFpEF	Mixed	Primary: Mortality Secondary end points: CVA and HF events	6 years	Positive—ablation ↓ mortality (9.2% vs. 20.5%). No difference in stroke	Real-world, propensity matched
Zylla et al. (2024, Women HFpEF)[41]	102 women (20 HFpEF vs. 22 no HF)	Women + HFpEF	Mixed	Symptoms, QoL, and AF recurrence	≥12 months	Negative—HFpEF women had ↑ rehospitalization, persistent symptoms	Subanalysis of AFFECT study
CABANA–HFpEF (2025, Martens et al.)[42]	1,763 (CABANA patients with HFpEF probability)	AF with high likelihood of HFpEF (modified H_2FPEF ≥6, LVEF >50%)	Paroxysmal, persistent, long-standing	Composite of CV hospitalization or all-cause death or AF recurrence or functional status	Median ~4 years	Ablation reduced events in high-likelihood HFpEF (HR: 0.82, 95% CI: 0.69–0.98, $p = 0.025$); no benefit in low-likelihood HFpEF	Post hoc CABANA analysis; also showed greater AF recurrence reduction and NYHA improvement in HFpEF subgroup

TABLE 4: Meta-analyses of AF ablation in HFpEF and related HF phenotypes.

First author/ Year	N (studies/ patients)	Population	Comparison	Follow-up	Key findings
Kroshian 2024 (JCE)[2]	22 studies, 248,323 patients	AF + HF (HFrEF 49.7%, HFmrEF 16.5%, and HFpEF 33.8%)	AF vs. sinus rhythm (risk of outcomes by HF type)	Up to 6 years (registry-based)	AF ↑ mortality in HFmrEF (HR 1.25) and HFpEF (HR 1.16), not HFrEF. ↑ HF hospitalization in HFmrEF (HR 1.64) and HFpEF (HR 1.46). Stroke risk ↑ in all groups
Siddiqui 2022 (JOA)[44]	7 observational studies, 2,554 HFpEF patients	AF + HFpEF undergoing ablation	CA vs. HFrEF/ no HF	Mean 2.6 years (1–5 years)	No difference in arrhythmia recurrence, repeat ablation, mortality, hospitalization, or stroke between HFpEF vs. HFrEF/no HF. Safety (tamponade, stroke) similar
Bulhões 2024 (Heart Rhythm)[45]	8 studies, 20,257 patients (RCTs + observational)	AF + HFpEF	Ablation vs. medical therapy	24.6–61.2 months (median ~3–5 years)	Ablation ↓ death or HF hospitalization (HR 0.62), all-cause death (HR 0.68), CV death (HR 0.42), and HF hospitalization (HR 0.43) vs. medical therapy. Stronger benefit in CV outcomes
Oraii 2024 (JAMA Cardiol)[46]	12 RCTs, 2,465 patients (913 HFpEF, 1,552 HFrEF)	AF + HF (NYHA ≥ II)	Ablation vs. conventional therapy	6–60 months (trial dependent)	Ablation ↓ HF events in HFrEF (RR: 0.59) but no benefit in HFpEF (RR: 0.93). No mortality benefit in HFpEF (CV death RR: 0.91; all-cause RR: 0.95). Suggests phenotype-specific effect

TABLE 5: Planned/ongoing prospective trials evaluating rhythm versus rate control in AF and HFpEF.

Trial (ClinicalTrials.gov ID)	Comparison	PAF and PrsAF with	Primary endpoint
CABA-HFPEF (NCT05508256); recruiting	Catheter ablation vs. usual care	HFpEF or HFmrEF (41–49%) and HF hospitalization within 6 months	Composite of cardiovascular death, stroke, and total CV hospitalization for HF or ACS
STABLE-SR IV (NCT06125925); recruiting	Catheter ablation vs. AAD	HFpEF	Composite of worsening HF and cardiovascular death
TAP-CHF (NCT04160000); two-phase pilot study, recruiting	Catheter ablation vs. AAD (with or without wireless PA pressure monitoring)	HFpEF (EF > 50%) with hospitalization in last 12 months diuretic use, or evidence of structural heart disease. They will undergo a catheter ablation procedure within 14 days of randomization	Composite of HF hospitalization or cardiovascular death
AMPERE (NCT04282850); pilot study, not yet recruiting	Catheter ablation vs. medical management	HFpEF with prior hospitalization within past 12 months	Change in AF burden
CAPHF-AF (NCT06740539); not yet recruiting	Catheter ablation vs. AAD	HFpEF with prior HF hospitalization. NYHA II–IV and EF >50% and raised natriuretic peptides. At least one of following: LVH, LAE or diastolic dysfunction	Composite of all-cause death or hospitalization for worsening HF

atrial tachycardia recurrences.[47] The STABLE-SR-II trial found substrate ablation was not universally superior, but in abnormal LA substrate, additional LVA ablation trended toward better outcomes.[48]

Tailored Ablation

In hypertrophic cardiomyopathy and other structural diseases, substrate mapping and ablation can be tailored based on genetic and anatomical markers to improve outcomes.[49]

MARSHALL Plan (Vein of Marshall Alcohol Ablation)

The PROMPT-AF trial showed that adding ethanol infusion of the vein of Marshall and targeted linear ablation (mitral isthmus, LA roof) to PVI significantly improved arrhythmia-free survival in persistent AF. These benefits were achieved without an increase in serious adverse events.[50]

Left Atrial Posterior Wall Isolation

A meta-analysis has shown that posterior wall isolation could reduce AF recurrence in persistent AF.[51] Although observational and smaller studies previously suggested that PWI might be beneficial in HF populations due to the higher prevalence of low-voltage tissue and scar in the posterior wall, the randomized CAPLA data do not support routine empirical PWI in this group.[52] But a substudy of the CAPLA trial showed better outcomes when LA posterior wall isolation was performed for patients with rapid electrogram activity in the posterior wall (shortest cycle length <140 ms).[53]

■ Ablating Nonpulmonary Vein Triggers

Non-PV triggers such as those from the LA posterior wall, septum, superior vena cava, and coronary sinus are more common in persistent AF and in patients with atrial tissue degeneration and HF, who have larger low-voltage areas.[54] Zhao et al. have shown that about 70% of PAF patients with LV systolic dysfunction (LVEF ≤ 35%) have non-PV triggers. Outcomes with PV isolation alone are poorer, but adding ablation of non-PV triggers significantly improves long-term success, making results comparable to patients with normal LVEF. The most common source in this study was the coronary sinus.[55]

Though these studies did not specifically test these additional lesions in AF with HF, it could be conceived that they may be of benefit in HF, which is associated with an abnormal atrial substrate.

■ Early versus Delayed Ablation

Studies have suggested that long delays to CA of AF adversely impacted procedural success and increased HF and mortality.[56] A subanalysis of the EAST-AFNET4 has also suggested that recently diagnosed AF with a CHA_2DS_2-VASc score >4 should be considered for early rhythm control.[57] Importantly, there is a vulnerable phase following a decompensated HF, which lasts 3–6 months when the rehospitalizations are increased. Lador et al. have shown that in AF patients with HF, AF ablation was associated with better outcomes when done within 6 months.[58] In a multicenter Japanese cohort o 543 patients with AF and HF undergoing cryoballoon ablation (CBA), those treated within 6 months of AF diagnosis had significantly lower AF recurrence (24% vs. 34% with delayed ablation) over ~21 months of follow-up. Early ablation independently reduced recurrence risk (HR 0.58), particularly in patients with preserved LVEF, whereas differences in mortality and HF hospitalization were not significant.[59] Rillig et al. from a subanalysis of the EAST-AFNET4 trial have shown a significant benefit of early rhythm control when started within 1 year of AF in patients with HF.[33] DeLuca et al. in a retrospective cohort study showed that CA was associated with lower mortality and acute HF with HFrEF.[40] A meta-analysis of 10 observational studies concluded that early ablation in AF with HF was associated with lower AF recurrence, reduced HF hospitalizations, and a nonsignificant trend toward lower mortality.[60] In the nationwide JROAD-HF registry, early CA (within 90 days of hospitalization for HF with AF) was associated with significantly lower long-term all-cause mortality, cardiovascular death, and HF-related death compared with patients who did not undergo early ablation.[61] These findings suggest that performing ablation soon after an HF admission may interrupt the vicious cycle of AF and HF, improving prognosis beyond conventional therapy. Overall, there appears to be a significant benefit of early ablation in AF patients with HF, especially when performed within 6 months of diagnosis.

ALTERNATIVE ENERGY SOURCES

Radiofrequency ablation has been commonly employed in AF ablation over the years. Currently, two alternative energy sources are available for CA of AF: Pulsed field ablation and cryotherapy.

■ Cryoballoon Ablation

Cryoballoon ablation has been established as a safe and effective strategy for AF in patients with HF, particularly HFrEF. Due to its procedural simplicity, CB may be advantageous in achieving quick and durable PVI in patients with borderline hemodynamics. Meta-analyses show that CBA yields significant improvements in LV ejection fraction (≈10–13% absolute increase), NYHA functional class, and arrhythmia-free survival rates of ~60–65% at 1 year, comparable to radiofrequency ablation. Major complications occur in about 6%, most often transient phrenic nerve injury, with very low procedure-related mortality. While outcomes in HFrEF are consistent, evidence in HFpEF is limited, with lower arrhythmia-free survival and less clear benefit on remodeling.[62]

■ Pulsed-field Ablation

Potential advantages of pulsed-field ablation (PFA) in HF are: (1) Myocardial selectivity with sparing of adjacent structures such as esophagus and nerves, thereby reducing complications in sick HF patients. (2) Shorter procedure times with lesser myocardial depressant effects of anesthesia. This may help patients with impaired hemodynamics by achieving a quicker isolation. (3) Better hemodynamic stability and less char formation.[63] (4) Potential for less fibroelastic scarring and less atrial remodeling. Limiting additional fibrosis could help preserve atrial compliance and ventricular filling, resulting in a lower incidence of stiff left atrium.[64]

The MANIFEST-PF multicenter registry established the safety of PFA in AF patients with HF with similar adverse events.[65] An ongoing study CABA-HFpEF-DZHK27 aims to determine the long-term benefits of PF ablation in HFpEF.

COMPLICATIONS

Atrial fibrillation ablation can be associated with major complications such as periprocedural death, atrioesophageal fistula, stroke, and cardiac perforation. These complications are now very uncommon, with life-threatening events reported in <1% of cases across contemporary studies.[66] Crowley et al. showed that the major complication rates with ablation were similar in patients with low EF and preserved EF, but patients with low EF had a higher incidence of LAA thrombus, periprocedural hypotension, and bradycardia and HF decompensation.[67] These authors proposed the following steps for HF patients undergoing ablation:

1. Holding HF medications and antiarrhythmic medications before the procedure to avoid hypotension and bradycardia.
2. Preprocedural imaging for LAA thrombus.
3. Using low-volume irrigated catheters or PFA to reduce fluid overload.
4. Monitoring input/output strictly and use of diuretics.
5. Overnight hospitalization and hemodynamic monitoring.

GUIDELINE PERSPECTIVES

- For HFrEF, the ACC/AHA guidelines give a *Class I, Level B* recommendation for AF ablation, supported by strong evidence of improved outcomes.[68] The ESC guidelines provide a *Class I, Level B* recommendation for ablation in AF-related tachycardiomyopathy and a *Class IIa, Level B* recommendation for ablation in selected HFrEF patients.[69]
- For HFpEF, the ACC/AHA guidelines give a *Class IIa* recommendation, acknowledging potential benefit but with less robust evidence. The ESC guidelines do not provide a distinct prognostic indication for ablation in HFpEF, instead applying general AF ablation criteria, and note that unlike HFrEF, randomized trials have not shown clear prognostic benefit.
- Patients most likely to benefit from AF ablation include those with mild LA fibrosis and smaller atria, no scar on CMR, suspected arrhythmia-mediated cardiomyopathy, paroxysmal or early persistent AF, and younger age with few comorbidities. Those less likely to benefit include patients with advanced HF, large ventricular scar on CMR, long-standing AF, advanced age, multiple comorbidities, or prior failed ablation.[70]

Atrial Flutter

The prevalence of HF in patients with atrial flutter ranges from 6% to 56%, though most studies do not distinguish from AF or HF phenotype.[71] Evidence—including a retrospective cohort showing lower 1-year mortality and reduced HF readmissions after AFL ablation in HFrEF, but not in HFpEF—supports ablation as first-line therapy at index presentation for typical cavotricuspid isthmus flutter, while atypical circuits require individualized decisions.

CONCLUSION

Catheter ablation is strongly supported in AF with HFrEF, where RCTs show reductions in mortality, HF hospitalizations, and improvements in LV function and QoL. There is data suggesting that in selected patients with an AF-induced cardiomyopathy, HF therapy may be withdrawn after successful rhythm control. In HFpEF, AF is highly prevalent and mechanistically linked; while early evidence suggests CA reduces AF burden, improves QoL, and lowers admissions, definitive RCT data are still awaited. Future studies will highlight the value of alternate energy sources and optimal ablation lesions in patients with HF and AF.

REFERENCES

1. Chelikam N, Katapadi A, Venkata Pothineni N, et al. Epidemiology of Atrial Fibrillation in Heart Failure. Card Electrophysiol Clin. 2025;17(1):1-11.
2. Kroshian G, Joseph J, Kinlay S, et al. Atrial fibrillation and risk of adverse outcomes in heart failure with reduced, mildly reduced, and preserved ejection fraction: A systematic review and meta-analysis. J Cardiovasc Electrophysiol. 2024;35(4):715-26.
3. Newman JD, O'Meara E, Böhm M, et al. Implications of Atrial Fibrillation for Guideline-Directed Therapy in Patients With Heart Failure: JACC State-of-the-Art Review. J Am Coll Cardiol. 2024;83(9):932-50.
4. Gopinathannair R, Chen LY, Chung MK, et al. Managing Atrial Fibrillation in Patients With Heart Failure and Reduced Ejection Fraction: A Scientific Statement From the American Heart Association. Circ Arrhythm Electrophysiol. 2021;14(6): HAE0000000000000078. Erratum in: Circ Arrhythm Electrophysiol. 2021;14(11):e000080.
5. Zou F, Levine H, Mohanty S, et al. Atrial Fibrillation-Induced Cardiomyopathy. Card Electrophysiol Clin. 2025;17(1):13-18.
6. Pabel S, Knierim M, Stehle T, et al. Effects of Atrial Fibrillation on the Human Ventricle. Circ Res. 2022;130(7):994-1010.
7. Takahashi Y, Yamaguchi T, Otsubo T, et al. Histological validation of atrial structural remodelling in patients with atrial fibrillation. Eur Heart J. 2023;44(35):3339-53.
8. Khan MN, Jaïs P, Cummings J, et al. Pulmonary-vein isolation for atrial fibrillation in patients with heart failure. N Engl J Med. 2008;359(17):1778-85.
9. MacDonald MR, Connelly DT, Hawkins NM, et al. Radiofrequency ablation for persistent atrial fibrillation in patients with advanced heart failure and severe left ventricular systolic dysfunction: a randomised controlled trial. Heart. 2011;97(9):740-7.
10. Jones DG, Haldar SK, Hussain W, et al. A randomized trial to assess catheter ablation versus rate control in the management

of persistent atrial fibrillation in heart failure. J Am Coll Cardiol. 2013;61(18):1894-903.

11. Hunter RJ, Berriman TJ, Diab I, et al. A randomized controlled trial of catheter ablation versus medical treatment of atrial fibrillation in heart failure (the CAMTAF trial). Circ Arrhythm Electrophysiol. 2014;7(1):31-8.
12. Di Biase L, Mohanty P, Mohanty S, et al. Ablation Versus Amiodarone for Treatment of Persistent Atrial Fibrillation in Patients With Congestive Heart Failure and an Implanted Device: Results From the AATAC Multicenter Randomized Trial. Circulation. 2016;133(17):1637-44.
13. Prabhu S, Taylor AJ, Costello BT, et al. Catheter Ablation Versus Medical Rate Control in Atrial Fibrillation and Systolic Dysfunction: The CAMERA-MRI Study. J Am Coll Cardiol. 2017;70(16):1949-61.
14. Marrouche NF, Brachmann J, Andresen D, et al. Catheter Ablation for Atrial Fibrillation with Heart Failure. N Engl J Med. 2018;378(5):417-27.
15. Kuck KH, Merkely B, Zahn R, et al. Catheter Ablation Versus Best Medical Therapy in Patients With Persistent Atrial Fibrillation and Congestive Heart Failure: The Randomized AMICA Trial. Circ Arrhythm Electrophysiol. 2019;12(12):e007731.
16. Parkash R, Wells GA, Rouleau J, et al. Randomized Ablation-Based Rhythm-Control Versus Rate-Control Trial in Patients With Heart Failure and Atrial Fibrillation: Results from the RAFT-AF trial. Circulation. 2022;145(23):1693-704.
17. Packer DL, Piccini JP, Monahan KH, et al. Ablation Versus Drug Therapy for Atrial Fibrillation in Heart Failure: Results From the CABANA Trial. Circulation. 2021;143(14):1377-90.
18. Zakeri R, Ahluwalia N, Tindale A, et al. Long-term outcomes following catheter ablation versus medical therapy in patients with persistent atrial fibrillation and heart failure with reduced ejection fraction. Eur J Heart Fail. 2023;25(1):77-86.
19. Sohns C, Fox H, Marrouche NF, et al. Catheter Ablation in End-Stage Heart Failure with Atrial Fibrillation. N Engl J Med. 2023;389(15):1380-9.
20. Chen S, Pürerfellner H, Meyer C, et al. Rhythm control for patients with atrial fibrillation complicated with heart failure in the contemporary era of catheter ablation: a stratified pooled analysis of randomized data. Eur Heart J. 2020;41(30):2863-73.
21. Pan KL, Wu YL, Lee M, et al. Catheter Ablation Compared with Medical Therapy for Atrial Fibrillation with Heart Failure: A Systematic Review and Meta-analysis of Randomized Controlled Trials. Int J Med Sci. 2021;18(6):1325-31.
22. Pasqualotto E, Ternes CMP, Chavez MP, et al. Catheter ablation for atrial fibrillation in heart failure with reduced ejection fraction patients: A meta-analysis. Heart Rhythm. 2024;21(9):1604-12.
23. Zhang Z, Zheng Y, He W, et al. Efficacy of catheter ablation for atrial fibrillation in heart failure: a meta-analysis of randomized controlled trials. ESC Heart Fail. 2024;11(5):2684-93.
24. Schach C, Körtl T, Zeman F, et al. Clinical Characterization of Arrhythmia-Induced Cardiomyopathy in Patients With Tachyarrhythmia and Idiopathic Heart Failure. JACC Clin Electrophysiol. 2024;10(5):870-81.
25. Segan L, Kistler PM, Nanayakkara S, et al. Withdrawal of heart failure therapy after atrial fibrillation rhythm control with ejection fraction normalization: the WITHDRAW-AF trial. Eur Heart J. 2025:ehaf563.
26. Fukui A, Tanino T, Yamaguchi T, et al. Catheter ablation of atrial fibrillation reduces heart failure rehospitalization in patients with heart failure with preserved ejection fraction. J Cardiovasc Electrophysiol. 2020;31(3):682-8.
27. Krishnamurthy A, Goyal P, Markowitz SM, et al. Outcomes of patients with heart failure with preserved ejection fraction undergoing catheter ablation of atrial fibrillation. Heart Rhythm O_2. 2022;3(5):501-8.
28. Zylla MM, Leiner J, Rahm AK, et al. Catheter Ablation of Atrial Fibrillation in Patients With Heart Failure and Preserved Ejection Fraction. Circ Heart Fail. 2022;15(9):e009281.
29. Aldaas OM, Malladi CL, Mylavarapu PS, et al. Comparison of Outcomes After Ablation of Atrial Fibrillation in Patients With Heart Failure With Preserved Versus Reduced Ejection Fraction. Am J Cardiol. 2020;136:62-70.
30. Zhang P, Chamberlain AM, Hodge DO, et al. Outcomes of incident atrial fibrillation in heart failure with preserved or reduced ejection fraction: A community-based study. J Cardiovasc Electrophysiol. 2020;31(9):2275-83.
31. Arora S, Jaswaney R, Jani C, et al. Catheter Ablation for Atrial Fibrillation in Patients With Concurrent Heart Failure. Am J Cardiol. 2020;137:45-54.
32. Sugumar H, Nanayakkara S, Vizi D, et al. A prospective STudy using invAsive haemodynamic measurements foLLowing catheter ablation for AF and early HFpEF: STALL AF-HFpEF. Eur J Heart Fail. 2021;23(5):785-96.
33. Rillig A, Magnussen C, Ozga AK, et al. Early Rhythm Control Therapy in Patients With Atrial Fibrillation and Heart Failure. Circulation. 2021;144(11):845-58.
34. Rattka M, Kühberger A, Pott A, et al. Catheter ablation for atrial fibrillation in HFpEF patients-A propensity-score-matched analysis. J Cardiovasc Electrophysiol. 2021;32(9):2357-67.
35. Yamauchi R, Morishima I, Okumura K, et al. Catheter ablation for non-paroxysmal atrial fibrillation accompanied by heart failure with preserved ejection fraction: feasibility and benefits in functions and B-type natriuretic peptide. Europace. 2021;23(8):1252-61.
36. von Olshausen G, Benson L, Dahlström U, et al. Catheter ablation for patients with atrial fibrillation and heart failure: insights from the Swedish Heart Failure Registry. Eur J Heart Fail. 2022;24(9):1636-46.
37. Chieng D, Sugumar H, Segan L, et al. Atrial Fibrillation Ablation for Heart Failure With Preserved Ejection Fraction: A Randomized Controlled Trial. JACC Heart Fail. 2023;11(6):646-58.
38. Tsuda T, Kato T, Usuda K, et al. Effect of Catheter Ablation for Atrial Fibrillation in Heart Failure With Mid-Range or Preserved Ejection Fraction-Pooled Analysis of the AF Frontier Ablation Registry and Hokuriku-Plus AF Registry. Circ J. 2023;87(7):939-46.
39. Xie Z, Qi B, Wang Z, et al. Ablation for atrial fibrillation improves the outcomes in patients with heart failure with preserved ejection fraction. Europace. 2023;26(1):euad363.
40. DeLuca MR, Ali B, Tarabichi Y, et al. Catheter ablation vs antiarrhythmic therapy for atrial fibrillation in heart failure with preserved ejection fraction. Heart Rhythm. 2024:S1547-5271(24)03460-X.
41. Zylla MM, Leiner J, Rahm AK, et al. Catheter ablation of atrial fibrillation in women with heart failure with preserved ejection fraction. Front Cardiovasc Med. 2024;11:1463815.
42. Martens P, Augusto SN Jr, Erzeel J, et al. Effects of Atrial Fibrillation Ablation for Heart Failure With Preserved Ejection Fraction: Insights From CABANA. JACC Heart Fail. 2025;13(5):785-94.
43. La Fazia VM, Pierucci N, Mohanty S, et al. Atrial Fibrillation Ablation in Heart Failure with Preserved Ejection Fraction. Card Electrophysiol Clin. 2025;17(1):53-62.
44. Siddiqui MU, Junarta J, Riley JM, et al. Catheter ablation in patients with atrial fibrillation and heart failure with preserved ejection fraction: A systematic review and meta-analysis. J Arrhythm. 2022;38(6):981-90.

45. Bulhões E, Antunes VLJ, Mazetto R, et al. Catheter ablation versus medical therapy for atrial fibrillation in patients with heart failure with preserved ejection fraction: A systematic review and meta-analysis. Heart Rhythm. 2024;21(9):1595-603.
46. Oraii A, McIntyre WF, Parkash R, et al. Atrial Fibrillation Ablation in Heart Failure With Reduced vs Preserved Ejection Fraction: A Systematic Review and Meta-Analysis. JAMA Cardiol. 2024;9(6):545-55.
47. Rivera A, Gewehr DM, Braga MAP, et al. Adjunctive low-voltage area ablation for patients with atrial fibrillation: An updated meta-analysis of randomized controlled trials. J Cardiovasc Electrophysiol. 2024;35(7):1329-39.
48. Yang G, Zheng L, Jiang C, et al. Circumferential Pulmonary Vein Isolation Plus Low-Voltage Area Modification in Persistent Atrial Fibrillation: The STABLE-SR-II Trial. JACC Clin Electrophysiol. 2022;8(7):882-91.
49. El-Harasis MA, Yoneda ZT, Anderson KC, et al. Ablation for Atrial Fibrillation in Patients With Rare Pathogenic Variants in Cardiomyopathy and Arrhythmia Genes. JACC Clin Electrophysiol. 2024;10(11):2359-70.
50. Sang C, Liu Q, Lai Y, et al. Pulmonary Vein Isolation With Optimized Linear Ablation vs Pulmonary Vein Isolation Alone for Persistent AF: The PROMPT-AF Randomized Clinical Trial. JAMA. 2025;333(5):381-9.
51. Kanitsoraphan C, Rattanawong P, Techorueangwiwat C, et al. The efficacy of posterior wall isolation in atrial fibrillation ablation: A systematic review and meta-analysis of randomized controlled trials. J Arrhythm. 2022;38(3):275-86.
52. Kistler PM, Chieng D, Sugumar H, et al. Effect of Catheter Ablation Using Pulmonary Vein Isolation With vs Without Posterior Left Atrial Wall Isolation on Atrial Arrhythmia Recurrence in Patients With Persistent Atrial Fibrillation: The CAPLA Randomized Clinical Trial. JAMA. 2023;329(2):127-35.
53. Segan L, Chieng D, Prabhu S, et al. Posterior Wall Isolation Improves Outcomes for Persistent AF With Rapid Posterior Wall Activity: CAPLA Substudy. JACC Clin Electrophysiol. 2023;9(12):2536-46.
54. Della Rocca DG, Di Biase L, Mohanty S, et al. Targeting non-pulmonary vein triggers in persistent atrial fibrillation: results from a prospective, multicentre, observational registry. Europace. 2021;23(12):1939-49.
55. Zhao Y, Di Biase L, Trivedi C, et al. Importance of non-pulmonary vein triggers ablation to achieve long-term freedom from paroxysmal atrial fibrillation in patients with low ejection fraction. Heart Rhythm. 2016;13(1):141-9.
56. Sessions AJ, May HT, Crandall BG, et al. Increasing time between first diagnosis of atrial fibrillation and catheter ablation adversely affects long-term outcomes in patients with and without structural heart disease. J Cardiovasc Electrophysiol. 2023;34(3):507-15.
57. Rillig A, Borof K, Breithardt G, et al. Early Rhythm Control in Patients With Atrial Fibrillation and High Comorbidity Burden. Circulation. 2022;146(11):836-47.
58. Lador A, Maccioni S, Khanna R, et al. Influence of time to ablation on outcomes among patients with atrial fibrillation with pre-existing heart failure. Heart Rhythm O_2. 2024;5(9):606-13.
59. Ando M, Yanagisawa S, Suzuki H, et al. Early Cryoablation After First Diagnosis of Atrial Fibrillation Reduces Arrhythmia Recurrence in Heart Failure Patients. JACC Asia. 2024;4(11):857-71.
60. Kilic ME, Arayici ME, Yilancioglu YR, et al. Early versus delayed catheter ablation in atrial fibrillation and heart failure: A systematic review and meta-analysis. Heart Rhythm. 2025;22(10):e882-e893.
61. Sakamoto K, Tohyama T, Ide T, et al. Efficacy of Early Catheter Ablation for Atrial Fibrillation After Admission for Heart Failure. JACC Clin Electrophysiol. 2023;9(9):1948-59.
62. Taha AM, Hendi NI, Elwekel AB, et al. Cryoballoon ablation for atrial fibrillation in patients with heart failure and reduced left ventricular ejection fraction: A systematic review and meta-analysis. Clin Cardiol. 2024;47(1):e24177.
63. Schoof L, Lemoine MD, Söffker G, et al. Pulsed field ablation for rhythm control in acute heart failure and extracorporeal membrane oxygenation: a case report. Eur Heart J Case Rep. 2025;9(8):ytaf373.
64. Parwani AS, Kossmann B, Schweiger V. Targeting atrial fibrillation in HFpEF: the emerging role of pulsed field ablation. Front Physiol. 2025;16:1621118.
65. Turagam MK, Neuzil P, Schmidt B, et al. Safety and Effectiveness of Pulsed Field Ablation for Atrial Fibrillation in Patients With Heart Failure. JACC Clin Electrophysiol. 2024:S2405-500X(24)00351-7.
66. Tzeis S, Gerstenfeld EP, Kalman J, et al. 2024 European Heart Rhythm Association/Heart Rhythm Society/Asia Pacific Heart Rhythm Society/Latin American Heart Rhythm Society expert consensus statement on catheter and surgical ablation of atrial fibrillation. Europace. 2024;26(4):euae043. Corrected and republished in: Heart Rhythm. 2024;21(9):e31-e149.
67. Crowley R, Ma J, Morton MB, et al. Complications of catheter ablation for atrial fibrillation: Important differences in patients with systolic heart failure. Heart Rhythm. 2025;22(6):1437-39.
68. Joglar JA, Chung MK, Armbruster AL, et al. 2023 ACC/AHA/ACCP/HRS Guideline for the Diagnosis and Management of Atrial Fibrillation: A Report of the American College of Cardiology/American Heart Association Joint Committee on Clinical Practice Guidelines. Circulation. 2024;149(1):e1-e156. Erratum in: Circulation. 2024;149(1):e167. Erratum in: Circulation. 2024;149(9):e936. Erratum in: Circulation. 2024;149(24):e1413.
69. Van Gelder IC, Rienstra M, Bunting KV, et al. 2024 ESC Guidelines for the management of atrial fibrillation developed in collaboration with the European Association for Cardio-Thoracic Surgery (EACTS). Eur Heart J. 2024;45(36):3314-414. Erratum in: Eur Heart J. 2025:ehaf306.
70. Diamant MJ, Andrade JG, Virani SA, et al. Heart failure and atrial flutter: a systematic review of current knowledge and practices. ESC Heart Fail. 2021;8(6):4484-96.
71. Jani C, Arora S, Zuzek Z, et al. Impact of catheter ablation in patients with atrial flutter and concurrent heart failure. Heart Rhythm O_2. 2020;2(1):53-63. Erratum in: Heart Rhythm O_2. 2021;2(3):309.

CHAPTER

84

Ventricular Tachycardia Ablation in the Emergency Setting

Aditya Mulgaonkar, Deepak Padmanabhan

ABSTRACT

Ventricular tachycardia (VT) storm, also known as electrical storm (ES) and incessant VT, represents a life-threatening arrhythmia that often requires urgent management. While initial stabilization relies on antiarrhythmic drugs, autonomic modulation and circulatory support, catheter ablation (CA) has emerged as a pivotal therapy in the emergency setting. Recent guideline updates from the ESC (2022) and European Heart Rhythm Association (EHRA) (2024) emphasize ablation as the treatment of choice for drug-refractory monomorphic VT in ES, highlighting its role in reducing arrhythmia recurrence, implantable cardioverter-defibrillator (ICD) shocks, and hospitalizations. Evidence from randomized trials, registries, and meta-analyses indicates significant reductions in arrhythmic burden, although mortality benefits remain less conclusive. Outcomes vary by underlying substrate, with ischemic cardiomyopathy (CMP) patients demonstrating more favorable results than those with nonischemic or inherited cardiomyopathies. Evolving strategies such as prophylactic mechanical circulatory support (MCS) and epicardial ablation in selected populations further strengthen the role of ablation in this high-risk group. This chapter reviews current pathophysiology, acute and long-term management, and evidence-based applications of catheter ablation in VT storm, underscoring its central role in modern arrhythmia care.

Keywords: Ventricular tachycardia, electrical storm, catheter ablation (CA), incessant VT, monomorphic VT, implantable cardioverter-defibrillator (ICD), mechanical circulatory support (MCS), ischemic cardiomyopathy (CMP), nonischemic CMP, primary electrical disease.

INTRODUCTION

Catheter ablation (CA) of cardiac arrhythmias using radiofrequency energy was first introduced by Huang and colleagues in 1985.[1] As different research groups contemporaneously evaluated the use of radiofrequency ablation (RFA) for various arrhythmias, the first reports of RF ablation for ventricular arrhythmias (VAs) in the emergency setting were published in the 1990s.[2,3] Since then, catheter ablation has emerged as a promising treatment option for certain patients presenting with electrical storm (ES) or incessant ventricular tachycardia (VT), especially when the storm is due to sustained monomorphic ventricular tachycardia (SMVT) or due to recurrent ventricular fibrillation by a similar PVC.

Electrical storm is defined as three or more episodes of sustained VAs occurring within 24 hours, requiring either antitachycardia pacing (ATP) or cardioversion/defibrillation, with each event separated by at least 5 minutes.[4]

The 2022 ESC guidelines for the management of patients with VAs and the prevention of sudden cardiac death, as well as the EHRA 2024 Consensus Statement on Management of patients with an ES or clustered VAs, provide the most recent guidance on the management of ES.

DEFINITIONS

Table 1 provides definitions of various terms as per the EHRA 2024 guidelines.[5]

PATHOPHYSIOLOGY

The mechanisms of ES vary depending upon the underlying substrate (i.e., structural heart disease or primary electrical disease). Most mechanistic insights have come from animal studies. Interrogation of implantable cardioverter-defibrillators (ICDs) in patients having these devices provides valuable clues to the origin of recurrent VAs. **Figure 1** summarizes our current knowledge on this aspect.

TABLE 1: Definitions.

Incessant VT	Continuous sustained VT that recurs promptly despite repeated intervention for termination over several hours
Sustained VT	VT for at least 30 seconds or which requires an acute intervention for termination
Nonsustained VT	Run of consecutive ventricular beats persisting for at least 3 beats to <30 seconds duration
Monomorphic VT	VT with the same QRS morphology from beat to beat
PVT (pleomorphic)	VT showing an abrupt morphological change of the 12-lead ECG VT morphology during an ongoing VT episode
Bidirectional VT	VT with beat-to-beat alternation of the frontal QRS axis
PVT (Polymorphic)	VT with continually changing QRS morphology
TdP	Subtype of a PVT in the context of QT prolongation, with continually changing QRS complexes that appear to spiral around the baseline of the ECG lead in a sinusoidal pattern
Short-coupled ventricular complexes	A PVC that interrupts the T-wave of the preceding conducted beat
VF	A chaotic rhythm with undulations that are irregular in timing and morphology, without discrete QRS complexes on the surface ECG
ES	Three or more episodes of sustained VA occurring within 24 hours, separated by at least 5 minutes, each requiring termination by an intervention
Clustered VAs	Two or more sustained VA events within 3 months

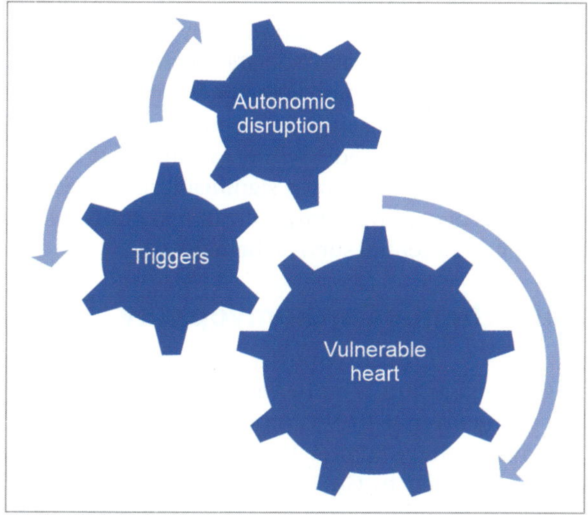

FIG. 1: The three contributing factors of ES.

Electrical storm arises from a vulnerable myocardium—due to scar, fibrosis, or genetic channelopathies—combined with external triggers such as ischemia, inflammation, fever, drugs, stress, exertion, or electrolyte imbalance. Autonomic dysregulation, regional catecholamine hypersensitivity, and repolarization heterogeneity facilitate arrhythmia initiation and perpetuation.

GENERAL PRINCIPLES IN MANAGING ELECTRICAL STORM

Patients presenting with ES require immediate stabilization. A focused history should include underlying cardiac disease, comorbidities, family history of sudden cardiac death, and drug exposures such as QT-prolonging agents. On arrival, hemodynamic and neurological assessment is crucial, with resuscitation per ACLS guidelines if arrest occurs.

A 12-lead ECG can identify arrhythmia mechanisms (e.g., bidirectional VT in CPVT, Brugada, ischemia, or electrolyte imbalance). Interrogation of an implantable cardioverter defibrillator (ICD), if present, provides details on arrhythmia burden and appropriateness of shocks; ICD therapies should initially be disabled to prevent worsening instability. Laboratory testing should prioritize electrolytes, renal, liver, and thyroid function, as well as troponins to rule out acute coronary syndrome, although elevations may result from the arrhythmia itself. Imaging—echocardiography, coronary angiography, or cardiac MRI—helps identify structural disease, ischemia, or inflammatory substrates, such as myocarditis.

Acute Therapy

Unstable VT/VF mandates prompt defibrillation. External cardioversion requires sedation in conscious patients, with paddles placed at least 8 cm away from the ICD pulse generator.[6] Urgent revascularization is indicated for early post-STEMI arrhythmias, while revascularization in a non-ACS setting may not be beneficial.[7] Fever and acute illness must be treated aggressively, especially in Brugada syndrome. Deep sedation and mechanical ventilation have been shown to be highly effective in treatment-refractory ES, achieving complete suppression of VT/VF within minutes to hours[8,9] and allowing time for definitive therapy. Electrolyte correction and avoidance of QT-prolonging drugs are essential.

Implantable cardioverter-defibrillator programming should be adjusted to prevent recurrent shocks, and deep sedation with ventilation may suppress refractory arrhythmias.

Pharmacotherapy

- In structural heart disease, first-line therapy is sympathetic blockade with non-selective beta-blockers, supplemented by IV amiodarone. Procainamide may be used if VT is tolerated, while lignocaine is useful in acute ischemia.
- In primary electrical syndromes, treatment is disease-specific: Isoproterenol and quinidine for Brugada or idiopathic VF; beta-blockers and mexiletine for long QT; pacing for certain LQTS types; and potassium/magnesium repletion across variants.

Autonomic modulation techniques (stellate ganglion block, thoracic epidural, or surgical denervation) may be considered in refractory cases.

Mechanical circulatory support (MCS) can stabilize patients with shock from refractory arrhythmias,[10] allow safer catheter ablation, or be deployed prophylactically[11] in high-risk procedures, though its use is limited by availability, cost, and complications.

ROLE OF CATHETER ABLATION

Catheter ablation (CA) can be done either in the acute setting (i.e., ongoing VT storm or incessant VT) or as an elective procedure in a stabilized patient (to prevent ES recurrence).

Box 1 summarizes the recommendations of the ESC 2022 guidelines[4] relevant to the role of CA.

ACUTE ABLATION

According to the EHRA 2024 guidelines, catheter ablation is the treatment of choice for monomorphic VT refractory to drug therapy in the acute phase and is advised in all eligible patients to reduce ES recurrence. Catheter ablation aims to suppress VA and to prevent a prolonged low-output state that can lead to acute multiorgan failure. Hemodynamic stabilization and arrhythmia suppression before proceeding with catheter ablation should be attempted, but may not always be possible.

A recent meta-analysis[10] by Mariani et al. concluded that prophylactic temporary mechanical circulatory support (tMCS) is associated with improved survival as compared to rescue or non-tMCS in patients with life-threatening arrhythmia. The PAINESD risk score[11] may be used to predict high risk of hemodynamic deterioration and initiate prophylactic MCS before the ablation procedure **(Fig. 2)**.

The PAUSE-SCD trial[12] investigated the role of catheter ablation as early first-line therapy in 180 patients with cardiomyopathy (CMP) and monomorphic VT with an indication for ICD implantation. Patient distribution was: Ischemic CMP—35%, nonischemic CMP—30% and arrhythmogenic CMP—35%. The authors concluded that early catheter ablation performed at the time of ICD implantation significantly reduced the composite primary outcome of VT recurrence, cardiovascular hospitalization, or death, predominantly due to a reduction in ICD therapies.

In a multicenter study[13] by Candil et al., catheter ablation for ES done beyond 48 hours after admission significantly reduced mortality at 30 days (in comparison to no CA), but catheter ablation done before 48 hours did not reach significance. Also, in the group who underwent catheter ablation after 48 hours, use of ECMO support during the procedure resulted in a higher rate of noninducibility, implying that hemodynamic support using ECMO may contribute to catheter ablation procedural success.

ABLATION TO PREVENT ES RECURRENCE IN THE STABILIZED PATIENT

Ischemic Heart Disease

A meta-analysis[14] of 6 RCTs (791 patients) concluded that radiofrequency catheter ablation for VT in patients with ischemic heart disease was associated with a reduced risk of VT storm, ICD therapies, and ICD shocks.

Evidence regarding mortality reduction with catheter ablation in ES is limited;[5] while randomized trials and meta-analyses have not shown significant improvements in survival or cardiovascular hospitalizations, nonrandomized studies suggest potential survival benefits.

Nonischemic Cardiomyopathy

Nonischemic cardiomyopathy (NICM) comprises a heterogeneous group. The benefit of catheter ablation to prevent ES recurrence in NICM patients lacks data. Overall, NICM patients have higher VA recurrence after catheter ablation compared to CAD patients. Hypertrophic CMP, inherited DCM, active cardiac sarcoidosis, and valvular heart disease have poorer outcomes. Combined epicardial-endocardial ablation may be needed for ARVC and Chagas CMP (as epicardial scars are more extensive). Treatment at high-volume, experienced centers is advisable.

Primary Electrical Disease

For ES in the context of PED, catheter ablation is not a first-line treatment. Research is still ongoing, and long-term data and RCTs are lacking. Epicardia RVOT substrate is a well-studied target in Brugada syndrome, with the recent report on long-term outcomes of ablation in BrS (BRAVO registry)[15] demonstrating the effectiveness of catheter ablation in preventing VF recurrence in high-risk BrS patients. Of note, 81% of the patients were free from VF recurrence at a mean follow-up of 48 months after just a single ablation procedure.

BOX 1: Recommendations on catheter ablation as per ESC 2022 guidelines on VA and SCD.

Class I recommendations:

- Catheter ablation is recommended in patients presenting with incessant VT or electrical storm due to SMVT refractory to AADs
- Catheter ablation is recommended for ICD patients with recurrent SVT resulting in inappropriate ICD therapies
- Pharmacological treatment or catheter ablation is recommended in patients with AF-related inappropriate ICD therapies despite optimal ICD programming
- In patients with CAD and recurrent, symptomatic SMVT, or ICD shocks for SMVT despite chronic amiodarone therapy, catheter ablation is recommended in preference to escalating AAD therapy
- Catheter ablation as first-line treatment is recommended for symptomatic idiopathic VT/PVCs from the RVOT or the left fascicles
- In symptomatic patients with BBR-VT, catheter ablation is recommended
- PES with standby catheter ablation is recommended in patients with aortic valve disease and SMVT to identify and ablate BBR-VT, especially if it occurs following a valve intervention
- In patients with ventricular preexcitation and symptomatic AVRT, catheter ablation is recommended

Class IIa recommendations:

- Catheter ablation should be considered in patients with recurrent episodes of PVT/VF triggered by a similar PVC, nonresponsive to medical treatment or coronary revascularization
- Catheter ablation should be considered in patients with recurrent episodes of PVT/VF triggered by a similar PVC nonresponsive to medical treatment or coronary revascularization in the subacute phase of MI
- In patients with CAD and hemodynamically well-tolerated SMVT and LVEF ≥ 40%, catheter ablation in experienced centers should be considered as an alternative to ICD therapy, provided that established endpoints have been reached
- Catheter ablation should be considered in patients with CAD and recurrent, symptomatic SMVT, or ICD shocks for SMVT despite beta-blockers or sotalol treatment
- Catheter ablation or flecainide should be considered in symptomatic patients with idiopathic VT/PVCs from an origin other than the RVOT or the left fascicles
- Catheter ablation in specialized centers should be considered in patients with DCM/HNDCM and recurrent, symptomatic SMVT or ICD shocks for SMVT, in whom AADs are ineffective, contraindicated, or not tolerated
- In patients with ARVC and recurrent, symptomatic SMVT or ICD shocks for SMVT despite beta-blockers, catheter ablation in specialized centers should be considered
- Catheter ablation, performed in specialized centers, should be considered in postmyocarditis patients with recurrent, symptomatic SMVT or ICD shocks for SMVT in whom AADs are ineffective, not tolerated, or not desired
- In patients with congenital heart disease and recurrent, symptomatic SMVT or ICD shocks for SMVT not manageable by medical therapy or ICD reprogramming, catheter ablation performed in specialized centers should be considered
- Catheter ablation by experienced electrophysiologists should be considered in idiopathic VF patients with recurrent episodes of VF triggered by a similar PVC nonresponsive to medical treatment
- Catheter ablation of triggering PVCs and/or RVOT epicardial substrate should be considered in BrS patients with recurrent appropriate ICD shocks refractory to drug therapy
- Catheter ablation using nonfluoroscopic mapping systems should be considered, preferably after the first trimester, in women with highly symptomatic recurrent SMVT refractory or who are intolerant to AADs

Class IIb recommendations:

- In patients with SMVT or SPVT/VF triggered by a PVC with similar morphology and an indication for ICD, catheter ablation may be considered when an ICD is not available, contraindicated for concurrent medical reasons, or declined by the patient
- In patients with CAD eligible for ICD implantation, catheter ablation may be considered just before (or immediately after) ICD implantation to decrease subsequent VT burden and ICD shocks
- Catheter ablation may be considered for idiopathic VT/PVCs in asymptomatic patients with repeatedly > 20% of PVCs per day at follow-up
- Catheter ablation in specialized centers may be considered in selected patients with HCM and recurrent, symptomatic SMVT or ICD shocks for SMVT, in whom AAD are ineffective, contraindicated, or not tolerated
- In patients with hemodynamically well-tolerated SMVT occurring in the chronic phase of myocarditis, preserved LV function and a limited scar amenable to ablation, catheter ablation may be considered as an alternative to ICD therapy, after discussion with the patient and provided that established endpoints have been reached
- Catheter ablation, in specialized centers, may be considered in cardiac sarcoidosis ICD-recipients with recurrent, symptomatic SMVT or ICD shocks for SMVT, in whom AADs are ineffective, contraindicated, or not tolerated

Class III recommendations:

- Catheter ablation of idiopathic VT/PVCs is not recommended in children < 5 years of age or <10 kg weight except when previous medical therapy fails or when VT is not hemodynamically tolerated
- Catheter ablation in asymptomatic BrS patients is not recommended

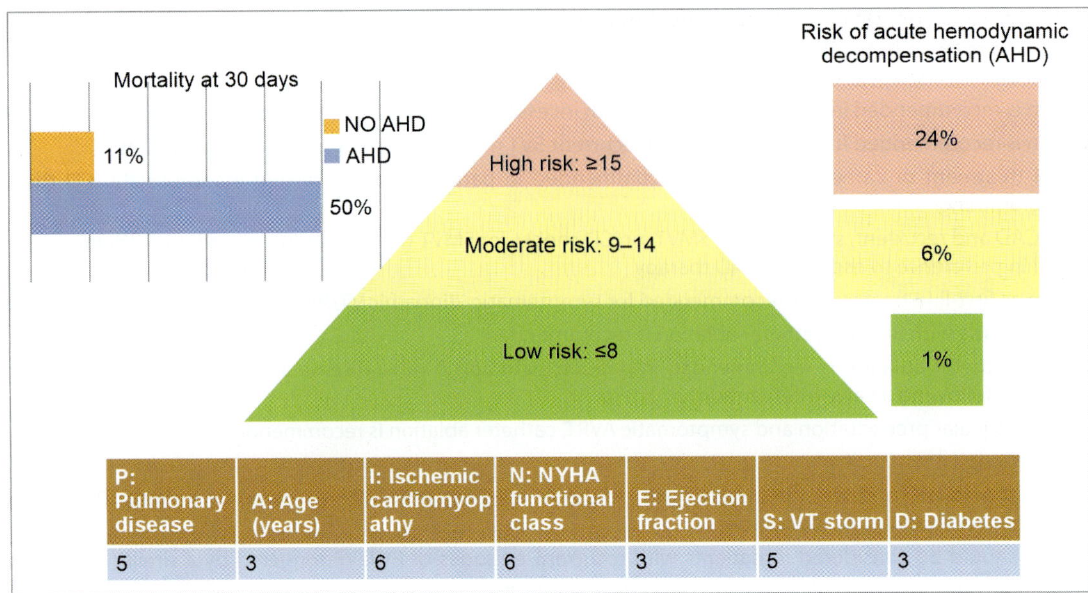

FIG. 2: The PAINESD score for selecting patients for prophylactic MCS before catheter ablation of ES.

In the case of LQTS, abnormally fragmented, low-voltage, and prolonged electrograms were exclusively localized in the right ventricular epicardium.[16]

For CPVT, a recent genetic knock-out study in mice[17] revealed that ectopic beats are likely generated at the Purkinje–myocardial junction via an as yet unrecognized mechanism, whereby DADs in the ventricular myocardium trigger full action potentials in adjacent Purkinje cells.

PROCEDURAL ASPECTS OF CATHETER ABLATION

Principles and Planning

Effective planning is the foundation of VT ablation. The process begins with a detailed review of 12-lead ECGs, arrhythmia cycle length, and device electrograms to distinguish between clinical and procedure-induced rhythms. Imaging tools add value by mapping scarred myocardium and locating arrhythmogenic zones, enabling precise identification of targets for ablation.

Catheter Ablation Approaches

The primary goal of VT ablation is to interrupt re-entry circuits or eliminate focal sites driving arrhythmias, such as ventricular premature depolarizations (VPDs). Four mapping strategies guide the procedure: *Activation mapping, entrainment mapping, pace mapping, and substrate mapping.*

Activation Mapping

This method is feasible when VT is hemodynamically tolerated. By recording electrograms across the ventricles and comparing them with QRS onset, clinicians can identify the earliest activation site. Electrograms preceding the QRS by >20 milliseconds often pinpoint focal origins. In scar-related circuits, diastolic low-amplitude or fractionated signals reveal slow-conduction isthmuses. While powerful, activation mapping alone can misidentify bystander sites; therefore, it is often combined with entrainment mapping.

Entrainment Mapping

Entrainment examines stable reentry loops by pacing slightly faster than the tachycardia. The pacing wavefront resets the circuit, allowing identification of essential elements such as entry, isthmus, and exit sites. Successful ablation at these locations usually terminates VT, whereas targeting peripheral or bystander zones does not. Matching postpacing intervals and QRS morphology helps confirm circuit participation. However, this approach is only possible in hemodynamically stable patients and may not detect deeply intramyocardial circuits.

Pace Mapping

When VT is noninducible or unstable, pace mapping provides an alternative. By pacing the myocardium during sinus rhythm and comparing the resulting QRS pattern to the clinical VT, the operator can approximate the origin or exit site. Although less precise than activation mapping, it is useful in both focal and reentrant arrhythmias, especially when activation or entrainment mapping is limited.

Substrate Mapping

In patients with unstable or noninducible VT, substrate mapping offers a practical solution. Conducted during sinus or paced rhythm, it relies on 3D electroanatomical mapping (EAM) to define scar regions. Normal myocardium typically exhibits voltages > 1.5 mV, while values < 0.5 mV indicate dense scar. Current EAM platforms—*CARTO, NavX, and Rhythmia*—combine voltage with activation data to identify potential conduction channels.

- *CARTO* uses magnetic localization for high-resolution chamber geometry and voltage maps.
- *NavX* employs electrical fields generated by surface patches, enabling nonfluoroscopic catheter visualization and intracardiac ultrasound guidance.
- *Rhythmia* collects simultaneous signals from 64 electrodes, producing ultradense maps with minimal manual annotation.

Substrate-based techniques include linear lesion creation, elimination of late or abnormal potentials, scar homogenization, dechanneling, and core isolation.

Endpoints of VT Ablation

Defining endpoints is essential for procedural success. The conventional standard is *noninducibility of VT* during programmed ventricular stimulation (PVS). While reproducibility is imperfect, it remains the most widely accepted benchmark. Additional physiological endpoints include:

- Isolation of critical substrate
- Demonstrated exit block or non-excitability
- Elimination of late/fractionated electrograms
- Scar dechanneling

Noninvasive postablation PVS via implanted defibrillators can help confirm outcomes. However, the necessity of repeat procedures for early inducible VT remains uncertain.

For linear lesions, failure to capture with high-output pacing and altered conduction patterns are proposed markers. For late-potential ablation, disappearance of abnormal signals or failure of pacing capture are considered valid endpoints.

CASE STUDY

A 45-year-old male presented to our institute with hemodynamically tolerated VT storm on a background of ischemic dilated cardiomyopathy with LV ejection fraction 25% and LV apical aneurysm. Conservative measures (including AADs, general anesthesia with mechanical ventilation, and bilateral stellate ganglion block) failed to control the VT. Catheter ablation was done on an emergency basis, with scar VT as the likely diagnosis and probable site of origin localized to the LV apical scar. During activation mapping of the LV via transseptal approach VT isthmus was localized to the midapical interventricular septum, which corresponded to the scar area demarcated by voltage mapping. Irrigated RF ablation at that site terminated the tachycardia. The patient later received a single-chamber ICD for secondary prevention of SCD. This case highlights the immense value of catheter ablation as a rescue modality when conservative measures fail to control ventricular arrhythmias.

Figures 3 and 4 illustrate the discussed case.

For ES consequential to PVC-triggered PVT/VF, trigger elimination is effective both in the short and long term. Epicardial approach may be needed in refractory cases.

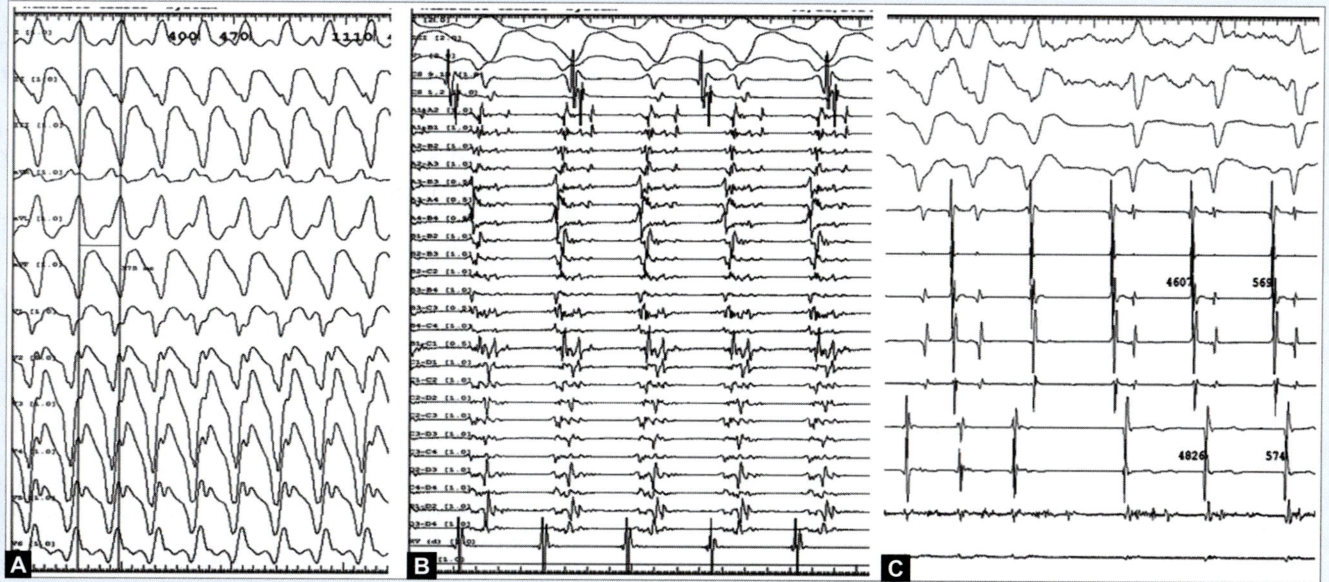

FIGS. 3A TO C: Ablation of the VT described above (See "case study" in the box). (A) 12-lead ECG of the VT ongoing during the procedure; (B) VT mapping using a multipolar catheter; and (C) VT termination on RF ablation.

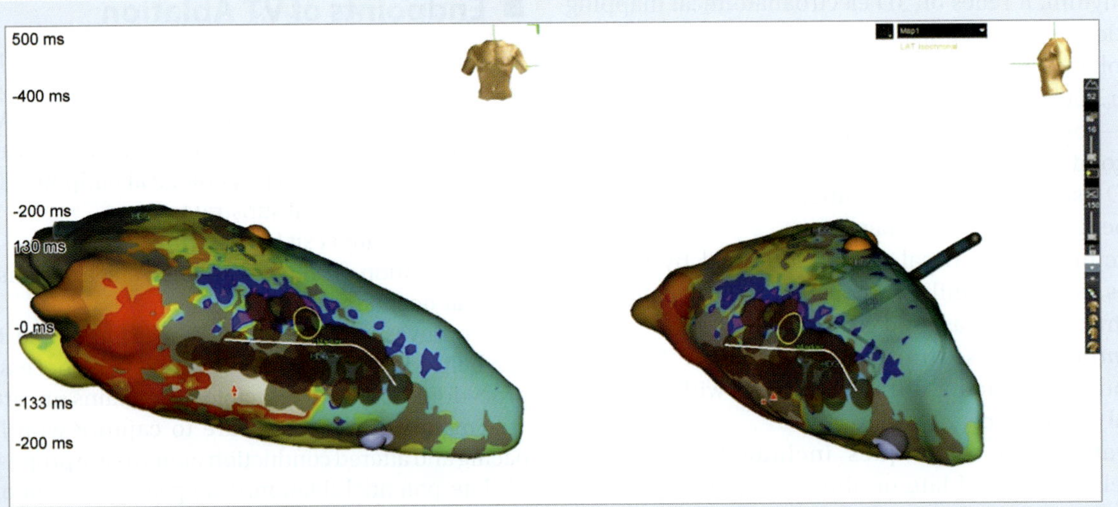

FIG. 4: Electroanatomic 3D activation map shows activation with a color-coded sequence, whereby white corresponds to the earliest activation, followed by red, and progressing to blue and purple (latest activation). Grey areas correspond to scar. The cluster of dark brown spots corresponds to ablation lesions in the isthmus of the VT.

CONCLUSION

Catheter ablation has transitioned from a rescue option to a cornerstone of therapy for ES and incessant VT, particularly when conventional therapies fail. It provides durable arrhythmia control, reduces ICD therapies, and improves quality of life, although consistent survival benefits are yet to be firmly established. Patient selection, procedural timing, and availability of hemodynamic support remain critical determinants of success, especially in complex substrates such as nonischemic cardiomyopathies and primary electrical diseases. Ongoing advances in mapping, ablation strategies, and adjunctive support devices are likely to refine outcomes further. In carefully selected patients and specialized centers, ablation offers the best chance of stabilizing this critically ill population and preventing recurrent ESs.

REFERENCES

1. Huang SK, Jordan N, Graham A, et al. Closed-chest catheter desiccation of atrioventricular junction using radiofrequency energy: a new method of catheter ablation [abstract]. Circulation. 1985;72:III-1389.
2. Guiraudon GM, Klein GJ, Sharma AD, et al. Surgical and catheter ablation of incessant ventricular tachycardia. Circulation. 1990;82(6):2259-68.
3. Timmermans C, Rodriguez LM, Smeets JL, et al. Catheter ablation of ventricular fibrillation and ventricular tachycardia storm in patients with coronary artery disease. J Cardiovasc Electrophysiol. 1998;9(5):465-70.
4. Zeppenfeld K, Tfelt-Hansen J, de Riva M, et al. 2022 ESC guidelines for the management of patients with ventricular arrhythmias and the prevention of sudden cardiac death. Eur Heart J. 2022;43(40):3997-4126.
5. Radosław Lenarczyk, Katja Zeppenfeld, Jacob Tfelt-Hansen, et al. Management of patients with an electrical storm or clustered ventricular arrhythmias: a clinical consensus statement of the European Heart Rhythm Association of the ESC-endorsed by the Asia-Pacific Heart Rhythm Society, Heart Rhythm Society, and Latin-American Heart Rhythm Society. Europace. 2024;26(4):euae049.
6. Soar J, Bottiger BW, Carli P, et al. European resuscitation council guidelines 2021: adult advanced life support. Resuscitation. 2021;161:115-51.
7. Alkhalaileh F, Wazni OM, Kiang A, et al. Ischemic or coronary evaluations in patients with monomorphic VT electrical storm undergoing VT ablation. JACC Clin Electrophysiol. 2023;9(9): 1890-9.
8. Martins RP, Urien JM, Barbarot N, et al. Effectiveness of deep sedation for patients with intractable electrical storm refractory to antiarrhythmic drugs. Circulation. 2020;142(16):1599-601.
9. Bundgaard JS, Jacobsen PK, Grand J, et al. Deep sedation as a temporary bridge to definitive treatment of ventricular arrhythmia storm. Eur Heart J Acute Cardiovasc Care. 2020;9(6):657-64.
10. Mariani S, Napp LC, Lo Coco V, et al. Mechanical circulatory support for life-threatening arrhythmia: a systematic review. Int J Cardiol. 2020;308:42-9.
11. Muser D, Castro SA, Liang JJ, Santangeli P. Identifying Risk and Management of Acute Haemodynamic Decompensation During Catheter Ablation of Ventricular Tachycardia. Arrhythm Electrophysiol Rev. 2018;7(4):282-7.
12. Tung R, Xue Y, Chen M, Jiang C, et al; PAUSE-SCD Investigators. First-Line Catheter Ablation of Monomorphic Ventricular Tachycardia in Cardiomyopathy Concurrent With Defibrillator Implantation: The PAUSE-SCD Randomized Trial. Circulation. 2022;145(25):1839-49.
13. Jiménez Candil J, Castro JC, Hernández J, et al. Timing of Ablation and Prognosis of Patients With Electrical Storm and Scar-Related Left Ventricular Dysfunction. Am J Cardiol. 2020;136:87-93.

14. Lima da Silva G, Nunes-Ferreira A, Cortez-Dias N, et al. Radiofrequency catheter ablation of ventricular tachycardia in ischemic heart disease in light of current practice: a systematic review and meta-analysis of randomized controlled trials. J Interv Card Electrophysiol. 2020;59(3):603-16.
15. Nademanee K, Chung FP, Sacher F, et al. Long-term outcomes of Brugada substrate ablation: a report from BRAVO (Brugada ablation of VF substrate ongoing multicenter registry). Circulation 2023;147(21):1568-78.
16. Pappone C, Ciconte G, Anastasia L, et al. Right ventricular epicardial arrhythmogenic substrate in long-QT syndrome patients at risk of sudden death. Europace 2023;25(3):948-55.
17. Blackwell DJ, Faggioni M, Wleklinski MJ, et al. The Purkinje-myocardial junction is the anatomic origin of ventricular arrhythmia in CPVT. JCI Insight. 2022;7(3):e151893.

CHAPTER 85

Prevention of Sudden Cardiac Death beyond Automated External Defibrillators and Implantable Cardioverter Defibrillators

Girish B Navasundi

ABSTRACT

Sudden cardiac death (SCD) remains a major cause of mortality worldwide despite advancements in diagnostic tools and therapeutic strategies. While automated external defibrillators (AEDs) and implantable cardioverter defibrillators (ICDs) have been cornerstone interventions, they are primarily reactive measures. Preventive strategies extending beyond these devices are critical to reduce the global burden of SCD. This chapter explores novel preventive strategies, risk stratification, lifestyle interventions, pharmacotherapy, genetic screening, and emerging therapies that go beyond AEDs and ICDs.

Keywords: Sudden cardiac death, prevention, risk stratification, genetics, pharmacotherapy.

INTRODUCTION

Sudden cardiac death (SCD) accounts for approximately 4–5 million deaths annually worldwide, posing a significant public health burden. Traditionally, the use of automated external defibrillators (AEDs) in community settings and implantable cardioverter defibrillators (ICDs) in high-risk patients has reduced mortality but is limited by accessibility, costs, and patient's eligibility. Hence, the emphasis has shifted toward prevention strategies aimed at identifying and mitigating risk before the onset of fatal arrhythmias.

EPIDEMIOLOGY AND RISK STRATIFICATION

The burden of SCD varies across populations, with the highest risk seen in individuals with coronary artery disease, structural heart disease, cardiomyopathies, and inherited arrhythmia syndromes.

Risk stratification **(Table 1)** approaches include the following:

- *Electrocardiography and Holter monitoring* for arrhythmic risk detection **(Flowchart 1)**
- *Echocardiography and cardiac MRI* for structural abnormalities
- *Biomarkers* such as high-sensitivity troponins and natriuretic peptides
- *Genetic testing* for inherited syndromes (long QT, Brugada, and CPVT)
- *AI-based algorithms* integrating clinical, imaging, and genomic data

TABLE 1: Key methods for sudden cardiac death (SCD) risk stratification.

Category	Key parameters/tools	Clinical role in SCD prevention
Clinical risk factors	LVEF < 35%, prior myocardial infarction, symptomatic heart failure	Identifies high-risk patients traditionally eligible for ICDs
Advanced imaging	Cardiac MRI (late-gadolinium enhancement), echocardiography	Detects myocardial scar, fibrosis, and remodeling
Ambulatory monitoring	Holter monitoring, event recorders, wearables	Detects silent arrhythmias and transient ischemic episodes
Genetic testing	Inherited arrhythmia syndromes (LQTS, Brugada, ARVC, and HCM)	Enables early family screening and precision therapy

(ARVC: arrhythmogenic right ventricular cardiomyopathy; HCM: hypertrophic cardiomyopathy; ICDs: implantable cardioverter defibrillators)

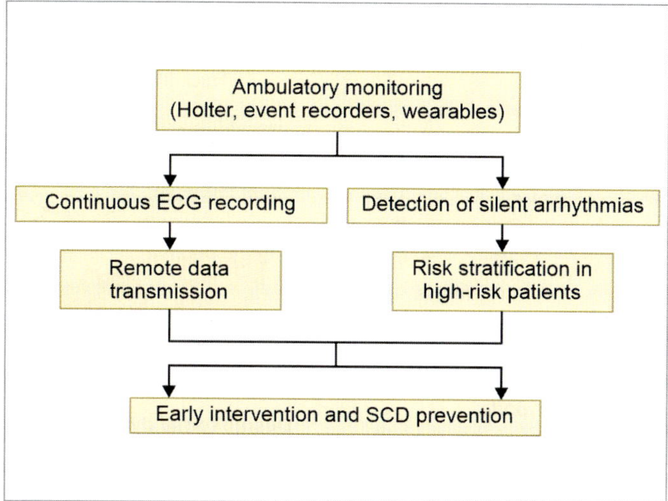

FLOWCHART 1: Ambulatory monitoring in SCD prevention.
(ECG: echocardiography; SCD: sudden cardiac death)

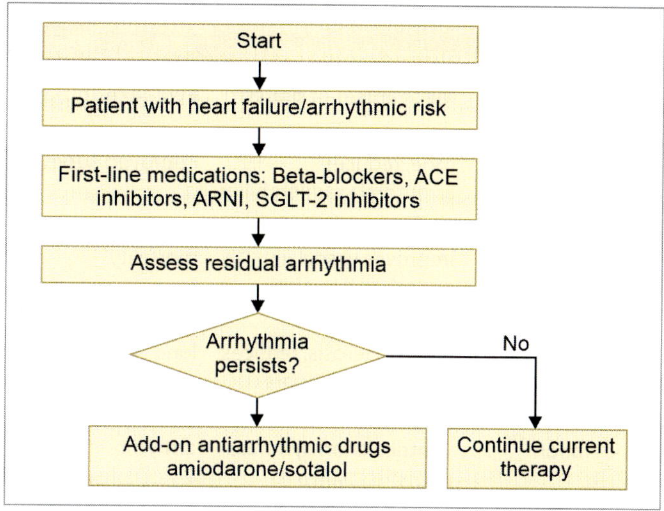

FLOWCHART 2: Pharmacological approach to reduce arrhythmic risk.

PHARMACOLOGICAL STRATEGIES

Medication Strategies for Heart Problems and Arrhythmias

Medications are very important for lowering the risk of dangerous heart rhythms. Some medicines, such as beta-blockers, ACE inhibitors, ARNI, and SGLT-2 inhibitors,[1,2] do two things:

1. Help the heart work better in heart failure[3]
2. Reduce the chances of serious abnormal heart rhythms

Other medicines, called antiarrhythmics (such as amiodarone and sotalol), can also help control irregular heartbeats. But these are usually added only when needed because they can cause side effects **(Flowchart 2 and Table 2)**.

TABLE 2: Pharmacotherapy for prevention of sudden cardiac death.

Drug type	Examples	Purpose/ Benefit	Notes/ Limitations
Heart failure + antiarrhythmic benefit	Beta-blockers, ACE inhibitors, ARNI, SGLT-2 inhibitors	Improve heart function and reduce risk of serious arrhythmias	First-line therapy
Antiarrhythmic drugs	Amiodarone, Sotalol	Control irregular heartbeats	Used as add-on therapy; may cause side effects

Lifestyle and Behavioral Interventions in Sudden Cardiac Death Prevention

Lifestyle and behavioral interventions form the foundation of primary prevention of SCD **(Flowchart 3 and Table 3)**.[4,5] While devices and pharmacotherapy target high-risk individuals, population-wide modification of risk factors can significantly reduce incidence.

- Regular exercise improves heart strength and lowers the chance of dangerous heart rhythms.
- Eating a healthy diet, like the Mediterranean diet, supports heart health by reducing inflammation.
- Avoiding smoking and limiting alcohol prevents damage to blood vessels and heart rhythm disturbances.
- Managing weight, controlling diabetes, reducing stress, and getting good sleep all contribute to a healthier heart.
- Community efforts such as CPR training and AED[6] access also improve survival in cardiac emergencies.

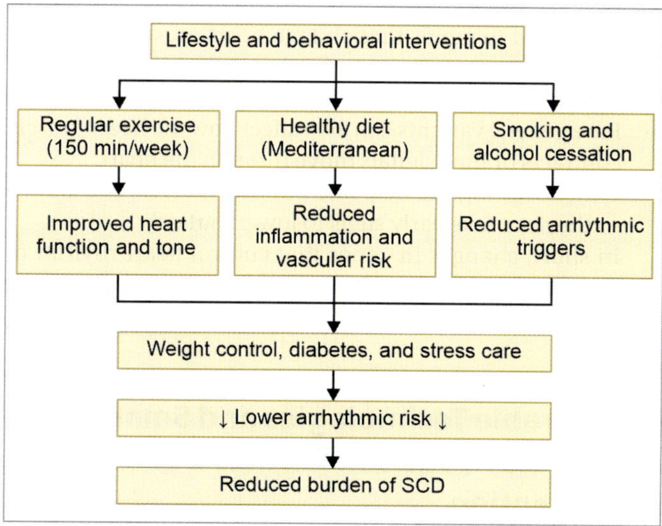

FLOWCHART 3: Lifestyle and behavioral interventions in SCD prevention.
(SCD: sudden cardiac death)

TABLE 3: Lifestyle and behavioral interventions to prevent sudden cardiac death (SCD).

Intervention	Mechanism of benefit	Evidence/Impact
Regular physical activity	Improves autonomic tone, reduces arrhythmia vulnerability	↓ SCD incidence, improved survival
Mediterranean-style diet	Reduces inflammation, improves vascular/ endothelial health	↓ Cardiac events, mortality
Smoking cessation	Prevents atherosclerosis, reduces arrhythmic triggers	Significant ↓ in long-term SCD risk
Alcohol moderation	Prevents atrial/ ventricular arrhythmias	↓ Risk of sudden arrhythmic death
Weight management	Improves blood pressure, sleep apnea, metabolic health	↓ Risk of HF and arrhythmias
Diabetes control	Prevents autonomic dysfunction, ischemia	↓ SCD risk in diabetics
Stress reduction and sleep	Lowers sympathetic drive, stabilizes heart rhythm	Adjunct benefit in high-risk patients
Community-level measures	CPR training, AED deployment	↑ Survival after cardiac arrest

(AED: automated external defibrillator; HF: heart failure)

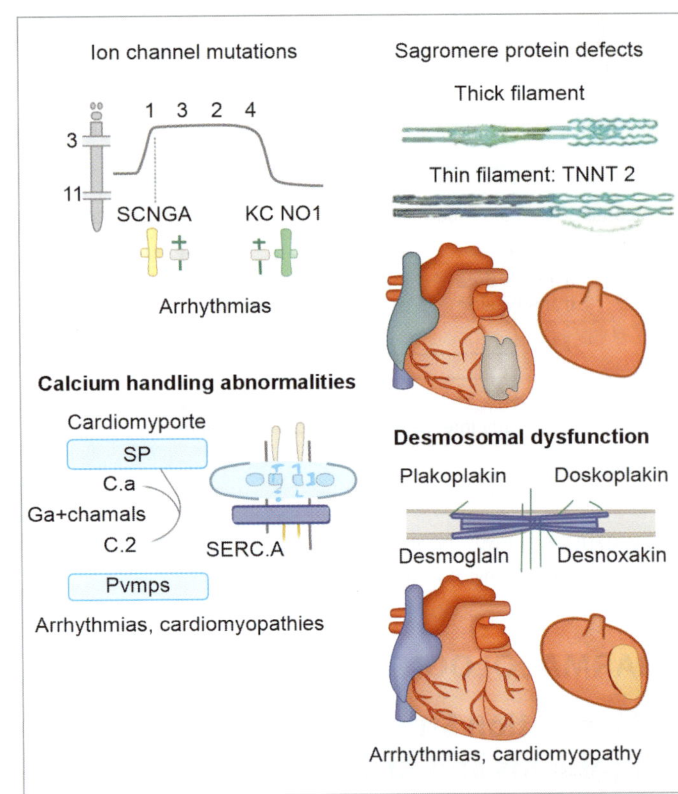

FIG. 1: Genetic and molecular mechanisms in sudden cardiac death.

Genetic and Molecular Insights in Sudden Cardiac Death

- Certain inherited conditions, such as long QT syndrome and Brugada syndrome, are caused by gene changes that disrupt the heart's electrical signals, leading to dangerous rhythms.
- Other problems, such as hypertrophic cardiomyopathy, are linked to genes that change heart muscle structure, making the heart more likely to develop abnormal rhythms.
- Rare genetic variants can also affect how the heart muscle contracts or how signals move through the heart.
- Genetic testing can help find out who is at risk in a family, so they can take early steps to lower that risk.

In short, changes in genes that control heart rhythm or structure can increase the risk of SCD, especially in young people and families with a history of heart disease **(Fig. 1 and Table 4)**.

Wearable Technologies and Smart Devices in Sudden Cardiac Death Prevention

Wearable technologies, like smartwatches[7] and special patches, can help prevent SCD by monitoring heart rhythms all day. These devices can detect irregular or dangerous heartbeats and alert people or doctors, so action can be taken early **(Flowchart 4 and Table 5)**.

- Some wearables, like the wearable defibrillator vest, can even deliver a shock to the heart if a life-threatening rhythm is found.[8-10]
- Using these technologies can catch problems before they become emergencies and help people manage their heart health better.

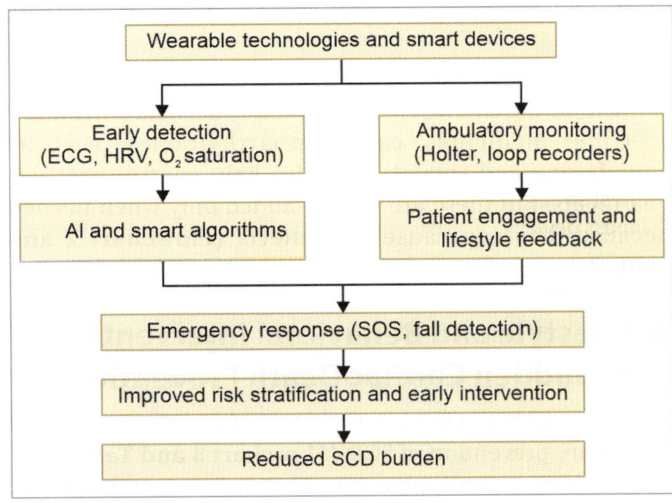

FLOWCHART 4: Wearable technologies and smart devices in SCD prevention.

(ECG: echocardiography; SCD: sudden cardiac death)

TABLE 4: Genetic and molecular insights in sudden cardiac death (SCD).

Condition	Key genes involved	Molecular mechanism	Clinical implication
Long QT syndrome (LQTS)	*KCNQ1, KCNH2, SCN5A*	Abnormal ion channel function → delayed repolarization	Risk of torsades de pointes, syncope, SCD
Brugada syndrome	*SCN5A, CACNA1C, GPD1L*	Sodium channel dysfunction → ventricular fibrillation	SCD in structurally normal hearts, often nocturnal
Catecholaminergic polymorphic ventricular tachycardia (CPVT)	*RYR2, CASQ2*	Abnormal calcium handling → adrenergic-triggered arrhythmias	Exercise/stress-induced VT, high SCD risk in children and young adults
Hypertrophic cardiomyopathy (HCM)	*MYH7, MYBPC3, TNNT2*	Sarcomeric protein mutations → hypertrophy, fibrosis	Substrate for ventricular arrhythmias, SCD in athletes
Arrhythmogenic right ventricular cardiomyopathy (ARVC)	*PKP2, DSG2, DSP, JUP*	Defective desmosomes → fibrofatty myocardial replacement	Ventricular arrhythmias, SCD in young adults/athletes
Dilated cardiomyopathy (DCM)	*TTN, LMNA, DSP*	Structural protein mutations → ventricular dysfunction	Progressive HF, arrhythmia, SCD risk
Polygenic risk	Multiple SNPs across ion channel, and structural genes	Combined small effects increase arrhythmic risk	Precision risk stratification beyond monogenic syndromes
Molecular biomarkers	Circulating microRNAs, inflammatory mediators	Reflect myocardial stress/ remodeling	Potential early detection and monitoring tools

(HF: heart failure)

TABLE 5: Wearable and smart device technologies in SCD prevention.

Device type	Examples	Clinical use	Strengths	Limitations
Smartwatches	Apple watch, Fitbit, Samsung Galaxy watch	Detection of AFib, irregular heart rhythms, activity tracking	Widely available, user-friendly, continuous monitoring	Limited ECG leads, false positives
Adhesive ECG patches	Zio Patch, VitalPatch	Continuous rhythm monitoring (1–14 days)	Comfortable, extended monitoring, higher accuracy	Cannot be reused, cost considerations
Chest straps and fitness devices	Polar H10, Garmin HRM	Accurate HR/HRV monitoring during exercise	High accuracy during activity, useful in athletes	Limited arrhythmia detection
Implantable loop recorders (ILRs)	Medtronic reveal LINQ, Biotronik BioMonitor	Long-term monitoring (months–years) for unexplained syncope/ arrhythmias	Gold standard for continuous detection, automatic alerts	Invasive, costly
Smart rings and biosensors	Oura ring, Withings ScanWatch	Sleep, stress, HRV, oxygen saturation	Noninvasive, continuous lifestyle data	Limited arrhythmia-specific detection
AI-integrated platforms	AliveCor Kardia mobile, cloud- interpretation, physician based ECG	Real-time ECG alerts systems	AI enhances diagnostic yield, remote access	Requires internet, regulatory challenges

(ECG: echocardiography; SCD: sudden cardiac death)

CONCLUSION

Preventing SCD requires a multifaceted strategy that goes beyond AEDs and ICDs. Risk stratification, evidence-based pharmacology (notably SGLT-2 inhibitors), genetic insights, lifestyle modifications, and wearable/AI-driven technologies together represent the future of prevention.

A paradigm shift from reactive interventions to proactive, personalized prevention will be key in reducing the global burden of SCD.

REFERENCES

1. Sato T, Kouzu H, Yano T, et al. Potential favorable action of sodium-glucose cotransporter-2 inhibitors on sudden cardiac death: a brief overview. Front Cardiovasc Med. 2023;10:1159953.
2. Bae JW. Clinical impact and practical use of sodium-glucose cotransporter 2 inhibitors for patients with chronic kidney disease. Cardiovasc Prev Pharmacother. 2025;7:44-9.
3. Crispino SP, Segreti A, Nafisio V, et al. The role of SGLT2-inhibitors across all stages of heart failure and mechanisms of early clinical benefit: from prevention to advanced heart failure. Biomedicines. 2025;13:608.
4. Chaphalkar SR. (2024). SGLT2 inhibitors: a game-changer in preventing heart failure and sudden cardiac deaths. [online] Available from https://www.news-medical.net/news/20240409/SGLT2-inhibitors-A-game-changer-in-preventing-heart-failure-and-sudden-cardiac-deaths.aspx [Last accessed November, 2025].
5. Marijon E, Garcia R, Narayanan K, et al. Fighting against sudden cardiac death: need for a paradigm shift—adding near-term prevention and pre-emptive action to long-term prevention. Eur Heart J. 2022;43(15):1457-67.
6. Chugh SS. Prevention of sudden cardiac death: beyond automated external defibrillators and implantable cardioverter defibrillators. Circulation. 2024;149:1059-61.
7. Xiang E, Wang T, Poddar V. High-throughput detection of risk factors to sudden cardiac arrest in youth athletes: a smartwatch-based screening platform. arXiv preprint. 2024;18:35.
8. Wikipedia contributors. (2025). Wearable cardioverter defibrillator. [online] Available from https://en.wikipedia.org/wiki/Wearable_cardioverter_defibrillator [Last accessed November, 2025].
9. Wikipedia contributors. (2025). Cardiac arrest. [online] Available from https://en.wikipedia.org/wiki/Cardiac_arrest [Last accessed November, 2025].
10. Wikipedia contributors. (2025). Chain of survival. [online] Available from https://en.wikipedia.org/wiki/Chain_of_survival [Last accessed November, 2025].

CHAPTER 86

Pulsed Field Ablation—in Present Perspective

Vadivelu Ramalingam, Atul Verma, KK Talwar

ABSTRACT

Catheter ablation (CA) is an established therapy for symptomatic atrial fibrillation (AF), with superior efficacy to antiarrhythmic drugs. Yet, recurrence after ablation is common with conventional thermal modalities such as radiofrequency and cryoablation. This limitation has spurred interest in nonthermal technologies that can achieve durable rhythm control with fewer complications. Pulsed field ablation (PFA), which delivers short bursts of high-intensity electric fields, has emerged as a promising approach.

Pulsed field ablation induces irreversible electroporation (IRE), selectively targeting myocardium while sparing adjacent structures. This confers an excellent safety profile, with complications such as esophageal injury, phrenic nerve palsy, and pulmonary vein stenosis being extremely rare or virtually absent compared with thermal ablation. The low collateral risk also permits broader lesion sets, including posterior wall isolation, with greater procedural confidence.

Preclinical studies consistently support the efficiency and selectivity of PFA, while early clinical trials confirm its feasibility, speed, and safety in both paroxysmal and persistent AF. Several catheter platforms—including Farapulse, PulseSelect, Varipulse, and Volt—are currently being evaluated in pivotal trials. Remaining challenges include long-term durability beyond 3–5 years, performance outside AF, such as in ventricular tachycardia, and variability across operators. Practical aspects such as cost and integration into practice will also guide adoption. This review outlines the biophysics, mechanisms, procedural workflow, and clinical evidence for PFA, highlighting its potential to transform AF ablation by combining efficacy with better safety profile.

Keywords: Pulsed field ablation, atrial fibrillation, catheter ablation.

INTRODUCTION

Atrial fibrillation (AF), the most common arrhythmia in adults, is poorly controlled with antiarrhythmic drugs, establishing catheter ablation (CA), especially pulmonary vein isolation, as the standard therapy for symptomatic and drug-refractory patients.[1-3] As first-line therapy, CA yields high acute success and quality of life improvement, though recurrence may reach 50% at 18 months.[4] Radiofrequency ablation (RFA), the gold standard, requires point-by-point delivery and risks collateral injury. Cryoballoon ablation enables single-shot PVI but shares similar safety issues,[5] while ultra-low temperature cryo creates deeper lesions but remains under evaluation.[6] All thermal methods are nonselective, with risks including atrioesophageal fistula (0.02–0.1%), phrenic nerve palsy (≤0.4%), and PV stenosis (<1%).[7] Laser balloon ablation has seen limited use.[8]

Pulsed field ablation (PFA), in contrast, employs nonthermal electroporation, selectively ablating myocardium while sparing adjacent structures. Its safety, tissue selectivity, and rapid single-shot application make it a potentially transformative option for AF ablation **(Table 1)**.

HISTORY OF PULSED FIELD ABLATION

Pulsed field ablation evolved from electroporation, first described in the 1970s, when electric fields made cell membranes transiently permeable.[9] By the early 2000s, irreversible electroporation (IRE) was applied for oncologic ablation, producing cell death while sparing connective tissue and vessels.[10] Preclinical cardiac studies then showed cardiomyocytes have lower electroporation thresholds than surrounding tissues, allowing targeted ablation with minimal

TABLE 1: Comparison summary of different technologies for AF ablation.

Characteristics	PFA	RFA	Cryoablation	ULTC
Energy type	Nonthermal and electric fields	Thermal heating (50–60°C)	Cryogenic N_2O (–40°C to –80°C)	LN_2 freezing (–130°C to –140°C)
Mechanism	Irreversible electroporation	Coagulation necrosis	Cryogenic necrosis Ice crystals and osmotic shifts	Similar to cryo
Lesion formation	Nanopores → apoptosis/necrosis	Protein denaturation	Cell swelling, vacuolization, and membrane disruption	Similar to cryo, and deeper lesions
Histopathology	Minimal inflammation; preserved ECM; selective myocyte death	Eosinophilic cytoplasm, nuclear loss	Microvascular injury and cell disruption	Similar to cryoablation
Tissue selectivity	High—spares nerves, vessels, and esophagus	Low—collateral injury risk	Moderate—phrenic/esophagus/PV stenosis risk	Similar risks; deeper lesions
Durability	High acute; long term under study	High, but gaps possible	Variable; balloon position dependent	Very high—deep and homogeneous
Acute success (PVI)	~99% (major studies)	~95–98%	~95–98%	~99% (early studies)
AF recurrence (1 year)	~15–25%	~20–25%	~20–25%	≤20% (early data)
Safety	Few collateral injuries (hemolysis, coronary spasm, and effusion)	Risk of esophageal injury, PV stenosis, and tamponade	Risk of phrenic/esophageal injury and PV stenosis	Similar to cryo; safety pending
Limitations	Durability data limited; early adoption	Thermal complications	Anatomical limits (PV size/branching)	Few trials; availability; long-term safety unknown

(AF: atrial fibrillation; PFA: pulsed field ablation; RFA: radiofrequency ablation; ULTC: ultra-low temperature cryoablation)

collateral injury.[11] These findings led to the first-in-human PFA trial in 2018, demonstrating rapid pulmonary vein isolation with excellent acute safety.[12]

BIOPHYSICS AND MECHANISM OF PULSED FIELD ABLATION

Pulsed field ablation is based on IRE, a nonthermal process in which ultrashort, high-intensity electric fields create nanopores in the cell membrane, leading to ionic imbalance, loss of homeostasis, and cardiomyocyte death. The biological effect depends on field strength: <200 V/cm has no effect, 200–400 V/cm induces reversible electroporation, >400–800 V/cm causes IRE (therapeutic range), and >1,500 V/cm risks thermal injury. Clinically, biphasic pulses of ~1,000–2,000 V generate tissue fields of ~500–800 V/cm, within the IRE range. Monophasic pulses produce strong skeletal muscle contractions, arrhythmia risk, and charge accumulation with possible thermal effects, whereas biphasic or multiphasic pulses achieve charge balance, minimize muscle stimulation, avoid arrhythmogenicity, and create homogeneous lesions within seconds—far faster than thermal ablation.

Unlike radiofrequency (coagulation necrosis) or cryoablation (freeze–thaw necrosis), PFA spares extracellular matrix, vasculature, and connective tissue while inducing sharply demarcated fibrotic replacement of myocardium. Importantly, cardiomyocytes have lower electroporation thresholds than surrounding tissues, enabling rapid antral pulmonary vein isolation with high acute success. This myocardial selectivity underlies the consistently observed safety profile: minimal esophageal injury, rare phrenic nerve involvement, and negligible risk of pulmonary vein stenosis.[13] **Figure 1** illustrates the mechanism, tissue selectivity, and safety of PFA.

PRECLINICAL STUDIES

Animal studies confirmed the mechanistic basis, feasibility, durability, and safety of intracardiac PFA. The first chronic model demonstrated sharply demarcated lesions.[14] Subsequent work showed consistent pulmonary vein and linear atrial isolation with preserved vasculature and minimal extracardiac injury.[15,16] PFA lesion size was independent of contact force, unlike RF.[17] In ventricular models, PFA produced deep lesions penetrating infarct scar with low arrhythmogenic risk when gated, and effective ablation of papillary muscles and trabeculae without vascular damage.[18,19] Collectively, these studies highlight PFAs myocardial selectivity, reproducibility, and translational potential.

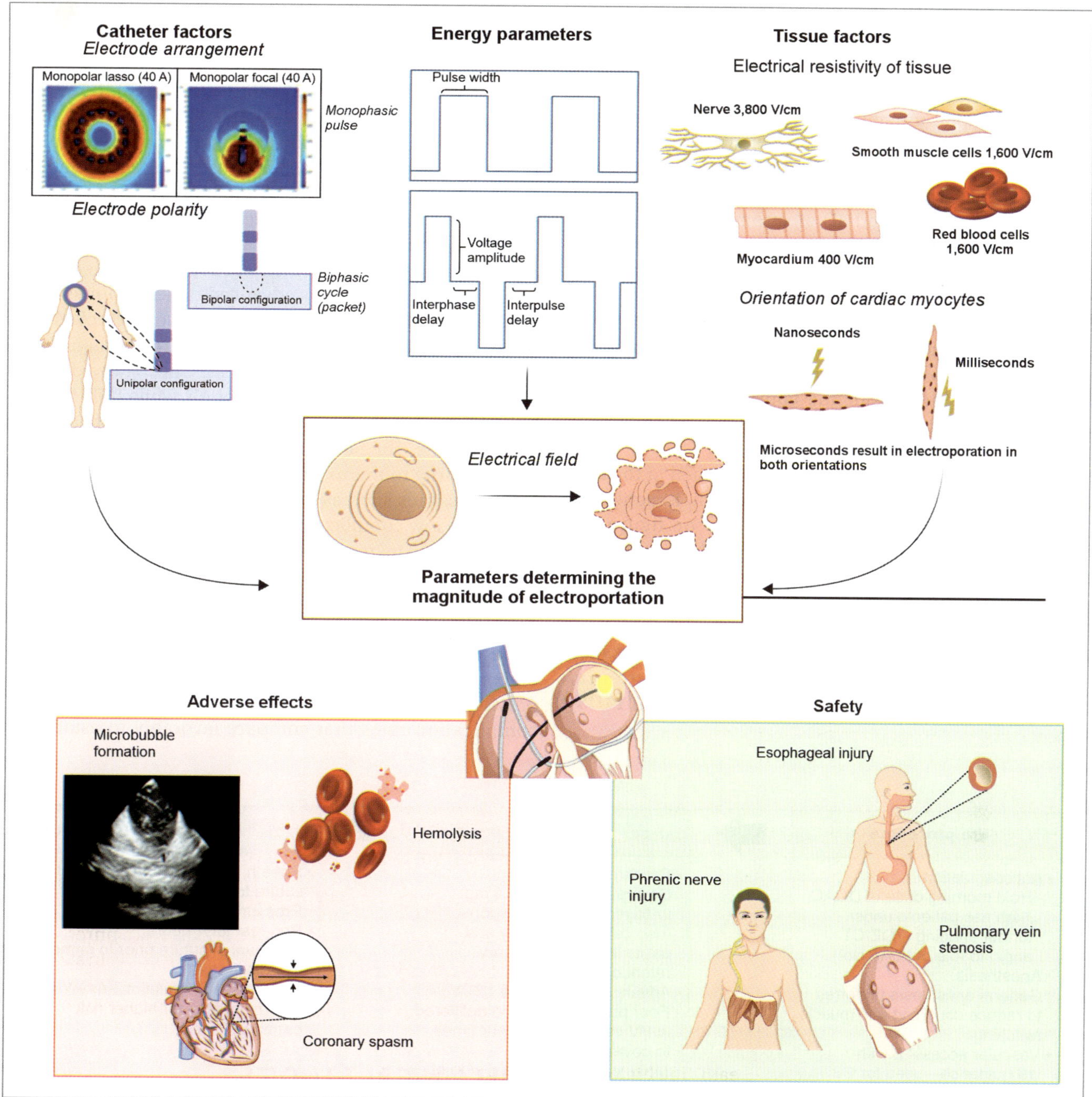

FIG. 1: Biophysics, mechanism, tissue selectivity, safety, and adverse effects of pulsed field ablation (PFA). *Left panel*: PFA catheter electrode arrangement. *Middle panel top:* Monophasic and biphasic waveforms; biphasic pulses are used clinically to achieve charge balance and minimize muscle stimulation. *Middle center panel*: PFA electric field inducing membrane pore formation and increasing membrane permeability. *Right panel:* PFA selectivity showing cellular responses to electric fields, enabling effective myocardial ablation while sparing adjacent tissues. *Bottom panel*: Adverse effects and safety features of PFA.

Histopathology of PFA lesions demonstrates cell swelling, vacuolization, and membrane disruption with preserved collagen and vascular structures, reducing risks of PV stenosis and collateral injury. Compared with thermal ablation, inflammation is minimal, and healing is characterized by sharply demarcated fibrotic replacement while sparing connective tissue and large vessels.[15,16]

PROCEDURAL STEPS OF PULSED FIELD ABLATION FOR AF ABLATION

Pulmonary vein isolation with PFA is usually performed under general anesthesia (preferred to minimize cough/ twitching), though deep sedation is an alternative. Morning DOAC is withheld, and high-risk patients undergo TEE or

CTA to exclude LAA thrombus. Vascular access is obtained conventionally or under ultrasound guidance, typically with three venous punctures for the coronary sinus, ablation, and intracardiac echocardiography (ICE) catheters, followed by a single transseptal puncture. The mapping catheter may be used for voltage mapping, then exchanged for the PFA catheter. Glycopyrrolate (0.2–0.4 mg IV) is given at this stage to reduce vagal responses **(Fig. 2)**. Mutimodality imaging using fluoroscopy, ICE, and 3D electroanatomic mapping (EAM) is typically used in the PFA procedure to enhance success **(Fig. 3)**. Ablation begins in the LSPV with four pulses per lesion, applied circumferentially at ostial and antral sites, and repeated for all PVs; posterior wall, septum, or roof may be targeted if needed. Phrenic pacing is used during right PV ablation, and entrance/exit block confirmed. Post ablation, 3D mapping is repeated for the completion of ablation, and look for any conduction gaps, in which case additional lesions are performed **(Fig. 4)**.

Intracardiac echocardiography is performed at the end to exclude pericardial effusion. Hemostasis is achieved with local pressure at the puncture site or figure-of-eight suture and pressure dressing as per the operator's preference, followed by 4 hours of bed rest. Anticoagulation is restarted the same day, with same-day discharge feasible in most patients; overnight stay is reserved for higher-risk cases. Postprocedure monitoring includes checks for effusion, vascular complications, and rhythm recurrence, with anticoagulation continued per stroke risk by $CHADS_2$ score.

CLINICAL EVIDENCE OF PFA: A SUMMARY OF KEY CLINICAL TRIALS

Several dedicated PFA systems **(Table 2)** have been developed with distinct designs. Farapulse employs a pentaspline multielectrode catheter for single-shot PVI with biphasic pulses; PulseSelect uses a circular mapping-ablation catheter for precise PV targeting; Varipulse features a variable-loop system adaptable to diverse atrial anatomies; and Volt applies a lattice-tip catheter for focal and linear lesions across atrial and ventricular substrates.

Clinical evaluation has advanced rapidly from feasibility to pivotal trials. The first-in-human study achieved 100% acute PVI with ~87% 1-year arrhythmia freedom and no PV stenosis or esophageal injury.[12] PersAFOne[20] showed durable posterior wall isolation in persistent AF, while IMPULSE and PEFCAT[21] confirmed high acute success and encouraging 1-year results. The landmark ADVENT trial[22] demonstrated noninferiority to thermal ablation with lower PV narrowing. Large registries such as EU-PORIA[23] and MANIFEST-17K[24] confirmed low complication rates (<1–2%) across thousands of patients. Device-specific pivotal studies, including PULSED AF[25] and inspire,[26] demonstrated consistent safety and efficacy in paroxysmal and persistent AF, and ADVANTAGE-AF[27] extended evidence with continuous monitoring in persistent AF, showing favorable rhythm outcomes. Collectively, these trials **(Table 3)** show that PFA provides rapid, effective, and tissue-selective ablation with complication rates that compare favorably to established

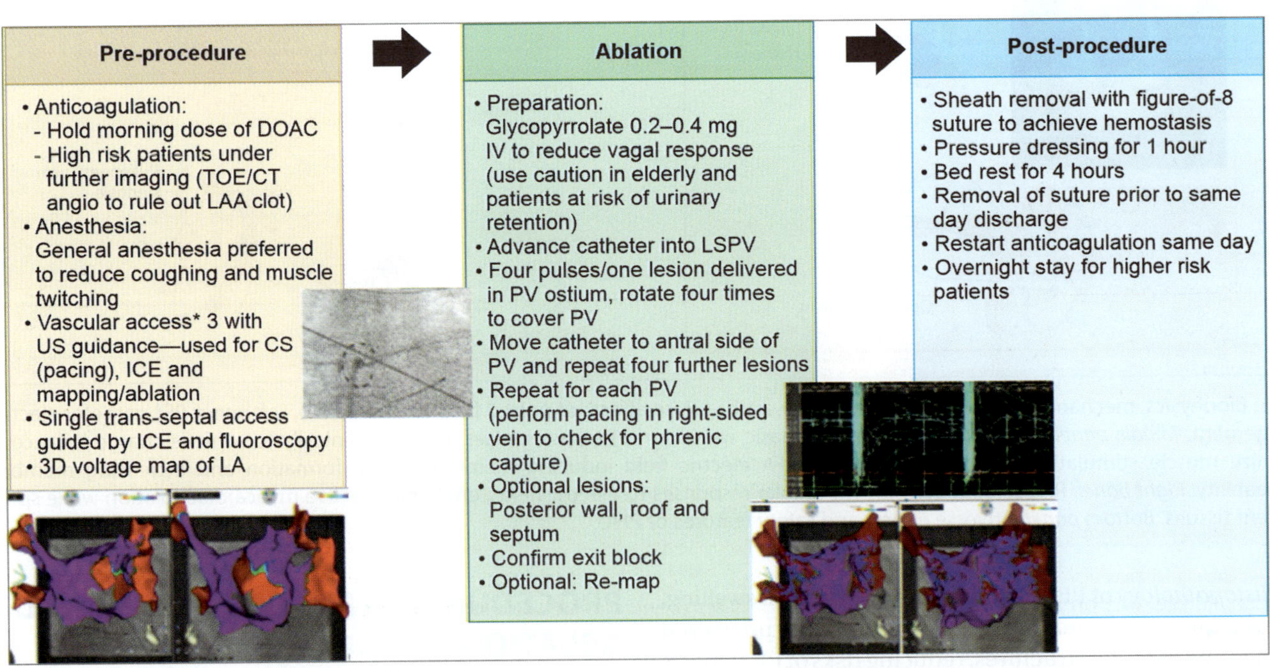

*Vascular access × 3.

FIG. 2: Workflow of pulsed field ablation (PFA) procedure.

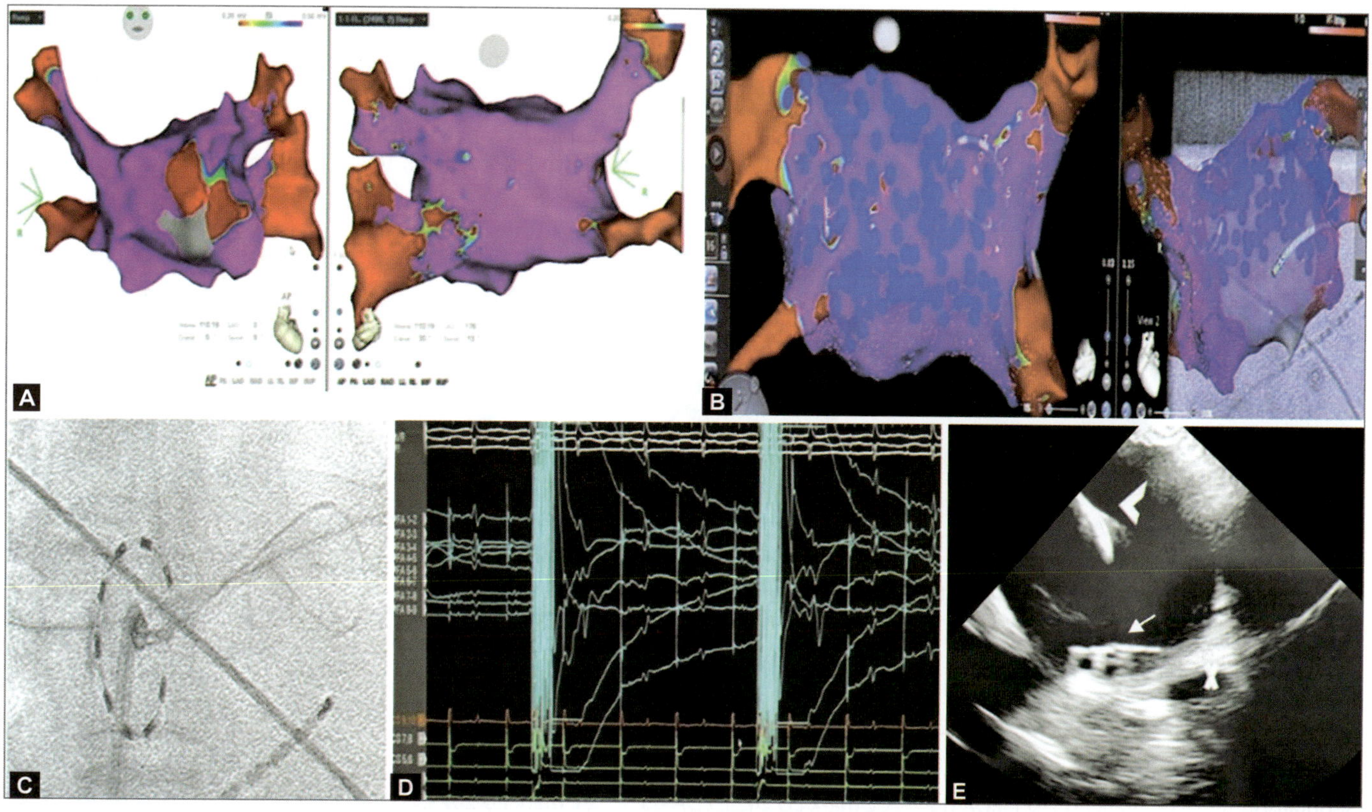

FIGS. 3A TO E: (A) Preablation anteroposterior (AP) and posteroanterior (PA) 3D EAM images. (B) PA and LAO 3D EAM images during pulsed field ablation (PFA) ablation. (C) X-ray showing PFA catheter positioned in posterior wall. (D) EGM images showing artifacts during PFA application. (E) Intracardiac echo image showing PFA catheter in contact with posterior LA wall (white arrowhead: PFA catheter shaft; white arrow: PFA catheter tip; x: esophagus).

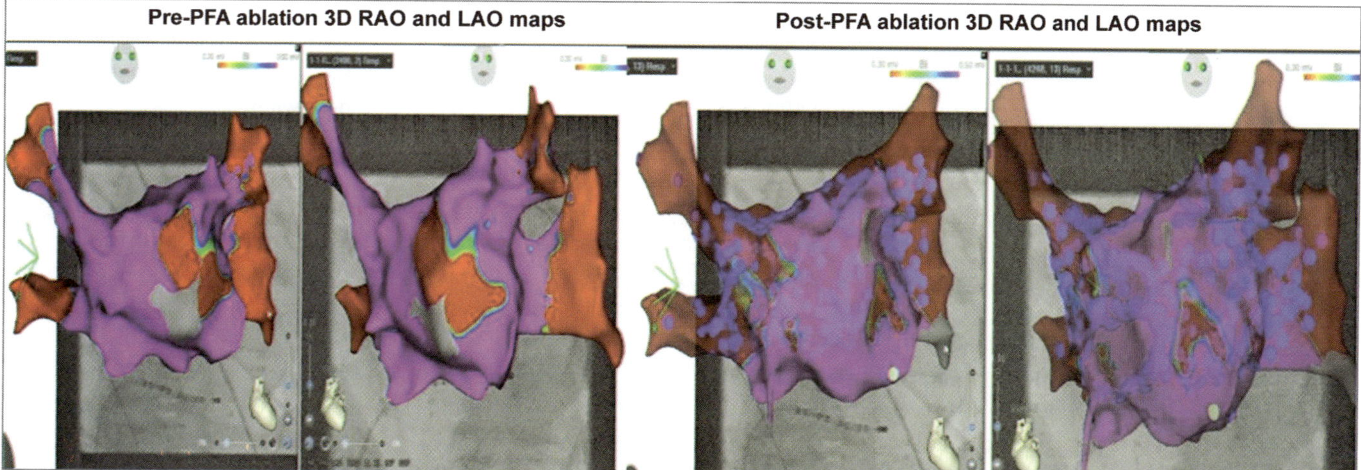

FIG. 4: Pre- and postablation 3D EAM images of pulsed field ablation (PFA) ablation procedure of pulmonary vein and posterior wall isolation. Purple dots on the right side indicate ablation lesions and can be seen in the antrum of all four pulmonary veins and in the posterior wall, septum, and roof.

TABLE 2: Comparison of different vendors of the PFA system.

Feature	Farapulse™ (Boston Scientific)	PulseSelect™ (Medtronic)	Varipulse™ (Biosense Webster/J&J)	Volt PFA™ (Abbott)
Catheter design	Five splines "flower" and "basket" catheter, 20 electrodes (5 × 4)[3]	Horseshoe, 25 mm loop, nine electrodes, 3.75 mm electrode spacing, 20° tilt[4]	Variable-loop (25–35 mm) "lasso-like" catheter, 10 electrodes[5]	Balloon-basket with eight splines[6]
Catheter				
Sheath	16.8 Fr Faradrive™	10 Fr FlexCath Contour™	8.5 Fr CartoVizigo™	13 Fr Agilis™ NxT Dual Reach™
Generator and waveform	FARASTAR generator, biphasic pulses[3]	PulseSelect generator, biphasic R-wave gated[4]	TRUPULSE generator, high-voltage bipolar[5]	Current™ PFA generator, alternating pulses[6]
Energy delivery	Single-shot circumferential PV isolation in seconds[1,3]	Overlapping circular lesions with rotation[4]	Pulse trains, catheter rotation for overlap[2,5]	Balloon-based circumferential[6]
Mapping integration	OPAL HDx Faraview[3]	Integrated mapping + ablation[4]	Full CARTO 3 compatibility[5]	EnSite X compatibility[6]
Voltage	~1,800–2,000 V[3]	~1,200–1,500 V[4]	~1,500–1,800 V[5]	~1,800 V[6]
Pulse duration	~100–200 µs[3]	~100 µs, gated[4]	~250 µs[5]	~100 µs[6]
Regulatory status	CE mark EU 2021; FDA US 2023[3]	CE mark EU 2023; FDA US 2023[4]	CE mark EU 2023; US IDE ongoing[5]	CE mark EU 2024; US IDE ongoing[6]

TABLE 3: Clinical evidence and key trials of pulsed field ablation (PFA) for atrial fibrillation.

Study (Author, Year)	*n* (patients)	Follow-up	Acute success (PVI)	Arrhythmia-free survival/ effectiveness	Complications
First-in-human trial, 2019[12]	81	12 months	100% PVs	87.4% arrhythmia-free at 12 months	1.2% tamponade; no stroke, PV stenosis, or esophageal injury
PersAFOne[20]	25	2–3 months remap, clinical FU	100% PVI and LAPW	Durability: PV 96%, LAPW 100%	No esophageal injury or PV narrowing
IMPULSE/PEFCAT/ PEFCAT II[21]	121	12 months	100% PVs	78.5% arrhythmia-free (overall); 84.5% with biphasic	2.5% primary adverse events
ADVENT[7]	607 (PFA vs. thermal)	12 months	99.6% PFA vs. 99.8% thermal	73.3% PFA vs. 71.3% thermal (noninferior)	Safety 2.1% PFA vs. 1.5% thermal; less PV narrowing with PFA
EU-PORIA registry[23]	1,233	≈12 months	Procedural success across centers	1-year AF/AT-free: 74% overall; 80% paroxysmal; 66% persistent	Major complications 1.7% (tamponade 1.1%, stroke 0.41%)
PULSED AF[28]	300 (150 PAF, 150 PerAF)	12 months	High acute success	66.2% paroxysmal; 55.1% persistent at 12 months	Primary safety 0.7% in each cohort
inspIRE[26]	226 (PAF)	12 months	97.1% veins isolated; 100% entrance block	78.9% arrhythmia-free (pivotal); 70.9% (interim)	No primary AEs in pivotal phase; workflow changes reduced SCLs
MANIFEST-17K Registry[24]	17,642	Registry (real-world)	—	— (safety-focused registry)	Major AEs 0.98%; tamponade 0.36%; stroke 0.12%; no AEF, PV stenosis, persistent phrenic palsy
ADVANTAGE-AF, 2025[27]	255 (PerAF)	15 months	—	Event-free survival 81% at 15 months; 70% <1 h AA burden	Safety 2.4%; no PV stenosis or AEF

thermal modalities, laying the foundation for widespread adoption in AF ablation.

PULSED FIELD ABLATION FOR VENTRICULAR TACHYCARDIA ABLATION

In idiopathic ventricular arrhythmias, PFA created lesions of similar depth but greater width than RFA in the septum, and consistently deeper, wider lesions in papillary muscles, LV summit, and epicardium, without steam pops or proarrhythmia. Epicardial PFA away from coronaries caused only transient ST changes without coronary injury.[29] Clinically, small feasibility reports show high acute success: a two-center study (n = 44) reported 84% success [PVC suppression 81%, ventricular tachycardia (VT) noninducibility 83%] with 52% arrhythmia-free survival at 4 months and only transient conduction disturbances.[30] Other series (n = 20 and n = 24) showed 85–91% acute success, 85–93% short-term arrhythmia-free survival, and minor complications.[31,32] At ~9 months, success was 75% for PVCs and 45% for VTs; 26% experienced complications (20% minor, 6% major, including two strokes).[32] Overall, PFA appears effective and safe, though evidence remains limited to small cohorts with short follow-up.

PULSED FIELD ABLATION FOR SUPRAVENTRICULAR TACHYCARDIA ABLATION

Pulsed field ablation has been investigated in the context of supraventricular tachycardia (SVT) ablation as an experimental approach; however, its clinical application in this setting remains limited and is not part of routine practice. Studies have shown a 97.6% acute success rate, with outcomes of 99.8% in AVNRT, 98.7% in AVRT, and 96.1% in AT. Transient AV block occurred in ~19% (mostly AVNRT slow pathway ablation), resolving within 24 hours, and no permanent block or major complications were seen. At 6 months, recurrence was 9.6% overall, highest in AT (21.4%). Lesion durability, especially for linear ablations, was limited, occasionally requiring adjunctive RF. PFAs tissue selectivity was advantageous in challenging SVTs near structures such as the phrenic nerve and right atrial appendage.[33]

SPECIFIC COMPLICATIONS

Hemolysis: With current PFA systems, >90% of patients show biochemical hemolysis (elevated plasma-free Hb, fHb), and 36% develop hemoglobinuria, but clinically relevant events (hemolytic anemia needing transfusion or AKI requiring dialysis) are extremely uncommon.[34,35] Markers include ↑fHb, LDH, bilirubin, reticulocytes, and ↓haptoglobin. Risk factors are GFR < 50 mL/min, ≥54 deliveries, posterior wall ablation, hypovolemia, and poor catheter contact.[34] AKI occurs in ~1% with PFA versus 1.8% with cryoballoon and 4.3% with RF.[35] Prevention includes optimal contact (ICE), hydration, limiting deliveries, and patient selection.

Coronary vasospasm: Typically, proximity-related (CTI and mitral isthmus), vasospasm is universal in swine but rare in humans (<0.2% overall; 0.02% generalized, 0.14% proximity-related in MANIFEST-17K).[24,36] It results from smooth muscle stimulation rather than ischemia, is transient/reversible with nitroglycerin, and is prevented by prophylactic nitrates. Catheter awareness is key.[37]

Pericardial effusion: Mostly mild/self-limiting; clinically significant effusion/tamponade occurs in 1–2% (ADVENT 2.1%,[22] EU-PORIA 1.1%,[23] MANIFEST-17K 0.36%[24]). Importantly, no cases of delayed tamponade or effusion-related mortality have been reported in major PFA trials or registries.[22-24]

Pro-arrhythmogenicity: In an animal study using bipolar PFA, sustained ventricular fibrillation requiring defibrillation occurred in three (1.6%) ungated applications. Gating of PFA applications eliminated the risk of VT/VF.[18] With *monophasic waveforms,* PFA delivery during the T wave consistently induced ventricular fibrillation (7/7 applications). In contrast, *biphasic waveforms* did not provoke any ventricular arrhythmias, even when applied throughout the T-wave interval.[38] The arrhythmogenicity is practically nonexistent in clinical studies using biphasic waveforms and ECG gating.[38]

LATEST DEVELOPMENTS IN PULSED FIELD ABLATION

Pulse-field cryoablation (PFCA) integrates PFA with ultra-low temperature cryotherapy (–130° to –140°C) to improve lesion formation and safety. Precooling the tissue prior to pulse application reduces muscle contractions and microbubble generation, resulting in broader, deeper lesions with minimal collateral injury. Preclinical data show PFCA produces a more favorable thermal profile than cryo alone, halving the ablation time and slightly greater depth (20.5 mm vs. 17 mm) with similar width (22 mm).[39]

Dual-energy PFA-RF ablation alternates pulsed field and radiofrequency to create deeper, contiguous lesions with minimal scar attenuation. Two systems—TRUPULSE™ (J&J) and Affera™ (Medtronic)—are available, enabling efficient PV and posterior wall isolation in AF and substrate modification in VT. The SPHERE PER-AF trial demonstrated noninferiority to RF in persistent AF (arrhythmia-free survival 73.8% vs. 65.8%, $p < 0.0001$) with no excess complications.[40] Preclinical swine models showed larger, deeper lesions with a thermal necrosis core and PF transition zone,[41] while early VT studies are promising and the Dual VT trial (NCT06816368) is ongoing.[42]

LIMITATIONS AND KNOWLEDGE GAPS

- Long-term durability (>3–5 years) is still unknown.[22]
- Limited data in persistent AF[20,27]

- Concerns about coronary vasospasm, hemolysis: Extremely rare[34]
- Cost and availability

CONCLUSION

Pulsed field ablation is a transformative modality in electrophysiology, offering myocardial selectivity, efficiency, and a favorable safety profile compared to thermal ablation. Important gaps remain regarding durability beyond 3–5 years, the limited evidence in VT, and infrequent safety signals such as coronary spasm or hemolysis. Practical factors such as cost, device accessibility, and operator expertise will also influence widespread adoption. Current evidence supports PFA in AF ablation, while ongoing trials and registries will clarify its long-term safety, efficacy, and role in broader practice.

Funding: None

Acknowledgment: Deepti Ranganathan.

REFERENCES

1. Raatikainen MJ, Hakalahti A, Uusimaa P, et al. Radiofrequency catheter ablation maintains its efficacy better than antiarrhythmic medication in patients with paroxysmal atrial fibrillation: On-treatment analysis. Int J Cardiol. 2015;198:108-14.
2. Pappone C, Augello G, Sala S, et al. A randomized trial of circumferential pulmonary vein ablation versus antiarrhythmic drug therapy in paroxysmal atrial fibrillation (APAF). J Am Coll Cardiol. 2006;48(11):2340-7.
3. Willems S, Borof K, Brandes A, et al. Systematic, early rhythm control strategy for atrial fibrillation in patients with or without symptoms: EAST–AFNET 4. Eur Heart J. 2022;43(12):1219-28.
4. Verma A, Jiang CY, Betts TR, et al. Approaches to catheter ablation for persistent atrial fibrillation. N Engl J Med. 2015;372(19):1812-22.
5. Kuck KH, Brugada J, Fürnkranz A, et al. Cryoballoon or radiofrequency ablation for paroxysmal atrial fibrillation. N Engl J Med. 2016;374:2235-45.
6. De Potter T, Klaver M, Babkin A, et al. Ultra-low temperature cryoablation for atrial fibrillation: primary outcomes for efficacy and safety (CRYOCURE-2). JACC Clin Electrophysiol. 2022;8(8):1034-9.
7. Reddy VY, Gerstenfeld EP, Natale A, et al. Pulsed field or conventional thermal ablation for paroxysmal atrial fibrillation (ADVENT). N Engl J Med. 2023;389(18):1660-71.
8. Dukkipati SR, Kuck KH, Neuzil P, et al. Pulmonary vein isolation using a visually guided laser balloon catheter: the first 200-patient multicenter experience. Circ Arrhythm Electrophysiol. 2013;6(3):467-72.
9. Neumann E, Schaefer-Ridder M, Wang Y, et al. Gene transfer into mouse lyoma cells by electroporation in high electric fields. EMBO J. 1982;1(7):841-5.
10. Davalos RV, Mir LM, Rubinsky B. Tissue ablation with irreversible electroporation. Ann Biomed Eng. 2005;33(2):223-31.
11. Koruth J, Kuroki K, Iwasawa J, et al. Preclinical evaluation of pulsed field ablation: electrophysiological and histological assessment of thoracic vein isolation. Circ Arrhythm Electrophysiol. 2019;12(12):e007781.
12. Reddy VY, Neuzil P, Koruth JS, et al. Pulsed field ablation for pulmonary vein isolation in atrial fibrillation. J Am Coll Cardiol. 2019;74(3):315-26.
13. Benali K, Vlachos K, Reddy V, et al. Pulsed field ablation for atrial fibrillation: efficacy, safety and lesion durability in patients with recurrences. Europace. 2024;26(Suppl 1):euae102.162.
14. Stewart M, Haines DE, Verma A, et al. Intracardiac pulsed field ablation: proof of feasibility in a chronic porcine model. Heart Rhythm. 2019;16:1031-9.
15. Grimaldi M, Di Monaco A, Gomez T, et al. Time course of irreversible electroporation lesion development through short- and long-term follow-up in pulsed-field ablation–treated hearts. Circ Arrhythm Electrophysiol. 2022;15(7):e010661.
16. Koruth JS, Kuroki K, Kawamura I, et al. Focal pulsed field ablation for pulmonary vein isolation and linear atrial lesions: safety and durability in a preclinical model. Circ Arrhythm Electrophysiol. 2020;13(6):e008716.
17. Nakagawa H, Castellvi Q, Neal R, et al. Effects of contact force on lesion size during pulsed field catheter ablation: histochemical characterization of ventricular lesion boundaries. Circ Arrhythm Electrophysiol. 2024;17(1):11-23.
18. Kawamura I, Reddy VY, Santos-Gallego CG, et al. Electrophysiology, pathology, and imaging of pulsed field ablation of scarred and healthy ventricles in swine. Circ Arrhythm Electrophysiol. 2023;16(1):e011369.
19. Nies M, Watanabe K, Kawamura I, et al. Pulsed field ablation of difficult ventricular targets: papillary muscles, trabeculae, septum, and LV free wall in swine. Circ Arrhythm Electrophysiol. 2024;17(6):e012734.
20. Reddy VY, Anic A, Koruth J, et al. Pulsed field ablation in patients with persistent atrial fibrillation. J Am Coll Cardiol. 2020;76(9):1068-80.
21. Reddy VY, Dukkipati SR, Neuzil P, et al. Pulsed field ablation of paroxysmal atrial fibrillation: 1-year outcomes of IMPULSE, PEFCAT, and PEFCAT II. JACC Clin Electrophysiol. 2021;7(5):614-27.
22. Reddy VY, Lehmann JW, Gerstenfeld EP, et al. A randomized controlled trial of pulsed field ablation versus standard-of-care ablation for paroxysmal atrial fibrillation: ADVENT trial rationale and design. Heart Rhythm O2. 2023;4(5):317-28.
23. Schmidt B, Bordignon S, Neven K, et al. European real-world outcomes with pulsed field ablation in symptomatic atrial fibrillation: the EU-PORIA registry. Europace. 2023;25(7):euad185.
24. Ekanem E, Neuzil P, Reichlin T, et al. Safety of pulsed field ablation in more than 17,000 patients with atrial fibrillation: the MANIFEST-17K study. Nat Med. 2024;30(7):2020-9.
25. Verma A, Boersma L, Haines DE, et al. First-in-human experience using a novel pulsed field ablation system: PULSED AF pilot trial. Circ Arrhythm Electrophysiol. 2022;15(1):e010168.
26. De Potter T, Grimaldi M, Duytschaever M, et al. Predictors of success for pulmonary vein isolation with pulsed-field ablation using a variable-loop catheter with 3D mapping: 12-month outcomes from inspIRE. Circ Arrhythm Electrophysiol. 2024;17(5):e012667.
27. Reddy VY, Gerstenfeld EP, Schmidt B, et al. Pulsed field ablation of persistent atrial fibrillation with continuous ECG monitoring: ADVANTAGE-AF phase 2. Circulation. 2025;152(1):27-40.
28. Verma A, Haines DE, Boersma LV, et al. Pulsed field ablation for the treatment of atrial fibrillation: PULSED AF pivotal trial. Circulation. 2023;147(19):1422-32.

29. Younis A, Tabaja C, Kleve R, et al. Comparative efficacy and safety of pulsed field ablation versus radiofrequency ablation of idiopathic LV arrhythmias. JACC Clin Electrophysiol. 2024;10(9):1998-2009.
30. Peichl P, Bulava A, Wichterle D, et al. Efficacy and safety of focal pulsed-field ablation for ventricular arrhythmias: two-centre experience. Europace. 2024;26(7):euae192.
31. Della Rocca DG, Cespón-Fernández M, Keelani A, et al. Focal pulsed field ablation for premature ventricular contractions: a multicenter experience. Circ Arrhythm Electrophysiol. 2024;17(9):e012826.
32. Ruwald MH, Johannessen A, Worck R, et al. Feasibility and midterm effectiveness of focal pulsed field ablation for ventricular arrhythmias. Heart Rhythm. 2025:S1547-5271(25)00129-8.
33. Sawalha K, Pundlik S, Khawaja U, et al. Safety and outcomes of pulsed field ablation in the management of supraventricular arrhythmia: a systematic review. Trends Cardiovasc Med. 2025:S1050-1738(25)00100-8.
34. Popa MA, Venier S, Menè R, et al. Hemolysis after pulsed field ablation for atrial fibrillation: multicenter analysis. Circ Arrhythm Electrophysiol. 2024;17(10):e012732.
35. Jordan F, Knecht S, Isenegger C, et al. Acute kidney injury after catheter ablation of atrial fibrillation: comparison between energy sources. Heart Rhythm. 2024;21(8):1248-9.
36. Ramirez DA, Garrott K, Garlitski A, et al. Coronary spasm due to pulsed field ablation: a state-of-the-art review. Pacing Clin Electrophysiol. 2024.
37. Reddy VY, Petru J, Funasako M, et al. Coronary arterial spasm during pulsed field ablation to treat atrial fibrillation. Circulation. 2022;146(24):1808-19.
38. Kumru HT, Mattison L, Tarakji KG, et al. Arrhythmogenicity of monophasic and biphasic PFA waveforms in a porcine model. J Cardiovasc Electrophysiol. 2024;35(12):2487-90.
39. Dewland TA, Higuchi S, Venkateswaran R, et al. Ultra-low temperature cryoablation versus ultra-low temperature cryoablation combined with pulsed field ablation in a swine ventricular model. Heart Rhythm. 2023;20(5 Suppl):S92-3.
40. Anter E, Mansour M, Nair DG, et al. Dual-energy lattice-tip ablation system for persistent atrial fibrillation: a randomized trial. Nat Med. 2024;30(8):2303-10.
41. Verma A, Maffre J, Sharma T, et al. Effect of sequential, colocalized radiofrequency and pulsed field ablation on cardiac lesion size and histology. Circ Arrhythm Electrophysiol. 2025;18(2): e013143.
42. Peichl P, Wichterle D, Schlosser F, et al. Mapping and ablation of ventricular tachycardia using a dual-energy lattice-tip focal catheter: early feasibility and safety. Europace. 2024;26(11).

CHAPTER 87

Para-Hisian Ventricular Arrhythmias

Sathish S Reddy, Priyanka Agarwal

ABSTRACT

Most cases of idiopathic ventricular arrhythmias (VAs), such as ventricular tachycardia (VT) and premature ventricular complexes (PVC), originate from the heart muscle surrounding the outflow tract. Idiopathic VAs that arise near the His bundle, commonly referred to as para-Hisian VAs, account for 3–9% of all idiopathic VAs.[1] The classic ECG characteristics of these para-hisian VAs include relatively narrow QRS complexes <150 msec, discordance between the aVR and aVL leads, where aVR is predominantly negative and aVL is predominantly monophasic and positive, inferior lead discordance, R wave taller in II>III, and a predominantly negative V1 with QS and early transition.[2,3] Cardiac MRI is crucial for ruling out structural heart disease, as the management approach may differ from that of patients with a structurally normal heart. These VAs can be medically treated, and radiofrequency catheter ablation (RFCA) may be considered if medical treatment is unsuccessful or if the patient chooses it as a treatment option. However, RFCA for this subset of arrhythmias poses a significant risk of atrioventricular (AV) block because of the proximity of ablation site to the conduction system.

Keywords: Premature ventricular complexes, para-Hisian ventricular arrhythmia, radiofrequency catheter ablation.

INTRODUCTION

Idiopathic ventricular arrhythmias (VAs) are a significant cause of morbidity and occasionally mortality in patients with a structurally normal heart. Most idiopathic VAs originate from the right ventricular outflow tract (RVOT), left ventricular outflow tract (LVOT), aortic sinuses, left ventricular (LV) summit, or fascicles. However, some idiopathic VAs may originate near the His bundle region, referred to as para-hisian ventricular arrhythmias (PHVAs). It represents 3–9% of all idiopathic VAs.[1] They may also occur in patients with structural heart disease, in which myocardial scar tissue may or may not be related to the origin of the arrhythmia.[2,3] However, QRS morphology can vary owing to the presence of a scar, resulting in a wider QRS and notching.[4] Previous studies have demonstrated that radiofrequency catheter ablation (RFCA) of frequent PHVAs reduces VA burden, improves LV function, and enhances the quality of life. A well-established fact is that a wider QRS duration of VAs ≥ 150 ms is an independent predictor of impaired LV function, possibly related to greater ventricular dyssynchrony. Although, PHVAs typically have a narrower QRS duration (133 ± 19 ms) than other VA types, they can still contribute to LV dysfunction.[4]

Para-Hisian ventricular arrhythmias can be defined as those in which the earliest activation of the premature ventricular complex (PVC) after complete mapping is recorded in the presence of a His potential or within 10 mm from the His cloud.[5] These arrhythmias can originate from the right ventricle (RV) or left ventricle (LV) septum, near the His bundle area.

They can be further divided into supra-hisian or infra-hisian categories, based on whether they originate above or below the His Cloud, and whether they are positioned on the right or left side of the septum: Right supra-hisian, right infra-hisian, left supra-hisian and left infra-hisian.[4] This classification is clinically significant, because it guides the ablation strategy and helps assess the risk of AV block.

ANATOMICAL CONSIDERATIONS

The compact atrioventricular (AV) node is situated at the apex of the triangle of Koch within the right atrium (RA) **(Fig. 1)**. It extends anterosuperiorly as the His bundle, which traverses the membranous septum via the central fibrous tissue. At the crest of the muscular septum, it is divided into the left and right bundle branches. The membranous septum is a crucial

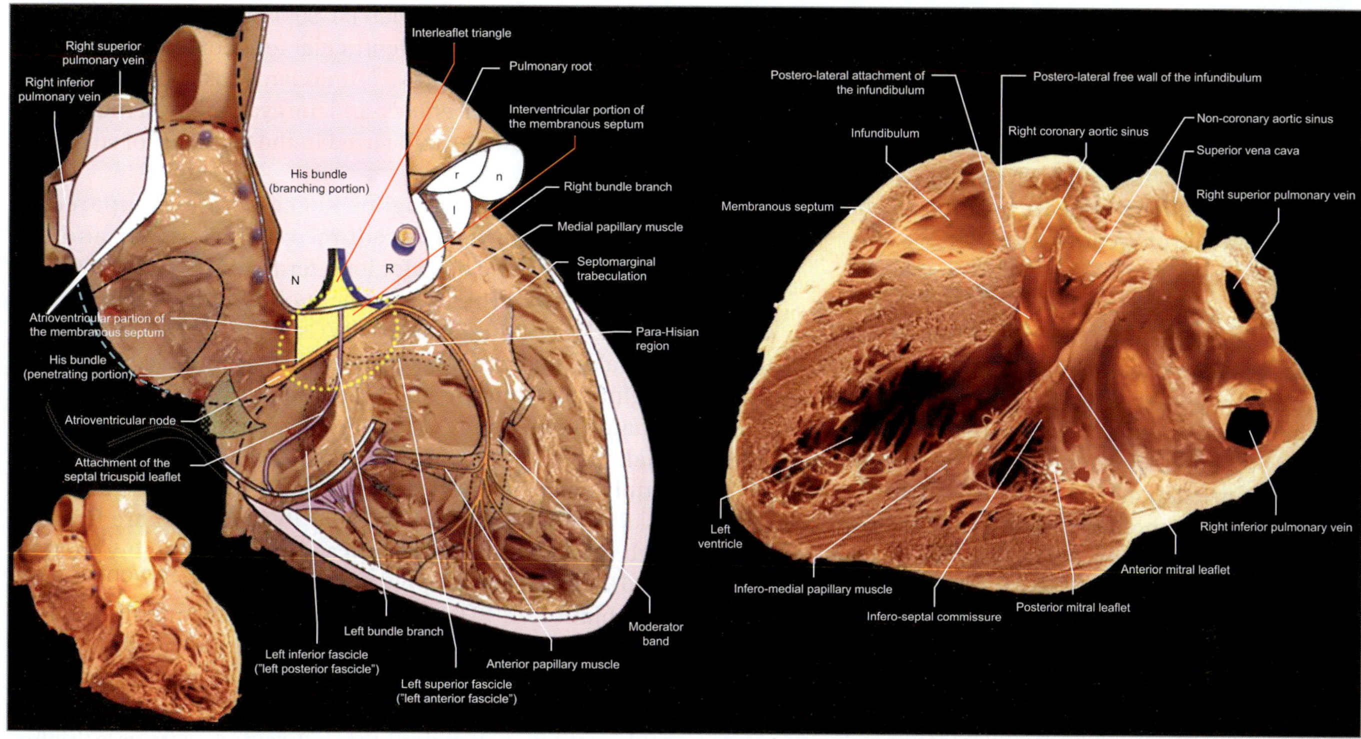

FIG. 1: The para-hisian region and its close anatomic relationship with the right coronary cusp (RCC) and noncoronary cusp (NCC) from the right and left sides of the septum.

Source: Kalyanam Shivkumar (Ed). Atlas of Interventional Electrophysiology (Anatomical Basis of Cardiac Interventions), Volume 2.

structure that extends obliquely downward and leftward from its upper attachment to the aortic annulus. It reaches the upper and posterior edges of the muscular septum and merges with the subendocardium, covering both the right and left sides of the ventricular septum. On the right side, it is covered by the septal leaflet of the tricuspid valve, dividing it into an interventricular section (between the RV and LV) and an AV section (between the RA and LV). It is located on the left side, beneath the junction of the right coronary cusp (RCC) and noncoronary cusp (NCC) of the aortic valve.[6]

ECG CHARACTERISTICS

Because the His bundle region is located in the rightward, posterior, and inferior position within the RVOT, the ECG features of PHVA resemble those of the lower septal RVOT.

The RVOT and LVOT are anatomically proximate and situated at the base of the heart. VPCs from these sites exhibit an inferiorly directed axis, characterized by positive deflections in leads II and III and negative deflections in leads aVL and aVR. Typically, they display a left bundle branch block (LBBB) pattern in lead V1, with variations in the precordial transition depending on the specific site of origin of the arrhythmia.[7]

Key features of PHVA include QRS complexes that are narrower than those typically seen in RVOT VA, frequent discordance in inferior leads, the presence of an R wave in

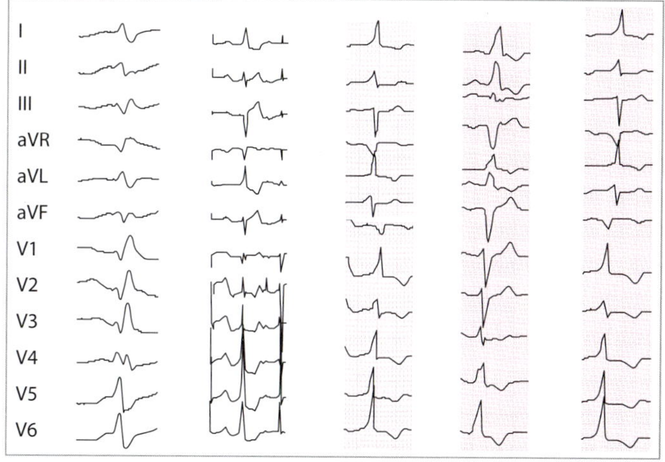

FIG. 2: A 12-lead ECG of para-hisian PVC ablated from the para-hisian region. First case was ablated from the LV septum, and the remaining cases were ablated from the RV septal side and the aortic sinus.

lead aVL and Qs in aVR, indicating discordance between aVR and aVL, an early R-wave transition in V1–V2 for left PHVAs compared to those on the right side, and an inferior axis with a taller R wave in lead II than in lead III or inferior lead discordance with a positive lead II and a negative lead III **(Fig. 2)**. When compared with sinus beats, right PHVAs displayed larger S-waves in V1 and aVR, and left PHVAs showed a larger R-wave in lead V2.[4]

The QRS complexes of the VAs can also be compared with those of the preceding sinus beats. The location, rotation, and horizontal position of the heart within the chest can vary among individuals, which can affect surface ECG characteristics. Therefore, the comparison of QRS complexes between sinus rhythm and VAs would correct for such anatomical variations in heart position to some extent in predicting the site of VA origin.

MANAGEMENT

It is necessary to review all the ECGs and the 12-lead Holters to confirm whether PVC is monomorphic or multiple morphologies were observed. Holter helps in quantifying the PVC burden, to look for diurnal variation in the burden, complex ventricular ectopics, and to assess the response to treatment. C-MRI should be done in patients with suspected PVC-induced cardiomyopathy to rule out other causes of LV dysfunction. C-MRI can be done in these patients after adequate suppression of PVCs.[8] The most significant independent factor predicting PVC-induced cardiomyopathy is the PVC burden. Although patients monitored for more than 14 days exhibit daily variations in PVC burden, most studies rely on 24-hour recordings. A PVC burden of 10% is considered the minimum threshold for the onset of PVC-induced cardiomyopathy, with the risk increasing when the burden exceeds 20%.[9] The likelihood of developing PVC-induced cardiomyopathy is heightened by factors such as a superior PVC axis, epicardial origin, NSVT, shorter coupling interval, and male sex.

When dealing with a patient with PVCs, a physician can offer reassurance as a form of intervention. Additional management depends on symptoms, the burden of PVCs on Holter monitoring, and the presence or absence of structural heart disease. Beta-blockers or nondihydropyridine calcium channel blockers (diltiazem or verapamil) are considered first-line drugs for PVCs. Although better than placebo, randomized controlled clinical trials have demonstrated that β-blockers result in a clinically meaningful reduction in symptomatic outflow tract PVCs in only 12–24% of patients. Nondihydropyridine calcium channel blockers have similarly demonstrated effectiveness in outflow tract PVCs and are considered particularly useful for fascicular VAs. Flecainide, a class IC antiarrhythmic agent, is often used to manage symptomatic or frequent ventricular premature complexes (VPCs), especially those arising from the ventricular outflow tract. Its mechanism involves blocking cardiac sodium channels and inhibiting ryanodine receptor-mediated calcium release, which may explain its effectiveness in suppressing VPCs caused by the delayed afterdepolarizations typical of outflow tract arrhythmias. It is important to emphasize that flecainide should not be used in patients with underlying structural heart disease due to the higher risk of proarrhythmias. Clinical studies have shown that flecainide can significantly decrease the burden of PVCs, often by more than 80–90%, relieve symptoms, and sometimes improve left ventricular function in cases of PVC-induced cardiomyopathy.[10] Amiodarone is avoided because of its long-term side effects, and the availability of much safer drugs and ablation can be used in the presence of structural heart disease.

Considering its higher success rate compared to medication, fewer procedural complications, and the elimination of the need for long-term drug use, RFCA can be regarded as a primary treatment option for typical outflow tract PVCs.[11] Right-sided PVCs generally exhibit more favorable outcomes in terms of efficacy and risk than those originating from the left. Epicardial PVCs, as well as those situated in proximity to the coronary arteries, present greater challenges in terms of accessibility and treatment, often requiring specialized techniques and entailing additional risks. While the success rates for PVC ablation are typically high across various anatomical locations, ranging from 80 to 95%, this does not apply to PHVAs.

Ablation of PHVAs is technically challenging because of the high risk of AV block. A systematic approach is essential to improve outcomes and minimize complications. Radiofrequency (RF) energy application at the RV mid-septum, just below the HB region, carries a higher risk of inadvertent AV conduction block than that at the RV anteroseptum, just above the HB region, because of the close anatomic relation of its location to the AV node. VAs originating from the RCC or NCC adjacent to the membranous septum may exhibit electrocardiographic and electrophysiological characteristics similar to those originating near the HB region in the RV. Activation from the RCC or NCC origin is conducted across the septum to the peri-Hisian RV breakthrough sites. Owing to rapid transseptal conduction, RV activation mapping alone cannot differentiate between right- and left-sided VA origins. Therefore, when RV mapping reveals the earliest ventricular activation in the HB region, mapping in the RCC and NCC should also be performed before ablation to identify the VA origin and decrease the risk of inadvertent damage to the AV conduction system.[1]

Ablation strategies to reduce the risk of inadvertent AV block in PHVAs include gradual uptitration of RF energy delivery, use of cryoablation to allow reversible lesions, pacing techniques to differentiate near-field from far-field His bundle potentials, subvalvular approaches (e.g., reversed C-curve technique) for right infra-Hisian VAs, and ablation from adjacent aortic cusps (RCC or NCC) when mapping suggests earliest activation in these regions **(Fig. 3)**.[4]

Simson et al. reported an acute procedural success rate of 69% for PHVA ablation, corresponding to 33 out of 48 patients.[12] The procedure resulted in the complete elimination of clinical PVCs immediately after ablation; however, some patients experienced recurrence during follow-up. Partial success, characterized by a reduction in PVC frequency without complete elimination, was observed in 8 out of 48 patients (17%), with one patient developing

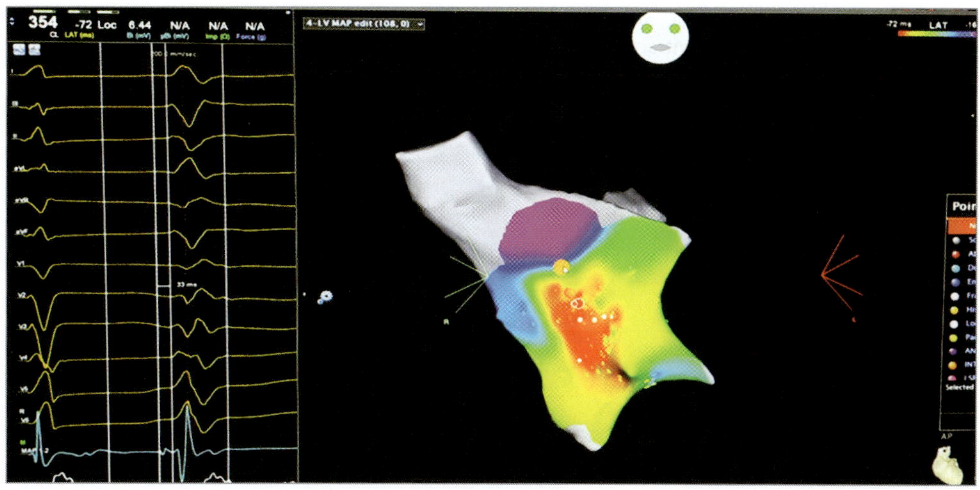

FIG. 3: Intracardiac recordings at the successful ablation site of ventricular arrhythmia originating from the left ventricular (LV) septum just inferior to the His bundle (HB), as there was no earlier site in the coronary cusps.

complete AV block. Notably, the presence or absence of late gadolinium-enhanced cardiac magnetic resonance (LGE-CMR) scar did not significantly influence long-term outcomes, as the postablation PVC burden was comparable between patients with and without scar. In the scar group, ablation was performed on both sides of the septum, and extensive ablation was performed. An intramural LGE-CMR scar was identified in 33 of 48 (69%) patients.

Miyamoto et al. demonstrated in their study that cryoablation effectively eliminated VAs in 7 out of 10 patients, achieving a procedural success rate of 70%.[13] During the follow-up period, four patients (50%) remained free of VA recurrence. Complete AV block occurred in one patient, and transient AV block was observed in two patients. The advantages of cryoablation over RF ablation include a reduced risk of damage to surrounding structures, enhanced catheter stability, and improved energy delivery in challenging anatomical sites.

CONCLUSION

Para-Hisian ventricular arrhythmias constitute a small yet clinically significant subset of idiopathic VAs. The classic ECG characteristics of these para-Hisian arrhythmias include relatively narrow QRS complexes <150 ms, discordance between the aVR and aVL leads, inferior lead discordance with R wave taller in II > III, and a predominantly negative V1 with QS and early transition. Owing to their proximity to the conduction system, ablation poses a considerable risk of AV block. Therefore, comprehensive mapping, consideration of alternative ablation sites (such as the RCC or NCC), right atria, and implementation of risk-reduction strategies are crucial for safe and effective management.

REFERENCES

1. Yamada T, McElderry HT, Doppalapudi H, et al. Catheter ablation of ventricular arrhythmias originating in the vicinity of the His bundle: Significance of mapping the aortic sinus cusp. Heart Rhythm. 2008;5(1):37-42.
2. Pathak R, Kochar A, Enriquez A, et al Ventricular Tachycardia Originating Near the His-Bundle: Electrocardiographic and Catheter Ablation Characteristics. Heart, Lung Circulation. 2017;26:S196.
3. Yamauchi Y, Iesaka Y, Yokoyama Y, et al. Electrocardiographic Characteristics of Repetitive Monomorphic Right Ventricular Tachycardia Originating Near the His-Bundle. Cardiovasc Electrophysiol. 2005;16(10):1041-8.
4. Nair A, Mehta A, Sanders P, et al. Electrocardiographic Characteristics and Ablation Outcomes Associated with Para-Hisian Ventricular Arrhythmias. JACC Asia. 2025;5(2):299-312.
5. Ban JE, Chen YL, Park HC, et al. Idiopathic ventricular arrhythmia originating from the para-Hisian area: prevalence, electrocardiographic and electrophysiological characteristics. J Arrhyth. 2014;30:48-54.
6. Walmsley R, Sinclair D. Anatomy of the membranous ventricular septum in the human heart. Clin Anat. 1994;7(5):305-14.
7. Hutchinson MD, Garcia FC. An Organized Approach to the Localization, Mapping, and Ablation of Outflow Tract Ventricular Arrhythmias. Cardiovasc Electrophysiol. 2013;24(10):1189-97.
8. Yokokawa M, Siontis KC, Kim HM, et al. Value of cardiac magnetic resonance imaging and programmed ventricular stimulation in patients with frequent premature ventricular complexes undergoing radiofrequency ablation. Heart Rhythm. 2017;14(11):1695-701.
9. Baman TS, Lange DC, Ilg KJ, et al. Relationship between burden of premature ventricular complexes and left ventricular function. Heart Rhythm. 2010;7(7):865-9.

10. Hyman MC, Mustin D, Supple G, et al. Class IC antiarrhythmic drugs for suspected premature ventricular contraction-induced cardiomyopathy. Heart Rhythm. 2018;15:159-63.
11. Zang M, Zhang T, Mao J, et al. Beneficial effects of catheter ablation of frequent premature ventricular complexes on left ventricular function. Heart. 2014;100(10):787-93.
12. Simpson J, Al-Sadawi M, Deshmukh A, et al. Catheter ablation of parahisian premature ventricular complexes in patients with and without cardiac scar. Heart Rhythm. 2024;21(10):1845-52.
13. Miyamoto K, Kapa S, Munger TM, et al. Safety and Efficacy of Cryoablation in Patients with Ventricular Arrhythmias Originating From the Para-Hisian Region. JACC Clinical Electrophysiology. 2018;4(3):366-73.

SECTION

12

Imaging

Section Outline

88. **Risk Stratification with Coronary Computed Tomography Angiography-derived Fractional Flow Reserve and Fractional Flow Reserve Gradient**
Lekha Adik Pathak, Ronak V Ruparelia

89. **Role of Multimodality Imaging in Multivalvular Heart Disease**
Rajendra Kumar Jain, Sanjana R Badami

90. **Role of Left Atrial Indices in Management of Chronic Severe Asymptomatic Aortic Regurgitation**
Satish K Parashar

91. **Application of Emerging Hybrid Intracoronary Imaging Technologies in Clinical Practice and Research**
Harilalith Kovvuri, Nagendra Boopathy Senguttuvan

92. **Current Concepts and Clinical Implications of Coronary Artery Calcification**
Satyavan Sharma

93. **Cardiac CT: Emerging Role in Microvascular Dysfunction**
VS Prakash, Varsha Rakshitha Prakash

94. **Role of Cardiac Imaging for Optimizing Medical Therapy**
Vilas Magarkar

CHAPTER

88

Risk Stratification with Coronary Computed Tomography Angiography-derived Fractional Flow Reserve and Fractional Flow Reserve Gradient

Lekha Adik Pathak, Ronak V Ruparelia

ABSTRACT

Coronary artery disease (CAD) remains the leading cause of global morbidity and mortality. Optimal diagnosis and treatment require an accurate understanding of both the anatomical and functional significance of coronary lesions. While coronary computed tomography angiography (CCTA) has transformed noninvasive imaging, it is limited by its inability to assess ischemia. Computed tomography-derived fractional flow reserve (CT-FFR) integrates anatomical imaging with physiological assessment, overcoming these limitations. Furthermore, the CT-FFR gradient—quantifying the pressure drop along a coronary artery—enables distinction between focal and diffuse atherosclerosis, refining risk stratification and treatment planning. This review discusses the pathophysiological basis, technical principles, clinical applications, trial evidence, limitations, future perspectives, and includes a step-by-step clinical case and algorithm to aid practical understanding.

Keywords: Coronary artery disease, CCTA, CT-FFR, ischemia assessment, risk stratification.

INTRODUCTION

Coronary artery disease (CAD) is a progressive atherosclerotic condition characterized by plaque accumulation within coronary arteries, potentially resulting in myocardial ischemia and infarction. Global data show CAD accounts for nearly 9 million deaths annually. Despite significant advances in medical therapy and revascularization techniques, accurate diagnosis remains pivotal for improving outcomes.

Invasive coronary angiography (ICA) has long been the reference standard for anatomical assessment of CAD. However, angiography is limited in its ability to identify lesions responsible for ischemia, often leading to overtreatment of anatomically moderate but physiologically insignificant lesions and undertreatment of truly ischemic segments. Fractional flow reserve (FFR)—an invasive pressure-derived index—revolutionized functional assessment by providing a lesion-specific measure of ischemia. Landmark trials such as FAME demonstrated that FFR-guided percutaneous coronary intervention (PCI) reduces major adverse cardiovascular events (MACEs) compared with angiography-guided PCI.

Despite these advantages, invasive FFR has limitations—procedural risk, need for adenosine, patient discomfort, and cost. This led to the development of computed tomography-derived fractional flow reserve (CT-FFR), a noninvasive alternative derived from coronary computed tomography angiography (CCTA). CT-FFR combines detailed anatomical imaging with computational modeling of blood flow, providing a comprehensive assessment of both stenosis severity and physiological impact. Beyond CT-FFR, the CT-FFR gradient offers additional insights into disease phenotype by distinguishing focal obstructive lesions, typically treatable with percutaneous coronary intervention (PCI), from diffuse disease, better managed medically.[1-4]

PATHOPHYSIOLOGICAL BASIS OF CT-FFR AND CT-FFR GRADIENT

Myocardial ischemia develops when myocardial oxygen demand exceeds supply. In healthy vessels, the coronary microvasculature dynamically regulates blood flow to match oxygen demand. A significant epicardial stenosis increases resistance to flow, particularly under hyperemic conditions, leading to ischemia.

Computed tomography-derived fractional flow reserve calculates the ratio of distal coronary pressure to aortic pressure during maximal hyperemia. Using high-resolution CCTA, 3D coronary models are reconstructed. These models undergo either:

- *Computational fluid dynamics (CFD):* Solves Navier–Stokes equations to simulate hyperemic flow.
- *Machine learning (ML):* Predicts pressure-flow relationships using large datasets correlating CCTA with invasive FFR.[5]

Computed tomography-derived fractional flow reserve gradient quantifies the rate of pressure loss along a vessel, identifying the hemodynamic pattern:

- *Focal disease:* Abrupt, localized pressure drop due to discrete plaque—ideal for PCI.[1,2,4]
- *Diffuse disease:* Gradual, distributed pressure decline typical of long-segment atherosclerosis—best managed with optimal medical therapy (OMT).[1,3,6]

CT-FFR: Principles and Technical Aspects

- *Patient preparation and CCTA acquisition:* Accurate CT-FFR begins with high-quality CCTA, as image artifacts significantly affect computational modeling.[5]
- *Patient preparation:* Heart rate control (<60 bpm) with oral or IV β-blockers (e.g., metoprolol) and sublingual nitrates to ensure coronary vasodilation.[5]
- *Scanning protocol:* Retrospective or prospective ECG-gated acquisition on ≥64-slice CT scanners, ideally 256–320-detector-row systems for superior temporal and spatial resolution.[5] Contrast injection is optimized for homogenous opacification with bolus tracking.
- *Artifact avoidance:* Breath-holding instructions, arrhythmia detection, and avoiding severe coronary calcification are critical, as blooming artifacts hinder lumen visualization.[5]
- *Data processing workflow:* CT-FFR employs 3D anatomical reconstruction of the coronary tree and physiological simulation. Two main approaches exist:
    1. *CFD:* Utilizes Navier–Stokes equations to simulate hyperemic coronary flow. Requires segmentation of coronary lumen, application of boundary conditions (aortic pressure and microvascular resistance), and solving flow equations in supercomputing environments. Examples: HeartFlow FFRct and Siemens cFFR.
    2. *ML-based CT-FFR:* Employs AI models trained on large datasets of CCTA and invasive FFR pairs. Provides rapid, on-site results without heavy computational load. Examples: cFFR (Philips) and Medis Suite FFR.
- *Quality control:* Images must be checked for segmentation errors, lumen misregistration, and boundary condition anomalies.
- *Interpretation:*
    - *Thresholds:* CT-FFR ≤0.80 indicates hemodynamically significant stenosis.
    - *Integration with CCTA:* CT-FFR localizes ischemia-causing lesions, avoiding overestimation from angiographic stenosis severity alone.
- *Clinical workflow:* CT-FFR can triage patients to medical therapy, invasive angiography with PCI, or further functional testing **(Flowchart 1)**.[7,8]
- *Advantages over traditional imaging:* CT-FFR noninvasively combines anatomy and physiology, reducing unnecessary invasive angiography by up to 60% as shown in the PLATFORM trial.[7]

CT-FFR Gradient: Concept and Clinical Significance

- *Conceptual framework:* CT-FFR provides a single distal vessel value but cannot differentiate why ischemia occurs. The CT-FFR gradient—the rate of pressure drop ($\Delta P/\Delta L$) along the vessel—solves this by distinguishing between focal stenosis and diffuse disease.[1-4]
    - *Focal disease:* Abrupt pressure drop localized to a short segment.
    - *Diffuse disease:* Gradual, continuous pressure loss over long segments, often in diabetics and elderly patients.[1,3,6]

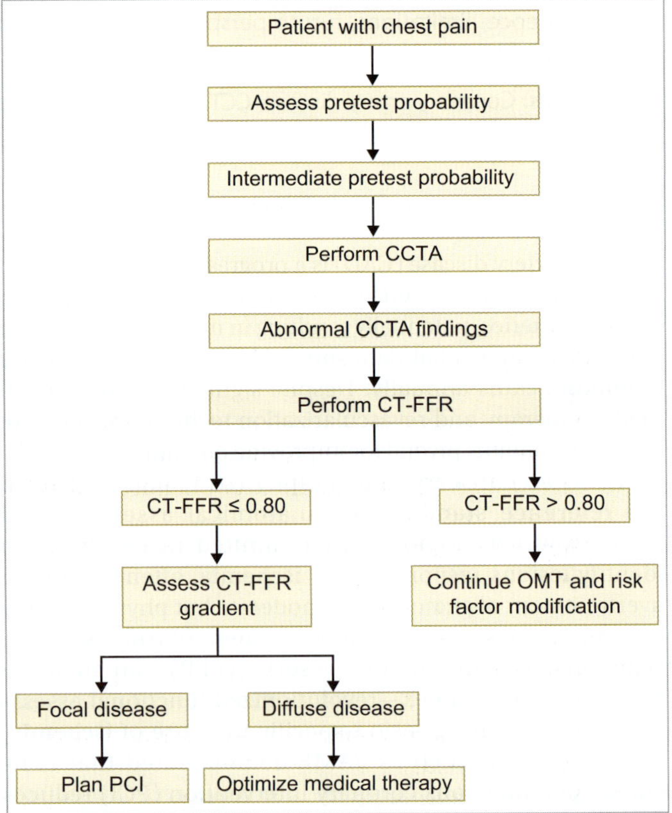

FLOWCHART 1: CT-FFR: clinical workflow.

(CCTA: coronary computed tomography angiography; CT-FFR: computed tomography-derived fractional flow reserve; OMT: optimal medical therapy; PCI: percutaneous coronary intervention)

TABLE 1: Evidence from landmark CT-FFR trials.

Trial (year)	Population	Methods	Key results	Clinical significance
DISCOVER-FLOW (2010)	103 patients, 159 vessels	Prospective multicenter comparison of CT-FFR vs. invasive FFR	Sensitivity 88%, specificity 82%; superior to CCTA alone	First robust validation of CT-FFR as noninvasive physiology
DeFACTO (2012)	252 patients	Multinational trial comparing CT-FFR with invasive FFR	Accuracy 73%, specificity improved (67% vs. 40% for CCTA)	Established CT-FFRs ability to reduce false positives
NXT (2014)	251 patients, 484 vessels	Optimized imaging and CFD modeling	AUC 0.90 vs. 0.81 (CCTA)	Cemented CT-FFR as reference noninvasive physiology
PLATFORM (2016)	584 patients	Randomized to standard care vs. CT-FFR-guided care	Reduced unnecessary ICA by 61%; cost-effective	Demonstrated clinical and economic value of CT-FFR
TARGET (2023)	348 patients	On-site ML-based CT-FFR validation	AUC > 0.90, strong correlation with invasive FFR	Supports real-time, in-laboratory CT-FFR use
Li et al. (2025)	2,457 patients	Long-term registry on prognostic value	CT-FFR ≤ 0.80 predicts 5-year MACE	Provides robust prognostic evidence for CT-FFR
DESTINY (2024)	245 vessels	CT-FFR gradient for focal vs. diffuse disease	Gradient predicts events even when CT-FFR >0.80	Highlights prognostic and therapeutic value of gradient

(CCTA: coronary computed tomography angiography; CT-FFR: computed tomography-derived fractional flow reserve; ICA: invasive coronary angiography; MACE: major adverse cardiovascular event)

- *Calculation methodology:* Gradient derived from multiple CT-FFR sampling points along the vessel.[1,3] A steep negative slope (>0.05/mm) indicates focal disease, while a mild continuous slope (<0.02/mm) suggests diffuse disease.[1,4,6]
- *Clinical utility:*
  - *PCI planning:* Focal disease benefits from stenting, with post-PCI normalization of pressure profiles.[1,3]
  - Diffuse disease often does not improve with focal stenting and should be treated with OMT or CABG if multivessel.[4,6]
- *Prognostication:* Gradient predicts adverse events independent of CT-FFR value; vessels with mild ischemia (CT-FFR 0.81–0.85) but steep gradients have high future event rates.[3,4,6]
- *Integration into clinical decision-making:*
  - *Step 1:* Assess CCTA for plaque burden
  - *Step 2:* Apply CT-FFR to detect ischemia
  - *Step 3:* Use CT-FFR gradient to phenotype disease (focal vs. diffuse)
  - *Step 4:* Tailor therapy—PCI for focal and OMT/CABG for diffuse[1,3,6]
- *Pitfalls and limitations:*
  - *Calcification:* Can mask lesion geometry, distorting gradient analysis.[5]
  - *Microvascular dysfunction:* Gradient assumes normal microvascular resistance; false negatives may occur in microvascular disease.
  - *Standardization:* Lack of universally accepted gradient thresholds limits routine adoption.[1,4]
- *Evidence base:*
  - *DESTINY trial:* CT-FFR gradient predicted vessel-specific MACE beyond CT-FFR alone.[6]
  - *Yang et al.:* Demonstrated real-time on-site CT-FFR gradient improves decision-making in stable CAD.[3]

Evidence from key trials: The clinical utility of CT-FFR and CT-FFR gradient has been validated in multiple landmark studies **(Table 1)**.

COMPARISON WITH OTHER FUNCTIONAL IMAGING MODALITIES

Stress cardiac magnetic resonance (CMR): Stress CMR provides excellent spatial resolution and accurate assessment of myocardial perfusion and viability without ionizing radiation. It can identify subendocardial ischemia missed by other modalities and quantify ischemic burden precisely. However, its use is limited by high cost, long examination times, contraindications (implanted devices and claustrophobia), and limited availability outside specialized centers.

Nuclear perfusion (SPECT/PET): Nuclear imaging with SPECT and PET is widely available and extensively validated for ischemia detection. PET offers superior resolution and absolute flow quantification compared to SPECT, but both involve ionizing radiation and provide poor correlation with coronary anatomy. Attenuation artifacts, especially in obese patients, and inability to identify specific culprit lesions reduce specificity.

Stress echocardiography: This modality is cost-effective, noninvasive, and widely available, using either exercise or pharmacologic stress to detect wall motion abnormalities. It allows rapid bedside assessment, making it useful in acute care settings. However, it is highly operator-dependent, limited by poor acoustic windows in some patients, and less sensitive in multivessel or balanced ischemia.

LIMITATIONS AND CHALLENGES

Image quality dependence: CT-FFR accuracy relies heavily on optimal CCTA images; motion artifacts, heavy calcification, and suboptimal contrast can produce errors.[5] Blooming from calcium often overestimates stenosis severity, reducing diagnostic reliability in elderly or diabetic populations with diffuse disease. Ongoing advances in iterative reconstruction and dual-energy CT aim to mitigate these issues.[5]

Lack of direct assessment of microvascular dysfunction: CT-FFR and CT-FFR gradient evaluate epicardial flow limitation but do not assess microvascular dysfunction, a key cause of angina in up to 40% of patients with nonobstructive CAD. This can lead to false reassurance in patients with ischemia due to microvascular disease, necessitating adjunctive testing such as stress CMR or invasive microvascular assessment.

Need for gradient threshold validation: Although CT-FFR gradient has shown promise in distinguishing focal versus diffuse disease and predicting outcomes, standardized cut-off values and large-scale validation are still lacking.[1,4] Variability in gradient algorithms across vendors further complicates clinical adoption and regulatory approval.[1,4]

Cost and availability: While CT-FFR can reduce downstream costs by preventing unnecessary invasive angiography, its upfront cost and inconsistent availability limit widespread adoption.[7] Broader economic analyses and healthcare policy support are needed to expand accessibility.[7]

FUTURE PERSPECTIVES

Artificial intelligence (AI)-driven on-site CT-FFR: Emerging AI-based software allows real-time CT-FFR computation within the catheterization laboratory, eliminating delays from off-site processing.[9] This enables immediate functional assessment during clinical decision-making and supports wider adoption in busy clinical settings.[9]

Integration with plaque characterization: Combining CT-FFR with advanced plaque analysis (low-attenuation plaque, positive remodeling, and perivascular fat attenuation index) provides comprehensive risk profiling.[5] Such integration could identify high risk but non-flow-limiting plaques, guiding early intervention to prevent events.[5]

Machine-learning models for predicting PCI benefit: Beyond current physiological thresholds, machine-learning models integrating CT-FFR, plaque morphology, and patient-specific data are being developed to predict which patients will derive the greatest symptomatic and prognostic benefit from PCI. These personalized approaches represent the future of precision cardiology.

STEP-BY-STEP CLINICAL CASE EXAMPLE

Patient presentation: A 63-year-old male with hypertension, dyslipidemia, and exertional angina (CCS class II) presents for evaluation. Resting ECG shows nonspecific ST-T changes; troponin is negative.

- *Step 1:* CCTA acquisition—CCTA reveals moderate (50–70%) stenosis in the proximal left anterior descending (LAD) artery and diffuse noncalcified plaques in the right coronary artery (RCA). Plaque characterization suggests high-risk features (low-attenuation plaque and positive remodeling).
- *Step 2: CT-FFR analysis—*
  - *Proximal LAD lesion:* CT-FFR value = 0.76.
  - *RCA diffusely diseased:* Vessel-level CT-FFR = 0.83. Interpretation: LAD lesion is physiologically significant (≤0.80), RCA is borderline but not clearly ischemic.
- *Step 3: CT-FFR gradient analysis—*
  - *LAD:* Abrupt pressure drops from 0.93 to 0.76 over a short 8 mm segment, indicating a focal obstructive plaque suitable for PCI.
  - *RCA:* Gradual decline from 0.95 to 0.83 across 80 mm, consistent with diffuse disease.
- *Step 4: Clinical decision-making—*
  - Proceed with PCI of the LAD lesion
  - Optimize medical therapy (statins, antiplatelet agents, and risk factor control) for RCA diffuse disease.
- *Step 5:* Outcome—patient undergoes LAD PCI with DES placement. Postprocedure, symptoms resolve. Follow-up at 12 months shows no recurrent angina or adverse events.

  Learning points:
  - CT-FFR accurately identified the ischemia-producing LAD lesion, avoiding unnecessary RCA intervention.
  - CT-FFR gradient distinguished focal versus diffuse disease, guiding optimal treatment strategy.
  - Comprehensive noninvasive assessment can streamline patient care and improve outcomes.[3,4,6,7,10]

CONCLUSION

Computed tomography-derived fractional flow reserve and CT-FFR gradient have transformed noninvasive CAD assessment by integrating anatomy and physiology into a single, comprehensive modality. CT-FFR improves diagnostic accuracy, optimizes management, and predicts outcomes, while CT-FFR gradient refines risk stratification by identifying high-risk lesion patterns. Together, they represent the future of precision cardiology, enabling better patient selection, efficient resource utilization, and potentially improved clinical outcomes. Ongoing advancements in AI and wider clinical adoption promise to solidify their role in routine care.[3-10]

REFERENCES

1. Zhao Y, Li J, Li S, et al. Risk stratification with fractional flow reserve and fractional flow reserve gradient from CCTA. J Cardiovasc Comput Tomogr. 2025;19(2):155-67.
2. Hong SJ, Lee J, Kim J, et al. Fractional flow reserve and fractional flow reserve gradient from CCTA for predicting future coronary events. JACC Cardiovasc Imaging. 2024;17(1):45-57.
3. Yang DH, Kim YH, Roh JH, et al. On-site computed tomography-derived fractional flow reserve to guide management of patients with stable chest pain: A prospective, multicenter, outcome study. Eur Heart J. 2024;45(6):789-800.
4. Han D, Lee JH, Park GM, et al. Prognostic value of CT-derived fractional flow reserve gradient in predicting long-term outcomes. JACC Cardiovasc Imaging. 2024;17(3):523-35.
5. Nørgaard BL, Terkelsen CJ, Mathiassen ON, et al. Noninvasive assessment of coronary artery disease with CT fractional flow reserve and plaque characterization. J Am Coll Cardiol. 2019; 74(15):1958-70.
6. Ito K, Takahashi K, et al. Clinical utility of CT-FFR gradient for phenotyping coronary artery disease: DESTINY trial. Circ Cardiovasc Imaging. 2024;17(4):e015324.
7. Douglas PS, Pontone G, Hlatky MA, et al. Clinical outcomes of fractional flow reserve CT-guided versus usual care in suspected CAD: the PLATFORM trial. J Am Coll Cardiol. 2016; 68(5):435-45.
8. Douglas PS, Patel MR, Bailey SR, et al. 1-year outcomes of FFRCT-guided care in patients with suspected coronary disease. Eur Heart J. 2023;44(3):335-48.
9. Tang CX, Liu CY, Xu L, et al. Real-time on-site CT-derived fractional flow reserve in the catheterization lab: the TARGET trial. J Am Coll Cardiol. 2023;81(2):174-86.
10. Li S, Zhao Y, Wang C, et al. Prognostic significance of computed tomography-derived fractional flow reserve for long-term outcomes in patients with stable CAD. J Cardiovasc Comput Tomogr. 2025;19(3):245-57.

CHAPTER 89

Role of Multimodality Imaging in Multivalvular Heart Disease

Rajendra Kumar Jain, Sanjana R Badami

ABSTRACT

The evaluation and management of multivalvular heart disease (MVHD) are challenging. While echocardiography remains the primary diagnostic tool, the presence of MVHD alters cardiac loading and flow dynamics, potentially compromising the accuracy of conventional echocardiographic parameters used to evaluate isolated valve lesions. The primary objectives of clinicians are to accurately diagnose severe valvular pathology and to identify high-risk features of early adverse ventricular remodeling through a systematic approach using various imaging techniques. Multimodality imaging plays a pivotal role in providing a comprehensive evaluation, characterizing disease mechanisms, and guiding appropriate therapeutic strategies.

Keywords: Multivalvular heart disease, echocardiography, cardiac remodeling, valvular pathology, multimodality imaging, hemodynamics, ventricular function, diagnostic imaging, risk assessment, cardiac valve disorders.

INTRODUCTION

Multivalvular heart disease (MVHD) is defined as the presence of a regurgitant and/or a stenotic lesion affecting at least two cardiac valves.[1] Echocardiographic parameters that are dependent on flow or loading conditions represent potential sources of error in the evaluation of patients with MVHDs.[2] Rheumatic heart disease and degenerative heart disease are the most common etiologies of MVHDs in developing and developed nations, respectively.[3]

CONVENTIONAL TWO-DIMENSIONAL TRANSTHORACIC ECHO AND DOPPLER-DERIVED MEASUREMENTS

Two-dimensional echocardiography remains the primary and most practical imaging modality for evaluating valvular pathology, offering excellent visualization of valve anatomy while combining wide availability, noninvasiveness, and ease of use **(Flowchart 1)**.

- Low-flow, low-gradient (LFLG) stenosis is common, making severity assessment difficult.
- Increased forward flow and transvalvular gradients potentially leading to overestimation of stenosis severity.
- The continuity equation becomes unreliable when flow across different valves is unequal.[4]

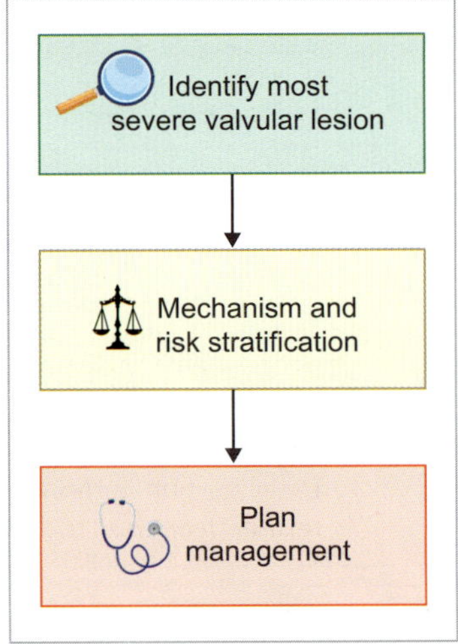

FLOWCHART 1: Conventional two-dimensional TTE.
(TTE: transthoracic echo)

- Severe lesions in one valve can cause or worsen regurgitation [mitral regurgitation (MR) or tricuspid regurgitation (TR)] in upstream valves.
- Methods based on pressure half-time (PHT) may be inaccurate if left ventricular (LV) compliance or filling is altered **(Table 1)**.

TABLE 1: Echocardiographic limitations and recommendations in diagnosis of multivalvular heart disease.

Severe lesion	Association	Hemodynamics	Transthoracic echo—limitations	Recommendation
AS	MR	Reduced forward cardiac output and marked pulmonary venous hypertension	• Significant MR decreases aortic V_{max} and mean gradient, which may lead to underestimation of AS[5,6] • Classical low-flow, low-gradient AS/paradoxical low-flow, low-gradient AS • Continuity equation unreliable	CT-AVC score
	MS	Reduced forward cardiac output	• Underestimation of AS severity using aortic V_{max} and mean PG[7] • Classical low-flow, low-gradient AS[8]	CT-AVC score
MS	AS	Reduced stroke volume	• Mitral PHT unreliable. Altered left ventricular compliance due to AS disrupts diastolic pressure equilibration, shortening PHT, and hence, overestimating MVA[9] • Low-flow, low-gradient MS	3D echo for MVA/CT
	AR	Reduced stroke volume	Shortens mitral PHT—overestimation of MVA[10]	3D echo—direct planimetry, PISA
	TR	RV volume overload—IVS flattening—reduces transmitral flow	Overestimates PHT—underestimates MVA[11]	3D TEE—planimetry
	TS	Low forward flow due to TS limits transmitral flow	PHT overestimation—underestimation of MVA	3D TEE—planimetry
AR	MR	Regurgitant flows disrupt the equality of mitral and aortic stroke volumes	Continuity equation and Doppler volumetric method using left-sided assessment of net forward flow invalid[12] PHT unreliable	PISA, 3D VCA (for eccentric jets),[13] 3D TTE/TEE, CMR
	MS	Forward stroke volume across the mitral valve does not equal that across the aortic valve when AR is present. MS can blunt the increase in pulse pressure and ventricular dilation	Continuity method and PHT invalid[14]	3D VC—TEE, CMR, and CT for evaluation of aortic root and ascending aorta
MR	AS	Increase in LV pressure and regurgitant volume- reduced stroke volume[15]	MR jet area is unreliable	EROA by PISA, 3D TTE/TEE, CMR-MR volume, and regurgitant fraction
	AR	Regurgitant flows disrupt the equality of mitral and aortic stroke volumes	Continuity equation and Doppler volumetric method using left-sided assessment of net forward flow invalid[12]	3D VCA, PISA, CMR-MR volume and fraction
	TR	Decrease pulmonary venous return- decreased transmitral flow[11]	Underestimates severity—Doppler derived like regurgitant volume is not reliable	3D TTE/3D TEE

(AR: aortic regurgitation; AS: aortic stenosis; AVC: aortic valve calcium; LV: left ventricle; MR: mitral regurgitation; MS: mitral stenosis; MVA: mitral valve area; PG: pressure gradient; PHT: pressure half time; PISA: proximal isovelocity surface area; RV: right ventricle; TEE: transesophageal echocardiography; TR: tricuspid regurgitation; TS: tricuspid stenosis; TTE: transthoracic echocardiography; VCA: vena contracta area)

Aortic Stenosis with Mitral Regurgitation

In patients with severe aortic stenosis (AS), chronic pressure overload leads to LV hypertrophic remodeling, dilatation, and dysfunction.

The increased afterload from AS elevates the transmitral systolic pressure gradient, thereby amplifying the mitral regurgitant volume for a given effective regurgitant orifice area (EROA). Significant MR can reduce forward stroke volume, diminishing the transaortic gradient and leading to underestimation of AS severity. This scenario may present as either classical LFLG AS [with reduced left ventricular ejection fraction (LVEF)] or paradoxical LFLG AS (with preserved LVEF). In such cases, dobutamine stress echocardiography (DSE) may be inconclusive, as MR-related low flow may limit contractile reserve. Multidetector computed tomography (CT)-based aortic valve calcium scoring can assist in distinguishing true-severe from pseudosevere AS.

In patients with LFLG AS (regardless of LVEF) and concomitant MR, cardiac CT-based calcium scoring of the aortic valve offers flow-independent anatomical insights that support differentiation between true severe and pseudosevere AS.[16]

Cardiac magnetic resonance (CMR), while less available, serves as the gold standard for assessing LV volumes, function, and myocardial fibrosis. It also enables direct quantification of transvalvular flow using phase-contrast imaging, which is especially useful when echocardiographic findings are discordant **(Table 2)**.

Aortic Stenosis with Mitral Stenosis

The coexistence of mitral stenosis (MS) and AS is uncommon; however, when present, it is often poorly tolerated because of the significant reduction in cardiac output resulting from combined valvular obstruction. Low cardiac output often results in deceptively low transvalvular gradients across both aortic and mitral valves. This diminished pressure gradient can lead to underestimation of stenosis severity in both AS and MS, particularly in low-flow states **(Table 3)**.

Aortic Regurgitation with Mitral Regurgitation

The presence of a primary aortic regurgitation (AR) that leads to LV dilation and thus secondary MR is the most common phenotype, resulting in progressive LV dysfunction.[17]

Transthoracic and transesophageal echocardiography remain the first-line tool for initial diagnosis, including jet characteristics, vena contracta (VC), and proximal isovelocity surface area (PISA). However, in complex or borderline cases—especially with multiple jets, eccentric flow, or suboptimal acoustic windows—CMR provides superior quantification of regurgitant volume and fraction, with high reproducibility. Cardiac CT aids in anatomical delineation, particularly for preprocedural valve planning.

Multiple jets often produce noncircular EROA, influenced by the orientation of the echocardiographic imaging plane. When multiple regurgitant jets are observed, averaging the 3D VC width measured in the apical four- and two-chamber views can provide useful information. Among quantitative techniques, the PISA method remains the most commonly used, despite its recognized limitations.

Aortic Regurgitation and Mitral Stenosis

The coexistence of MS and AR imposes discordant loading conditions—MS diminishes preload while AR increases it—which attenuates LV dilation and blunts stroke volume augmentation typically observed in isolated AR.[18]

Accurate assessment of MS becomes particularly challenging in the presence of concomitant AR. AR leads to elevated LV diastolic pressure, which shortens the PHT, resulting in an overestimation of the mitral valve area (MVA).

TABLE 2: Comparison of various imaging techniques in evaluation aortic valve.

Parameter	Echocardiography	Cardiac CT	Cardiac MRI
Aortic valve area (AVA)	• Aortic valve planimetry by TEE • Continuity equation unreliable	Planimetry CT-AVA	Direct planimetry
Calcium quantification (AVC score)		Gold standard	
Flow assessment	Doppler-based (load and flow dependent)	Not feasible	Accurate, flow-independent (phase contrast)
LV function and mass	Visual and Simpson-based EF	Limited	Gold standard for volume and mass assessment
Tissue characterization	Not possible	Not possible	Late gadolinium enhancement, ECV (fibrosis)
Bicuspid aortic valve detection	Possible	Excellent valve morphology and cusp separation	Good for valve morphology
Use in low-flow, low-gradient AS	Limited role	AVC helps confirm severity (flow-independent)	Differentiates true vs. pseudosevere with flow

(AS: aortic stenosis; AVC: aortic valve calcium; ECV: extracellular volume; LV: left ventricle)

TABLE 3: Hemodynamic and appropriate imaging strategy in AS + MS.

Feature	Importance in AS + MS	Recommended imaging
Low-flow, low-gradient	Mask severity of AS and MS	CT (AVC) and CMR planimetry
Valve area	Flow-dependent echocardiographic errors	3D TEE for MS, CT, or CMR for AS
LV response and fibrosis	Prognosis	CMR for remodeling and fibrosis quantification

(AS: aortic stenosis; CMR: cardiac magnetic resonance; LV: left ventricle; MS: mitral stenosis)

Similarly, the use of the continuity equation to calculate MVA is unreliable in this context due to differing flow volumes across the mitral and aortic valves. Therefore, whenever feasible, direct planimetry is the preferred method for MVA assessment, preferably 3D echocardiography.

In cases where planimetry is not feasible, the PISA method provides a more accurate alternative to PHT in evaluating MVA in patients with combined MS and AR.

In the evaluation of AR severity, the VC area—preferably assessed using 3D imaging, and ideally via transesophageal echocardiography (TEE)—is a valuable tool. CMR with phase-contrast imaging can further support AR severity grading, offering accurate quantification regardless of coexisting MS. Additionally, as with all significant AR cases, assessment of the aortic root and ascending aorta is essential. Cross-sectional imaging modalities like CT should be employed to detect and measure aortic dilation, with regular follow-up recommended to monitor for progressive enlargement.

Tricuspid Regurgitation

Tricuspid regurgitation hemodynamics are often influenced by complex interactions between right- and left-sided valvular lesions. Functional TR is the most common mechanism, resulting from right ventricular (RV) and tricuspid annular dilation secondary to chronic pressure or volume overload **(Table 4)**.

TABLE 4: Hemodynamics and imaging techniques in the presence of significant TR.

Valvular lesion	Key hemodynamic effects	Multimodality imaging approach
TR + AS	• Severe AS ↑ LV afterload → ↑ LVEDP → pulmonary hypertension → RV pressure overload → functional TR. TR causes regurgitant RV output → ↓ effective pulmonary flow, may mask AS low-flow states • Low SVI can cause underestimation of AS severity[19]	• TTE: AS gradients/AVA, TR vena contracta/PISA, RVSP • TEE: Better leaflet and annulus assessment • 3D echo: Annular sizing for repair feasibility • CMR: RV volumes/function, TR regurgitant volume • RHC: PAP, RA pressure, cardiac output • CT: Pre-TAVR sizing/planning
TR + MS	• MS → ↑ LA pressure → pulmonary venous congestion → pulmonary hypertension → RV dilation/dysfunction → TR • Severe TR ↓ forward pulmonary flow → affects MS gradient measurement. Low-flow state may underestimate MS severity	• TTE: MVA (PHT, planimetry), TR severity • TEE: Detailed valve morphology • 3D echo: MS orifice shape, TR annulus • CMR: RV volume/TR quantification • RHC: Gradient across MV, PAP, and RA pressure • CT: LA anatomy—chamber morphology, annular calcification, and surrounding structures[20] • TTE: MR severity (EROA, regurgitant volume), TR quantification • TEE: Detailed leaflet pathology • *3D echo*: 3D vena contracta area (noncircular shape in case of TR), tricuspid valve anatomy (annulus geometry and dimension, leaflet tenting), quantification of RV and RA size and function
TR + MR	• MR → volume overload of LA and LV → pulmonary venous hypertension → RV afterload ↑ → TR • Severe TR ↓ pulmonary flow, may lower MR forward volume fraction—underestimate MR	• RV–arterial coupling (TAPSE/sPAP < 0.4 mm/mm Hg) • CMR: Accurate MR and TR quantification • RHC: PAP and cardiac output • CT: Planning tricuspid annuloplasty or replacement
TR + AR	• AR → LV volume overload → ↑ LVEDP → pulmonary hypertension → RV dysfunction → TR • TR ↓ effective forward stroke volume → affects AR regurgitant fraction calculation	• TTE: AR severity (vena contracta, PISA), TR quantification • TEE: AR jet origin, TR leaflet coaptation • 3D echo: Aortic root sizing, TR annulus • CMR: Phase-contrast imaging for AR regardless of TR • RHC: PAP • CT: Aortic root/ascending aorta sizing
	Opposed loading conditions in chronic AR + TR—volume overload from AR counterbalanced by the TR causes reduction in effective forward flow—may attenuate LV dilation[18]	

(AS: aortic stenosis; AVA: aortic valve area; CMR: cardiac magnetic resonance; LA: left atrial; LV: left ventricle; MR: mitral regurgitation; MS: mitral stenosis; RV: right ventricle; TAVR: transcatheter aortic valve replacement; TTE: transthoracic echo; TR: tricuspid regurgitation)

GLOBAL LONGITUDINAL STRAIN—TWO-DIMENSIONAL TRANSTHORACIC ECHO

Global longitudinal strain (GLS) provides additional insight into myocardial performance beyond conventional measures in MVHD.

By detecting subtle ventricular dysfunction in MVHD, such as AS + MR, MS + AR, or AR + TR, where opposing or additive preload and afterload effects may obscure true LV function.

A reduced GLS is associated with worse prognosis, faster symptom progression, and earlier need for intervention. Even in asymptomatic patients with preserved LVEF, a progressive decline in GLS may signal early contractile dysfunction, supporting timely surgical or transcatheter treatment decisions.

THREE-DIMENSIONAL TRANSTHORACIC ECHO/TEE

Mitral Valve

- Anatomic features of the leaflets—better delineation of leaflet segmentation and identification of the zone of coaptation.
- MVA by planimetry
- Suitability of customized prosthesis or other repair strategies aimed at restoring or maintaining the saddle shape of the annulus results in less leaflet stress and improves durability of prosthetic valve.
- Detailed quantification of the mitral annulus—including area, circumference, and nonplanarity indices—allows comprehensive assessment of disease complexity, assists in tailoring repair strategies, and helps predict postoperative outcomes.[21]
- Quantification of MR—anatomic regurgitant orifice area, 3D PISA-derived EROA, and regurgitant volumes—is suitable in eccentric jets.

Aortic Valve

- 3DE measurements of the aortic root align closely with CT and CMR dimensions.[22]
- Analysis of 3DE images has demonstrated that the LVOT cross-section is not always circular but often elliptical, and use of direct volumetric measurements of stroke volume results in accurate aortic valve area (AVA) calculation.
- Assessment of AR by allowing direct measurement of the VC cross-sectional area, which serves as a surrogate for the EROA **(Figs. 1 and 2)**.

DOBUTAMINE STRESS ECHOCARDIOGRAPHY

Stress echocardiography plays a well-established role not only in ruling out myocardial ischemia but also in dynamically assessing LV interaction with valvular structures and function under physiological (exercise) or pharmacological (inotropic or vasodilator) stress conditions **(Flowchart 2)**. Current guidelines recommend stress echocardiography when there is a discrepancy between the presenting symptoms and the findings of baseline echocardiography as well as in patients with asymptomatic severe AS who may not be aware of subtle changes to their effort tolerance.

- True LFLG AS with reduced LVEF (LVEF < 50%) is characterized by a fixed AVA (AVA <1.0 cm^2), reduced stroke volume (<35 mL/m^2), and a mean gradient <40 mm Hg. This form reflects advanced disease with increased afterload and declining contractility, but it may improve with valve intervention.
  Pseudosevere AS, on the other hand, mimics severe AS due to impaired LV systolic function, which leads to reduced valve opening despite a potentially nonsevere fixed lesion.
  Low-dose DSE helps distinguish between the two. In true severe AS, dobutamine increases stroke volume (≥20%) and raises the mean transvalvular gradient above 40 mm Hg without significantly increasing AVA (remains <1.0 cm^2). In pseudosevere AS, improved contractility increases both gradient and AVA (>1.0 cm^2), confirming a nonsevere stenosis.
- Flow reserve assessment during DSE is a key component in evaluating patients with LFLG AS. Flow reserve is defined as a ≥20% increase in stroke volume in response to dobutamine infusion. The presence of flow reserve is associated with a more favorable prognosis and suggests

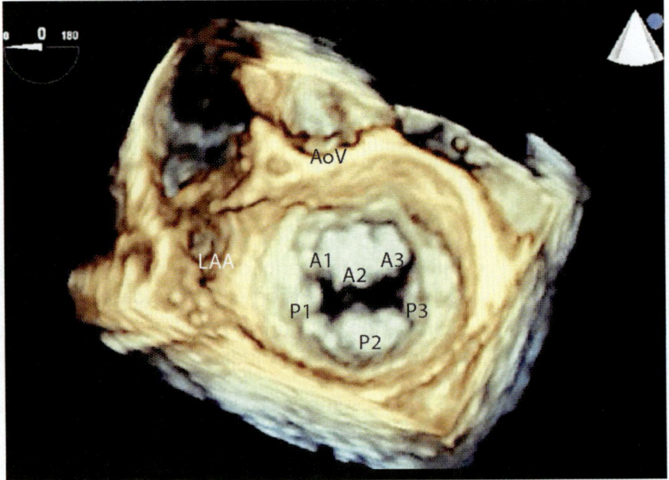

FIG. 1: Three-dimensional TEE showing scallops of mitral valve. The mitral valve has two leaflets: The anterior and posterior leaflets. Each leaflet is further subdivided into three different scallops with the A1 and P1 scallops closest to the left atrial appendage. This view of the mitral valve is referred to as the surgeons view with the aortic valve oriented at the top of the image.

(AoV: aortic valve; LAA: left atrial appendage).

Source: Quader N, Rigolin VH. Two and three-dimensional echocardiography for pre-operative assessment of mitral valve regurgitation. Cardiovasc Ultrasound. 2014;12:42.

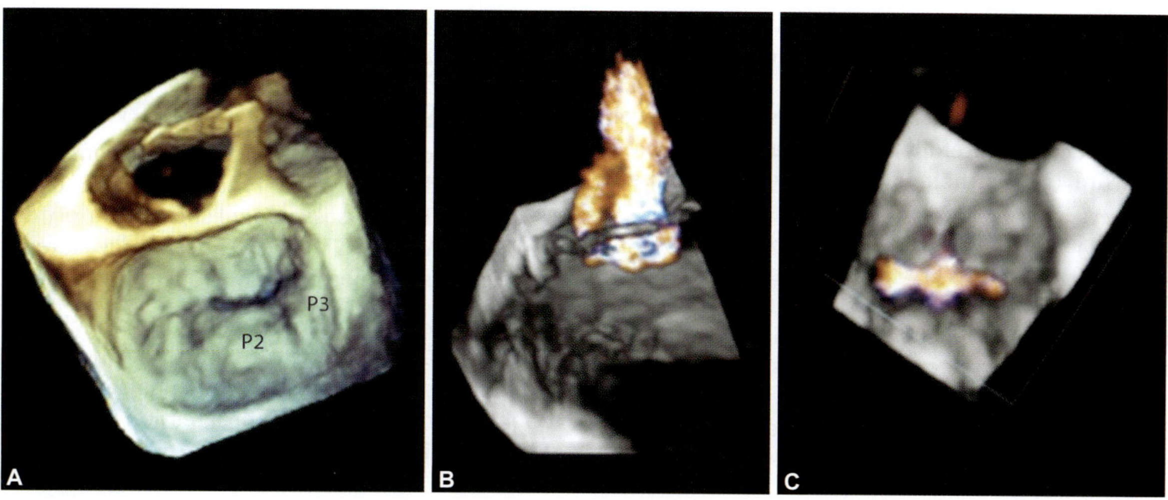

FIGS. 2A TO C: (A) En-face view of the mitral valve. Ischemic mitral regurgitation due to the tethering of posteromedial part of the valve. (B) The proximal isovelocity surface area (PISA). (C) 3D TEE full volume color Doppler image of "vena contracta."

Source: Drąsutienė A, Aidietienė S, Zakarkaitė D. The role of real time three-dimensional transoesophageal echocardiography in acquired mitral valve disease. Semin Cardiovasc Med. 2015;21(2):16-26.

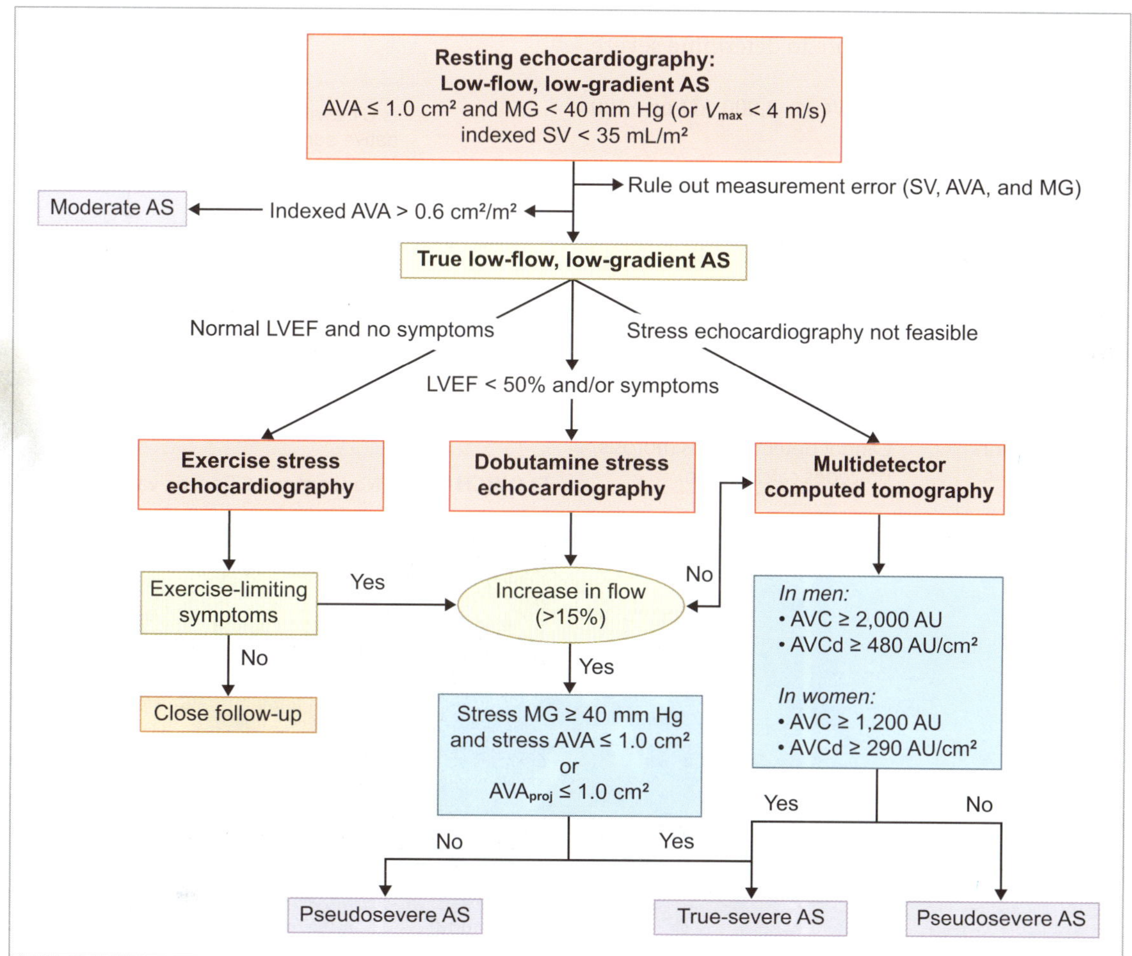

FLOWCHART 2: Approach to diagnosis of true severe and pseudosevere AS.

(AVA: aortic valve area; AVC: aortic valve calcification; AVCd: AVC density, i.e., AVC divided by aortic annulus cross-sectional area; AS: aortic stenosis; LVEF: left ventricular ejection fraction)

Source: Clavel and Pibarot.[5]

that the patient is more likely to experience improvement in LV function following valve intervention. Conversely, the absence of flow reserve indicates a higher surgical risk due to poor myocardial contractile reserve. However, even in such cases, carefully selected patients may still benefit from transcatheter aortic valve replacement (TAVR).[23]

- In paradoxical LFLG AS (AVA < 1.0 cm^2, SVI < 35 mL/m^2, mean PG < 40 mm Hg, LVEF > 50%) with preserved LVEF, DSE has a limited role.
- In patients with significant MR or MS, DSE may fail to elicit the necessary increase in transvalvular stroke volume because the low flow is due to the valve pathology rather than impaired myocardial contractility, making the test inconclusive for confirming AS severity.[24]

COMPUTED TOMOGRAPHY

Noncontrast Computed Tomography Aortic Valve Calcification (Table 5 and Flowchart 3)

- Cutoff values of aortic calcium score to determine severe AS **(Figs. 3 and 4)**.
- *Men*: Aortic valve calcification (AVC) ≥ 2,000 AU or ≥480 AU/cm^2.
- *Women*: AVC ≥ 1,200 AU or ≥290 AU/cm^2.[25]

TABLE 5: Advantages and limitations of noncontrast computed tomography.

Advantages	Limitations
Anatomical, flow-independent, and quantitative measurement of valve calcium	Limited information about valve morphology
Tracks disease progression	Cannot detect fibrosis (fibrosis precedes calcification)

Contrast-enhanced Computed Tomography and Computed Tomography Angiography

- Quantification of both calcific and fibrotic leaflet tissue
- Bicuspid aortic valve—classification and detection of aortopathy.[26] Assessment of coronary artery disease
- Hybrid AVA by CTA—LVOT area is measured by CT and velocities are measured by echocardiography.[27]

New technique: The aortic valve fibrocalcific volume by automated Gaussian mixture model (GMM)-generated HU thresholds for fibrotic tissue, blood pool, and calcific tissue.[28] It helps in tracking disease progression with high precision **(Figs. 5A to D)**.

CARDIAC MAGNETIC RESONANCE IMAGING

Aortic Valve

Cardiac magnetic resonance can provide high-resolution, 3D datasets for direct planimetry of the aortic valve orifice in

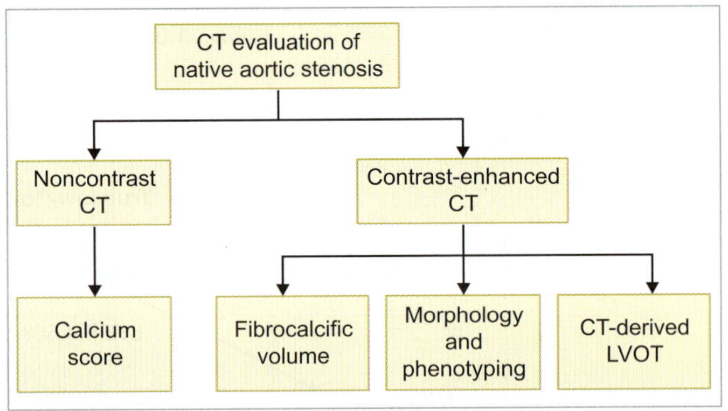

FLOWCHART 3: Noncontrast CT aortic valve calcification.

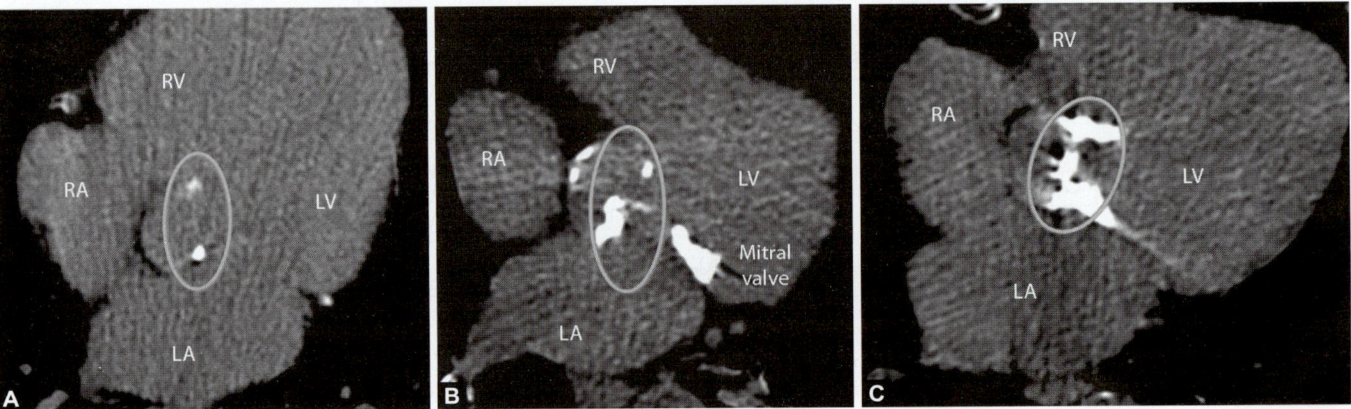

FIGS. 3A TO C: Aortic valve calcium (AVC) assessment by multidetector computed tomography. (A) Mild AVC score = 200 AU. (B) Moderate AVC score = 800 AU. (C) Severe AVC score = 2,000 AU.

(LA: left atrial; LV: left ventricular; RV: right ventricular)

Source: Bax JJ, Delgado V, Bapat V, Baumgartner H. Open issues in transcatheter aortic valve implantation. Part 1: patient selection and treatment strategy for transcatheter aortic valve implantation. Eur Heart J. 2014;35(38):2627-38.

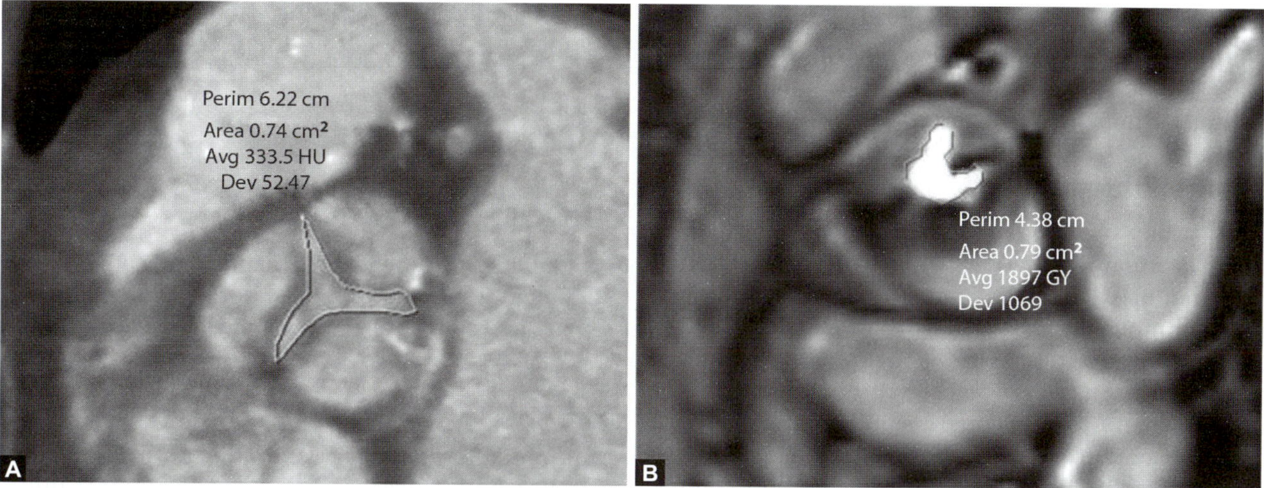

FIGS. 4A AND B: Measurement of aortic valve area in patients with severe aortic stenosis. Cross-sectional view of severely stenotic tricuspid valve is used for measurement of aortic valve area in systolic phase of ECG-gated multidetector CT image (A) and MRI (B).
Source: Chun EJ, Choi SI, Lim C, et al. Aortic stenosis: Evaluation with multidetector CT angiography and MR imaging. Korean J Radiol. 2008;9(5):439-48.

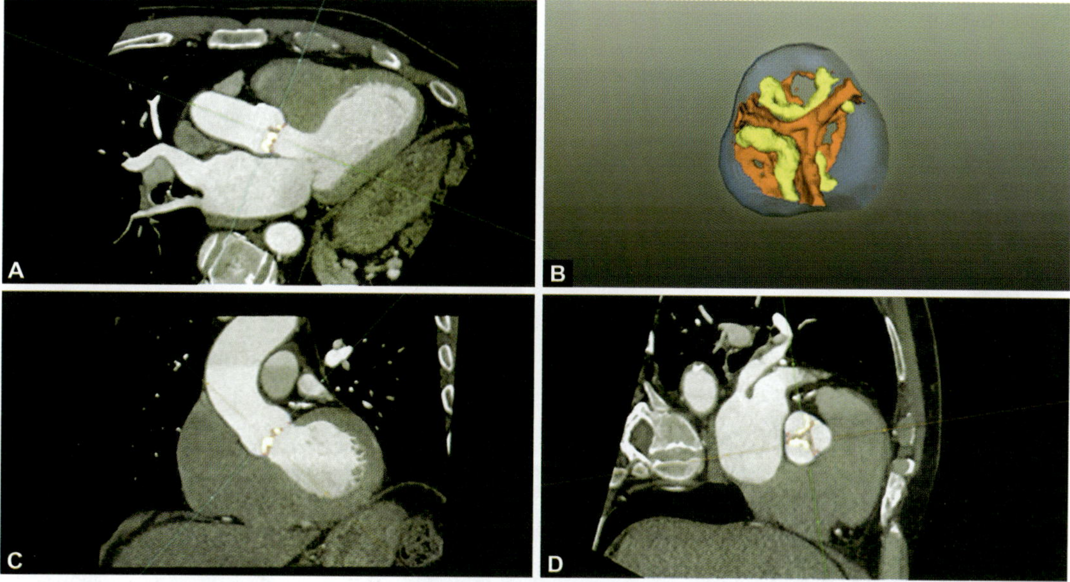

FIGS. 5A TO D: The aortic valve fibrocalcific volume by automated GMM (Gaussian mixture model); red—fibrosis and yellow—calcium.[25]

systole, especially with balanced steady-state free precession (bSSFP) or contrast-enhanced 3D MR angiography. It is particularly helpful when echocardiographic windows are poor or when LVOT measurement is uncertain. However, its temporal resolution is lower than echocardiography, so very rapid leaflet motion may be challenging to capture.

Cine CMR provides gold-standard quantification of LV volumes, mass, and geometry, remodeling patterns (concentric/eccentric), subtle changes in LV mass/volume ratio (typically SSFP sequences) even in patients with preserved LVEF.

Using phase-contrast velocity mapping in the ascending aorta, CMR directly measures forward and reverse flow, allowing accurate calculation of regurgitant volume and regurgitant fraction—considered the gold standard for noninvasive AR quantification.

Role in Myocardial Fibrosis Quantification

Late gadolinium enhancement (LGE)

Detects focal replacement fibrosis, typically in a midwall distribution in AS, linked to worse outcomes, higher postoperative mortality, and less reverse remodeling after AVR.

T1 mapping and extracellular volume (ECV)

Identify diffuse interstitial fibrosis not seen on LGE. Elevated native T1 and ECV predict adverse events and may indicate subclinical decompensation before LVEF falls.

Mitral Valve

Balanced steady-state free precession cine imaging enables clear visualization of mitral leaflet morphology, restricted motion, commissural fusion, and subvalvular thickening. Direct planimetry of the mitral orifice in mid-diastole can be performed without the geometric assumptions of echocardiography. It is less affected by PHT errors that occur in multivalvular disease or altered loading conditions.

Quantification of ventricular volumes, thicknesses, and ejection fraction distinguishes pressure and volume overload.[29]

Myocardial tissue characterization includes assessment of replacement fibrosis via LGE and diffuse fibrosis through ECV quantification.

Cardiac magnetic resonance quantifies MR by calculating regurgitant volume as the difference between LV stroke volume, measured using cine SSFP imaging, and forward aortic flow determined by phase-contrast imaging **(Figs. 6A to D)**.[30]

PROSTHETIC VALVES

Evaluation of prosthetic valves in the setting of MVHD is often challenging due to acoustic shadowing, overlapping flow signals, and complex hemodynamic interactions **(Table 6)**.

CONCLUSION

Multimodality imaging (MMI) has an expanded role in valvular heart disease (VHD) management, informing decision-making and long-term care. Imaging-guided planning plays a pivotal role in surgical and percutaneous interventions by enabling accurate risk stratification and improving clinical outcomes.

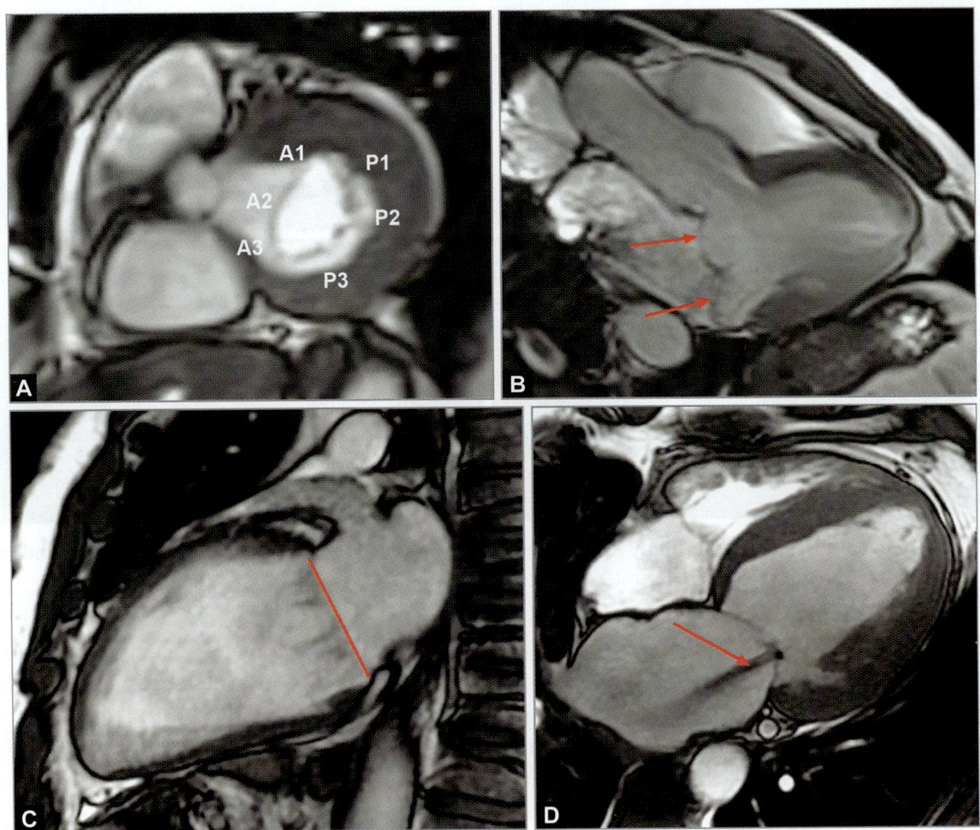

FIGS. 6A TO D: Anterior and posterior mitral valves and their scallops (A1, A2, and A3 and P1, P2, and P3) visualized in diastole using balanced steady-state free precession (bSSFP) cine images in the plane of the mitral valve (A). Cine 4 chamber view in a patient with posterior and anterior mitral valve prolapse (red arrows) (B). Example of mitral annular measurement from the anterior commissure to the posterior commissure (red line) in the two-chamber view (C). A central mitral regurgitation (flow voiding the left atrium, red arrow) secondary to mitral annular dilatation visualized in the four-chamber view (D).[31]

TABLE 6: Modality, strengths, and limitations of prosthetic valves.

Modality	Strengths	Limitations
2D transthoracic echo (TTE)	First-line, widely available	*Reverberation artifact*: Suboptimal visualization of pannus/thrombus
Transesophageal echo (TEE, 2D/3D)	• High spatial and temporal resolution • Measurement of gradients, identification of vegetations, abscesses, or dehiscence • Differentiate trans- vs. paravalvular regurgitation and pannus vs. thrombus	Reverberation artifact
Cardiac MRI (CMRI)	• Quantification of volumes and regurgitant fraction • Anatomical valve area in bioprosthetic valves • Identify paravalvular abscess, dehiscence, and pseudoaneurysm	• Artifacts • Difficult in unstable cardiac status
Cardiac CT (MDCT)	• Excellent spatial resolution—3D anatomy leaflet motion, calcification, pannus vs. thrombus • Identify paravalvular abscess, dehiscence, and pseudoaneurysm useful imaging modality in multiple prosthetic valves	Beam hardening artifact

(CMRI: cardiac magnetic resonance imaging)

REFERENCES

1. Lancellotti P, Pibarot P, Chambers J, et al. Multimodality imaging in valvular heart disease: an expert consensus from the European Association of Cardiovascular Imaging. Eur Heart J Cardiovasc Imaging. 2025;26(4):593-608.
2. Vahanian A, Beyersdorf F, Praz F, et al. 2021 ESC/EACTS Guidelines for the management of valvular heart disease. Eur Heart J. 2022;43:561-632.
3. Tribouilloy C, Bohbot Y, Kubala M, et al. Characteristics, management, and outcomes of patients with multiple native valvular heart disease: a substudy of the EURObservational research programme valvular heart disease II survey. Eur Heart J. 2022;43:2756-66.
4. Mascherbauer J, Beatty AL, Wessely M, et al. Multiple and mixed valvular heart disease: state-of-the-art. Heart Lung Circ. 2025;34(3):350-64.
5. Clavel MA, Pibarot P. Assessment of low-flow, low-gradient aortic stenosis: multimodality imaging is the key to success. EuroIntervention. 2022;18(Suppl. V):V10-2.
6. Praz F, Taramasso M, Stortecky S, et al. Concomitant mitral stenosis in patients undergoing transcatheter aortic valve implantation: impact on outcomes and hemodynamics. Circulation. 2020;141(16):1290-301.
7. Ring L, Shah BN, Bhattacharyya S, et al. Echocardiographic assessment of aortic stenosis: a practical guideline from the British Society of Echocardiography. Echo Res Pract. 2021;8(1):G19-59.
8. Alaa M, Mohamed M, Lu H, et al. Impact of concomitant mitral regurgitation on hemodynamic assessment of aortic stenosis and outcomes in low-flow, low-gradient settings. J Am Heart Assoc. 2022;11(3):e025648.
9. Ong P, Pibarot P. When aortic stenosis is not alone: challenges in echocardiographic evaluation of multivalvular heart disease. Front Cardiovasc Med. 2021;8:744497.
10. De Zan G, van der Bilt IAC, Broekhuizen LN, et al. Non-invasive assessment of multivalvular heart disease: echocardiographic pitfalls in mixed lesions. Rev Cardiovasc Med. 2024;25(1):29.
11. Panidapu N, Sen B, Poduval D, et al. Severe tricuspid regurgitation leads to underestimation of the severity of mitral stenosis by Doppler. CASE (Phila). 2024;8(11):496-9.
12. Chioncel O, Adamo M, Nikolaou M, et al. Acute heart failure and valvular heart disease: a scientific statement of the Heart Failure Association, the Association for Acute CardioVascular Care and the European Association of Percutaneous Cardiovascular Interventions of the European Society of Cardiology. Eur J Heart Fail. 2023;25:1025-48.
13. Poduval D, Jose RL, Madathil T, et al. Intraoperative transoesophageal echocardiography quantification of mitral regurgitation by regurgitant volume and fraction using 2D and 3D techniques. Ann Cardiac Anaesth. 2025;28(2):161-9.
14. Baumgartner H, Falk V, Bax JJ, et al. 2021 ESC/EACTS Guidelines for the management of valvular heart disease. Eur Heart J. 2022;43(7):561-632.
15. Katte F, Franz M, Jung C, et al. Impact of concomitant mitral regurgitation on transvalvular gradient and flow in severe aortic stenosis: a systematic ex vivo analysis of a subentity of low-flow, low-gradient aortic stenosis. EuroIntervention. 2018;13(14):1635-44.
16. Otto CM, Nishimura RA, Bonow RO, et al. 2020 ACC/AHA guideline for the management of patients with valvular heart disease: a report of the American College of Cardiology/American Heart Association Joint Committee on Clinical Practice Guidelines. Circulation. 2021;143(5):e35-71.
17. Patel KM, Desai RG, Krishnan S. Mitral regurgitation in patients with coexisting chronic aortic regurgitation: an evidence-based narrative review. J Cardiothorac Vasc Anesth. 2021;35:3404-15.
18. de Castro Rodrigues AB, Bernardez-Pereira S, Lanna GJN, et al. Mixed-valve disease and its pathophysiological impact: insights from advanced echocardiography. Circ Cardiovasc Imaging. 2019;12(3):e007862.
19. Vieitez JM, Monteagudo JM, Mahia P, et al. New insights of tricuspid regurgitation: a large-scale prospective cohort study. Eur Heart J Cardiovasc Imaging. 2021;22:196-202.

20. Schuijf JD, Vliegenthart R, Zijlstra F, et al. Cardiac CT beyond coronaries: focus on structural heart disease. Curr Heart Fail Rep. 2023;20(3):115-25.
21. Mantegazza V, Gripari P, Tamborini G, et al. 3D echocardiography in mitral valve prolapse: anatomy, dysfunction, and surgical planning. Front Cardiovasc Med. 2023;9:1050476.
22. Voormolen EHJ, Schafers HJ, van der Steen AFW, et al. Extension and validation of aortic root volumetric quantification using 3D echocardiography: comparison with multislice CT in patients with tricuspid aortic anatomy. Sci Rep. 2022;12:19461.
23. Rahman F, Mehta HH, Resar JR, et al. Outcomes among patients undergoing transcatheter aortic valve replacement with very low baseline gradients. Front Cardiovasc Med. 2023;10:1194360.
24. Zhou D, Wang X, Liu Y, et al. Diagnostic advances in valvular heart disease: current state and future perspectives. Rev Cardiovasc Med. 2024;25(1):29.
25. Lembo M, Joshi SS, Geers J, et al. Quantitative computed tomography angiography for the evaluation of valvular fibrocalcific volume in aortic stenosis. JACC Cardiovasc Imaging. 2024;17(11):1351-62.
26. Ali M, Córdova S, Michelena HI, et al. Multimodality imaging in bicuspid aortic valve: an evolving role for computed tomography. JACC Cardiovasc Imaging. 2023;16(5):758-71.
27. Ash J, Sandhu GS, Arriola-Montenegro J, et al. Performance of computed tomographic angiography-based aortic valve area for assessment of aortic stenosis. J Am Heart Assoc. 2023;12:e030055.
28. Joshi S, Lembo M, Bing R, et al. 140 fibrocalcific volume in aortic valve stenosis using contrast-enhanced computed tomography. Heart. 2022;108:A106-8.
29. Tsampasian V, Hothi SS, Ravindrarajah T, et al. Valvular cardiomyopathy: the value of cardiovascular magnetic resonance imaging. Cardiol Res Pract. 2022;2022:3144386.
30. Goldfarb JW, Krishnam M, McCulloch ML, et al. Cardiovascular magnetic resonance for quantification of mitral regurgitation: techniques and clinical implications. J Cardiovasc Magn Reson. 2025;23:12.
31. Vermes E, Iacuzio L, Levy F, et al. Role of cardiovascular magnetic resonance in native valvular regurgitation: a comprehensive review of protocols, grading of severity, and prediction of valve surgery. Front Cardiovasc Med. 2022;9:881141.

CHAPTER

90

Role of Left Atrial Indices in Management of Chronic Severe Asymptomatic Aortic Regurgitation

Satish K Parashar

ABSTRACT

Chronic aortic regurgitation (AR) is the third most common valvular heart disease. It typically has an insidious clinical course, with a prolonged asymptomatic phase where a progressive left ventricular (LV) remodeling takes place before the onset of symptoms and/or overt LV dysfunction. It is an important cause for morbidity and mortality if not intervened at the right time. Echocardiography plays a significant role in assessing the severity of AR and guiding intervention. Initial conventional criteria for surgical intervention in patients with asymptomatic AR have been LVEF ≤50–55%, LVESD ≥25 mm/m^2, progressive decline in LVEF, or increase in LVEDD to >65 mm. However, to reduce morbidity and mortality in asymptomatic patients, the identification of more sensitive and accurate markers of cardiac damage has gained attention. Studies have focused on reassessing the ideal LV lower thresholds of end-systolic diameter index, LV end-systolic volume index, etc. Other recommended end points have been reviewed. In spite of numerous parameters, the severity of AR still remains unclear in some patients. In AR, left atrial (LA) mechanics can be affected in time and LA strain variations can be illuminating for the grading of AR. Values proposed for guiding intervention are, namely, LA volume index of ≥37 mL/m^2 and LA reservoir strain ≤35%, and longer-term follow-up studies with hard endpoints will be needed to establish the role of LAS in the preoperative evaluation of patients with AR.

Keywords: Aortic regurgitation, intervention, LA mechanics, LV dimensions and volumes.

INTRODUCTION

Aortic regurgitation (AR) is the third most common native valvular heart disease with a prevalence of approximately 0.5% of the total population. Clinically significant AR (≥ moderate or 3+) is estimated to account for 1.6–15% of the AR population. Severe AR is an important cause of morbidity and mortality. If left untreated, the risk of death is approximately one third over 10 years, and almost a half of all patients will develop heart failure. Even in asymptomatic patients, severe AR carries a noteworthy annual mortality risk of up to 2.2%. It may be secondary to abnormalities of the AV leaflets, the structure or geometry of the aortic root or the ascending aorta, or a combination of the two.

Chronic AR typically has an insidious clinical course, with a prolonged asymptomatic phase where a progressive left ventricular (LV) remodeling takes place before the onset of symptoms and/or overt LV dysfunction. Echocardiography is the primary imaging modality for assessment of AR severity; a comprehensive TTE examination provides the mechanism and severity of the valve lesion, the hemodynamic impact of the valve lesion on the cardiac chambers, and the presence of other cardiac pathology. When data is incongruent or incomplete, cardiac magnetic resonance may be helpful.

HEMODYNAMICS

Chronic severe AR imposes a combined volume and pressure overload on the LV. The volume overload is a consequence of the regurgitant volume itself and is therefore directly related to the severity of the leak. Over time excessive preload and afterload portend to eccentric LV hypertrophy and dilation. The eccentric hypertrophy increases LV mass and LV ejection fraction (LVEF) is maintained by increased preload. In turn, this leads to diastolic and microvascular dysfunction and interstitial cellular changes. The long-standing pressure and volume overload can result in marked LV dilation and irreversible LV systolic dysfunction, all of which are associated with poor prognosis. At some stage in AR, accompanied by decreased LV diastolic compliance as a result of hypertrophy and fibrosis, it leads to high filling pressures and thereby affecting LA dynamics.

STAGES OF AORTIC REGURGITATION

Similar to other valvular diseases, the stages of AR range from patients at risk of AR (stage A) or with progressive mild-to-moderate AR (stage B) to severe asymptomatic (stage C) and symptomatic (stage D) AR. Each of these stages is defined by valve anatomy, valve hemodynamics, severity of LV dilation, and LV systolic function, as well as by patient symptoms and the effects of valve dysfunction on ventricular and vascular function (e.g., end-organ damage).

ROLE OF ECHOCARDIOGRAPHY IN ASSESSMENT OF SEVERITY IN CHRONIC AORTIC REGURGITATION

Grading the severity of AR is very important for clinical follow-up and determining an optimal time for intervention. As mentioned earlier, echocardiography is the key examination. A combination of various echo methods is employed for assessing AR severity since relying on a single method is often insufficient and has limitations. The usual findings supporting severe AR are as follows:

- *Supportive data:* LV enlargement as per BSA
- *Specific data (>90% specific)*:
  - Pan diastolic reversal of flow in the descending aorta with end diastolic velocity of >20 cm/s) and VTI >15 cm **(Figs. 1 and 2)**; it is more diagnostic, especially in study of proximal abdominal aorta
  - Vena contracta width >0.6 cm **(Fig. 3)**
  - % LVOT occupied by AR jet ≥65% **(Fig. 4)**; jet length and jet area are much dependent on LV compliance and diastolic pressure and do not reflect the severity of the AR; hence, are usually not recommended for use.

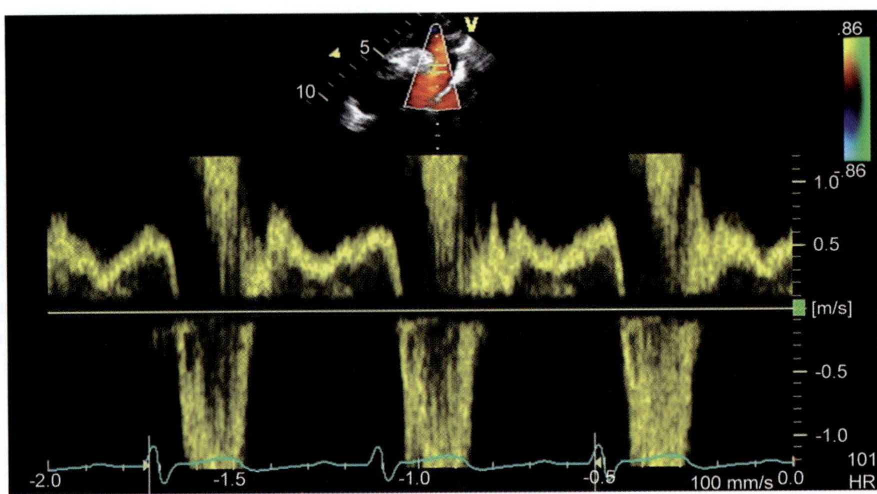

FIG. 1: Pandiastolic reversal of flow from descending aorta.

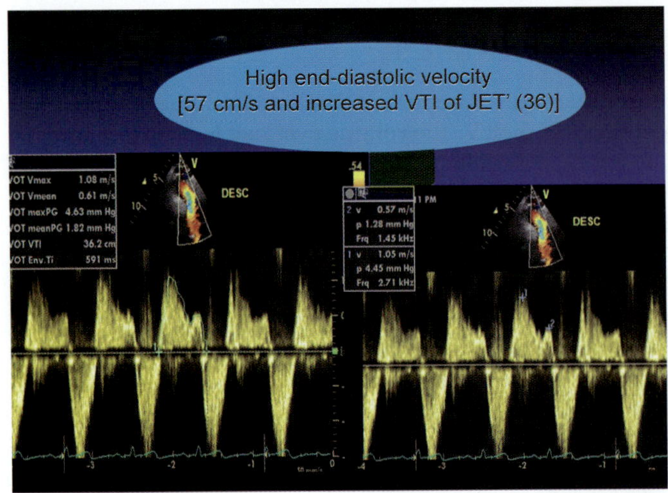

FIG. 2: High end-diastolic velocity and VTI of flow.

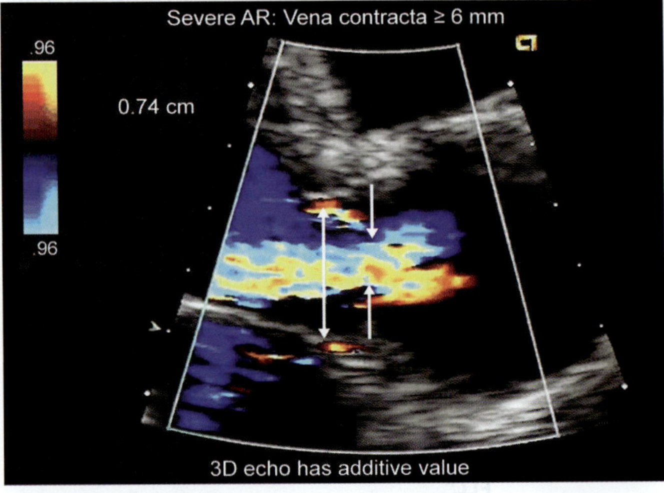

FIG. 3: Vena contracta suggestive of severe AR.

- *Quantitative data: 2D and 3D* regurgitant volume ≥60 mL, regurgitant fraction ≥50%, effective regurgitation orifice area (EROA) ≥0.30 cm/m^2; a general guideline is shown in **(Flowchart 1)**.

USUAL INDICES FOR INTERVENTION

The challenge of determining the optimal timing for valvular intervention has been a long-standing focus of clinical investigation. The incorporation of GLS and LA indices into the planning of such an intervention has garnered interest due to their improved sensitivity in the early prediction of mortality and symptom progression even in patients with preserved EF. Ideally, aortic valve intervention is performed before the onset of irreversible remodeling and/or LV systolic dysfunction. The ACC/AHA and ESC guidelines recommend surgical intervention for patients with severe AR and impaired LV systolic function (LVEF ≤ 50%) or significantly dilated LV [LV end-systolic diameter (LVESD) > 50 mm, indexed LV end-systolic diameter > 25 mm/m^2 or LV end-diastolic diameter > 65 mm], even in the absence of symptoms. The ESC guidelines, however, suggest intervention when the LVESD index reaches 20 mm/m^2, provided that the surgical risk is low. Some recent retrospective, non-randomized studies emphasized the role of indexed LVESD and proposed a lower cut-off value of 20 or 22 mm/m^2 BSA.

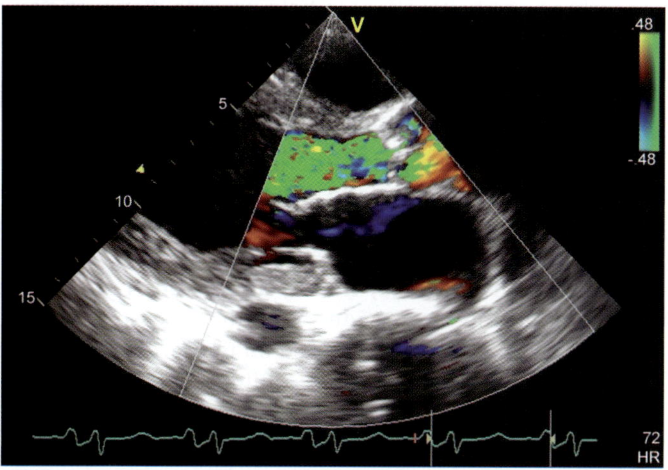

FIG. 4: A case of severe AR, with jet occupying whole of LVOT.

De Meester et al.[1] in a study of 356 patients with severe AR with minimal or no symptoms and a follow-up of up to 10 years reported that LVEF < 55% and LVESDi > 20–22 mm/m^2 were markers of increased 10-year mortality. LV end-diastolic dimensions did not influence outcomes. *Yang* et al.[2], in a study of 748 patients with significant AR, of whom 361 patients had AVR, observed that LVESDi was the only LV parameter independently associated with all-cause mortality. Compared with patients having LVESDi <20 mm/m^2, those with LVESDi 20–25 mm/m^2 had increased risks of death. In another study by *Yang* et al.,[3] in 1259 patients, all-cause and cardiovascular mortality were increased when LVEF ≤53%, LVESDi ≥22 mm/m^2, and LVESVi ≥of 46 mL/m^2. *Malahfji* et al.[4] in a multicentric MRI study on 458 patients of AR had

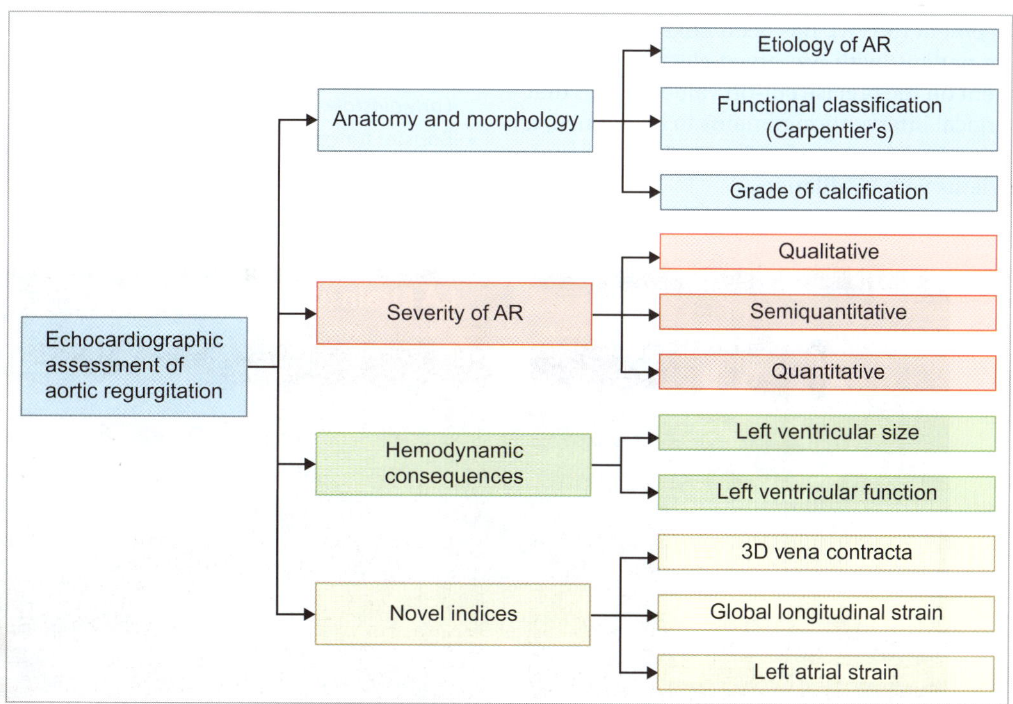

FLOWCHART 1: Summary of all the parameters of significance in the echocardiographic assessment of AR.

a similar observation but supported the use of LV volumes over LV diameters in patients with moderate or severe AR. The threshold of indexed LVES diameter identified by CMR was 2.0 cm/m^2, and the threshold of indexed LVES volume was 43 mL/m^2. 25% patients in their series met the threshold of LVES volume while not meeting the threshold of LVES diameter, and these patients were at a significantly increased hazard for AVR/death compared with those who met the diameter threshold but not the volume threshold. *Mentias* et al.[5] studied 1,417 patients with grade 3+AR with preserved EF, and it was one of the largest study. One of the aims of this study was to reassess the threshold of LV dimension, beyond which mortality significantly increases. It was observed that there was a significant and continuous increase in the risk of death beyond an iLVESD >2 cm/m^2. As such, LVESDi in the range of 20–25 mm/m^2 has been suggested as a threshold for surgical referral in patients with asymptomatic severe AR and preserved LVEF. Based on the current data available, we cannot establish causality but only associations between these thresholds (LVEF <60%, GLS worse than –15 to –19, LVESDi >20 mm/m^2, LVESVi >45 mL/m^2) and worse prognosis; therefore, no single imaging-based early threshold is absolute.[6] However, recently, published role of additional factors, especially, global longitudinal strain and left atrial dynamics have gained significance in determining their role in intervention in severe AR and are worthy of future investigation.

Left ventricular global longitudinal strain (GLS) has emerged as an exceedingly sensitive marker of subclinical LV dysfunction and prognostic indicator in patients with AR. A worsening of GLS, both before and after surgical aortic valve replacement (SAVR), has been linked to adverse outcomes, even in patients with preserved ejection fraction. Although agreement on the precise cut-off value for GLS that would prompt surgical intervention remains to be defined, a depressed GLS value in the range of –15% to –18% is useful, particularly in patients with LV dilation.

CLINICAL UTILITY OF LEFT ATRIAL STRAIN INDICES IN TIMING OF INTERVENTION IN CHRONIC SEVERE ASYMPTOMATIC AORTIC REGURGITATION

The LA is directly exposed to LV vacuum pressure during diastole. Hence, in AR, LA mechanics can be affected in time in parallel with the elevated LV end-diastolic pressure (LVEDP) and LA strain variations can be illuminating for the grading of AR. The strain evaluation of the LA has emerged recently as an exciting tool to help provide diagnostic and prognostic information for patients with a broad range of cardiovascular pathologies, including AR.[7] Perhaps due to the LA's relatively thin-walled architecture compared with the more muscular structure of the left ventricle (LV), functional changes in the left atrium often precede changes in the LV, making LA strain (LAS) an earlier marker for underlying pathology than many conventional echocardiographic parameters.

As seen in **Figure 5, Box 1, and Table 1** the strain evaluation of the LA provides a unique assessment of the three phases of LA function based on the cardiac cycle. The reservoir phase describes the LA filling by the pulmonary

BOX 1: Different components of left atrial strain.

LA modulates LV filling by 3 functions:

- Reservoir function (LA expansion index)
  Systole: 40%
- Conduit function (passive emptying index)
  Early diastole: 35%
- Booster function (active emptying index)
  Late diastole: 25%

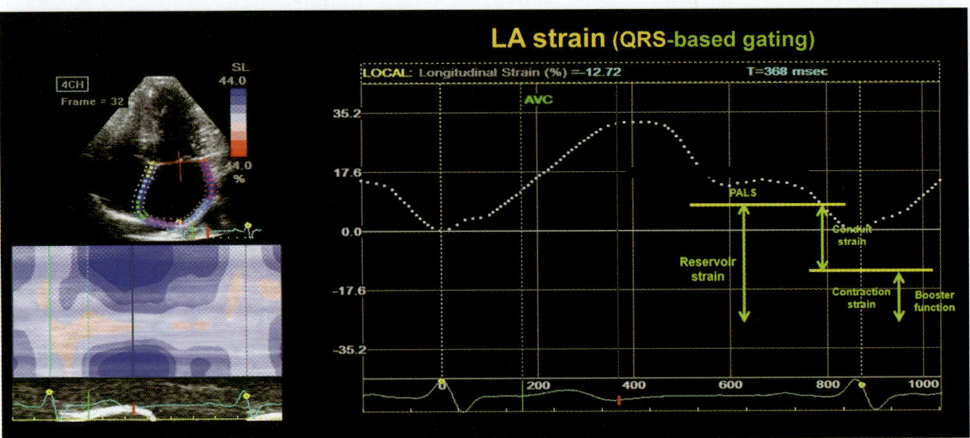

FIG. 5: Three phases of LA strain as per cardiac cycle.

TABLE 1: Normal values of strain components.

Strain component	*Mean*	*95% CI*
Reservoir	39.4	38–40.8
Conduit	23	20.7–25.2
Contractile	17.4	16–19

Source: Adapted from Pathan F, D'Elia N, Nolan MT, et al. Normal ranges of left atrial strain by speckle-tracking echocardiography: A systematic review and meta-analysis. J Am Soc Echocardiogr. 2017;30(1):59-70.e8.

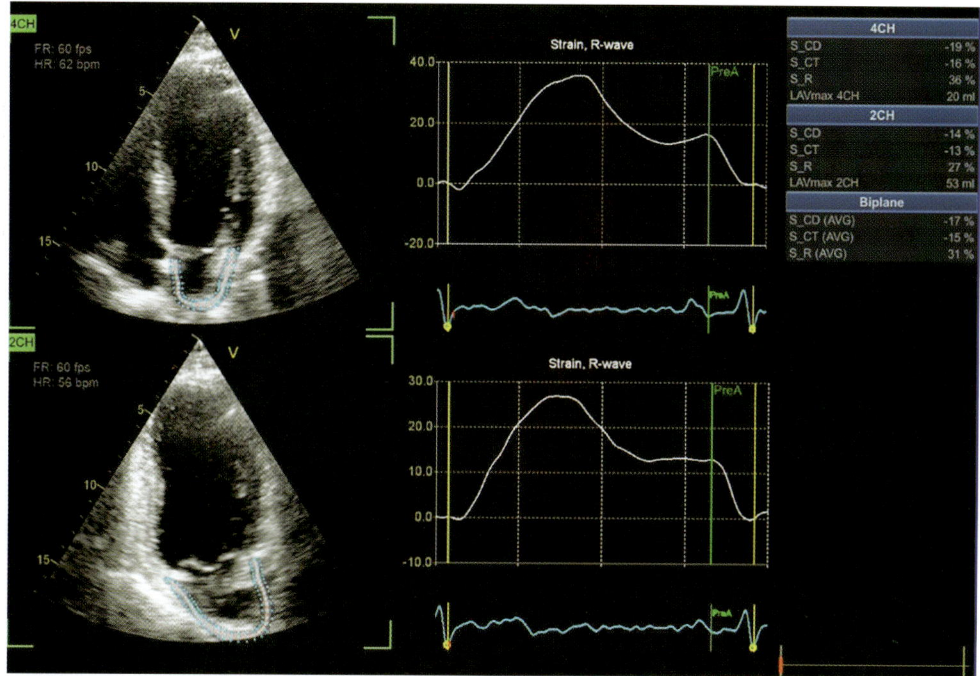

FIG. 6: A patient with severe AR having an LAr of 31%.

veins during LV systole before the opening of mitral valve. This is the phase where the left atrium enlarges. The conduit phase describes the passive LV filling from the LA during early LV diastole. The booster-pump phase describes the atrial kick whereby the LA ejects blood as a form of active LV filling during late LV diastole. Conduit strain is defined as the difference between booster and reservoir strain. Among these indices, left atrial reservoir (LAr) strain has been most extensively studied. It reflects instantaneous LA function and LV filling pressure. Left atrial volume index (LAVI) is another studied parameter. LAr has been documented to be impaired in patients with chronic asymptomatic severe AR, but lower values of LA strain are associated with adverse prognosis and show promise in risk stratification of patients with severe AR. *Kalkan* et al.,[8] in a study of 64 patients with varying grades of AR, showed that LAr and LA pump parameters of the patients with severe AR significantly decreased compared to those of the mild and moderate AR group. Hence, it could be a supplementary contribution to the present parameters in the grading of AR. Contrary to the other parameters, *Jenner* et al.[9] observed that preoperative LA strain during the conduit phase added to LVESVi for the prediction of impaired LV functional and structural recovery after aortic valve replacement. In one of the studies by García Martín et al.,[10] their aim was to analyze the prognostic significance of the diastolic function evaluated by echocardiography, in asymptomatic patients with severe AR. They concluded that in these group of asymptomatic patients, baseline diastolic parameters were prognostic markers of cardiovascular events; among them, LAr played a significant predictor role. **Figure 6** is the LA strain imaging of a 34-year-old asymptomatic individual with reduced LAr of 31%. Though the value is decreased, different studies have taken variable figures for normal or decreased LAr. However, this value corresponds to severe AR and will need frequent follow-up prior to intervention.

Akintoye et al.[11] highlighted the importance of LA anatomical and functional remodeling in patients with

TABLE 2: Progressive decline in LA strain values with increasing severity of AR. Values of strain rates are not statistically significant.

Parameter	Mild	Moderate	Severe
LA Reservoir	42.0 ± 18.0	41.4 ± 14.8	29.2 ± 6.0
LA Pump	21.2 ± 8.7	19.3 ± 7.4	13.1 ± 4.4
LA SRs	2.0 ± 0.8	2.0 ± 0.6	2.0 ± 0.6
LA SRe	−1.7 ± 0.8	−1.5 ± 0.8	−1.7 ± 0.8
LA SRa	−2.5 ± 1.2	−2.4 ± 0.9	−1.9 ± 1.3

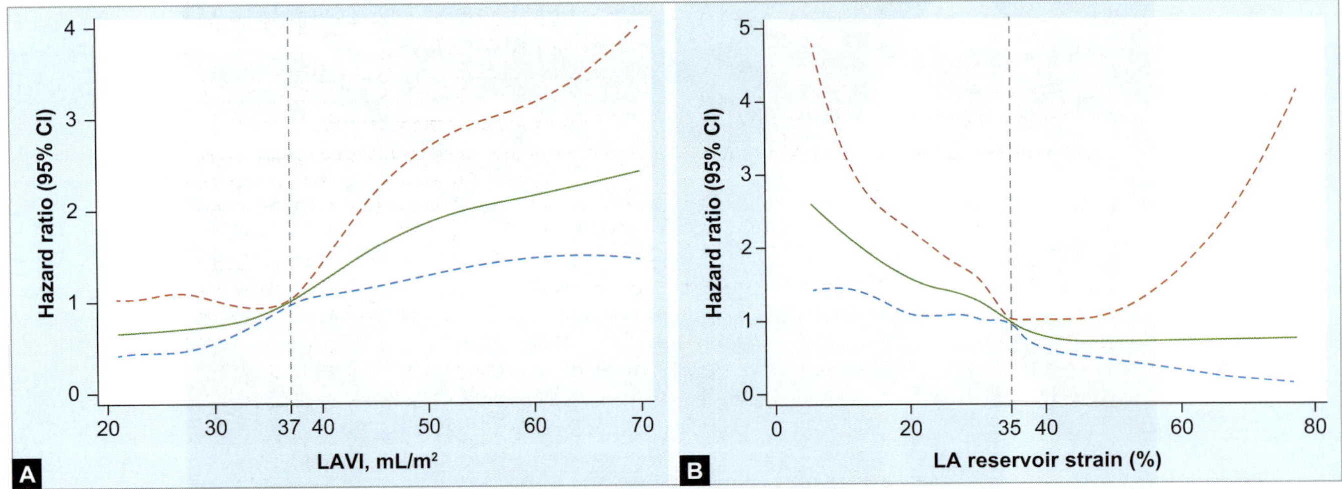

FIGS. 7A AND B: Spline curve showing HR (95% CI) of adverse events.
Source: Adapted from Akintoye et al. (2024).[11]

moderate-to-severe or severe AR in their retrospective analysis. The study's 3 main findings were as follows:

1. Unlike the LV, the rate of LA remodeling progression was consistent across different sexes and age groups.
2. Remodeling provided incremental prognostic value over traditional LV parameters.
3. The authors proposed optimal cut-off values for guiding intervention, namely, LAVI ≥37 mL/m^2 and LAr ≤35% **(Fig. 6)**.

Negishi et al.[12], in their editorial comments, compared guidelines of ACC/AHA, ESC, and Japanese societies and questioned the validity of LV size as criteria for intervention. Notably, many deaths occur in patients whose LV dimensions are below the guideline-recommended LV dimension cut-off values. Researchers from the Cleveland Clinic have reported significant interactions between LV dimensions and factors such as sex or age, indicating that older patients and women experience adverse events at lower LV volumes.[11] They commented that integration of LA volume and LA strain analysis into therapeutic interventions for chronic severe AR holds promise but cautioned that it requires further validation **(Table 2 and Figs. 7A and B)**.

CONCLUSION

Echocardiography plays a key role in diagnosis, assessment of severity and mechanism, risk stratification, and evaluation of the timing for surgery in patients with AR. A comprehensive assessment of valve morphology, severity, and LV remodeling is essential for the adequate evaluation of these patients. The usual indications for surgery were earlier confined to symptoms/LVEF <55%, LVESD >50 mm, LVESDi >25 mm/m^2, which was later addressed to 20–25 mm/m^2, LVESVi >45 mL/m^2, etc. In last few years, LA strain imaging has demonstrated exciting potential to assist in diagnosis, categorization, and prognosis in various cardiac disorders including AR, which have been described earlier. Large-scale studies are still needed, however, to verify and standardize some of the findings discussed in this chapter; there is a need for standardization in LA strain measurement techniques and software platforms to ensure consistent and reproducible results across different clinical settings. While the use of machine learning and artificial intelligence in LAS imaging is still in its early stages, there is clear potential to leverage these technologies to identify subtle differences among a range of pathologies. As such further research in this area with larger, longer-term follow-up studies with hard endpoints will be needed to establish the role of LAS in the preoperative evaluation of patients with AR.

REFERENCES

1. de Meester C, Gerber BL, Vancraeynest D, et al. Do guideline-based indications result in an outcome penalty for patients with severe aortic regurgitation? JACC Cardiovasc Imaging. 2019;12:2126-38.
2. Yang LT, Michelena HI, Scott CG, et al. Outcomes in chronic hemodynamically significant aortic regurgitation and limitations of current guidelines. JACC. 2019;73(14):1741-52.
3. Yang LT, Lee CC, Su CH, et al. Analysis of left ventricular indexes and mortality among Asian adults with hemodynamically significant chronic aortic regurgitation. JAMA Netw Open. 2023;6(3):e234632.
4. Malahfji M, Crudo V, Kaolawanich Y, et al. Influence of cardiac remodeling on clinical outcomes in patients with aortic regurgitation. JACC. 2023;81(19):1885-98.
5. Mentias A, Feng K, Alashi A, et al. Long-term outcomes in patients with aortic regurgitation and preserved left ventricular ejection fraction. J Am Coll Cardiol. 2016;68(20):2144-53.
6. Ranard LS, Bonow RO, Nishimura R, et al. Imaging methods for evaluation of chronic aortic regurgitation in adults: JACC State-of-the-Art Review. JACC. 2023;82(20):1953-66.
7. O'Neill T, Kang P, Hagendorff A, et al. The clinical applications of left atrial strain: A comprehensive review. Medicina (Kaunas). 2024;60(5):693.
8. Kalkan S, Efe SC, Tasar O, et al. The role of the left atrial strain parameters on grading of aortic regurgitation. J Cardiovasc Echogr. 2021;31(3):151-6.
9. Jenner J, Ilami A, Petrini J, et al. Pre- and postoperative left atrial and ventricular volumetric and deformation analyses in severe aortic regurgitation. Cardiovasc Ultrasound. 2021;19(1):14.
10. García Martín A, Abellás Sequeiros M, González Gómez AG, et al. Prognostic value of diastolic function parameters in significant aortic regurgitation: The role of the left atrial strain. J Echocardiogr. 2022;20(4):216-23
11. Akintoye E, El Dahdah J, Dabbagh MM, et al. Longitudinal Assessment of Left Atrial Remodelling in Patients with Chronic Severe Aortic Regurgitation. JACC Cardiovascular Imaging. 2024;17(10):1133-45.
12. Negishi K, Ozawa K. Clinical Utility of LA Indices in chronic severe aortic regurgitation: A Comes before V. JACC: Cardiovascular Imaging. 2024;17(10):1146-8.

CHAPTER

91

Application of Emerging Hybrid Intracoronary Imaging Technologies in Clinical Practice and Research

Harilalith Kovvuri, Nagendra Boopathy Senguttuvan

ABSTRACT

Intracoronary imaging (ICI) has reshaped how we understand and treat coronary artery disease over the last three decades. Tools such as intravascular ultrasound (IVUS), optical coherence tomography (OCT), and near-infrared spectroscopy (NIRS) provide unparalleled insights into plaque morphology and poststent complications. Yet, routine use remains limited, largely due to procedural complexity and the training required to interpret images. Recent developments in automation and multimodality imaging are beginning to change this landscape.

IVUS and OCT remain the workhorses of ICI. IVUS excels at assessing vessel size and plaque burden, while OCT offers unmatched resolution for stent optimization and plaque characterization. New-generation systems aim to simplify interpretation and reduce intra- and interobserver variability. AVVIGO+ (The Boston Scientific, USA) uses Automated Lesion Assessment (ALA™) to trace lumen and vessel borders, identify reference segments, and provide instant measurements with expert-level accuracy. Ultreon™ 2.0 (Abbott, USA) builds on OCT's strengths by adding automated calcium assessment, external elastic lamina visualization, and real-time angiographic coregistration through the MLD MAX workflow, supporting informed decision-making before, during, and after PCI. NIRS adds a compositional layer, detecting lipid-rich plaques linked to future adverse events through measures such as maxLCBI4 mm.

Integrating IVUS, OCT, and NIRS gives a more complete picture of complex lesions, whether in left main disease, bifurcations, or heavily calcified segments. New phenotyping systems, incorporating plaque burden (L1), lipid content (L2), and minimal lumen area (L3), have shown predictive value in studies such as PROSPECT II, identifying lesions at risk of causing future events.

ICI is evolving from a specialized diagnostic tool to a cornerstone of personalized PCI. With automation, multimodality integration, and risk-based strategies, it has the potential to make precision coronary intervention both practical and impactful in routine clinical care.

Keywords: Intracoronary imaging (ICI), intravascular ultrasound (IVUS), optical coherence tomography (OCT), near-infrared spectroscopy (NIRS), plaque morphology, stent optimization, automated lesion assessment (ALA™), AVVIGO+, Ultreon™ 2.0, calcium assessment, angiographic coregistration, lipid-rich plaques, maxLCBI4mm, multimodality imaging, risk stratification, PROSPECT II, personalized PCI, complex lesions, left main disease, bifurcation lesions, calcified lesions.

INTRODUCTION

Intracoronary imaging (ICI) was introduced almost 30 years ago to assess atherosclerosis.[1] This has provided unique insights into a better understanding of plaque progression. Many prospective studies have been conducted to identify lesions prone to progression and cause future events.[2] Existing intravascular ultrasound (IVUS) and optical coherence tomography (OCT) are undeniably powerful, changed the way we diagnose, and treat coronary artery disease patients. So, do we really need updates to existing modalities? Are they not perfect as they are now? Yes, indeed they are really good; however, they had steep learning curve, which demands lot of practice from young interventional cardiologists (IC), that being one of the main reasons for low adaptability around the world. With artificial intelligence (AI), coming up like storm, and challenging a lot of other professions, for ICs it is a boon. With these AI-based software, automatic plaque identification, automatic minimal lumen area (MLA), appropriate landing zones, minimal stent area (MSA) identification, makes day-to-day practice less time consuming and thereby improving the outcomes of patients.

COMMONLY USED INTRACORONARY IMAGING MODALITIES

Till date, most commonly used ICI modalities are IVUS and OCT predominantly by The Boston Scientific and Abbott Vascular, respectively. The available software predominantly focus on operator expertise in identifying the type of plaque, minimal lumen area (MLA), and post-DES minimal stent area (MSA), under expansion and any other complications. The biggest challenge for IVUS is no angiographic coregistration. Hence, the latest innovations focused predominantly on this. Now that, ICI guidance is recommended for performing PCI on anatomically complex lesions, in particular, left main stem, true bifurcations, and long lesions (Class IA),[3] these enhancements are of paramount importance.

The AVVIGO+ Intravascular Ultrasound Imaging

The AVVIGO+ Multi-Modality Guidance System (Boston Scientific, USA) directly addresses the points. At its heart lies Automated Lesion Assessment (ALA™), a machine learning algorithm that automatically traces the lumen and vessel borders on every frame. It highlights the MLA, identifies reference segments, and generates precise area and diameter measurements instantly. No more manual contouring, "eyeballing" MLA, and second-guessing stent sizing. Validation data are impressive. ALA™ matches expert cardiologists with 92.4% agreement on balloon sizing and shows a near-perfect intraclass correlation (>0.99) for vessel and lumen dimensions **(Fig. 1A)**.[4]

Standardized automated pullback adds another layer of precision. With speeds from 0.5 to 8 mm/s and crystal-clear HD images even at the fastest pullback, operators can scan long, complex lesions in seconds without losing quality. This consistency enables accurate length measurements and complete visualization of disease, solving a long-standing limitation of manual pullback. Although there is an option of manual pullback, this ALA algorithm works only in automatic pullbacks. Finally, tableside control makes the entire system more practical. Operators can manipulate IVUS and ALA™ directly from the sterile field, reducing interruptions and keeping focus on the patient. It is a small change with a big impact: Smoother workflow, fewer delays, and more efficient procedures.

Optical Coherence Tomography Reimagined: Ultreon™ 2.0

While IVUS excels in vessel sizing and depth, OCT's resolution is unmatched, revealing details as small as microcalcifications. Until date, one key advantage of OCT over IVUS is that it automatically measures the MSA and

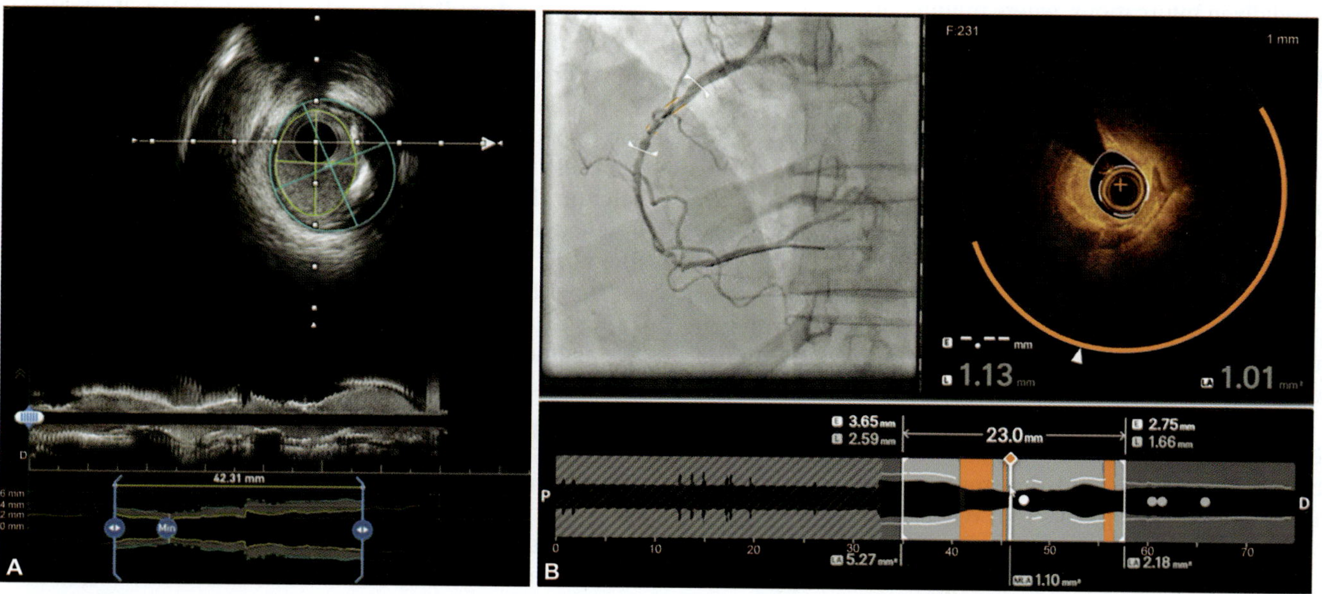

FIGS. 1A AND B: (A) IVUS pull back showing ALA technology in AVIGO+ (B) OCT pull back with angiographic coregistration in latest ULTREON2.0 software.

clearly shows the expansion of stents. 3D view helps in achieving good MSA even in bifurcation lesions and also the ability to visualize the distal strut wire crossing. These features are further enhanced with Ultreon™ 2.0 (Abbott, USA).

One of its most powerful features is automated detection of the calcium directly on coregistered angiography image. In real time, the system highlights the arc and thickness and length of calcium, enabling operators to decide whether to modify the lesion before stenting and how best to do it, based on Rule of 5 (>5 mm thickness, >5 mm length, and >50% vessel size arc). This is crucial, as inadequate preparation of heavily calcified lesions remains a leading cause of stent failure **(Fig. 1B)**.

The platform also automatically visualizes the external elastic lamina (EEL), by revealing the true vessel size consistently, thereby removing the of under sizing, a major reason linked to restenosis and thrombosis.

At the core of this system is the MLD MAX (Morphology, Length, Diameter, Medial Dissection, Apposition, Expansion) workflow. Think of it as a structured checklist:

- Before PCI, it identifies calcium burden, lipid pools, and ideal landing zones.
- During PCI, it integrates with angiography for precise positioning.
- After PCI, it automatically flags under expansion, malapposition, and dissections, all in a single, easy-to-read view.

This approach brings clarity and efficiency to complex decision-making, particularly valuable for operators still climbing the learning curve. Dynamic Angio, which coregisters OCT with angiography in real time, completes the picture. By overlaying intravascular findings onto the angiogram, it eliminates guesswork in stent positioning, especially in bifurcations, where millimeters matter.

Near-infrared Spectroscopy: Understanding Plaque Biology in Real Time

Intravascular ultrasound and OCT show us the structure of the artery. NIRS goes one step further by showing us its composition. Vulnerable plaques, those rich in lipid and prone to rupture, are the major cause of acute coronary syndromes. NIRS allows us to detect them in vivo, providing insights that neither angiography, IVUS, nor OCT alone can deliver.

NIRS works by measuring how near-infrared light is absorbed by different tissue components, generating a chemogram where lipid-rich regions appear yellow and more stable tissue appears red. When combined with IVUS (NIRS-IVUS), the result is a comprehensive map of both plaque structure and composition. Beyond its visuals, NIRS offers powerful quantitative data. The Lipid Core Burden Index (LCBI) reflects the proportion of lipid-rich plaque within a segment. It is calculated by using the formula, LCBI = Yellow pixels × 1,000/ Total valid pixels with a score range from 0 to 1,000. The maxLCBI4mm, the highest LCBI in any 4 mm segment, is a strong predictor of future adverse events **(Fig. 3B)**. A maxLCBI4mm >400 is widely regarded as indicative of a high-risk plaque, often corresponding to thin-cap fibroatheromas (TCFAs) that can trigger myocardial infarction.[5] The ability to identify these plaques has clear clinical implications: guiding intensified medical therapy, informing stenting decisions, and potentially flagging patients for closer surveillance **(Fig. 2A)**.

COMBINATION OF THESE TECHNOLOGIES

Is IVUS or OCT not sufficient? Do we need dual modalities? OCT has been associated with smaller stent sizing, largely due to its limited penetration and inability to visualize the external elastic membrane (EEM) in diffusely diseased vessels. In contrast, IVUS provides deeper penetration, allowing more accurate assessment of vessel dimensions and plaque burden, although it remains less reliable in identifying lipid-rich tissue. This distinction is clinically relevant, since stent deployment within lipid-laden segments has been linked to higher rates of restenosis, thrombosis, and major adverse cardiovascular events. Hence, currently, combination modalities are gaining popularity, and at present, 5 dual probe catheters are available: NIRS IVUS, IVUS OCT, OCT NIRS, OCT NIRF, and FLim OCT.

Out of these most promising are IVUS/OCT in combination with NIRS, because of its ability to identify the lipid plaque **(Figs. 2B and C)**.

Concerning lesions, IVUS does well for ostial LM lesion,[6] while OCT is better for distal LM bifurcation lesions, and both IVUS and OCT have their limitations for identifying calcium thickness and predicting stent underexpansion. Theoretically, if we combine IVUS-OCT, it will provide a synergistic role; however, clinical RCTs have yet to be conducted.

Similarly, while imaging a densely calcified lesion, IVUS can visualize calcium, but it neither provides proper calcium thickness nor visualizes EEM. In contrast, OCT gives detailed calcium thickness, but it lacks information about EEM, in lipidic plaque due to poor penetration. However, neither of them can detect lipid in those calcified lesions. Combining these with NIRS will give better information about lipid. **Table 1** summarizes the best imaging modality for a respective plaque.

PLAQUE PHENOTYPES

Over the decades, intravascular imaging has evolved and classified the lesions into lipidic, fibrotic and calcified, thereby deciding on the management pathway. However, are these nomenclatures prognostically relevant?

Apart from identifying plaque morphology, a new nomenclature was proposed by Héctor M. García-García et al.[6] which includes L1: Large (>70%) plaque burden; L2:

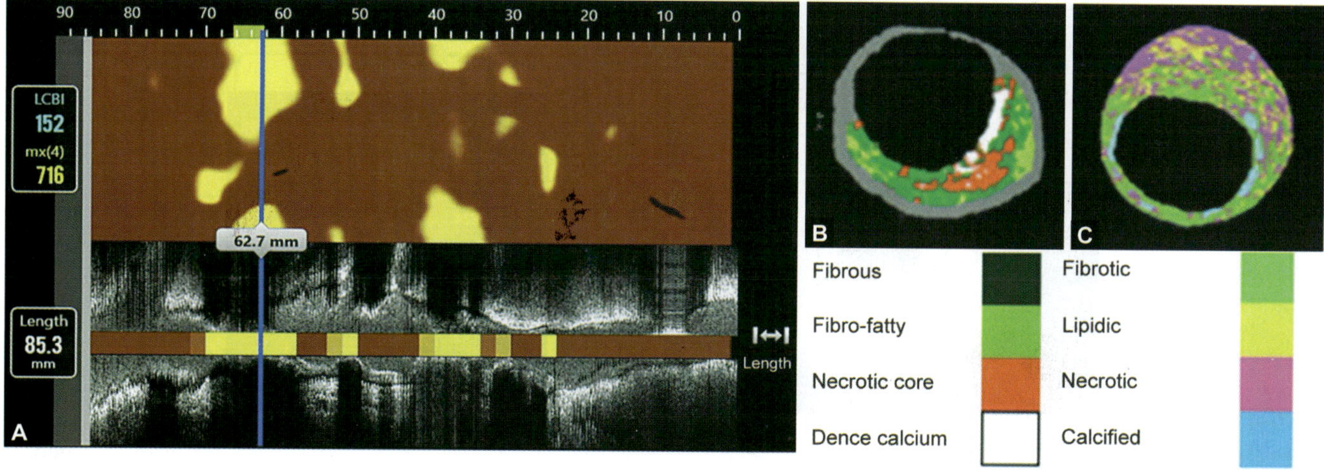

FIGS. 2A TO C: (A): IVUS-NIRS pull back showing lipid (B) VH-IVUS; (C) iMAP IVUS.

TABLE 1: Best imaging modality for respective imaging parameter.

Imaging parameter	Best imaging modality
Plaque burden	IVUS
Lipid burden	NIRS
Calcium/Nodule	IVUS/OCT
Cap thickness	OCT-NIRF
Stent under expansion	IVUS > OCT
Stent Mal-apposition	OCT
Stent edge dissection	OCT
Stent edge plaque	IVUS
Stent edge lipid	NIRS > IVUS-NIRS > OCT-NIRS
Ostial LM	IVUS > OCT
Distal LM and LAD, LCX bifurcation	OCT > IVUS

(IVUS: intravascular ultrasound; NIRS: near-infrared spectroscopy; OCT: optical coherence tomography)

Lipid-rich composition (hyporeflective/hypoechoic by OCT/IVUS, LCBI >400 by NIRS); L3: MLA <4 mm^2. By IVUS or OCT, identify the type of lesion, fibrotic, fibroatheroma (thin cap vs. thick cap by OCT), fibrocalcific, plaque rupture (by OCT), and then add L1/L2/L3 if any of the above features are present **(Figs. 3A and B)**.

In the PROSPECT trial,[7] with 697 acute coronary syndrome patients, IVUS was done to all epicardial vessel after PCI to the culprit. These patients had a median follow-up of 3 years, MACE events due to nonculprit vessel were predominantly of these three phenotypes. So, while reporting intracoronary imaging, plaque morphology, along with high-risk features such as L1/L2/L3, to be reported to prognosticate future events.

PROSPECT II trial,[8] done using IVUS-NIRS, in all epicardial vessels after treating culprit in recent MI patients. 898 patients (3,629 nonculprit lesions) were followed for a median of 3.7 years and highly lipidic lesions, present in 24% of lesions and 59% of patients, independently predicted nonculprit lesion-related MACEs (adjusted OR 2.27; 95% CI 1.25–4.13 at the patient level and 7.83; 95% CI 4.12–14.89 at the lesion level). Similarly, large plaque burden (22% of lesions; 59% of patients) was a significant predictor. Lesions with both large plaque burden and lipid-rich cores had a 4-year MACE risk of 7.0% (95% CI 4.0–10.0), rising to 13.2% (95% CI 9.4–17.6) in patients with ≥1 such lesion. So, these new advanced imaging features and new plaque phenotypes will aid ICs in better classifying the lesion and strategic management of them.

FUTURE: TAILORED TREATMENT BY IMAGING STRATEGY

The PREVENT trial[9] evaluated whether preventive PCI, in addition to optimal medical therapy, offers benefit in patients

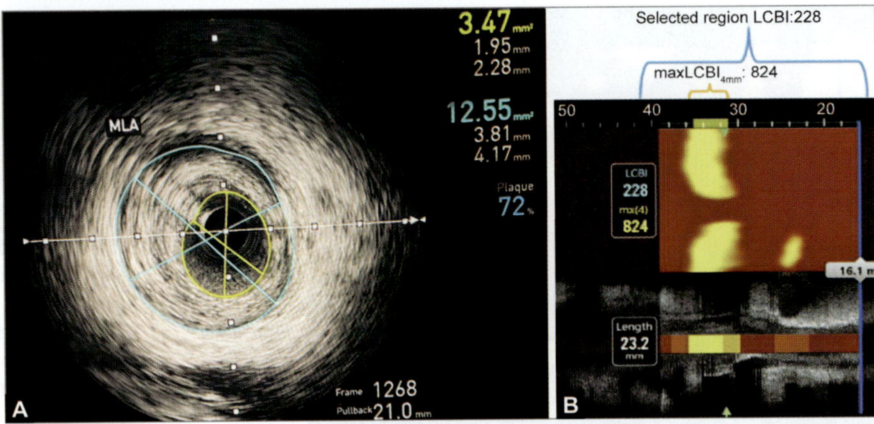

FIGS. 3A AND B: (A) Showing IVUS pullback with two high-risk features, L1—plaque burden >70%, L3—MLA <4 mm^2; (B) IVUS-NIRS showing maxLCBI4 mm >400.

with functionally nonsignificant yet high-risk coronary plaques (FFR >0.80) identified by IVUS, NIRS, or OCT. Among 1,606 patients, preventive PCI significantly reduced the composite endpoint of cardiac death, target-vessel MI, revascularization, or unstable angina at 2 years (0.4% vs. 3.4%; absolute risk reduction –3.0%, 95% CI –4.4 to –1.8; p = 0.0003), reflecting number needed to treat is 33 lesions. This suggests that preemptive PCI in nonflow limiting vulnerable coronary plaques may reduce adverse cardiac events when compared to optimal medical therapy alone.

Imaging has shown plaque rupture not only in the culprit vessel but also in nonculprit arteries (17% in AMI, 5% in stable angina),[10] which rarely require intervention or lead to MACE. The EROSION (Effective Anti-Thrombotic Therapy Without Stenting: Intravascular Optical Coherence Tomography Based Management in Plaque Erosion study),[11] 53 ACS patients with plaque erosion as cause of events, treated with aspirin and ticagrelor alone, underwent repeat OCT after 1 year showed, 46.9% had no residual thrombus at 1 year and minimal effective flow area remained unchanged [2.1 mm^2 (1.5–3.8 mm^2) versus 2.1 mm^2 (1.6–4.0 mm^2); p = 0.152] and 49 (92.5%) patients remained event-free at 1 year.

EROSION III,[12] enrolled patients with STEMI with angiographic stenosis <70% with TIMI III flow either at presentation or after antegrade flow restoration, were randomized to either OCT or angiographic guidance. Among 246 randomized patients, 226 (91.9%) comprised the per-protocol population (112 OCT-guided and 114 angiography-guided). The rate of stent implantation was significantly lower with OCT guidance compared with angiographic guidance [43.8% vs. 58.8%; relative risk (RR) 0.74; 95% CI 0.57–0.97; p = 0.024], representing a 15.0% absolute risk reduction. Among patients receiving stents, OCT guidance achieved superior postprocedural optimization with lower residual angiographic diameter stenosis (8.7 ± 3.7% vs. 11.8 ± 4.6%; p < 0.001). Larger RCTs are needed to validate these approaches and thereby change the way we address these lesions.

CONCLUSION

Intravascular imaging has enhanced understanding of atherosclerosis, guided personalized therapies, and enabled long-term treatment evaluation. Multimodality ICI is increasingly feasible with emerging commercial and research platforms. Ongoing trials will define their role in routine practice.

REFERENCES

1. Bourantas C, Tenekecioglu E, Radu M, et al. State of the art: role of intravascular imaging in the evolution of percutaneous coronary intervention–a 30-year review. EuroIntervention. 2017;13(6):644-53.
2. Stone PH, Saito S, Takahashi S, et al. Prediction of Progression of Coronary Artery Disease and Clinical Outcomes Using Vascular Profiling of Endothelial Shear Stress and Arterial Plaque Characteristics: The PREDICTION Study. Circulation. 2012;126(2):172-81.
3. Biccirè FG, Gatto L, Prati F. Intracoronary imaging to guide percutaneous coronary intervention: from evidence to guidelines. Eur Heart J Suppl. 2024;26(Supplement_1):i11-4.
4. Matsumura M, Mintz GS, Dohi T, et al. Accuracy of IVUS-based machine learning segmentation for the assessment of coronary artery vessel and lumen dimensions and balloon sizing. J Am Coll Cardiol. 2023;81(8):1353.
5. Terada K, Wakana N, Kubo T, et al. Clinical outcomes of acute myocardial infarction arising from non-lipid-rich plaque determined by NIRS-IVUS. Sci Rep. 2023;13:11544.
6. Ladwiniec A, Walsh SJ, Holm NR, et al. Intravascular ultrasound to guide left main stem intervention: a NOBLE trial substudy. EuroIntervention. 2020;16(3):201-9.

7. Stone GW, Maehara A, Lansky AJ, et al. A Prospective Natural-History Study of Coronary Atherosclerosis. N Engl J Med. 2011;364(3):226-35.
8. Erlinge D, Maehara A, Ben-Yehuda O, et al. Identification of vulnerable plaques and patients by intracoronary near-infrared spectroscopy and ultrasound (PROSPECT II): a prospective natural history study. Lancet. 2021;397(10278):985-95.
9. Park SJ, Ahn JM, Kang DY, et al. Preventive percutaneous coronary intervention versus optimal medical therapy alone for the treatment of vulnerable atherosclerotic coronary plaques (PREVENT): a multicentre, open-label, randomised controlled trial. Lancet. 2024;403(10438):1753-65.
10. Hong MK, Mintz GS, Lee CW, et al. Comparison of Coronary Plaque Rupture Between Stable Angina and Acute Myocardial Infarction: A Three-Vessel Intravascular Ultrasound Study in 235 Patients. Circulation. 2004;110(8):928-33.
11. Xing L, Yamamoto E, Sugiyama T, et al. EROSION Study (Effective Anti-Thrombotic Therapy Without Stenting: Intravascular Optical Coherence Tomography–Based Management in Plaque Erosion): A 1-Year Follow-Up Report. Circ Cardiovasc Interv. 2017;10(12):e005860.
12. Jia H, Dai J, He L, et al. EROSION III. JACC Cardiovasc Interv. 2022;15(8):846-56.

CHAPTER 92

Current Concepts and Clinical Implications of Coronary Artery Calcification

Satyavan Sharma

ABSTRACT

The prevalence of coronary artery calcification (CAC) is increasing with aging of the population and enormous burden of atherosclerotic risk factors. CAC accompanies the advent of advanced atherosclerosis; however, the prediction of adverse coronary events remains challenging. Noninvasive techniques using novel coronary computed tomography angiography (CCTA) focus on the atherosclerotic plaque. Assessment of plaque burden, plaque type, disease activity, and plaque thrombosis hold promise in risk stratification as well as in planning preventive and therapeutic strategies. Invasive intracoronary imaging and range of technologies and devices have revolutionized the treatment of calcific atherosclerotic coronary artery disease.

Keywords: Coronary artery calcification, coronary calcium score, plaque imaging, coronary computed tomography angiography (CCTA), intracoronary imaging.

INTRODUCTION

Coronary artery calcification (CAC) is an important marker of coronary artery disease (CAD) and correlates with degree of atherosclerosis. CAC results in alteration in vascular compliance, vasomotor function and can impair myocardial function.[1] Patients with CAC are at a high risk of major adverse coronary events (MACEs). Its presence has also been correlated with unfavorable outcomes in patients undergoing percutaneous coronary intervention.[2]

There have been a phenomenal progress in our understanding, early diagnosis, and treatment of CAC. The chapter will be discussed under the following heads:

- Prevalence and risk factors
- Histopathology of calcification
- Diagnosis
- Plaque morphology and imaging
- Therapies for CAC
- Clinical implications
- Conclusion

PREVALENCE AND RISK FACTORS

Atherosclerosis remains a leading cause of morbidity and mortality around the world. Globally, 17.9 million deaths were attributed to cardiovascular disease (CVD) in 2019.[3] There are two recognized types of CAC: Atherosclerotic and medial artery calcification (Monckeberg). The latter variety of CAC results from crystallization of calcium and phosphate in extracellular matrix of the arterial wall. This primarily affects the tunica media of peripheral arteries of individuals with long standing diabetes mellitus (DM) and chronic kidney disease (CKD). High calcium, phosphorus, prolonged dialysis, and secondary parathyroidism in CKD contribute to medial CAC. Reduced arterial stiffness caused by medial calcification increases risk of CVD events.

Atherosclerotic CAC is an active process and primarily intimal. The main discussion in this manuscript is focused on atherosclerotic intimal CAC. There are several risk factors which contribute to development of CAC (**Box 1**). The prevalence of CAC is age and sex dependent and is observed in over 90% of men and >67% of women >70 years of age. Conventional risk factors such as DM, hypertension, CKD, and abnormal lipids play an important role. In addition, there are local, metabolic, and chromosomal factors which play a role. It is important to recognize that there is no relationship between dietary calcium intake and atherosclerotic calcification. Studies suggest that calcification results from aberrant regulatory mechanism rather than calcium overload.

Coronary artery calcification might be inherited through chromosomal variants, rare mutation, and dysregulation in microribonucleic acid. Intimal calcification results from the chondrocyte like cells by an inflammatory cascade, activated by macrophage and local cytokine release, death of inflammatory cells within atheroma. These mechanisms promote oxidative stress and inflammation and consequent calcification within atheroma. In advanced atherosclerosis, there is significant CAC, and its extent usually predicts MACE.

HISTOPATHOLOGY OF CALCIFICATION

The histopathology of CAC has been studied extensively during the last two decades.[4,5] The classification depends on diameter of calcium in the atheroma and includes:

- Microcalcification (0.5–15 μm)
- Punctate calcification (15–1 mm)
- Fragment calcification (>1 mm)
- Sheet calcification (>3 mm)
- Nodular calcification

The process of calcification typically starts with microcalcification, which grows into large fragments forming spotty calcification and eventually diffuse sheet like. The sheet calcification may fracture and lead to calcific nodules. However, the calcification in the plaque can change from one variety to another depending on activity of inflammation and lipid lowering therapies. The extent of CAC correlates with plaque burden. Microcalcification in fibrous cap might provoke plaque rupture. Calcific nodules can disrupt the fibrous cap and lead to thrombosis. Recurrent plaque rupture with hemorrhage with subsequent healing might result in obstructive fibrocalcific lesions often seen in stable angina and sudden cardiac death.

There have been great advances in technology for histopathological analysis and visualization of CAC. Micro computed tomography (CT) is an imaging modality which permits greater spatial resolution up to 1–10 μm.

This technique is still not available for clinical use and allows better understanding of calcium progression, especially when interpreted along with histological and radiological images. It has capability to differentiate between microscopic and macroscopic calcification. High resolution micro-CT study of human arteries at autopsy has shown excellent correlation with histology and can differentiate nodular from sheet calcification.[6]

BOX 1: Risk factors for coronary artery calcification (CAC).

- Advanced age, male sex
- Diabetes mellitus, hypertension
- Dyslipidemia
- Smoking
- Renal dysfunction (mostly causes medial calcification)
- Aberrant regulatory mechanisms
- Chromosomal variants

DIAGNOSIS

Box 2 outlines the various methods for diagnosis of CAC. Noninvasive or invasive imaging remains essential for diagnosis of CAC.

Serum Biomarkers

Recent studies have explored the potential role of specific biomarkers such as alkaline phosphatase (ALP), 1.5 AG (1.5 anhydrous D-glucitol), MMP (metalloproteases), and Lp(a) in diagnosing pattern and progression of CAC.[6] Aberrant calcium regulatory mechanisms that affect bone formation and growth also influence CAC, and ALP has been considered a molecular biomarker of vascular calcification. Elevated Lp(a) is a well-recognized genetic risk factor for CVD and correlates positively with CAC. Lp(a) has been shown to be associated with rapid CAC progression and increase in CAC volume, especially in patients with higher levels of inflammation and coagulation parameters.

Computed Tomography

Computed tomography is extensively utilized noninvasive modality with high sensitivity and specificity for detection and quantification of CAC. The CT technologies evolved very rapidly from electron beam CT (EBCT) to multidetector ultrafast CT to ECG gated spiral acquisition technique. CAC scoring has emerged as a widely available and useful tool for stratifying CV risk, predicting patient outcomes, and preventing therapy. There are currently three CAC scoring methods: Agatston score, volume score, and mass score. Agatston score is quite imperfect and was developed during the EBCT era; however, this continues to be used widely due to its robust validation.[7] The score represents a weighted sum of calcified lesions, accounting for the total area and maximal attenuation of calcification. A CAC score of zero means no calcium is visualized in the heart, and there is low chance of developing a heart attack in the future. CAC score between 1 and 99 suggests mildly increased, 100–299 moderately increased, and moderate to severely enhanced risk if score is >300. CAC score > 1,000 indicates higher all cause and CVD mortality.

Coronary CT angiography (CCTA) has assumed an important diagnostic role in patients evaluated for chest pain

BOX 2: Modalities for diagnosis of coronary artery calcification (CAC).

- Serum biomarkers
- Electron beam computed tomography (EBCT)
- Coronary computed tomography angiography (CCTA)
- Invasive coronary angiography
- Enhanced angiography techniques (stent boost)
- Intravascular ultrasound (IVUS)
- Optical coherence tomography (OCT)

and suspected to have CAD. Calcification on CCTA appears as bright areas with Hounsfield units >130 due to significant X-ray attenuation within a typical coronary distribution. CCTA offers a noninvasive approach to identify CAC with an accuracy rate of 94%. It can provide useful information about calcium eccentricity and longitudinal extension similar to optical coherence tomography (OCT). CCTA has several limitations due to blooming artefacts. The technique can overestimate calcium volume and fails to differentiate between nodular and nonnodular calcification. Newer generation CT scanners and deblooming computer software can minimize artefacts and enhance quality.[8] At this point, CCTA is of great values in providing an overview of calcium burden and distribution.

Coronary Angiography

Coronary angiography (CAG) has historically been the first modality used to detect CAC. On angiogram, CAC can be visualized as areas of linear X-ray attenuation along the course of a coronary artery. It has low to moderate sensitivity for detecting CAC compared to intravascular ultrasound (IVUS) and CCTA but is very specific (high positive predictive value). Angiographic CAC is classified into three: None/mild, moderate, and severe. Severe CAC is defined as radio-opacities seen without cardiac motion before contrast injection and affecting both sides of the arterial wall **(Fig. 1)**. Moderate CAC refers to radio-opacities noted only during the cardiac cycle before contrast injection.

The diagnostic accuracy of CAG depends on the pattern of the CAC. The detection is enhanced if calcium is superficial, eccentricity is >180°, and length is >6 mm. Accuracy rates are lower if CAC is deep with less eccentricity and lower length. Conventional CAG may be used to detect presence of significant CAC, but it fails to diagnose a specific pattern of CAC and fails to determine whether CAC has been modified by interventional treatment.

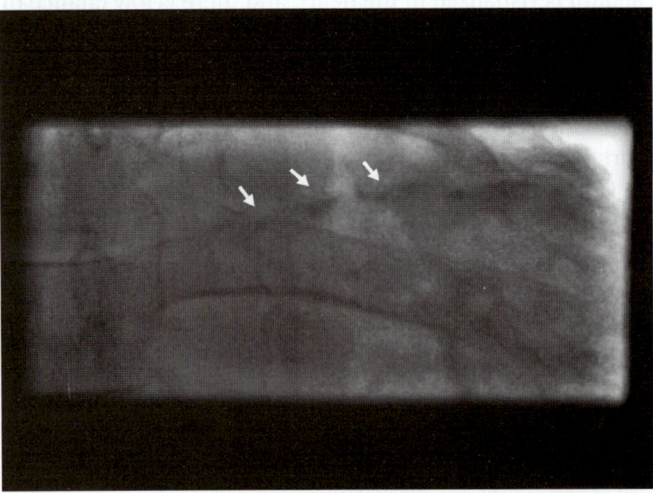

FIG. 1: Cine-fluoroscopy during coronary angiography shows dense calcification in left main coronary artery and left anterior descending artery (arrows).

Enhanced angiographic techniques such as ClearStent (Siemens) or Stent boost (Philips) can be useful in circumstances where IVUS or OCT is not available. These techniques can give insight about total calcium burden, its symmetry, and about stent expansion.

INTRAVASCULAR ULTRASOUND

Intravascular ultrasound is distinctly superior to CAG for detection of CAC with sensitivity of over 90% and specificity of 99–100%. CAC on grayscale IVUS is diagnosed by documenting bright echoes with acoustic shadowing. The extent of CAC is categorized as none, 1 quadrant (0–90°), 2 quadrants (91–180°), 3 quadrants (181–270°), and 4 quadrants (271–360°).

The CAC is labeled as superficial when confined to intimal-luminal interface and deep if present in the medial-adventitial border or closer to adventitia. The calcium length can be measured but not the thickness and volume.

Radiofrequency analysis of the IVUS signal allows for characterization of coronary plaque components into fibrous, fibrofatty, necrotic core, and dense calcium. IVUS studies have shown that patients with highest dense calcium volume exhibited high-risk atherosclerotic features and highest 3-year MACE.

Stent underexpansion is a cause of stent thrombosis and in-stent restenosis. CAC often inhibits stent expansion. A recent study developed an IVUS-based risk score to enable interventional cardiologist to identify calcified lesion at risk of underexpansion and adapt necessary adjunctive calcium modification strategy before stent deployment. Calcification angle of <270°, circumferential or long calcium, calcific nodule, and small vessels defined adverse outcomes.[9] **Figures 2A and B** delineate circumferential calcification often associated with stent underexpansion.

OPTICAL COHERENCE TOMOGRAPHY

Optical coherence tomography provides higher resolution using imaging (10–20 μm) compared to grayscale IVUS (150–200 μm). It detects CAC as low-intensity, low-attenuation areas with sharp borders. The sensitivity (95–100%) and specificity of 97–100% are akin to IVUS. OCT is light based and can penetrate calcium and provide better information on thickness and measure calcium volume. However, OCT has a reduced capacity to detect deep calcium with a limit to within 1.5 mm of the vessel wall. Three distinctive entities were described according to OCT imaging: Superficial calcified plates (SCP), eruptive calcified nodule (CN), and calcified profusion (CP).[10] Eruptive nodule is an established mechanism of plaque instability and observed in up to 8% of acute coronary syndrome (ACS). **Figures 3A and B** show extensive calcification and calcific nodules.

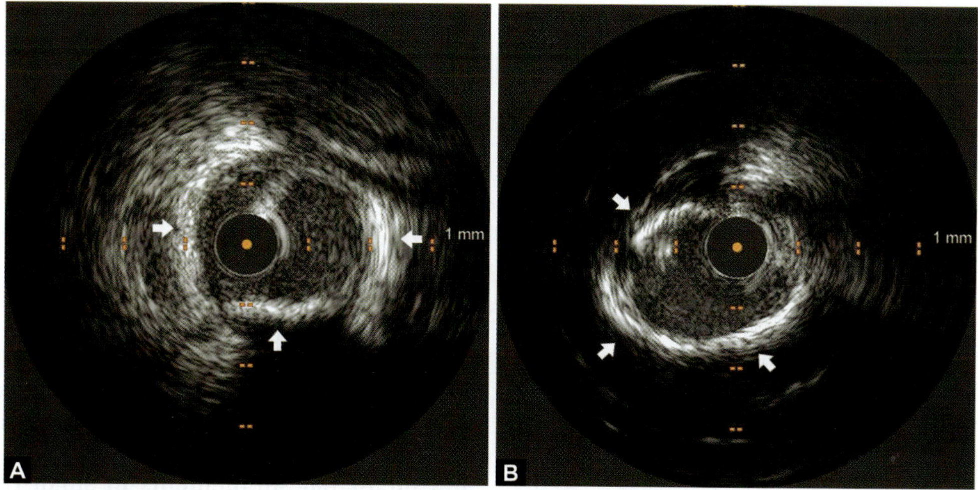

FIGS. 2A AND B: IVUS images—(A) and (B) demonstrate circumferential calcification (shown by arrows).

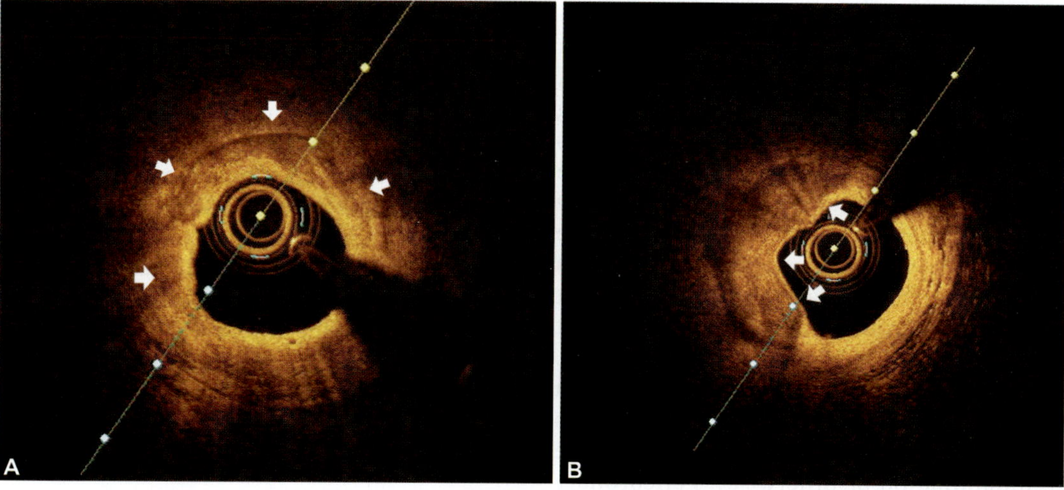

FIGS. 3A AND B: OCT images: (A) extensive calcification in 3 quadrants (arrows) whereas (B) reveals calcific nodules (arrows).

PLAQUE MORPHOLOGY AND IMAGING

Almost all stages of atherosclerotic lesions can be complicated by one or the other type of calcification. An in-depth review of the CAC is available.[6] The morphological categories are as follows:

- *Intimal thickening:* Deposition of smooth muscle cell (SMC) and lipid near intimal-media border (foci of micro or mixed micro/punctate calcification)
- *Fibroatheroma (early or late):* Macrophage accumulation in lipid core. Punctate or fragmented calcification
- *Thin cap atheroma:* Fibrous cap <65 µm thick, large necrotic core (>10%) along with calcification with or without hemorrhage
- *Plaque rupture:* Degradation of fibrous cap, microcalcification + thrombosis
- *Plaque erosion:* Thickening of fibroatheroma
- *Calcified nodule (2.5 mm):* Fibrous plaque with nodular calcification, protrudes into lumen
- *Healed plaque:* SMC, large calcium (fractured or sheet), and small necrotic core

Plaque Imaging

For many decades, myocardial ischemia imaging has been used to identify and manage patients with CAD. This rationale was supported by robust evidence demonstrating association between symptoms, ischemia documented on various tests, and future risk of myocardial infarction (MI). The post-hoc analysis of ISCHEMIA trial has demonstrated that extent of ischemia is a poor discriminator of clinical end points like all-cause mortality and CVD death. The superiority of anatomical plaque assessments over functional testing suggests that to improve outcomes in CAD, a greater emphasis should be placed on coronary plaque.

Initial efforts for plaque imaging were based around invasive techniques such as IVUS and OCT. Plaque imaging with CCTA developed rapidly and provided incredible qualitative and quantitative information about plaque morphology. The lack of high spatial resolution and blooming artefacts make assessment of microcalcification, distinction between various types of calcification and degree of stenosis difficult. High spatial resolution (0.2–0.33 mm) CCTA scanners reduce partial volume and beam hardening artefacts and provide better assessment of calcific lesions. Further step forward in CCTA-based characterization of CAC might come from the latest technology. Photon counting CT (PCCT) allows better accuracy in images, lower image noise, high temporal resolution, and significant reduction in residual motion artefacts.[11] Dual source CT (DECT) or spiral CT enhances plaque visualization and enables better assessment of high risk plaques.[12] Another advance is F-Na F PET/CT imaging, a useful tool to detect molecular calcification during early stages of atherosclerosis. The technique is also useful for diagnosing inflammation.

Four factors emerge as the key players to the overall risk of MI. The key determinants are plaque burden, plaque type, its activity, and thrombosis.[8] Comprehensive plaque imaging is feasible with availability of advanced CCTA technologies which are described in **Table 1**. These novel techniques are still in research domain and beyond the reach of day-to-day clinical practice. Assessment of plaque burden is feasible with contrast CT using novel image analysis and provides superior diagnostic information than calcium score. Most of the obstructive plaques display a large plaque burden. It is feasible to identify plaque type by newer CT technologies. Features such as positive remodeling and low attenuation identify plaques with enhanced risk of adverse events such as MI. PET/CT scanners with 18F-Na F tracer can evaluate plaque activity (active inflammation or otherwise). Pericoronary adipose tissue (PCAT) density assessment on CCTA is also used as a surrogate marker for inflammation. Noninvasive recognition of plaque thrombosis is still a challenge but can be attempted using molecular PET imaging or T1 deficient cardiac magnetic resonance imaging (CMRI).

Plaque Imaging by Invasive Modalities

Invasive imaging by IVUS and OCT have been utilized to understand and correlate atherosclerotic plaque changes with clinical events. It is worth knowing that presence of calcification was exclusion criteria from early progression/regression studies. However, it is interesting to know that culprit lesions and ruptured plaques exhibit more spotty calcification. This type of calcification may represent a marker of ruptured and subsequently healed plaques.

TABLE 1: Noninvasive coronary plaque imaging.

	Modality	Application
Plaque burden	Contrast CT	Guiding therapy
Plaque type	CT	Treatment response
Plaque activity	PET-CT	Active or burnt out
Plaque thrombosis	PET-CT and CMRI	Predicting mace

(CMRI: cardiac magnetic resonance imaging; CT: computed tomography; PET-CT: positron emission tomography-computed tomography)

THERAPIES FOR CORONARY ARTERY CALCIFICATION

Medical Therapies

Several studies have explored whether medical therapy can halt or even reverse CAC progression. ACE inhibitor, calcium channel blocker, hormone therapy, phosphate binders, and medicinal supplements in small randomized trials and observational studies have shown benefits. However, large randomized studies are lacking to formulate any recommendations.

The impact of statins on CAC has been extensively investigated using Agatston score, CCTA, and IVUS studies. An excellent study evaluated the impact of statin therapy on coronary plaque using serial CCTA.[13] Statin use was associated with an increased progression of calcified coronary plaque and reduced progression of noncalcified plaque. It has been hypothesized that the increase in coronary calcium represents a healing mechanism of statins, whereas calcified plaques become more stabilized through calcification of necrotic core. Statins result in plaque stabilization. This study also emphasized the need to intensify preventive treatment of patients with hypertension and diabetes to slow and stabilize the CAD progression and improve clinical outcomes.

Percutaneous Coronary Interventions

Coronary artery calcification continues to be an obstacle for PCI with higher rates of procedural challenges, postintervention complications, and overall unfavorable long-term outcomes. Identification and appropriate management of calcific lesions is important to improve patient outcomes after PCI. As explained earlier, the ability of CAG to identify morphological features of CAC is limited, and this drawback can lead to suboptimal stent implantation. In contrast, intravascular imaging, particularly OCT, is able to identify and quantitate CAC facilitating lesion preparation techniques prior to stent deployment. In the ILUMEN IV trial, OCT-guided PCI in patients with moderately or severely calcified lesions reduced the 2-year rate of target vessel failure compared with angiography-guided PCI.[14] OCT guidance is recommended in calcified lesions as it improves procedural safety, efficacy, and long-term results.

There are several calcification modification techniques **(Box 3)**. They are divided into debulking techniques (rotational atherectomy, orbital atherectomy, and excimer laser) and nondebulking or "balloon-based techniques" (cutting balloon, scoring balloon, super high-noncompliant

BOX 3: Coronary artery calcification (CAC) modifications tools.

Ablation techniques:
- Rotational atherectomy
- Orbital atherectomy
- Excimer laser

Balloon-based techniques:
- Cutting balloon
- Scoring balloon
- Super high compliant balloon
- Lithotripsy balloon

balloon, and lithotripsy balloon).[15] Imaging derived data on pattern and characteristics of CAC enables the interventional cardiologist to choose an appropriate technique

CLINICAL IMPLICATIONS

The identification of high-risk coronary plaque features through noninvasive imaging carry important clinical implications for accurate identification of patients at risk of acute CV events. In those with high-risk features, preventive measures such as lifestyle changes and risk factor control should be intensified.

CONFIRM registry observed that a fine line separates primary and secondary prevention among patients with high CAC score.[16] It was demonstrated that individuals without CAD with CAC score >300 have similar incidence of MACE as in stable high-risk CAD patients after MI. These observations carry a significant message because high-risk post-MI patients are treated with high intensity statin and other nonstatin lipid-lowering agents. On the other hand, there are no recommendations for using nonstatin therapies in patients with high CAC and no CAD. Further studies are needed to refine the role of CAC score in prevention and treatment strategies.

Coronary computed tomography angiography can assess and define the features with greater likelihood of ACS. CAC predicts future risks of ACS better than any biochemical test. On plaque imaging, high-risk features prone to ACS are: Positive remodeling, noncalcified plaque or low attenuation plaques (<30 HU), and spotty calcification (<3 mm). Out of the three, positive remodeling has the highest accuracy for ACS. The ongoing trials: SCOT HEART, ROBINSCA, and CAC PREVENTABLE will define the role of CAC in guiding preventive therapies.[6]

Percutaneous treatment in individuals with calcified CAD is demanding with unpredictable outcomes. A significant advance in this field comes from noninvasive imaging by CCTA and invasive imaging by IVUS and OCT. Imaging allows the operator to delineate the pattern of CAC and adapt appropriate modification techniques and stent optimization.

CONCLUSION

Coronary artery calcification has emerged as an additional risk marker of CV events in patients with atherosclerotic CAD. The extent and pattern of calcification have prognostic and therapeutic implications. Advances in noninvasive CCTA technologies have made plaque imaging a reality. Assessment of high-risk plaques and vulnerable patients holds promise for novel preventive therapies. Multimodality imaging and calcium modifying technologies have revolutionized the percutaneous interventions in cardiac catheterization laboratory.

REFERENCES

1. Wang L, Jerosch-Harold M, Jacobs DR Jr, et al. Coronary artery calcification and myocardial perfusion in asymptomatic adults: the MESA (Multi-Ethnic Study of Atherosclerosis). L Am Coll Cardiol. 2006;48:1018-26.
2. Vavuranakis M, Toutouzas K, Stenfadis C, et al. Stent deployment in calcified lesions; can we overcome calcification restraint with high pressure balloon inflations? Cathet Cardiovascular Interv. 2001;52:164-72.
3. Roth GA, Mensah GA, Johnson CA, et al. Global burden of cardiovascular diseases and risk factors 1990-2019: update from the GBD 2019 study. J Am Coll Cardiol. 2020;22:2982-30.
4. Burke AP, Weber DK, Kologie FD, et al. Pathophysiology of calcium deposition in coronary arteries. Herz. 2001;26:239-44.
5. Sorin DC, Nardi G, Ristalli F, et al. Contemporary approach to calcified coronary lesions. Interv Cardiol. 2019;14:754-63.
6. Onnis C, Virmani R, Kawai K, et al. Coronary artery calcification: current concepts and clinical implications. Circulation. 2024;149:251-66.
7. Agatston AS, Janowitz WR, Hildner PJ, et al. Quantification of coronary artery using ultrafast computed tomography. J Am Coll Cardiol. 1990;15:827-32.
8. Kwiecinski J, Tzolos E, William MC, et al. Non-invasive coronary atherosclerotic imaging. J Am Coll Cardiol Imaging. 2023;16: 1608-22.
9. Zhang M, Matsumura M, Usui E, et al. IVUS derived calcium score to predict stent under-expansion in severe calcified lesions. Circ Cardiovascular Interv. 2021;1:14210296.
10. Onea HL, Olinc M, Lazar FI, et al. A review paper on optical coherence tomography evaluation of coronary calcification pattern: Is it relevant today? J Cardiovascular Dev Dis. 2024;11(8):231.
11. Si-Mohamed SA, Boccalini S, Lacombe H, et al. Coronary CT angiography with photon counting CT: first in human results. Radiology. 2022;303:303-13.
12. Tarkowski P, Czekajskg-Chebab E. Dual energy heart CT: beyond better angiography—review. J Clin Med. 2021;10:5193.

13. Smit JM, Vam Rosendael AR, El Mahdiui M, et al. Impact of clinical characteristics and statins on coronary plaque progression by serial computed tomography angiography. Cir Cardiovasc Imaging, 2020;13:e009750.
14. Ali ZA, Shin D, Vijayvergiya R, et al. Optical coherence tomography -vs angiography-guided coronary stent implantation in calcified lesions: the ILUMEN IV trial. Eur Heart J. 2025;46(32): 3201-10.
15. Wopperer SB, Kotronias R, Marin F, et al. The role of invasive and non-invasive imaging technologies and calcium modification therapies in the evaluation and management of coronary artery calcification. Front Cardiovasc Med. 2023;10:1133510.
16. Budoff MJ, Kinninger A, Gransar H, et al.; CONFIRM investigators. When does a calcium score equivalent to secondary prevention? Insights from the multinational CONFIRM Registry. JACC Cardiovasc Imaging. 2023;16:1181-9.

CHAPTER 93

Cardiac CT: Emerging Role in Microvascular Dysfunction

VS Prakash, Varsha Rakshitha Prakash

ABSTRACT

Coronary microvascular dysfunction (CMD) is one of the key contributing etiologies for myocardial infarction with nonobstructive coronary arteries. Coronary microvascular dysfunction occurs due to an imbalance between the vasodilatory and vasoconstrictive properties of the coronary microvasculature, which are mainly constituted by the prearterioles, arterioles, and capillaries. Oxidative stress, along with the ensuing inflammatory response are important contributing factors for the occurrence of CMD. The occurrence of CMD portends a worse prognosis in patients, and hence early diagnosis and treatment are of utmost importance. Both invasive and noninvasive methods exist for the diagnosis of CMD, with noninvasive methods being preferred due to safety concerns. The current noninvasive methods used are transthoracic echo, CT, cardiac MRI, positron emission tomography (PET), and single photon emission CT (SPECT). CT, due to its ability to offer anatomic and functional assessment in the same sitting, is gaining preference. Unlike other noninvasive imaging modalities, CT also has the ability to detect epicardial stenosis and CMD. The most commonly used methods for diagnosis of CMD are CT-myocardial perfusion imaging (static and dynamic) and derived coronary artery lumen volume-to-myocardial mass ratio (V/M ratio) from CT angiography. Its drawbacks include radiation exposure and risk of contrast induced nephropathy. However, newer modalities in CT are being developed, and this method of imaging is growing as an effective method for evaluating CMD, especially when paired with perfusion imaging to assess both anatomical and functional aspects of coronary circulation.

Keywords: Myocardial infarction with nonobstructive coronary arteries, coronary microvascular dysfunction, computed tomography, CT-myocardial perfusion imaging, CT-fractional flow reserve, CT coronary angiography, coronary artery lumen volume-to-myocardial mass ratio (V/M ratio).

INTRODUCTION

Acute myocardial infarction (MI) with <50% stenosis on coronary angiography (CAG) (without significant obstruction) is a heterogeneous condition known as myocardial infarction with nonobstructive coronary arteries (MINOCA). The diagnostic criteria for MINOCA are (1) features consistent with the Fourth Universal definition of *acute MI*, (2) the presence of nonobstructive infarct-related artery on CAG, (3) the *absence* of any other alternate cause for the presentation, and (4) absence of nonischemic causes of myocardial *injury.*[1]

In patients diagnosed with MINOCA, nearly 60% of symptomatic individuals undergoing CAG do not exhibit obstructive coronary artery disease (CAD).[2]

Although it varies, the current rate of this condition is approximately 15%.[2] Numerous pathophysiological factors can lead to the phenomenon of MINOCA, which is frequently misdiagnosed.[1] One of the important factors causing MINOCA is microvascular dysfunction, which will further be discussed in detail in the following section.

CORONARY MICROVASCULAR DYSFUNCTION

The phrase "microvascular angina" was first used by Cannon and Epstein in 1985 to refer to the clinical presentation of myocardial ischemia brought on by structural or functional alterations in the coronary microvasculature.[3]

As the name indicates, coronary microvascular dysfunction affects the coronary microvasculature, that is, blood vessels < 0.5 mm in diameter, which in the absence of obstructive CAD disease constitute up to 70% of the coronary arterial resistance.[1] According to invasive flow evaluation, coronary microvascular dysfunction (CMD) may be present in up to two-thirds of the patients with MINOCA.[2]

Apart from having a higher risk of serious cardiovascular events such as heart failure, sudden cardiac death, and acute coronary syndrome, CMD is acknowledged as a critical component in a number of clinical situations, such as Takotsubo syndrome and heart failure.[3] Additionally, CMD is linked to poor clinical outcomes and is an early indicator of cardiovascular disease.[4]

The following paragraphs give an overview regarding coronary microvascular circulation, to have a comprehensive understanding of the coronary circulation's functional anatomy before delving into the imaging modalities useful for the diagnosis of CMD.

OVERVIEW OF CORONARY MICROVASCULAR CIRCULATION

The network of coronary arteries is a continuous network made up of functionally separate vascular segments, each of which has a specific purpose in modulating coronary blood flow. The epicardial coronary arteries, intramural arterioles, and prearteriole vessels constitute the coronary artery vasculature. The latter two play a crucial role in coordinating blood flow with myocardial oxygen consumption. Dynamic and simultaneous alterations in the microcirculation and epicardial coronary arteries control myocardial perfusion.[2]

Under normal circumstances, the proximal epicardial coronary arteries (diameter > 500 µm) mostly function as conduits with little resistance to blood flow. The system changes from conductance to resistance as these arteries divide into smaller prearterioles (100–500 µm) and then intramural arterioles (<100 µm). The majority of the heart's resistance circuit is made up of intramural arterioles, which are essential for regulating coronary blood flow in response to metabolic signals from the myocardium and balancing the myocardial blood supply with oxygen demand.[3] While the distal component of the prearterioles (150–100 µm) are more sensitive to changes in pressure, the proximal component (500–150 µm) responds more quickly to changes in flow **(Table 1)**.[4,5]

The metabolic modulation of coronary blood flow (CBF) in response to myocardial oxygen demand (autoregulation) is carried out by the intramyocardial arterioles (<100 µm), which have the highest resistance. Finally, because of their enormous surface area and relatively high permeability, capillaries (<10 µm) serve as exchange channels. The capillaries, intramyocardial arterioles, and epicardial prearterioles are all included in the coronary microcirculation.[4]

The **Figure 1** shows the network of coronary arteries and the coronary microvasculature.

Seventy-five percent of blood oxygen is extracted by the myocardium when at rest, therefore any increase in oxygen intake raises oxygen demand, which in turn raises myocardial blood flow (MBF).[2]

The volume of blood delivered per gram of cardiac tissue over a specified time period is a typical way to quantify MBF, which is the rate at which blood flows through the coronary arteries[3] and is primarily controlled by microcirculation through a number of processes, such as arterial diameter and tone.[2]

Numerous variables, such as endothelial dysfunction, coronary spasm, inflammation, atherosclerosis, microvascular rarefaction, and diffuse fibrosis, cause these systems to be disrupted in the context of CMD. Changes in the distribution of the blood supply and the resulting chest discomfort are determined by these abnormalities.[2]

PATHOPHYSIOLOGY OF CORONARY MICROVASCULAR DYSFUNCTION

The phrase CMD refers to any disease that affects microvasculature in the absence of obstructive CAD. This includes atherosclerosis, inflammation, endothelial dysfunction, and coronary spasm, all of which might impede the heart's ability to increase coronary blood flow in response to stress and jeopardize autoregulatory systems. A reduced ability for microvascular vasodilation and an exaggerated response of the coronary microcirculation to vasoconstrictor stimuli are characteristics of CMD. Due to a mismatch between oxygen supply and demand, this results in an inadequate vasodilatory response during physical activity or pharmacological stress, which can produce myocardial ischemia, whether it be subtle or obvious.[3]

Oxidative stress, brought on by cellular reactive oxygen species (ROS) overproduction and buildup, together with the ensuing inflammatory response, are thought to be important

TABLE 1: Components of the coronary vasculature and microvasculature.

Epicardial vessel	Prearterioles	Arterioles	Capillaries
• Conduit vessel • > 500 µm • 5% of total resistance	• Metabolic control and flow regulation • Resistance vessel • 100–500 µm • 20% of total resistance Distal component (150–100 µm)—more sensitive to changes in pressure, proximal component (500–150 µm) responds more quickly to changes in flow	• Metabolic control and flow regulation • Resistance vessel • < 100 µm • 60% of total resistance	• Exchange vessels • <10 µm • 15% of total resistance

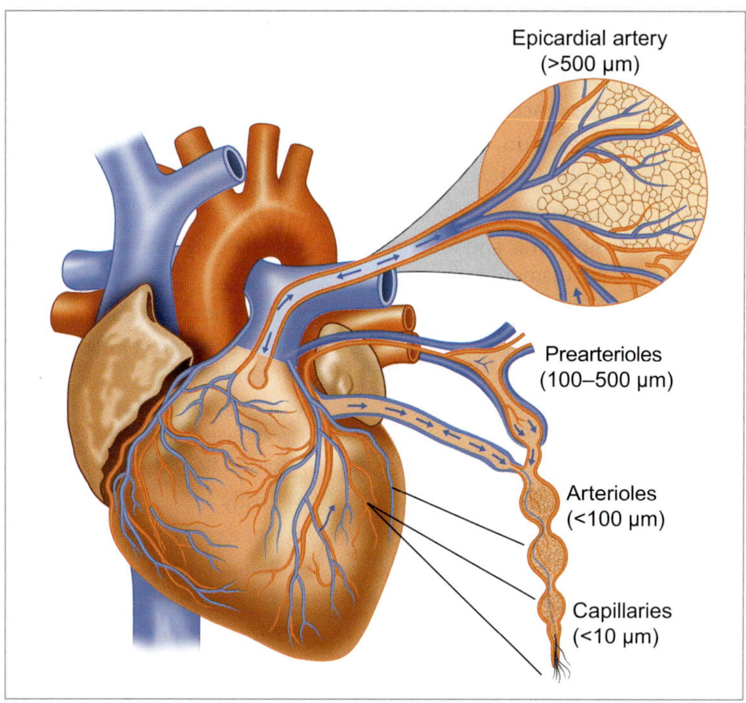

FIG. 1: Network of coronary arteries and the coronary microvasculature.

pathogenic processes for the development of CMD, even though the exact mechanisms causing it are not fully understood.[5]

By modulating vasorelaxant chemicals such as prostacyclin (PGI2), nitric oxide (NO), and endothelium-derived hyperpolarizing factors (EDHF), the endothelium plays a crucial role in controlling CBF. When pathological vasoconstrictive chemicals (such as endothelin-1, superoxide, hydrogen peroxide, and thromboxane) alter the vascular steady state, the endothelium becomes dysfunctional. Furthermore, endothelial dysfunction is intimately associated with microvascular spasm, which entails the disruption of vasomotion (physiological rhythmical contractions). Vascular smooth muscle cell (VSMC) failure and a preponderance of vasoconstrictive metabolites in the context of elevated Rho-kinase activity are hallmarks of its intricate pathogenesis. By blocking the myosin-binding submit (MBS), increased Rho-kinase activity causes excessive myosin light chain phosphorylation, which in turn causes hypercontractility. Moreover, excessive autonomic nervous system activity and persistent low-grade inflammation might also be causative factors.[4]

The onset and advancement of coronary atherosclerosis are significantly influenced by chronic inflammation. According to recent data,[3] autoimmune rheumatic diseases and other systemic inflammatory disorders may possibly have a role in the development of CMD. Impaired coronary vasodilator reserve has been associated with worse cardiovascular outcomes and a higher all-cause mortality rate in patients with systemic inflammatory diseases. Furthermore, there is mounting proof that coronary vasomotor problems are significantly influenced by psychological stress.[3]

ASSESSMENT OF CORONARY MICROVASCULAR DYSFUNCTION

Invasive and noninvasive methods exist for the assessment of CMD, of which the noninvasive methods are elaborated in **Table 2**.

CARDIAC COMPUTED TOMOGRAPHY EMERGING ROLE IN MICROVASCULAR DYSFUNCTION

One common imaging technique for the diagnosis of cardiovascular disorders is computed tomography (CT). Over the past few decades, dramatic improvements in CT technologies have greatly increased the diagnostic usefulness of cardiovascular CT by enabling the capture of high-resolution images with minimal radiation doses. The diagnostic utility of cardiovascular CT in the context of numerous cardiovascular disorders is further increased by the increasing availability of dual-source and dual-energy CT in the majority of modern multi-slice CT scanners, in addition to the common use of single-energy CT in daily practice.[6]

In addition to conventional and invasive diagnostic pathways, CT, especially sophisticated modalities such as coronary CT angiography (CCTA) and CT myocardial perfusion (CT-MP), is becoming more and more important in the identification, description, and risk assessment of microvascular dysfunction in cardiac patients. Despite its acknowledged limitations and growing usefulness, recent research has examined how these noninvasive technologies

TABLE 2: Noninvasive methods of assessment of CMD.

Method	Sensitivity/specificity	Advantages	Disadvantages	Diagnostic parameter
Transthoracic echo	+/++	• Easily accessible • Easy to do • Cost effective • Low risk	• Interobserver variability+ • Acoustic window limitations • Artifacts	• Coronary flow • Velocity ratio
Cardiac CT	++/+++	• Anatomic and functional assessment in the same sitting • Assessment of epicardial stenosis in the same sitting	• Not easily available • Costly • Radiation exposure • Risk of contrast induced nephropathy • Higher chance of overestimating myocardial blood flow	• Coronary volume-to-myocardial mass ratio (V/M) • CT-myocardial perfusion imaging (CT-MPI)
PET	+++/+++	• Most sensitive and specific modality • Most validated modality • Highly reproducible and accurate modality • Not restricted by renal derangement	• Costly • Not easily available • Radiation exposure • Time consuming • No assessment of epicardial stenosis	Coronary flow reserve (CFR)
SPECT	+/++	Promising modality for the diagnosis of CMD	• Requires more research for validation • Limited availability • Radiation exposure • Requires new generation cameras • Costly	CFR
CMR	+++/++	• High tissue characterization and spatial resolution • No exposure to radiation • Validated and compared with PET and invasive techniques	• Costly • Limited availability • Risk of contrast associated side effects • Time consuming • No assessment of epicardial stenosis	Myocardial perfusion reserve index (MPRI)

evaluate the anatomical and functional characteristics of microvasculature.[2,3,7-11]

ROLE OF COMPUTED TOMOGRAPHY: MYOCARDIAL PERFUSION IMAGING IN DIAGNOSIS OF CORONARY MICROVASCULAR DYSFUNCTION

In evaluating microvascular illness, CT angiography combined with CT perfusion/CT-myocardial perfusion imaging (CTP/CT-MPI) has shown strength, because it offers cardiac perfusion data and comprehensive coronary anatomical information in a single examination.[2,3,7-11]

The assessment of the flow of contrast material from the vascular to the myocardial compartment both at rest and following adenosine injection makes up CT-MPI. The amount of the contrast agent determines how much radiation it attenuates. Consequently, areas of decreased density, whether hypoenhanced or nonenhanced, indicate areas of the myocardium with decreased perfusion.[2]

Two types of CT-MPI are currently available—the static type and the dynamic CT-MPI.

By analyzing a single dataset obtained during the first-pass contrast enhancement, static CT-MPI evaluates myocardial perfusion and allows for a qualitative assessment of regional variations in contrast uptake throughout the myocardium. When comparing hypoenhanced regions to normal distant myocardial segments, the deficiencies are evaluated qualitatively. Stress pictures are compared to baseline perfusion, much like nuclear myocardial perfusion imaging, in order to identify myocardial ischemia and evaluate reversibility. This qualitative approach's main drawback is that it may mask globally decreased myocardial perfusion because it relies on a region that is typically perfused for comparison, and diffuse ischemia may manifest as uniformly low attenuation across the myocardium. Furthermore, inaccurate bolus timing may result in peak myocardial attenuation being missed, which could make it more difficult to distinguish between ischemia and normal regions.[3]

By taking several consecutive CT images after a contrast bolus injection, dynamic CT-MPI offers a quantitative evaluation. This enables the development of time-attenuation curves that track the arrival of the contrast and its washout from the myocardium and aorta. It offers diagnostic precision on par with PET and CMR. Myocardial perfusion can be measured in absolute terms by mathematically modeling these patterns, providing a more accurate assessment of perfusion dynamics. Microvascular ischemia is indicated by an MBF in at least one left ventricular segment that is <100 mL/min/100 mL.[3]

More sensitivity has been shown by dynamic CT-MPI in conjunction with CTA than by static CT-MPI in determining inducible ischemia in individuals whose angiography shows nonobstructive coronary stenosis. Nevertheless, dynamic CT-MPI has significant drawbacks, such as a higher radiation dosage than static CT-MPI and the need for extended breath-holding, which calls for sophisticated motion correction algorithms.[3] Territories with CMD exhibit substantially lower hyperemic MBF on CT-MP than those without, according to studies.[10]

COMPUTED TOMOGRAPHY DERIVED VOLUME-TO-MYOCARDIAL MASS RATIO IN THE DIAGNOSIS OF CORONARY MICROVASCULAR DYSFUNCTION

A measure of supply-demand mismatch that might shed light on cardiac physiology is the coronary artery lumen volume-to-myocardial mass ratio (V/M). Improved coronary reserve and a lower risk of ischemia are implied by higher coronary volume to unchanged myocardial mass, and therefore higher V/M. When circumstances that increase oxygen demand arise, a low V/M increases the risk of ischemia because it indicates insufficient coronary supply for a given cardiac demand. Ischemia can result from a supply-demand imbalance brought on by either a decrease in coronary volume, as in atherosclerosis, or an increase in myocardial mass, as in myocardial hypertrophy. V/M can be utilized as a prognostic sign, according to recent research, which can influence clinical care and comprehension of the patient's cardiovascular risk.[12]

Low V/M may be a possible sign of CMD and is an independent predictor of ischemia. V/M can be obtained noninvasively from clinical imaging in contrast to coronary flow reserve (CFR) and index of microcirculatory resistance (IMR). A typical noninvasive test that reveals anatomical features of the myocardium and coronary arteries is coronary computed tomography angiography (CCTA).[13]

The V/M ratio can be obtained by estimating the mass of the left ventricle and the coronary artery volume using three-dimensional reconstruction of CCTA images. Furthermore, computational fluid dynamics simulation of patient-specific hemodynamic parameters (such as flow rate and FFR) can be performed using CCTA-reconstructed three-dimensional geometry of coronary arteries to evaluate the risk of myocardial ischemia in patients with CMD.[13]

The **Table 3** summarizes the important recent trials on V/M ratio in CMD.

STRENGTHS OF USING COMPUTED TOMOGRAPHY FOR THE DIAGNOSIS OF CORONARY MICROVASCULAR DYSFUNCTION

- *Combined anatomical-functional data:* CT captures both epicardial and microvascular disease in a single examination, enabling the simultaneous evaluation of CAD and myocardial perfusion.[7,16]

TABLE 3: Recent trials on CT-derived volume/myocardial mass ratio (V/M ratio) in CMD.

Trial/author name	Study details	Outcomes
Collet et al. (2024)[14]	The study included 68 patients who had CMD. Lumen volume and vessel-specific myocardial mass were assessed using coronary computed tomography angiography (CTA). CMD was defined as coronary flow reserve < 2.5 and high minimal microvascular resistance as > 470 WU	Epicardial vessels were observed to be smaller in patients with CMD than in individuals without the condition. Coronary CTA detected high minimal microvascular resistance with very good diagnostic capacity
Sun et al. (2025)[13]	The study was done in 23 patients with suspected CMD and 25 controls in the Chinese population. CT-derived fractional flow reserve (CT-FFR) and patient-specific and vessel-specific V/M were estimated by three-dimensionally reconstructing the computed tomography (CT) images	The abnormally decreased V/M value in patients with CMD could serve as a potential biomarker in Chinese population
Grover et al. (2017)[15]	A retrospective case-control analysis was done in 30 patients with confirmed CMD and 32 controls. V/M ratio was extracted, and the FFR-CT values were calculated from the major epicardial coronary arteries	Patients with CMD demonstrated a significantly lower coronary CTA-derived coronary volume/myocardial mass ratio compared to asymptomatic controls

- *Noninvasive imaging modality:* Although radiation and contrast exposure are still issues, noninvasiveness eliminates the procedural dangers associated with invasive coronary reactivity testing.[7,10]
- *Quantitative indices:* Advanced, quantitative assessment pertinent to microvascular disease is made possible by novel techniques such as the coronary luminal V/M ratio and CT-derived FFR.[7,9]
- *Role in the diagnosis of CMD:* Coronary CTA, a recognized first-line test for assessing chest discomfort, has been proven to advance beyond stenosis diagnosis and offer information on general "coronary health," including microvascular physiology.

Patients with ANOCA who may also have CMD can be identified with the aid of this expanded capability, which is simple to integrate into standard practice. Due to the widespread availability of cardiac CT, this method could hasten the diagnosis of CMD and revolutionize the treatment of the sizable group of ANOCA patients who nevertheless suffer from excruciating angina symptoms even when they do not have obstructive CAD.[17]

LIMITATIONS

- *Resolution limitations:* The majority of results are inferential or dependent on functional surrogates because standard CTCA frequently lacks the resolution necessary to directly scan the microvasculature.[11]
- *Radiation and contrast:* The necessity of iodinated contrast and repetitive imaging in dynamic perfusion CT raises the danger of radiation exposure and nephropathy, particularly for patients with coexisting medical conditions.[7,9,10]
- *Physiological confounders:* Perfusion measures may be distorted by rapid contrast flow, vasodilation, and wall thinning (such as in dilated cardiomyopathy).[7]

EMERGING ROLES OF COMPUTED TOMOGRAPHY IN DIAGNOSIS OF CORONARY MICROVASCULAR DYSFUNCTION

- *CT-derived myocardial strain analysis in the diagnosis of CMD:* A combination of circumferential, longitudinal, and radial strain will be used for the diagnosis of CMD.
- *CT-FFR:* Currently CT-FFR has excelled in the diagnosis of epicardial CAD, its role in the diagnosis of CMD is still underway.
- *CT-derived pericoronary adipose tissue attenuation (PCAT):* PCAT has been proven to be associated with increased risk of vulnerable plaque and microvascular dysfunction. Studies on the role of CT-derived PCAT in the diagnosis/prognostication of CMD are still being studied.

CONCLUSION

Despite the possibility that this technology can detect CMD, CTA is not frequently used at present for CMD evaluation due to its drawbacks, which include radiation exposure, the need to exercise caution when using iodinated contrast agents in cases of renal insufficiency, and the possibility that contrast-mediated vasodilation will overestimate the MBF. However, newer modalities in CT imaging are being developed, and this modality is advancing as a powerful noninvasive method for evaluating microvascular dysfunction, especially when paired with perfusion imaging to assess both anatomical and functional aspects of the coronary circulation.

REFERENCES

1. Ezhumalai B, Modi R, Chidambaram S. A comprehensive review on myocardial infarction with non-obstructive coronary arteries (MINOCA): One size does not fit all. Indian Heart J. 2025;77(4):318-25.
2. Tonet E, Pompei G, Faragasso E, et al. Coronary microvascular dysfunction: PET, CMR and CT assessment. J Clin Med. 2021;10(9):1848.
3. Martins AM, Nobre Menezes M, Alves da Silva P, et al. Multimodality imaging in the diagnosis of coronary microvascular disease: An update. J Pers Med. 2025;15(2):75.
4. Rehan R, Yong A, Ng M, et al. Coronary microvascular dysfunction: A review of recent progress and clinical implications. Front Cardiovasc Med. 2023;10:1111721.
5. Del Buono MG, Montone RA, Camilli M, et al. Coronary microvascular dysfunction across the spectrum of cardiovascular diseases. J Am Coll Cardiol. 2021;78(13):1352-71.
6. Sun Z, Silberstein J, Vaccarezza M. Cardiovascular computed tomography in the diagnosis of cardiovascular disease: Beyond lumen assessment. J Cardiovasc Dev Dis. 2024;11(1):22.
7. Ayub MT, Kalra D. Coronary microvascular dysfunction and the role of noninvasive cardiovascular imaging. Diagnostics. 2020;10(9):679.
8. Serruys PW, Kotoku N, Nørgaard BL, et al. Computed tomographic angiography in coronary artery disease. EuroIntervention. 2023;18(16):e1307-27.
9. Aldiwani H, Mahdai S, Alhatemi G, et al. Microvascular angina: Diagnosis and management. Eur Cardiol. 2021;16:e46.
10. Hada M, Hoshino M, Sugiyama T, et al. Diagnostic value of computed tomography myocardial perfusion imaging to detect coexisting microvascular dysfunction in patients with obstructive epicardial coronary artery disease. Quant Imaging Med Surg. 2023;13(12):8423-34.

11. Berry C, Kramer CM, Kunadian V, et al. Great debate: Computed tomography coronary angiography should be the initial diagnostic test in suspected angina. Eur Heart J. 2023;44(26):2366-75.
12. van Assen M, Onnis C. Coronary volume–to–myocardial mass ratio giving additional insights in coronary artery disease pathophysiology. Radiology: Cardiothoracic Imaging. 2024;6(2):e240049.
13. Sun L, Yu Y, Li X, et al. Coronary artery volume to left ventricular myocardial mass ratio in detecting primary microvascular angina: A retrospective observational study in Chinese population. BMC Cardiovascular Disorders. 2025;25(1):552.
14. Collet C, Sakai K, Mizukami T, et al. Vascular remodeling in coronary microvascular dysfunction. JACC Cardiovasc Imag. 2024;17(12):1463-76.
15. Grover R, Leipsic JA, Mooney J, et al. Coronary lumen volume to myocardial mass ratio in primary microvascular angina. J Cardiovasc Comput Tomogr. 2017;11(6):423-8.
16. Mathew RC, Bourque JM, Salerno M, et al. Cardiovascular imaging techniques to assess microvascular dysfunction. JACC: Cardiovasc Imag. 2020;13(7):1577-90.
17. Ihdayhid AR, Gahungu N. Looking beyond stenosis. JACC: Cardiovasc Imag. 2024;17(12):1477-9.

CHAPTER 94

Role of Cardiac Imaging for Optimizing Medical Therapy

Vilas Magarkar

ABSTRACT

Contemporary cardiac imaging: Coronary CT angiography (CCTA), functional ischemia testing (stress echocardiography, SPECT, PET, and stress CMR), and echocardiography are the most important imaging modalities, which help in structural and functional cardiac evaluation. Thoughtful use of imaging helps in optimizing medical therapy by delineating actionable disease characteristics such as plaque burden, ischemia, microvascular dysfunction, myocardial scar, ventricular/valvular mechanics, pulmonary vascular coupling, and therapy related toxicity. It ultimately helps the physician in redefining the cardiac risk, which enables the initiation and intensification of therapies. Randomized trials and guidelines showed that an imaging-guided strategy increases the use of preventive therapies, improves symptom control, avoids nonessential interventions and in some settings reduces myocardial damage. This chapter focuses on informed decision making in lipid-lowering, antithrombotic, heart failure therapies, pulmonary hypertension regimens and timing or deferral of revascularization with the help of cardiac imaging. It provides practical evidence based *"Imaging-To-Therapy"* approach.

Keywords: CCTA, CAC, SPECT, PET, stress CMR, echocardiography, GLS, CT-FFR, microvascular angina, HF, INOCA, pulmonary hypertension.

INTRODUCTION

Contemporary cardiac imaging techniques play a pivotal role in diagnosing and managing heart diseases. Advanced modalities provide precise insights into cardiac structure and function, guiding personalized therapies. By enhancing diagnostic accuracy and treatment planning, these technologies significantly improve patient outcomes, marking a transformative shift in cardiovascular care.

WHY "IMAGING-TO-THERAPY" MATTERS

Across major cardiovascular syndromes, most of the medical decisions depend on:

- How much atherosclerosis?
- Is there flow-limiting CAD?
- Is there any microvascular ischemia?
- Is the myocardium viable?
- What is LV/RV EF, strain, filling pressures?
- Is the right ventricular-pulmonary vascular coupling preserved?

In most cases, cardiac imaging addresses these queries and facilitates precise, targeted therapy.

Preventive Cardiology

Coronary CT angiography (CCTA) and coronary artery calcium (CAC) define ASCVD risk thereby identifying patients eligible for statin and antiplatelet therapy. It has been clearly demonstrated that long-term follow-up shows lesser incidence of cardiac events, when CCTA is embedded in chest pain pathways.[1-3]

Stable Angina/Ischemia with No Obstructive Coronary Arteries

The ISCHEMIA trial demonstrated that, in patients with moderate-to-severe ischemia, optimized medical therapy (OMT) is as effective as an initial invasive strategy in reducing hard clinical outcomes. This reserves the revascularization for symptomatic select patients. Imaging is *"The Gatekeeper"* that identifies ischemia mechanism and severity to tailor OMT.[4]

HEART FAILURE

Echocardiography and CMR determine ventricular ejection fraction and etiology. It helps in initiation and titration of quadruple GDMT (ARNI/ACEi/ARB, beta-blocker, MRA, SGLT-2 inhibitor) and also in flagging phenotypes (amyloid, sarcoid, and valvular).[5]

CORONARY COMPUTED TOMOGRAPHY ANGIOGRAPHY AND CORONARY ARTERY CALCIUM: ROLE IN DIAGNOSIS AND MANAGEMENT

Risk, Prevention, and Chest Pain Strategies

Guidelines now endorse CCTA (and stress imaging) as first-line in intermediate-to-high risk stable chest pain. CCTA clarifies obstructive versus nonobstructive CAD and total plaque burden, enabling targeted statin intensification, addition of ezetimibe/PCSK9 in very-high risk substrates and lifestyle prescriptions.[6-9]

SCOT-HEART: Incorporating CCTA into the evaluation of stable chest pain led to preventive use (statins/antiplatelets) and lower incidence of cardiac events over long-term follow-up. This implicates the medical optimization and avoids unwarranted revascularization.[1-3]

PROMISE: An anatomic (CCTA) versus functional testing strategy showed similar hard clinical outcomes at 2 years; however, CCTA improved diagnostic certainty and downstream preventive care in many analyses.[10,11]

Coronary artery calcium (CAC) scoring (noncontrast CT) is guideline-endorsed to resolve statin uncertainty:

CAC = 0 can suggest avoidance of statins in selected intermediate-risk adults (absent diabetes, smoking, and strong family history).

CAC ≥100 or ≥75th percentile favors/intensified statin therapy. Higher the calcium score also more is the need of lipid lowering agents as LDL-C threshold is low.[8,9,12,13]

Beyond Stenosis: Computed Tomography-derived Fractional Flow Reserve and Plaque Features

Computed tomography-derived FFR reclassifies lesion physiology and guides anti-anginal versus invasive strategy. Comparative studies proved improvement in the patient management, cost-benefit, and quality of life when computed tomography-derived fractional flow reserve (CT-FFR) is combined with CCTA.[14-16]

High-risk plaque on CCTA (low-attenuation, positive remodeling, and napkin-ring) identifies patients who may benefit from statin intensification and aggressive risk factor modification even without severe stenosis.[17]

Imaging-to-therapy Pathway (Coronary CT Angiography/Coronary Artery Calcium)

No plaque/CAC= 0: Emphasize lifestyle; defer statin, if truly low risk; avoid aspirin in primary prevention.

Non-obstructive CAD or CAC 1–99: Start/intensify statin, optimize medical management for hypertension, obesity, nicotine addiction. If LDL-C above the goals, then consider for adding ezetimibe/bempedoic acid. Aspirin is usually not for primary prevention unless indicated.

Obstructive CAD or high-risk plaque/CAC ≥100: High-intensity statin, consider ezetimibe/PCSK9 to reach guideline LDL-C targets; add antianginals; pursue ischemia testing or CT-FFR to decide on revascularization versus OMT.

FUNCTIONAL IMAGING (SPECT, PET, STRESS CMR, STRESS ECHOCARDIOGRAPHY): GUIDING ANTI-ANGINALS, REVASCULARIZATION, AND INOCA CARE

Choosing a Functional Modality

Guidelines treat stress imaging [echocardiography, single photon emission computed tomography (SPECT), positron emission tomography (PET), cardiovascular magnetic resonance (CMR)] as equivalent first-line options for intermediate to high-risk chest pain; selection rests on availability, patient factors, and the need for quantitative perfusion or flow.[6,18,19]

What Ischemia Suggests About Future Therapy Options

The severity of ischemia guides the intensification of anti-anginal therapy (beta-blocker, CCB, nitrates, ranolazine), aggressive lipid-lowering therapy and optimal blood pressure control, and if required, revascularization for symptomatic relief.

ISCHEMIA reframed expectations: For patients with moderate to severe ischemia with preserved LV function, initial OMT (high-intensity statin, antiplatelet when indicated, anti-anginals and lifestyle) matches early invasive strategy for hard endpoints like death and MI at 3–5 years; revascularization primarily improves angina and quality of life.[4]

Positron Emission Tomography with Myocardial Blood Flow/Myocardial Flow Reserve Quantification

By enabling physiology-based personalization of therapy, PET uniquely quantifies myocardial blood flow (MBF) and myocardial flow reserve (MFR), exposing microvascular dysfunction (CMD) and diffuse atherosclerosis. Low MFR predicts adverse outcomes and prompts therapy intensification even with non-obstructive coronaries (statins, ACEi/ARB, SGLT2i/GLP-1RA, symptom-directed anti-anginals, exercise, and weight loss).[20-23]

Stress Cardiovascular Magnetic Resonance

Anatomy + ischemia + tissue for tailored OMT

Stress CMR reveals high-resolution perfusion, ventricular function, and scar/edema mapping. MR-INFORM trial showed a stress-CMR-guided strategy was non-inferior to an invasive FFR-guided strategy for MACE. It also highlights the capacity of CMR to optimize medical therapy without compromising safety.[24-26]

Stress Echocardiography

Stress echo remains accessible, radiation-free, and excellent tool for ischemia and valve evaluation (e.g., dynamic MR, exercise-induced gradients). It effectively guides anti-anginal management and referral for revascularization when wall-motion ischemia is extensive.

Imaging-to-therapy Pathway (Functional Imaging) (Table 1)

No ischemia: Emphasize prevention; if symptomatic, evaluate for INOCA/CMD (consider PET MFR), adjust anti-anginals (e.g., CCBs/ranolazine/trimetazidine).

Mild-moderate ischemia: Prioritize OMT; adjust anti-anginals; consider CT-FFR or invasive physiology if symptoms persist.

Severe ischemia or high-risk features (LV dysfunction, extensive scar): Optimize OMT and consider revascularization for symptoms/selected prognostic scenarios.

ECHOCARDIOGRAPHY ACROSS THE THERAPEUTIC JOURNEY

Heart failure [Heart Failure with Reduced Ejection Fraction/ Heart Failure with Mid-range (Or Mildly Reduced) Ejection Fraction/Heart Failure with Preserved Ejection Fraction]

Echocardiography is the first-line tool to determine EF, mechanics, filling pressures, and right-sided function—

TABLE 1: Imaging to therapy approach.

Condition	Assessment	Management
Stable chest pain (no known CAD) with intermediate–high pretest risk	CCT (± CT-FFR)	• No plaque/CAC = 0 → Lifestyle changes; defer statin if appropriate • Non-obstructive plaque → Start/intensify statin, risk-factor control, GLP-1RA/SGLT-2i in diabetes, avoid aspirin in primary prevention • Obstructive CAD → OMT (high-intensity statin, antiplatelet if indicated, anti-anginals), ischemia assessment for revascularization
	Stress imaging	• No/minimal ischemia → OMT; evaluate INOCA/CMD if symptoms persist (consider PET MFR) • Moderate–severe ischemia → OMT first; revascularize for refractory symptoms or specific anatomies
Chronic coronary syndrome with angina	Guided by ischemia burden and mechanism	• *Antianginals*: beta-blocker → CCB/long-acting nitrates → ranolazine/ ivabradine - Titrate to symptom relief with BP/HR targets • Consider revascularization for QoL or prognostic subsets (e.g., left main, extensive ischemia + LV dysfunction)
Heart failure	Echo (± CMR) to define EF and etiology	• *Initiate/up-titrate*: ARNI/ACEi/ARB, beta-blocker, MRA, SGLT-2i • Use echo to monitor reverse remodeling and functional CMR • Add devices if criteria met
Cardio-Oncology	Baseline echo + GLS - surveillance every 3–6 cycles	• If >15% GLS drop or EF decline → Start ACEi/ARB and beta-blocker • Oncologic dose modifications
Pulmonary hypertension	Echo + biomarkers + 6MWD/ CPET for risk stratification	• Initial combination therapy • Repeat echo at 3–6 months for further guidance

measurements that help in initiating, titrating, and monitoring GDMT. The 2022 AHA/ACC/HFSA guideline recommends quadruple therapy in HFrEF and emphasizes imaging to detect etiologies (ischemic vs. non-ischemic), concomitant valvular disease, and pulmonary pressures. Serial echocardiographic evaluation supports up-titration and evaluates response (reverse remodeling and MR reduction).[5]

Global longitudinal strain (GLS) detects subclinical systolic dysfunction and can motivate earlier ACEi/ARB/ARNI or cardio-toxicity mitigation. Emerging consensus documents codify GLS thresholds and use cases.[27]

Valvular Heart Disease

For mitral, aortic, and tricuspid valve stenotic and regurgitation lesions, echo characterizes severity, mechanism, and hemodynamic impact. Even when the definitive therapy is interventional, echo optimizes medical therapy (e.g., diuretics and afterload reduction in MR/AR; blood pressure control in AS; diuretics and pulmonary vasodilators where indicated in TR) and identifies timing for referral.

ESC/EACTS 2021 VHD guidelines highlight "echocardiography" as the key modality for serial follow-up and decision-making.[28,29]

Cardio-Oncology

In patients receiving potentially cardio-toxic therapy (anthracyclines, HER2-targeted agents, TKIs), GLS declines >15% from baseline signals subclinical cardiotoxicity and triggers early cardioprotective therapy (ACEi/ARB, beta-blocker) or treatment modification.[30,31]

Pulmonary Hypertension/Right Heart Failure

Echo estimates pulmonary pressures, RV size/function, and RV-PA coupling (TAPSE/PASP), informing risk-based initiation and escalation of PAH therapies. The 2022 ESC/ERS PH guideline endorses serial imaging as part of comprehensive risk assessment guiding combination therapy and escalation.[32,33]

SPECIAL SITUATIONS WHERE IMAGING PIVOTS THERAPY

INOCA and Microvascular Angina

Positron emission tomography MFR <2 (or markedly reduced hyperemic MBF) supports endotype-specific therapy CCB/nitrates for vasospasm; beta-blocker or ranolazine for microvascular dysfunction and aggressive preventive therapy regardless of coronary stenosis.[20,23]

Myocardial Scar/Viability

Cardiovascular magnetic resonance late gadolinium enhancement (LGE) and PET FDG scan identify scar burden and non-viable myocardium directs OMT versus device therapy decisions.

Infiltrative Disease (e.g., Amyloidosis)

Echo strain apical-sparing pattern plus CMR T1/extracellular volume and bone-tracer scintigraphy directs the disease-modifying therapy (e.g., tafamidis in ATTR-CM) and HF regimen tailoring.

Hypertension and Left Ventricular Hypertrophy

Echo-detected concentric left ventricular hypertrophy (LVH) and diastolic dysfunction support tighter BP targets and agent selection (RAAS blockade, SGLT-2i in diabetic hypertension) with regression of LVH as a trackable target.

Athlete's Heart Versus Pathology

Strain, diastolic indices, and RV parameters separate physiology from cardiomyopathy, preventing over-treatment or unwarranted restrictions.

PUTTING IT INTO PRACTICE: CONCISE IMAGING-TO-THERAPY ALGORITHMS

Stable Chest Pain (No Known CAD)

- Pretest risk intermediate–high → CCTA (± CT-FFR) or stress imaging per guideline.[6,18]
- *CCTA*: No plaque/CAC = 0 → lifestyle; defer statin if appropriate.

Nonobstructive plaque → start or intensify statin; risk-factor blitz; consider GLP-1RA/SGLT-2i in diabetes; usually avoid aspirin in primary prevention.

Obstructive CAD → OMT (high-intensity statin, antiplatelet if indicated, antianginals); ischemia assessment (CT-FFR or stress imaging) for revascularization decisions.

- *Stress imaging*: No/minimal ischemia → OMT; evaluate INOCA/CMD if symptoms persist (consider PET MFR).

Moderate–severe ischemia → OMT first; revascularize for refractory symptoms or specific anatomies.

Chronic Coronary Syndrome with Angina

Antianginal therapy guided by ischemia burden and mechanism: Beta-blocker → CCB/long-acting nitrates → ranolazine/ivabradine; titrate to symptom relief with BP/HR targets; consider revascularization for QoL or prognostic subsets (left main, extensive ischemia + LV dysfunction).

Heart Failure

Echo (± CMR) defines EF and etiology → initiate and up-titrate ARNI/ACEi/ARB, beta-blocker, MRA, SGLT-2i; use echo to track reverse remodeling and functional MR improvement; add devices if criteria met.

Cardio-Oncology

Baseline echo + GLS → q3–6 cycle surveillance; >15% GLS drop or EF decline → start ACEi/ARB and beta-blocker, coordinate oncologic dose modifications per guideline.[30]

Pulmonary Hypertension

Echo + biomarkers + 6MWD/CPET → risk stratification → initial combination therapy; repeat echo at 3–6 months to decide escalation or de-escalation.[32]

PRACTICAL TIPS, PITFALLS, AND STEWARDSHIP

Match the question to the modality: Anatomy (CCTA/CAC), physiology (PET/SPECT/CMR/echo), tissue (CMR/PET), hemodynamics (echo).

Use quantitative metrics when available: MFR on PET; GLS on echo; extracellular volume on CMR; plaque burden on CCTA. Numbers drive therapy.

Beware of "treating the test": Tie every imaging finding to a specific medication action and a follow-up plan (e.g., LDL-C target, antianginal titration, GDMT up-titration).

Equity and access: Where PET/CMR are not available, stress echo or SPECT remain excellent for ischemia; CAC is widely accessible and inexpensive for risk decisions.

Radiation and contrast safety: Prefer stress echo/CMR in younger patients or when cumulative dose is a concern; check renal function for iodinated or gadolinium contrast.

Reassessment matters: Schedule time-bound follow-up (e.g., 6–12 weeks after therapy change) with repeat imaging only when it will change management.

FUTURE DIRECTIONS

Artificial intelligence (AI)-assisted CCTA (automated plaque quantification and on-site CT-FFR) to standardize who needs intensification versus invasive testing.[16,34]

Routine MBF/MFR in PET (and emerging dynamic SPECT) to phenotype CMD and guide therapies under study (endothelial agents and metabolic modulators).[21,26]

Strain-guided HF and cardio-oncology protocols using GLS to trigger earlier GDMT or cardioprotection.[27,31]

CONCLUSION

Thoughtful integration of contemporary cardiac imaging, including CCTA, functional ischemia testing, and echocardiography, optimizes medical therapy by identifying actionable disease characteristics and redefining cardiac risk. Imaging-guided strategies enhance preventive therapy use, improve symptom control, and avoid unnecessary interventions. An evidence-based "imaging-to-therapy" approach enables informed decisions in lipid-lowering, antithrombotic, heart failure, and pulmonary hypertension management, ensuring precise, patient-centered cardiovascular care.

REFERENCES

1. Williams MC, Wereski R, Tuck C, et al. Coronary CT angiography-guided management of patients with stable chest pain: 10-year outcomes from the SCOT-HEART randomised controlled trial in Scotland. Lancet. 2025;405(10475):329-37.
2. Newby DE, Adamson PD, Berry C, et al. Coronary CT angiography and MI prevention in patients with stable chest pain. N Engl J Med. 2018;379:924-33.
3. Generoso G, Agarwal V, Shaw LJ, Changes in use of preventive medications after assessment of chest pain by coronary computed tomography angiography: A meta-analysis. J Cardiovasc Comput Tomogr. 2024;18(3):233-42.
4. Maron DJ, Hochman JS, Reynolds HR, et al. Initial invasive vs conservative management for stable ischemic heart disease. N Engl J Med. 2020;382(1):1395-407.
5. Heidenreich PA, Bozkurt B, Aguilar D, et al. 2022 AHA/ACC/HFSA Guideline for the Management of Heart Failure. J Am Coll Cardiol. 2022;79:e263-e421.
6. Gulati M, Levy PD, Mukherjee D, et al. 021AHA/ACC/ASE/SAEM/SCCT/SCMR Guideline for the Evaluation and Diagnosis of Chest Pain. Circulation. 2021;144:e368-e454.
7. Blankstein, R, Gulati, M, Jaber, W. et al. The 2021 Chest Pain Guideline: A Revolutionary New Paradigm for Cardiac Testing. JACC Cardiovasc Imaging. 2022;15(1):140-4.
8. Grundy SM, Stone NJ, Bailey AL, et al. 2018 AHA/ACC Multisociety Guideline on the Management of Blood Cholesterol. Circulation. 2019;139:e1082-143.
9. Bittner V. New ACC-AHA cholesterol guidelines significantly increase potential eligibility for statin treatment. Evid Based Med. 2014;19(5):198.
10. Douglas PS, Hoffmann U, Patel MR, et al. Anatomic vs functional testing for suspected CAD. N Engl J Med. 2015;372(14):1291-300.
11. Hoffmann U, Ferencik M, Udelson JE, et al. Prognostic Value of Noninvasive Cardiovascular Testing in Patients With Stable Chest Pain: Insights From the PROMISE Trial (Prospective Multicenter Imaging Study for Evaluation of Chest Pain). Circulation. 2017;135(24):2320-32.
12. Taron J, Lyass A, Mahoney TF, et al. Coronary Artery Calcium Score-Directed Primary Prevention With Statins on the Basis of the 2018 American College of Cardiology/American Heart Association/Multisociety Cholesterol Guidelines. J Am Heart Assoc. 2021;10(1):e018342.
13. Golub IS, Termeie OG, Kristo S, et al. Major Global Coronary Artery Calcium Guidelines. JACC Cardiovasc Imaging. 2023;16(1):98-117.
14. Douglas PS, Bruyne BD, Pontone G, et al. 1-Year Outcomes of FFRCT-Guided Care in Patients With Suspected Coronary Disease: The PLATFORM Study. J Am Coll Cardiol. 2016;68(5):435-45.

15. Nørgaard BL, Leipsic J, Gaur S, et al. Diagnostic performance of noninvasive fractional flow reserve derived from coronary computed tomography angiography in suspected coronary artery disease: the NXT trial (Analysis of Coronary Blood Flow Using CT Angiography: Next Steps). J Am Coll Cardiol. 2014;63(12):1145-55.
16. Coenen A, Kim YH, Kruk M, et al. Diagnostic Accuracy of a Machine-Learning Approach to Coronary Computed Tomographic Angiography-Based Fractional Flow Reserve: Result From the MACHINE Consortium. Circ Cardiovasc Imaging. 2018;11(6):e007217.
17. Lee SE, Sung JM, Andreini D, et al. Differences in Progression to Obstructive Lesions per High-Risk Plaque Features and Plaque Volumes With CCTA. JACC Cardiovasc Imaging. 2020;13(6): 1409-1417.
18. Gulati M, Levy PD, Mukherjee D, et al. 2021 AHA/ACC/ASE/CHEST/SAEM/SCCT/SCMR guideline for the evaluation and diagnosis of chest pain: a report of the American College of Cardiology/American Heart Association Joint Committee on Clinical Practice Guidelines. J Am Coll Cardiol . 2021:78:e187-e285
19. Zhou W, Sin J, Yan AT, et al. Qualitative and Quantitative Stress Perfusion Cardiac Magnetic Resonance in Clinical Practice: A Comprehensive Review. Diagnostics (Basel). 2023;13(3):524.
20. Murthy, Venkatesh L, Beanlands RS, et al. Clinical Quantification of Myocardial Blood Flow Using PET: Joint Position Paper of the SNMMI Cardiovascular Council and the ASNC. J Nucl Med. 2018;59(2):273-93.
21. Pelletier-Galarneau M, Martineau P, El Fakhri G. Quantification of PET Myocardial Blood Flow. Curr Cardiol Rep. 2019;21(3):11.
22. Rasmussen LD, Gormsen LC, Ejlersen JA, et al. Impact of absolute MBF quantification on clinical decision-making. Circ Cardiovasc Imaging. 2024;17(1):e016138.
23. Taqueti VR, Di Carli MF. Coronary Microvascular Disease Pathogenic Mechanisms and Therapeutic Options: JACC State-of-the-Art Review. J Am Coll Cardiol. 2018;72(21):2625-41.
24. Hamilton-Craig C, Ugander M, Greenwood JP, et al. Stress perfusion cardiovascular magnetic resonance imaging: a guide for the general cardiologist. Heart. 2023;109(6):428-433.
25. Nagel E, Greenwood JP, McCann GP, et al. Magnetic resonance perfusion or fractional flow reserve in coronary disease. N Engl J Med. 2019;380:2418-28.
26. Yuka Otaki. Beyond perfusion imaging: the growing clinical role of myocardial blood flow quantification by SPECT. J Cardiol. 2025:S0914-5087(25)00136-4.
27. Mihos CG, Liu JE, Anderson KM, et al. Speckle-Tracking Strain Echocardiography for the Assessment of Left Ventricular Structure and Function: A Scientific Statement From the American Heart Association. Circulation. 2025;152(10):e96-e109.
28. Vahanian A, Beyersdorf F, Praz F, et al. 2021 ESC/EACTS Guidelines for management of valvular heart disease. Eur Heart J. 2022;43:561-632.
29. Vahanian A, Beyersdorf F, Praz F, et al. 2021 ESC/EACTS Guidelines for the management of valvular heart disease. Eur Heart J. 2022;43(7):561-632.
30. Lyon AR, López-Fernández T, Couch LS, et al. 2022 ESC Cardio-Oncology Guidelines. Eur Heart J. 2022;43:4229-4361.
31. Sławiński G, Hawryszko M, Liżewska-Springer A, et al. Global Longitudinal Strain in Cardio-Oncology: A Review. Cancers (Basel). 2023;15(3):986.
32. Humbert M, Kovacs G, Hoeper MM, et al. 2022 ESC/ERS Guidelines for pulmonary hypertension. Eur Heart J. 2022;43:3618-731.
33. Humbert M, Kovacs G, Hoeper MM, et al. 2022 ESC/ERS Guidelines for the diagnosis and treatment of pulmonary hypertension. Eur Respir J. 2023;61(1):2200879.
34. Zhang LJ, Chen Q, Tang CX, et al. Consensus on the research and application of artificial intelligence in coronary computed tomography angiography. Intelligent Med. 2025;5(3): 234-42.

Index

Page numbers followed by *b* refer to box, *f* refer to figure, *fc* refer to flowchart, and *t* refer to table.

A

Ablation, acute 614
Abnormal cardiac function 132
Acamprosate 330
Acetaldehyde 327*f*
Acetazolamide 246, 249
Acetylsalicylic acid 141
Actin myosin complex 222*f*
Activated partial thromboplastin time 533
Activates nucleotide oligomerization 139*f*
Active cellular processes 474
Acute coronary syndrome 141, 237, 540
  whole spectrum of 540
Acute heart failure 158, 199*t*, 246, 250, 269
  management of 248, 510*f*
  risk models for 158
  risk scores 157, 160*t*
  syndromes 236
Acute kidney injury 250
Acute myocardial infarction 232, 677
Acute rheumatic fever 456-458, 460, 460*fc*, 486
  manifestations of 461, 463
  pathophysiology of 458
  prevention of 464
  secondary prophylaxis of 467
Adipokines 142*f*
Adipose tissue, subcutaneous 538
Adiposity management 73
Adjunctive therapies 228
Adrenal hyperplasia, bilateral 37
Adrenal incidentalomas 38
Adrenal vein sampling 37, 39
Adrenalectomy 37
Advanced echocardiographic assessment 421
Advanced heart failure 160, 164, 165*t*, 378
  long-term management of 167
  pathophysiology of 164
  risk scores 161*t*
  therapies 129
  treatment strategies of 164
Advanced hemodynamic modeling 270
Advanced therapy risk assessment 269
AI-enhanced hypertension management 31, 31*t*
Air pollution 8, 9, 73
  burden 8
  changing ecology of 8
  composition 9
Air-quality index 73
Albuminuria 136
Alcohol 60
  abstinence 330, 331
  consumption, cardiovascular effects of 326
  direct toxic effect of 327*f*
  moderation 622
Alcoholic cardiomyopathy 326, 327*f*, 329*f*, 331*f*, 331*fc*
  comprehensive assessment of 328*fc*
  pathogenesis of 327
  pathophysiology of 327*f*
  prevalence of 326
  signs of 328
  symptoms of 328
Alcoholism, chronic 327
Aldehyde dehydrogenase inhibitor 330
Aldosterone synthase inhibitors 56, 62
Aldosteronism, primary 37, 38*t*, 39*fc*
Ambulatory rhythm monitoring 434
American College of Cardiology 96, 165
  Foundation Risk-based Framework 279
American College of Obstetricians and Gynecologists 512
American Heart Association 96, 165, 279, 467, 468, 468*fc*, 512
Amiodarone 566
  higher dosage of 566
Amplatzer duct occlude 390
Amplatzer vascular plugs 390
Amyloid 208
Amyloidosis 687
Anchor stent 340
Anemia, classification of 150
Anesthesia, general 348
Aneurysms 550*b*
  aortic 20
  apical 284, 285
  coronary 551*f*
  multiple 552*f*
  transcatheter management of 551*f*
  types of 549*f*
Angina 686, 687
  microvascular 571, 677, 687
  stable 684
  unstable 141
Angiography
  invasive 85
  techniques 671
Angiotensin 47, 228
Angiotensin-converting enzyme inhibitor 47, 379
Angiotensin-receptor
  blockers 47
  neprilysin inhibitor 61, 169, 171, 172, 192, 255, 256, 379
Anomalous coronary artery 387
Anorexia 148
Antepartum cardiovascular risk assessment 505, 506
Anti-anginal therapy, intensification of 685
Antiapoptotic B-cell lymphoma 47
Antiarrhythmic drugs 320
Antibiotics 243
Anticoagulant 528, 530, 533*t*
  therapies 529
  treatment 512*t*
Anticoagulation 278*f*, 509, 509*t*, 512, 517, 572
  inadequate use of 573
  management of 512*t*, 533
  oral 481
  regimen 530, 530*t*
Anti-inflammatory
  agents 141*t*
  therapy 74, 554
Antiplatelet 525, 685
  therapy 545
Aorta 434, 465
  coarctation of 365*f*, 402
Aortic diameter 508, 508*t*
Aortic dissection 554, 559
Aortic jet velocity 440
Aortic regurgitation 262, 458, 465, 647, 648
  acute 261*f*
  chronic 261*f*, 657, 658, 660
  grading severity of 658
  stages of 658
Aortic sinus 634, 635*f*

Aortic stenosis 155, 260, 262, 419, 439, 443, 448*f*, 451, 465, 473, 500, 647-649, 651
  asymptomatic 419, 420
  catheterization evaluation of 477
  early 444
  echocardiographic evaluation of 476
  grading severity of 476*t*
  high-gradient 439, 441
  mild 446
  natural history of 419
  pathophysiology of 419
  severe 261*f*, 440, 653*f*
  severity 440
    echocardiographic assessment of 439
  staging classification 444*f*
Aortic syndromes 560*t*
Aortic vagal nerve stimulation 194
Aortic valve 465, 473*f*, 474*f*, 648*t*, 650, 650*f*, 652
  area 262, 439, 465, 476, 649, 651
    calculation of 440
    measurement of 653*f*
  calcification 651, 652*fc*
  calcium 647, 648, 652*f*
    score 465
  fibrocalcific volume 653*f*
  pathophysiology 473
  replacement 439, 448
  stenosis 508
Aortopulmonary shunt 349, 350
Apolipoprotein B 90, 102
Apoptosis 49, 212
Arrhythmia 79, 292, 298*f*, 308, 318, 320, 343, 394, 399, 408, 510, 621, 630
  cardiac 563
  management 331, 565
  origin of 634
  ventricular 275, 394, 433, 637*f*
Arrhythmia-induced cardiomyopathy 318, 319*f*, 320, 324*fc*, 599
  classification of 318*f*
Arrhythmic risk 620, 621*fc*
Arrhythmogenesis 575
Arrhythmogenic right ventricular cardiomyopathy 294, 297, 620
Arterial hypertension, severe pulmonary 398
Arterial stiffness 69
Arterial wall thickening 555*f*
Arterioles 678
Artery
  disease, peripheral 554
  pulmonary 387
Arthritis 461
Artificial intelligence 29, 30, 32, 69, 73, 162, 228, 270, 353, 367, 447
  fundamentals of 29
  limitations of 367
Aspirin, low-dose 525, 530
Asymptomatic left ventricular dysfunction 132
Atherogenic lipid control 73
Atherogenicity 101
Atherosclerosis 9, 48, 105, 108*f*, 139*f*, 554, 555*f*, 556, 556*t*, 557, 571, 684
  advanced 670
  initiation 106*f*
  prevention 112*f*
Atherosclerotic cardiovascular disease 79, 95, 101
  adult 113*t*
  risk 101, 102
Atherothrombosis 545
Athlete's heart 687
Atrial arrhythmias 346, 346*t*, 394
Atrial dyssynchrony 576
Atrial fibrillation 128, 155, 185, 186, 189, 276, 283, 318, 570-572, 598, 626, 630*t*
  ablation 599
    trials of 600*t*, 604*t*
  phenotype 572
Atrial flutter 609
Atrial functional mitral regurgitation 429*f*
Atrial regions perturbs, relaxation of 576
Atrial secondary mitral regurgitation 427
  management of 428
  phenotypes of 428*f*
Atrial septal defects 343, 353, 355*f*, 357*f*, 387, 390, 398-401
  closure 346
  secundum 355*f*
Atrial strain 575
Atrioventricular coupling index 207
Atrioventricular nodal
  ablation 320
  re-entrant tachycardia 320
Atrioventricular node 634
Atrioventricular valve regurgitation 374
Autoinflammatory diseases 313
Automated external defibrillators 620, 622
Automatic plaque identification 665
Autonomic nervous system imbalance 322

B

B cells 142
Balloon
  diameter of 338
  inflation 339*f*
  pulmonary valvuloplasty 348
  valvotomy 499
Balloon-assisted atrial septal defect device deployment 390
Baroreceptor activation therapy 192
Baroreflex activation therapy 56, 63, 124, 195
Barrier dysfunction 242
Barth syndrome 394
Baseline therapy, optimization of 61
Benzathine penicillin G 456, 468
Beta 2-stimulated glycolysis 223
Beta-blockers 169, 255, 320, 560, 636, 685
Bethesda disease complexity classification 344
Bicuspid aortic valve 356*f*, 451
Bile acid metabolites 242
Bileaflet mitral valve prolapse 434*f*, 435*f*
Biomolecular techniques, use of 585
Bioprosthetic valves 533
Bioresorbable pacemakers 591
Biplane transesophageal echocardiogram 586*f*
Bleeding, postpartum 532
Blood
  loss, occult 148
  oxygen level 47
  pressure 29, 47, 237
    control 25, 73
    measurement 30
    monitoring 30
    systolic 159, 233, 260
    variability 27
  urea nitrogen 159
Body mass index 73
  category 77
Brain natriuretic peptide 237, 506
Branch pulmonary arteries 349*f*
  reconstruction of 408
Breast cancer treatments 541
Breastfeeding 524
Bromocriptine 517
Bromodomain 143
Bull's eye map 215*f*, 216*f*
Bupropion 19

C

Calcification 465, 474
  histopathology of 671
Calcified aortic valve pathology 475*f*
Calcitropes, mechanism of action of 222*fc*
Calcium
  deposits 465
  sensitizers 224
California Maternal Quality Care Collaborative 505
Calorie consumption, high 77*fc*
Carbonic anhydrase inhibitors 248
Cardiac arrest, resuscitated 141

Cardiac biomarkers 84
Cardiac computed tomography 353, 360, 578, 648, 677, 679
 electrocardiography-gated 336
Cardiac contractility modulation 117, 124
Cardiac cycle 660*f*
Cardiac damage 443, 444, 446
 extent of 444*f*
 potential determinants of 448*f*
 stage, evolution of 445, 629*f*
Cardiac delivery, high-risk 505
Cardiac dysfunction 142*f*
Cardiac fibroblastic activity assessment 208
Cardiac imaging 282
Cardiac implantable electronic device 188, 189, 584
 extraction 587
  hardware, nonavailability of 589
 infection
  guideline directed management of 584
  management protocol 587*fc*
 reimplantation plan 590
Cardiac index 260, 262
Cardiac injury 142*f*
Cardiac interventions 499, 500, 501*t*
 indications for 500
Cardiac involvement, assessment of 314
Cardiac magnetic resonance 141, 205-207, 276, 278, 281, 283, 284, 294, 297, 353, 434, 465, 648, 649
 abnormalities 285*t*
 finger printing 363
 imaging 85, 329, 337, 361, 362, 411*f*, 419, 436*f*, 577, 648, 652, 655, 674
Cardiac myocytes 213*f*, 222
Cardiac output 230, 233, 267, 374
Cardiac perforation 595
Cardiac resynchronization therapy 206, 381, 575, 578, 579
 role of 383
 selection 209
Cardiac shear wave elastography 208
Cardiac transplant 267
Cardiac troponin levels 132
Cardiac valve disorders 646
Cardiogenic shock 174, 176, 177, 220, 221, 221*f*, 225*t*, 230, 232, 232*t*, 233, 260, 263, 269, 542
 classification of 229*t*
 evaluation of 233
 features of 220*t*
 management of 227*fc*, 233
 medical therapy of 220
 pathophysiology of 221*fc*
 pharmacological management of 263
 risk stratifying continuum of 232
 treatment 228*t*
Cardiological Society of India 10
Cardiometabolic drugs 243
Cardiometabolic health 69
Cardiomyocytes 212
Cardiomyopathy 82, 135, 273, 292, 294, 309, 318, 320*t*, 505, 510*f*
 abnormal conduction induced 320
 alcoholic 326, 327*f*, 329*f*, 331*f*, 331*fc*
 arrhythmia-induced 318, 319*f*, 320, 324*fc*, 599
 atrial fibrillation-induced 321
 causes of 328
 clinical diagnostic workflow of 294*f*
 dilated 206, 292, 294, 297, 306-309, 310*t*, 313, 326
 dual 292
 end-stage hypertrophic 279
 hypertrophic 275-281, 283-285, 285*t*, 289, 289*fc*, 294, 297, 510, 620
 inherited 294
 ischemic 84, 154, 209, 292, 566, 612
 management of 297*f*
 pediatric 393
 peripartum 320, 500, 510, 515, 517
 restrictive 297
 reversible causes of 320*t*
 severe peripartum 517
 stress-induced 320
 tachycardia-induced 318, 570
Cardioneuroablation therapy 300, 304
Cardio-obstetrics 497
 team 505
Cardio-oncology 216, 686-688
Cardiopulmonary bypass 348
Cardiopulmonary exercise testing 155
Cardiorenal cachexia 537
Cardiovascular aging
 drivers of 71*f*
 epigenetic determinants of 71
Cardiovascular changes 523*t*
Cardiovascular death 523
Cardiovascular disease 3, 4, 8, 17, 18, 25, 29, 76, 78*f*, 79, 105, 106, 109*f*, 307, 505, 506, 520, 554, 556
 acute 175
 escalating burden of 3
 prompt recognition of 506
 risk 13
Cardiovascular disorders 528
Cardiovascular effect 70, 70*t*
Cardiovascular health 520, 525*f*
 risks 524
Cardiovascular implantable electronic device 183-185
Cardiovascular implications 70
Cardiovascular outcome, long-term 520, 571
Cardiovascular relevance 72, 72*t*
Cardiovascular risk 12, 13, 76, 520, 523
 assessment 524
 factors 78
Carditis 461
 classification of 457
CardShock risk score 232*t*
Catecholamines 222
Catheter ablation 292, 570, 572, 598, 603, 612, 615*b*, 625
 approaches 616
 procedural aspects of 616
 role of 598, 614
Catheter-directed pulmonary thrombectomy 503
Cavoatrial incision 335
Cell-based therapies 51
Cellular mechanisms 420
Centor criteria, modified 466*f*
Central venous pressure 260
Cerebrovascular accident 141
Cervical vagal nerve stimulation 193
Chemokine receptor 143
Chest
 pain
  stable 687
  strategies 685
 X-ray 400*f*, 403*f*
Chimeric antigen receptors T-cell therapy 310
Chin method 395*f*
Cholesterol
 lipoproteins 105, 111*f*
 Z-scores 109*f*
Chronic coronary syndrome 686, 687
Chronic heart failure 146, 147, 373
 acute decompensation of 236
 evaluation of 373
 management of 373
 severity grading of 375*t*
Chronic heavy alcohol consumption, history of 328
Chronic inflammatory disease 555*f*
Chronic kidney disease 12, 13, 71, 98, 136, 151
Chronic loop diuretic exposure 200
Chronic obstructive pulmonary disease 71, 159
Chronic total occlusion 390
Churg-Strauss syndrome 313
Chylomicrons, remnants of 95
Clonal burden 307
Clonal hematopoiesis 306-308, 310, 556, 557, 559
 mutations 306, 309
 overview of 307
 role of 306, 306*fc*
 therapy-related 309

Cold clammy extremities 220
Communities heart failure risk score, atherosclerosis risk in 158
Complex congenital heart diseases 401
Complex premature ventricular complexes 436*f*
Computed tomography 434, 465, 652, 671, 674, 677, 681
angiography 652, 677
derived fractional flow reserve 641-643, 677, 685
derived myocardial strain analysis 682
emerging roles of 682
myocardial perfusion imaging 677
role of 85, 680
Concomitant valve lesion 465
Conduction
defects 394
system pacing 591
Congenital cardiac research collaborative cohort study 351, 351*t*
Congenital heart disease 292, 333, 342, 343, 345*t*, 353, 373-375, 375*t*, 378, 381, 386, 387, 387*t*, 388*fc*, 389*f*, 391*fc*, 398, 404, 511*t*
across lifespan 342
acyanotic 401
adult 381, 398
assessment of 354
complexity of 343
cyanotic 398, 400
estimates of 386, 387
factors influencing lifetime risk of 343, 343*f*
functional index 344
imaging 367
novel imaging techniques for 353
pediatric 373
Congestion 166, 198, 199
clinical relevance of 199
management of 123, 123*f*, 124*t*
Consciousness, transient loss of 300
Contrast-enhanced computed tomography 652
Conventional two-dimensional transthoracic echo 646, 646*fc*
Coronary angiography 330, 542, 672, 672*f*, 677
Coronary artery
aneurysm 549
complications 550
diagnosis 550
formation 550*b*
management 550
pathophysiology 550
risk factors 550
bypass
grafting 503
surgery 576*f*
calcification 670, 674
clinical implications of 670
current concepts of 670
diagnosis of 671*b*
modifications tools 675*b*
risk factors for 671*b*
calcium 685
scoring 685
disease 20, 105, 141, 155, 293, 327, 535, 641
premature 89, 93*f*
lumen volume-to-myocardial mass ratio 677, 681
network of 679*f*
Coronary atherosclerosis, advancement of 679
Coronary calcium score 670
Coronary computed tomography angiography 641-643, 670, 671, 681, 684, 685
Coronary flow reserve 681
Coronary microvascular circulation, overview of 678
Coronary microvascular dysfunction 139, 209, 537, 677
assessment of 679
diagnosis of 680-682
pathophysiology of 678
types of 538
Coronary revascularization 292
Coronary vasculature, components of 678*t*
Coronary vasospasm 631
C-reactive protein 460
high-sensitivity 141
Creatine kinase-muscle brain 141
Critical Care Cardiology Trials Network 233
Cryoablation 626
Cryoballoon 598
ablation 608
Cumulative valvular injury 456
Cyanosis, reduces duration of 348
Cyclic guanosine monophosphate 143
Cytokine 44, 139, 139*t*
driven myocardial dysfunction 228

D

Dapagliflozin 228
de novo heart failure, clinical profile of 199*b*
Death
causes of 276
rate 488, 489
Decongestion 250
Deep intertrabecular recesses 393
Deep learning 29, 353
Deep myocardial critical channels 568*f*
Delivery planning 511
Dendritic cells 140, 142
Dermatomyositis 313
Device therapy 62, 205
role of 136
Diabetes 78, 84, 98
control 622
management of 136
mellitus 83, 135, 141, 155, 523, 671
Diabetic cardiomyopathy 84
mechanism of development of 84*fc*
Dietary
interventions 80
modulation 243
pattern 72
strategies 59
Diffuse fibrosis 285
identification of 207
Digital health 69, 73
and system solutions 99
Digitoxin 117
role of 121
Dilated cardiomyopathy 206, 292, 294, 297, 306-309, 310*t*, 313, 326
cohorts 307
phenotype 328
pathogenesis of 306, 306*fc*
Dilated dysfunctional right ventricular outflow tract 410*f*
Diltiazem 636
Dimensionless velocity index 465
Direct myocyte toxicity 327
Disability-adjusted life years 486, 487*t*
Distal convoluted tubule 247
Distal tubular hypertrophy 200
Disulfiram 330
Diuretic
classes, sites of action of 248*t*
potentiation strategies 246, 251*fc*
resistance 166, 198, 200, 246
mechanism of 247
therapy 117
monitoring of 250
titration strategy 202*t*
types of 247
Dobutamine 224, 225
stress echocardiography 650
Dopamine 223, 225
Doppler echocardiography 440
Double outlet right ventricle 387
Drug 77, 121, 124, 225, 250, 303, 379, 463
class 171, 248
therapies, novel 121*t*
type 621
Dual-chamber pacemaker 586*f*, 594*f*
Dual-pathway inhibition 554, 560
Ductal stent 348-350

Dysbiosis 241
pathophysiologic consequences of 241
Dyslipidemia 76, 78, 95, 101, 523, 671
management 87
prevalence of 89
screening guidelines for 90

E

Ebstein's anomaly 404
Echocardiographic abnormalities 283*t*
Echocardiography 84, 282, 328, 353, 393, 434, 490*t*, 621-623, 648
across therapeutic journey 686
role of 658
three-dimensional 353, 354, 356, 577
transesophageal 336, 390, 647
E-cigarettes 20
Edema 200
Effective regurgitant orifice area 465, 659
Eisenmenger syndrome 398, 400
Ejection fraction 141, 218, 262, 374
Electrical conduction abnormalities 576
Electrical disease, primary 612, 614
Electrical storm 612, 613
Electrocardiogram 281, 294, 576, 578
Electrocardiographic abnormalities 281*t*
Electrocardiography 328, 434, 436*f*, 620
Electron beam computed tomography 671
Electrophysiologic virtual heart models 205, 210
Electrophysiological abnormalities 343
Electroporation 625
Elevated natriuretic peptide 132
Embolism, coronary 542
Embryology 393
Emergent transcatheter aortic valve implantation 259
Emerging hybrid intracoronary imaging technologies, application of 664
Empagliflozin 228
Endocarditis 584, 585
infective 413
Endocardium 296*f*
Endocrine 320
Endomyocardial biopsy 315*f*, 330
End-organ hypoperfusion, evidence of 260
Endothelial cells 555*f*
Endothelial dysfunction 49, 58, 69, 139*f*, 559
modulation 130
Endothelial nitric oxide synthase 139, 143
Endothelial progenitor cells 47
Endothelial-to-mesenchymal transition 556
Endothelin receptor antagonists 62
Endothelin system 58
Endovascular coiling 552
Eosinophilic granulomatosis 313, 315*f*
Epicardial adipose tissue 208
Epicardial critical sites 567
Epicardial enhancement 296
Epicardial vessel 678
Epigenetic modulation 73
Epigenetic therapies 74
Epinephrine 46, 223, 225
Erythema marginatum 463
Erythrocyte sedimentation rate 460
Erythropoiesis-impaired iron utilization 148
Estimated glomerular filtration rate 171, 172
European Association of Cardiothoracic Surgery 481
European Society of Cardiology 201, 481
guidelines 531
European Society of Cardiology Risk-Sudden Cardiac Death Model 279
Euvolemia, challenge of 200
Excess cardiovascular risk, pathophysiology of 12
Experimental therapy 517
Extracardiac organs 142, 142*f*
Extracellular matrix 143, 213*f*
components 555*f*
Extracellular volume 206, 285, 648, 654
fraction 208
Extracorporeal cardiopulmonary resuscitation 260
Extracorporeal membrane oxygenation 167, 381

F

Fallot tetralogy 345, 348, 353, 381, 387, 398, 400, 404, 408, 409, 409*fc*
Farapulse 630
Fatty acid oxidation 222*fc*
Fecal microbiota transplantation 243
Ferric carboxymaltose 146, 153, 155
Ferric derisomaltose 146
Fibrillation 542
Fibroatheroma 673
Fibrocalcific aortic stenosis 473, 478
pathology of 474
Fibrocalcific aortic valve
disease 473
stenosis, imaging of 476
Fibrocalcific disease 473
Fibrogenic pathways 48
Fibromuscular dysplasia 542
Fibrosed aortic valve pathology 475*f*
Fibrosis 212, 298*f*, 322, 436*f*, 474
assessment of 45
diagnosis of 45
diffuse 285
mechanism of 44
Fibrous aortic valve stenosis 473
Fibrous caps, formation of 555*f*
Flow-dependent hemodynamic parameters 420
Fluid
management 177
retention, pathophysiology of 246
Foam cells 555*f*
Focal replacement fibrosis 207
Fontan
circulation 381, 405
completion, percutaneous 390
fenestration occlusion test 365*f*
Fractional shortening 374
Fragile heath systems 391
Fragment calcification 671
Fragmented QRS complexes 281
Free wall papillary muscles, displacement of 408
Functioning single ventricle physiology 405
Furosemide 249, 249*t*

G

G stimulatory receptor 222
Gadolinium-filled balloon 365*f*
Gastrointestinal comorbidities 148
Gastrointestinal malabsorption 148
Gastrointestinal tract 149
Gaussian mixture model 653*f*
Genes 394
Genetic 394
mutations 285*t*
predisposition 541
risk markers 285
screening 437
susceptibility 327
syndrome 343
testing 377, 620
Genomic technologies 309
Genotype directed therapy 40
Germline dilated cardiomyopathy mutations 308
Giant negative T waves 281
Global longitudinal strain 85, 206, 212, 280, 650
Glomerular filtration rate 47, 200
Glucagon-like peptide 1 256
Glycemia 74
Glycopyrrolate 628
Gorlin equation 477
Granulocyte-colony stimulating factor 47
Granulomatosis 316

Great arteries
congenitally corrected transposition of 381, 403
dextro-transposition of 381
transposition of 381, 390, 405
Group A *Streptococcus* 456
infection, autoimmune sequelae of 486
pharyngitis, nonsuppurative complication of 456
Grown-up congenital heart disease 398
Growth
factors 44
issues 350
Guanosine triphosphate 143
Guideline-directed heart failure therapy 129
Guideline-directed medical therapy 155, 170-172, 189, 190, 202, 297, 331, 424, 426, 427, 572
primary goals of 170
Gut microbiota 241
derived metabolites, role of 241
disorder 142*f*

H

Hazard ratio range 346
Head-up tilt table test 300
Health
benefits 18
timeline of 18*t*
disparities 386
economics 152
education 3
policy 99
social determinants of 343
span 69
Healthcare
intervention strategies 5
system 98
Heart 149
catheterization 267, 267*f*, 268*t*, 270
basics of 268
disease 128*fc*
congenital 292, 333, 342, 343, 345*t*, 353, 373-375, 375*t*, 378, 381, 386, 387, 387*t*, 388*fc*, 389*f*, 391*fc*, 398, 404, 511*t*
hypertensive 43, 44, 45*fc*, 327
ischemic 510, 614
multivalvular 465*t*, 646
rheumatic 456, 456*f*, 457, 458*fc*, 463, 467, 469, 486, 487*t*, 488, 488*t*, 493, 494
structural 132
valvular 80, 190*fc*, 327, 417, 481, 509*f*, 657, 687
failure 20, 26, 79, 83, 84*f*, 85*b*, 115, 117*f*, 118, 123*f*, 124*t*, 126-128, 134*f*, 135*fc*, 138, 139*t*, 140*t*, 141*t*, 142*f*, 147, 148*fc*, 148*t*, 150, 151*t*, 154*t*, 157, 167, 180, 181*fc*, 182*t*, 183, 188, 192, 206, 212, 217*f*, 233, 241, 254, 267, 283, 292, 308, 318, 381, 373, 408, 505, 515, 517, 570, 571, 575, 584, 598, 600*t*, 622, 623, 685-687
acute 158, 199*t*, 246, 250, 269
acute decompensated 147, 152, 153, 155, 236, 237
advanced 160, 164, 165*t*, 378
associated pulmonary hypertension 126
burden of 246
chronic 146, 147, 373
congestive 152, 269
development of 515
etiology of 381
features 394
gut hypothesis of 241
hospitalization 118, 236, 250, 345*t*, 419
immunology of 138
management of 120*f*, 123, 157, 169, 192, 267
mechanism of 381
medication 379*t*, 516
microbial dysbiosis in 241
pathogenesis of 149*fc*
predictor of 216
progression of 181*f*
progressive 276
risk-guided management of 162*fc*
severity 375, 375*t*
stages of 83, 133, 133*t*, 375
studies, major 147*t*
subclinical 132
subtypes 269*t*
symptomatic 134
treatment 270*t*
triage scale 239*fc*
type of 374
injury, inflammation-driven 143*f*
lung transplant 400
pressure 267
problems 621
rate 159, 237
services, congenital 388
stress 132
transplantation 380
valve 528, 533*t*
choice of 530
management of 530
Heart failure with
mildly reduced ejection fraction 182, 254
preserved ejection fraction 128, 139*f*, 143, 147, 154, 182, 183, 189, 193, 254, 269, 280*f*, 374, 537, 598, 599, 686
score 161, 161*t*
reduced ejection fraction 146, 147, 152, 153, 155, 169, 182, 183, 188, 189, 192, 193, 206, 269, 279*f*, 326, 373, 374*t*, 599, 686
HELLP syndrome 520, 521
Hematopoietic stem cells 556
Hemodynamic 464, 646, 647, 657
adaptations 505
classification 126
consequences 474
effects 225
impairment 322
metrics 269
monitoring 174, 233
parameters 267
pattern 262
valve-specific 260
profiles 269
stabilization, achievement of 121
Hemolysis 631
Hepcidin–ferroportin axis 149
High velocity systolic waves 435*f*
High-density lipoprotein-cholesterol 141
High-risk cardiac delivery 505
antepartum cardiovascular risk assessment of 505
His bundle 635, 637*f*
Holter monitoring 620
Hormone replacement therapy 541
Hridyam model 392
Hybrid stent 340
Hydrochlorthiazide 250
Hydroxyephedrine 206, 207
Hypercholesterolemia, familial 90
Hypersensitivity testing 151
Hypertension 23, 25, 29, 38, 43, 56, 59, 76, 78, 128*fc*, 403, 523, 687
detection of 31
diagnosis of 29
gestational 521
management 29, 30*f*, 34*f*
phenotyping of 32
pregnancy-associated 522
primary 32
pulmonary 126-128, 183, 188, 189, 269, 329*f*, 399, 686-688
refractory 56, 63
renovascular 47
resistant 38, 56, 62
risk prediction of 31
secondary 32, 37
uncontrolled 320

Hypertensive disorder 520, 521*t*, 522*f*, 523-525
Hypertensive emergencies 403
Hypertriglyceridemia, persistent 92*fc*
Hypertrophic cardiomyopathy 275-281, 283-285, 285*t*, 289, 289*fc*, 294, 297, 510, 620
Hypertrophy 212
Hypoalbuminemia 200
Hypokalemia 38
Hypoperfusion, clinical evidence of 237
Hypotension, isolated 233
Hypoxia 50
HySyn vasovagal syncope protocol 301

I

Ideal pulmonary valve 413
Idiopathic pulmonary arterial hypertension 399
Immune
activation 44, 242
cells 140
role of 140
injury mechanisms 459
Immunity 556, 557
metabolic control of 557
Immunometabolism 557
Immunomodulation 558
Impaired coronary microcirculation 571
Impaired ventricular mechanics 419
Impella 234, 263
ventricular support systems 167
Impetigo 456
Implantable cardioverter-defibrillator 181, 206, 209, 277, 278, 292, 297, 437, 517, 612, 620
implantation 565
Implantable hemodynamic monitoring, role of 383
Inferior vena cava 390
Infiltrative disease 687
Inflammation 44, 48, 130, 176, 212, 241, 307, 556, 558, 560, 571
chronic 148, 555*f*
targeted therapies 228
Inflammatory biomarkers 138
Inflammatory cytokines, role of 138
Inflammatory mediators 555*f*
Inflammatory pathways 139*f*, 327
Innominate vein
injection 338*f*
obstruction 340
Innovative pediatric cardiac interventions 390*b*
Inotropes 220, 517
contemporary use of 220
mechanism of action of 222, 223*fc*
Integrated care pathway 186
Intensive care unit 237
Intercellular adhesion molecule-1 139
Interferon-gamma 555
Interleukin 139-142, 555
beta 139
receptor 143
Intermittent levosimendan, key clinical trials of 122
Internal jugular vein 595
International Cardiac Implantable Electrical Device Infection Criteria 586
Interstitial fibrosis, diffuse 208
Interventional cardio-obstetrics team care 499
Interventricular septum 278*f*
Intestinal barrier 241
Intestinal fatty acid-binding protein 242
Intra-aortic balloon pump 167, 234, 263
Intracardiac echocardiography 628
catheters 628
Intracoronary imaging 664, 670
modalities 665
Intravascular ultrasound 540, 542, 664, 667, 671, 672
Intravenous iron
formulations 151*t*
supplementation 153*t*, 154*t*
therapy 150
Intrinsic atrial cardiomyopathy 576
Invasive cardiovascular magnetic resonance imaging 364, 365*f*
Invasive coronary angiography 643, 671
Invasive procedure 267
Investigational Device Exemption Study 592
Investigational interventional therapies 130
Iron
deficiency 146-148, 148*t*, 149*fc*, 154
anemia 151-153, 155
global burden of 147
mechanism of 148*fc*
prevalence of 147*t*
staging of 150
states 146
symptoms of 150
oral 151*t*
role 149
supplementation 146, 150
therapy 154
Irreversible left ventricular damage 419
Ischemia 208, 540, 684, 685
assessment 641
guides, severity of 685
microvascular 681
reframed expectations 685
testing, functional 684
transient 320
Ischemic disease 296*f*
Ischemic mitral regurgitation 651*f*
mechanism of 426*f*

J

Jaccoud's arthropathy 461
Jenni method 393, 395, 395*f*
Jones criteria, modified 460, 460*t*, 461*t*
Jugular suture control technique 340
Jugular venous pressure 199

K

Kansas City Cardiomyopathy Questionnaire 155, 250
Kaplan–Meier
analysis 346
curves 580*f*
Kawasaki disease 550
Kidney 150
disease
acute 250
chronic 12, 13, 71, 98, 136, 151
Kinetics 107
Knowledge, attitudes, practices surveys 4

L

Late gadolinium enhancement 206, 207, 275, 276, 278, 283, 284, 653
Lead extraction 584
Leadless devices, newer generation of 593*f*
Leadless pacemakers 591, 593-596
first-generation 592*f*
Leadless pacing, timeline of 596*f*
Leadless self-rechargeable devices 596
Leadless wise cardiac resynchronization therapy system 595*ff*
Left anterior descending artery 672*f*
Left atrial 649, 652
appendage 650
dyssynchrony 575, 578, 581
effect of 575
origins of 576
enlargement 282
posterior wall isolation 608
strain 282
different components of 660*b*
Left atrioventricular coupling index 206
Left atrium 181, 262, 335, 465, 576
Left main coronary artery 672*f*
Left ventricle 184, 188, 189, 283, 353, 426, 465, 576, 647-649
ejection fraction 517

Left ventricular 206, 262, 276, 280, 283, 284, 634, 652
apical aneurysm 278
assist device 167, 182, 269
management 270
diastolic dysfunction 400
dilatation 206, 328
dysfunction 326, 408, 515, 565
dyssynchrony 322
ejection fraction 141, 152, 153, 155, 164, 205, 206, 210, 218*f*, 232, 257, 426, 430, 468, 647, 651
insensitivity of 420
end-diastolic diameter 205, 206, 262, 375
end-systolic volume 141
function 598
marker of 214
recovery 518
global longitudinal strain 284, 660
assessment of 214
hemodynamic overload 420
hypertrophy 329*f*, 443, 465, 687
noncompaction 393, 394
childhood 393
pediatric 396
outflow tract 283, 465, 634
obstruction 280, 282, 297
peak systolic longitudinal strain 215*f*
systolic dysfunction 279, 515
wall strain predict heart failure 212
Lepodisiran 101
Lesion
formation 626
severe 647
Levosimendan 117, 224, 225
Lifelong pulmonary valve, quest for 408
LION-HEART 122
Lipid-lowering therapy 89, 92
implications of 89
Lipoprotein 102, 560
A 91, 101, 558
associated phospholipase A2 141
characteristics of 101
cholesterol
high-density 141
non-high density 95, 97, 105-108, 110
concentrations 90*t*
intermediate-density 95
levels, impact of 92
low-density 89, 101, 106*f*, 555
metabolism 558
particle, high atherogenicity of 103
remnants of 95
very low-density 95, 107
Live birth rate 530
Liver 149
disease, Fontan-associated 405
Loop diuretics 198, 246, 248
Low muscle strength 537
Low-density lipoprotein 89, 101, 106*f*, 555
cholesterol 95, 105-107, 110
biochemistry of 106
childhood 105, 107
pathophysiology of 106
kinetics 106
Lower insulin sensitivity 538
Low-molecular-weight heparin 528, 530-533
Lusitropy 182

M

Machine learning 29, 162, 228, 353, 367
Macrophages 140
Magnetic resonance
imaging 151, 214*f*
four-dimensional 363
three-dimensional 363
lymphangiography 363
Major adverse cardiovascular events 25, 141, 206, 643
Marshall alcohol ablation, vein of 607
Marshall plan 607
Mast cells 140, 141
Maternal cardiovascular
adaptations 520
risk, classification of 506
Matrix metalloproteinase inhibition 560
Maximal wall thickness 282
Maximum left ventricular wall thickness 277
Mean arterial pressure 260
Mean transvalvular gradient 465
Mechanical circulatory
devices, role of 383
support 164, 174, 177, 228, 230, 233, 234, 259, 260, 297, 381, 517, 612
Mechanical pulmonary valve 412
Mechanical valve 531*t*, 532*t*, 533
management of 531*fc*, 532*fc*
Medical management 40, 377, 550
Medical therapy 429, 478, 531, 674, 684
follow-up 41
Mediterranean diets 59, 622
Mesenchymal stem cells 47
Metabolic dysfunction associated steatotic liver disease 71
Metabolic modulation 241, 559
Metabolic syndrome 98, 523
Metaiodobenzylguanidine 206
Methylene blue 228
Mexiletine, addition of 566
Micra longitudinal coverage with evidence development study 592
Microbial enzyme inhibitors 243
Microbial metabolites 242, 558
Microbiome modulation 559
Microcalcification 671
Microcirculatory resistance, index of 681
Microvascular disease 49
Microvascular dysfunction 677, 679, 684
Midmyocardial enhancement 295
Midventricular aneurysms 285
Milrinone 224, 225
Mineralocorticoid receptor antagonists 61, 169, 171, 201, 250, 255, 256, 379
Minimal extracardiac injury 626
Mitochondrial cytopathies 394
Mitochondrial dysfunction 327, 327*f*
Mitochondrial injury 50
Mitochondrial physiology 149
Mitotropes, mechanism of action of 222*fc*
Mitral annular 434*f*
dimension 435*f*
disjunction 433, 435*f*, 436*f*
displacement of 434*f*
posterior 436*f*
Mitral leaflet tethering 426*f*
Mitral regurgitation 260, 262, 425, 426, 430, 458, 465, 646-649
acute severe 261, 261*f*
atrial 429*f*
chronic 261, 261*f*
ischemic 651*f*
secondary 206, 329*f*, 424, 426, 426*t*, 430*f*, 465
Mitral stenosis 260, 262, 465, 500, 508, 647-649
Mitral transcatheter edge-to-edge repair 424, 426, 430
Mitral valve 465, 650, 650*f*, 654
anterior 654*f*
area 262, 465, 647
closure 578
en-face view of 651*f*
geometry 426*f*
opening 578
prolapse 433
Mixed shock 174, 177
different phenotypes of 175*f*
evaluation of 176
management of 178*f*
proposed phenotypes of 174
Molecular mechanism 420, 623
Molecular pathways 149
Molecular structure 106
Molecular target 559
Monocyte chemoattractant protein 47
Monomorphic ventricular tachycardia 567, 612
Mortality rate contribution, anticipated trend of 488*t*

Multidetector computed tomography 652*f*
Multidisciplinary cardio-obstetric teamwork 505
Multidisciplinary postpartum team
  approach 524
  key members of 524*b*
Multifactorial model 290
Multimodality imaging 420, 421, 646
  approach 649
  role of 646
Multimodality preprocedural planning 336
Multiorgan failure 220
Multiparametric risk stratification 419, 420
Multiple lipoprotein components 97
Multiple mutation model 290
Multivalvular heart disease 465*t*, 646
  diagnosis of 647*t*
  evaluation of 646
  management of 646
Muscle protein homeostasis dysregulation 537
Muscle wasting 537
Mycotic coronary aneurysms, treatment of 552
Myeloperoxidase 143
Myocardial abnormalities 83
Myocardial blood flow 685
Myocardial bridging 542
Myocardial changes
  functional 319
  structural 319
Myocardial deformation indices 206
Myocardial dysfunction 213*f*, 327*f*
Myocardial fibrosis 292, 433
  clinical consequences of 44
  histopathological basis of 44
  pathogenesis of 45*fc*
  quantification 653
Myocardial flow reserve 686
  quantification 685
Myocardial function, intrinsic determinants of 213*f*
Myocardial infarction 96, 141, 218*f*, 232, 677
  acute 232, 677
Myocardial injury, subclinical 419
Myocardial interstitial fibrosis 43
  implications of 43
Myocardial involvement 313, 316*fc*
Myocardial mass ratio 681*t*
Myocardial oxygen consumption 375
Myocardial perfusion imaging 680
Myocardial scar 684, 687
Myocardial strain 212
  vectors of 212*f*
Myocardial substrate 294, 295*f*
Myocarditis 315*f*
Myocardium 142*f*
Myotonic dystrophy 394
Myotropes 222*f*

N

Naltrexone 330
Nanostim device 592
National Programme for Prevention and Control of Cancer, Diabetes, Cardiovascular Diseases and Stroke 488
Natriuretic peptides 58, 132, 155
Natural killer cells 140, 142
Near-infrared spectroscopy 664, 666, 667
Necrosis 212
Neurohormonal activation 200, 327
Neurohormonal modulators 166
Neuromodulation 192
  interventions 192
Neutrophils 142
  extracellular traps 547
New Vasovagal Syncope International Study Classification 301
New York Heart Association 152, 153, 155, 210, 375, 468, 501
  classification system 375
Nicotinamide-adenine dinucleotide phosphate 47
Nicotine
  consumption 73
  replacement therapy 19
Nitrates 685
Nitric oxide 47, 139, 143
  synthase inhibitors 228
Nodular calcification 671
Nodules, subcutaneous 463
Noncontrast computed tomography 652*t*
  aortic valve calcification 652
Nondihydropyridine calcium channel blockers 636
Non-dilated left ventricular cardiomyopathy 294, 297
Non-high density lipoprotein cholesterol 95, 97, 105-108, 110
  biochemistry of 107
  composition of 95
  pathophysiology of 107
  role of 95
Noninvasive adjunctive imaging 542
Noninvasive coronary plaque imaging 674*t*
Noninvasive surrogates 270
Noninvasive ventilation 517
Nonischemic cardiomyopathy 292, 293, 295*f*, 612, 614
  causes of 294
  triggers of 294
Nonobstructive coronary arteries 677
Nonpharmacological therapy 300, 302
Nonsteroidal mineralocorticoid receptor antagonists 40
Nonsustained ventricular tachycardia 276, 281
Norepinephrine 220, 223, 225
N-terminal pro-B-type natriuretic peptide 375
Nuclear factor-kappa B 47
Nucleotide oligomerization 143
Nutritional deficiencies 148, 327

O

Obesity 76, 78, 78*f*, 79, 80, 128*fc*
  abdominal 76
  management of 80
  visceral 76
Obstetric bleeding, delayed 532
Obstetrical care 505
Obstructive coronary arteries 684
Obstructive sleep apnea 61, 73, 79
Oliguria 220
Olpasiran 101
Omecamtiv mecarbil 117, 122
Optical coherence tomography 540, 542, 664, 665, 667, 671, 672
Optimal medical therapy 642, 684
Oral iron therapy 150
Organ level dysfunction 149
Orphan status 492
Ostium secundum 355*f*
Outflow tract obstruction 374
Oxidative phosphorylation 556
Oxidative stress 48, 327, 327*f*, 559
Oxidized phospholipids 558
Oxygen consumption 152, 153, 155

P

Pace mapping 616
Pacemaker
  implantation 303, 503
  therapy 300
PAINESD score 616*f*
Papillary muscles 426*f*
Para-Hisian ventricular arrhythmias 634, 637
Paravalvular leak 479
Patent ductus arteriosus 387, 390, 398, 400, 402
Pathologic valve dysfunction 462*t*

Peak atrial longitudinal strain 577
Peak jet velocity 465, 476
Pelacarsen 101
Penicillin 469
  subcutaneous 468
Percutaneous balloon
  aortic valvuloplasty 502
  pulmonic valvuloplasty 502
Percutaneous coronary intervention 141, 499, 502, 503, 642, 674
Percutaneous mitral balloon commissurotomy 501
Percutaneous pulmonic valve implantation 502
Percutaneous transvenous mitral commissurotomy 390
Perfusion status 199
Perhexiline 228
Pericardial effusion 595, 631
Pericardial valves 412
Perimembranous ventricular septal defect 357*f*
Peripartum cardiomyopathy 320, 500, 510, 515, 517
  management of 515, 517*t*
  moderate 517
  pathogenesis of 516*f*
Peripheral artery disease 554, 560
  progression 572
Peripheral organ hypoperfusion 142*f*
Persistent culture-negative status 585
Personalized antihypertensive therapy 32
Pharmacotherapy 378, 614
  historical context of 221
Phenotype-guided therapy 226
Phosphodiesterase 143, 222
  inhibitors 224
Phospholamban 222
Phospholipase A2 inhibitors 141
Phospholipokinase C 223
Physiological cardiovascular changes 506
Pickelhaube sign 435*f*
Pirfenidone 43
Plantar flexion 303*f*
Plaque
  advancement 555*f*
  burden 684
  ecosystem model 558
  erosion 545, 547, 547*t*, 673
  imaging 670, 673, 674
  morphology 546, 664, 673
  phenotypes 666
  rupture 545, 547, 547*t*, 673
  type of 665
Plasminogen activator inhibitor 47, 139
Platelet
  activation 545
  biology 545
  function 545
Platform 467
Point-of-care ultrasound 233
Polyangiitis 313, 315*f*, 316
Polygenic inheritance 289
Polygenic model 290
Polymyositis 313
Positron emission tomography 207, 674, 685
  scan 296
Post-adrenalectomy monitoring 41
Postcardiac arrest 176
Posterior basal
  mitral annulus 435*f*
  papillary muscle 436*f*
Posterior mitral valve 654*f*
  leaflet, hamstringing of 428*f*
Posterior wall isolation 629*f*
Post-Fontan operation 345
Postmyocardial infarction 565
Postpartum hypertensive clinics 524
Post-tricuspid shunts 399
Potassium supplementation 59
Potent vasoconstrictor 228
Potential immunomodulatory treatment targets 309
Prearterioles 678
Preeclampsia 520, 521, 523
  early-onset 524, 524*t*
  late-onset 524, 524*t*
Pregnancy 343, 505, 510, 515, 528, 533
  hypertensive disorder of 520, 522*f*, 523-525
  normal 523, 524
  subsequent 515, 518
  termination 541
Pre-heart failure 132, 134, 136
  classification of 133
  continuum of 133
Premature atherosclerotic cardiovascular disease, prevention of 92
Premature ventricular
  complexes 634
  contraction 318
    cardiomyopathy 321, 322
    epidemiology of 321
Prepregnancy counseling 533
Preshock state 230
Pressure
  gradients 440, 647
  half time 647, 465
  strain loop 217*f*
  volume loop 221*f*, 261*f*
Primary aldosteronism 37, 38*t*, 39*fc*
  clinical management of 37
Primary care partner-heart failure score 158
Pro-arrhythmogenicity 631
Probiotics 241, 243
Procizumab 228
Prosthetic valve 509, 528, 654, 655*t*
  management 530
Protein kinase A 222
Proximal convoluted tubule 247
Proximal isovelocity surface area 465, 647, 651*f*
Pseudoinfarction patterns 281
Pseudo-mitral annular disjunction 434*f*
Psychological interventions 80
Public health 25
  policy 8
Pulmonary arterial hypertension 128
Pulmonary artery 387
  catheterization effectiveness trial 269
  wedge pressure 128
Pulmonary blood flow, type of 350
Pulmonary capillary wedge pressure 260, 262
Pulmonary edema, weaning-induced 227
Pulmonary embolism 500
Pulmonary hypertension 126-128, 183, 188, 189, 269, 329*f*, 399, 686-688
  regimens 684
Pulmonary pressures 208
Pulmonary regurgitation 408, 409
  pathophysiology of 409*fc*
Pulmonary stenosis 403
Pulmonary valve 412
  replacement 408, 411
Pulmonary vascular
  coupling 684
  resistance 297
Pulmonary vasodilator therapies 129
Pulmonary vein 338*f*, 629*f*
  balloon rescue technique 340
  isolation 320, 340, 598, 627
  stenosis, risk of 626
  stent rescue technique 340
Pulse Doppler, midsystolic notching of 399
Pulsed-field ablation 598, 608, 625, 626, 627*f*, 629*f*, 630*t*, 631, 632
  biophysics of 626
  clinical evidence of 628
  history of 625
  mechanism of 626
  procedure, workflow of 628*f*
Pump strain 577*f*
Punctate calcification 671
P-value 351
P-wave abnormalities 282
Pyrophosphate 206
Pyroptosis 212

Q

Q waves 281
QRS complex 411
Quadriceps, isometric contraction of 303*f*
Quality of life 153, 155
Quantitative data 659

R

Radial strain 213*f*
Radiation 499, 688
 exposure 350, 500
Radiofrequency ablation 503, 625, 626, 634
Randomized controlled trial 152, 153, 155, 599
Ranolazine 685
Rashtriya Bal Swasthya Karyakram 391
Reactive oxygen species 47, 71, 139
Reflex vasovagal syncope 300
Refractory vasodilatory shock 228
Regurgitant
 fraction 465
 lesions 508
Regurgitation, aortic 262, 458, 465, 647, 648
Remote hemodynamic monitoring 269
Renal artery stenosis 47
Renal denervation 56, 62, 192, 193
Renal dysfunction 142*f*, 148, 671
Renin–angiotensin–aldosterone system 47, 57, 171, 192
 activation 49
 inhibition 46
Replacement fibrosis 419
Resistant hypertension 38, 56, 62
 management of 60*fc*
 pathogenesis of 57, 57*f*
Respiratory failure 236
Resuscitation, cardiopulmonary 260
Reverse remodeling therapies 164, 166
Rheumatic cardiac involvement span 457
Rheumatic carditis, classification of 458*fc*
Rheumatic fever 463*t*, 486
 acute 456-458, 460, 460*fc*, 486
 primary prevention of 467*t*
Rheumatic heart disease 456, 456*f*, 457, 458*fc*, 463, 467, 469, 486, 487*t*, 488, 488*t*, 493, 494
 burden 488
  state-level 489*t*
 classification 458
 confirmatory morphologic criteria 462*t*
 global burden of 486, 487*f*
 latent 461
 multivalvular 463
 pathophysiology of 458
 prevention of 464, 491
 revised classification of 491*t*
 state-level burden of 488
 subclinical 491
Rheumatic valvulitis 462
Rheumatoid arthritis 313, 315*f*, 316
Rhythm control 572, 598
Right atrial
 pressure 262
 remodeling 182
Right atrium 181, 183-186, 188, 335
Right ventricle 181, 183-186, 188-190, 353, 465, 647, 649
 global longitudinal strain 206
Right ventricular 206, 260, 652
 dysfunction 126, 182, 183
  classification of 182
 failure 227, 269
 function 208
 outflow tract 349*f*, 390, 408, 409, 410*f*, 634
  dysfunction 408
  stenting 348, 350
 systolic pressure 262
Rotational angiography, three-dimensional 365
Rynadine receptor 222

S

Sacubitril 256
Sahajanand laser technology 340
Sandwich stent 340
Saphenous vein graft 141
Sarcoidosis 313, 315, 315*f*
Sarcopenia 537, 538
Scar
 border zone, quantification of 207
 density estimation 207
 identification 207
 quantification 207
Seattle heart failure model 158, 165
Second hit hypothesis 308
Secondary hypertension 32, 37
 causes of 59*t*
Secondary mitral regurgitation 206, 329*f*, 424, 426, 426*t*, 430*f*, 465
 phenotypes 425*f*
Secundum atrial septal defect 355*f*
Self-rechargeable devices 591
Semaglutide 256
Sensitivity 396, 680
Sequential nephron blockade 246, 248
Serum sodium 159
Sex hormones 541
Shock 226*f*
 cardiogenic 174, 176, 177, 220, 221, 221*f*, 225*t*, 230, 232, 232*t*, 233, 260, 263, 269, 542
  vasodilatory 175
 classic cardiogenic 230, 231
 early cardiogenic 231
 mixed 174, 177
 postcardiotomy 176
 refractory vasodilatory 228
 state 221
 teams 234
 valvular cardiogenic 259, 264
 vasodilatory 174
Short-chain fatty acids 241, 242, 556
Single transseptal puncture 628
Single-photon emission computed tomography 207, 685
Sinus tachycardia 320, 328
Sinus venosus atrial septal defect 335, 340
 balloon interrogation of 338
 closure 335
 correction of 335
Six-minute walk distance 152, 153, 155
Sjögren's syndrome 313
Skeletal muscle catabolism 142*f*
Sleep
 apnea 61
 lack of 73
Smoking 18, 60
 cessation 17, 18, 18*t*, 20
Society for Cardiovascular Angiography and Interventions 232, 233
 shock
  classification 230
  staging system 220*b*, 232*t*, 233, 260, 260*t*
Society of Thoracic Surgeons risk score 444*t*
Sodium
 glucose cotransporter-2 47, 171, 172, 255
  inhibitors 51, 62, 169, 198, 201, 228, 249, 256, 379
 hydrogen exchanger 3 247
 restriction 59
Soluble guanylate cyclase 143
Somatic mutations 307
Sore throat, natural history of 459*fc*
Sotagliflozin 117, 122
Speckle-tracking echocardiography 207, 575, 576, 581
Spinal cord stimulation 194
Spironolactone 37, 46
Splanchnic hypoperfusion 223
Splanchnic nerve modulation 195

Splenic monocytes 142*f*
Spline curve 662*f*
Spondyloarthropathies 313
Spontaneous coronary artery dissection 500, 540, 541
  accurate diagnosis of 542
  epidemiology of 541
  management 542
  types 541
Statins 525, 685, 686
  therapy 95
ST-elevation myocardial infarction 141
Stenosis 685
Stenotic tricuspid valve 653*f*
Stents
  choice of 340
  optimization 664
Steroid metabolite profiling 40
Stöllberger criteria 395
Stöllberger method 396*f*
Strain
  biophysics of 213
  component 661
    normal values of 661*t*
  echocardiography 85
  vectors 213, 214*f*
Streptococcus vaccine, scope of 492
Stress 60, 73, 85
  cardiovascular magnetic resonance 686
  echocardiography 684-686
  imaging 622, 685, 686
Stroke 276
  prevention 572
  volume 221*f*, 439
Sudden cardiac death 79, 206, 275-277, 281*t*, 283, 285, 285*t*, 292, 297, 419, 572, 620-622, 622*f*, 622*t*, 623, 623*t*
  family history of 276
  increased risk of 399
  mechanisms of 276
  pathophysiology of 276
  prevention of 584, 620, 621, 621*t*, 622
  risk assessment 276
  risk stratification 620*t*
Suicide, factor associated 139
Superior sinus venosus atrial septal defect, anatomy of 335
Superior vena cava
  rims 355*f*
  stenting 349
Supraventricular tachycardia 318, 510
  ablation 631
Surgical aortic valve replacement 155, 443, 451, 479
Surgical pulmonary valve replacement 413
Swan–Ganz catheter, course of 267*f*
Sydenham's chorea 462
Sympathetic nervous system 58
Synbiotics 243
Syncope 302*f*
  near 302*f*
  neurocardiogenic 300
  treatment of 303*t*
  unexplained 276, 278
Systemic immune-mediated disease 313, 315*f*, 316
  cardiomyopathy, management of 316
Systemic inflammation, low-grade 139*f*
Systemic inflammatory connective tissue diseases 542
Systemic lupus erythematosus 313, 314
Systemic sclerosis 314, 315*f*
Systemic vascular resistance 202, 260, 262, 522
Systolic blood pressure 159, 233, 260
  time, implications of 25

T

T cells 142
Tachyarrhythmia 223, 320*t*
  atrial 576
  ventricular 236
Tachycardia 515
  supraventricular 318, 510
  ventricular 155, 275, 542, 565, 568*f*, 612
Tachycardia-induced cardiomyopathy 318, 570
  treatment options of 320*t*
Tachypnea 515
Tadasana 300
  steps 303*f*
Takotsubo cardiomyopathy 227, 542
Tandem heart 167
Target organ damage
  detection of 32
  imaging of 32
Temporary mechanical circulatory support 167
Tetralogy of Fallot 345, 348, 353, 381, 387, 398, 400, 404, 408, 409, 409*fc*
Therapeutic targets, novel 558, 559*t*, 560
Therapeutic window 185
Thermal ablation 632
Thiazides 246, 248
Thick ascending limb 247
Thin cap atheroma 673
Thromboembolic phenomena 394
Thromboembolic stroke 570
Thromboembolism 530, 571
  competing risks of 532
Thrombogenicity 479, 531
Thrombosis, valve-associated 413
Thrombus composition 545, 546
Thyrotoxicosis 320
Time-to-peak strain 577
Tissue
  characterization 207
  Doppler imaging 435*f*, 577
  engineered heart valve 413
    need for 413
  inhibitor matrix metalloproteinase 47
  selectivity 626
Toll-like receptor 139
Torsemide 249, 249*t*
Total anomalous pulmonary venous
  communication 387
  connection 390, 401
Total iron binding capacity 148
Total particle atherosclerotic cardiovascular disease risk 104*f*
Traditional blood pressure measurement, limitations of 25
Transannular patch 349
  placement 408
Transcatheter 350
  aortic valve
    implantation 263
    replacement 155, 451, 452, 479, 481, 501, 502, 649
  initial palliation 350*t*
  interventions 351
  management 551, 551*f*
  mitral valve
    edge-to-edge repair 264, 425*f*, 430
    replacement 481
  palliation 348, 351
    approaches 350*t*
  pulmonary valve 390, 408
    implants 412*t*
    long-term outcomes 412
    replacement 413
  techniques 408
  tricuspid valve intervention 186, 187, 189
  valve
    replacement 381
    therapy 259
Transcutaneous aortic valve replacement 443
Transesophageal echocardiography 336, 390, 647
Transferrin saturation 152, 155
Translational animal model 321*f*
Transoesophageal echocardiography 465
Transthoracic echocardiogram 336, 357*f*, 646, 647, 649
  three-dimensional 650
  two-dimensional 650
Transthyretin amyloidosis 206
Transvenous pacemakers 591
  achilles heel of 591

Tricuspid annular peak systolic excursion 206
Tricuspid regurgitation 180, 181, 184, 184*f*, 185-190, 262, 465, 646, 647, 649
  grading of 187*f*
  pathophysiology of 181*fc*
  phenotypes 182
Tricuspid stenosis 647
Tricuspid valve 186, 189, 190
  dilatation of 408
  management of 190*fc*
  replacement 180
Triglycerides 90, 91, 107
Trimetazidine 228
Trimethylamine N-oxide 241, 242, 556
  pathway 557
Troponin 141
Tumor necrosis factor 138, 139, 142
  alpha 47, 139, 555
  receptor 143

U

Ultra-low temperature cryoablation 626
Unfractionated heparin 528, 530-533
Unilateral aldosterone-producing adenoma 37
Unilateral renovascular disease 47
Uremic toxins 241, 242
  influence inflammation 241
Urine albumin 135

V

Vaccine development 465
Vagal nerve stimulation 192, 193
Validation data 665
Valsalva ruptured sinus 390
Valsartan 256
Valve 462
  area calculation 477
  cusp changes 474
  diameter 413
  durability 451
  evaluation 686
  interventions, need for 209
  involvement 461
  leaflet changes 475
  lesion 262, 465
  longevity 413
  material 412
  models 412
  replacement 419
  thrombosis 532
Valvular cardiogenic shock 259, 264
  outcomes of 264
Valvular disease 292, 505
Valvular dysfunction
  acute 259
  acute on chronic 259
Valvular heart disease 80, 190*fc*, 327, 417, 481, 509*f*, 657, 687
  management 481
  subacute 320
Valvular lesion 649
Valvular pathology 646
  severe 646
Valvular shock specifics 260
Varenicline 19
Variant allele frequency 306, 307
Vascular aging rationale 74
Vascular anti-aging potential 73
Vascular cell adhesion molecule 139
Vascular disease, atherosclerotic 542
Vascular injury 139*f*
Vascular smooth muscle 222
  cell 139, 547, 555, 556
    phenotypic switching 557
Vasoactive medications 177
Vasopressin 225, 247
  antagonists 246, 248, 249
Vasopressors 174, 220, 223*fc*, 225*t*
  contemporary use of 220
  efficacy of 226*f*
Vasovagal syncope 300
  management of 301, 301*t*
Vasovagal syncope International Study classification 301*t*
Velocity-time integral 465
Vena cava
  inferior 390
  superior 355*f*
Vena contracta 465, 651*f*, 658*f*
  area 647
  width 658
Venoarterial-extracorporeal membrane oxygenation 263
Venous thromboembolism 80
Ventricular arrhythmia 275, 394, 433, 637*f*
  pathophysiology of 434
Ventricular assist devices 267
Ventricular dysfunction 399
Ventricular dyssynchrony 576
Ventricular fibrillation 275
Ventricular function 646
Ventricular interdependence 465
Ventricular quadrigeminy 436*f*
Ventricular septal defect 343, 353, 387, 390, 398, 400, 402
Ventricular tachycardia 155, 275, 542, 565, 568*f*, 612
  ablation 566, 567, 569, 612, 631
Ventricular volume 221*f*
Verapamil 636
Vericiguat 117, 122
Very low-density lipoproteins 95, 107
Virtual heart modeling 210*t*
Visceral adipose tissue 538
Vitamin K antagonist 530-533
  use of 528
Voltage-guided substrate modification 603

W

Waist circumference 73, 77*t*
Warfarin 528
Wegener's granulomatosis 316
Weight
  control therapy 74
  loss, pharmacological interventions for 80
  management 59, 622
  reduction 60
World Health Organization 468
World Heart Federation 486
  guidelines, new features of 491
Worsening heart failure 117, 118, 118*t*, 119*t*, 121, 122, 198, 200, 236
  clinical impact of 199*fc*
  management 117, 202
  pathophysiology of 199*fc*
Worsening valvular heart disease 571

Y

Yoga 302

Z

ZASP protein 394
Zephyr stent 390